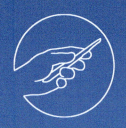

Master Techniques in Orthopaedic Surgery®

The Foot and Ankle

Fourth Edition

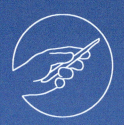

Master Techniques in Orthopaedic Surgery®

The Foot and Ankle

Fourth Edition

Scott Ellis, MD
Professor of Orthopaedic Surgery
Weill Cornell Medical College
Treasurer, American Orthopaedic Foot and Ankle Society
Hospital for Special Surgery
New York, New York

Section Editors

A. Holly Johnson, MD
Associate Professor
Department of Orthopedic Surgery
Weill-Cornell Medical School
Hospital for Special Surgery
New York, New York

Constantine A. Demetracopoulos, MD
Associate Professor of Orthopaedic Surgery
Weill Cornell Medical College
Associate Attending
Foot and Ankle Service
Hospital for Special Surgery
New York, New York

Mark Drakos, BA, MD
Attending Orthopedic Surgeon
Foot and Ankle Service, Sports Medicine
Hospital for Special Surgery
New York, New York

Cesar de Cesar Netto, MD, PhD
Associate Professor
Division of Orthopedic Foot and Ankle Surgery
Department of Orthopedic Surgery
Duke University
Durham, North Carolina

John Y. Kwon, MD
Associate Chief, Foot and Ankle Service
Department of Orthopaedics
Massachusetts General Hospital
Boston, Massachusetts

Series Editor
Bernard F. Morrey, MD

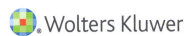

Philadelphia • Baltimore • New York • London
Buenos Aires • Hong Kong • Sydney • Tokyo

Senior Acquisitions Editor: Tulie McKay
Senior Development Editor: Stacey Sebring
Editorial Coordinator: Varshaanaa SM
Editorial Assistant: Kristen Kardoley
Marketing Manager: Kirsten Watrud
Production Project Manager: Kirstin Johnson
Manager, Graphic Arts & Design: Stephen Druding
Manufacturing Coordinator: Lisa Bowling
Prepress Vendor: Straive

Fourth edition

Copyright © 2025 Wolters Kluwer.

Copyright © 2013 by LIPPINCOTT WILLIAMS & WILKINS, a WOLTERS KLUWER business. All rights reserved. This book is protected by copyright. No part of this book may be reproduced or transmitted in any form or by any means, including as photocopies or scanned-in or other electronic copies, or utilized by any information storage and retrieval system without written permission from the copyright owner, except for brief quotations embodied in critical articles and reviews. Materials appearing in this book prepared by individuals as part of their official duties as U.S. government employees are not covered by the above-mentioned copyright. To request permission, please contact Wolters Kluwer at Two Commerce Square, 2001 Market Street, Philadelphia, PA 19103, via email at permissions@lww.com, or via our website at shop.lww.com (products and services).

The views expressed in this work are the private views of the authors and do not purport to reflect the official policy or position of the Food and Drug Administration or any part of the US Government, nor were the materials prepared as part of official government duties.

9 8 7 6 5 4 3 2 1

Printed in United States of America

Cataloging-in-Publication Data available on request from the Publisher

ISBN: 978-1-9751-9941-8

This work is provided "as is," and the publisher disclaims any and all warranties, express or implied, including any warranties as to accuracy, comprehensiveness, or currency of the content of this work.

This work is no substitute for individual patient assessment based upon healthcare professionals' examination of each patient and consideration of, among other things, age, weight, gender, current or prior medical conditions, medication history, laboratory data and other factors unique to the patient. The publisher does not provide medical advice or guidance and this work is merely a reference tool. Healthcare professionals, and not the publisher, are solely responsible for the use of this work including all medical judgments and for any resulting diagnosis and treatments.

Given continuous, rapid advances in medical science and health information, independent professional verification of medical diagnoses, indications, appropriate pharmaceutical selections and dosages, and treatment options should be made and healthcare professionals should consult a variety of sources. When prescribing medication, healthcare professionals are advised to consult the product information sheet (the manufacturer's package insert) accompanying each drug to verify, among other things, conditions of use, warnings and side effects and identify any changes in dosage schedule or contraindications, particularly if the medication to be administered is new, infrequently used or has a narrow therapeutic range. To the maximum extent permitted under applicable law, no responsibility is assumed by the publisher for any injury and/or damage to persons or property, as a matter of products liability, negligence law or otherwise, or from any reference to or use by any person of this work.

shop.lww.com

Contributors

Amiethab Aiyer, MD, FAAOS, FAOA
Chief, Foot and Ankle Service
Associate Professor, Department of Orthopaedics
Faculty Affiliate, Center for Innovative Leadership
Johns Hopkins University Carey Business School
Director, Orthopaedic Medical Student Education
Director, UME to GME Transition
The Johns Hopkins University School of Medicine
Baltimore, Maryland

Tonya An, MA, MD
Clinical Assistant Professor, Orthopedic Surgery
Department of Orthopedic Surgery
Stanford University
Redwood City, California

Albert T. Anastasio, MD
Resident Orthopaedic Surgeon
Division of Foot and Ankle
Department of Orthopaedic Surgery
Duke University Hospital
Durham, North Carolina

Michael Aronow, MD, FAAOS, FACS
Clinical Professor
Department of Orthopaedic Surgery
School of Medicine
University of Connecticut
Hartford Hospital Bone and Joint Institute
Orthopedic Associates of Hartford, PC
Hartford, Connecticut

Ahmed Khalil Attia, MD
Foot and Ankle Fellow
Department of Orthopedic Surgery
University of Pittsburgh
Pittsburgh, Pennsylvania

Jonathon Backus, MD
Assistant Professor
Department of Orthopaedic Surgery
Washington University in St. Louis
St. Louis, Missouri

Daniel Baumfeld, MD, PHD
Adjunct Professor
Federal University of Minas Gerais
Foot and Ankle Surgeon
Head, Foot and Ankle Clinic
Felicio Rocho Hospital
Belo Horizonte, Brazil

Judy Baumhauer, MD, MPH, FAAOS, FAOA
Professor of Orthopaedic Surgery
Senior Associate Dean for Academic Affairs
University of Rochester School of Medicine and Dentistry
Director, University of Rochester Clinical Health Informatics Core
University of Rochester Medical Center
Rochester, New York

Clayton C. Bettin, MD, FAAOS
Assistant Professor
Foot and Ankle Fellowship Director
Associate Residency Program Director
Department of Orthopaedic Surgery and Biomedical Engineering
University of Tennessee–Campbell Clinic
Memphis, Tennessee

Braden Boyer, MD
Orthopedic Surgeon
Department of Orthopedics
Campbell Clinic
Memphis, Tennessee

James W. Brodsky, MD
Professor of Surgery, Orthopaedics
Texas A&M University HSC College of Medicine
Founder, Foot and Ankle Surgery Fellowship Program
Baylor University Medical Center
Fellowship Director
Clinical Professor of Orthopaedic Surgery
University of Texas Southwestern Medical School
Dallas, Texas

John Wunn Cancian Sr, MD
Staff Orthopedic Surgeon
Bone and Joint Sports Medicine Institute
Naval Medical Center Portsmouth
Portsmouth, Virginia

Rebecca Cerrato, MD
Director, Fellowship Program
The Institute for Foot and Ankle Reconstruction
Mercy Medical Center
Baltimore, Maryland

Elizabeth A. Cody, MD
Assistant Professor of Orthopedic Surgery
Weill Cornell Medical College
Assistant Attending Orthopedic Surgeon
Hospital for Special Surgery and New York Presbyterian Hospital
New York, New York
Stamford Hospital
Stamford, Connecticut

J. Chris Coetzee, MD
Orthopedic Foot and Ankle Surgeon
Past President, American Orthopedic Foot and Ankle Society
Twin Cities Orthopedics
Eagan, Minnesota

Matthew S. Conti, MD
Assistant Attending Orthopedic Surgeon
Hospital for Special Surgery
Assistant Professor of Orthopedic Surgery
Weill Cornell Medical College
New York, New York

Miki Dalmau-Pastor, PhD
Associate Professor
Pathology and Experimental Therapeutics
Human Anatomy and Embryology Unit
University of Barcelona
Barcelona, Spain

Constantine A. Demetracopoulos, MD
Associate Professor of Orthopaedic Surgery
Weill Cornell Medical College
Associate Attending
Foot and Ankle Service
Hospital for Special Surgery
New York, New York

W. Hodges Davis, MD
Senior Partner, OrthoCarolina Foot & Ankle Institute
Foot and Ankle Section Chief
Atrium Health
Charlotte, North Carolina

James S. Davitt, MD, FAAOS
Orthopedic and Fracture Specialists, PC
Portland, Oregon

Paul Dayton, DPM, MS
Foot and Ankle Surgeon
Foot and Ankle Center of Iowa
Ankeny, Iowa

Kepler Alencar Mendes de Carvalho, MD
Visiting Associate
Foot and Ankle Surgery
Orthopedic Functional Imaging Research Laboratory
Department of Orthopedics and Rehabilitation
Carver College of Medicine
University of Iowa
Iowa City, Iowa

William T. DeCarbo, DPM
Foot and Ankle Surgeon
Department of Surgery
Greater Pittsburgh Foot and Ankle Center
Wexford, Pennsylvania

Jonathan Deland, MD
Attending Surgeon
Orthopaedic Surgery
Hospital for Special Surgery
New York, New York

Mark Drakos, BA, MD
Attending Orthopedic Surgeon
Foot and Ankle Service, Sports Medicine
Hospital for Special Surgery
New York, New York

Mark E. Easley, MD
Associate Professor
Chief, Division of Foot and Ankle
Department of Orthopaedic Surgery
Duke University Medical Center
Durham, North Carolina

M. Pierce Ebaugh, DO
Attending Orthopedic Surgeon
Jewett Orthopedic Institute at Orlando Health
Orlando, Florida

Benjamin Ebben, MD
Bellin Health Titletown Sports Medicine and Orthopedics
Green Bay, Wisconsin

J. Kent Ellington, MD, MS, FAAOS
OrthoCarolina
Medical Director of the Foot and Ankle Institute
Assistant Professor of Orthopaedic Surgery Atrium Health
Adjunct Assistant Professor of Biology UNC Charlotte
Co-Founder, Pressio Spine, Inc.
Charlotte, North Carolina

Contributors

Scott Ellis, MD
Professor of Orthopaedic Surgery
Weill Cornell Medical College
Treasurer, American Orthopaedic Foot and Ankle Society
Hospital for Special Surgery
New York, New York

Norman Espinosa, MD
Head of FussInstitut Zürich AG
Institute for Foot and Ankle Reconstruction
Zurich, Switzerland

Richard D. Ferkel, MD
Assistant Clinic Professor
Department of Orthopedic Surgery
University of California, Los Angeles
Los Angeles, California
Program Director, Sports Medicine Fellowship
Southern California Orthopedic Institute
Van Nuys, California

Brian M. Fisher, MD
Assistant Professor
Department of Orthopaedic Surgery
School of Medicine Greenville
University of South Carolina
Prisma Health Blue Ridge Orthopedics
Easley, South Carolina

Amanda N. Fletcher, MD, MSc
Orthopaedic Surgeon, Foot and Ankle Fellowship Trained
Orthopaedic Surgery, Foot and Ankle
Institute of Foot and Ankle Reconstruction
Mercy Medical Center
Baltimore, Maryland

Austin T. Fragomen, MD
Professor of Clinical Orthopaedic Surgery
Weill Medical College of Cornell University
Director, Limb Salvage and Amputation Reconstruction Center
Fellowship Director, Limb Salvage and Amputation Reconstruction Center
Hospital for Special Surgery
New York, New York

Daniel Fuchs, MD
Assistant Professor
Department of Orthopaedic Surgery
Rothman Orthopaedics at Jefferson University
Philadelphia, Pennsylvania

Oliver J. Gagne, MDCM, MSc, FRCSC
Clinical Instructor
University of British Columbia
Foot and Ankle Orthopedic Surgeon
Saint-Paul's Hospital
Vancouver, British Columbia

Stephanie S. Gardner, MD
Foot and Ankle Clinical Fellow
Department of Orthopedics
Campbell Clinic
Memphis, Tennessee

Arianna L. Gianakos, DO
Assistant Professor of Orthopaedic Surgery
Foot and Ankle Division
Department of Orthopaedic Surgery
Yale Orthopaedics and Rehabilitation
New Haven, Connecticut

Christopher E. Gross, MD
Professor of Orthopaedic Surgery
Department of Orthopaedic Surgery
Medical University of South Carolina
Director, Foot and Ankle Surgery
Fellowship Director
Charleston, South Carolina

Matteo Guelfi, MD, PhD
Consultant
Foot and Ankle Unit
Casa di Cura Villa Montallegro
Genoa, Italy

Ajay N. Gurbani, MD
Assistant Professor
Department of Orthopaedic Surgery
David Geffen School of Medicine at UCLA
Los Angeles, California

Gregory P. Guyton, MD
Division Chief of Foot and Ankle Surgery, and the Fellowship Director
Department of Orthopaedic Surgery
MedStar Union Memorial Hospital
Baltimore, Maryland

Daniel J. Hatch, DPM
Director, Foot and Ankle Surgery–Podiatry Residency
Department of Surgery
North Colorado Medical Center
Greenly, Colorado

Jensen K. Henry, MD
Assistant Attending Surgeon
Orthopaedic Foot and Ankle Surgery
Hospital for Special Surgery
New York, New York

McCalus V. Hogan, MD, MBA, FAAOS, FAOA
Professor and Chair Chief
Division of Foot and Ankle Surgery
Department of Orthopaedic Surgery
University of Pittsburgh
Pittsburgh, Pennsylvania

James R. Holmes, MD
Associate Professor
Chief of Foot and Ankle Service
Department of Orthopaedic Surgery
University of Michigan
Ann Arbor, Michigan

Kenneth J. Hunt, MD
Associate Professor and Chief
Foot and Ankle Surgery
Vice Chair, Quality, Patient Safety and Outcomes
Medical Director
UCHealth Foot and Ankle Center
Department of Orthopaedic Surgery
University of Colorado School of Medicine
Denver, Colorado

Kelly K. Hynes, MScBMI, MD, FRCSC
Associate Professor
Department of Orthopedic Surgery
The University of Chicago
Chicago, Illinois

Eitan M. Ingall, MD
Fellow
OrthoCarolina Foot & Ankle Institute
Charlotte, North Carolina

A. Holly Johnson, MD
Associate Professor
Department of Orthopedic Surgery
Weill-Cornell Medical School
Hospital for Special Surgery
New York, New York

Anish R. Kadakia, MD
Professor of Orthopaedic Surgery
Northwestern Center for Comprehensive Orthopaedic and Spine Care
Fellowship Director, Foot and Ankle
Department of Orthopaedic Surgery
Northwestern Memorial Hospital
Primary Specialty Foot and Ankle Surgery
Chicago, Illinois

Sarang P. Kasture, FRCS (T&O)
Consultant Foot and Ankle Surgeon
Department of Trauma and Orthopaedics
University Hospitals of Derby and Burton
Burton upon Trent, United Kingdom

Jaeyoung Kim, MD
Research Fellow
Foot and Ankle Service
Orthopaedic Surgery
Hospital for Special Surgery
New York, New York

Georg C. Klammer, MD
Deputy Head of FussInstitut Zürich AG
Institute for Foot and Ankle Reconstruction
Zurich, Switzerland

Kimberly Koury, MD
Department of Orthopedic Surgery
Englewood Hospital
Englewood, New Jersey

John Y. Kwon, MD
Associate Chief, Foot and Ankle Service
Department of Orthopaedics
Massachusetts General Hospital
Boston, Massachusetts

L. Daniel Latt, MD, PhD
Associate Professor
Orthopaedic Surgery and Biomedical Engineering
Director of Clinical Research
Department of Orthopaedic Surgery
University of Arizona
Tucson, Arizona

Woo-Chun Lee, MD, PhD
Director, Fellowship Training Program
Seoul Foot and Ankle Center
Department of Orthopaedic Surgery
Dubalo Hospital
Seoul, South Korea

Shuyuan Li, MD, PhD
International Program Director
Steps2Walk, Inc.
Denver, Colorado

Stephanie Maestre, MD
Foot and Ankle Orthopaedic Surgeon
Department of Orthopaedic Surgery and Sports Medicine
Excela Health System
Greensburg, Pennsylvania

Nacime Salomao Barbachan Mansur, MD, PhD
Visiting Associate
Orthopedic Functional Imaging Research Laboratory
Department of Orthopedics and Rehabilitation
Carver College of Medicine
University of Iowa
Iowa City, Iowa
Foot and Ankle Surgeon
Department of Orthopedics and Traumatology
Paulista School of Medicine
Federal University of Sao Paulo
Sao Paulo, Brazil

Jody P. McAleer, DPM, FACFAS
Foot and Ankle Surgeon
Department of Podiatry
Jefferson City Medical Group
Jefferson City, Missouri

Jeremy J. McCormick, MD
Associate Professor of Orthopaedic Surgery
Chief, Foot and Ankle Surgery
Director, Foot and Ankle Fellowship Program
Washington University in St. Louis
St. Louis, Missouri

Contributors

William C. McGarvey, MD
Professor and Vice Chairman
Department of Orthopedic Surgery
University of Texas Health Science Center–Houston
Residency Program Director
Department of Orthopedic Surgery
Fellowship Program Director–Orthopedic Foot and
    Ankle Fellowship
University of Texas Health Science Center–Houston
Past President, American Orthopedic Foot and Ankle Society
Houston, Texas

Max P. Michalski, MD, MSc
Assistant Professor
Department of Orthopaedic Surgery
Cedars-Sinai Medical Center
Los Angeles, California

Andrew Molloy, MBChB, MRCS, FRCS Tr&Orth
Consultant Orthopaedic Surgeon
Spire Liverpool Hospital
Consultant Orthopaedic Surgeon
Liverpool University Hospitals Foundation Trust
Honorary Clinical Senior Lecturer
Department of Musculoskeletal Biology and Ageing
University of Liverpool
Liverpool, Merseyside, United Kingdom

Drew Murphy, MD
Professor
Department of Orthopedic Surgery
University of Tennessee–Campbell Clinic
Memphis, Tennessee

Mark S. Myerson, MD
Professor of Orthopedics
University of Colorado
President and Founder
Steps2Walk, Inc.
Denver, Colorado

Justin Orr, MD
Associate Clinical Professor
Department of Orthopaedic Surgery
Texas Tech University of Health Sciences
El Paso, Texas

Caio Nery, MD, PhD
Associate Professor
Department of Orthopedics and Traumatology
Foot and Ankle Clinic
Escola Paulista de Medicina
Federal University of São Paulo
São Paulo, Brazil

Cesar de Cesar Netto, MD, PhD
Associate Professor
Division of Orthopedic Foot and Ankle Surgery
Department of Orthopedic Surgery
Duke University
Durham, North Carolina

Martin O'Malley, MD
Orthopaedic Surgeon
Foot and Ankle
Sports Medicine
Hospital for Special Surgery
Associate Professor of Orthopaedic Surgery
Weill Cornell Medical College
New York, New York

Brian Joseph Page, MD
Clinical Fellow
Limb Lengthening and Complex Reconstruction
    Service
Hospital for Special Surgery
New York, New York

Selene G. Parekh, MBA, MD
Professor of Orthopaedic Surgery
Rothman Orthopaedic Institute
Sidney Kimmel College of Medicine at Thomas Jefferson
    University
Philadelphia, Pennsylvania

Vandan D. Patel, MD
Foot and Ankle Fellow
Institute for Foot and Ankle Reconstruction
Mercy Medical Center
Baltimore, Maryland

David Pedowitz, MS, MD
Chief, Division of Foot and Ankle
Professor of Orthopaedic Surgery
Director, Foot and Ankle Fellowship
Sidney Kimmel Medical College
Thomas Jefferson University
Rothman Orthopedics
Philadelphia, Pennsylvania

Alexander B. Peterson, MD
Assistant Professor of Clinical Orthopedic
    Surgery
Department of Orthopedics
Keck School of Medicine of USC
Los Angeles, California

Phinit Phisitkul, MD, MHA, FAAOS
Orthopedic Surgeon
Center for Neurosciences, Orthopaedics,
    and Spine
Dakota Dunes, South Dakota
Medical Director
Riverview Surgical Center
South Sioux City, Nebraska
Adjunct Assistant Professor
College of Allied Health Professions
University of Nebraska Medical Center
Omaha, Nebraska

Fernando Raduan, MD
Foot and Ankle Division
Massachusetts General Hospital
Harvard Medical School
Boston, Massachusetts

John M. Rawlings, MD
Orthopedic Sports Medicine Surgeon
Western Orthopedics & Sports Medicine
Community Hospital
Grand Junction, Colorado

Carson Rider, MD
Instructor of Orthopaedic Surgery
University of Tennessee Health Science Center
Campbell Clinic
Memphis, Tennessee

Matthew M. Roberts, MD
Chief, Foot and Ankle Service
Hospital for Special Surgery
Associate Professor of Clinical Orthopedic Surgery
Weill Medical College of Cornell University
New York, New York

Andrew J. Rosenbaum, MD
Vice-Chairman, Research
Associate Professor
Department of Orthopaedic Surgery
Albany Medical College
Albany, New York

Robert D. Santrock, MD
Clinical Associate Professor
Orthopaedics
Duke University
Durham, North Carolina

Ian Savage-Elliott, MD
Fellow
Department of Orthopedics
Washington University in St. Louis
St. Louis, Missouri

Kevin A. Schafer, MD
Fellow
Department of Orthopedic Surgery
Mercy Medical Center
Baltimore, Maryland

Lew C. Schon, MD, FACS, FAAOS
Director of Orthopaedic Innovation
Institute of Foot and Ankle Reconstruction
Mercy Medical Center
Professor of Orthopaedics
New York University Langone
Professor of Orthopaedics & BME Johns Hopkins School of Medicine
Associate Professor of Orthopaedics
Georgetown School of Medicine
Adjunct Professor and Fischell Literati Faculty
Department of Bioengineering
University of Maryland Orthopaedics
Baltimore, Maryland

Daniel J. Scott, MD, MBA
Associate Professor
Department of Orthopaedic Surgery
Medical University of South Carolina
Charleston, South Carolina

W. Bret Smith, DO, MSc
Director of Foot and Ankle Center
Mercy Orthopedic Associates
Mercy Hospital
Durango, Colorado

Niall Smyth, MD
Orthopaedic Surgeon
Department of Orthopaedic Surgery
Cleveland Clinic Florida
Weston, Florida

Nelson F. SooHoo, MD
Associate Dean for Graduate Medical Education
Professor of Orthopaedic Surgery
UCLA School of Medicine
Los Angeles, California

Andrew P. Thome Jr, MD
Assistant Professor
Foot and Ankle Division
Department of Orthopaedic Surgery
Washington University School of Medicine
St. Louis, Missouri

David B. Thordarson, MD
Professor, Department of Orthopedic Surgery
Director of Orthopedic Research
Cedars-Sinai Medical Center
Los Angeles, California

Contributors

Justin Tsai, MD
Orthopaedic Surgeon
Department of Orthopaedic Surgery
Rothman Orthopaedic Institute
Philadelphia, Pennsylvania

Jordi Vega, MD
Associate Professor
Laboratory of Arthroscopic and Surgical Anatomy
Human Anatomy Unit
Department of Pathology and Experimental Therapeutics
University of Barcelona
Orthopaedic Surgeon
Foot and Ankle Unit
iMove Traumatology–Clinica Tres Torres
Barcelona, Spain

Emilio Wagner, MD
Associate Professor
Department of Foot and Ankle Surgery
Clinica Alemana de Santiago—Universidad del Desarrol
Universidad del Desarrollo
Santiago, Chile

Pablo Wagner, MD, MPH
Associate Professor
Clinica Alemana de Santiago—Universidad del Desarrollo
Associate Professor
Hospital Militar de Santiago—Universidad de los Andes
Foot and Ankle Staff
Department of Orthopedic Surgery
Clinica Alemana de Santiago
Hospital Militar de Santiago
Santiago, Chile

David M. Walton, MD
Assistant Professor
Department of Orthopaedic Surgery
University of Michigan Medical Center
Ann Arbor, Michigan

Alastair S. E. Younger, MB, ChB, MSc, ChM, FRCSC
Orthopaedic Foot and Ankle Surgeon
Professor
Head of Distal Extremities
Department of Orthopaedics
University of British Columbia
Director of Foot and Ankle Research
St. Paul's Hospital
Past President
British Columbia Orthopaedic Association
Partner
Footbridge Centre for Integrated Orthopaedic Care Inc.
Surgeon Scientist, CHEOS
Department of Orthopaedics
St. Paul's Hospital
Vancouver, British Columbia, Canada

John Z. Zhao, MD
Foot and Ankle Clinical Fellow
Department of Orthopedics
Campbell Clinic
Memphis, Tennessee

Series Preface

Since its inception 1994, the *Master Techniques in Orthopaedic Surgery* series has become the gold standard for both physicians in training and experienced surgeons. Its exceptional success may be traced to the leadership of the original series editor, Roby Thompson, whose clarity of thought and focused vision sought "to provide direct, detailed access to techniques preferred by orthopaedic surgeons who are recognized by their colleagues as 'masters' in their specialty," as he stated in his series preface. It is personally very rewarding to hear testimonials from both residents and practicing surgeons on the value of these volumes to their training and practice. A key element of the success of the series is its format. Of note, this format was inspired by Dr. Kenneth Johnson, a foot and ankle orthopaedic surgeon from the Mayo Clinic. Ken was a personal friend of mine. This fourth edition of *Master Techniques* series is, in my opinion, a testament to his vision and individuality. He wanted to prepare a book about the way he did foot and ankle surgery. He was not interested in presenting the world's experience, but rather, "here's how I do it." The effectiveness of this format is reflected by the fact that it is now being replicated by other publishers. Among other strengths, an essential feature of the *Master Techniques* series is the standardized presentation and illustration of information with tips and pearls shared by experts with years of experience. Abundant color photographs and drawings guide the reader through the procedures step-by-step.

The second key to the success of the *Master Techniques* series rests in the reputation and experience of our volume editors. The editors are truly dedicated and recognized "masters" with a commitment to share their rich experience through these texts. We are proud of the progress made in formulating the fourth edition volumes and are particularly pleased with the expanded context of this series. Since its inception, new volumes have been added in an effort to remain relevant and to cover topics that are exciting and useful to a broad cross-section of our profession. While we have expanded the *Master Techniques* topics and editors with additional titles, we have remained true to the now classic format.

The first of the new volumes was *Relevant Surgical Exposures*, edited with my son, Matthew. Additional volumes include *Essential Procedures in Pediatrics, Soft Tissue Reconstruction, Advanced Techniques in Joint Reconstruction,* and *Essential Procedures in Sports Medicine*. The full library consists of useful and relevant titles covering the full spectrum of our profession.

I am pleased to be involved as the series editor, as I feel strongly about the value of the series in educating the surgeon in the full array of expert surgical procedures. The true worth of this endeavor will continue to be measured by the ever-increasing success and critical acceptance of the series. I remain indebted to Dr. Thompson for his inaugural leadership as well as to the *Master Techniques* volume editors and numerous contributors who have been true to the series style and vision. The words of William Mayo are especially relevant to characterize the ultimate goal of this endeavor. "The best interest of the patient is the only interest to be considered." We are confident that the information in the expanded *Master Techniques* offers the surgeon an opportunity to realize the patient-centric view of our surgical practice.

Bernard F. Morrey, MD
Series Editor

Preface

I still remember reading the second edition of *Master Techniques in Foot and Ankle Surgery* as a resident and fellow as I prepared for my cases on the foot and ankle service each day. I found myself ready each morning to carry out surgeries that my attendings scheduled, no matter what the calendar might have held. The vast array of types and techniques of surgery, described by leaders in the field I would later come to know, drew me to my ultimate decision to specialize in this exciting field. When Dr. Morrey and Dr. Kitaoka asked me edit the fourth edition of *Master Techniques in Orthopaedic Surgery*, I felt honored and motivated to contribute, but knew I would need help. After all, it was their insight and hard work that brought the book to its current level. However, much has changed as the field rapidly evolves.

I have leveraged expertise by colleagues from all over the world to capitalize on the latest advances in our field. While cutting edge research and data drives much of our decision-making in surgery, having a trusted colleague take you through a case presents the most valuable opportunity to learn and improve patient outcomes that I know. I have chosen the subsection editors carefully for this series given their international reputation, research, and expertise: A. Holly Johnson (forefoot and MIS), Mark Drakos (sports and Achilles), Constantine A. Demetracopoulos (total ankle), Cesar de Cesar Netto (flatfoot), and John Kwon (trauma and neuromuscular disorder) have provided countless hours to create a book that will serve both as a teaching manual and reference for both trainees and experienced surgeons alike.

The vast majority of chapters present new material and, in particular, even new techniques not performed at the time the last edition came out over 10 years ago. This holds true for each subsection, but especially for total ankle and minimally invasive approaches. Chapters on deformity reconstruction, bunion, and tendon/ligament reconstruction also reflect the latest advances. I am confident that in another 10 years we will all read a different book as well.

I have tried to balance opinions, strategies, and approaches across all techniques. For example, all current total ankle replacement prostheses have their own chapter, each highlighting positive design features along with tips and pearls from the experts that use them regularly. The same holds true for traditional versus more minimally invasive approaches. Because nothing comes easy in foot and ankle surgery, topics run from the simple to most complex.

I hope that you learn as much as I have when reading these techniques, written by the masters in our field. I thank the authors for their tireless efforts despite running busy practices, spending time away from their families, and competing with other academic duties such as teaching and research. I encourage our colleagues in foot and ankle surgery to use these to update their knowledge and as a reference for the cases you perform. I am confident that those reading the chapters will likely be the next ones writing them in the coming years.

Scott Ellis, MD

Contents

Contributors v

Series Preface xiii

Preface xv

PART 1 Forefoot/Bunion 1
Section Editor: A. Holly Johnson

CHAPTER 1
Lapidus With Akin   1
Matthew S. Conti and W. Hodges Davis

CHAPTER 2
Scarf First Metatarsal Osteotomy   19
Andrew Molloy and Sarang P. Kasture

CHAPTER 3
Minimally Invasive Surgical (MIS) Bunionectomy   31
Tonya An and A. Holly Johnson

CHAPTER 4
Correction of Hallux Valgus With and Without Metatarsus Adductus   53
Mark E. Easley, Paul Dayton, William T. DeCarbo, Daniel J. Hatch, Jody P. McAleer, W. Bret Smith, and Robert D. Santrock

CHAPTER 5
Proximal Rotational Metatarsal Osteotomy (PROMO)   101
Emilio Wagner and Pablo Wagner

PART 2 Forefoot/Hallux Rigidus 113

Section Editor: A. Holly Johnson

CHAPTER 6
Cheilectomy/Moberg 113
Kimberly Koury and Judy Baumhauer

CHAPTER 7
Minimally Invasive Surgery (MIS) Cheilectomy With Moberg Osteotomy 129
Vandan D. Patel and Rebecca Cerrato

PART 3 Total Ankle Replacement 143

Section Editor: Constantine A. Demetracopoulos

CHAPTER 8
Salto Talaris Total Ankle Replacement 143
James S. Davitt

CHAPTER 9
Paragon 28 APEX 3D Fixed-Bearing Total Ankle Replacement 163
Christopher E. Gross and Daniel J. Scott

CHAPTER 10
Infinity Total Ankle Replacement 179
Brian M. Fisher and Jeremy J. McCormick

CHAPTER 11
Lateral Approach Total Ankle Arthroplasty 199
Kevin A. Schafer and Lew C. Schon

CHAPTER 12
The Stryker INBONE II Total Ankle Arthroplasty System 219
M. Pierce Ebaugh and William C. McGarvey

CHAPTER 13
Exactech Vantage Fixed-Bearing Total Ankle Replacement 233
Jensen K. Henry and Constantine A. Demetracopoulos

CHAPTER 14
Cadence Total Ankle Replacement 251
Justin Tsai, Daniel Fuchs, and David Pedowitz

CHAPTER 15
The Kinos Axiom Total Ankle System 263
Eitan M. Ingall and J. Kent Ellington

Contents

PART 4 Sports 275
Section Editor: Mark Drakos

CHAPTER 16
Hamstring Peroneals 275
Mark Drakos

CHAPTER 17
Lateral Ankle Ligament Repair and Reconstruction 285
L. Daniel Latt

CHAPTER 18
Débridement, Repair, and Regeneration of Osteochondral Lesions of the Talus 299
John M. Rawlings and Richard D. Ferkel

CHAPTER 19
Osteochondral Autologous Transfer Systems (OATS) for the Treatment of Talar Osteochondral Lesions: The OATS Procedure 317
Ahmed Khalil Attia and McCalus V. Hogan

CHAPTER 20
Open Reduction and Internal Fixation Fifth Metatarsal 337
Kenneth J. Hunt and Benjamin Ebben

CHAPTER 21
Open Reduction and Internal Fixation of Navicular Stress Fractures 349
Andrew J. Rosenbaum and Martin O'Malley

CHAPTER 22
Os Trigonum Resection 359
J. Chris Coetzee

PART 5 Achilles 367
Section Editor: Mark Drakos

CHAPTER 23
Graft Reconstruction for Treatment of Chronic Achilles Tendon Ruptures 367
Carson Rider, Drew Murphy, Stephanie S. Gardner, and John Z. Zhao

CHAPTER 24
Haglund Deformity With Flexor Hallucis Longus Tendon Transfer 377
Kelly K. Hynes

CHAPTER 25
Endoscopic Treatment of Insertional Achilles Deformity   389
Jordi Vega, Matteo Guelfi, and Miki Dalmau-Pastor

CHAPTER 26
Minimally Invasive (MIS) Repair of Achilles Tendon Ruptures   403
Ian Savage-Elliott and Jonathon Backus

PART 6   Flatfoot   417
Section Editor: Cesar de Cesar Netto

CHAPTER 27
Lateral Column Lengthening and Medial Displacement Calcaneal Osteotomies for Progressive Collapsing Foot Deformity   417
Michael Aronow

CHAPTER 28
First Ray Procedures in Progressive Collapsing Foot Deformity: Cotton, Lapidus, and Lapicotton   429
Nacime Salomao Barbachan Mansur, Kepler Alencar Mendes de Carvalho, and Cesar de Cesar Netto

CHAPTER 29
Subtalar Fusion for Progressive Collapsing Foot Deformity   453
Tonya An, Scott Ellis, and Matthew M. Roberts

CHAPTER 30
Minimally Invasive Osteotomies of the Calcaneus   471
Gregory P. Guyton

CHAPTER 31
Spring Ligament Reconstruction   481
Jaeyoung Kim and Jonathan Deland

CHAPTER 32
Double/Triple Arthrodesis   491
James W. Brodsky and Andrew P. Thome Jr

PART 7   Ankle Osteoarthritis   513
Section Editor: Constantine A. Demetracopoulos

CHAPTER 33
Ankle Distraction Arthroplasty   513
Austin T. Fragomen and Brian Joseph Page

CHAPTER 34
Open Ankle Arthrodesis Utilizing Anterior Plating   527
David M. Walton and James R. Holmes

Contents

CHAPTER 35
Ankle Fusion With External Fixation 539
Justin Orr

CHAPTER 36
Arthroscopic Ankle Arthrodesis 567
Oliver J. Gagne and Alastair S. E. Younger

CHAPTER 37
Supramalleolar Osteotomy 577
Jaeyoung Kim and Woo-Chun Lee

CHAPTER 38
Tibiotalocalcaneal Fusion 595
Braden Boyer, John Wunn Cancian, and Clayton C. Bettin

CHAPTER 39
Total Talus Replacement 615
Albert T. Anastasio, Amanda N. Fletcher, and Selene G. Parekh

PART 8 Forefoot/Lesser Toes 629
Section Editor: A. Holly Johnson

CHAPTER 40
Crossover Toe Correction 629
Phinit Phisitkul

CHAPTER 41
Lesser Toes Metatarsophalangeal Plantar Plate Tears: Dorsal Direct Repair in Combination With Weil Osteotomy 647
Caio Nery and Daniel Baumfeld

PART 9 Trauma 663
Section Editor: John Y. Kwon

CHAPTER 42
Ankle Fracture Late Syndesmosis Repair 663
Fernando Raduan and John Y. Kwon

CHAPTER 43
Arthroscopic-Assisted Open Reduction and Internal Fixation Ankle 677
Arianna L. Gianakos, Stephanie Maestre, Niall Smyth, and Amiethab Aiyer

CHAPTER 44
Minimally Invasive Open Reduction and Internal Fixation Calcaneus 689
Alexander B. Peterson, Max P. Michalski, and David B. Thordarson

PART 10 Neuromuscular 703
Section Editor: John Y. Kwon

CHAPTER 45
Posterior Tibial Tendon Transfer 703
Ajay N. Gurbani and Nelson F. SooHoo

CHAPTER 46
The Malerba Osteotomy and First Metatarsal Dorsiflexion Osteotomy 711
Elizabeth A. Cody

CHAPTER 47
Reconstruction in Charcot-Marie-Tooth Disease 719
Norman Espinosa, Anish R. Kadakia, and Georg C. Klammer

CHAPTER 48
Salvage of Over/Undercorrected Neuromuscular Foot 739
Shuyuan Li and Mark S. Myerson

Index 765

PART ONE
FOREFOOT/BUNION

1 Lapidus With Akin

Matthew S. Conti and W. Hodges Davis

INTRODUCTION

Hallux valgus is a triplanar deformity of the first ray in which there is metatarsus primus varus and valgus of the great toe, first metatarsal dorsiflexion, and pronation of the first metatarsal.[1] The apex of the deformity occurs at the first tarsometatarsal (TMT) joint with recent literature suggesting that there is instability between the medial and middle cuneiforms.[2] Arthrodesis of the first TMT joint in conjunction with a distal soft tissue procedure for the correction of a hallux valgus deformity was promoted by Lapidus during the 1930s through the 1960s.[3-5]

Although not the originator of this technique, Lapidus reported on it to stress his perception of the mechanical importance of metatarsus primus varus as one of the most common causes and most prominent factors of the hallux valgus deformity. His original description of the procedure involved arthrodesis of the first TMT joint with the creation of a bony bridge between the bases of the first and second metatarsals and a distal soft tissue release. In the past six decades since Lapidus last reported his work, the indications for performing this surgery have significantly changed and many modifications to the procedure have been proposed.[6-12] Nonetheless, the goals of this operation have remained the same: to correct and stabilize the first metatarsal at the apex of the deformity.

While the Lapidus procedure is a powerful tool that allows for correction of hallux valgus in all three planes with recent work demonstrating its effectiveness in correcting the rotational component,[13] it is often used in combination with a medial closing wedge osteotomy of the proximal phalanx (Akin osteotomy) to correct hallux valgus interphalangeus or residual hallux valgus deformity. The Akin osteotomy was described by Akin in 1925 for the correction of hallux valgus.[14] The concomitant use of an Akin osteotomy with a first TMT joint arthrodesis results in excellent postoperative alignment of the foot, low rates of recurrence, and high patient-reported outcomes.[6]

INDICATIONS AND CONTRAINDICATIONS

The primary indication for the Lapidus procedure remains hallux valgus deformity associated with metatarsus primus varus and a hypermobile first ray. Historically, first TMT arthrodesis was generally performed for moderate to severe hallux valgus deformity with a hallux valgus angle of greater than 30° and an intermetatarsal (IM) angle of 14° or more. If metatarsus adductus is present, however, the IM 1 to 2 angle may measure less than 14°, even though the position of the first metatarsal with respect to the longitudinal axis of the foot is in marked varus. Isolated first TMT arthrodesis in the setting of metatarsus adductus has demonstrated good results.[15]

It is the authors' opinion that evidence of hypermobility at the first TMT joint as an indication for the Lapidus procedure outweighs using the severity of the deformity measured on anteroposterior (AP) radiographs as the sole criterion for patient selection. Patients with clinical or radiographic hypermobility at the first TMT joint may benefit from a Lapidus procedure to decrease the risk of recurrence.

Other indications for this operation are hallux valgus and severe metatarsus primus varus associated with generalized ligamentous laxity or first TMT arthritis. The adolescent bunion with moderate to severe deformity is at a high risk for recurrence and has been successfully treated with a first TMT arthrodesis when the epiphysis has closed. Additionally, patients who have failed previous bunionectomy are often good candidates for the procedure. Severe deformities that occur in osteopenic feet may fare better with fixation at the TMT level than the proximal aspect of the first metatarsal. Historically, a relative contraindication for the Lapidus procedure was the elderly population due to the need for patients to be non–weight bearing until the arthrodesis had healed. However, modern fixation techniques that allow earlier weight bearing have expanded the indications for this procedure.

This procedure may be contraindicated in dancers or elite athletes, who typically require maximum joint flexibility during their desired activities. That said, recreational athletes have been found to have a high rate of return to sports including high-impact activities.[16] Additionally, this procedure is contraindicated in juvenile patients with an open epiphysis, noncompliant patients, or those with Charcot arthropathy. In patients with symptomatic arthritis of the first metatarsophalangeal (MTP) joint, fusion of both the TMT and MTP joints is often avoided due to increased stiffness of the medial column but may be performed in select cases. In most patients with symptomatic first MTP joint arthritis, an isolated first MTP arthrodesis may result in a more predictable outcome and frequently obviates the need for fusion at the first TMT joint. Patients who have short first metatarsals may suffer from additional shortening from the Lapidus procedure that may precipitate symptoms from second MTP overload. In these cases, if a first TMT arthrodesis is planned, a concomitant procedure to lengthen the first metatarsal or to shorten the lesser metatarsals should be considered. Alternatively, length can be obtained through a bone block distraction arthrodesis at the first MTP joint. At times, plantar translation or plantarflexion through the first TMT joint could permit better weight bearing when there is less severe shortening.

PREOPERATIVE PLANNING

A general assessment of a patient's alertness and mental status will help determine his or her compliance for the surgical reconstruction. Ligamentous laxity observed throughout the musculoskeletal system as tested using the Beighton score lends support to choosing a first TMT arthrodesis over a proximal or distal first metatarsal osteotomy.

Overall alignment of the lower extremity should be observed statically and dynamically to identify etiologic factors that may influence the outcome. Hallux valgus is often present in patients with progressive collapsing foot deformity. Patients with collapse of the medial longitudinal arch do not routinely require reconstruction of their deformity unless they are symptomatic.[17] Additionally, pronation of the hallux may be present. Although recent studies have demonstrated that rotation of the hallux is not necessarily correlated with rotation of the first metatarsal,[18] severe hallux pronation with medial rotation of the nailbed should be noted and corrected at the time of surgery (Fig. 1.1A). A callus on the medial aspect of the hallux may also be suggestive of a pronation deformity of the great toe (Fig. 1.1B). Palpation of the pulses is critical to determine whether there is adequate vascularity and to assess the position of the dorsalis pedis relative to the first TMT joint. It may be possible to palpate the medial dorsal cutaneous nerve, which is vulnerable to iatrogenic injury.

In addition to observing parameters such as the size and shape of the foot, it is helpful to assess the range of motion of the entire foot and ankle. A Silfverskiold test should be performed to examine for an equinus contracture and gastrocnemius tightness. A proximal medial gastrocnemius recession[19] or more distal gastrocnemius recession may be indicated in the setting of an equinus contracture. While a first TMT arthrodesis may exacerbate preexisting symptoms in adjacent joints, motion at this joint is limited and fusion rarely causes issues in surrounding joints. The second and third TMT joints should be evaluated, especially in cases of arthritis or more severe deformity, because it is occasionally necessary to extend the fusion to incorporate these joints.

Hypermobility of the first ray is evaluated in a position of neutral ankle dorsiflexion by grasping the first metatarsal with the examiner's hand while stabilizing the rest of the foot with the other hand.[20,21] While the midfoot is held stable, the thumb and forefinger of the opposite hand manipulate

1 Lapidus With Akin

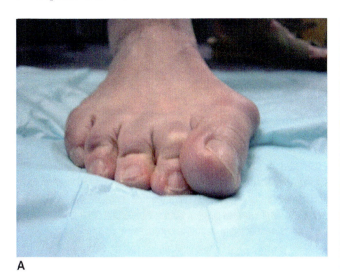
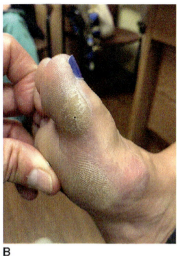

FIGURE 1.1 **A.** Clinical photograph of a patient with hallux valgus and pronation of the nailbed of the great toe. The deformity should be noted preoperatively, and attention should be paid to correcting the rotation of the toe intraoperatively. **B.** Clinical photograph of a patient with a callus on the medial aspect of their hallux suggesting pronation deformity of the hallux.

the first metatarsal in the dorsal-plantar plane (Fig. 1.2). The joint is then placed through a rotational arc (supination-pronation). Particular attention is paid to the increased arc of motion in the dorsal direction, which is associated with dorsal elevation or prominence of the first metatarsal and weight transfer to the second metatarsal. By abducting and adducting the metatarsal, medial-lateral stability is checked.

In cases of first TMT hypermobility, it is important to assess first MTP motion with the first metatarsal reduced to proper alignment. This will allow for an estimate of postoperative first MTP range of motion and congruency. Additionally, first TMT hypermobility can present as transfer metatarsalgia to the second ray, causing plantar callus formation and second MTP joint synovitis with subsequent subluxation and hammer toe or crossover toe formation.

Weight-bearing AP and lateral radiographs should be obtained. On AP radiographs, measurements of the 1 to 2 IM and hallux valgus angles are made. The presence of metatarsus adductus, hallux valgus interphalangeus, the lengths of the first and second metatarsals, the position of the sesamoids, and the congruity of the hallux MTP joint are noted. On lateral weight-bearing radiographs, several findings are indicative of first TMT instability (hypermobility), including loss of alignment between the first metatarsal and the medial cuneiform resulting in medial or dorsal translation of the first metatarsal and a break in the axis of the medial column that occurs at the first

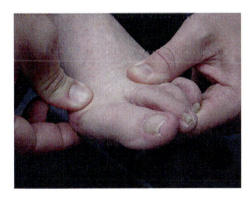
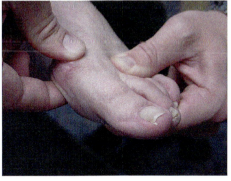

FIGURE 1.2 Clinical examination of hypermobility at the first tarsometatarsal (TMT) joint. The examiner holds the lesser toes with one hand while the other hand moves the first metatarsal dorsally and plantarly. Excessive motion at the first TMT joint suggests hypermobility of the first ray.

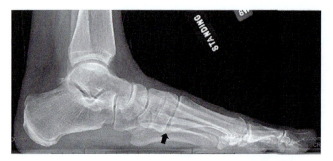

FIGURE 1.3 Lateral weight-bearing radiographs of the foot demonstrating instability at the first tarsometatarsal (TMT) joint. The *black arrow* points to a plantar gap at the base of the first TMT joint.

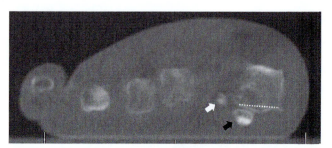

FIGURE 1.4 Coronal image of a weight-bearing computed tomography scan in a patient with hallux valgus. The *dashed white line* demonstrates mild pronation of the first metatarsal head. The *black* and *white arrows* point to subluxation of the tibial and fibular sesamoids, respectively, from their grooves.

metatarsal-medial cuneiform joint resulting in a plantar gap (Fig. 1.3) or widening between the joint surfaces, although some authors have argued against plantar gapping as a reliable sign of first TMT joint hypermobility.[22] Hypermobility may also be suggested radiographically as increased cortical hypertrophy along the medial border of the second metatarsal shaft.

Incongruity of the first MTP joint and/or tightness of the lateral capsule may contribute to restricted motion. This incongruity, sometimes caused by a distal metatarsal articular surface (DMAA) angle of more than 15°, will cause a decrease in the first MTP joint range of motion postoperatively. Recent studies have suggested that an increase in the DMAA is the result of both distal obliquity of the first metatarsal head articular surface and rotation of the first metatarsal.[23] If substantial incongruity is present, correction may rarely require a medial closing wedge distal metatarsal osteotomy or a proximal phalangeal medial closing wedge osteotomy (Akin osteotomy).

Preoperative weight-bearing computed tomography (WBCT) scans may help to assess rotational deformity of the first metatarsal and subluxation of the sesamoids.[24] No association between the 1 to 2 IM angle or hallux valgus angle and first metatarsal pronation has been found, so weight-bearing three-dimensional imaging modalities may be necessary to correctly understand the magnitude of the first metatarsal rotational deformity.[13] Studies have demonstrated that judging sesamoid position on radiographs alone is inaccurate as the sesamoids may sit in their grooves but appear subluxated due to pronation of the first metatarsal.[24] The coronal view of a WBCT scan can be used to evaluate first metatarsal pronation by comparing the sesamoid grooves and intersesamoidal ridge (crista) to a reference such as the floor (Fig. 1.4).[24] This may provide an estimation of the degree of rotational correction necessary when performing the Lapidus procedure. The relative position of the sesamoids from their grooves may also be assessed on this view, which can help with planning for reduction of the sesamoids at the time of surgery. The sagittal view may be used to better judge plantar gapping and first TMT instability.

Preoperatively, it is important to educate the patient as to the nature of this operation as well as to alternative treatments. Patients need to be aware of the potential for complications including prolonged recovery time and swelling, recurrent deformity, nonunion, and malunion. Anecdotally, after a first TMT arthrodesis, we have found that patients experience more discomfort and swelling than with other procedures for severe hallux valgus. We tell patients that, by 3 months postoperatively, the bone is 75% healed, and by 6 months, it is 90% healed (Fig. 1.5). Swelling is the last symptom to improve, and various aches and pains may take more than a year for resolution. Joint stiffness and pain beneath the sesamoids, problems with wound healing, infection, incisional neuromas, and the need for hardware removal should be discussed and are otherwise similar to other bunion operations that require internal fixation.

SURGICAL TECHNIQUE

- Careful preoperative planning is essential to obtain appropriate correction (Fig. 1.6).
- The patient is positioned supine on the operating table with a bump under the ipsilateral hip. If other concomitant procedures are being performed, initial positioning may be different. Bilateral procedures are rarely performed simultaneously.

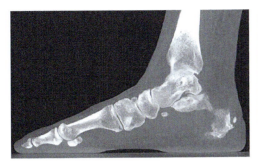 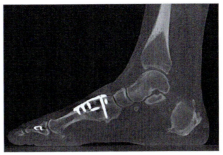

FIGURE 1.5 Preoperative and postoperative sagittal weight-bearing computed tomography scans. The 6-month postoperative sagittal view demonstrates bony bridging across the first tarsometatarsal joint.

- This procedure can be performed with general anesthetic or under intravenous sedation with an ankle block analgesia using a mixture of 1.0% lidocaine and 0.5% bupivacaine without epinephrine (equal amounts). About 30 to 40 mL is used. Alternatively, a popliteal block and/or a spinal anesthetic may be used.
- The procedure is performed with an Esmarch bandage around the ankle or a thigh tourniquet or lower leg tourniquet, or without a tourniquet. If performing hammer toe or crossover toe correction, we prefer a thigh tourniquet to prevent tension on the flexor and extensor tendons of the toes.

Calcaneal Bone Graft

- The authors routinely use calcaneal bone graft in all Lapidus procedures. We prefer to pack the bone graft in the joint space prior to compression across the first TMT joint.
- A 1-cm incision is made in the center of the calcaneal tuberosity. It is located approximately 1 cm dorsal to the glabrous skin and 1 cm anterior to the posterior border of the calcaneus.
- The incision is made through skin and then a hemostat is used to spread to bone.
- An 8-mm bone graft reamer or trephine is used to obtain bone graft (Fig. 1.7). We typically make one pass across the calcaneus with care not to violate the far cortex. The bone graft is removed from the reamer at this point. If additional bone graft is required, an additional pass dorsally and/or anteriorly may be used.

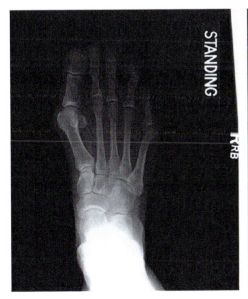 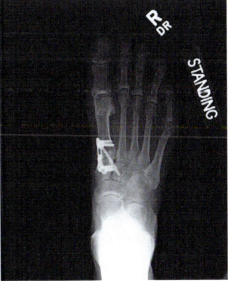

FIGURE 1.6 Preoperative and postoperative anteroposterior (AP) radiographs of a patient with a high intermetatarsal angle and significant hallux valgus deformity. The postoperative AP radiograph demonstrates correction of the deformity with the Lapidus procedure.

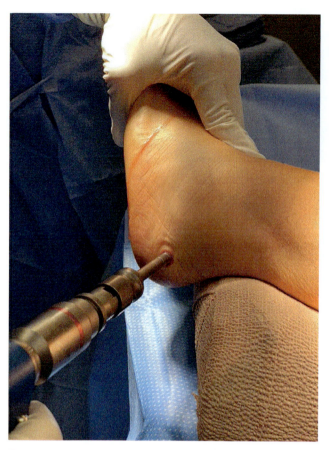

FIGURE 1.7 Obtaining calcaneal bone graft. An 8-mm bone graft reamer is used to obtain graft from the calcaneus.

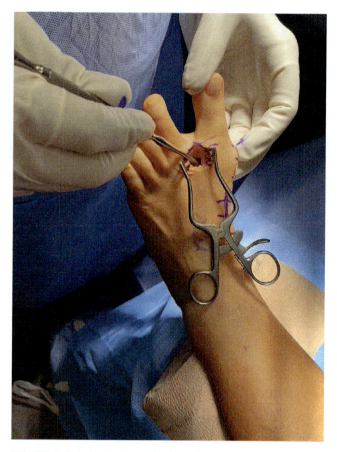

FIGURE 1.8 Lateral release via dorsal first web space incision. Through the dorsal first web space incision, the metatarsosesamoid ligament was released. The surgeon then places a varus stress on the hallux to ensure that it can be manipulated into slight varus, which confirms adequate soft tissue release.

Intermetatarsal Incision

- A 3-cm dorsal incision in the first web space is performed.
- The incision is made through skin with blunt dissection down to the lateral aspect of the first metatarsal head. A freer is used to palpate the space between the metatarsal head and fibular sesamoid (ie, the metatarsosesamoid ligament) (Fig. 1.8).
- A scalpel is used to release the metatarsosesamoid ligament longitudinally. This release facilitates reduction of the sesamoids under the metatarsal head.
- The hallux is then manipulated into varus. If the hallux can be manually manipulated into varus, no further release is performed. It has been our experience that routine release of the adductor tendon may result in postoperative hallux varus deformity. If the hallux cannot be manipulated into varus, partial release of the adductor tendon from the fibular sesamoid may be performed. We avoid fully releasing the adductor tendon.
- A hemostat clamp is then used to bluntly dissect over the second metatarsal neck. This will allow a distal reduction clamp to reduce the 1 to 2 IM angle by wrapping around the second metatarsal distally.

Medial Incision

- Attention is then turned to the medial first MTP capsulotomy and medial eminence resection. A midmedial longitudinal incision is made over the hallux MTP joint. Care is taken to identify the dorsal medial cutaneous nerve that courses dorsomedially across the MTP joint. This nerve

is often seen just dorsal to the incision. Skin flaps are then developed to better visualize the joint capsule.
- The medial joint capsule and first MTP joint are then identified. We prefer a V to Y capsulotomy. The two limbs of the V are divergent distally and converge proximally just proximal to the MTP joint. The capsulotomy is extended proximally to form the Y portion (Fig. 1.9).
- The capsule is then peeled off the medial eminence, and the entire medial eminence is exposed (Fig. 1.10).
- Following capsulotomy and exposure of the medial eminence, we prefer to perform the correction at the first TMT joint before completing our medial eminence resection.

Dorsal Incision Over the First TMT Joint

- A dorsomedial incision is made over the first TMT joint and medial to the extensor hallucis longus (EHL) tendon (Fig. 1.11). Care should be taken to avoid injury to the distal branch of the dorsal medial cutaneous nerve, which originates proximally from the superficial peroneal nerve.
- The EHL tendon is retracted laterally, and the first TMT joint capsule exposed. The first TMT joint may be identified with a needle or scalpel. An incision is made through the first TMT joint capsule, and the capsule peeled off the bone.
- A pin-based retractor is then placed with the pins on either side of the first TMT joint in the medial cuneiform and first metatarsal base. The wires are placed parallel to each other in the coronal and sagittal planes (Fig. 1.12). Care is taken to place the pins parallel in the coronal plane as this can help the surgeon to judge changes in rotational alignment of the first metatarsal. It is important to

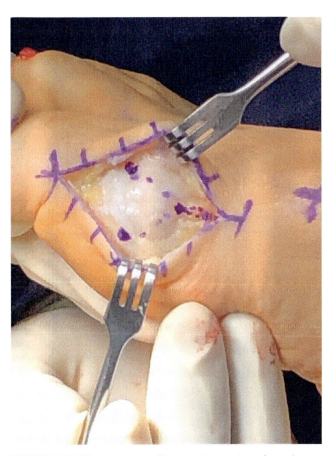

FIGURE 1.9 V-Y capsulotomy. The capsulotomy is performed in line with the markings shown here on the medial joint capsule. Additionally, tissue can be removed from the "V" or "Y" components of the capsule in order to provide a soft tissue restraint to valgus drift of the hallux.

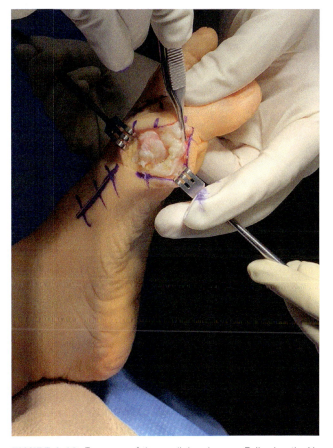

FIGURE 1.10 Exposure of the medial eminence. Following the V to Y capsulotomy, the capsule is carefully peeled from the medial eminence.

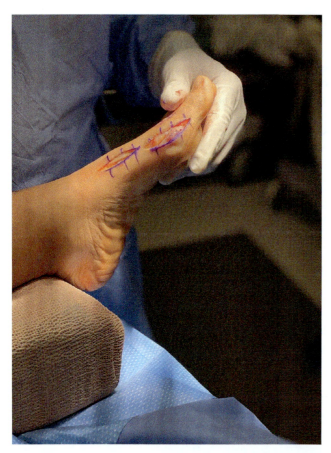

FIGURE 1.11 Dorsomedial incision over the first tarsometatarsal joint. The incision is made just medial to the extensor hallucis longus tendon.

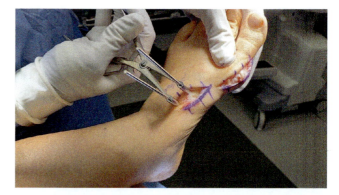

FIGURE 1.12 Pin-based distractor placement. The pins for the distractor are then placed. They are placed parallel in the coronal and sagittal planes in order to later determine changes in first metatarsal pronation.

  note that there are a number of commercially available products to assist the surgeon in obtaining appropriate triplanar correction.
- The pin-based distractor is then used to allow access to the joint.
- To minimize bone resection and shortening of the first metatarsal, an osteotome is employed to denude the cartilage from the joint surfaces (Fig. 1.13). A curette is used to remove cartilage from the outer rim as well as débride the joint of cartilage pushed plantarly. The natural contour of the joint surfaces may be preserved by carefully resecting cartilage with the use of sharp chisels. Because of the unusual shape of the joint, optimal correction of deformity is not always easy to achieve. The correction depends on the presence of the slight concave-convex configuration, which can also be saddle-shaped or bean-shaped but not flat. Numerous configurations of the joint surfaces are encountered, some of which enhance and some block the repositioning of the metatarsal. Occasionally, there are two separate facets on the base of the metatarsal. The plane of this concavity is toward the second cuneiform, and the convexity faces medially. The depth of the articular surface is deep and sometimes difficult to reach even with a long curette. Alternatively, flat cuts with a saw blade may be performed in order to maintain the most surface area for correction. Care must be taken to avoid shortening or dorsiflexing the first metatarsal when performing the cuts.
- The first TMT joint is about 3 cm in depth, and it is important to ensure that the plantar cartilage is removed. There is a tendency to remove insufficient cartilage from the deeper (plantar) metatarsal and cuneiform joint surfaces, and careful inspection is needed when removing the deeper parts of the metatarsal with a long pituitary rongeur, curette, or thin chisel.
- The joint is then gently irrigated to remove any remaining cartilage or bone fragments that may prevent appropriate reduction.
- A 2.5-mm drill is used to prepare the joint surfaces. The bone graft from the calcaneus is then packed into the joint. Alternatively, burr holes at the site of the arthrodesis can be made and bone graft packed into these holes.

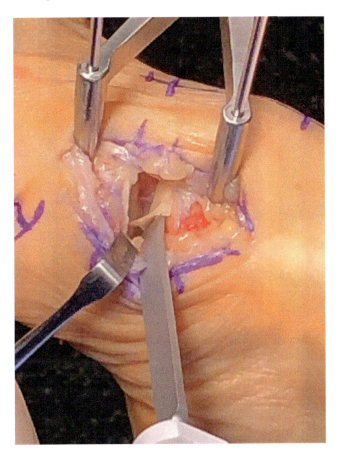

FIGURE 1.13 Removing cartilage from the first tarsometatarsal (TMT) joint. Following placement of the pin-based distractor, an osteotome is used to denude the first TMT joint cartilage. This may help to avoid shortening the first metatarsal.

- The reduction is then performed. A clamp is placed distally from the first metatarsal head and around the second metatarsal neck (Fig. 1.14). This clamp is used to reduce the 1 to 2 IM angle. Care should be taken to assess rotational changes of the first metatarsal in the coronal plane by judging the divergence of the distractor pins. Special attention should be paid to correcting the first metatarsal pronation deformity (Fig. 1.15).
- An AP fluoroscopic view of the foot may help to assess the 1 to 2 IM angle as well as the position of the sesamoids (Fig. 1.16). Manual palpation of the first metatarsal head may be performed to ensure that the first metatarsal is appropriately plantarflexed. Dorsiflexion of the first metatarsal may lead to subsequent overload of the second metatarsal.
- If the correction cannot be achieved by simply rotating the metatarsal on the cuneiform, then a small wedge may be resected from the joint. The wedge is biplanar with the openings lateral and plantar. Care must be taken not to overcorrect the first metatarsal; if a negative IM angle is created, a hallux varus deformity may result.

Plate Fixation

- Once the appropriate reduction has been obtained, a guidewire for a 4.0-mm cannulated screw is then placed plantarly and medially in the first metatarsal base. This guidewire starts medially in the first metatarsal base (at the plantar third) and aims proximally and dorsally to the far proximal and lateral corner of the middle cuneiform. Intraoperative AP and lateral fluoroscopic views are obtained to ensure that the guidewire is in the appropriate trajectory (Fig. 1.17).
- A 4.0-mm cannulated screw with a washer is then placed over the guidewire to hold reduction of the hallux valgus deformity. A washer is used due to the soft bone at the base of the first metatarsal.
- A five- or six-hole low-profile plate with locking screw options is then used with 3.5-mm screws. Often, the plate requires a small offset due to the step-off and incongruency that is created when the first metatarsal is rotated. The plate sits dorsomedially over the first TMT joint (Fig. 1.18).
- Two locking screws are placed in the proximal aspect of the plate. The plate is then eccentrically loaded distally with a cortical screw to create additional compression across the first TMT joint. Two additional locking screws are placed distally to stabilize the construct.

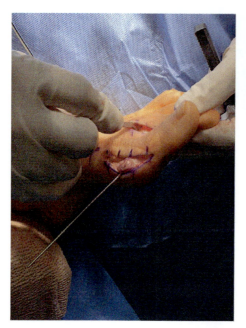
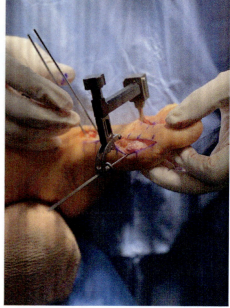

FIGURE 1.14 Distal reduction clamp placement. The guidewire for the clamp in the first metatarsal head is placed perpendicular to the second metatarsal shaft to facilitate the reduction. A clamp is then placed distally to reduce the 1 to 2 IM angle by bringing the first and second metatarsal heads together.

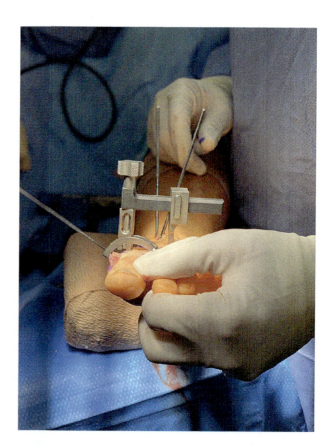

FIGURE 1.15 Rotational changes of the first metatarsal. The distal pin can be rotated laterally in order to supinate the first metatarsal and correct the pronation deformity. The pins should initially be placed parallel in order to determine the amount of first metatarsal rotational correction that has been achieved.

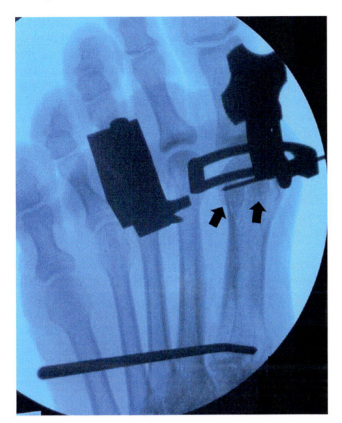

FIGURE 1.16 Correction of the sesamoids on an anteroposterior fluoroscopic view. Two *black arrows* point to appropriate correction of the sesamoids beneath the first metatarsal head. The pin at the base of the first metatarsal has been supinated to reduce the pronation deformity. The distal clamp helps correct rotation as well as the intermetatarsal angle. Adequate correction of the deformity allows reduction of the sesamoids beneath the first metatarsal head.

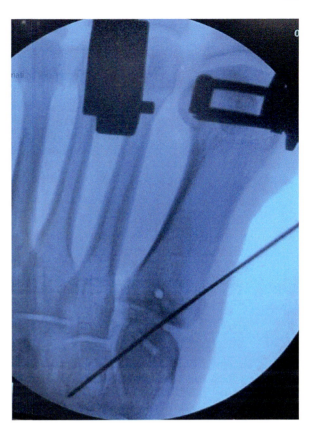

FIGURE 1.17 Trajectory of the guidewire for the cannulated screw. Following correction of the 1 to 2 IM angle and rotational deformity of the first metatarsal, a 4.0-mm cannulated screw is placed from the base of the first metatarsal to the proximal lateral corner of the middle cuneiform. The wire typically starts plantar medially on the first metatarsal base and aims slightly dorsally.

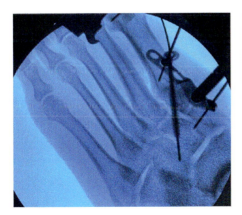 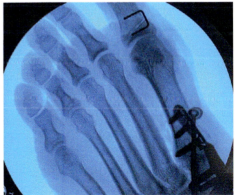

FIGURE 1.18 Position of the first tarsometatarsal (TMT) joint plate. The plate should be placed dorsomedially over the first TMT joint. The plate usually requires a step-off due to deformity correction at the first TMT joint.

- If additional stability is required, a screw can be placed from the base of the first metatarsal to the base of the second metatarsal (Fig. 1.19). This should be done with the clamp still in place. In order to place this screw, the compression cortical screw from the dorsomedial plate may need to be removed at this time. Because the plate construct has been stabilized with locking screws proximally and distally at this point, compression through the first TMT joint has already been achieved and removal of the compression screw does not affect compression across the joint. It is important to ensure that the 1 to 2 metatarsal base screw does not widen the 1 to 2 IM angle, which can occur if the screw does not follow the original trajectory of the drill. Intraoperative AP and lateral fluoroscopic views will confirm screw position.

Alternative Methods of Fixation

- Although not routinely used by the authors, alternative forms of first TMT joint fixation have been employed. Crossing screws, Nitinol staples, and intramedullary implants have been successfully used.
- Crossing screws using 4.0- or 4.5-mm cannulated screws are a common construct for first TMT arthrodesis.[25-28]
- Additionally, a biologic such as concentrated bone marrow aspirate either from the ipsilateral calcaneus or iliac crest can be applied to the arthrodesis site either at this point or mixed with calcaneal autograft.

Medial Eminence Resection

- Once the metatarsal has been stabilized, attention is again directed toward the distal alignment.
- The metatarsal head is again evaluated, and the necessary amount of medial eminence resection can be judged. We strongly recommend that the medial eminence resection be performed after the proximal correction.
- The medial sulcus of the first metatarsal head is identified. The amount of first metatarsal head that is excised is never lateral to the medial sulcus of the first metatarsal head. Care should be taken to avoid continuing the cut into the first metatarsal shaft. The ostectomy site can be marked with a marking pen or electrocautery to avoid over resection of the medial eminence.
- A sagittal saw is then used to perform the medial eminence resection. We prefer to cut from dorsally to plantarly in order to avoid extending our cut into the metatarsal shaft (Fig. 1.20); however, the cut can also be performed from anteriorly to posteriorly.
- The congruity of the MTP joint is again evaluated. If the range of motion of the MTP joint is diminished in the corrected position, this indicates that here is a potential for medial impingement and incongruity. It is then preferable to leave the metatarsal in this position and perform a closing wedge osteotomy at the base of the proximal phalanx or neck of the metatarsal.

Capsular Imbrication

- Ideally, the hallux should rest in a neutral position and closure made without relying on the capsulorrhaphy to realign the toe. Redundant capsule from the "V" aspect of the capsulotomy should be excised in order to provide a soft tissue restraint to valgus drift of the hallux.
- If slight valgus or pronation of the hallux exists after bony realignment, additional capsule may be removed from the "V" component of the capsule. A sponge is placed in the first web space in order to push the hallux out of valgus. Sutures (eg, 2-0 braided absorbable) are then used to tighten the two distal limbs of the "V."
- Excess capsule is then removed from the "Y" component, and sutures (eg, 2-0 braided absorbable) are used to imbricate this part of the capsule.

Akin Osteotomy

- The decision to perform an Akin osteotomy is driven primarily by the clinical position of the toe following the Lapidus procedure, medial eminence resection, and capsular imbrication. Performing the Akin osteotomy prior to closing the capsule may result in hallux varus or inadequate correction of the hallux valgus deformity. An intraoperative AP fluoroscopic image of the foot will assist the surgeon if there is residual hallux valgus or excessive hallux valgus interphalangeus, which may require additional correction through an Akin osteotomy. The Akin osteotomy, however, is not a substitute for adequate correction of the 1 to 2 IM angle or first metatarsal rotation.

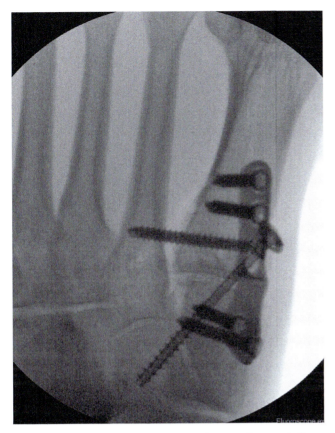

FIGURE 1.19 First to second metatarsal screw placement. If additional stability is required, a screw can be placed from the base of the first metatarsal to the second metatarsal. This often necessitates removal of the compression screw from the plate.

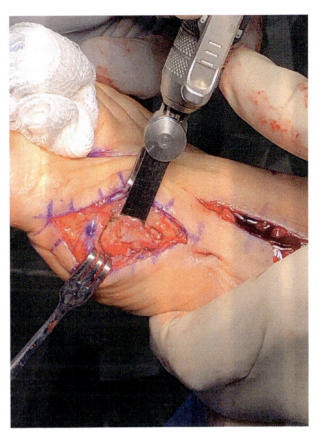

FIGURE 1.20 Medial eminence resection. Following placement of the first tarsometatarsal joint plate, the medial eminence resection is performed using an oscillating saw blade from dorsal to plantar to avoid extending the cut into the metatarsal shaft.

We have a low threshold to add an Akin osteotomy as there is often some recurrence of the hallux valgus deformity.
- Once the decision to perform an Akin osteotomy is made, the medial incision over the first MTP joint is extended distally (Fig. 1.21). Care is taken to protect the plantar and dorsal cutaneous nerves to the hallux.
- The periosteum is elevated medially only as much as is necessary to expose the flexor hallucis longus (FHL) and EHL tendons so that they can be protected with a small Hohmann retractor during the osteotomy.
- To guide the osteotomy, a 0.062-inch Kirschner wire (K-wire) can be passed from medial to lateral just proximal to the intended site of the osteotomy. The position of the K-wire can be checked on fluoroscopy and should be distal to the apex of the concavity of the base of the proximal phalanx. The pin is then cut so that it does not interference with the saw blade during the osteotomy.
- A saw blade is then used to cut parallel to the K-wire from medial to lateral. It is important to avoid penetrating the far cortex as this decreases the stability of the osteotomy.
- The second cut is made 2 to 5 mm from the first (depending on the amount of deformity to be corrected) and angled toward the same point on the lateral cortex (Fig. 1.22). Again, care is taken to avoid penetrating the lateral cortex. The lateral cortex does need to be weakened in order for the osteotomy site to close.
- After the osteotomy is closed medially, the osteotomy is stabilized using fixation. A variety of fixation choices may be used including sutures, staples, screws, wires, or a plate-screw combination. We typically secure the osteotomy with a 9 × 9 mm staple if the far lateral cortex has not been violated (Fig. 1.23). If the far lateral cortex has been violated, then the authors prefer to use screw fixation from the proximal medial base of the proximal phalanx aiming distally and laterally across the osteotomy site.

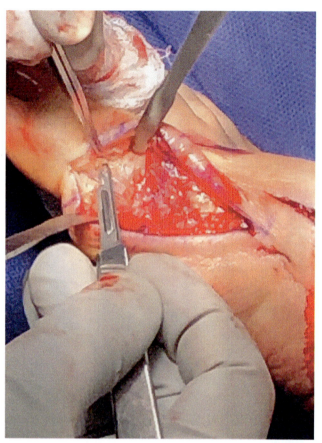

FIGURE 1.21 Approach for the Akin osteotomy. The incision over the medial capsule is extended distally and care is taken to protect the plantar and dorsal cutaneous nerves to the hallux.

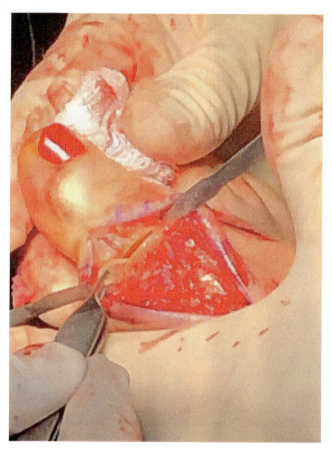

FIGURE 1.22 Akin osteotomy wedge. A saw blade is used to remove a wedge of bone from the proximal phalanx. The lateral cortex should not be violated.

Closure and Dressing

- Copious irrigation should be used. All incisions can be closed with inverted 3-0 absorbable suture with either nylon mattress sutures on the skin or a running absorbable subcuticular stitch.
- 4 × 4s are unfolded and then refolded lengthwise. Two 4 × 4s are placed in the first web space and wrapped medially around the hallux in order to hold the toe straight while the medial capsule imbrication heals (Fig. 1.24).
- The patient is then placed into a soft dressing or splint depending on surgeon preference.

PEARLS AND PITFALLS

- A common mistake is failure to adequately denude the more plantar cartilage in the first TMT joint. The first TMT joint is approximately 3 cm in depth, and the surgeon must remove cartilage plantarly in order to decrease the risk for nonunion and a dorsiflexion malunion of the first metatarsal.
- Avoid shortening the first metatarsal. We prefer to prepare the first TMT joint using osteotomes, curettes, and a rongeur. Flat cuts with a saw blade may result in excessive shortening of the first metatarsal.
- Failure to obtain an adequate reduction at the first TMT joint and appropriately correct the 1 to 2 IM angle may lead to recurrence of the deformity.
- Additionally, failure to adequately address the pronation deformity of the first metatarsal or reduce the sesamoids may also lead to a high recurrence rate (Fig. 1.25).[29,30]

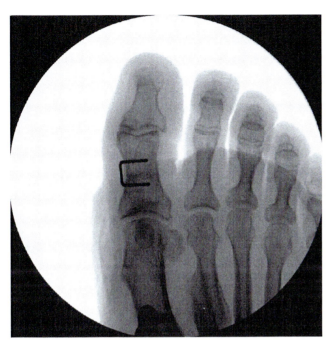

FIGURE 1.23 Staple for Akin osteotomy. The Akin osteotomy is made just distal to the apex of the concavity of the base of the proximal phalanx. The lateral cortex is not violated, and the osteotomy is closed medially. A staple is then placed across the osteotomy site.

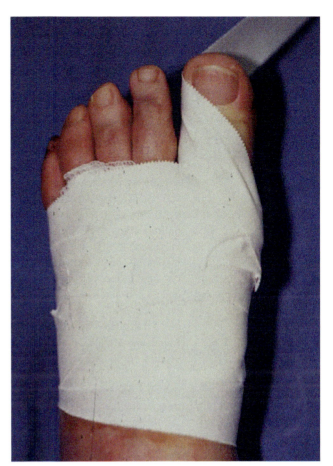

FIGURE 1.24 Bunion dressing. A soft dressing is applied to the foot. Gauze is wrapped laterally around the hallux in order to hold the position of the toe out of valgus while the soft tissue repair heals.

POSTOPERATIVE MANAGEMENT

- Unless the patient is very active and noncompliant, a postoperative shoe is used. The patient is made heel weight bearing in a postoperative shoe for 2 weeks. Sutures are then removed at 2 weeks, and the wound is redressed for another 2 weeks.
- After the first 2 weeks, the patient begins passive range of motion of the first MTP joint.
- The patient is then allowed to be full weight bearing in a short boot for 4 to 5 weeks. They may then wean to a regular shoe as swelling allows.

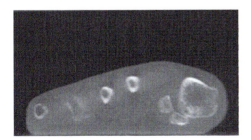 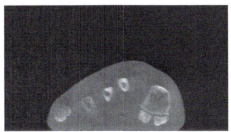

FIGURE 1.25 Preoperative and postoperative weight-bearing computed tomography scan demonstrating reduction of the sesamoids following a Lapidus procedure.

- A soft bunion splint or a narrow elastic bandage is used until 3 months from the surgery to maintain the hallux in neutral alignment.
- Some patients are able to advance into a comfortable sneaker by 8 to 10 weeks, typically bearing weight on the lateral side of the foot. As healing progresses, they apply more weight medially.
- In the last few weeks of the 3-month postoperative period, they often wear a shoe with a spacer placed between the first and second toes to help maintain the position of the hallux.

RESULTS AND COMPLICATIONS

Kopp et al[6] reported the results of the Lapidus procedure in 29 patients (35 feet). Average age at surgery was 54 years, and average follow-up was 42 months. Improvements in visual analog pain score and American Orthopaedic Foot and Ankle Society hallux metatarsophalangeal-interphalangeal score were reported. The average preoperative IM angle was 16°, and the average preoperative hallux valgus angle was 34°. Postoperatively, the average IM angle was 6° and the average hallux valgus angle 11°. There were no cases of nonunion or malunion. Complications included symptomatic hallux varus in two, recurrence of hallux valgus deformity in one, deep venous thrombosis in one, and failure of fixation in one patient. Twenty-four percent of patients noted midfoot stiffness, and 34% noted forefoot stiffness. Ninety percent of patients were satisfied. Coetzee and Wickum[7] prospectively looked at the functional outcome of patients with moderate and severe hallux valgus deformities (IM angle of more than 14° and a hallux valgus angle of more than 30°) after the Lapidus procedure. One hundred and five feet in 91 patients were followed for an average of 3.7 years. Complications included TMT nonunion in seven patients. Five patients lost correction, and all seven patients had a revision procedure done for pain. Removal of hardware was necessary in eight patients; minor wound problems occurred in two patients, superficial neuroma in two patients, and transfer metatarsalgia in four patients.

MacMahon et al retrospectively reviewed patients' return to physical activity, including high-impact activities, following a modified Lapidus procedure in 48 patients less than 50 years old (average age 37.3 years old).[16] Forty percent of patients stated that their participation in physical activities was improved postoperatively, 41% of patients said that their participation in physical was the same postoperatively as preoperatively, and 19% of patients had impaired physical activity postoperatively.[16] Complications included scarring around the EHL tendon in one patient, draining hematoma requiring irrigation and débridement in one patient, complex regional pain syndrome in one patient, second MTP joint metatarsalgia in one patient, anterior tibial tendonitis in one patient, numbness in the third through fifth toes in one patient, and neuritic symptoms of the superficial peroneal nerve and numbness of sural nerve following a postoperative nerve block and calcaneal bone grafting. In this series, there were no cases of nonunion or malunion. Bednarz and Manoli[8] reported the intermediate outcome of 31 feet in 26 patients who underwent a modified Lapidus procedure. All working patients (100%) returned to full-time work. There was an average of 8 months until sports or unlimited activities were performed, and an average 16 weeks until conventional shoes could be worn.

Recent emphasis has been placed on correcting the pronation deformity using the Lapidus procedure. Conti et al[29] investigated the effect of rotational correction on the outcomes of 39 consecutive hallux valgus patients who underwent a modified Lapidus procedure with two crossing screws and had a minimum 2-year postoperative follow-up. They found that patients who had a decrease in first metatarsal rotation had significantly greater improvement in the Patient-Reported Outcomes Measurement Information System physical function and a lower rate of recurrence of the deformity. A secondary analysis found that patients who had a 2° to 8° decrease in first metatarsal pronation had greater improvements in patient-reported outcomes than patients with more or less change in their first metatarsal rotation.

Complications of this operation include loss of correction, dorsal malunion or metatarsal shortening resulting in transfer metatarsalgia, hallux varus, nonunion, and delayed union. The majority of these complications can be avoided with careful attention during the operative procedure. It has been the authors' experience that the rate of reoperation for these complications is very low. The most prevalent postoperative complaint in our hands is prolonged swelling. Symptomatic hardware is rare. A revision arthrodesis is rarely warranted. Although it may seem that revision of the arthrodesis is a major undertaking, it is easily accomplished by a simple opening wedge osteotomy of the arthrodesis site and interposition of a tricortical bone graft. This osteotomy/arthrodesis is quite stable, and patients tend to recover quickly.

ACKNOWLEDGMENTS

The authors would like to thank Dr. Lew C. Schon and Dr. Samuel B. Adams Jr. who wrote a previous version of this chapter.

REFERENCES

1. Coughlin MJ. Hallux valgus. *J Bone Joint Surg Am.* 1997;78(6):932-966.
2. Kimura T, Kubota M, Suzuki N, Hattori A, Marumo K. Comparison of intercuneiform 1-2 joint mobility between hallux valgus and normal feet using weightbearing computed tomography and 3-dimensional analysis. *Foot Ankle Int.* 2018;39(3):355-360.
3. Lapidus P. The operative correction of the metatarsus varus primus in hallux valgus. *Surg Gynecol Obstet.* 1934;58:183-191.
4. Lapidus PW. A quarter of a century of experience with the operative correction of the metatarsus varus primus in hallux valgus. *Bull Hosp Joint Dis.* 1956;17(2):404-421.
5. Lapidus P. The author's bunion operation from 1931 to 1959. *Clin Orthop.* 1960;16:119-135.
6. Kopp FJ, Patel MM, Levine DS, Deland JT. The modified Lapidus procedure for hallux valgus: a clinical and radiographic analysis. *Foot Ankle Int.* 2005;26(11):913-917.
7. Coetzee JC, Wickum D. The Lapidus procedure: a prospective cohort outcome study. *Foot Ankle Int.* 2004;25(8):526-531.
8. Bednarz PA, Manoli A. Modified Lapidus procedure for the treatment of hypermobile hallux valgus. *Foot Ankle Int.* 2000;21(10):816-821.
9. Catanzariti AR, Mendicino RW, Lee MS, Gallina MR. The modified Lapidus arthrodesis: a retrospective analysis. *J Foot Ankle Surg.* 1999;38(5):322-332.
10. Clark HR, Veith RG, Hansen ST. Adolescent bunions treated by the modified Lapidus procedure. *Bull Hosp Jt Dis Orthop Inst.* 1987;47(2):109-122.
11. Myerson M. Metatarsocuneiform arthrodesis for treatment of hallux valgus and metatarsus primus varus. *Orthopedics.* 1990;13(9):1025-1031.
12. Myerson M, Allon S, McGarvey W. Metatarsocuneiform arthrodesis for management of hallux valgus and metatarsus primus varus. *Foot Ankle.* 1992;13(3):107-115.
13. Conti MS, Willett JF, Garfinkel JH, et al. Effect of the modified Lapidus procedure on pronation of the first ray in hallux valgus. *Foot Ankle Int.* 2020;41(2):125-132.
14. Akin O. The treatment of hallux valgus—a new operative procedure and its results. *Med Sentinel.* 1925;33:678.
15. Conti MS, Caolo KC, Ellis SJ, Cody EA. Radiographic and clinical outcomes of hallux valgus and metatarsus adductus treated with a modified Lapidus procedure. *Foot Ankle Int.* 2021;42(1):38-45.
16. MacMahon A, Karbassi J, Burket JC, et al. Return to sports and physical activities after the modified lapidus procedure for hallux valgus in young patients. *Foot Ankle Int.* 2016;37(4):378-385.
17. Rajan L, Kim J, Fuller R, et al. Impact of asymptomatic flatfoot on clinical and radiographic outcomes of the modified Lapidus procedure in patients with hallux valgus. *Foot Ankle Orthop.* 2022;7(2):247301142210999.
18. Campbell B, Miller MC, Williams L, Conti SF. Pilot study of a 3-dimensional method for analysis of pronation of the first metatarsal of hallux valgus patients. *Foot Ankle Int.* 2018;39(12):1449-1456.
19. Gamba C, Álvarez Gomez C, Martínez Zaragoza J, Leal Alexandre C, Bianco Adames D, Ginés-Cespedosa A. Proximal medial gastrocnemius release. *JBJS Essent Surg Tech.* 2022;12(1).
20. Faber FW, Kleinrensink GJ, Verhoog MW, et al. Mobility of the first tarsometatarsal joint in relation to hallux valgus deformity: anatomical and biomechanical aspects. *Foot Ankle Int.* 1999;20(10):651-656.
21. Klaue K, Hansen ST, Masquelet AC. Clinical, quantitative assessment of first tarsometatarsal mobility in the sagittal plane and its relation to hallux valgus deformity. *Foot Ankle Int.* 1994;15(1):9-13.
22. Coughlin MJ, Jones CP. Hallux valgus and first ray mobility—a prospective study. *J Bone Joint Surg Am.* 2007;89(9):1887-1898.
23. Lalevée M, Barbachan Mansur NS, Lee HY, et al. Distal metatarsal articular angle in hallux valgus deformity. Fact or fiction? A 3-dimensional weightbearing CT assessment. *Foot Ankle Int.* 2022;43(4):495-503.
24. Kim Y, Kim JS, Young KW, Naraghi R, Cho HK, Lee SY. A new measure of tibial sesamoid position in hallux valgus in relation to the coronal rotation of the first metatarsal in CT scans. *Foot Ankle Int.* 2015;36(8):944-952.
25. Gruber F, Sinkov VS, Bae SY, Parks BG, Schon LC. Crossed screws versus dorsomedial locking plate with compression screw for first metatarsocuneiform arthrodesis: a cadaver study. *Foot Ankle Int.* 2008;29(9):927-930.
26. Cohen DA, Parks BG, Schon LC. Screw fixation compared to H-locking plate fixation for first metatarsocuneiform arthrodesis: a biomechanical study. *Foot Ankle Int.* 2005;26(11):984-989.
27. Scranton PE, Coetzee JC, Carreira D. Arthrodesis of the first metatarsocuneiform joint: a comparative study of fixation methods. *Foot Ankle Int.* 2009;30(4):341-345.
28. Klos K, Gueorguiev B, Mückley T, et al. Stability of medial locking plate and compression screw versus two crossed screws for Lapidus arthrodesis. *Foot Ankle Int.* 2010;31(2):158-163.
29. Conti MS, Patel TJ, Zhu J, Elliott AJ, Conti SF, Ellis SJ. Association of first metatarsal pronation correction with patient-reported outcomes and recurrence rates in hallux valgus. *Foot Ankle Int.* 2022;43(3):309-320.
30. Okuda R, Kinoshita M, Yasuda T, Jotoku T, Kitano N, Shima H. Postoperative incomplete reduction of the sesamoids as a risk factor for recurrence of hallux valgus. *J Bone Joint Surg Am.* 2009;91(7):1637-1645.

2 Scarf First Metatarsal Osteotomy

Andrew Molloy and Sarang P. Kasture

BACKGROUND

Hallux valgus is one of the most common pathologies presented in foot and ankle practice. Various intrinsic and extrinsic causative factors have been discussed in the literature.[1] About 60% to 90% patients reveal familial tendency indicating genetic association. Females are more likely to be affected and seek treatment compared to male counterparts.[2] The speculated reason for this is multifactorial with higher prevalence of ligament and first ray laxity in females.

Pes planus is thought to increase the rate of deformity progression by causing increased medial loading of the hallux secondary to excessive pronation. Also, tight plantar fascia on weight bearing cause exacerbation of valgus and pronation deforming force of the hallux due to windlass mechanism.[3,4]

Nonoperative management still forms the mainstay of the treatment. It does not correct the deformity but can relieve the symptoms. This includes footwear modification such as accommodating shoes with a wide toe box, padding over the medial eminence, toe spacer devices, adjustments to the shoe, night splints, or physical therapy and insoles. Successful surgical correction provides better outcomes compared to conservative treatment.[5]

Choice of surgical treatment depends on various factors such as joint congruency, extent of the deformity, and presence or absence of arthritis. Osteotomy of the first metatarsal aims to correct intermetatarsal angle (IMA), align the sesamoids under the metatarsal head, and alleviate dynamic deforming forces. The level of the osteotomy depends on the severity of the deformity, surgeon training and experience, and the presence or absence of tarsometatarsal laxity. The scarf osteotomy is a diaphyseal osteotomy to correct mild to moderate hallux valgus deformity. Various modifications in the orientation and length of the bone cuts make it a powerful and versatile tool to address the deformity.

"Scarf" is a carpentry term describing beveling the ends of two pieces of wood and securely fastening them so that they overlap creating one continuous piece. Burutaran first described a Z-shaped osteotomy in 1976.[6] This was later popularized by Weil and Barouk as a method to correct the hallux valgus while maintaining the blood supply of the metatarsal and allow early mobilization from the inherent stability.[7,8] Despite its versatility, it is vital to understand that the scarf osteotomy itself is only one of the four steps for correction of hallux valgus deformity. Lateral release, medial capsulorrhaphy, and proximal phalanx osteotomy (Akin osteotomy), if required, are other key elements to achieve and maintain good correction.

Multiple studies have confirmed favorable results after scarf osteotomy.[9-11] The outcome measures studied were clinical (appearance, range of motion at metatarsophalangeal joint [MTPJ], and recurrence), radiological (weight-bearing anteroposterior [AP] and lateral radiographs to measure IMA, hallux valgus angle [HVA], distal metatarsal articular angle [DMAA], and sesamoid position), and recently pedobarography (peak pressure, mean pressure, pressure/time, force/time).[10] Versatility, early functional recovery, preservation of the first MTPJ motion, and long-term reliability are the main advantages of scarf osteotomy compared to other techniques.[7]

INDICATIONS AND CONTRADICTIONS

The scarf osteotomy can be performed in symptomatic moderate to severe hallux valgus deformity. In severe cases, one should ensure that the width of the metatarsal is sufficient to allow correction.

Displacement of the sesamoid is a good marker for this. Age or presence of osteoporosis is not a limiting factor, but one should be cautious of iatrogenic fractures that could make various types of fixation less stable. Asymptomatic deformity should be approached with caution. Early compliance after surgery is essential to maintain correction as the osteotomies heal. Use of footwear that forces the big toe back into a valgus position may be associated with recurrence.

Contraindications to scarf osteotomy are poor skin and soft tissue envelope, presence of ongoing infection, and arthritis of the MTPJ or tarsometatarsal joint. Instability or frank hypermobility of the first tarsometatarsal joint has a higher recurrence rate.[11,12] Peripheral vascular assessment from vascular surgeons is sought for patients with peripheral vascular disease.

PREOPERATIVE PLANNING

The appropriateness of the indication of scarf osteotomy should be determined by detailed history, symptoms, and examination of the foot. Diabetics with or without peripheral neuropathy and those with history of smoking have increased incidence of wound breakdown, infection, and delayed union. HBA1c test is routinely performed in diabetic patients to determine the blood glucose over a period. Good diabetic control is a prerequisite for surgery. Similarly, patients are strongly advised to quit smoking at least a few weeks prior to surgery though there is no evidence to suggest that the risk of wound breakdown or infection is reduced with short-term smoking cessation.[13]

Severe pain in the forefoot other than the bunion region should prompt further evaluation. Many patients benefit from concurrent lesser toe procedures. Similarly, patients with limited range of motion at the MTPJ preoperatively will continue to experience increased stiffness after the surgery and a possible unfavorable outcome. In our practice, a grind test is routinely performed in all patients to assess pain due to arthritis and if positive, scarf osteotomy is not offered. Overall alignment of the foot in a weight-bearing position should be assessed. Patients with flat foot deformity are prone to recurrence. If symptomatic, flat foot reconstruction should precede the forefoot surgery.

Preoperative planning of the osteotomy is essential. Weight-bearing anteroposterior foot radiographs are used for templating (Fig. 2.1A through C). Measurement of IMA and HVA is key to

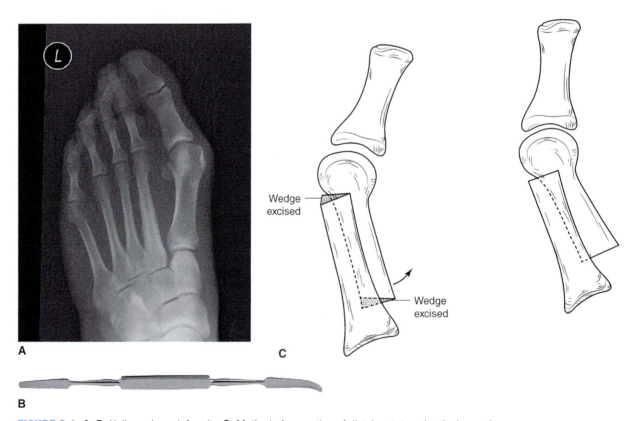

FIGURE 2.1 **A, B.** Hallux valgus deformity. **C.** Method of correction of distal metatarsal articular angle.

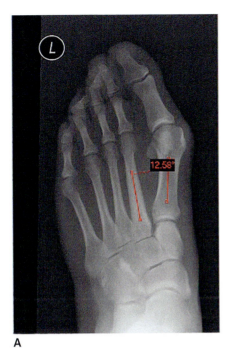
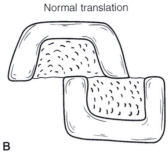
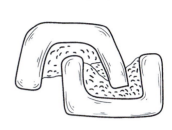

FIGURE 2.2 A. Radiographic measurement of intermetatarsal angle (12.58°). **B.** Schematic representation of troughing.

determine the severity of the deformity and to plan the osteotomy (Figs. 2.2A, B and 2.3). The amount of translation required can be determined by measuring the extent of the uncovered fibular sesamoid on an AP view (Fig. 2.4). In severe deformities, complete relocation of the sesamoids under the metatarsal head may not be possible with translation alone. A maximum of 75% translation can be attained to allow at least cortex to cortex contact along the length of the osteotomy. Lateral release with medial capsular reefing in such cases is paramount. The proximal plantar and distal dorsal sagittal cuts are parallel, which is planned on the AP radiograph perpendicular to the second metatarsal to prevent lengthening or shortening of the first metatarsal (Fig. 2.5).

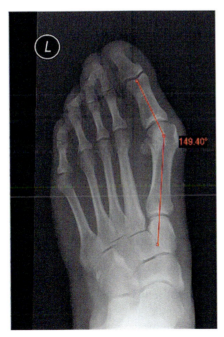

FIGURE 2.3 Radiographic measurement of hallux valgus angle (30.60°).

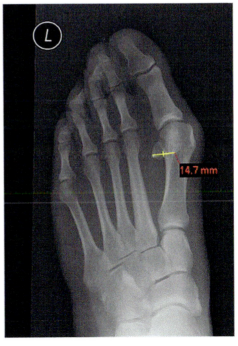

FIGURE 2.4 Amount of translation of the osteotomy required to achieve sesamoid coverage.

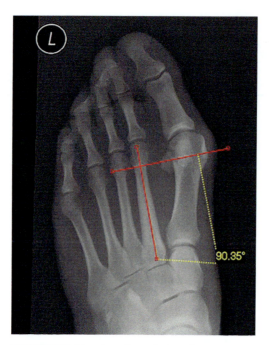

FIGURE 2.5 Direction of translation of the transverse distal dorsal and proximal plantar osteotomy, which is perpendicular to the second metatarsal.

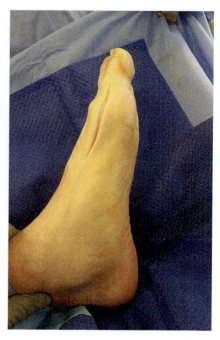

FIGURE 2.6 Medial longitudinal incision centering over the metatarsophalangeal joint.

SURGICAL TECHNIQUE

- Most of the patients in the authors' practice have surgery under general anesthesia or regional anesthesia.
- We use a thigh tourniquet with pressure of 120 mm Hg above the systolic blood pressure.
- Ankle block is administered with a mixture of 10 mL of 0.5% levobupivacaine and 10 mL of 1% lidocaine.
- The authors prefer to stand on the same side of the operating foot, turning the leg into external rotation. This ensures that the medial side faces upward to facilitate correct plantarflexion of the longitudinal osteotomy.
- A medial longitudinal incision is centered over the MTPJ and extends from the middle of the proximal phalanx to mid shaft or the base of the first metatarsal (Fig. 2.6).
- The medial capsule is exposed protecting the dorsomedial cutaneous nerve to the hallux (Fig. 2.7)
- The capsule is incised longitudinally and peeled off the dorsal metatarsal and the proximal phalanx. The attachment to the plantar aspect of the metatarsal neck is left intact to preserve the blood supply to the head of the metatarsal (Fig. 2.8).
- In most of the cases, a lateral release is performed through the medial incision over the top of the metatarsal, though in severe cases a separate lateral incision in the first web space can be used.
- Blunt dissection to the lateral aspect of the MTPJ is performed to release the lateral sesamoid suspensory ligament and the lateral capsule. The adductor hallucis tendon insertion is released in severe cases and the hallux is stressed in varus stress to ensure adequate release (Figs. 2.9 and 2.10).
- The medial eminence is resected dorsal to plantar with a saw to provide a flat surface for the distal osteotomy (Figs. 2.11 and 2.12).
- The distal and proximal apex of the osteotomy are then determined. The distal apex lies 7 to 8 mm proximal to the articular surface at the junction of the dorsal third and plantar two-third of the metatarsal head. The proximal apex lies at the junction of dorsal two-third and plantar one-third of the metatarsal shaft. In the majority of the cases, a short scarf of 3 to 3.5 cm achieves sufficient translation and avoids exit of the osteotomy more proximally along the medial vessels.
- The risk of fracture at the junction of longitudinal and transverse limb of the osteotomy can be avoided by placing K-wires along the apex.

2 Scarf First Metatarsal Osteotomy

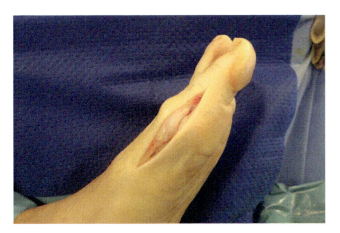

FIGURE 2.7 Medial capsule incision.

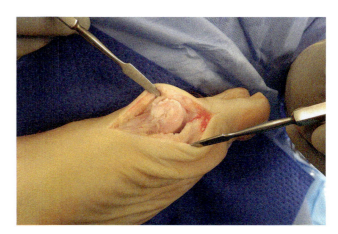

FIGURE 2.8 Capsule peeled from the dorsal metatarsal and the phalanx. Intact plantar attachment at the metatarsal neck.

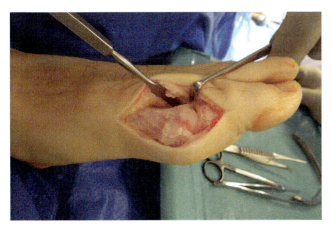

FIGURE 2.9 Blunt dissection extended to lateral aspect of the metatarsophalangeal joint.

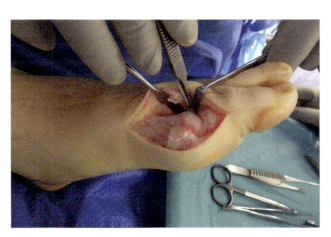

FIGURE 2.10 Release of the lateral sesamoid suspensory ligament, lateral capsule, and adductor hallucis tendon.

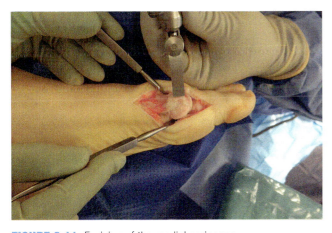

FIGURE 2.11 Excision of the medial eminence.

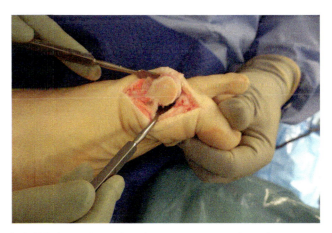

FIGURE 2.12 Flat surface for distal transverse limb of the osteotomy.

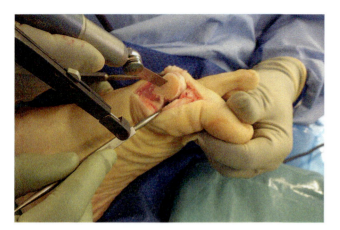

FIGURE 2.13 Orientation of the distal aspect of the longitudinal osteotomy with 10° of inclination to achieve planarization.

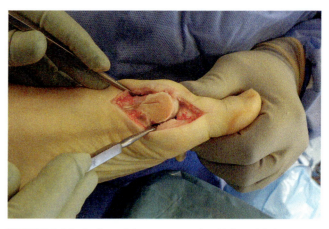

FIGURE 2.14 Outline of the osteotomy by ridging with the saw.

- The longitudinal osteotomy line is outlined by ridging the medial cortex with the saw. Around 10° inclination is provided to ensure planarization of the metatarsal head. The plantar cortex of the metatarsal shaft serves as a guide. The osteotomy of the near cortex is completed along the length, then progressing to the far cortex (Figs. 2.13 and 2.14).
- The transverse cut of the distal osteotomy is perpendicular to the second metatarsal as planned in the template. This usually points to the fourth metatarsal head (Figs. 2.15 and 2.16). The proximal transverse osteotomy is made parallel to the distal osteotomy to facilitate smooth translation.
- The fragments should be mobilized completely before any attempt to translate is made. No leverage should be needed. The intact lateral periosteum can sometimes hinder mobilization and, therefore, be released (Fig. 2.17).
- The translation is achieved by push and pull method with the metatarsal head pushed lateral with the thumb and the proximal fragment pulled medially grasped with a pointed clamp.
- Up to 75% of the width of the metatarsal can be achieved without compromising the stability.

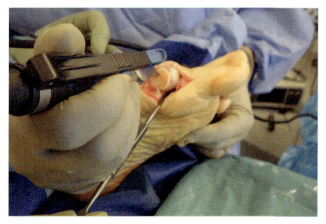

FIGURE 2.15 Orientation of the distal transverse osteotomy perpendicular to the second metatarsal.

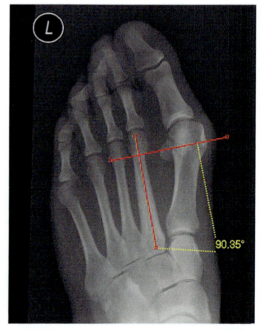

FIGURE 2.16 Distal transverse osteotomy perpendicular to second metatarsal, which clinically corresponds to the fourth metatarsal head.

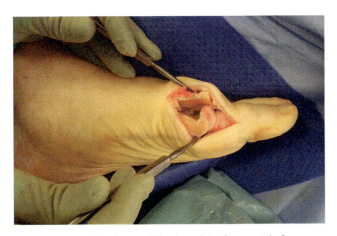

FIGURE 2.17 Complete mobilization of the fragment before translation.

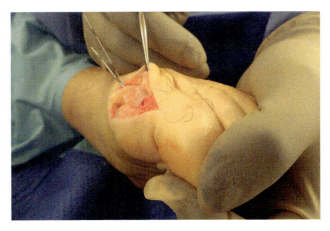

FIGURE 2.18 Translation of the fragments as seen tangentially.

- If indicated in the preoperative planning, the correction of DMMA can be attempted at this stage. This is done by resecting a medial wedge from the distal and/or proximal osteotomy and translating the proximal osteotomy fragment more to correct the DMMA (see Fig. 2.1C).
- Once translation is achieved, the fragments are held secure with a clamp and reduction of sesamoids under the metatarsal head is assessed with image intensifier. One should ensure that there is no troughing of the fragments (see Fig. 2.2B). Troughing is seen intraoperatively when cortex of the osteotomy is wedged into the soft cancellous bone of the other osteotomy fragment. This can cause elevation of the metatarsal head and instability of the construct.
- The 1.0-mm guidewire used for provisional fixation is inserted 7 to 8 mm from the distal osteotomy directed to the center of the metatarsal head. The second guidewire is inserted 7 to 8 mm distal to the proximal osteotomy cut engaging both the cortices (Figs. 2.18 and 2.19). The fixation is achieved by 3-mm cannulated compression screws (Fig. 2.20).
- Before insertion of the screw, weight simulation assessment is done to ensure alignment is satisfactory, and there is no elevation of the metatarsal head (see Figs. 2.1C and 2.2B). One should also assess the correction under image intensifier to ensure relocation of the sesamoids, correction of DMMA, and metatarsal length are maintained.
- The translation of the osteotomy could be lost with the final turns of the screw, and one should be vigilant about maintaining fixation without overtightening. Similarly, one should check there is no troughing of the limbs of the osteotomy as this is a cause for elevation of the metatarsal head.
- The proximal fragment overhang on the medial side is excised and the edges are smoothened with a saw (Figs. 2.21 through 2.24).

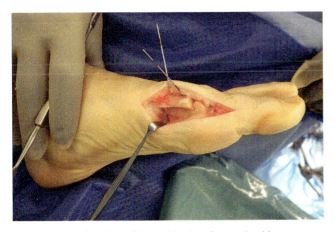

FIGURE 2.19 Position of the guidewires for maximal bone purchase.

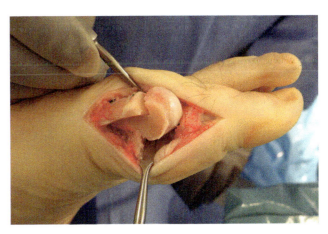

FIGURE 2.20 Position of the screws.

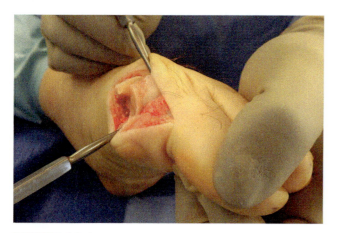

FIGURE 2.21 Overhang of the proximal fragment after fixation of the osteotomy.

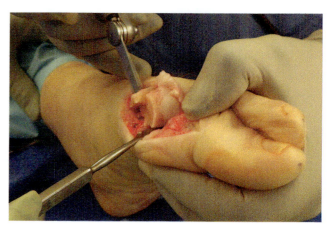

FIGURE 2.22 Excision of the medial bony overhang

- An Akin osteotomy fixed with a headless compression screw is added to improve correction if persistent hallux interphalangeus is present (Fig. 2.25).
- No capsule is excised. A medial capsulorrhaphy is performed with an absorbable suture holding the hallux in varus and plantar flexion. The first plantar stitch is placed adjacent to the medial sesamoid and passed 5 mm distal in the dorsal capsule (Figs. 2.26 and 2.27).
- Another capsular stitch is placed distally followed by subcutaneous and skin stitches (Figs. 2.28 through 2.30).
- A nonadhesive dressing is then applied to the wound.
- A soft dressing bandage is applied to maintain plantar flexion and varus position of the big toe (Figs. 2.31 and 2.32).

PEARLS AND PITFALLS

- It is vital to assess the extent of the deformity from preoperative planning on the weight-bearing radiographs. It is useful to measure the distance from the lateral sesamoid to its expected position to give an estimate of correction required. There is a limit to the amount of translation that can be achieved and if the deformity is excessive. If severe, alternate options should be considered.
- The adequacy of lateral release is confirmed by passing a freer retractor from medial to lateral aspect through the capsule to ensure the suspensory ligament is released. Inadequate release of this ligament will prevent relocation of the sesamoids under the metatarsal head.
- The transverse cuts should be parallel to each other to ensure smooth translation of the fragments. If convergent, the translation will be limited due to wedging of the bone. This could be addressed by taking out a small wedge of the bone from the proximal aspect of the plantar distal fragment.

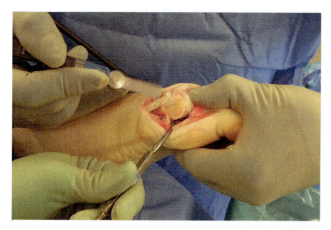

FIGURE 2.23 Smoothening of the sharp edges after excision of overhang.

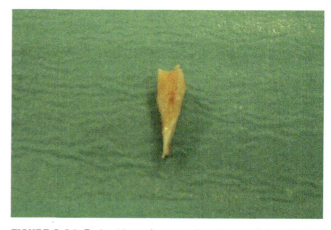

FIGURE 2.24 Excised bone fragment from the medial overhang.

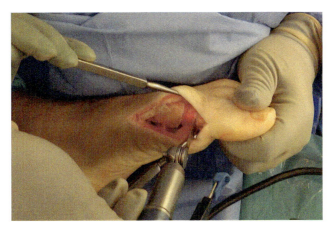

FIGURE 2.25 Akin osteotomy if required for hallux interphalangeus.

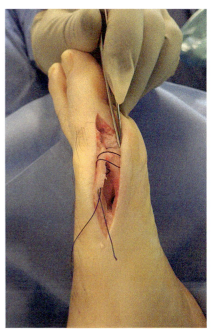

FIGURE 2.26 Medial capsulorrhaphy holding hallux in varus and plantar flexion.

- Ensure that all soft tissue and periosteum from the lateral aspect of the osteotomy are released to allow smooth translation of the fragments.
- McDonald retractor is placed in the osteotomy site to check if the fragments are free to translate without levering on any of them.
- In osteoporotic bone, caution should be exerted while holding the translated fragments with the clamp as inadvertent troughing will cause elevation of the head.
- The position of the distal screw should be as vertical as possible aiming toward the center of the metatarsal head to avoid loss of translation during final tightening.
- There is a substantial learning curve in correction of complex three-dimensional deformities with this osteotomy.

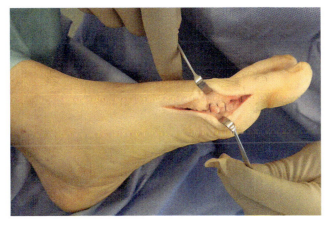

FIGURE 2.27 Completion of the capsular stitch.

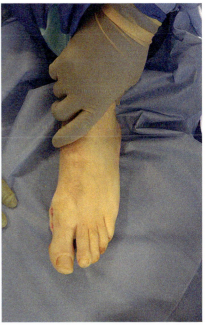

FIGURE 2.28 Clinical correction after capsular stitch.

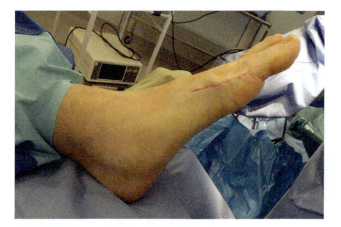

FIGURE 2.29 Subcutaneous sutures.

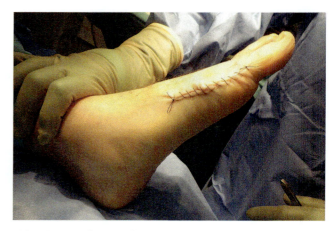

FIGURE 2.30 Closure of the skin.

POSTOPERATIVE MANAGEMENT

- In the author's practice, all patients are assessed by physiotherapists prior to the surgery to teach the details of the postoperative rehabilitation process.
- All patients ambulate weight bearing as tolerated immediately after surgery in a postoperative hard-sole shoe for 6 weeks.
- Patients are encouraged to elevate the limb to control swelling for the first 2 to 3 weeks.
- An experienced foot and ankle nurse specialist sees the patient at 2 weeks to assess the wound and remove the sutures.
- At 6 weeks, a radiograph is performed to assess bony healing and the patient may progress into comfortable footwear to accommodate swelling.

RESULTS AND COMPLICATIONS

De Vil reported on the longest prospective study available in the literature for scarf osteotomies. In this study, there was a mean improvement of the IMA of 6° and HVA of 19°.[14] The American Orthopaedic Foot and Ankle Society score improved from 47 to 83 at 1 year, and results were maintained at 8 years with no recurrence. Though a very powerful tool to correct all components of hallux valgus deformity, the scarf osteotomy has a steep learning curve. Coetzee in initial studies reported 47% complication in his series with troughing in 35% cases.[15] Other studies have reported a complication rate of 4% to 19%.[10,16] Troughing is a serious complication that can not only lead to elevation of the metatarsal but also rotational deformity, which is difficult to treat. Murawski portrayed a reduction in troughing if a rotational scarf was performed and the proximal end of the dorsal and distal end of the plantar bone was left very thin in order to reduce the trough in comparison to a traditional scarf.[17]

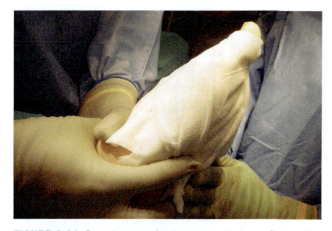

FIGURE 2.31 Dressing to maintain varus and plantar flexion of the big toe.

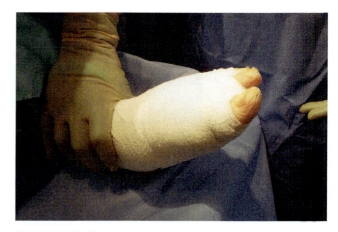

FIGURE 2.32 Final bandage.

Stress fracture of the first metatarsal is also reported though relatively rare. Intraoperatively, incomplete osteotomy and excessive stress during screw insertion is the cause. There is wide variation in recurrence of hallux valgus after scarf osteotomy ranging 0% to 78%. This is largely attributed to a variation in the definition of recurrence adopted in literature. Based on the results of a recent systematic review, it is reasonable to conclude that, in appropriately selected patients and in the hands of surgeons with sufficient expertise performing the scarf procedure, HV recurrence rates at a minimum of 24 months' follow-up would be expected to range from 0% to 10%.[17,18] Patients with flatfoot deformity are prone to recurrence. Similarly, other factors like systemic diseases (inflammatory arthritis, gout), anatomic predisposition (flat foot, metatarsus adductus), compliance with postcorrection directions, and surgical factors such as the suitability of the procedure and the technical expertise of the surgeons also predispose to recurrence. Avascular necrosis of the metatarsal head is a very rare complication.

Overall, the scarf osteotomy is a safe, versatile, and reliable tool to correct hallux valgus deformity. There is a steep learning curve and awareness of the possible pitfalls is essential to achieve a good outcome.

REFERENCES

1. Pique-Vidal C, Sole MT, Antich J. Hallux valgus inheritance: pedigree research in 350 patients with bunion deformity. *J Foot Ankle Surg*. 2007;46:149-154.
2. Saro C, Andre B, Wildemyr Z, Fellander-Tsai L. Outcome after distal metatarsal osteotomy for hallux valgus: a prospective randomized controlled trial of two methods. *Foot Ankle Int*. 2007;28:778-787.
3. Perera AM, Mason L, Stephens MM. The pathogenesis of hallux valgus. *J Bone Joint Surg Am*. 2011;93(17):1650-1661.
4. Atbaşı Z, Erdem Y, Kose O, Demiralp B, Ilkbahar S, Tekin HO. Relationship between hallux valgus and pes planus: real or fiction? *J Foot Ankle Surg*. 2020;59(3):513-517. Erratum in: *J Foot Ankle Surg*. 2020;59(4):873.
5. Torkki M, Malmivaara A, Seitsalo S, et al. Surgery vs orthosis vs watchful waiting for hallux valgus: a randomized controlled trial. *JAMA*. 2001;285(19):2474-2480.
6. Burutaran JM. Hallux valgus y cortedad anatomica del primer metatarsano (correction quirugica). *Actual Med Chir Pied XIII*. 1976;13:261-266.
7. Weil LS. Scarf osteotomy for correction of hallux valgus. Historical perspective, surgical technique and results. *Foot Ankle Clin*. 2000;5:559-580.
8. Barouk LS. Scarf osteotomy of the first metatarsal in the treatment of hallux valgus. *Foot Dis*. 1991;2:35-48.
9. Adam SP, Choung SC, Gu Y, O'Malley MJ. Outcomes after scarf osteotomy for treatment of adult hallux valgus deformity. *Clin Orthop Relat Res*. 2011;469(3):854-859.
10. Lipscombe S, Molloy A, Sirikonda S, Hennessy MS. Scarf osteotomy for the correction of hallux valgus: midterm clinical outcome. *J Foot Ankle Surg*. 2008;47(4):273-277.
11. Heyes GJ, Vosoughi AR, Weigelt L, Mason L, Molloy A. Pes planus deformity and its association with hallux valgus recurrence following scarf osteotomy. *Foot Ankle Int*. 2020;41(10):1212-1218.
12. Barouk LS. Scarf osteotomy for hallux valgus correction. Local anatomy, surgical technique, and combination with other forefoot procedures. *Foot Ankle Clin*. 2000;5(3):525-558.
13. Beahrs TR, Reagan J, Bettin CC, Grear BJ, Murphy GA, Richardson DR. Smoking effects in foot and ankle surgery: an evidence-based review. *Foot Ankle Int*. 2019;40(10):1226-1232.
14. De Vil JJ, Van Seymortier P, Bongaerts W, De Roo PJ, Boone B, Verdonk R. Scarf osteotomy for hallux valgus deformity: a prospective study with 8 years of clinical and radiologic follow-up. *J Am Podiatr Med Assoc*. 2010;100(1):35-40.
15. Coetzee JC. Scarf osteotomy for hallux valgus repair: the dark side. *Foot Ankle Int*. 2003;24(1):29-33.
16. Garrido IM, Rubio ER, Bosch MN, Gonzalez MS, Paz GB, Llabres AJ. Scarf and Akin osteotomies for moderate and severe hallux valgus: clinical and radiographic results. *Foot Ankle Surg*. 2008;14(4):194-203.
17. Murawski CD, Egan CJ, Kennedy JG. A rotational scarf osteotomy decreases troughing when treating hallux valgus. *Clin Orthop Relat Res*. 2011;469(3):847-853.
18. Clarke TAC, Platt SR. Treatment of hallux valgus by Scarf osteotomy-rates and reasons for recurrence and rates of avascular necrosis: a systematic review. *Foot Ankle Surg*. 2021;27(6):622-628.

3 Minimally Invasive Surgical (MIS) Bunionectomy

Tonya An and A. Holly Johnson

INTRODUCTION

The minimally invasive surgical (MIS) bunionectomy is indicated for patients with a symptomatic hallux valgus deformity. While many types of minimally invasive osteotomies and fixation have been described for bunion correction, the distal chevron combined with a proximal phalanx osteotomy has recently gained wide acceptance. "This procedure is commonly referred to as percutaneous extracapsular chevron and Akin (PECA) or minimally invasive chevron Akin (MICA). It involves a V-shaped osteotomy of the first metatarsal and is frequently combined with an "Akin" medial closing wedge proximal phalanx osteotomy. Like open distal metatarsal osteotomies, this operation is most appropriate for mild to moderate bunion deformities without significant instability at the first tarsometatarsal (TMT) joint.[1,2] Recent studies have also suggested that this may also be a treatment option for select cases of severe deformity as well.[3] Compared with the open distal chevron procedure, the MIS osteotomy is considered extracapsular, occurring more proximally at the meta-diaphyseal junction of the metatarsal instead of the head. This osteotomy site preserves metatarsal head blood supply and facilitates fixation. The minimally invasive technique also offers the advantages of smaller, more cosmetic incisions, decreased scarring and soft tissue edema, and the option of earlier weight bearing and return to activity.

Minimally invasive surgical bunionectomy features specialized burr instruments to perform osteotomies or shave down bone through percutaneous incisions, avoiding excessive trauma to the surrounding tissues. All the components of the open procedure, including modified McBride release, medial eminence resection, and chevron type osteotomy at the distal metatarsal, can be performed with adapted minimally invasive techniques. Due to the lack of direct visualization, intricate knowledge of local anatomy is mandatory. In addition, fluoroscopy is critical to determine instrument location and orientation, as well as the desired correction parameters. Fixation using percutaneous cannulated screws is typical for the distal chevron osteotomy and Akin osteotomy. Beveled headless screws are preferred in order to ensure that hardware is flush with the cortex and, therefore, not palpable under the skin. Increasing evidence including comparisons to open osteotomy and large case series have demonstrated reliable correction and positive clinical outcomes associated with the MIS technique.[4]

INDICATIONS

- The indication for MIS bunionectomy, similar to any hallux valgus surgery, is a symptomatic bunion deformity that has failed conservative treatment. Clinical factors such as prior scars or poor soft tissues, along with the patient's preference for cosmetic incisions, are more specific reasons for MIS technique.

CONTRAINDICATIONS

- Similar to open distal chevron or scarf osteotomy, this technique is relatively contraindicated in severe hallux valgus deformities with a 1 to 2 intermetatarsal angle (IMA) greater than 16°. Nevertheless, some minimally invasive corrections have been performed in severe deformity cases with successful bony union despite more than 100% lateral translation of the metatarsal head.

- Preexisting arthritis of the first metatarsophalangeal (MTP) and/or TMT joint compromise the outcomes of a joint-sparing osteotomy for deformity correction. This must be elicited on preoperative history, physical exam, and radiographs, as these patients may be better served by addressing both arthritis and deformity with arthrodesis.
- Patients with clinical hypermobility at the first TMT joint are at risk of recurrence after minimally invasive bunionectomy through the TMT joint or the intercuneiform joint and should be treated with a modified Lapidus procedure to correct multiplanar deformity and eliminate instability. Although instability is difficult to quantify and frequently examiner dependent, subluxation and gapping at the plantar TMT joint or medial arch collapse seen on lateral weight-bearing radiographs are objective findings that support TMT fusion over an osteotomy.
- Underlying osteopenia or osteoporosis is a major risk factor for loss of fixation, malunion, and nonunion following minimally invasive bunionectomy. Poor bone quality poses challenges for achieving stability across the osteotomy site with percutaneous screws. A presurgical assessment of patient demographic factors and prior history of osteoporotic fractures may prompt a dedicated bone density evaluation if multiple risk factors are present. Postoperative protocols may need to be modified to prolong immobilization in a sturdier postoperative device such as a walking boot instead of a standard postoperative shoe. Patient inability to comply with postoperative protocols is also a relative contraindication.
- Poorly controlled systemic disease, active or latent infection, and skin wounds are further contraindications for any type of elective surgical hallux valgus treatment.

PREOPERATIVE PLANNING

The preoperative planning for a minimally invasive bunionectomy is unchanged from the algorithm used for open bunionectomy. The typical history involves symptoms related to the bunion deformity and failure of conservative treatment such as shoe modification and spacer devices. Clinical examination should reveal a hallux valgus deformity without significant first MTP joint pain or crepitus or first TMT joint instability with excessive forefoot pronation.

Radiographic evaluation with anteroposterior (AP) and lateral weight-bearing radiographs are key (Fig. 3.1A and B). The AP view will best demonstrate the coronal plane severity of hallux valgus by the 1 to 2 IMA and hallux valgus angle (HVA). Lesser toe pathology, hallux degenerative joint changes, sesamoid position, and metatarsus adductus or talonavicular abduction should be noted if present. The lateral radiograph is necessary to assess for forefoot alignment and planus or cavus deformity; gapping seen at the first TMT joint or first metatarsal elevation may suggest instability. We recommend taking a preoperative clinical photo of the foot for documentation that can be saved in the patient's electronic medical record (Fig. 3.1C).

MIS Instrumentation

The typical minimally invasive instruments required include (Fig. 3.2A and B):

- The no. 15 blade or beaver blade (not pictured) is used to make poke-hole incisions through epidermis and dermis only. Tenotomy scissors or a hemostat is then used to spread through subcutaneous tissues.
- Periosteal elevators—specialized instruments inserted through poke hole incisions that can raise and peel any adherent capsular tissue.
- Head shifting tool—this instrument has different design types depending on the manufacturer but is typically inserted retrograde into the first MT shaft through the osteotomy to facilitate the varus and lateral translation of the MT head. In this specific design, the head shifting tool has a flexible handle can be bent laterally to lever the bone to help hold the reduction.
- Irrigation—a bulb syringe (not pictured) is used by the assistant to continuously irrigate the burr and soft tissue any time the burr is running. The fluid dissipates heat and helps to prevent bony thermal necrosis.
- Screws—screws specifically designed for the MIS bunionectomy are typically 3.0 or 4.0 mm fully threaded, cannulated headless screws (Fig. 3.2C). Many screws feature an oblique bevel at the head, which minimizes any hardware prominence when the final screw threads are sunk into the near cortex of bone. Screws designed for percutaneous Akin osteotomy are cannulated 3.0 mm and also have a beveled head.

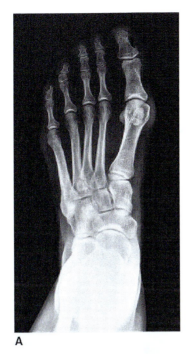
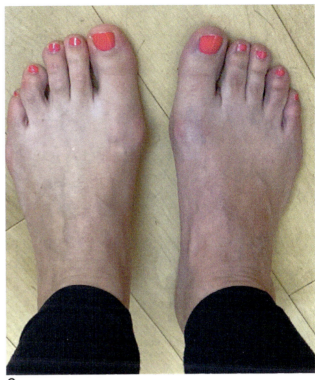

FIGURE 3.1 A, B. Anteroposterior and lateral weight-bearing radiographs demonstrating a moderate bunion deformity with 1 to 2 intermetatarsal angle of 13° and hallux valgus angle of 23°. **C.** A clinical photo of the bilateral feet in a weight-bearing stance is captured to document the appearance of hallux valgus preoperatively. The left foot is planned for surgical correction.

There are two categories of burrs used in particular for the MIS bunionectomy procedure.

- Shannon burr—this is a cutting burr. The sharp tip can pierce through the cortex to initiate the osteotomy and then rotational hand movements push the length of the burr to contact and cut through cortical bone. A 2 × 8 mm burr is used for lesser toe osteotomies, the 2 × 20 mm burr is used for the distal chevron osteotomy, the 2 × 12 mm burr is typically used for the Akin osteotomy.
- Wedge burr—this burr is designed for grinding down bone while minimizing damage to overlying soft tissues. A 3 × 13 mm burr is used for the medial eminence resection component of MIS bunionectomy.
- The burr tips are attached to a handpiece with either hand or foot pedal control. The recommended maximum revolution speed is 6,000 revolutions per minute to prevent thermal injury to bone.

SURGICAL TECHNIQUE

The MIS bunionectomy is typically performed as an outpatient procedure. Patients may receive general anesthesia, spinal anesthesia, or peripheral nerve block depending on patient comorbidities and surgeon preference.

Our preferred practice is sedation with a popliteal nerve block for perioperative pain control. The patient is positioned supine on the surgical table with the heel of the operative foot floating 3 to 4 inches off the end of the bed (Fig. 3.3). A tourniquet is typically not used given the small incisions and theoretical heat-dissipating effect of bone bleeding during osteotomy cuts. Positioning the

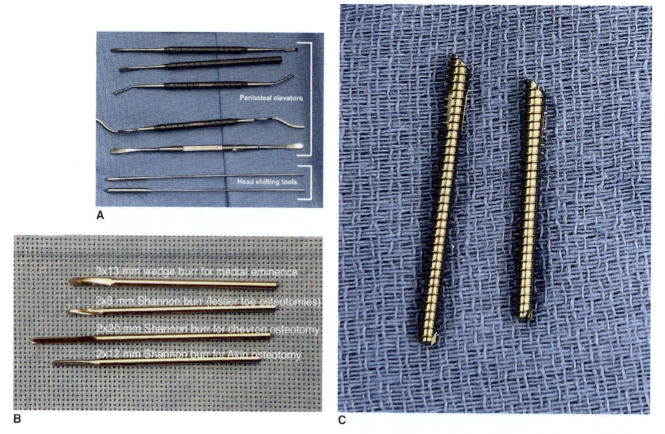

FIGURE 3.2 **A.** Common minimally invasive surgical (MIS) instruments, including periosteal elevators and two "bullet" head shifting tools. **B.** Various burr types for MIS bunionectomy. **C.** Screws specifically designed for MIS bunionectomy.

patient in some Trendelenburg can diminish the venous bleeding. However, an Esmarch bandage may be applied to the proximal calf region as a tourniquet if excessive bleeding is encountered.

For the right-handed surgeon, the mini C-arm is always positioned at the right side of the patient and the foot is resting on the C-arm image intensifier in an AP fashion. When working on the right foot, the surgeon stands at the end of the table facing proximal (Fig. 3.4A). Whereas for the left foot, the surgeon stands at the end of the table facing distal (Fig. 3.4B). An assistant may stand in the opposite position to deliver cooling irrigation and assist with fluoroscopy.

Medial Eminence Resection

- Using fluoroscopic localization, a poke-hole incision is made just proximal to the medial eminence, midline to avoid the dorsomedial cutaneous nerve (Fig. 3.5A). Soft tissues are spread with

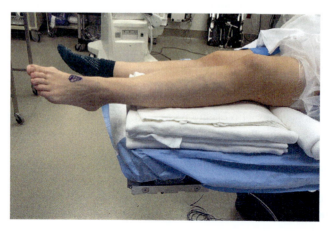

FIGURE 3.3 Patient positioning with the operative leg elevated on a stack of blankets, extending 3 to 4 inches off the end of the surgical table.

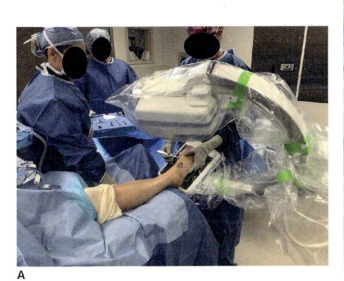
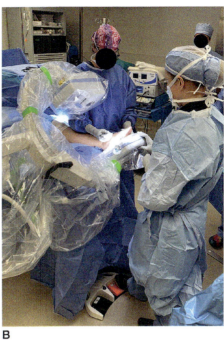

FIGURE 3.4 A. Mini C-arm and surgeon positioning for a right-sided procedure. **B.** Setup for a left-sided procedure.

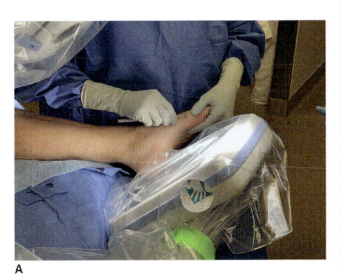
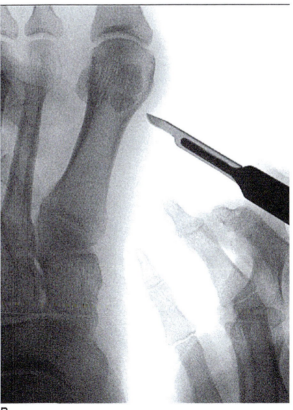

FIGURE 3.5 A. Fluoroscopic localization of the percutaneous incision site for the distal chevron osteotomy. **B.** After making a poke-hole incision, a periosteal elevator instrument is inserted to manually release the proximal metatarsophalangeal capsule from the medial eminence bone.

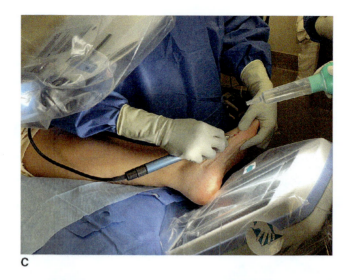

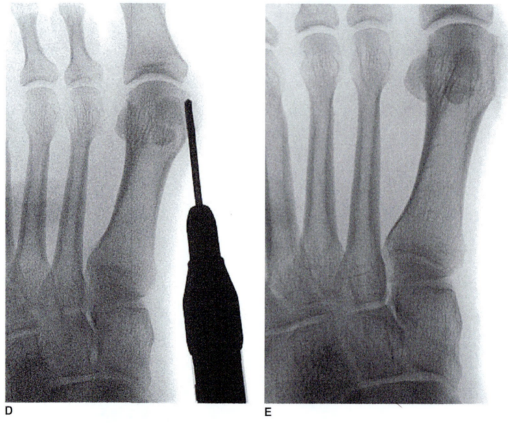

FIGURE 3.5 (*Continued*) **C.** The wedge burr is inserted to resect the bony medial eminence, under continuous cooling irrigation. This resection is easier when performed prior to osteotomy and correction of the bunion. **D.** Fluoroscopic verification of the position of the wedge burr for medial eminence resection. **E.** Fluoroscopic confirmation after completing the medial eminence resection.

tenotomy scissors or a hemostat. A capsular elevator is introduced through the incision to elevate the capsule off the medial eminence (Fig. 3.5B).
- The medial eminence may be resected initially or after the correction is complete. The 3 × 13 wedge burr is inserted parallel against the medial eminence on fluoroscopy. The handpiece is held against the medial arch of the foot using an "agricultural grip," which is an overhand grip like holding the handlebar of a bike. Then, the wedge burr tip is passed along the medial eminence in a dorsal and plantar fashion to shave down the bone. Check fluoroscopy intermittently to determine the amount of resection (Fig. 3.5C and D).

- Use copious normal saline irrigation with the bulb syringe any time the burr is running.
- The foot can be held in an everted position to allow better access to the medial eminence.
- The surgeon's contralateral hand palpates through the skin to guide burr position and detect residual bone.
- Bone paste is manually expressed through the percutaneous incision once the resection is complete and the resection is confirmed under fluoroscopy (Fig. 3.5E).

Distal Chevron Osteotomy

- A second poke-hole incision at the medial forefoot is made using fluoroscopy to localize it to the base of the sesamoids. After bluntly spreading through skin and subcutaneous tissues, the 2 × 22 burr is inserted to contact the bone (Fig. 3.6A and B).
- The orientation of the burr should be approximately 20° proximal to distal and slightly dorsal to plantar (Fig. 3.7A through D).
- The osteotomy trajectory is confirmed on fluoroscopy and the burr is pierced through the medial and subsequently the lateral cortex of the first metatarsal.
- The dorsal limb of the V-shaped osteotomy is performed by pushing the burr dorsal and proximal with a pronation or supination motion of the hand. The contralateral hand can be used to palpate when the cut is complete (Fig. 3.6C through F).
- The plantar limb is similarly created, with the burr exiting plantar and proximal at the shaft of the metatarsal.

Reduction and Fixation

- A head-shifting instrument is inserted into the metatarsal from distally at the osteotomy into the metatarsal shaft. Leverage on the instrument will translate the metatarsal head laterally on the metatarsal shaft (Fig. 3.8A and B).

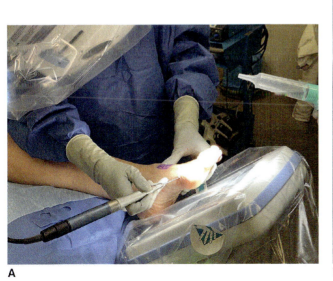
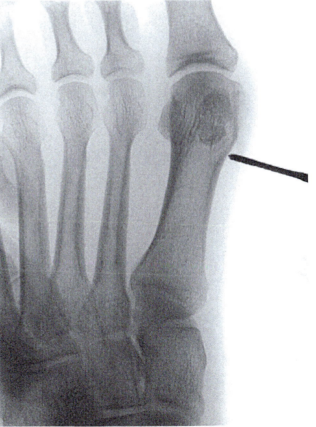

FIGURE 3.6 A, B. Clinical and fluoroscopic imaging of the entry point of the 2 × 20 mm Shannon burr used to perform the distal chevron osteotomy.

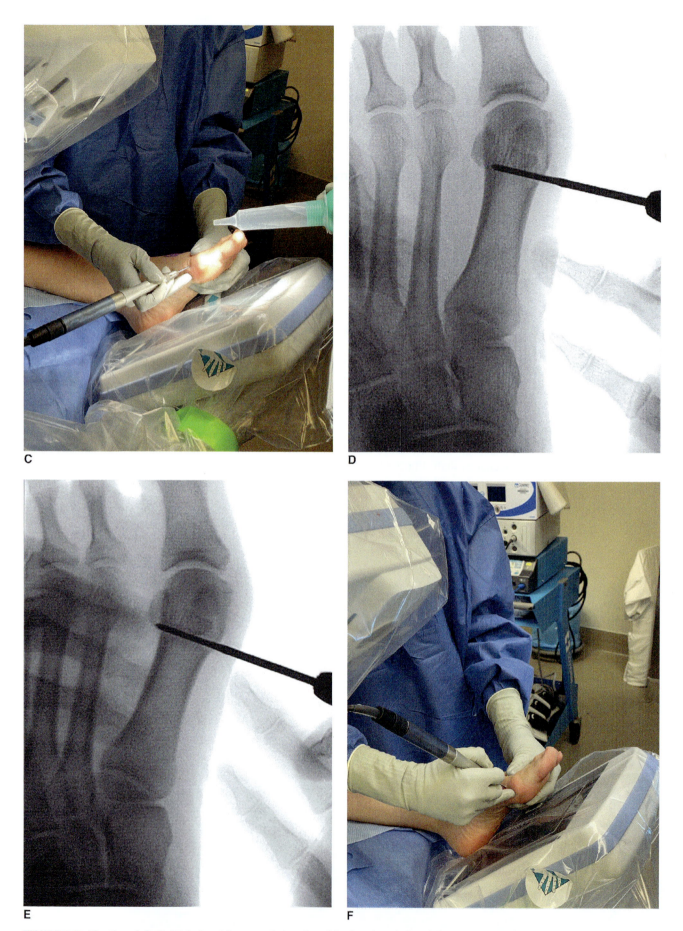

FIGURE 3.6 (Continued) **C, D.** Clinical and fluoroscopic imaging of the burr inserted straight across to the far cortex of the metatarsal neck. **E.** Fluoroscopic image as the burr penetrates the lateral cortical bone at the metatarsal neck and then can be pivoted dorsal and plantar to accomplish the two limbs of the chevron osteotomy cut. **F.** The clinical image illustrates the dorsal and distal movement of the hand to initiate the plantar limb of the chevron osteotomy.

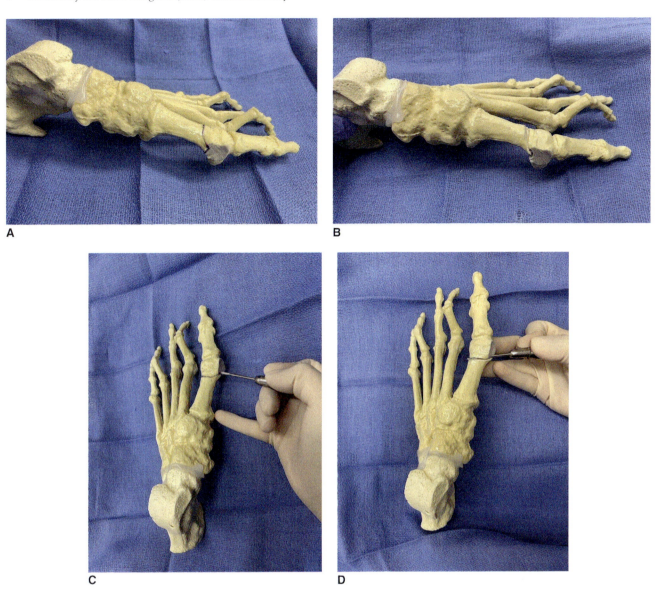

FIGURE 3.7 A. Sawbones model demonstrating the chevron osteotomy. The osteotomy is angled slightly proximal to distal to preserve length of the first metatarsal. The dorsal limb of the chevron is longer and flatter, while the plantar limb is short and transverse. **B.** The burr penetrates both the medial and lateral cortices. **C.** The dorsal limb of the osteotomy is created by pivoting the hand plantar and distal. **D.** The completed osteotomy is shown.

- Percutaneous guidewires for 4.0-mm cannulated screws are inserted under fluoroscopic guidance. Some surgeons prefer to use a 3.0-mm screw in the distal position, in which case the corresponding guidewire would be utilized. The most proximal wire should start as proximal as possible at the first metatarsal base and advanced obliquely, exiting the lateral cortex, aiming to the estimated position that the metatarsal head will end (Fig. 3.8C and D). On lateral fluoroscopy, the wire must match the declination of the metatarsal shaft.
- The second wire is started approximately 1 cm more distal to establish an adequate bony bridge and should parallel the first in all planes (Fig. 3.8F).
- With both wires primed, manual reduction of the metatarsal head is performed with varus leverage of the head shifting instrument, aka "bullet," pushing the head laterally and shaft medially. The surgeon must also support the metatarsal head to prevent plantarflexion or dorsiflexion malreduction and hold the toe in neutral rotation (Fig. 3.8E).
  - Only a limited amount of rotational correction can be achieved with the chevron osteotomy because of incongruity between the plantar and dorsal cuts. A transverse osteotomy is an alternative technique that facilitates derotation of the hallux but is less inherently stable. Varus and

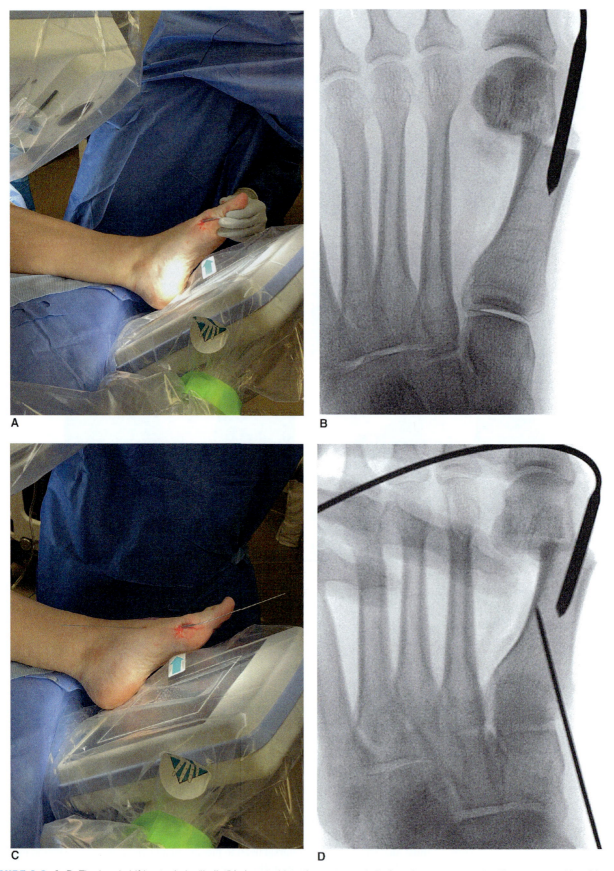

FIGURE 3.8 A, B. The head shifting tool aka "bullet" is inserted into the metatarsal shaft at the osteotomy site. The metatarsal head is reduced with varus force and levering on the shaft of the bullet to translate the metatarsal head laterally. The metatarsal head should be supported to prevent plantar or dorsal translation. **C, D.** After a provisional reduction, the appropriate guidewires for the percutaneous screws are inserted. Start the proximal wire at the base of the first metatarsal. The second wire is parallel but should be separated by a bridge of greater than 5 mm.

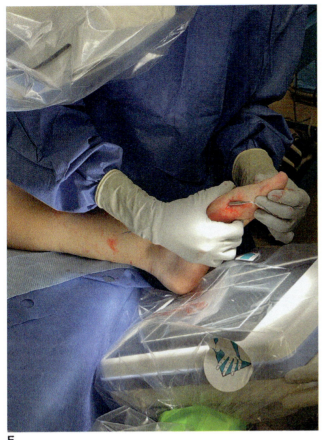 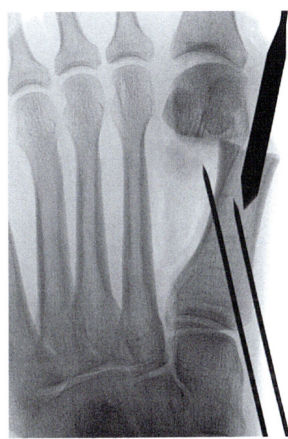

FIGURE 3.8 (*Continued*) **E, F.** The reduction maneuver is performed and the guidewires are advanced by an assistant into the metatarsal head.

- valgus angulation at the osteotomy site should be avoided as it changes the orientation of the joint and often lead to shortening.
- Up to 100% translation at the osteotomy can be achieved and confirmed with AP fluoroscopy. The first wire is advanced, ending in the lateral metatarsal head.
- If the correction is acceptable, the second wire is also advanced into the MT head and checked on orthogonal fluoroscopic views (Fig. 3.9A and B).
- A percutaneous incision is made at the starting site of each guidewire to allow for length measurement, and then overdrilling of 80% to 90% the length of the guidewire is performed.
- The more lateral and proximal screw is inserted while the osteotomy is manually held in a reduced position. The variable pitch of the screws should achieve some compression across the osteotomy. The second screw is inserted in a similar fashion. The final turn of the screw should ensure that the beveled head is flush with the near cortex of the bone.
- Fluoroscopy is used to confirm the fixation in AP and lateral planes (Fig. 3.10C and D).

Metatarsal Shaft Resection

- The metatarsal shaft distal to the screws typically feels prominent and contributes to the appearance of a widened forefoot.
- After the soft tissue is gently freed from the medial spike of bone using a percutaneous elevator, either a cutting burr or wedge burr is used to resect the bone. The senior author prefers resection of this bony segment with a 2 × 12 Shannon burr inserted from the more proximal percutaneous screw site (Fig. 3.11A and B).
- The burr is used to pierce the cortical bone of the shaft and then rotated dorsally and plantarly to create an osteotomy parallel to the screws.
- This shell of bone can be removed using a hemostat through the same percutaneous incision (Fig. 3.11C).

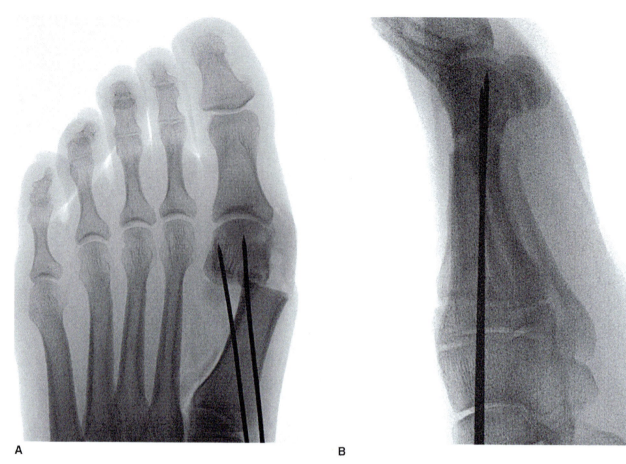

FIGURE 3.9 A, B. Fluoroscopic AP and lateral images showing 75% translation of the metatarsal head and the guidewires holding the reduction.

Akin Osteotomy

- An Akin proximal phalanx medial closing wedge osteotomy is performed in cases of residual hallux valgus interphalangeus. Only rarely is an Akin not indicated.
- After a medial poke-hole incision at the middle third of the proximal phalanx, the 2 × 12 mm Shannon burr is inserted to the near cortex of bone. This osteotomy is oriented distal to proximal by 15° to 20° and verified with fluoroscopy (Fig. 3.12A and B).
- The burr pierces the near cortex and hits the far cortex without passing through. Then, supination and pronation movements of the surgeon's hand push the burr through dorsal and plantar cortex bone (Fig. 3.12C and D). The contralateral hand may palpate through the skin to determine when the cut is completed.
- At this point, the osteotomy is hinged on the far lateral cortex and can be closed manually.
- A guidewire for a 3.0-mm cannulated screw is inserted from the medial base of the proximal phalanx, exiting the lateral cortex distal to the osteotomy (Fig. 3.12E).
- Check the fluoroscopic and clinical position of the toe with a flat plate to simulate weight bearing and confirm that the toe is in a neutral position, and that it is neither over nor under corrected.
- The wire is overdrilled with a cannulated drill and screw inserted, checking with fluoroscopy to ensure the medial side is closed and compressed.
- Final clinical position is assessed with a simulated weight bearing and multiplanar fluoroscopic views are checked for final correction and implant positioning (Fig. 3.13A through C).

Closure and Dressings

- The wounds are irrigated using a 14- or 16-gauge angiocatheter to remove bone paste from around the skin and under the capsule (Fig. 3.14A).
- All poke-hole incisions are irrigated and closed with 4-0 nylon stitches (Fig. 3.14B and C).

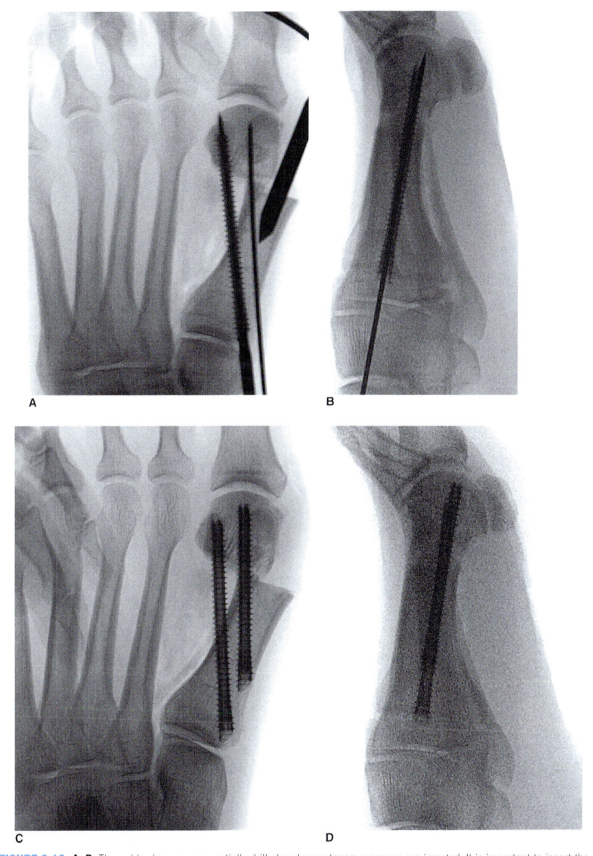

FIGURE 3.10 A, B. The guidewires are sequentially drilled and percutaneous screws are inserted. It is important to insert the lateral screw first. Reduction and hardware position are checked on anteroposterior (AP) and lateral fluoroscopic images. **C, D.** AP and lateral fluoroscopic views following fixation of the metatarsal osteotomy. Shown are 4.0 MIS percutaneous screws (Novastep), which are headless and have a bevel that matches the near cortex to minimize hardware irritation.

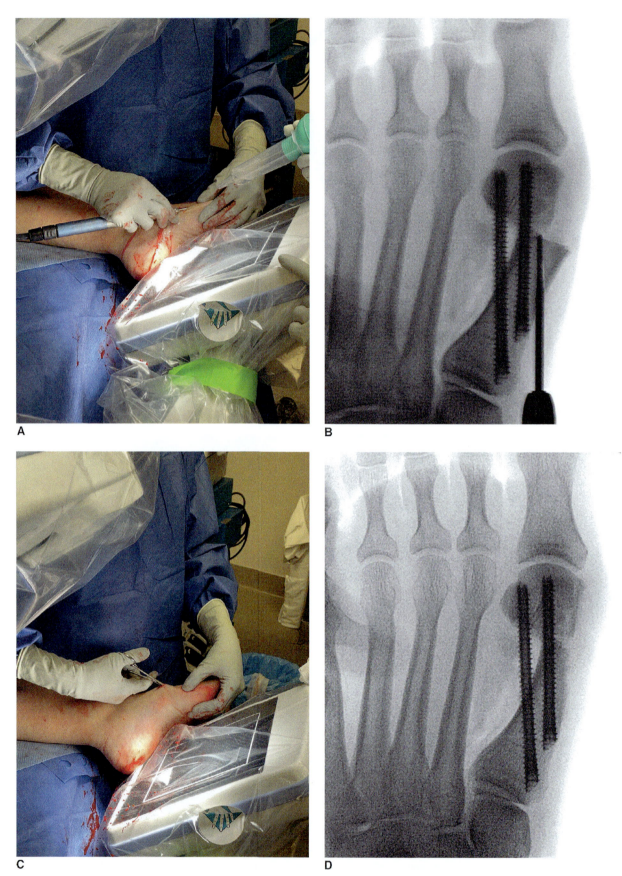

FIGURE 3.11 A, B. Clinical and fluoroscopic image of a 2 × 12 mm Shannon burr inserted through the same incision as the medial screw to resect the distal aspect of the medial metatarsal shaft. **C.** The bony piece is removed with a hemostat through the same incision. **D.** Fluoroscopy confirms that the prominent bony corner has been removed completely.

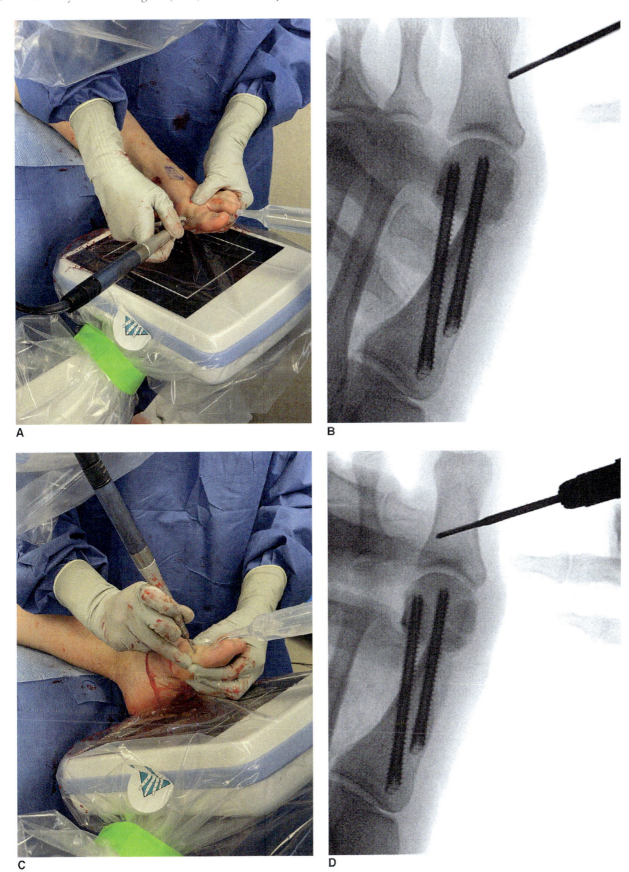

FIGURE 3.12 A, B. The 2 × 12 mm Shannon burr is introduced from the medial proximal phalanx under fluoroscopic guidance. **C, D.** This penetrates the near cortex of bone but does not disrupt the far cortex. Supination and pronation of the hand create an osteotomy cut at an oblique angle and approximately 2 mm wedge of bone is removed by the burr.

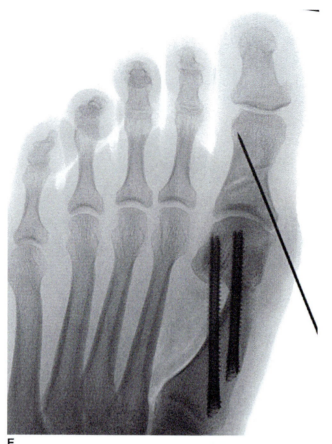

FIGURE 3.12 (Continued) **E.** A percutaneous guidewire is inserted from the medial base of the proximal phalanx transversely across the osteotomy.

- Nonadherent dressing (Xeroform or Adaptic) can be used to directly cover the incisions.
- A bunion dressing is applied using strips of saline-moistened gauze to splint the hallux in neutral to slight varus and lesser toes in the desired position. This is wrapped with additional cling or Kerlix dressing and a light layer elastic bandage overtop (Fig. 3.14D). The heel of the foot is typically left uncovered to allow for easier ambulation.

POSTOPERATIVE MANAGEMENT

- The patient is allowed to weight bear as tolerated immediately in a postoperative shoe or short walking boot. The dressing should be maintained until the first postoperative appointment at 2 weeks when dressings are removed.
- Weight-bearing radiographs are taken at the 2-week, 6-week, 3-month, and 6-month postoperative visits to ensure maintenance of correction and progression of bony healing (Fig. 3.15A and B).
- The patient is encouraged to perform passive flexion and extension exercises of the great toe immediately after the dressing is removed. Physical therapy is typically initiated after the first postoperative visit to help with range of motion, scar massage, and gait training.
- A prefabricated bunion splint or toe spacer is maintained for the first 6 weeks and then at night only until 3 months postoperatively (Fig. 3.16).
- The postoperative shoe or boot may be removed 5 to 6 weeks postoperatively and the patient may transition into a sneaker. As the swelling diminishes, other shoe wear is permitted.
- Physical activity may progress as tolerated postoperatively, though running, jumping, and other impact activity is restricted through 3 months postoperatively.

3   Minimally Invasive Surgical (MIS) Bunionectomy

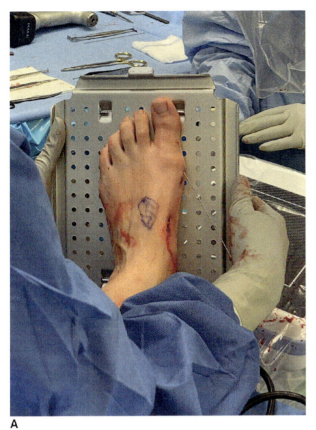

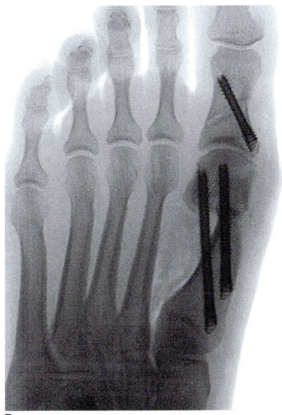

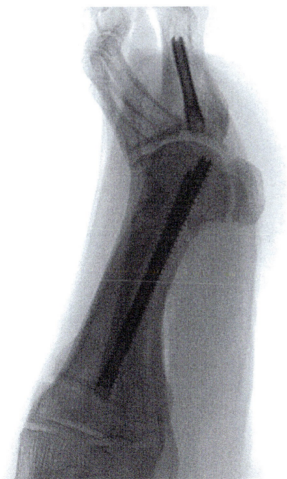

FIGURE 3.13 **A.** The clinical position of the foot is checked by simulating weight bearing on a flat plate. **B, C.** Final anteroposterior and lateral fluoroscopic images are taken.

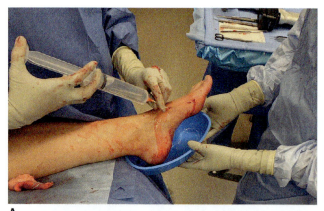
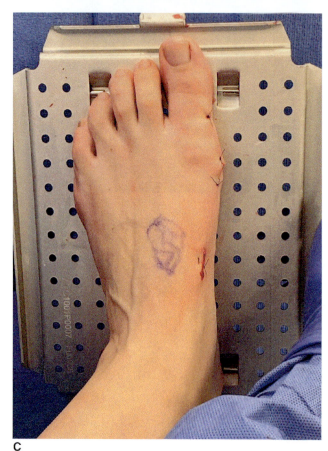
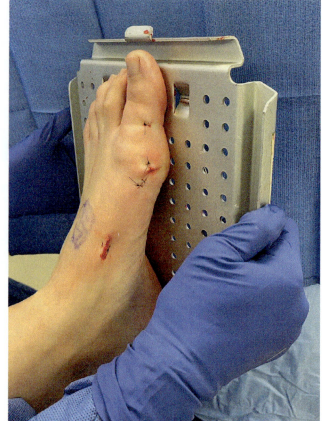
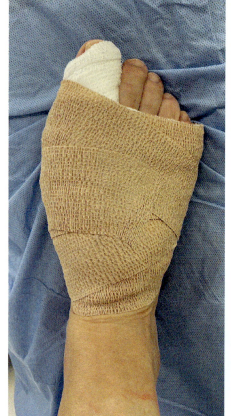

FIGURE 3.14 **A.** All incisions are irrigated with saline using an angiocatheter syringe tip. **B, C.** The poke-hole incisions are closed with 3-0 or 4-0 nylon simple sutures. **D.** A clinical photo of a surgical bunion dressing, using gauze to splint the hallux into slight varus and applying gentle compression with an outer wrap (Coban).

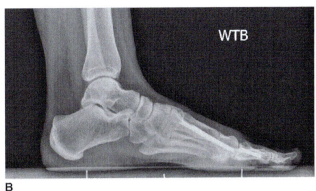
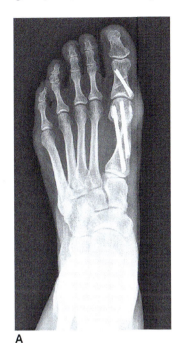

FIGURE 3.15 A, B. Anteroposterior and lateral radiographs of the patient 2 months postoperatively showing complete healing across the osteotomies and excellent deformity correction.

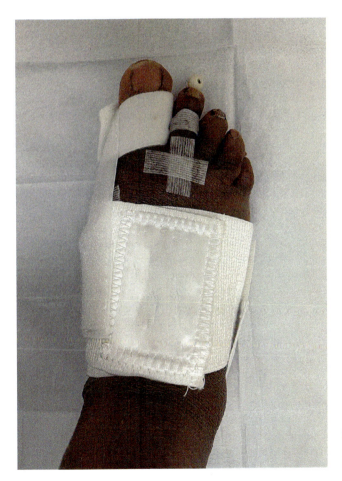

FIGURE 3.16 Prefabricated bunion splint worn fulltime for 6 weeks and then at nighttime only for 3 months.

PEARLS AND PITFALLS

- The MIS bunionectomy improves pain and deformity associated with hallux valgus. Postoperatively, patients typically advance activities more quickly and complain of fewer scar and swelling-related issues compared to open bunionectomy procedures.
- Medial eminence resection can be optional because this region will become less prominent once the lateral shift is performed. Some surgeons prefer to avoid this and stay extracapsular throughout the procedure.
- Lateral ligament release or modified McBride procedure is rarely required in conjunction with the MIS chevron osteotomy technique and should only be performed if necessary after the chevron and Akin are fixed. The lateral shift at the osteotomy usually corrects the head to the position of the sesamoids. If desired, a lateral ligament release can be performed percutaneously using a no. 64 beaver blade with a long handle. We do not routinely perform lateral ligament release, as it has been associated with overcorrection in our experience.
  - A poke-hole longitudinal incision is made dorsolateral after fluoroscopically localizing the joint level.
  - The beaver blade is inserted into the joint under fluoroscopy between the metatarsal head and sesamoid.
  - The metatarso-sesamoid ligament is released, along with some of plantar capsule. The abductor may also be released in some cases.
  - A dynamic exam using fluoroscopy should reveal a stable sesamoid position with varus manipulation of the hallux if release is complete.
- Typical though rare complications include burns to the skin or the bone. It is critical to maintain continuous and copious irrigation when the burr is running. This will also help avoid thermal necrosis, which can be associated with nonunion. Pronation and supination motions of the hand, which maintain the burr tip stationary at the percutaneous incision site, are key to preventing burning or ripping of the skin.
- New burrs, rather than resterilized used burrs, should be available for each case to ensure they are sharp and cut effectively through bone.
- Damage to cutaneous nerves can occur if incisions are not made in appropriate places, or if capsular tissues are not elevated to allow a space for the burr, as in the case of medial eminence resection.
- Fluoroscopy is a critical tool when direct visualization is not possible. Appropriate use of fluoroscopic localization will help facilitate proper burr position and orientation, as well as ensure the desired correction and stable fixation.
- Patients with significant osteopenia may not need overdrilling of the guidewires beyond the lateral cortex. These patients may also require sturdier support, that is, a walking boot postoperatively instead of a postoperative shoe alone.
- Radiographic healing will lag behind clinical healing. Typically bony consolidation of the metatarsal osteotomy will not be complete until 6 months postoperatively, though evidence of early bony bridging should be noted in earlier radiographs.

RESULTS AND COMPLICATIONS

The traditional open distal chevron osteotomy is associated with complications related to MTP joint stiffness, edema, and avascular necrosis to the metatarsal head associated with soft tissue stripping. The MIS bunionectomy is an alternative procedure that attempts to mitigate these problems and enhance recovery. While historical MIS bunionectomy involved no fixation or Kirschner wires to secure the osteotomy site, third-generation MIS techniques, which feature specialized burr instruments and rigid fixation with percutaneous screws, have demonstrated excellent clinical outcomes.[4-7] Lee et al published a prospective study with 50 total patients randomized to percutaneous chevron/Akin (PECA) versus open scarf and Akin.[8] The groups had comparable pre- and postoperative AOFAS scores, but the PECA group had significantly lower pain throughout the first 6 weeks postoperatively. Another randomized study between MIS and open scarf also reported similar deformity correction with lower postoperative VAS pain scores.[9] The operative time was shorter in the MIS group, 17 versus 26 minutes. A prospective single surgeon series by Lewis et al consisting of

333 consecutive feet reported improvement in multiple functional domains and preserved correction at 2-year follow-up.[10]

Although previously reserved for mild to moderate hallux valgus deformities, there is evidence for addressing even severe deformities with the MIS bunionectomy technique.[3] Lewis et al retrospectively assessed 50 patients with radiographic HVA greater than 40 and/or IMA greater than 20 with average 3 years follow-up. The average postoperative HVA and IMA were 11.5° and 5.1°, respectively. A total of 77% of patients were highly satisfied with their outcome, and 22% were satisfied. There were three cases of deformity recurrence. Even when compared with the open modified Lapidus procedure, Johnson et al observed similar radiographic correction in a retrospective matched cohort study.[11]

One of the disadvantages of MIS techniques is the lack of direct visualization of tissue layers and, therefore, dependence on intraoperative fluoroscopy. Even among surgeons highly experienced with the MIS technique, the radiation exposure was 14 times higher for MIS than open scarf osteotomy, 34 versus 2.4 mGy/cm^2.[9] There is a learning curve associated with the instrumentation and technique.[12] Approximately 20 cases were required before case duration and fluoroscopy time normalized.[13] In another series, the first 60 consecutive cases were found to be associated with poorer radiographic correction and higher rates of reoperation for hardware removal than the subsequent 60.[14] One of the proposed advantages of MIS bunionectomy is that the extracapsular osteotomy and minimal soft tissue dissection reduces stiffness at the MTP joint. However, a study of 50 open scarf patients and 48 MIS patients found similar low rate of moderate stiffness—3 cases in each group.[15] The MIS group gained an additional 10° of extension compared to preoperatively but was not significant relative to the scarf group. The authors concluded that a shorter scar length was the only notable outcome difference associated with MIS bunionectomy. Eleven MIS patients (27%) underwent elective hardware removal due to symptomatic hardware.

The rate of complications associated with MIS bunionectomy ranges widely depending on the report. Tendon injury is a known potential complication associated with using the MIS burr and no direct protection of the extensor hallucis longus (EHL) or flexor hallucis longus (FHL) tendons, but the rate is extremely low. One FHL injury was reported among a 292 case series.[10] Symptomatic hardware remains a prevalent complication requiring subsequent reoperation for hardware removal. This rate ranges from 2% to 27%.[15,16] In the largest series of MICA of 292 feet followed up for 30 months, all cause screw removal rate was 6.3%.[10] This event occurrence may be improved with specialized MIS screws featuring a beveled head to reduce hardware prominence.

In summary, the third-generation MIS bunionectomy technique featuring rigid internal fixation is gaining wide acceptance among surgeons and patients alike. The radiographic correction is comparable to open techniques, even for some severe hallux valgus deformities. Patients typically are weight bearing as tolerated immediately postoperatively without compromising healing at the osteotomies. The most common complication remains hardware irritation requiring removal. A learning curve associated with the first 20 to 60 cases but may be ameliorated with practice on sawbones and cadaver specimens. Current comparative studies are positive, but longer follow-up of clinical outcomes will further define the merits of this technique.

REFERENCES

1. Brogan K, Lindisfarne E, Akehurst H, Farook U, Shrier W, Palmer S. Minimally invasive and open distal chevron osteotomy for mild to moderate hallux valgus. *Foot Ankle Int.* 2016;37(11):1197-1204.
2. Kadakia AR, Smerek JP, Myerson MS. Radiographic results after percutaneous distal metatarsal osteotomy for correction of hallux valgus deformity. *Foot Ankle Int.* 2007;28(3):355-360.
3. Lewis TL, Ray R, Robinson P, et al. Percutaneous chevron and Akin (PECA) osteotomies for severe hallux valgus deformity with mean 3-year follow-up. *Foot Ankle Int.* 2021;42(10):1231-1240.
4. Kaufmann G, Dammerer D, Heyenbrock F, Braito M, Moertlbauer L, Liebensteiner M. Minimally invasive versus open chevron osteotomy for hallux valgus correction: a randomized controlled trial. *Int Orthop.* 2019;43(2):343-350.
5. Neufeld SK, Dean D, Hussaini S. Outcomes and surgical strategies of minimally invasive chevron/Akin procedures. *Foot Ankle Int.* 2021;42(6):676-688.
6. Trnka HJ, Krenn S, Schuh R. Minimally invasive hallux valgus surgery: a critical review of the evidence. *Int Orthop.* 2013;37(9):1731.
7. Holme TJ, Sivaloganathan SS, Patel B, Kunasingam K. Third-generation minimally invasive chevron Akin osteotomy for hallux valgus. *Foot Ankle Int.* 2020;41(1):50-56.
8. Lee M, Walsh J, Smith MM, Ling J, Wines A, Lam P. Hallux valgus correction comparing percutaneous chevron/Akin (PECA) and open scarf/Akin osteotomies. *Foot Ankle Int.* 2017;38(8):838-846.
9. Torrent J, Baduell A, Vega J, Malagelada F, Luna R, Rabat E. Open vs minimally invasive scarf osteotomy for hallux valgus correction: a randomized controlled trial. *Foot Ankle Int.* 2021;42(8):982-993.

10. Lewis TL, Ray R, Miller G, Gordon DJ. Third-generation minimally invasive chevron and Akin osteotomies (MICA) in hallux valgus surgery. *J Bone Jt Surg.* 2021;103(13):1203-1211.
11. Cody E, Caolo KC, Ellis SJ, Johnson A. Clinical and radiographic outcomes of minimally invasive chevron bunionectomy compared to the modified lapidus procedure. *Foot Ankle Orthop.* 2022;7(1).
12. Bedi H, Hickey B. Learning curve for minimally invasive surgery and how to minimize it. *Foot Ankle Clin.* 2020;25(3):361-371.
13. Palmanovich E, Ohana N, Atzmon R, et al. MICA: a learning curve. *J Foot Ankle Surg.* 2020;59(4):781-783.
14. Jowett CRJ, Bedi HS. Preliminary results and learning curve of the minimally invasive chevron Akin operation for hallux valgus. *J Foot Ankle Surg.* 2017;56(3):445-452.
15. Frigg A, Zaugg S, Maquieira G, Pellegrino A. Stiffness and range of motion after minimally invasive chevron-Akin and open scarf-Akin procedures. *Foot Ankle Int.* 2019;40(5):515-525.
16. Redfern D, Vernois J. Minimally invasive chevron Akin (MICA) for correction of hallux valgus. *Tech Foot Ankle Surg.* 2016;15(1):3-11.

4 Correction of Hallux Valgus With and Without Metatarsus Adductus

Mark E. Easley, Paul Dayton, William T. DeCarbo, Daniel J. Hatch, Jody P. McAleer, W. Bret Smith, and Robert D. Santrock*

INDICATIONS AND CONTRAINDICATIONS

Indications

Current studies indicate that metatarsal pronation is present in the majority of hallux valgus.[1-4] Reports suggest that incomplete correction of metatarsal pronation and/or metatarsus adductus may lead to hallux valgus recurrence.[5-7] The triplanar first tarsometatarsal (TMT) corrective arthrodesis is founded on a philosophy of three-dimensional anatomic realignment of the first metatarsal, sesamoids, and hallux that returns these structures to a physiologic position. This technique may be combined with triplanar correction of the lesser metatarsals in cases of metatarsus adductus through the implementation of a third, second, and first tarsometatarsal arthrodesis (3/2/1 TMT). Triplanar correction is indicated in all iterations of hallux valgus, which emphasizes the repositioning of a physiologically straight first metatarsal to a stable corrected position in the coronal, sagittal, and axial planes. Instrumented and reproducible metatarsal realignment in three planes, appropriate lateral first metatarsophalangeal (MTP) joint soft tissue release, and stabilization of the first metatarsal through TMT arthrodesis virtually eliminate the need for traditional radiographic measurements (ie, intermetatarsal angle [IMA], hallux valgus angle [HVA], and distal metatarsal articular angle [DMAA]). Whether the hallux valgus deformity is mild, moderate, or severe and regardless of the quantified angular relationships, we anatomically realign the first metatarsal with the same fundamental triplanar correction. Assessment of the first ray frontal plane position and osseous segment relationships is of greater importance and can be determined with a combination of anteroposterior (AP), lateral, and sesamoid axial plain films or through weight-bearing computed tomography (WBCT) assessment.

Contraindications

Absolute contraindications to the procedure are like any surgery and include inadequate vascular supply, active infection, metabolic conditions that impede bone healing, and neuropathy. Neuropathy poses a risk to the arthrodesis with potential for an insensate overload and stress failure of the hardware resulting in a loss of correction, malunion, or nonunion. With neuropathy, surgeons should consider dedicated, robust fixation intended for neuropathic patients. Other absolute contraindications include advanced first MTP joint arthritis and hallux valgus in skeletally immature patients.

Degenerative first MTP joint arthritis places the patient at risk for persistent pain and lack of appropriate joint function. Even when first MTP joint arthritis is not evident on AP radiographs, lateral radiographs, sesamoid views, and/or WBCT may identify the presence of advanced sesamoid

---

*Disclosure of financial interest: The authors of this chapter are paid consultants and/or royalty recipients for Treace Medical Concepts, Inc.

arthritis that can lead to persistent pain and limited MTP joint function despite appropriate metatarsal realignment. We counsel our patients and recommend first MTP joint arthrodesis for first MTP joint arthritis, and with a larger IMA, we suggest combining this approach with a first TMT joint arthrodesis. To optimize correction in these cases we also apply the principles of triplanar correction and biplanar plating to both the TMT and MTP joints.

Triplanar hallux valgus and metatarsus adductus correction techniques may be applied to juvenile hallux valgus, but, with the correction performed at the metatarsal bases and the distal poles of the cuneiforms, skeletal immaturity without physeal closure is an absolute contradiction (Videos 4.1 and 4.2). Relative contraindications are symptoms related to hallux valgus, second toe pathology, and patient compliance. Although the argument may be made that early intervention could potentially avert problems associated with worsening hallux valgus deformity, we reserve correction for patients with symptomatic concerns. In patients with an isolated symptomatic second toe deformity we recommend correcting asymptomatic hallux valgus due to crowding of the digits so that the area of chief complaint may be treated in an unimpeded manner. Our experience with these techniques suggests that the robust biplanar fixation constructs permit immediate protected postoperative weight bearing in a postoperative shoe or cast boot. However, if a patient advances prematurely to unprotected weight bearing there may be a risk of correction loss and delayed union.

PREOPERATIVE PLANNING

Triplanar First Tarsometatarsal Corrective Arthrodesis and Metatarsus Adductus Correction

Hallux valgus surgery warrants thorough clinical examination and radiographic evaluation. As for any procedure, we confirm intact vascular and neurologic status. We assess first MTP joint motion in the sagittal plane and in the coronal plane. Stiffness or incongruence in the sagittal plane may indicate arthritis to be assessed radiographically. Limitation to passive coronal plane correction suggests lateral soft tissue contracture that will most likely require lateral soft tissue release(s). Hallux alignment is less important since our preferred technique remains consistent irrespective of degree of deformity. Hallux pronation should be coordinated with radiographic evaluation, specifically sesamoid views and/or axial WBCT to determine metatarsal rotation and sesamoid position relative to the metatarsal head and crista. We correct hallux valgus in three planes through first TMT joint arthrodesis, so the presence of first TMT joint symptoms, arthrosis, and/or instability is noteworthy but less important in planning.

The first ray should not be viewed in isolation. Moderate to severe hallux valgus and valgus deviation of the lesser toes may be suggestive of metatarsus adductus and must be correlated with radiographic evaluation.[8-10] Hindfoot malalignment and equinus contracture, especially with pes planus, need to factor into planning; reports confirm that pes planus may contribute to hallux valgus and recurrence following isolated hallux valgus correction.[11-13]

Weight-bearing foot radiographs include standard AP, oblique, and lateral views, but we routinely obtain axial sesamoid views. The sesamoid view affords in-plane assessment of first metatarsal rotation and the first metatarsal (MT) head-sesamoid relationship[14] (Fig. 4.1A through C). If available, axial WBCT provides perhaps more meaningful detail of the first metatarsal head-sesamoid relationship. The sesamoid view is obtained with the hallux dorsiflexed, which tends to reduce the sesamoids on the crista, whereas the axial WBCT accurately assesses sesamoid position in natural stance phase.[3] Objective measurements may be obtained from these axial views to allow the surgeon to predict what degree of metatarsal derotation may be required for complete deformity correction.[15] As mentioned above, appropriate lateral first MTP joint soft tissue releases, metatarsal realignment in three planes, and first metatarsal stabilization with TMT arthrodesis, in our experience, render traditional radiographic measurements (ie, IMA, HVA, and DMAA) irrelevant in surgical planning.

Axial views may also confirm the presence of a dorsomedial metatarsal head prominence palpable on physical examination, one that typically becomes more prominent with correction of metatarsal pronation and may warrant an ancillary limited medial first MTP joint procedure to remove it (Fig. 4.2A and B).

In addition to lateral radiographs and sagittal CT, the sesamoid view and axial WBCT often provide greater detail of potential first MT head-sesamoid arthritis; first MTP joint arthritis, even if isolated to the first MT head-sesamoid articulation, may be an indication for first MTP arthrodesis.

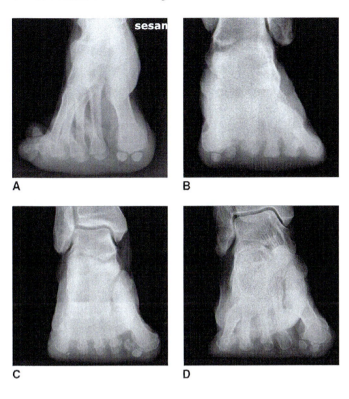

FIGURE 4.1 Axial sesamoid views. **A.** Normal without hallux valgus. **B.** Metatarsal head and sesamoid complex congruently pronated without sesamoid subluxation. **C.** Metatarsal head without pronation but sesamoid subluxation. **D.** Sesamoid subluxation with first metatarsal–sesamoid arthritis.

When the physical examination and plane radiographs suggest metatarsus adductus, we recommend applying dedicated radiographic measurements to determine the need for metatarsus adductus correction in addition to hallux valgus correction. Several authors have described intricate methods of measuring the metatarsus adductus angle.[9,16-18] While we apply these methods in our scientific work, we commonly assess the need for metatarsus adductus correction with a simplified plumb line technique (Fig. 4.3A through C). We assess the plumb line on standard, balanced weight-bearing AP radiographs. We recognize that a pronated or supinated foot position may impact the radiographic relationships and strive for a neutral foot position during image capture to obtain accurate measurements. A modified medial cuneiform reference line is drawn by identifying and linking two individual points marked at the medial aspects of the first TMT joint and the medial naviculo-cuneiform joint. A longitudinal line is subtended crossing these two established points. A third point is marked at the distal lateral apex of the medial cuneiform at the first TMT joint. The subtended line is translated to the lateral border of the medial cuneiform, crosses the third point, and extends distally to the level of the second metatarsal head. If the line intersects the second metatarsal head, it is considered a positive plumb line and indicates the presence of metatarsus adductus. Alternatively, a negative plumb line will remain tangential to the second metatarsal and will not intersect the ray, indicating that there is sufficient space to perform an isolated first metatarsal hallux valgus correction.

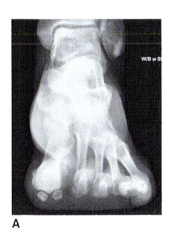
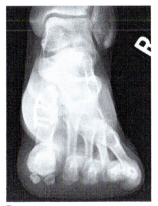

FIGURE 4.2 Axial views. **A.** Dorsomedial metatarsal head prominence preoperatively. **B.** Resected dorsomedial head prominence after hallux valgus correction.

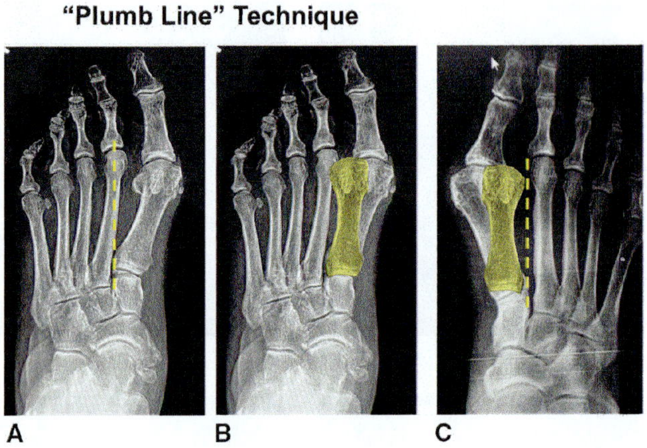

FIGURE 4.3 Plumb line method of assessing need for metatarsus adductus correction with hallux valgus correction. **A.** Plum line intersects second metatarsal (MT). **B.** Simulated hallux valgus correction confirms that desired first MT realignment would be limited by second metatarsal, indicating need for metatarsus adductus correction. **C.** Plumb line without second metatarsal intersection and simulated hallux valgus correction confirms no metatarsus adductus.

Should this line intersect with the second metatarsal head, we confirm metatarsus adductus (see Fig. 4.3A and B). Although our team believes that the plumb line technique is effective in determining the need for metatarsus adductus correction, we continue to study the validity of this method.

Theoretically, the plumb line mimics the longitudinal anatomic axis of the foot and provides a tangential reference to which the first metatarsal should be corrected. We believe that, like hallux valgus, metatarsus adductus is often a multiplanar deformity. Similar to our hallux valgus correction, our technique for correcting metatarsus adductus facilitates multiplanar correction at the metatarsal base(s). This approach reduces the lesser metatarsal deformity, uncovers the true 1 to 2 IMA, and subsequently produces space to perform hallux valgus correction in all three planes.

Hindfoot and midfoot malalignment syndromes, as seen in both pes planus and pes cavus, should be evaluated radiographically with dedicated hindfoot imaging and alignment views. First TMT joint stabilization may not suffice in correcting hallux valgus associated with pes planus, which may require concomitant hindfoot realignment procedures. Similarly, metatarsus adductus is often associated with pes cavus, and while concomitant hallux valgus and metatarsus adductus correction may afford considerable correction, hindfoot realignment may be warranted to achieve full correction.

SURGICAL TECHNIQUE

Triplanar First Tarsal-Metatarsal Corrective Arthrodesis (Lapiplasty)

We present a typical adult patient with hallux valgus as our case example (Fig. 4.4A through D). A video of the surgical technique is also available (see ▶ Video 4.1). We utilize a radiolucent operating room table, position the patient so the operative extremity is easily accessible, and use a proximal calf or thigh tourniquet. We prep and drape the operative extremity, exsanguinate the leg, and inflate the tourniquet. We prep and drape the operative extremity, exsanguinate the leg, and inflate the tourniquet. Taking the patient's blood pressure into consideration, we favor tourniquet pressure of 225 mm Hg or less, a pressure deemed safe, with a low wound complication rate, based upon findings reported by Olivecrona and colleagues.[19]

Triplanar hallux valgus correction procedure is image dependent with several key steps requiring image confirmation prior to proceeding to the next step. In our experience, both small C-arm and full-sized fluoroscopic units are effective.

A 3- to 4-cm incision is made over the dorsal aspect of the first TMT joint, just medial to the extensor hallucis longus (EHL) tendon (Fig. 4.4E). It is essential to keep the incision dorsal with this technique to position the guidance system properly. We avoid unnecessary soft tissue dissection, protect the overlying superficial peroneal nerve branches if possible, preserve crossing veins when possible, carefully mobilize the EHL tendon within its sheath and retract it laterally, and deepen the dorsal longitudinal incision to reflect the capsule and periosteum overlying the first TMT joint. Complete subperiosteal dissection is performed to expose the first TMT joint with care being taken to maintain the tibialis anterior tendon within the plantar medial soft tissue sleeve (Fig. 4.4F and G). With a dedicated oscillating saw and osteotome, the plantar flair of the first metatarsal base is resected and associated ligament releases are respectively performed to facilitate free, and smooth frontal plane metatarsal rotation through the TMT joint (Fig. 4.5A and B). The first TMT ligaments are carefully released, as the plantar-lateral and plantar-medial ligaments typically limit first metatarsal rotation and produce a tethering effect if left intact. A small soft tissue pocket at the proximal lateral first metatarsal base is also developed to allow for the introduction of fulcrum/seeker/cut guide instrumentation (Fig. 4.6A and B).

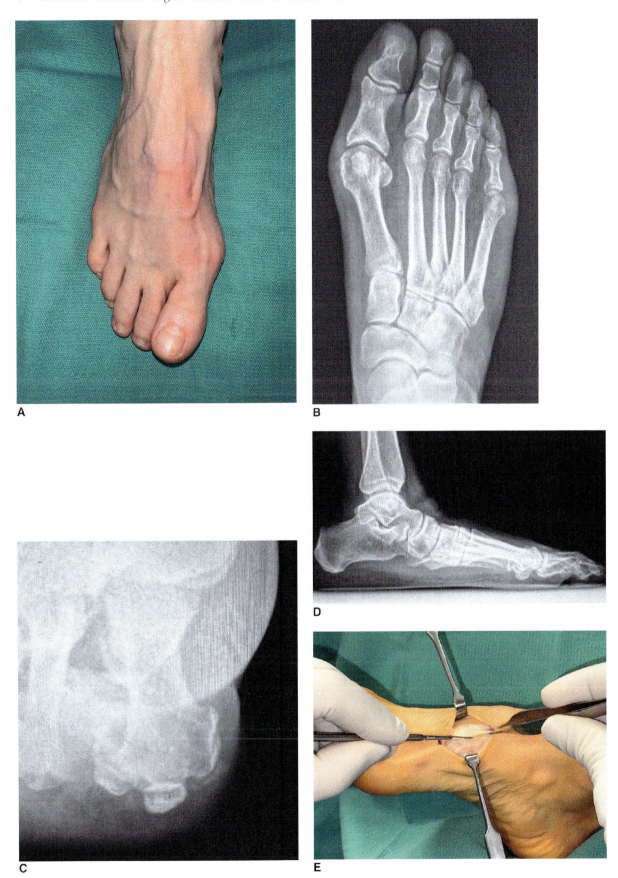

FIGURE 4.4 Case presentation and first tarsometatarsal (TMT) joint surgical approach. **A.** Dorsal clinical view of patient with hallux valgus. **B.** Weightbearing anteroposterior view of the foot. **C.** Axial sesamoid view with lateral sesamoid subluxation. **D.** Weightbearing lateral foot radiograph with suggestion of mild first TMT joint instability (dorsal subluxation). **E.** Dorsomedial approach, immediately medial to the extensor hallucis longus tendon. **F.** Dorsolateral subperiosteal dissection. **G.** Plantar medial subperiosteal dissection.

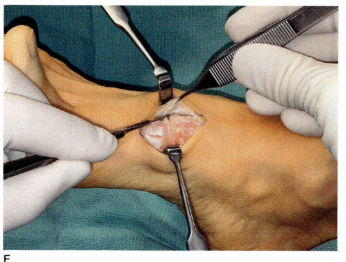
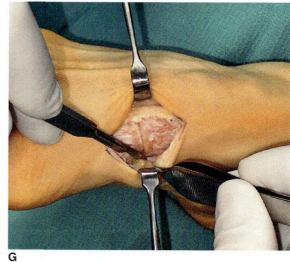

FIGURE 4.4 *(Continued)*

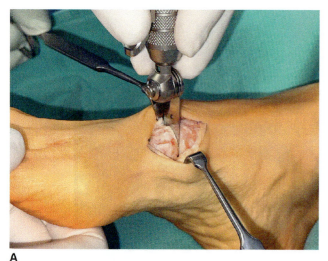
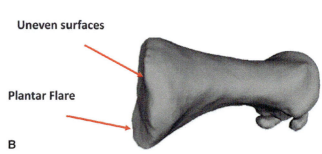

FIGURE 4.5 First tarsometatarsal (TMT) joint planing. **A.** Dedicated microsagittal blade carefully advanced from dorsal to plantar in the first TMT joint. **B.** Schematic of first metatarsal base highlighting the aim of planing; removing joint undulations to facilitate metatarsal base rotation.

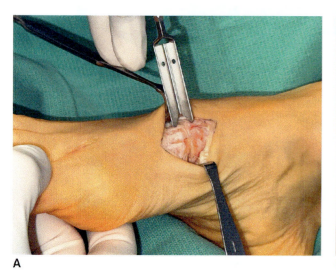
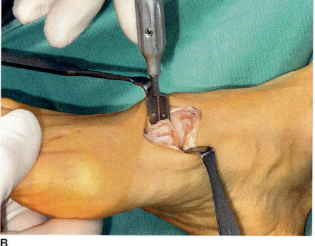

FIGURE 4.6 First tarsometatarsal (TMT) joint ligament release to allow metatarsal rotation and full insertion of the 3-in-1 cut guide. **A.** Dedicated corner chisel for lateral first TMT joint. **B.** Corner chisel advanced to release the dense plantar lateral TMT joint ligaments.

4 Correction of Hallux Valgus With and Without Metatarsus Adductus

Our emphasis in hallux valgus correction is reducing the sesamoids on a properly aligned first metatarsal. In our experience, successful sesamoid reduction routinely requires adequate and complete lateral soft tissue release, especially with sesamoid subluxation on preoperative imaging and/or a first MTP joint that does not allow passive correction of valgus. We recognize that the lateral soft tissue release may be performed though the joint from a medial approach. However, unless we identify a dorsomedial first metatarsal prominence that needs to be resected (see Fig. 4.2A), we favor performing the lateral release through a 1- to 1.5-cm dorsal webspace incision. In the majority of cases, we limit the lateral release to the suspensory ligament between the lateral capsule and lateral sesamoid. We have learned that the suspensory ligament release is more comprehensive than we originally considered, with fibers extending from the base of the proximal phalanx to at least 2 cm proximal to the proximal first metatarsal head (Fig. 4.7A). To limit the exposure and facilitate complete and safe suspensory ligament release, we developed a dedicated instrument, easily introduced between the lateral metatarsal head and lateral sesamoid via a minimal lateral capsular incision (Fig. 4.7B through E). With more severe contracture, we promote greater sesamoid mobility by releasing the adductor hallucis longus tendon and deep intermetatarsal ligament from the lateral sesamoid. In our experience a comprehensive lateral release does not lead to hallux varus following an anatomic first metatarsal correction. Moreover, we recommend against performing a medial capsulotomy as it may result in a destabilization of the MTP. If the surgeon is confident that the lateral release is necessary, then it may be performed prior to the first TMT joint preparation.

A temporary joystick pin may be placed in the proximal first metatarsal to confirm that the first metatarsal is free to rotate at the first TMT joint, and the lateral first MTP joint release is complete (Fig. 4.8A). The pin should be started at the dorsomedial metatarsal base and directed slightly distal as it is advanced through both cortices but with care taken to avoid the second metatarsal (Fig. 4.8B). This pin may be used to assist in coronal and axial plane correction of the metatarsal clinically and radiographically (Fig. 4.8C and D). Placing the pin along the recommended trajectory limits the risk of elevating the metatarsal with this manipulation. Provided the pin does not interfere with the cut guide, it may be used to rotate the metatarsal while the cut guide is positioned.

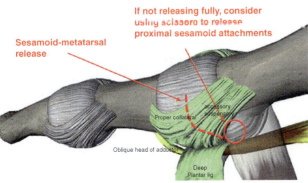
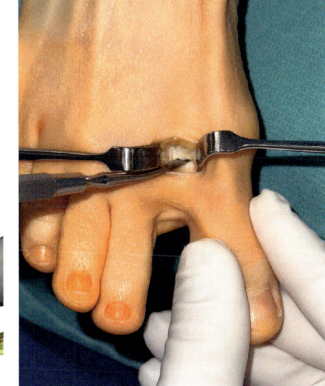

FIGURE 4.7 Lateral first MTP joint release. **A.** Schematic of lateral ligament structures. **B.** Dorsal first webspace approach with vertical lateral capsulotomy to allow access to the accessory suspensory ligament. **C.** Dedicated release tool. **D.** For complete release of the accessory suspensory ligament, release tool carefully introduced between metatarsal head and fibular sesamoid. **E.** To completely divide ligament, release tool advanced until resistance no longer experienced, at least 2 cm proximal to the metatarsal head.

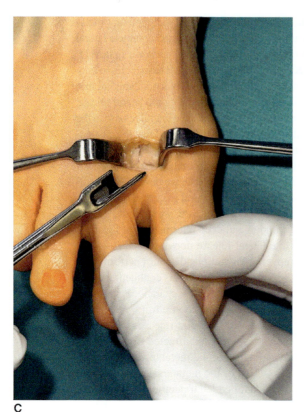
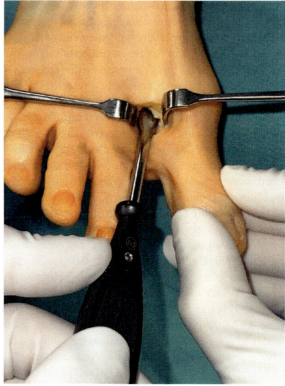
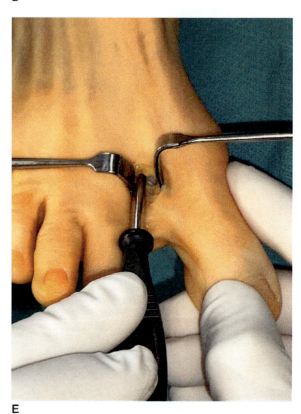

FIGURE 4.7 *(Continued)*

Multiple techniques have been described to prepare the first TMT joint for arthrodesis. Currently, we favor using a dedicated 3-in-1 cut guide over making free-hand cuts. To facilitate precise first TMT joint preparation, the 3-in-1 cut guide features three conjoined components: (1) a fulcrum between the first and second bases to promote optimal first metatarsal alignment in the coronal plane, (2) a joint seeker in the TMT joint to align the cut guide and minimize bone resection, and (3) cut

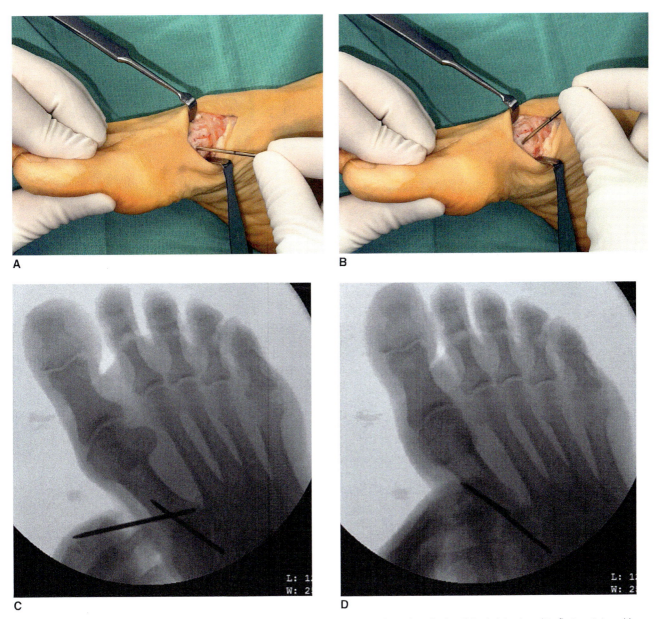

FIGURE 4.8 Confirming adequate soft tissue releases to allow adequate metatarsal rotation. **A.** Joystick pin introduced to first metatarsal base. **B.** Joystick being used to correct axial plane malrotation (pronation). **C.** Intraoperative fluoroscopic image prior to using joystick correct deformity. **D.** Intraoperative fluoroscopic image using joystick to confirm adequate ligament releases to allow full triplanar first metatarsal correction.

guide to allow for safe, captured and optimally directed saw blade preparations of the metatarsal base and distal cuneiform (Fig. 4.9A). Interference from the lateral soft tissues and the EHL tendon can bias the cut guide medially. It is imperative that the cut guide be properly positioned orthogonal to the TMT to develop the intended dorsal-to-plantar saw cuts (Fig. 4.9B and C). Prior to committing to the cut guide position, optimal alignment should be fluoroscopically confirmed on AP and lateral views.

With the 3-in-1 cut guide placed, a dedicated positioner device spanning the proximal first and second metatarsals is applied to the foot. The positioner has a small tine that engages the lateral cortex of the second metatarsal shaft through a small incision created at this level (Fig. 4.10A). The positioner has a saddle-shaped capture element that engages the medial first metatarsal. When using a longer incision, a lower profile internal positioner cup directly captures the first metatarsal's medial ridge (Fig. 4.10B). A larger profile external positioner cup has also been designed to rest on the skin overlying the medial ridge with a shorter incision (Fig. 4.10C). Both versions of the device promote triplane reduction of the first metatarsal when applied and engaged appropriately.

Adequate TMT and MTP joint mobilization and soft tissue releases promote a natural correction of the bone segments, often without the need to use the reduction joystick. Correction is confirmed

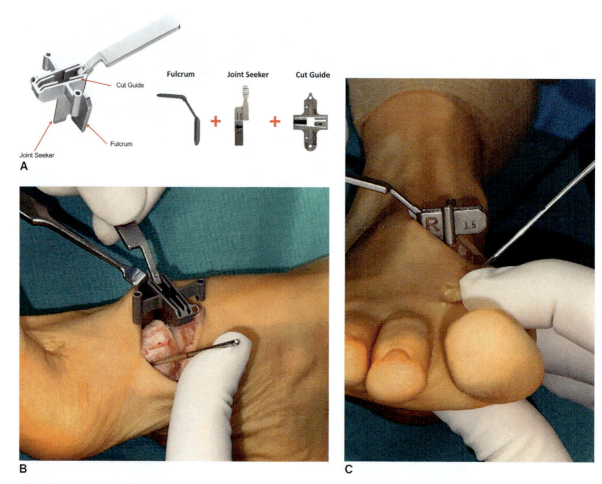

FIGURE 4.9 3-in-1 cut guide. **A.** The 3-in-1 cut guide combines three separate legacy instruments into one. **B.** While using the joystick to correct rotation the cut guide is introduced into the tarsometatarsal (TMT) joint. **C.** For the cut guide to direct accurate cuts, it must be positioned on the dorsal TMT joint.

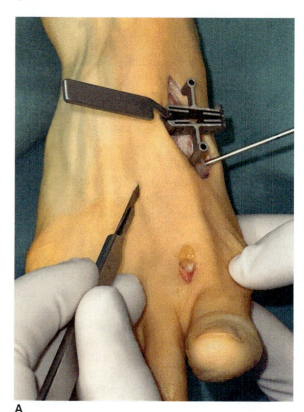

FIGURE 4.10 Positioner between first and second metatarsals. **A.** Small incision over second metatarsal (note that lateral soft tissues tend to force cut guide medially—key to maintain it on dorsal first tarsometatarsal joint). **B, C.** Positioner with smaller medial capture cup within a longer incision (note desirable medial joint space opening). **D.** Positioner with larger medial capture cup external to the shorter incision.

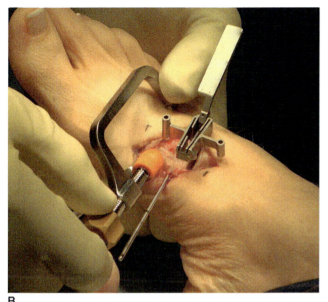

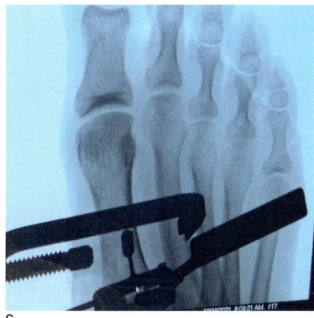

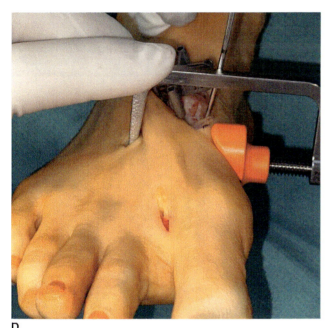

FIGURE 4.10 *(Continued)*

fluoroscopically, looking for parallelism of the first and second metatarsals, congruent TMT joint alignment in the lateral plane without plantar joint gapping, and sesamoids reduced under the first metatarsal head (Fig. 4.11A through D). An intraoperative sesamoid view may also be used to confirm satisfactory metatarsal axial plane correction (crista is in anatomic orientation) and satisfactory sesamoid correction (sesamoids centered over the crista) (Fig. 4.11E and F). Using traditional radiographic measurements, our goal is an IMA of 0° and a tibial sesamoid position (TSP) of 0. In the lateral fluoroscopic view plane, we aim for 0° of dorsal cortex change between the first metatarsal and first cuneiform on the lateral fluoroscopy. A transverse holding pin is placed through the cannulation in the positioner to temporarily stabilize the corrected metatarsal position, with the pin engaging the first and second metatarsals. Before pinning the cut guide, we confirm clinically and fluoroscopically that the cut guide is orthogonally positioned in the AP and lateral planes (see Fig. 4.11A through D). In the AP plane we ensure that the distal cut is congruent on the metatarsal base and the proximal cut positioned to remove more lateral bone from the cuneiform (see Fig. 4.11B). In the lateral plane, the joint seeker should be perfectly aligned with the axis of the TMT joint (see Fig. 4.11D). With proper cut guide position, the cut guide is pinned in place (see Fig. 4.11G). We recommend fluoroscopic confirmation of proper cut guide position after the introduction of bicortical metatarsal and

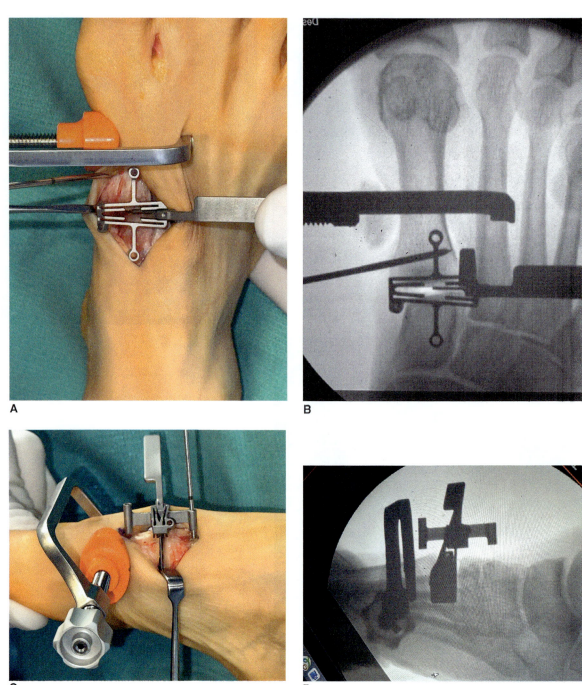

FIGURE 4.11 Clinical and fluoroscopic confirmation of anatomic first metatarsal correction and cut guide position. **A.** Clinical photo after anatomic first metatarsal reduction. **B.** Anteroposterior view of cut guide in optimal position, with anatomic first metatarsal alignment and first metatarsal head-sesamoid relationship (note distal capture guide directly over and perpendicular to metatarsal base and oblique cut planned for the cuneiform). **C.** Clinical lateral view after reduction confirming ideal medial tarsometatarsal (TMT) joint space opening and no plantar joint gapping. **D.** Fluoroscopic lateral view of joint seeker parallel to TMT joint and orthogonal sagittal plane cut guide position. **E.** Intraoperative fluoroscopic sesamoid view from case presentation suggesting proper sesamoid reduction under metatarsal head. **F.** Intraoperative fluoroscopic sesamoid view from different patient with better image angle demonstrating ideal sesamoid position after correction. **G.** With proper cut guide position confirmed clinically and radiographically, guide secured with pin fixation. **H.** Optimal cuts confirmed with orthogonal fluoroscopic view through the cut guide.

4 Correction of Hallux Valgus With and Without Metatarsus Adductus

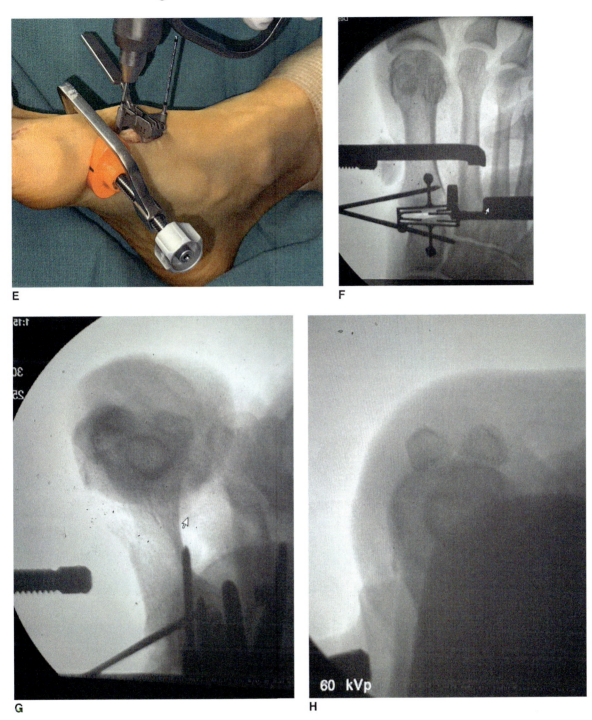

FIGURE 4.11 *(Continued)*

cuneiform pins across the cut guide outriggers (Fig. 4.11H). A third offset pin is introduced across the cut guide to reduce the risk of instrument migration produced by bone saw vibration.

Using the same dedicated microsagittal saw blade used for planing the TMT joint, the guide's cut slots direct optimal blade trajectory and help protect the adjacent bone and soft tissue structures (Fig. 4.12A through C). However, soft tissue retraction of the dorsal deep neurovascular bundle and the medial tibialis anterior tendon is recommended. Upon completion of the bone cuts, the offset pin is withdrawn and the cut guide is removed over the two remaining bicortical pins. The transverse positioner pin is removed, and the positioner is loosened or removed. The resected TMT joint slices are removed with a combination of osteotome and/or rongeur (Fig. 4.13A through D). To facilitate bone fragment removal, the joint may be distracted by placing a dedicated joint distractor/compressor over the bicortical pins used to secure the cut guide. As small fragments may remain plantarly, we recommend AP fluoroscopic confirmation to identify any residual fragments that could block satisfactory reduction of the metatarsal to the cuneiform (Fig. 4.14A through C). After joint irrigation, we use a small diameter drill bit to fenestrate the joint surfaces to a depth of approximately 2 mm; reamings created with this drilling serve as bone graft to promote fusion (Fig. 4.15A and B).

Using the compressor, we achieve axial apposition of the joint under direct visualization, ensuring congruent metatarsal contact to the cuneiform. The compressor has the option of adding 10

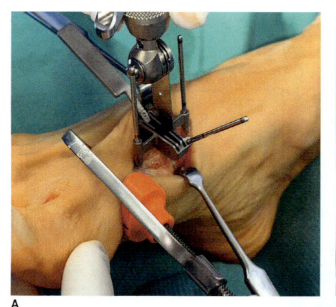
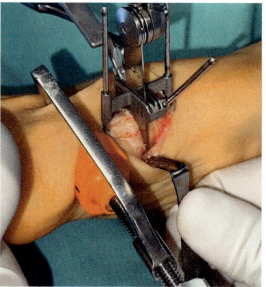
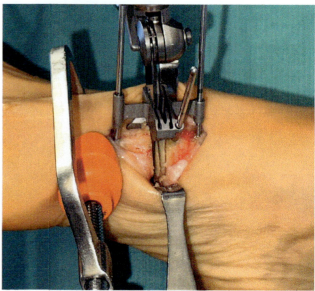

FIGURE 4.12 Tarsometatarsal (TMT) cuts through cut guide. **A.** Cuneiform cut. **B.** Metatarsal cut. **C.** Minimal resection with both cuts visible from medial TMT joint.

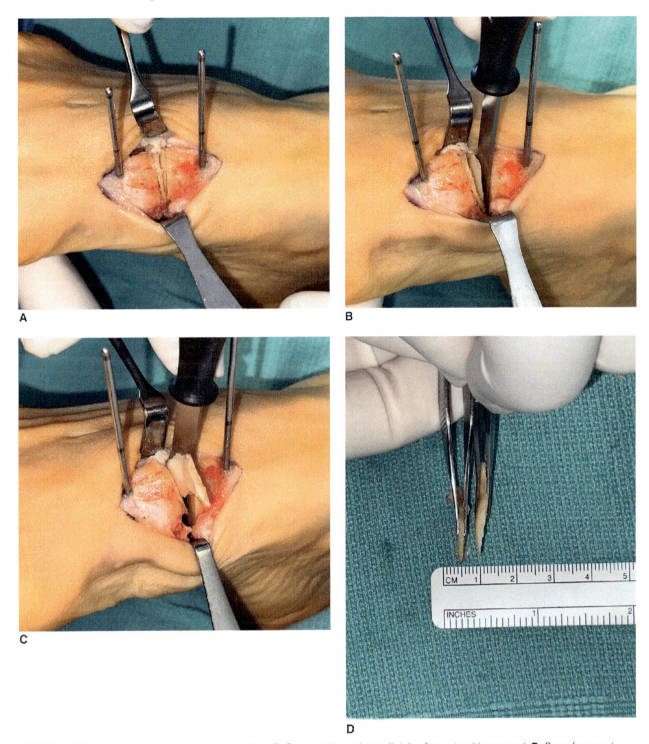

FIGURE 4.13 Tarsometatarsal joint bone extraction. **A.** Resected bone immediately after cut guide removal. **B.** Bone fragment mobilization with chisel. **C.** Bone extraction facilitated with specialized chisel. **D.** Minimal bone resection.

additional degrees of supination as the TMT arthrodesis is compressed, which can be used to achieve further axial plane rotational correction if desired (Fig. 4.16A and B). We add the additional rotational correction in the majority of cases. To maintain the parallelism of the first and second metatarsals, a dedicated fulcrum is placed lateral to the base of the first metatarsal during joint compression to avoid a convergence of the metatarsal bases, and the positioner may be reapplied without the transverse metatarsal pin to reinforce correction (see Fig. 4.16A and B). Satisfactory clinical correction is confirmed clinically and fluoroscopically: (1) anatomic first metatarsal head–sesamoid relationship (Fig. 4.16C), (2) parallelism between the first and second metatarsals (see Fig. 4.16C), (3) congruent

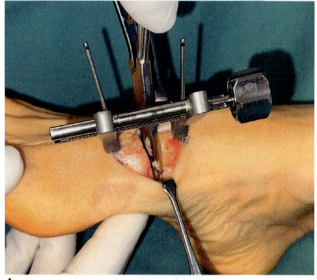

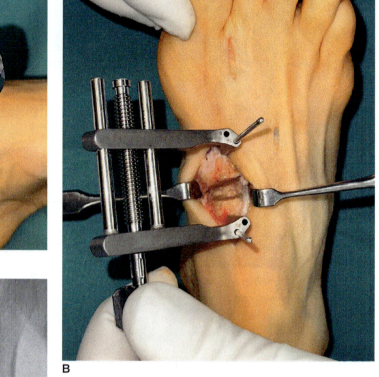

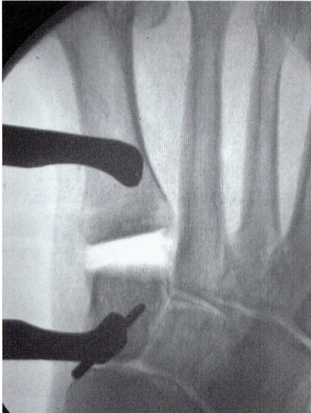

FIGURE 4.14 Residual bone in joint (that may limit optimal bone apposition). **A.** Rongeur used to remove residual bone in plantar joint. **B.** Bone cleared. **C.** Fluoroscopic confirmation that all resected bone evacuated from joint.

and complete bony TMT joint apposition, including plantar contact at the arthrodesis site (Fig. 4.16C through E), and (4) balance of the first metatarsal head and sesamoids relative to the lesser metatarsal heads (Fig. 4.16F). Crossing provisional wire fixation is introduced across the arthrodesis from the base of the first metatarsal into the first or second cuneiform (Fig. 4.17A and B). If a third wire is needed, it may be placed through the positioner to secure the first metatarsal to the second metatarsal.

4 Correction of Hallux Valgus With and Without Metatarsus Adductus

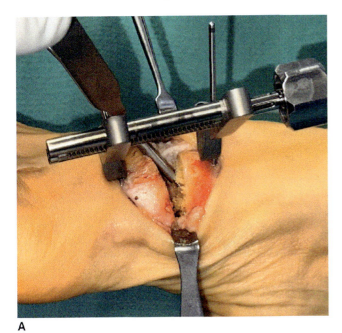
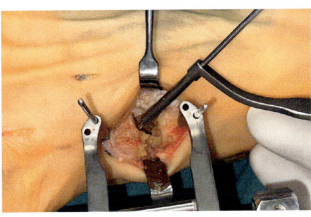

FIGURE 4.15 Subchondral bone fenestration to promote fusion. **A.** Prepping cuneiform. **B.** Prepping metatarsal.

The positioner and compressor are removed, and first ray correction is again confirmed fluoroscopically. The wire within the positioner may be cut shorter and the positioner opened fully to carefully remove the positioner while leaving the provisional metatarsal pin in place. To remove the compressor/distractor, the compression should not be released; instead, one of the pins is removed, allowing the compressor/distractor to slide from the remaining pin, after which that pin is also removed. With the compressor/distractor and its pins removed, there is ample space to place the definitive biplanar plate fixation. If there is concern that the provisional fixation is not maintaining correction of joint apposition, repeat fluoroscopic confirmation in two planes needs to be performed. In general, two of the three described provisional pins are adequate to maintain reduction; to be certain, all three may be used.

Permanent fixation includes the application of fixed-angle four-hole precontoured locking plates applied in a biplanar fashion to promote opposite cortex compression when secured with screw

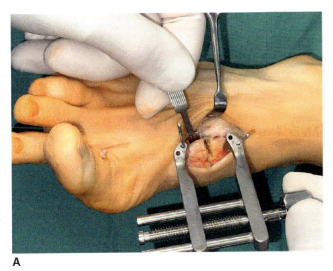
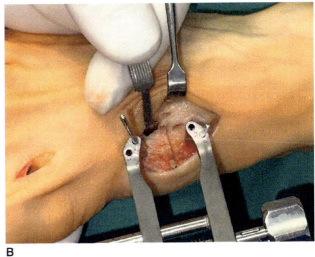

FIGURE 4.16 Tarsometatarsal joint compression. **A.** Ten degrees of additional axial-plane rotation added to the correction and standard fulcrum used to promote parallelism of first and second metatarsal. **B.** Joint surfaces apposed. **C.** Anteroposterior fluoroscopic confirmation. **D.** Clinical confirmation of plantar bone apposition. **E.** Fluoroscopic confirmation of plantar bone apposition (note compressor pins are bicortical and without overcompression that could lead to plantar gapping). **F.** Confirmation that the first ray is balanced with the transverse arch.

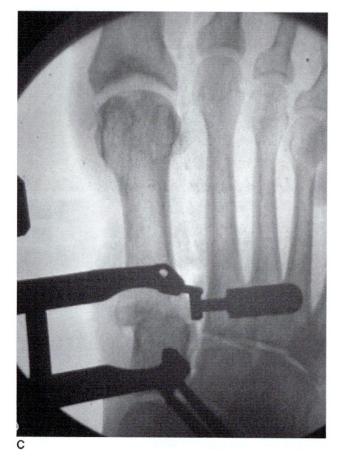
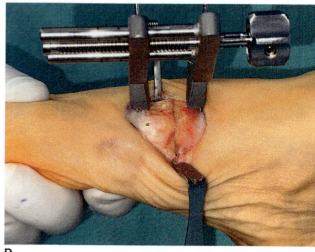
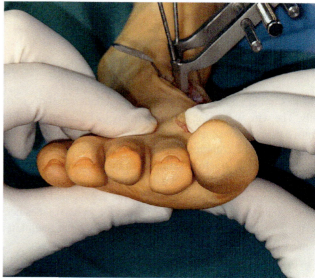
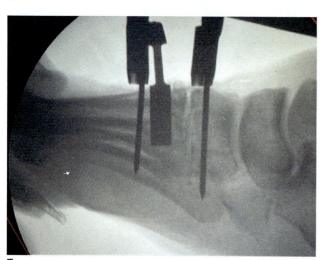

FIGURE 4.16 *(Continued)*

fixation. The unicortical locking plate and screw fixation provides reliable stability and allows for physiologic micromotion as described by Perren and colleagues that promotes healing.[20]

Achieving parallelism of the first and second metatarsals in the AP plane may result in a prominence of the medial first metatarsal base; we favor shaving this prominence with the microsagittal saw or carefully impacting it with a bone tamp (Fig. 4.18A through C).

We apply the dorsal plate first, as far lateral as possible (Fig. 4.19A). The intercuneiform joint's obliquity may lead to placing the most proximal of the four screws into the joint; therefore, a fluoroscopic check is recommended to confirm that the proximal screw trajectory will be in the cuneiform. Recent plate modifications include a slight bend to the proximal end of the plate, thereby matching the intercuneiform joint's obliquity and facilitating lateral plate positioning while still allowing the proximal screw to be secured into the cuneiform. With optimal position confirmed, the plate is provisionally

4 Correction of Hallux Valgus With and Without Metatarsus Adductus

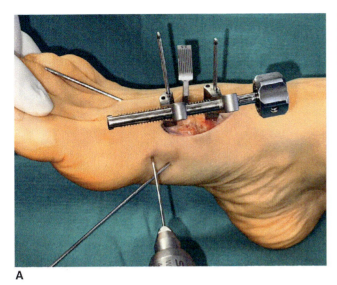

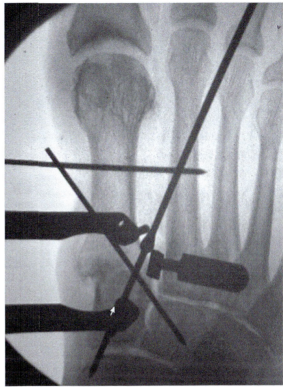

FIGURE 4.17 Confirmation of appropriate provisional pin fixation so that compressor may be removed. **A.** Clinical image of three points of fixation. **B.** Fluoroscopic image of the three points of fixation, including lateral threaded olive wire fixation.

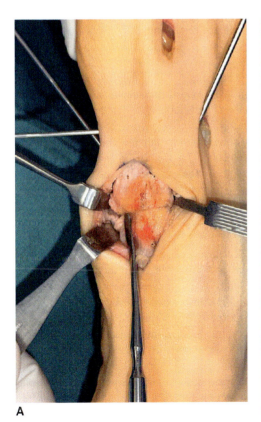

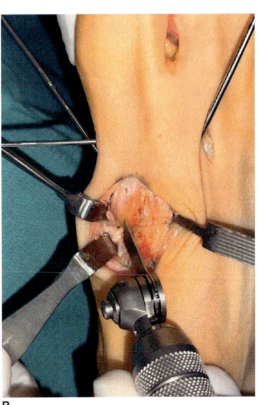

FIGURE 4.18 Routine medial metatarsal prominence anticipated with metatarsal rotation and desired metatarsal parallelism. **A.** Clinical appearance. **B.** Medial prominence shaving. **C.** Occasionally, dorsal prominence shaving required.

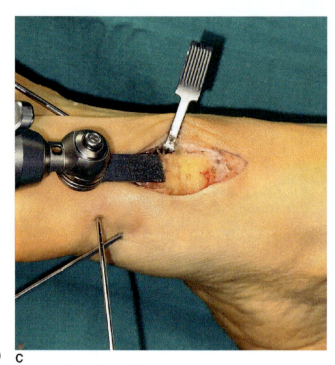

FIGURE 4.18 *(Continued)* **C**

pinned at the proximal and distal aspects with two dedicated plate tacks (Fig. 4.19B through D). The two central drill guides are drilled in preparation for screw placement (Fig. 4.19E). The drill guides are removed (Fig. 4.19F), and the locking screws are inserted. The screws are designed to pull the precontoured plate to the bone, thereby producing a far-sided joint compression to further stabilize the correction (Fig. 4.20A through C). The plate tacks are removed, the remaining drill guides are drilled, the drill guides are removed, and the final two locking screws are inserted to fully stabilize the plate to bone (Fig. 4.20D and E).

Optimal stability is produced when the second plate is applied across the medial first TMT joint at 90° to the dorsal lateral plate and just inferior to the mid-axial line of the metatarsal. Screw fixation at the medial plate uses the same stepwise process used for the dorsal lateral plate and, via plate precontour, the screws compress the lateral aspect of the arthrodesis and reinforce IMA reduction. The anatomic plate design matches the course of the tibialis anterior tendon, thereby limiting tendon and soft tissue dissection required to appropriately position the plate. Depending on anatomy, the medial plate may sit proud (Fig. 4.21A). If this is the case, we typically remove some of the plate precontour with dedicated plate benders (Fig. 4.21B). Provided some precontour remains, the desired opposite cortex compression will still occur, with the screws drawing medial plate to bone (Fig. 4.21C and D). Occasionally, the provisional wire fixation may interfere with screw placement. In this situation we achieve adequate stability by securing all other screws to the two plates, remove the provisional wire in question, and then fully seat the final screw. (Fig. 4.22A through C).

Once the biplanar plate construct is complete, a splay test should be performed to assess instability between the first and second ray. Thumb and index finger pressure between the first and second metatarsal heads determines splaying, with the IMA increasing readily in patients with a positive splay test. While relatively subjective, in our experience, surgeons readily learn to distinguish between a stable and unstable intercuneiform joint. Several investigators report that feet with hallux valgus have greater first to second intercuneiform mobility joint when compared to normal feet without hallux valgus; these same authors suggest that surgical outcomes for hallux valgus correction may be improved with intercuneiform arthrodesis in patients with a positive splay test.[21,22] We routinely use a 1 to 2 intercuneiform screw or a first metatarsal–second cuneiform screw when the splay test confirms first to second intercuneiform joint instability. Although the 1 to 2 intercuneiform joint may be prepared for fusion, in our experience, a countersunk 1 to 2 intercuneiform lag screw without intercuneiform preparation affords adequate medial-lateral stability between the first and second rays without sacrificing sagittal plane motion (Fig. 4.22A through C).

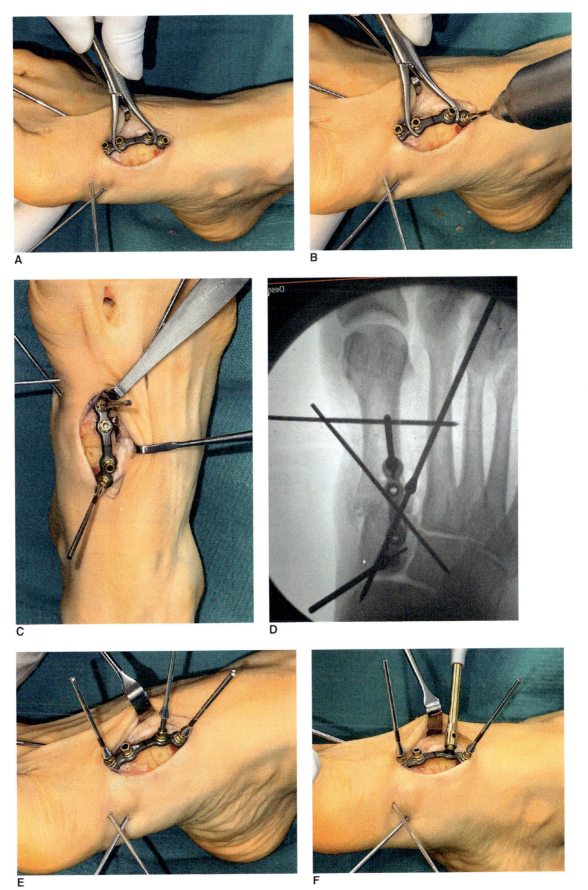

FIGURE 4.19 Dorsal tarsometatarsal joint plating. **A.** Plate positioning. **B.** Provisional pinning with plate tack. **C.** Plate is as dorsal and lateral as possible (to achieve 90-90 position with medial plate). **D.** Fluoroscopic confirmation of optimal dorsal plate position (note anatomic proximal plate contour that matches cuneiform architecture and avoids the intercuneiform joint). **E.** Drilling for screw placement. **F.** Removing drill sleeve.

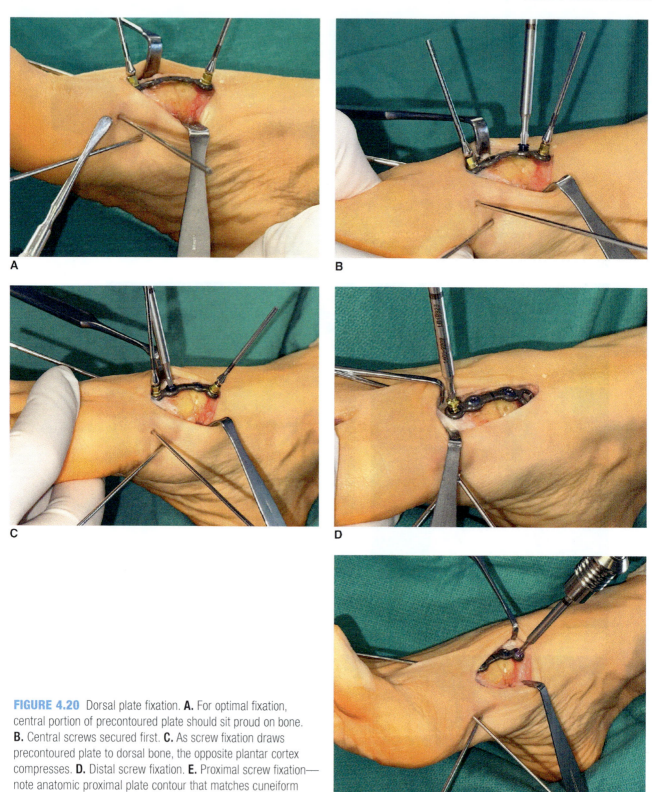

FIGURE 4.20 Dorsal plate fixation. **A.** For optimal fixation, central portion of precontoured plate should sit proud on bone. **B.** Central screws secured first. **C.** As screw fixation draws precontoured plate to dorsal bone, the opposite plantar cortex compresses. **D.** Distal screw fixation. **E.** Proximal screw fixation—note anatomic proximal plate contour that matches cuneiform anatomy.

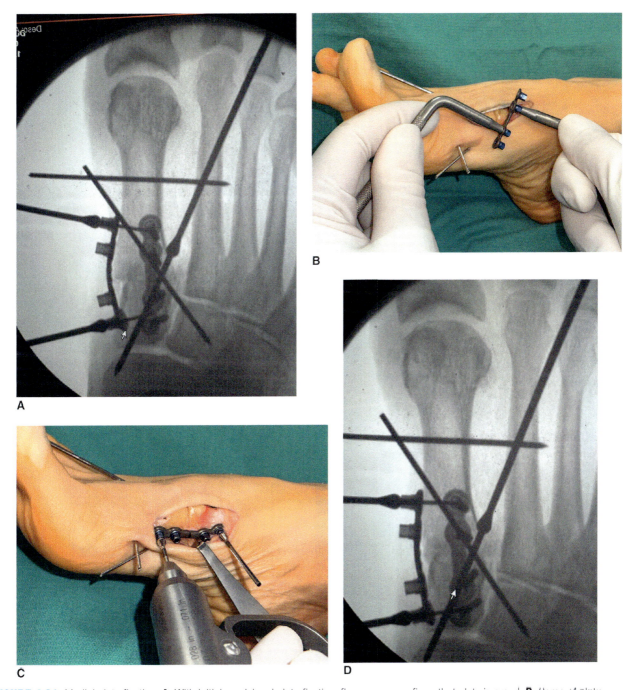

FIGURE 4.21 Medial plate fixation. **A.** With initial provisional plate fixation, fluoroscopy confirms that plate is proud. **B.** Some of plate precontour removed with dedicated plate benders. **C.** Improved clinical medial plate position (note anatomic proximal plate contour to limit tibialis anterior irritation). **D.** Fluoroscopic confirmation that medial plate is no longer proud.

After clinically confirming satisfactory MTP joint motion and toe position and fluoroscopically confirming optimal alignment and position of hardware, the surgical wounds are copiously irrigated and closed in standard fashion (Fig. 4.23A through F). A mildly compressive dressing is used over sterile wound dressings. With correction in three planes, a traditional bunion dressing is not required; if a bunion dressing is needed to achieve full correction, then we maintain that optimal triplanar correction was not achieved. Postoperatively, patients may immediately fully weight bear in either a stiff-soled postoperative shoe or a controlled ankle motion (CAM) walker boot. In general, this protected weight bearing is maintained for 6 weeks. Provided weight-bearing radiographs suggest adequate healing at 6 weeks, the patient is permitted to transition to supportive shoes. In our experience, a return to full athletic activities takes approximately 3 to 4 months.

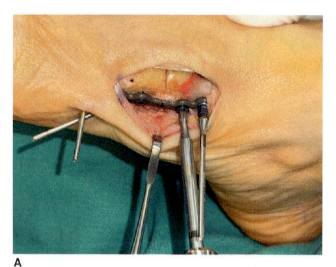
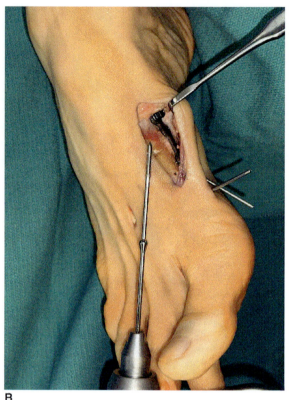
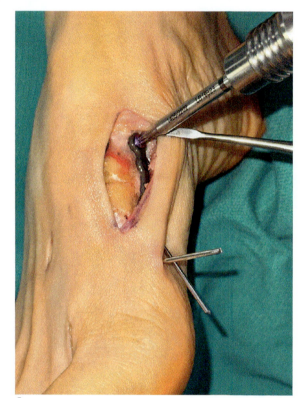

FIGURE 4.22 Provisional fixation interference with screw fixation. **A.** Screw cannot be fully seated due to olive wire obstruction. **B.** With three points of fixation and dorsal plate secured, the obstructing threaded olive wire may be removed without concern for loss if reduction or joint apposition; screw now fully seated. **C.** Medial plate now fully secured.

Correction of Metatarsus Adductus

On preoperative weight-bearing foot radiographs of our case example for this chapter, we determine if optimal hallux valgus correction may be limited by metatarsus adductus. As noted in the preoperative planning section above (see Fig. 4.3A through C), we designate a plumb line drawn from the lateral cuneiform to represent the longitudinal axis of the foot. Even if metatarsus adductus appears to be subtle, should the second metatarsal head interfere with this line, we consider metatarsus adductus correction to allow for full hallux valgus correction (Fig. 4.24A and B). We utilize a dorsal lateral incision centered along the longitudinal axis of the third metatarsal shaft; an oblique foot fluoroscopic image, with a Freer elevator or guide pin positioned on the skin, confirms ideal position for this incision. A video of the surgical technique is also available (see ▶ Video 4.2). This typically

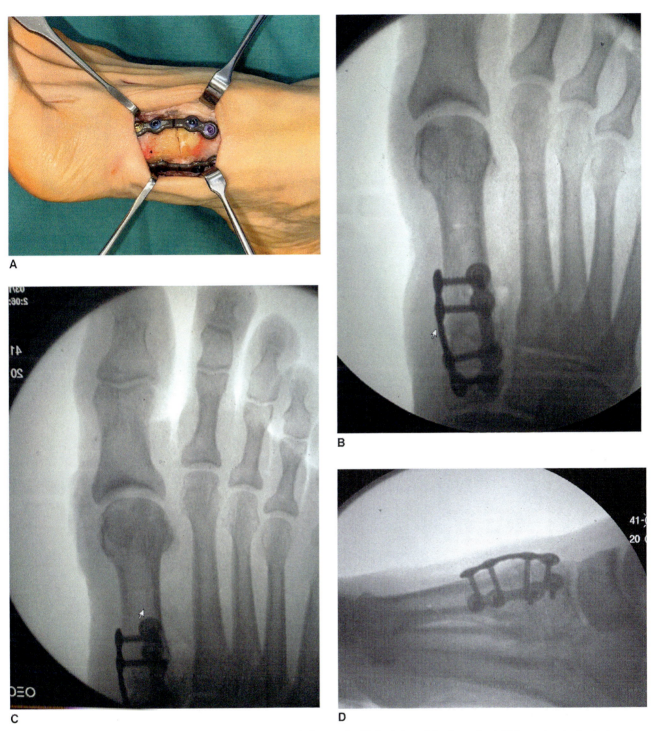

FIGURE 4.23 Final tarsometatarsal (TMT) joint construct and closure. **A.** Clinical view of final construct. Note anatomically designed plates, central portions of plates parallel, and 90-90 biplanar plate construct. **B.** Fluoroscopic confirmation of anteroposterior correction, satisfactory bone apposition at arthrodesis site, and optimal plate position. **C.** Fluoroscopic confirmation of satisfactory first metatarsal head–sesamoid relationship. **D.** Lateral fluoroscopic image confirms optimal plate position without TMT joint plantar gapping. **E.** Closure of deep fascial layer (the same one carefully elevated during approach) over the plates. **F.** Final clinical appearance.

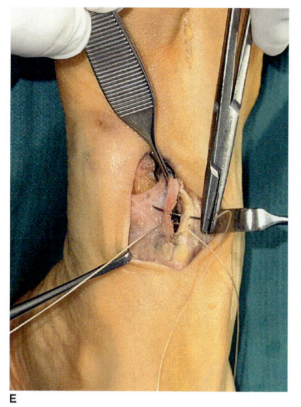
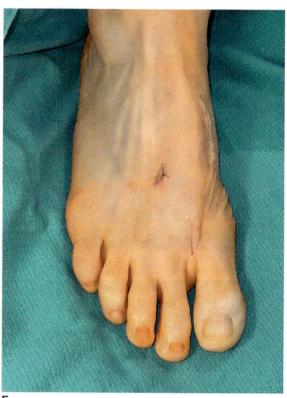

E F

FIGURE 4.23 *(Continued)*

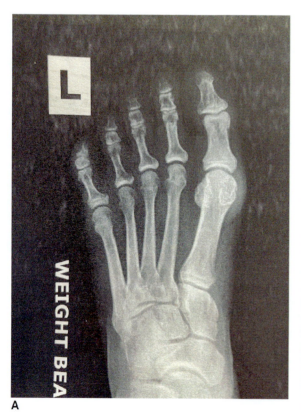
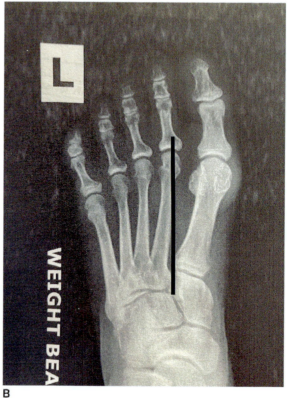

A B

FIGURE 4.24 Weight-bearing anteroposterior radiograph of hallux valgus with metatarsus adductus. While a more subtle example, adductus in the second metatarsal limits full correction of the first metatarsal. **A.** Standard radiograph. **B.** Radiograph with plumb line drawn from two points defining lateral first cuneiform along the axis of the foot demonstrating second metatarsal's limitation to optimal hallux valgus correction.

4 Correction of Hallux Valgus With and Without Metatarsus Adductus

leaves an adequate dorsal skin bridge to the preferred first TMT joint approach for hallux valgus correction (Fig. 4.25A). The first steps of hallux valgus correction, including lateral first MTP joint release (Fig. 4.25B), first TMT joint planing, and first TMT joint ligament release (Fig. 4.25C and D), may facilitate metatarsus adductus correction.

We divide the extensor retinaculum in line with the incision, carefully retract branches of the superficial peroneal nerve, and develop a deeper interval between the long extensor tendons (Fig. 4.26A). The extensor digitorum and extensor hallucis brevis muscles and tendons are reflected to expose the capsular tissue of the second and third TMT joints (Fig. 4.26B). The second and third TMT are fully exposed through a longitudinal incision followed by medial and lateral sharp subperiosteal and capsular dissection and elevation; with careful elevation, these soft tissues may be reapproximated after

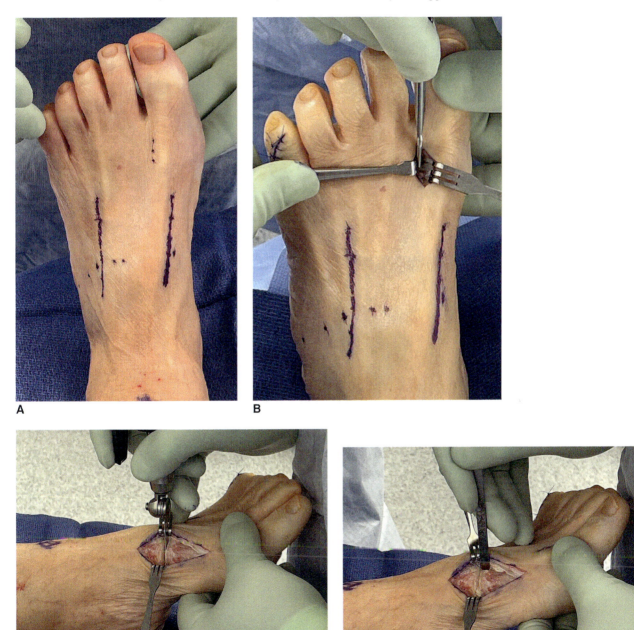

FIGURE 4.25 Combined hallux valgus and metatarsus adductus corrections and lateral release for the first metatarsophalangeal joint. **A.** Planned incisions. **B.** Lateral release of the first metatarsal phalangeal joint with dedicated release instrument. **C.** Planing the first tarsometatarsal (TMT) joint to facilitate metatarsus adductus correction. **D.** First TMT joint ligament release.

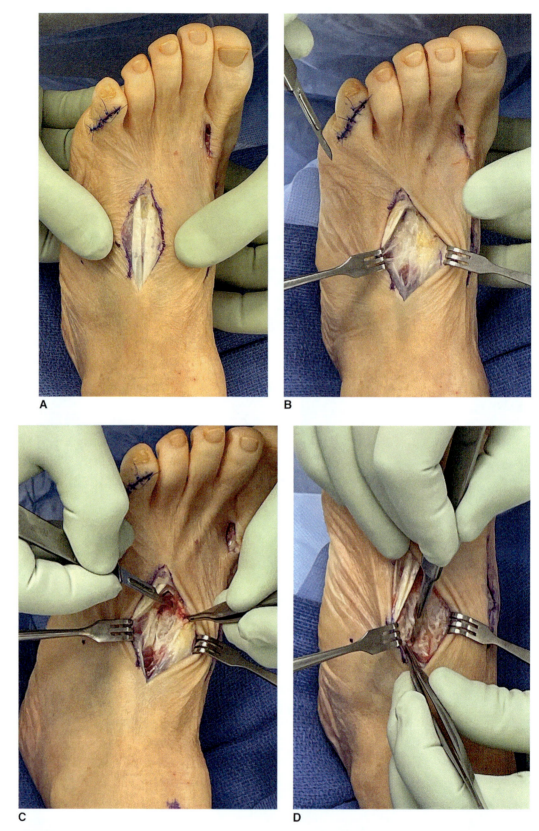

FIGURE 4.26 Approach to the second and third tarsometatarsal (TMT) joints to correct metatarsus adductus. **A.** Dorsolateral incision over the third TMT joint with superficial peroneal nerve retracted. **B.** Extensor tendons retracted to expose the TMT joint capsular tissue. **C.** Medial periosteal and capsular tissue elevation. **D.** Lateral periosteal elevation.

4   Correction of Hallux Valgus With and Without Metatarsus Adductus

correction and fixation (Fig. 4.26C and D). The ligaments between the second and third metatarsal bases should not be violated so that these two metatarsals may correct as a single unit.

With the capsule and periosteum reflected, the keystone architecture of the second and third TMT joints with the inherent offset between the two joints is easily visualized (Fig. 4.27A). We optimize metatarsus adductus correction and bony apposition at the TMT joints with comprehensive ligament release between the third and fourth metatarsal bases. In our experience, the fourth and fifth TMT joints do not need to be directly addressed to correct even severe metatarsus adductus. To allow the fourth and fifth metatarsals to shift with second and third TMT joint correction, the ligaments between the third and fourth metatarsal bases must be fully released. These ligaments are stout, and the release requires sharp dissection over 3 to 4 cm from the metatarsal bases distally until all ligamentous connections are freed. Since metatarsus adductus typically has a component of cavus, with the third metatarsal base positioned relatively dorsal to the fourth metatarsal, dissection requires oblique hand positioning to allow the scalpel blade or elevator entrance into the interval to completely free the ligamentous attachments. We favor a dedicated release instrument that facilitates this release essential to the success of metatarsus correction (Fig. 4.27B). An incomplete release between the third and fourth metatarsal bases will resist bony apposition of the third TMT joint and lead to incomplete metatarsus adductus correction. We place a dedicated retractor in the newly created third and fourth metatarsal base interval to provide additional protection beyond the dedicated adductoplasty cut guide for the lateral soft tissues, tendons, and fourth metatarsal during second and third TMT joint preparation with the microsagittal saw (Fig. 4.27C). To facilitate uniform correction of the second and third metatarsals, we use a microsagittal saw through a dedicated planing guide (Fig. 4.27D and E). The planing guide serves to direct the dedicated microsagittal saw to remove the step-off between the second and third TMT joints, creating uniform surfaces for the two metatarsal bases and the two cuneiforms (Fig. 4.27F). With the

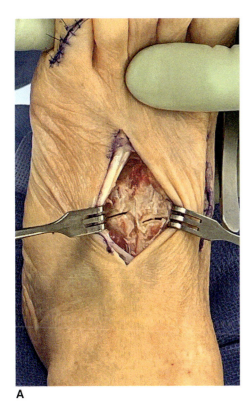
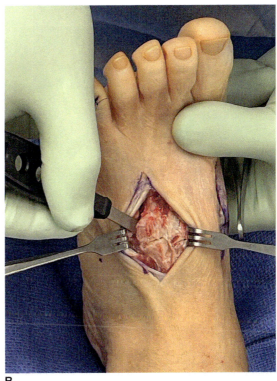

FIGURE 4.27 Initial second and third tarsometatarsal (TMT) joint preparation (planing). **A.** Full exposure of the second and third TMT joints (note the natural step-off between the two joints and that the ligaments between the second and third metatarsal bases remain intact). **B.** Release of the ligaments between the third and fourth metatarsal bases optimizes correction and TMT joint apposition (note use of a dedicated release tool). **C.** A retractor being used to maintain deep lateral soft tissue retraction. **D.** Planing guide positioned in the second and third TMT joints, spanning the step-off between these two joints. **E.** Microsagittal saw used to remove the step-off between the second and third TMT joints ("planing"). **F.** Second and third TMT joints converted into a single unit to be corrected in concert along a uniform plane.

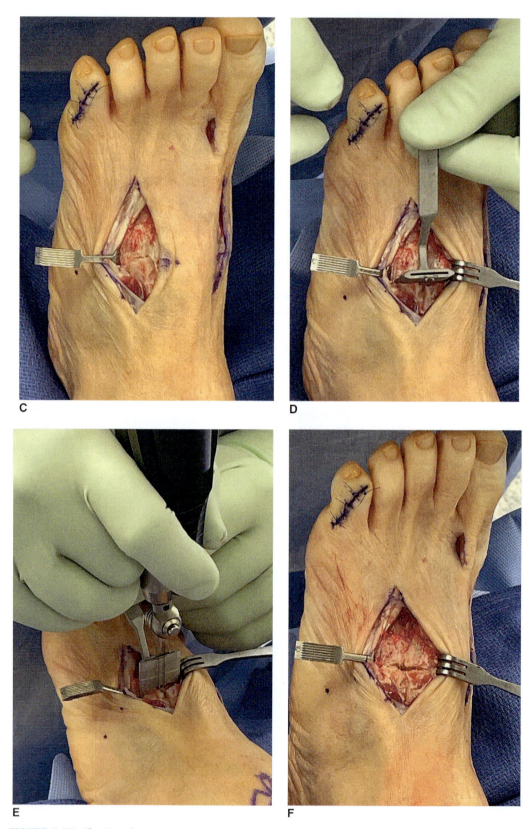

FIGURE 4.27 *(Continued)*

ligaments between the second and third metatarsal bases intact, in essence, planing converts the two TMT joints into a single unit that may be corrected in concert. We maintain that this method of correction confers greater control than attempting to correct each TMT joint independently.

Our dedicated metatarsus adductus cut guide features a design similar to that of the hallux valgus cut guide (Fig. 4.28A). In theory, it is a lateral extension of the hallux valgus cut guide. The joint seeker is

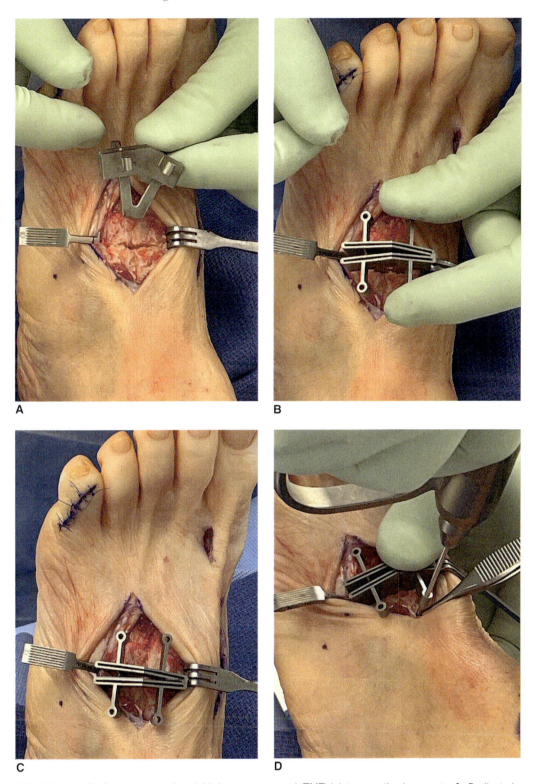

FIGURE 4.28 Performing second and third tarsometatarsal (TMT) joint corrective bone cuts. **A.** Dedicated cut guide. **B.** Positioning the cut guide in the planed second and third TMT joints. **C.** Cut guide fully seated. **D, E.** Cut guide secured with pins. **F.** Orthogonal fluoroscopic image of medial cut guide over second TMT joint, positioned correctly to avoid violation of first cuneiform. **G.** Orthogonal fluoroscopic image of lateral cut guide over third TMT joint, correctly positioned to avoid violation of fourth metatarsal. **H, I.** Performing corrective cuts through the cut guide with the microsagittal saw.

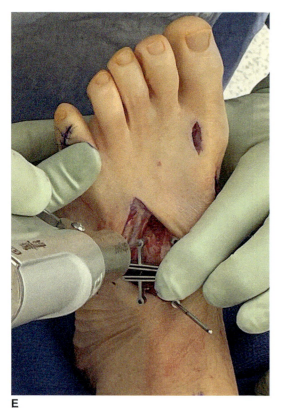

E

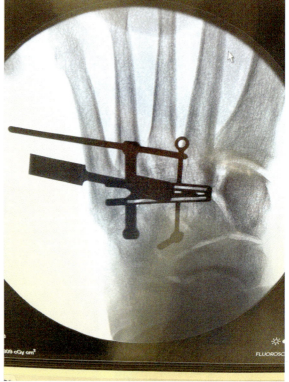

F

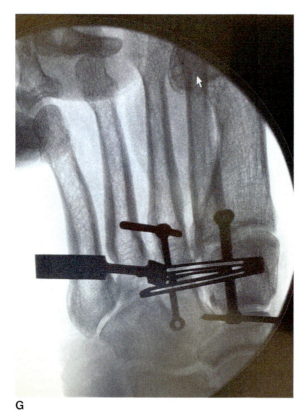

G

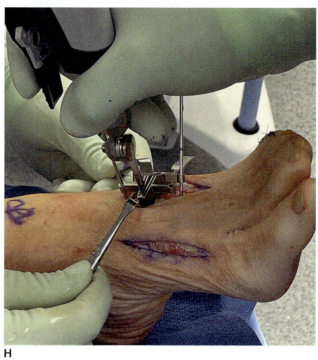

H

FIGURE 4.28 *(Continued)*

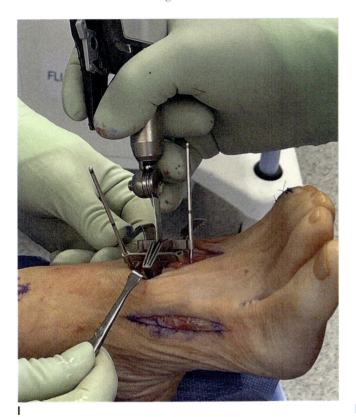

FIGURE 4.28 *(Continued)*

positioned in the uniform TMT space created through planing, and the guide's dual capture guides serve to direct the micro sagittal blade at a 6° angle from the medial extent of the second TMT joint to the lateral extent of the third TMT joint (Fig. 4.28B). The cut guide is available in 3 sizes so that the optimal cut guide size may be selected to safely complete cuts from the medial second to the lateral third TMT joints. Optimal cut guide position to ensure appropriate angulated wedge preparation is confirmed fluoroscopically, with care taken to avoid violating the medial cuneiform and fourth ray. Once optimal cut guide position is determined, it is secured with at least two pins in the four available pin hole options (Fig. 4.28D and E). The metatarsus adductus cut guide is designed to create orthogonal cuts on the second and third TMT joints, and to fluoroscopically confirm proper cut trajectory, an AP view is used for the second TMT joint and an oblique view is used for the third TMT joint (Fig. 4.28F and G).

The cut guide angle is available in 6° and 9° cut angles. We typically select the 6° cut guide when the plumb line intersects with the second metatarsal head only and consider using the 9° cut guide when the plumb line crosses into the third metatarsal. If the plumb line is in between the second and third metatarsals, then we recommend a graduated correction method. We first use the 6° cut guide for routine dual cuts, remove the resected bone, replace the cut guide, close the TMT joint unit on the cut guide's joint seeker, and recut the metatarsal side only. Rather than risking unnecessary resection of bone, this method allows a check to determine if the 6° cut alone allows for satisfactory correction and, if not, adding three more degrees to arrive at the appropriate correction in a controlled sequence. The microsagittal saw blade is used through the cut guide slots to resect the articular surfaces of the second and third TMT joints (Fig. 4.28H and I).

The outrigger pins and the cut guide are removed, and the resected bone slices are removed with dedicated instruments that facilitate bone extraction (Fig. 4.29A). We ensure that all bone fragments are removed and typically use fluoroscopy to confirm that no residual fragments that may not be visible on clinical examination are identified and extracted. If all resected fragments are not removed, satisfactory bone apposition and full correction may not be possible (Fig. 4.29B and C). Also, as noted above, without release of the third to fourth metatarsal ligaments, metatarsal-cuneiform bone apposition will not be possible (see Fig. 4.27B).

In our experience, metatarsus adductus is associated with a cavus foot alignment and optimal reduction of deformity is multiplanar. In addition to correcting adductus in the coronal plane, we use an up and out maneuver to correct the cavus in the sagittal plane (Fig. 4.30A through C). The cumulative effect

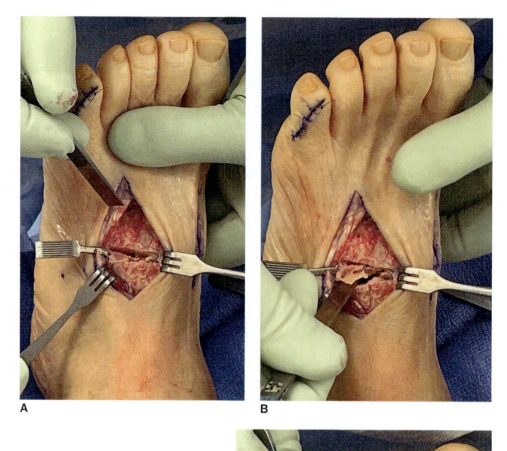

FIGURE 4.29 Removal of resected bone fragments. **A.** Second and third TMT joints after cut guide removal. **B, C.** Resected bone removal (important to remove all resected bone, especially any residual plantar bone fragments).

of this manual manipulation of the forefoot allows for full correction in two planes with optimal bony apposition of the realigned second and third TMT joints and full correction of the multiplanar deformity.

To promote fusion, we fenestrate the prepared metatarsal and cuneiform surfaces with a 2-mm drill bit; reamings from the drilling serve as bone graft (Fig. 4.31A and B). Additional bone graft, easily harvested from the calcaneus, may be considered, but, in our experience, proper planing and use of the dedicated cut guide tends to create uniform surfaces for fusion.

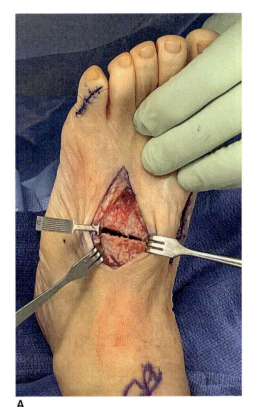
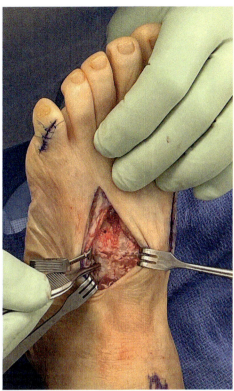
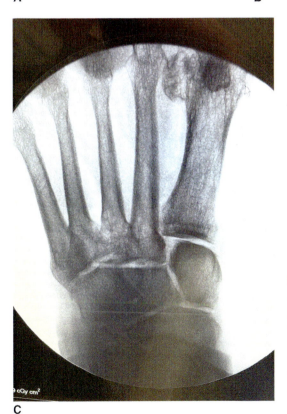

FIGURE 4.30 Confirming adequate metatarsus adductus correction (up-and-out maneuver). **A.** Second and third tarsometatarsal (TMT) joints after resected bone removal. **B.** Second and third TMT joint apposed with up-and-out maneuver. **C.** Fluoroscopic confirmation of adequate bone resection and satisfactory correction.

Following manually realigning the second and third TMT joints, we recommend maintaining correction and bony apposition with a dedicated compressor placed as lateral as possible across the third TMT joint (Fig. 4.32A through D). Compression wire fixation after manual reduction of the deformity is also possible, but we favor the effectiveness of the laterally placed compressor. The lateral compressor usually maintains satisfactory bony apposition of the second and third TMT joints. Occasionally, supplemental wire fixation is required to fully reduce the third and especially the

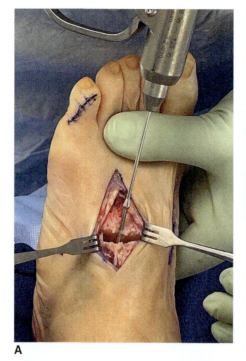
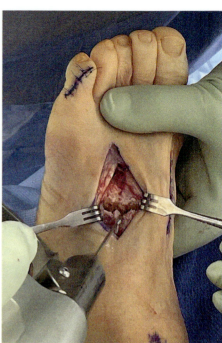

FIGURE 4.31 Arthrodesis site preparation. **A.** Proximal drilling of second and third cuneiforms. **B.** Distal drilling of second and third cuneiforms (note reamings created to serve as bone graft; additional bone graft may also be considered).

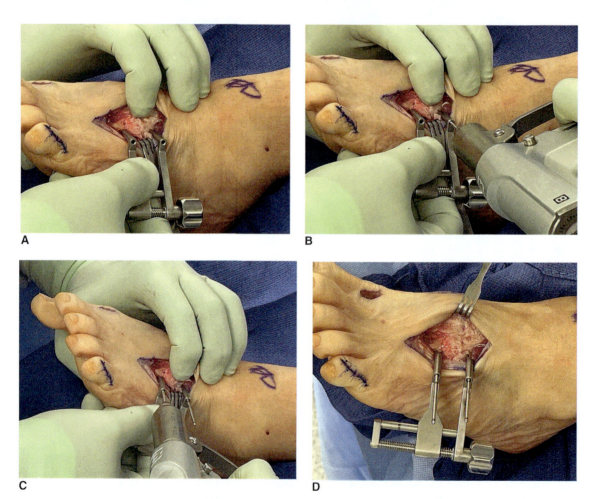

FIGURE 4.32 Optimizing metatarsus adductus correction and bone apposition. **A.** Placing a lateral compressor on third tarsometatarsal (TMT) joint (note compressor placed as far laterally as possible for optimal correction and to allow dorsal plate placement). **B, C.** Securing the compressor. **D.** Lateral third TMT joint compressed (avoiding overcompression). **E, F.** Supplemental pin fixation of second TMT joint (a compression or smooth pin may be used; note the lateral-to-medial trajectory to promote greatest correction and to avoid interference with dorsal plate placement). **G.** Fluoroscopic confirmation of adequate correction of metatarsus adductus (note that true first and second intermetatarsal ankle is now revealed).

4   Correction of Hallux Valgus With and Without Metatarsus Adductus

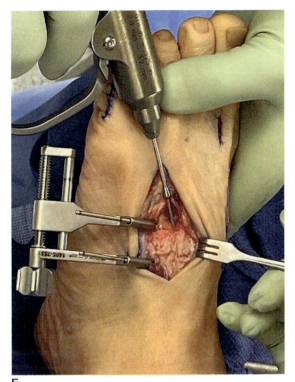
E

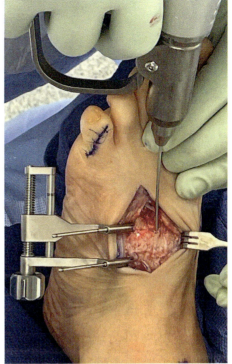
F

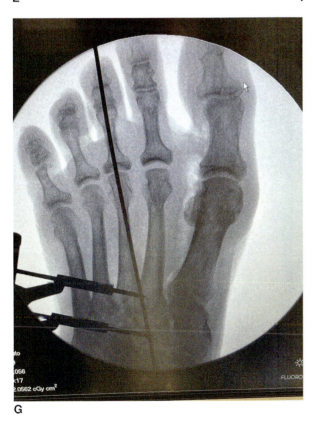
G

FIGURE 4.32 *(Continued)*

second TMT arthrodesis (Fig. 4.32E and F). After fluoroscopic confirmation of adequate reduction and bony apposition (Fig. 4.32G), we use dedicated fixed-angle locking plates across the third and second TMT joints to maintain correction (Fig. 4.33A through D). With fluoroscopic confirmation of optimal bone apposition and plate position (Fig. 4.34A and B), the provisional fixation wires and lateral compressor may be removed. Fluoroscopic imaging should be performed in the AP plane for the second TMT and oblique view for the third TMT to ensure satisfactory alignment and plate position. With the lesser metatarsals now corrected, the AP view should now uncover the true hallux

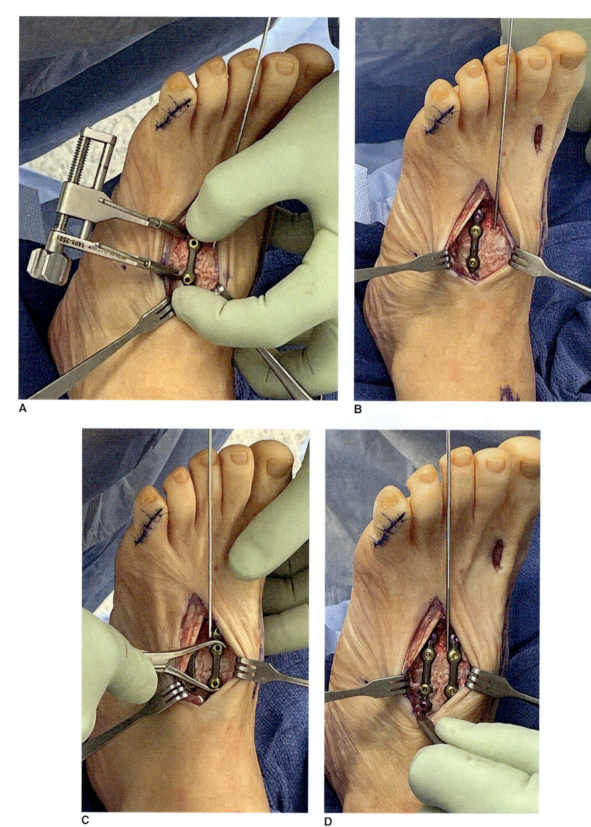

FIGURE 4.33 Definitive fixation for metatarsus adductus correction. **A.** Third tarsometatarsal (TMT) plate placement (note compressor still in place). **B.** Third TMT plate secured. **C.** Second TMT plate placed (note provisional wire fixation still in place). **D.** Second TMT plate secured.

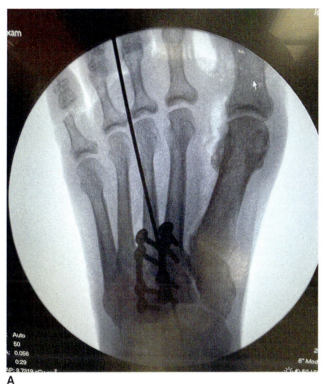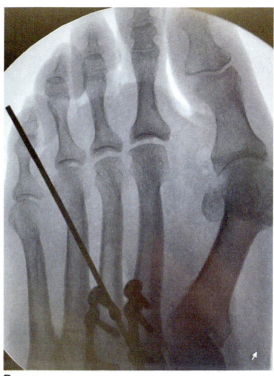

FIGURE 4.34 Fluoroscopic assessment after definitive fixation. **A.** Fluoroscopic confirmation of optimal correction, bone apposition, and plate position; note that with the true intermetatarsal angle (IMA) revealed after metatarsus adductus correction, satisfactory hallux valgus correction is possible. **B.** Fluoroscopic image from a different patient with an even more dramatic uncovering of the true IMA.

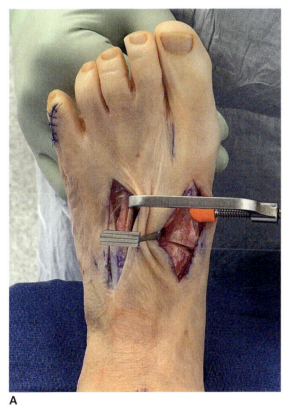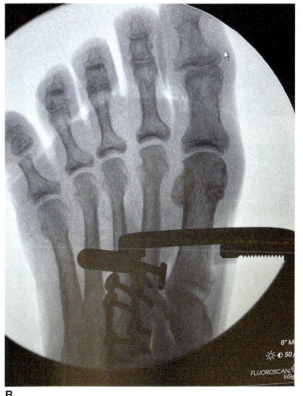

FIGURE 4.35 Following metatarsus adductus correction, routine and full hallux valgus correction is feasible. **A.** Initial correction. **B.** Fluoroscopic confirmation or correction. **C.** Final Fluoroscopic images demonstrating satisfactory correction of hallux valgus enabled by metatarsus adductus correction. **D.** Wound closures at completion of procedure (different patient).

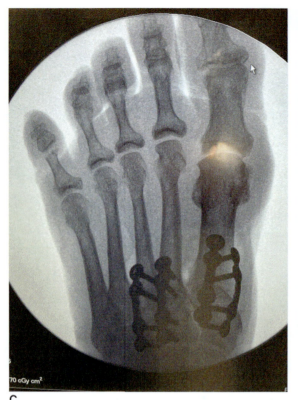
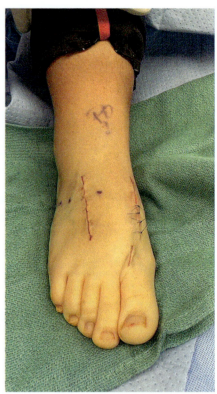

FIGURE 4.35 *(Continued)* **C**, **D**

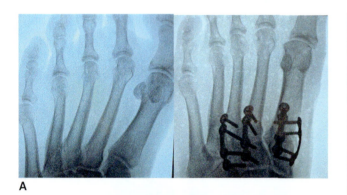

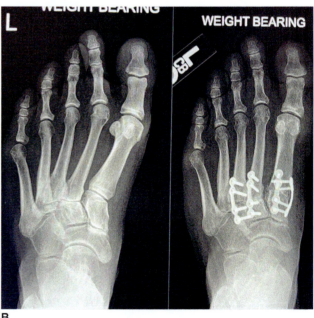

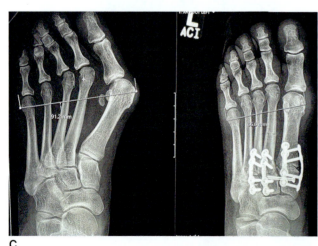

FIGURE 4.36 Before and after metatarsus adductus correction. **A.** Intraoperative fluoroscopic image before and after simultaneous hallux valgus and metatarsus adductus correction. **B.** Pre- and postoperative weight-bearing radiographs. **C.** Pre- and postoperative weight-bearing radiographs demonstrating not only metatarsus adductus and hallux valgus correction but also marked narrowing of the forefoot.

valgus deformity or, in traditional terms, the true IMA, and the hallux valgus deformity may be appropriately corrected (see Fig. 4.34A and B). We designed our hallux valgus correction system to complement our metatarsus adductus system (Fig. 4.35A through D). The combination of these two procedures has been found to provide a stable, reliable, and reproducible correction and narrowing of the wide forefoot[23] (Fig. 4.36A through C). Upon completion of the combined procedures, the incisions are copiously irrigated and closed in standard fashion.

PEARLS AND PITFALLS

Pearls

Distal Soft Tissue Release

Our technique for lateral distal soft tissue release is described in detail in the surgical technique above, but we wish to emphasize its importance here. Except for the rare hallux valgus patient without contracture, to enable the first metatarsal to laterally translate and rotate in its optimal anatomic position to center over the sesamoids, a limited lateral first MTP joint release is often required. Traditional teaching suggests that the sesamoids are in their anatomic position and it is the metatarsal head that needs to be reduced. In careful study of the axial first MTH-sesamoid relationship using sesamoid views and/or WBCT, in many patients with hallux valgus, the lateral soft tissue contracture displaces the sesamoid complex into a nonphysiologic position.[1] Whether using a scalpel or a dedicated lateral release tool, we give considerable attention to ensuring that the lateral soft tissue contracture is fully released; incomplete release will not allow a natural repositioning of the metatarsal head and, more importantly, the sesamoid complex. As noted earlier, the focus of the release is the accessory suspensory ligament. However, occasionally we must also release the adductor hallux tendon and deep intermetatarsal ligament from the lateral sesamoid and in some cases release the adductor tendon from the base of the proximal phalanx. In our experience, a comprehensive lateral release does not lead to hallux varus when anatomic realignment of the metatarsal head-sesamoid complex is reestablished (see Fig. 4.7A through E).

3-in-1 Cut Guide

As for many modern orthopedic procedures, dedicated instrumentation may improve accuracy, reliability, and reproducibility; we believe that instrumentation does the same for hallux valgus correction. To simplify our instrumentation, we have combined three key components of our legacy instrument system, the fulcrum, joint seeker, and cut guide, into a single 3-in-1 cut guide. In addition to the routine steps noted earlier in the surgical technique, we emphasize these finer points in using the 3-in-1 cut guide. The hinged connection between the fulcrum and joint seeker allows for accommodation of variable cuneiform slopes. Because of this connection, all soft tissues at the lateral first metatarsal base and lateral TMT joint must be fully released to properly insert the 3-in-1 cut guide. Although the cut guide's joint seeker typically allows it to self-center at the first TMT joint, following reduction we always confirm appropriately planned cuts with orthogonal fluoroscopic images before committing to pinning the cut guide in its final position. Even with the cut guide in the TMT joint, we routinely make subtle adjustments by twisting the guide's handle so that we may arrive at a flat cut on the metatarsal base perpendicular to the long axis of the metatarsal shaft and a laterally based wedge on the cuneiform. With lateral fluoroscopic view confirming full plantar TMT bone apposition and the seeker parallel to the TMT joint, the guide may be secured with pin fixation and cuts performed (see Figs. 4.9, 4.11 through 4.13).

Resection and Preparation of Subchondral Bone

Our instrumented technique minimizes the bone resection, thereby limiting first ray shortening and the risk for transfer metatarsalgia. With our cut guide, the planned saw cuts remain within the hard subchondral bone mantle. We recommend using a dedicated 40 mm saw blade that, in our experience, limits blade deflection in this harder subchondral bone; using a deliberate pecking sawing technique reduces the risk of blade deviation from its intended trajectory. To promote TMT joint fusion, we emphasize penetrating the entire hard subchondral bone surfaces on both sides of the arthrodesis site to a depth of 2 mm with a fluted drill bit. Drilling increases surface area for healing. The fluted bit creates reamings that serve as bone graft and limits heat generation that typically occurs with using a smooth K-wire (see Fig. 4.15).

Intercuneiform Stabilization

Fleming and colleagues reported that intercuneiform instability is present in 74% of cases of hallux valgus.[22] As noted in the surgical technique above, after stabilizing the first TMT joint, we perform a splay test under fluoroscopy.[21] While the splay test is designed to identify first to second intercuneiform instability, it also serves to identify sesamoid complex about the metatarsal head crista. If the splay test demonstrates instability either at the first metatarsal head–sesamoid complex or at the intercuneiform joint, we recommend placing a neutralization screw placed between the first and second rays, either between the first and second cuneiforms (C1-C2 screw) or from the first metatarsal base into the second cuneiform (M1-C2 screw).

The transverse C1-C2 screw theoretically acts as an axis about which the first ray may still plantarflex with the windlass mechanism but not allow splay in the transverse plane. After proper transverse-frontal reduction with manipulation or the positioner, we place the partially threaded C1-C2 screw perpendicular to the intercuneiform joint, either between the two plates or below the medial plate, ideally in the proximal half of the first cuneiform. We aim the screw from plantarmedial to dorsal-lateral to allow the screw threads to engage the widest portion of the second cuneiform's inverted pyramid bone configuration. In our experience, the optimal screw length is 23 mm if started between the plates and 26 mm if started below the medial plate. Even though this screw is partially threaded, we use it as a neutralization and not compression screw. The oblique M1-C2 screw confers greater stability than does the transverse C1-C2 screw,[24] while theoretically restricting first ray from plantarflexion with physiologic windlass mechanism activation and potentially forfeiting a physiologic first ray function. As for the transverse screw, after first to second ray reduction manually or with the positioner, we place the cannulated fully threaded M1-C2 screw obliquely from the medial first metatarsal into the second cuneiform, aiming to enter the cuneiform at the distal medial apex. To facilitate M1-C2 targeting, we identify the starting point as in the box, which is a fluoroscopic landmark on the AP view that comprises the medial plate, dorsal plate, and the two distal screws of the medial plate. We find that using this starting point and aiming for the distal medial apex of the cuneiform allows for accurate screw placement while avoiding the screws already positioned in the plates. Depending on patient size, the ideal M1-C2 screw length ranges from 36 to 42 mm.

When to Add a Phalanx Osteotomy

In our experience, reestablishing anatomic triplanar first metatarsal position and appropriate first metatarsal–sesamoid relationship obviates the need for a closing wedge medial proximal phalanx osteotomy. However, we do consider phalanx osteotomy with hallux valgus interphalangeus and in select revision cases. If at the completion of triplanar hallux valgus procedure, clinical and fluoroscopic assessment in a simulated weight-bearing position the hallux and second toe are contacting and/or hallux valgus interphalangeus is evident, we consider a phalanx osteotomy to promote EHL and flexor hallucis longus tendon forces in the optimal trajectory relative to the hallux.

The Third to Fourth Intermetatarsal Base Release

Although it has been covered in the surgical technique earlier, we emphasize the third to fourth metatarsal base release in metatarsus adductus correction. With cavus present in the majority of feet with metatarsus adductus, in the axial plane, the third TMT will often overload the fourth TMT joint. A standard scalpel blade or osteotome, even if angled appropriately, may not allow for full release of the deep ligaments between the third and fourth metatarsal. We developed a dedicated tool to facilitate complete transection of these stout interosseous and plantar ligaments (see Fig. 4.27B).

Bone Healing and Early Weight Bearing

Unicortical biplanar plate fixation in TMT joint arthrodesis with early weight bearing promotes fusion through secondary bone healing and follows current AO principles.[20] Our coauthors Dayton et al[25] reported on the observations made in a case series in which arthrodesis site lucency was initially noted with subsequent progressive callus formation, resulting in bone bridging and consolidation while maintaining deformity correction. Early protected weight bearing in a CAM boot or surgical shoe is encouraged and supported in a case series of subjects undergoing triplanar hallux valgus correction.[26] Early weight bearing stimulates secondary bone healing through controlled strain at the arthrodesis site.[20] While nonunion is a risk when performing any arthrodesis procedure, we encourage surgeons to remain patient, reserve final judgment, and continue with the prescribed postoperative course unless there are definitive signs of nonunion. Persistent surgical site pain that is out of proportion with what is typically expected during the recovery process and radiographic correction loss and/or hardware failure should not be ignored.

Pitfalls

Failure to Recognize First MTP–Sesamoid Arthritis

We emphasize performing a comprehensive radiographic assessment of the first ray deformity to determine if arthritic changes are noted at the TMT, MTP, or adjacent joints. Failure to identify MTP or sesamoid arthritis may leave the patient with persistent pain and limited MTP joint function despite adequate triplanar first ray repositioning via a TMT arthrodesis. We recommend first MTP joint arthrodesis to address both the first ray position and the degenerative nature of the MTP joint space.[27] Concomitant MTP joint arthritis and an IMA of greater than 15° prompts us to consider simultaneous MTP and TMT joint arthrodeses to fully reduce the deformity and to reestablish the optimal weight-bearing parabola. The triplanar philosophy of correction and biplanar plating techniques are performed at both the TMT and MTP joints to drive correction and realignment.

Failure to Recognize Metatarsus Adductus

Isolated attempts at hallux valgus correction surgery in patients with contaminant metatarsus adductus poses a significant risk of incomplete correction, recurrence, and failure.[7] In our experience, the plumb line evaluation simplifies the determination when metatarsus adductus correction should be considered. While metatarsus adductus adds complexity to otherwise relatively straightforward surgery of the first ray, we maintain that a highly instrumented and consistent technique allow effective and efficient simultaneous hallux valgus and metatarsus adductus correction and provide patients and surgeons with reproducible results (see Fig. 4.3).

Intraoperative Fluoroscopic Imaging

The techniques described in this chapter rely heavily on fluoroscopic guidance. Accurate correction of the first metatarsal–sesamoid complex, position of the cut guide, and placement of fixation demands precise imaging; in our opinion, these surgeries should not be performed without fluoroscopy confirmation. While a large fluoroscopy scanner may be used, we recommend the use of the lower radiation small C-arm for surgical efficiency and control of the image trajectory.

Addressing Atypical TMT Joint Morphology

A peaked cuneiform deformity is a relatively common anatomic variant (Fig. 4.37). This atavistic trait alters the anticipated lie of the 3-in-1 cut guide and forces the instrument to malposition with a medial bias at the first TMT joint. Occasionally, it may result in an excessive joint distraction that causes the saw blade to take an aberrant trajectory, thus producing misguided bone cuts. The peak of the cuneiform will often produce a binding effect at the instrumentation-bone interface resulting in challenges with correction of the first metatarsal in three planes. Due to these challenges, the TMT joint should be assessed for the presence of a peaked cuneiform prior to attempting correction or making bone cuts. Its presence can be identified with fluoroscopic assessment of the joint space. Projection of the beam parallel to the axis of the TMT joint will produce the desired image and will allow the surgeon to recognize the anatomy variant. The peak may be removed in a free-handed or instrumented fashion. The former can be carried out with a rongeur or saw blade while the latter may use the central slot in the 3-in-1 cut guide to direct the saw blade to its target. In both instances the bone is removed at the dorsal lateral aspect of the distal medial pole of the cuneiform and is approximately 1 to 2 mm in thickness. This bone removal is analogous to the initial planing step of the first TMT and helps to decompress the joint allowing the cut guide to sit in the proper orientation.

Another common anatomic variant of concern is an accessory articulating facet between the first and second metatarsal bases classified as a Romash III joint[28] (Fig. 4.38). This joint articulation can restrict proper fulcrum positioning at the lateral first metatarsal base and can result in a limitation of frontal plane correction when the positioner device is applied. The microsagittal saw is used to shave the lateral first

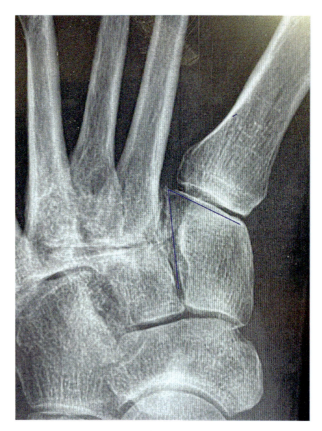

FIGURE 4.37 Peaked cuneiform at the first tarsometatarsal joint. The peak may need to be shaved to ensure optimal cut guide position.

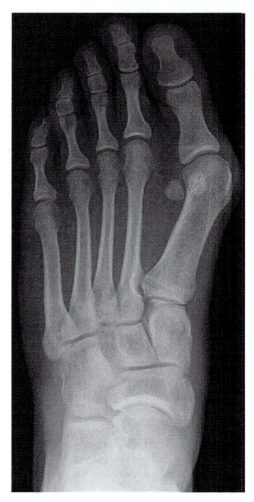

FIGURE 4.38 Abnormal lateral first and second metatarsal base articulation, Romash type III, that will most likely make it difficult to place the fulcrum.

metatarsal base in a free-handed manner to optimize sequential instrument cut guide orientation prior to TMT joint preparation. A bone slice approximately 1 to 2 mm in thickness is removed at this level.

Avoiding Excessive Compression With the Instruments

The dedicated positioner device applied from the first to second metatarsal and the compressor device used for first TMT joint apposition do not have a governor to restrict overzealous compression when engaging the jack screws specific to each of these instruments. The positioner should be used to naturally correct the first metatarsal to the longitudinal axis of the foot in a smooth and gradual manner, with care taken not to force the correction against resistance. Forced correction or overcorrection is typically a by-product of soft tissue tethering and a lack of appropriate soft tissue releases at the MTP and the TMT. A forced correction with the compressor will result in an elevation of the metatarsal that can lead to a destabilization of the weight-bearing parabola if maintained in this offset position.

The compressor gains its mechanical advantage over the first TMT joint through converging bicortical pins introduced through the cannulation of the device from dorsal-to-plantar at a 7° angle. This pin orientation results in the plantar first TMT cortices contacting followed by a gradual uniform compression along the more superior portion of the joint as the jack screw is advanced. Overcompression of the joint will produce a gap at the plantar TMT joint, will elevate the first metatarsal, and may lead to osteonecrosis at the bone interface due to the pressure imparted across the bone surfaces. Two-finger tightness, as recommended in standard AO technique, is a reasonable endpoint for optimal positioner and compressor utilization. In select cases, the hallux may be dorsiflexed to engage the windlass mechanism during positioner and especially compressor activation; the

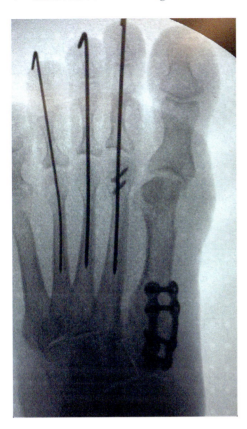

FIGURE 4.39 Unnecessary medial eminence correction with overresection may lead to hallux varus.

windlass mechanism contributes to ideal first metatarsal sagittal plane alignment and may enhance optimal plantar first TMT joint contact. First metatarsal correction and TMT joint apposition should always be confirmed fluoroscopically.

Avoiding Traditional Medial Metatarsal Head Resection

In our experience, triplanar hallux valgus correction typically obviates the need for medial eminence resection, as the bunion is eliminated with anatomic repositioning of the otherwise normal first metatarsal. The bunion, or "bump," usually resolves through triplanar repositioning of the first metatarsal. We acknowledge that occasionally there is medial bone overgrowth or relatively commonly a dorsomedial traction spur from long-standing malalignment that warrants judicious excision. However, we caution that routine medial eminence resection with appropriate triplanar correction typically leads to unnecessary and potentially detrimental removal of the physiologic medial metatarsal head and a portion of the MTP articular surface. This may also disrupt the medial MTP joint soft tissues, potentially lead to joint stiffness, alter the effectiveness of proximal metatarsal rotational correction, and risk varus deformity. Routine medial first MTP joint capsulotomy, eminence resection, or soft tissue plication are also not advised (Fig. 4.39).

OPTIMAL BIPLANAR PLATING

Effective biplanar plating demands that the central limbs of the plates be parallel/collinear and at 90° to one another. All eight of the fixed-angle unicortical locking screws should have satisfactory bone purchase and plate engagement. This plate configuration provides adequate stability to allow early weight bearing while avoiding excessive stiffness that could limit bone healing. The construct allows for limited micromotion, which promotes joint fusion through secondary bone healing.[29] In our experience, recurrence, malunion, and nonunion are risks when the plates are not parallel/collinear and at least 90° or more from one another. A convergence of the plates in a position where they are applied at less than 90° may result in hardware failure due to a loss of mechanical advantage during weight bearing. We typically place the dorsal plate first, as far lateral as possible. This allows the medial plate to be set at least 90° from the dorsal plate (see Fig. 4.23).

POSTOPERATIVE MANAGEMENT

We follow the protocol described by Feilmeier and colleagues.[30] The immediate postoperative dressing varies with the surgeon's preference. In general, we prefer a light-weight dressing with mild compression and recommend elevation and icing for edema control. We emphasize that anatomic triplane correction does not necessitate a traditional bunion strapping; in fact, we discourage the use of toe strapping as it limits postoperative hallux range of motion, which is encouraged in the immediate postoperative period. Meticulous layered closures are usually safe for dressing changes and shower water exposure within days. Early weight bearing in a CAM boot or stiff postsurgical shoe is encouraged for 6 weeks to help stimulate controlled micromotion and healing of the arthrodesis.[26] With appropriate patient education, we promote nonimpact exercise throughout the postoperative period that includes weight-training, elliptical trainer, exercise bike, and aquatic exercise/swimming with complete incision healing.

Four view weight-bearing plain films are taken at 6 weeks, 12 weeks, 16 weeks, 6 months, and 1 year. Progression from early TMT joint lucency, to callus formation, to fusion is anticipated as has been discussed above.[25] When available, WBCT may be used to more comprehensively assess the first MTP-sesamoid relationship, correction, and comprehensive 3D foot alignment than with conventional radiographs.[31]

Provided edema control has been rigorous and clinical and radiographic evaluation confirms satisfactory healing, we transition our patients to comfortable, supportive athletic shoes at 6 weeks following surgery. We recommend a standard running shoe with a wide toe box, and initially a one size larger shoe size may be required to accommodate anticipated residual edema. Other shoe considerations when making the transition from CAM boot or postoperative shoe include cork-bedded sandals and hiking shoes/boots. In our experience, by 3 to 4 months, most patients may transition to unrestricted shoewear, except perhaps for tight, ultra-high fashionable shoes. With satisfactory clinical and radiographic assessments at routine 16-week follow-up, most patients can gradually return to presurgical recreational and athletic activities.

RESULTS AND COMPLICATIONS

Although published long-term outcomes are not yet available, at just over 2-year average follow-up, Ray and colleagues reported triplane hallux valgus correction recurrence rate of 3%.[26] Dayton and colleagues reported a less than 1% recurrence rate at roughly 18-month follow-up for 109 triplane hallux valgus corrections.[32] The mean preoperative HVA, IMA, and TSP were 22.9°, 13.3°, and 4.6°; at mean follow-up of 17.4 months, the HVA, IMA, and TSP were 8.0, 5.6, and 2.0, respectively. Among bunions with MRA measurements, the mean difference was −12.3 (95% CI), and, without distal osteotomy and simple repositioning of the first metatarsal to an anatomic position, the DMAA decreased by a mean of −14.2°. Further study is needed to clarify both the outcomes and the mechanical effects found after triplane anatomic restoration of the first ray. A 15-site multicenter prospective outcome study of up to 200 patients undergoing triplane hallux valgus correction, ALIGN3D, was initiated 3 years ago; results are not yet published.

COMPLICATIONS

The success of the triplanar hallux valgus correction that we describe in this chapter requires full correction before the bone cuts are made. If correction is not anatomic in all three planes before temporary and final fixation, the first metatarsal will not be in optimal position and the first metatarsal head-sesamoid complex function will not be physiologic. In our experience, optimal bony correction requires appropriate soft tissue releases; failure to perform adequate releases will also compromise physiologic and anatomically correct sesamoid tracking.[14] Incomplete correction may lead to joint stiffness, continued pain, and recurrence.

With careful soft tissue management, we have experienced few wound healing problems. In the majority of cases, we are able to complete a three-layered closure over the plates. We maintain deep retraction and avoid superficial skin tension during the surgery. Moreover, we place one plate at a time, so that we do not tension the skin excessively, allowing the wound to gently shift dorsally for the dorsal plate application and medially for medial plate application. During dorsal plate application we limit retraction to the medial wound margin and limit dorsal (lateral) wound retraction when applying the medial plate.

Plate prominence is a concern. However, the plates are designed for the first TMT joint. Precontouring is typically eliminated with screw insertion as the screws draw the plate directly against the bone. For the medial first TMT joint, as described in the surgical technique above, we shave or impact the prominent medial first metatarsal base and may remove some of the plate's precontour to ensure flush plate apposition to bone (see Fig. 4.21). The plates are smooth and with the screws fully secured do not create any prominence that could irritate overlying soft tissue structures.

Delayed union or nonunion is always a risk. However, with proper joint preparation and properly performed biplanar plating, in our experience, the incidence of these complications is rare. In 195 cases of triplanar hallux valgus correction using biplanar plating, our authors reported a 97.4% union rate.[25]

Concern for first ray shortening has been an issue in hallux valgus correction through the first TMT joint. Again, in our experience, the dedicated cut guide properly positioned after appropriate deformity correction tends to minimize bone resection (see Fig. 4.13). In a recent study of triplanar hallux valgus correction, our authors reported an average shortening of 3.1 mm in the AP radiographic projection and 2.4 in the sagittal projection.[33]

REFERENCES

1. Kim Y, Kim JS, Young KW, Naraghi R, Cho HK, Lee SY. A new measure of tibial sesamoid position in hallux valgus in relation to the coronal rotation of the first metatarsal in CT scans. *Foot Ankle Int*. 2015;36:944-952.
2. Kimura T, Kubota M, Taguchi T, Suzuki N, Hattori A, Marumo K. Evaluation of first-ray mobility in patients with hallux valgus using weight-bearing CT and a 3-D analysis system: a comparison with normal feet. *J Bone Joint Surg Am*. 2017;99:247-255.
3. Najefi A-A, Katmeh R, Zaveri AK, et al. Imaging findings and first metatarsal rotation in hallux valgus. *Foot Ankle Int*. 2022;43(5):665-675.
4. Wei RX, Ko VM-C, Chui EC-S, et al. Investigation on the site of coronal deformities in hallux valgus. *Sci Rep*. 2023;13:1815.
5. Ferrari J, Malone-Lee J. A radiographic study of the relationship between metatarsus adductus and hallux valgus. *J Foot Ankle Surg*. 2003;42:9-14.
6. Sharma J, Aydogan U. Algorithm for severe hallux valgus associated with metatarsus adductus. *Foot Ankle Int*. 2015;36:1499-1503.
7. Aiyer A, Shub J, Shariff R, Ying L, Myerson M. Radiographic recurrence of deformity after hallux valgus surgery in patients with metatarsus adductus. *Foot Ankle Int*. 2016;37:165-171.
8. Marshall N, Ward E, Williams CM. The identification and appraisal of assessment tools used to evaluate metatarsus adductus: a systematic review of their measurement properties. *J Foot Ankle Res*. 2018;11:25.
9. Shima H, Okuda R, Yasuda T, et al. Operative treatment for hallux valgus with moderate to severe metatarsus adductus. *Foot Ankle Int*. 2019;40:641-647.
10. Reddy SC. Management of hallux valgus in metatarsus adductus. *Foot Ankle Clin*. 2020;25:59-68.
11. Najefi A-A, Malhotra K, Patel S, Cullen N, Welck M. Assessing the rotation of the first metatarsal on computed tomography scans: a systematic literature review. *Foot Ankle Int*. 2022;43(1):66-76.
12. Schmidt E, Silva T, Baumfeld D, et al. The rotational positioning of the bones in the medial column of the foot: a weight-bearing CT analysis. *Iowa Orthop J*. 2021;41:103-109.
13. Wagner P, Lescure N, Siddiqui N, Fink J, Wagner E. Validity and reliability of a new radiological method to estimate medial column internal rotation in hallux valgus using foot weight-bearing x-ray. *Foot Ankle Spec*. 2021;19386400211029162.
14. Shibuya N, Jasper J, Peterson B, Sessions J, Jupiter DC. Relationships between first metatarsal and sesamoid positions and other clinically relevant parameters for hallux valgus surgery. *J Foot Ankle Surg*. 2019;58:1095-1099.
15. Tejero S, González-Martín D, Martínez-Franco A, Jiménez-Diaz F, Gijón-Nogueron G, Herrera-Pérez M. Intraoperative checking of the first ray rotation and sesamoid position through sonographic assistance. *Arch Orthop Trauma Surg*. 2023;143(4):1915-1922. https://doi.org/10.1007/s00402-022-04359-8
16. Dawoodi AIS, Perera A. Radiological assessment of metatarsus adductus. *Foot Ankle Surg*. 2012;18:1-8.
17. Shibuya N, Jupiter DC, Plemmons BS, Martin L, Thorud JC. Correction of hallux valgus deformity in association with underlying metatarsus adductus deformity. *Foot Ankle Spec*. 2017;10(6):538-542.
18. Conti MS, Caolo KC, Ellis SJ, Cody EA. Radiographic and clinical outcomes of hallux valgus and metatarsus adductus treated with a modified Lapidus procedure. *Foot Ankle Int*. 2021;42:38-45.
19. Olivecrona C, Blomfeldt R, Ponzer S, Stanford BR, Nilsson BY. Tourniquet cuff pressure and nerve injury in knee arthroplasty in a bloodless field: a neurophysiological study. *Acta Orthop*. 2013;84:159-164.
20. Perren S. Evolution of the internal fixation of long bone fractures. *J Bone Joint Surg B*. 2002;84-B:1093-1110.
21. Weber AK, Hatch DJ, Jensen JL. Use of the first ray splay test to assess transverse plane instability before first metatarsocuneiform fusion. *J Foot Ankle Surg*. 2006;45:278-282.
22. Fleming JJ, Kwaadu KY, Brinkley JC, Ozuzu Y. Intraoperative evaluation of medial intercuneiform instability after lapidus arthrodesis: intercuneiform hook test. *J Foot Ankle Surg*. 2015;54:464-472.
23. McAleer JP, Dayton P, DeCarbo WT, Duke W, Hatch DJ, Smith WB, Santrock RD, Easley M. Radiographic outcomes following multi-joint triplanar tarsometatarsal arthrodesis of combined hallux valgus and metatarsus adductus deformities. 2023.
24. Feilmeier M, Dayton P, Kauwe M, et al. Comparison of transverse and coronal plane stability at the first tarsal-metatarsal joint with multiple screw orientations. *Foot Ankle Spec*. 2017;10:104-108.
25. Dayton P, Santrock R, Kauwe M, et al. Progression of healing on serial radiographs following first ray arthrodesis in the foot using a biplanar plating technique without compression. *J Foot Ankle Surg*. 2019;58:427-433.
26. Ray JJ, Friedmann AJ, Hanselman AE, et al. Hallux valgus. *Foot Ankle Orthop*. 2019;4:247301141983850.

27. Feilmeier M, Dayton P, Wienke JC Jr. Reduction of intermetatarsal angle after first metatarsophalangeal joint arthrodesis in patients with hallux valgus. *J Foot Ankle Surg*. 2014;53:29-31.
28. Romash MM, Fugate D, Yanklowitz B. Passive motion of the first metatarsal cuneiform joint: preoperative assessment. *Foot Ankle*. 1990;10:293-298.
29. Egol KA, Kubiak EN, Fulkerson E, Kummer FJ, Koval KJ. Biomechanics of locked plates and screws. *J Orthop Trauma*. 2004;18:488-493.
30. Feilmeier M, Dayton P, Sedberry S, Reimer RA. Incidence of surgical site infection in the foot and ankle with early exposure and showering of surgical sites: a prospective observation. *J Foot Ankle Surg*. 2014;53:173-175.
31. Lintz F, Beaudet P, Richardi G, Brilhault J. Weight-bearing CT in foot and ankle pathology. *Orthop Traumatol Surg Res*. 2021;107:102772.
32. Dayton P, Carvalho S, Egdorf R, Dayton M. Comparison of radiographic measurements before and after triplane tarsometatarsal arthrodesis for hallux valgus. *J Foot Ankle Surg*. 2020;59:291-297.
33. Hatch DJ, Dayton P, DeCarbo W, et al. Analysis of shortening and elevation of the first ray with instrumented triplane first tarsometatarsal arthrodesis. *Foot Ankle Orthop*. 2020;5:247301142096067.

5 Proximal Rotational Metatarsal Osteotomy (PROMO)

Emilio Wagner and Pablo Wagner

INTRODUCTION

Hallux valgus is a deformity, which include metatarsus varus, hallux valgus, and medial column pronation. Medial column external rotation (pronation) is present in most hallux valgus patients (87% according to Kim et al).[1,2] Operated hallux valgus patients have a relapse risk up to 70%.[3-5] Those with persistent pronation have worse functional scores and an increased deformity relapse risk compared with nonpronated hallux valgus cases.[6-8] The key in determining how to treat hallux valgus is to determine which deformities are present in a specific case, for example, metatarsus varus, medial ray pronation, and distal metatarsal articular angulation (altered distal metatarsal articular angle or DMAA).[6-14] All deformity parameters should be corrected to achieve the best possible outcome with the lowest achievable relapse rate.

Techniques to correct rotation include the Lapidus (tarsometatarsal arthrodesis) and the proximal dome osteotomy (known as Mann osteotomy). The Lapidus is an arthrodesis, that as such, may not be suitable or adequate for some active patients given the inevitable stiffness that may generate on the medial column. In addition, it is a demanding surgery, which makes it less favorable for some surgeons.[15,16]

The PROMO (proximal rotational metatarsal osteotomy) follows a geometrical concept whereby rotation of two segments on an oblique plane generates an angulation of one of them. Applying this concept to the hallux valgus, by performing an oblique osteotomy (dorsal-distal to proximal plantar) on the first metatarsal, pronation and varus correction can be achieved. The described osteotomy is stabilized using one interfragmentary screw and a medial locking metatarsal plate. Any combinations of metatarsal varus and medial column pronation can be corrected using this technique just by changing the osteotomy angulation. To facilitate this calculation, a table was published (Table 5.1) that shows what osteotomy should be performed to precisely correct a specific deformity.[17]

INDICATIONS AND CONTRAINDICATIONS

The indications for the PROMO technique are as follows. Regarding patient characteristics, an age younger than 65 years old is ideal to avoid poor bone quality and, therefore, minimize fixation failure risk.

Regarding the deformity parameters, it should be a hallux valgus with an intermetatarsal angle (IMA) below 18° and/or a hallux valgus angle below 40°. For greater deformities, a Lapidus would be the recommended technique. Medial ray pronation must be present to indicate this technique. Ways to measure pronation include weight-bearing computerized tomography (WBCT) or a weight-bearing anteroposterior (AP) foot view using the published staging system.[18] See images with progressive pronation as seen in radiographs and WBCT (Figs. 5.1 through 5.6).

The TMT joint is of paramount importance. It should not have any signs of arthritis to indicate a PROMO. In addition, no radiographic instability should be evident (such as joint space asymmetry

TABLE 5.1 PROMO Table

		Metatarsal Pronation		
		Mild	Moderate	Severe
IMA	9-12	42	33	28
	12-15	55	42	38
	15-18	55	47	42

This table represents what osteotomy (in degrees) should be performed to be able to correct shown combinations of intermetatarsal angles (IMAs) and metatarsal pronation values.

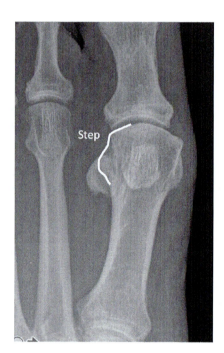

FIGURE 5.1 Anteroposterior foot weight-bearing radiograph showing a mild rotation or stage 1. A lateral head curvature can be seen that represents the metatarsal condyle barely appearing laterally in mild rotated metatarsals. There is an acute angle between the distal metatarsal joint line and condyle line. When this metatarsal head shape is evident, a rotation between 10° and 20° is present.

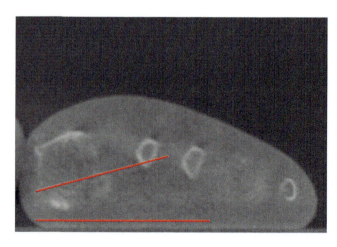

FIGURE 5.2 Weight-bearing computerized tomography showing a coronal cut at the first metatarsal head. Metatarsal rotation angle is measured between a line along the floor and one tangent to the sesamoid facets. In this case, 15° (same patient as in Figure 5.1).

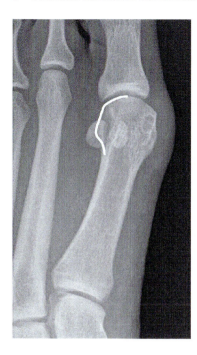

FIGURE 5.3 Anteroposterior foot weight-bearing radiograph showing a moderate metatarsal pronation or stage 2. A lateral head curvature that is in continuity with the distal metatarsal joint line can be seen. There is no acute angle present between the distal joint line and the condyle line. When this head shape is present, a rotation between 20° and 30° is present.

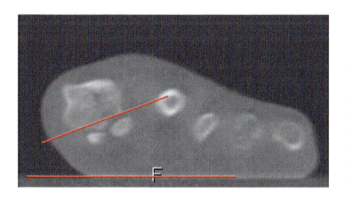

FIGURE 5.4 Weight-bearing computerized tomography showing a coronal cut at the first metatarsal head. Metatarsal rotation angle is measured between a line along the floor and one tangent to the sesamoid facets. In this case, 23° (same patient as in Figure 5.3).

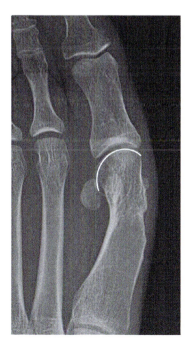

FIGURE 5.5 Anteroposterior foot weight-bearing radiograph showing a severe metatarsal pronation or stage 3. A lateral head curvature that is in completely round in continuity with the distal metatarsal joint line can be seen. When this head shape is present, a rotation above 30° is present.

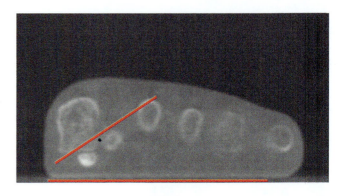

FIGURE 5.6 Weight-bearing computerized tomography showing a coronal cut at the first metatarsal head. Metatarsal rotation angle is measured between a line along the floor and one tangent to the sesamoid facets. In this case, 33° (same patient as in Figure 5.5).

or incongruency) on the frontal or lateral radiographic view. In both cases described (arthritis and/or unstable TMT), a Lapidus is recommended.

The contraindications are mainly a hallux valgus without pronation and a severe deformity with an unstable TMT. A symptomatic flatfoot with TMT synovitis should not be treated with a PROMO either.

PREOPERATIVE PLANNING

This technique corrects pronation and angulation through rotation on a single oblique proximal metatarsal osteotomy. The osteotomy angulation (dorsal/distal to plantar/proximal) varies according to the specific patient deformity parameters. If there is severe pronation and mild angulation, a more transverse osteotomy will be obtained from the calculations; if more angulation is needed to correct, a more horizontal osteotomy will be planned.

There is no need for a wedge resection. No undesired shortening occurs on the metatarsal (for moderate cases frequently shortening is needed).

Osteotomy Planning

To calculate the osteotomy angulation, the IMA and pronation angle stage have to be obtained. An AP weight-bearing foot radiograph or a WBCT are needed. Using the attached table, the osteotomy angulation can be obtained by entering the values into it Table 5.1.

SURGICAL TECHNIQUE

The hallux valgus that will be shown has 13° of IMA (metatarsus varus) and a moderate pronation (20° to 30°). See Figure 5.7. Position the patient supine on the operating table with no gluteal bumps and the usual bone prominences well padded. The incision starts at the TMT. It is approximately 4 cm long up to the metatarsal neck (Fig. 5.8). Proceed to remove the medial head eminence in cases where bone protrudes medially from the metatarsal neck. This is present in most adults but unfrequently seen in adolescents. Dissect all soft tissues dorsal and plantar of the metatarsal metaphysis. Drive a 1.6 K-wire 1 cm distal to the TMT at the metatarsal midline. This guidewire should be parallel to the weight-bearing plane and perpendicular to the metatarsal shaft (use fluoroscopy). A tray lid against the sole of the foot helps drive this wire parallel to a simulated weight-bearing surface (Fig. 5.9). Slide the positioning jig through its 0° hole on the K-wire. Add a 1.6 K-wire through the jig using the hole that matches the pronation measured in your preoperative planning (20° to 30°) (Fig. 5.10). Remove the 0° wire and positioning jig. Slide the osteotomy jig through the K-wire using the hole labeled with the osteotomy angulation previously chosen (42°). With a second 1.6 K-wire, fix the jig distally at the metatarsal equator. With an oscillating saw, perform the osteotomy using any jig slot, but avoid entering the TMT (Fig. 5.11). There are three slots available to be used. If the chosen slot enters the TMT, use a more distal one. Leave the lateral metatarsal cortex intact. Remove the osteotomy jig. Apply the rotation jig on the distal wire through its 0° hole. Add a second 1.6 K-wire using the pronation hole according to the pronation value previously measured (20° to 30°) (Fig. 5.12). Remove the 0° wire and the rotation jig. Using the saw blade, complete the osteotomy. Make sure to completely release the osteotomy laterally (periosteum and peroneus longus fibers are always present). Any soft tissue attachment

5 Proximal Rotational Metatarsal Osteotomy (PROMO)

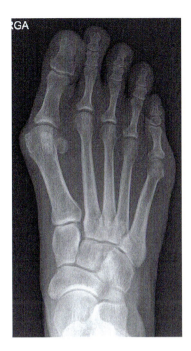

FIGURE 5.7 Anteroposterior foot weight-bearing radiograph for this example case. Intermetatarsal angle is 13°. Metatarsal rotation is moderate (stage 2), given that there is no acute angle between the condyle line and distal metatarsal joint line (what would be a stage 1) and the metatarsal head is not completely round (what would be a stage 3).

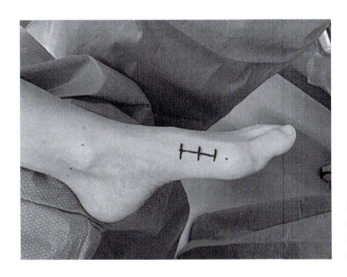

FIGURE 5.8 Medial foot view depicting the 3 to 4 cm approach to be performed for a proximal rotational metatarsal osteotomy.

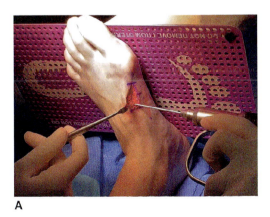
A
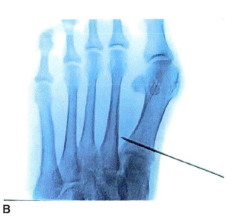
B

FIGURE 5.9 **A.** Intraoperative view of a hallux valgus patient. A tray lid is placed against the sole of the foot, helping drive the first wire parallel to the floor. **B.** Shows the fluoroscopic image of the same patient where the first K-wire must be placed perpendicular to the first metatarsal axis.

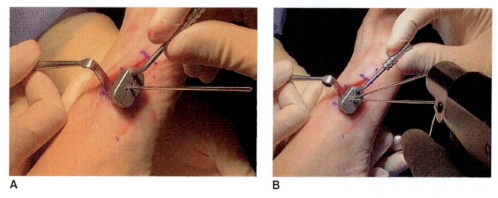

FIGURE 5.10 **A.** The positioning jig being slid over the first wire through the "0" degree hole. **B.** A second wire being placed through the 20° to 29° hole, representing the pronation estimated in this specific patient.

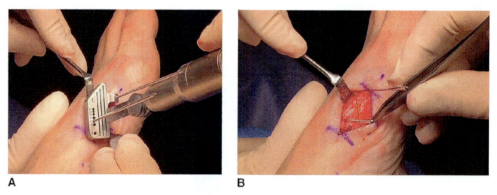

FIGURE 5.11 **A.** The osteotomy jig is seen placed through the last K-wire placed in the previous image and then fixed with an additional wire to the metatarsal equator/midline. **B.** An incomplete cut is demonstrated, keeping the lateral metatarsal cortex for temporal stability.

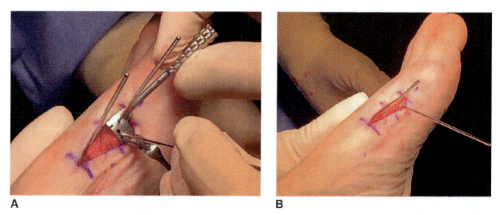

FIGURE 5.12 **A.** Demonstrates the rotational jig being slid over the distal K-wire through its "0" hole. A second wire is placed through the 20° to 29° hole replacing the wire in the "0" hole, representing the pronation estimated for this specific patient. **B.** The final position of the wires is shown, representing the amount of pronation the osteotomy will correct.

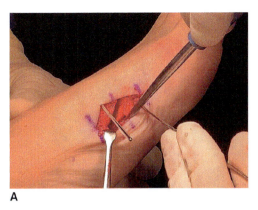 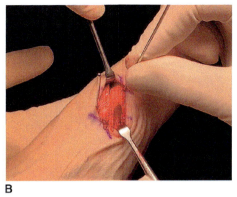

FIGURE 5.13 **A.** After finishing the osteotomy, the osteotomy site is dissected free from soft tissues, especially in the plantar aspect where the peroneus longus attachments lie. **B.** After the soft tissue dissection, the distal metatarsal bone fragment can be freely rotated relative to the proximal fragment.

will compromise an adequate metatarsal correction (Fig. 5.13). Using a clamp, internally rotate (supinate) the distal metatarsal segment until both K-wires are parallel. Always over-rotate the distal segment slightly, given that some rotation is normally lost during the next steps of the procedure. Medially, no step offs at the osteotomy should be present. Drive two wires perpendicular to the osteotomy for transient fixation (Fig. 5.14). The metatarsal head should have changed to a squared shaped laterally on a simulated weight-bearing fluoroscopic view. The sesamoids could be still slightly laterally subluxed given that the great toe is still in valgus and no capsular reefing has been performed.

If there is residual hallux valgus and/or the sesamoids are still laterally positioned, a percutaneous lateral release should be performed. By using a beaver blade, place the blade in the intermetatarsal space between the first and second metatarsal heads. Angle your hand 30° proximal and lateral to aim to the lateral aspect of the first metatarsophalangeal joint. Insert the beaver blade percutaneously in this angulation. Enter the metatarsophalangeal capsule and then release the adductor tendon by surrounding the lateral proximal phalangeal corner. After releasing the tendon, a lucent area where the tendon had inserted will be visualized on radiographs (Figs. 5.15 to 5.17).

Remove any bone step offs medially on the metatarsal that could prevent bone-plate apposition. Apply a locking plate medially. Fix the plate with 3 threaded olive wires to the metatarsal. Drive the recommended wire through the precision guide for interfragmentary screw placement.

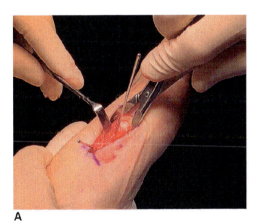 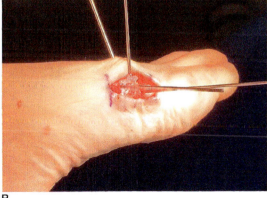

FIGURE 5.14 **A.** A bone clamp holding the distal metatarsal fragment, helping derotate the bone, achieving parallelism between the K-wires in place. As the osteotomy will correct both pronation and varus, the wires will diverge between them as the distal fragment is rotated relative to the proximal fragment. **B.** The temporal fixation of the osteotomy with two vertical K-wires. Please note the slight overcorrection of the pronation, represented by a more supinated position of the distal K-wire relative to the proximal wire.

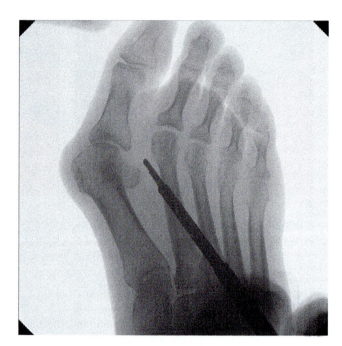

FIGURE 5.15 Intraoperative anteroposterior foot fluoroscopy. The image shows the beaver blade entering in an angled direction in the intermetatarsal space toward the metatarsophalangeal joint.

Measure the screw length using the supplied instruments. Drive the recommended wire through the precision guide for interfragmentary screw placement. Drive a 3.0- or 3.5-mm cannulated fully threaded screw across the osteotomy. After positioning this screw, replace one by one the plate olive wires by 2.5-mm locking screws (Fig. 5.18). Check under radiograph the correct metatarsal fixation and final position. Sometimes an abnormal DMAA is present. Do not hesitate to add a distal biplanar Chevron if necessary (Fig. 5.19). Close the subcutaneous layer with resorbable suture (3 to 4 stitches) and proceed with skin closure with intradermal technique. Postoperative radiographs are shown in Figure 5.20.

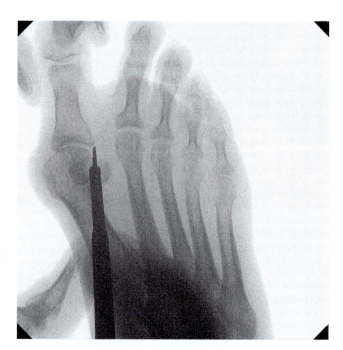

FIGURE 5.16 Intraoperative anteroposterior foot fluoroscopy. The image shows the beaver blade entering laterally at the metatarsophalangeal joint while holding the hallux in varus position. In this spot, perform a section of the adductor tendon and lateral collateral ligament.

5 Proximal Rotational Metatarsal Osteotomy (PROMO)

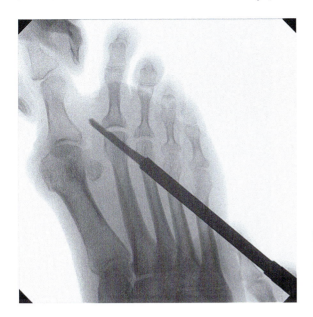

FIGURE 5.17 Intraoperative anteroposterior foot fluoroscopy. The image shows a lucency laterally at the proximal phalanx base, representing the adductor tendon and collateral ligament release.

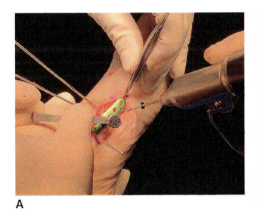 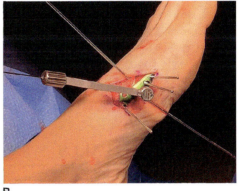

A B

FIGURE 5.18 A. Temporal positioning of the fixation plate, where a specifically designed locking plate is seen placed against the bone with the help of olive wires. **B.** The use of a precision guide locked to the plate to aid in the exact positioning of an interfragmentary screw. After this last screw is tightened, the rest of the holes of the plate are filled with locking screws (two proximal and two distal to the osteotomy).

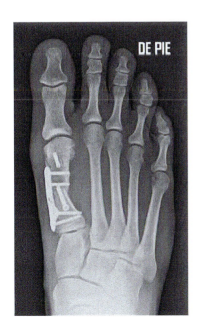

FIGURE 5.19 Anteroposterior foot weight-bearing radiograph showing a proximal rotational metatarsal osteotomy osteotomy in addition to a biplanar chevron osteotomy to correct for an altered distal metatarsal articular angle.

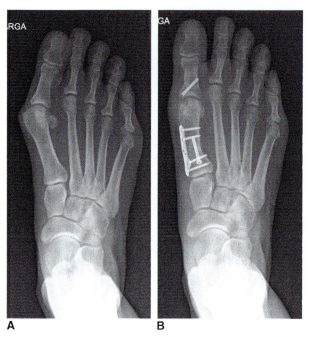

FIGURE 5.20 Weight-bearing radiographs of the same patient illustrated through the technical images is shown. **A.** The preoperative anteroposterior (AP) view is presented where an intermetatarsal angle of 15° was measured, with an estimated pronation of 20°. **B.** A final foot AP weight-bearing view is shown after bone union, showing the correction obtained.

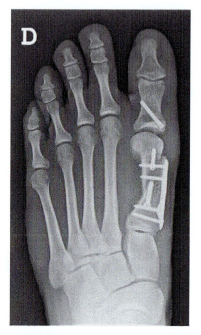

FIGURE 5.21 Anteroposterior foot weight-bearing radiograph showing a proximal rotational metatarsal osteotomy (PROMO) in addition to a chevron osteotomy. The chevron was used to compensate for an undercorrected intermetatarsal angle after the PROMO osteotomy.

PEARLS AND PITFALLS

If the osteotomy is rotating but not correcting IMA: this is because the osteotomy rotation was performed while not keeping the osteotomy closed. While the metatarsal is supinated, a simultaneous valgus deviation occurs only if the osteotomy apposition is maintained and congruent during rotation. If the metatarsal is exclusively rotated, the pronation will be corrected but the varus will not, resulting in an incongruent osteotomy. The surgeon should be conscious, that while rotating the metatarsal, a light valgus push should be applied to the metatarsal to keep a closed osteotomy and achieve an IMA correction.

If the osteotomy is not rotating and/or difficult to align: the soft tissues are still attached at the osteotomy level. The distal segment, including the peroneus longus and metatarsal periosteum, must be released.

If the osteotomy does not achieve full IMA correction, or desired rotation is not achieved: make sure the osteotomy is free of soft tissues. Frequently periosteum and peroneus longus fibers hold the distal fragment preventing an adequate rotation. If rotation was corrected, but there is an undercorrection of the IMA, translate the osteotomy laterally about 2 to 3 mm. This does not hinder the PROMO stability and improves the IMA correction (Fig. 5.21).

If correction is lost when the plate is applied: remove the plate, and over-rotate slightly during transient fixation. Once applying the plate, use Olive wires through the plate holes to aid holding correction before locking the plate. Make sure no bone step offs are present medially to avoid the plate reproducing the deformity (this plate first compresses and then locks).

If the sesamoids are still laterally displaced on the AP foot view after adequate IMA and pronation correction: a few millimeters of lateral sesamoids displacement will be self-corrected after medial closure and/or akin osteotomy. If the head recovered its squared shape, that means pronation was corrected. If sesamoids are obviously dislocated, perform a lateral metatarso-sesamoid ligament release (percutaneous or open) and push the sesamoid complex under the metatarsal head, making sure the IMA is completely corrected. Finally, medially re-tension the metatarsophalangeal capsule.

POSTOPERATIVE MANAGEMENT

One month of partial weight bearing (or weight bearing on the lateral border of the boot if bilateral surgery was performed) is necessary. Full weight bearing is allowed after 1 month, transitioning into sneakers or wide toe-box shoes. For postoperative medications, 10 days of acetaminophen and anti-inflammatories are preferred. Tramadol drops are prescribed as needed for pain. Oral antithrombotic prophylaxis is prescribed for 10 days using Dabigatran or Rivaroxaban. AP and lateral weight-bearing radiographs are taken preoperatively, at 6 weeks, 3 months, and 1 year postoperative. During the first month postoperatively, the foot is notably swollen. During the second- and third-month postoperative swelling rapidly decreases allowing to fit into smaller and thinner shoes. It may take a year for the swelling to completely resolve.

RESULTS AND COMPLICATIONS

Functional outcomes significantly improve over time after hallux valgus surgery. Lower Extremity Functional Scale score increase from 53 preoperative to 73 postoperative.[18]

Regarding radiologic correction, IMA improves from 15.5° to 5° and hallux valgus angle from 32° to 5°. Recurrence factors for operated hallux valgus were already described.[1,2,6-13]

Regarding complications the following are the most frequent: infection; deep venous thrombosis; wound dehiscence; deformity relapse 7% (3 years f/u); dorsal malunion 5%. Nonunion 1% (personal data, not published).

REFERENCES

1. Kim Y, Kim JS, Young KW, et al. A new measure of tibial sesamoid position in hallux valgus in relation to the coronal rotation of the first metatarsal in CT scans. *Foot Ankle Int.* 2015;36(8):944-952.
2. Kim JS, Young KW. Sesamoid position in hallux valgus in relation to the coronal rotation of the first metatarsal. *Foot Ankle Clin.* 2018;23(2):219-230.
3. Bock P, Kluger R, Kristen KH, et al. The scarf osteotomy with minimally invasive lateral release for treatment of hallux valgus deformity: intermediate and long-term results. *J Bone Joint Surg Am.* 2015;97(15):1238-1245.
4. Deveci A, Firat A, Yilmaz S, et al. Short-term clinical and radiologic results of the scarf osteotomy: what factors contribute to recurrence? *J Foot Ankle Surg.* 2013;52(6):771-775.
5. Jeuken RM, Schotanus MG, Kort NP, et al. Long-term follow-up of a randomized controlled trial comparing scarf to chevron osteotomy in hallux valgus correction. *Foot Ankle Int.* 2016;37(7):687-695.
6. Conti MS, Patel TJ, Zhu J, Elliott AJ, Conti SF, Ellis SJ. Association of first metatarsal pronation correction with patient-reported outcomes and recurrence rates in hallux valgus. *Foot Ankle Int.* 2022;43(3):309-320.
7. Okuda R, Kinoshita M, Yasuda T, et al. The shape of the lateral edge of the first metatarsal head as a risk factor for recurrence of hallux valgus. *J Bone Joint Surg Am.* 2007;89:2163-2172.
8. Okuda R, Kinoshita M, Yasuda T, et al. Postoperative incomplete reduction of the sesamoids as a risk factor for recurrence of hallux valgus. *J Bone Joint Surg Am.* 2009;91(7):1637-1645.
9. Aiyer A, Shub J, Shariff R, Ying L, Myerson M. Radiographic recurrence of deformity after hallux valgus surgery in patients with metatarsus adductus. *Foot Ankle Int.* 2016;37(2):165-171.
10. Coughlin MJ, Roger A, Award M. Juvenile hallux valgus: etiology and treatment. *Foot Ankle Int.* 1995;16(11):682-697.
11. Kaufmann G, Sinz S, Giesinger JM, et al. Loss of correction after chevron osteotomy for hallux valgus as a function of preoperative deformity. *Foot Ankle Int.* 2018;107.
12. Park CH, Lee WC. Recurrence of hallux valgus can be predicted from immediate postoperative non-weight bearing radiographs. *J Bone Joint Surg Am.* 2017;99(14):1190-1197.
13. Shibuya N, Kyprios EM, Panchani PN, et al. Factors associated with early loss of hallux valgus correction. *J Foot Ankle Surg.* 2018;57(2):236-240.
14. Wagner P, Wagner E. Is the rotational deformity important in our decision-making process for correction of hallux valgus deformity? *Foot Ankle Clin.* 2018;23(2):205-217.
15. Wang Y, Li Z, Zhang M. Biomechanical study of tarsometatarsal joint fusion using finite element analysis. *Med Eng Phys.* 2014;36:1394-1400.
16. Wong D, Zhang M, Yu J, Leung A. Biomechanics of first ray hypermobility: an investigation on joint force during walking using finite element analysis. *Med Eng Phys.* 2014;36:1388-1393.
17. Wagner P, Wagner E. Proximal rotational metatarsal osteotomy for hallux valgus (PROMO): short-term prospective case series with a novel technique and topic review. *Foot Ankle Orthop.* 2018;3(3):247301141879007.
18. Wagner P, Lescure N, Siddiqui N, Fink J, Wagner E. Validity and reliability of a new radiological method to estimate medial column internal rotation in hallux valgus using foot weight-bearing x-ray. *Foot Ankle Spec.* 2021;19386400211029162.

PART TWO
FOREFOOT/HALLUX RIGIDUS

6 Cheilectomy/Moberg

Kimberly Koury and Judy Baumhauer

INTRODUCTION

Hallux rigidus is a painful degenerative joint disease affecting the first metatarsophalangeal (MTP) joint and is associated with osteophyte formation and limitation of motion, especially in dorsiflexion. It was first described by Davies-Colley in 1887, and J. M. Cotterill later coined the term hallux rigidus.[1] After hallux valgus, it is the most common painful affliction of the great toe, occurring in approximately 2% of the population between the ages of 30 and 60 years. As the degenerative process progresses, proliferation of bone on the dorsal aspect of the metatarsal head increases the size of the joint and blocks dorsiflexion of the proximal phalanx (Fig. 6.1). These changes are possibly initiated by previous occult trauma.[1,2] Patients usually present with unilateral symptoms, but it is common for stiffness and the degenerative process to affect the opposite foot. Abnormal gait is common,[3] and patients may walk on the lateral border of the foot to minimize painful hallux MTP dorsiflexion.

Nonoperative treatment of hallux rigidus includes activity modification, administration of nonsteroidal anti-inflammatory medications, footwear alteration, and intra-articular injection of corticosteroids. Shoe modification includes wide and deep toe box to reduce skin abrasion from dorsal osteophytes and irritation of the dorsal-medial cutaneous nerve. A stiff-soled shoe with rocker-bottom, steel, fiberglass shank built in the sole, or full length rigid carbon fiber orthotic can also help by minimizing first MTP motion at toe-off.

When nonoperative treatment fails, surgical intervention with cheilectomy should be considered, for mild and selected cases of moderate hallux rigidus.[4] It improves pain related to the arthritic joint (see Fig. 6.1) or from skin ulceration or abrasion overlying large dorsal osteophytes. The goal of surgery is to excise the proliferative bone on the "lip" of the joint, thereby relieving pain with dorsiflexion motion. Cheilectomy offers the advantages of preserving the length, stability, and flexion-extension strength of the great toe that are often affected with other procedures. Other options have been described such as resection arthroplasty, interposition arthroplasty, implant arthroplasty or hemiarthroplasty with polyvinyl alcohol, and MTP arthrodesis.[5,6] Additionally, there are osteotomies about the first MTP joint that can be performed such as closing wedge proximal phalangeal osteotomy, proximal metatarsal osteotomy, and distal metatarsal osteotomy.[6,7]

Closing wedge osteotomy of the proximal phalanx for hallux rigidus was first proposed by Bonney and Macnab[8] in 1952, and short-term results were reported by Kessel and Bonney[9] in 1958. Closing wedge proximal phalanx osteotomy is, however, best known as the Moberg osteotomy since he popularized this technique.[10] The aim of the operation is to move the limited arc of motion at the affected joint to a more dorsiflexed position so that the function is improved. It is applicable in patients with mild to moderate degenerative disease of the first MTP joint with a proximal phalanx that sits in relative plantarflexion to the metatarsal head. Most authors recommend cheilectomy for the surgical treatment of Hattrup and Johnson grade I and II disease and arthrodesis for grade III disease (Fig. 6.2). However, there have been recent outcomes supporting joint preservation techniques in more severe stages as well.[11]

PART II Forefoot/Hallux Rigidus

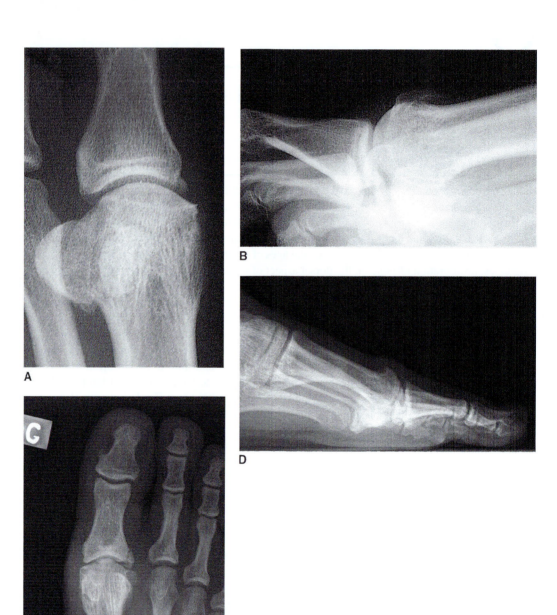

FIGURE 6.1 Medial view of a foot with hallux rigidus. Dorsal osteophytes on the first metatarsal head block normal dorsiflexion of the proximal phalanx.

FIGURE 6.2 A, B. Grade I or mild hallux rigidus with small osteophyte and no joint space narrowing. **C, D.** Grade II or moderate hallux rigidus with osteophytes dorsally and laterally and with joint space narrowing.

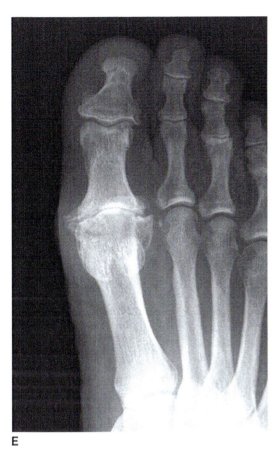
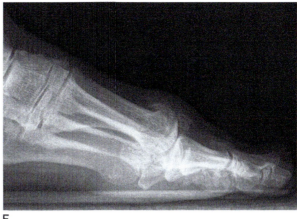

FIGURE 6.2 *(Continued)* **E, F.** Grade III or advanced hallux rigidus with osteophytes dorsally and laterally and with severe joint destruction with loss of joint space.

INDICATIONS AND CONTRAINDICATIONS

The indications for cheilectomy are hallux rigidus with dorsally based pain that is disabling and refractory to nonoperative treatment. Additional indications include stiff, painful range of motion (ROM) of the MTP joint, difficulty with footwear, and recurrent bursitis or skin callosity over prominent osteophytes (Fig. 6.3). It may be indicated for recurrent abrasion or skin ulceration over the prominent osteophytes once the ulcer is healed. The contraindications are a foot with vascular insufficiency, infection, or ulceration. Relative contraindications include sesamoid pain, pain and crepitus with grind testing, or pain with mid ROM indicating intra-articular symptoms, which are more effectively addressed with a joint sacrificing procedure such as arthrodesis.

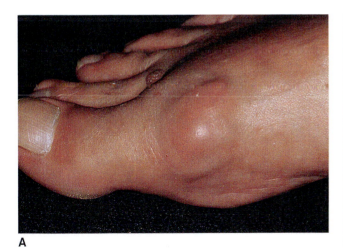
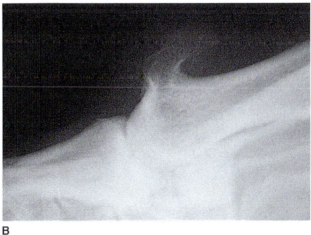

FIGURE 6.3 **A.** Enlargement about the metatarsophalangeal joint from soft tissue inflammation and osteophytes in a patient with hallux rigidus. **B.** A large, prominent dorsal osteophyte is observed on the lateral radiograph.

Cheilectomy with phalangeal osteotomy could be considered in a relatively young, active patient and/or athlete with pain and impairment due to moderate hallux rigidus with marked restriction of dorsiflexion and adequate plantarflexion.

PREOPERATIVE PLANNING

Painful motion and crepitus may occur with sagittal motion. The ROM of the first MTP should be measured with a goniometer and recorded. We use the plantar surface of the foot and the axis of the proximal phalanx for ROM measurements (Fig. 6.4). Others measure the position of the toe relative to the metatarsal axis, recognizing that the angular measurement obtained is influenced by the height of the arch. During clinical evaluation, care should be taken to note the posture and the ROM of the interphalangeal (IP) joint. This joint often develops compensatory hypermobility in dorsiflexion. Failure to recognize hyperextension of the IP joint can result in poor outcomes and patient dissatisfaction if this joint becomes painful and arthritic postoperatively. The IP joint should be held in a neutral position when measuring MTP motion (see Fig. 6.4), or the degree of the dorsiflexion will be overestimated.

Radiographs should be obtained to evaluate the severity of the joint degenerative disease and to determine the presence of concurrent pathology.[12] Radiograph evaluation should include standing anteroposterior and lateral views (Fig. 6.5). The anteroposterior view can be useful in evaluating medial and lateral osteophytes, toe alignment, joint space narrowing, and condition of the adjacent joints. The standing lateral view is helpful because it demonstrates the dorsal osteophytes and reveals the extent of joint space narrowing. Hyperextension of the IP joint can be appreciated in this view, but this usually is determined clinically. The oblique view of the foot can help visualize early joint space narrowing. Based on the radiographic findings, the grade of the hallux rigidus can be determined. There are a number of useful grading systems available (see Fig. 6.2),[13,14] and one can use a simple radiographic system described by Hattrup and Johnson[4]:

- Grade I: mild to moderate osteophytes formation but good joint space preservation
- Grade II: moderate osteophyte formation with joint space narrowing and subchondral sclerosis
- Grade III: marked osteophyte formation and loss of the visible joint space, with or without subchondral cyst formation

Coughlin and Shurnas modified this three-grade radiographic classification to a five-grade system that includes subjective clinical findings and is the most widely utilized classification system.[11] Under this classification system, grade 0 has normal radiographs with loss of 10% to 20% of passive motion compared to the opposite side. Grade I represents 20% to 50% loss of motion with dorsal spurring and minimal joint space narrowing on radiographs. Grade II involves 50% to 75% loss of motion and mild to moderate joint space loss. Whereas grade III and grade IV have 75% to 100% loss of motion with substantial loss of joint space with grade IV having pain at mid ROM on exam.

Some patients with an essentially normal joint space have severe stiffness and pain, while others with severe disease radiologically have no joint pain but only skin irritation from the prominence. Advanced diagnostic studies could be performed but are rarely indicated.

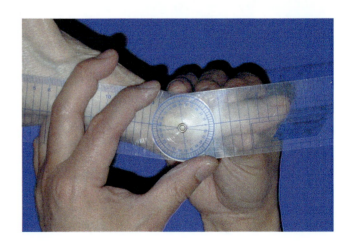

FIGURE 6.4 A patient with painful hallux rigidus has restriction of dorsiflexion as measured with a goniometer.

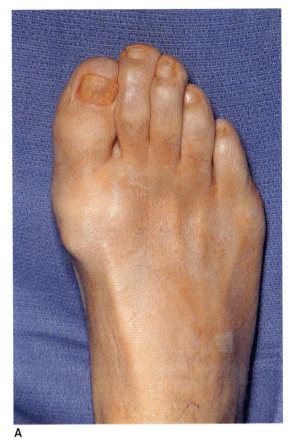
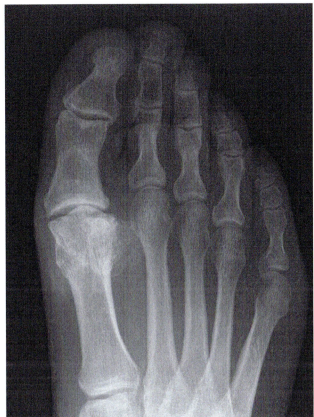
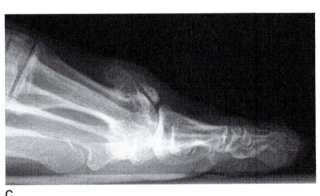

FIGURE 6.5 A. Photograph of a 60-year-old male with a prominence over the first metatarsophalangeal joint, which is painful with footwear, but he had no joint pain, and no painful joint motion. **B.** Anteroposterior foot radiograph shows hallux rigidus with large bony prominence. **C.** Lateral radiograph.

SURGICAL TECHNIQUE

Technique 1: Cheilectomy

- Local metatarsal block or an ankle block anesthesia is usually administered.
- Patient is placed supine, and the extremity is prepared and draped up to the knee.
- The extremity is exsanguinated over a sterile, double stockinet using a 4-inch rubber Esmarch bandage.
- In most cases, the rubber bandage is then wrapped at the ankle level several times for hemostasis. As an alternative, a tourniquet may be used at the calf.
- In patients who have general or spinal anesthesia, a thigh tourniquet may be used.
- Preoperative ROM in the first MTP joint is again tested.
- The 5- to 6-cm skin incision is centered over the dorsal aspect of the first MTP joint, or alternatively, a dorsal-medial incision can be made. Care is taken to identify and protect the extensor hallucis longus (EHL) tendon and avoid the dorsal-medial cutaneous nerve.

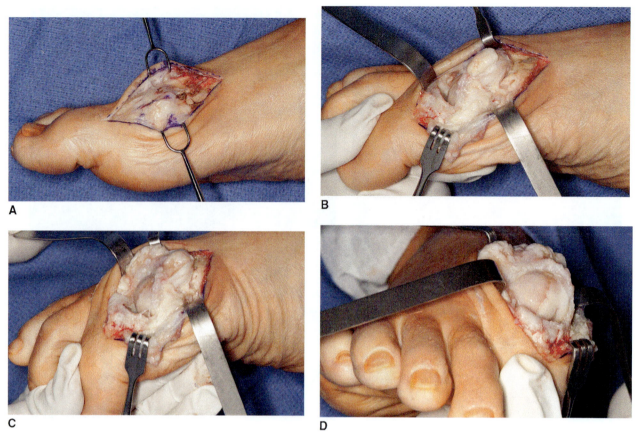

FIGURE 6.6 A. Medial capsule. Dorsal-medial cutaneous nerve is protected (*purple*). **B.** Following longitudinal capsulotomy, large bone mass observed and loose osteochondral fragment. **C.** With toe flexion, the extent of chondral degeneration is observed. **D.** Frontal view shows bare subchondral bone observed over much of the metatarsal joint surface.

- The capsule is then longitudinally incised leaving a 2-mm cuff along the EHL tendon to expose the underlying first MTP joint and the base of the proximal phalanx (Fig. 6.6A).
- The joint is examined, particularly the condition of the articular cartilage, and loose osteochondral fragments removed (Fig. 6.6B through D).
- Synovitis is débrided from the medial and lateral gutters of the joint.
- Osteophytes are removed from the base of the proximal phalanx dorsally, dorsomedially, and dorsolaterally.

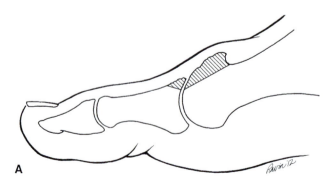
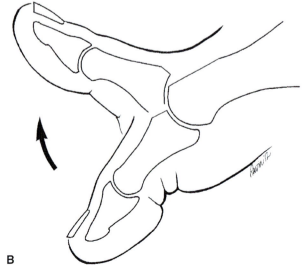

FIGURE 6.7 A. Line of resection of the metatarsal and phalangeal sides of the joint for cheilectomy. **B.** Adequate resection of the metatarsal head and phalangeal base is necessary to gain adequate motion.

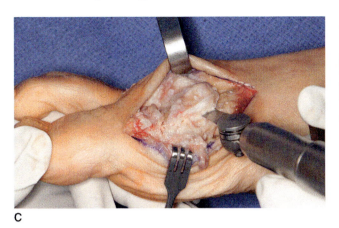
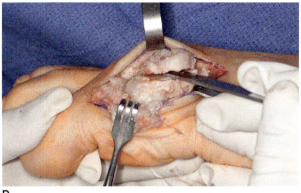

FIGURE 6.7 *(Continued)* **C.** Cheilectomy is performed with a microsagittal saw from medial to lateral. **D.** This cheilectomy was completed with osteotome, because of its large size.

- Cheilectomy can be performed with either an osteotome or microsagittal saw, resecting the dorsal 30% of the metatarsal head (Figs. 6.7 and 6.12).
- Osteophytes are removed from the metatarsal laterally and if needed the medial eminence is resected. The sharp margins of the metatarsal dorsomedially and dorsolaterally are beveled, as these are palpable prominences (Fig. 6.8).
- Copious irrigation is used to remove all bony debris from around the joint.

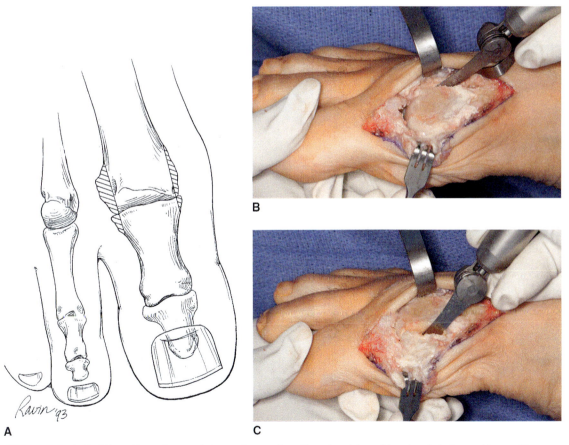

FIGURE 6.8 A. Excision of lateral osteophytes and a small portion of metatarsal head and phalangeal base with cartilage loss. Bony prominences are resected medially, and osteophyte is resected from the base of the proximal phalanx dorsally, dorsolaterally, and dorsomedially. **B.** Osteophytes along the lateral metatarsal head are excised with a saw. **C.** Osteophytes removed medially with a saw.

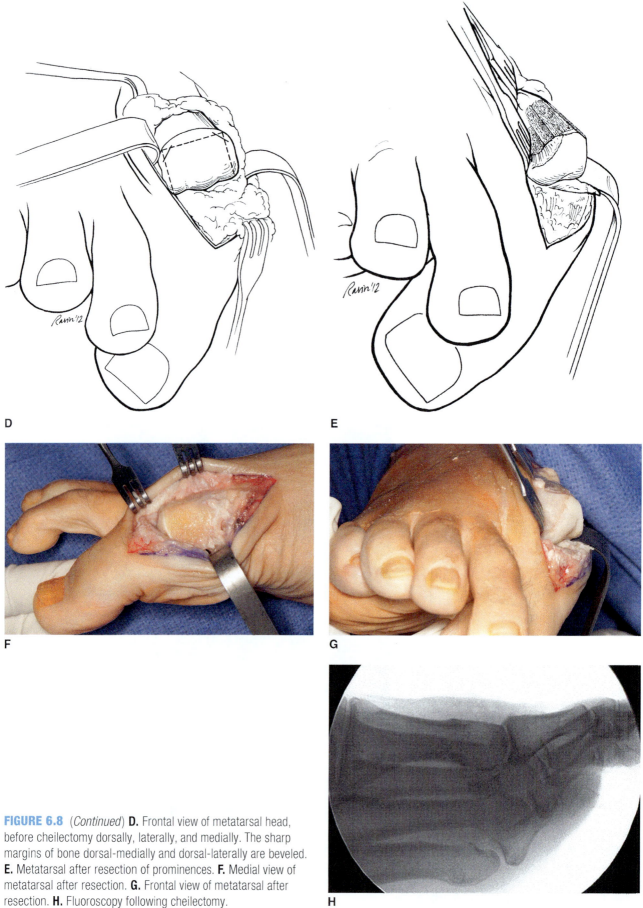

FIGURE 6.8 (Continued) **D.** Frontal view of metatarsal head, before cheilectomy dorsally, laterally, and medially. The sharp margins of bone dorsal-medially and dorsal-laterally are beveled. **E.** Metatarsal after resection of prominences. **F.** Medial view of metatarsal after resection. **G.** Frontal view of metatarsal after resection. **H.** Fluoroscopy following cheilectomy.

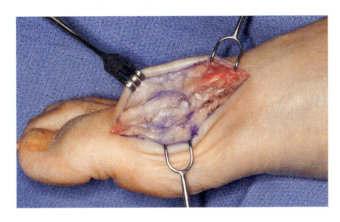

FIGURE 6.9 Capsulotomy closed.

- A careful capsular closure is recommended (Fig. 6.9).
- Skin is closed in usual fashion, and a soft dressing and postoperative shoe are applied.

Technique 2: Cheilectomy With Proximal Phalangeal Osteotomy (Moberg)

- Patient assessment is performed as described above (Figs. 6.3 and 6.10).
- The incision and longitudinal capsulotomy are performed (Fig. 6.11).
- The base of the proximal phalanx is exposed medially, dorsomedially, and dorsolaterally sharply with a no. 15 blade scalpel, avoiding circumferential dissection of the soft tissues from the base. Right-angle retractors, such as Senn retractors, are preferred (Fig. 6.12).
- A closing wedge osteotomy is marked at the meta-diaphyseal region of the bone, designed to remove approximately a 3-mm wedge of bone. This can be planned for a larger or smaller resection depending on preoperative examination of motion (Fig. 6.13A and B).
- Using a microsagittal saw with a thin, sharp blade, the osteotomy is performed from a dorsal to plantar direction. The cut can also be made from the medial side depending on surgeon preference.

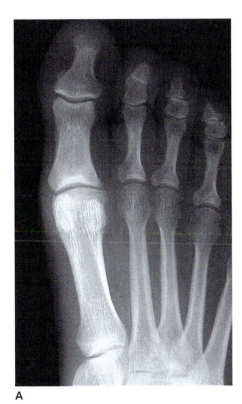
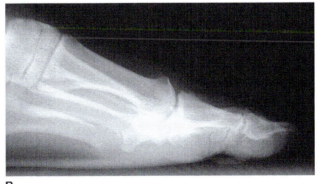

A   B

FIGURE 6.10 Radiographs of a 62-year-old man with painful grade II hallux rigidus and with prominent dorsal osteophytes. Anteroposterior **(A)** and lateral **(B)** standing radiographs of the foot.

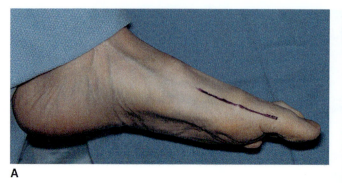
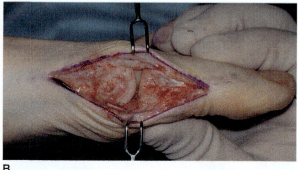
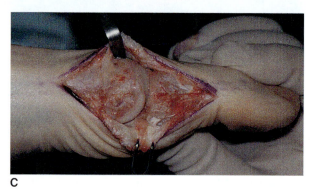

FIGURE 6.11 A. The medial longitudinal incision is marked. **B.** The capsule is incised longitudinally to expose the first metatarsophalangeal joint, the proximal phalanx, and metatarsal head. **C.** The soft tissues are carefully dissected from the metatarsal head and the base of proximal phalanx. The osteophytes then become visible.

- The proximal cut is aligned parallel with the phalangeal joint surface, and the distal cut is fashioned obliquely (Fig. 6.13C).
- The proximal cut should be placed at the junctional region of the diaphyseal and metaphyseal bone; the concave joint surface of the proximal phalanx and its preoperative radiographic morphology should be taken into account to avoid penetrating the joint surface (Fig. 6.13D).
- The osteotomy cuts should extend to but not through the plantar cortex, and the tendon of flexor hallucis longus should be protected during the osteotomy cuts with a retractor. The plantar cortex should be left intact at the completion of these cuts and excision of the wedge (Fig. 6.13E).
- Occasionally, we use a 0.045-inch K-wire to create multiple perforations in the plantar cortex that facilitate completion of the osteotomy (Fig. 6.13F). The osteotomy is then gently closed, hinging on the plantar cortex and the plantar periosteum (Fig. 6.13G).
- If there is concomitant hallux valgus interphalangeus deformity, the osteotomy is made with a medial closing wedge in addition to the dorsal closing wedge component to correct the deformity in both planes.
- The osteotomy site is then fixed with 0.045 threaded K-wire starting from the plantar medial base of the phalanx aiming slightly dorsally across the osteotomy site. The wire is then cut flush with the bone (Fig. 6.14E).
- Alternatively, a small diameter screw, 2.0 or 2.4 mm, a small staple, or suture wire (Fig. 6.14A through D) may be positioned across the osteotomy site for fixation.
- The toe is then tested for adequacy of motion, which should be approximately 70° to 75° of dorsiflexion relative to the plantar foot (Fig. 6.15).

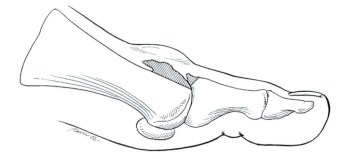

FIGURE 6.12 Cheilectomy performed prior to phalangeal osteotomy, removing the dorsal 20% to 25% of the metatarsal head. Osteophytes are removed from the metatarsal dorsolaterally and laterally as well as from the dorsal base of the proximal phalanx. Loose osteochondral fragments are removed.

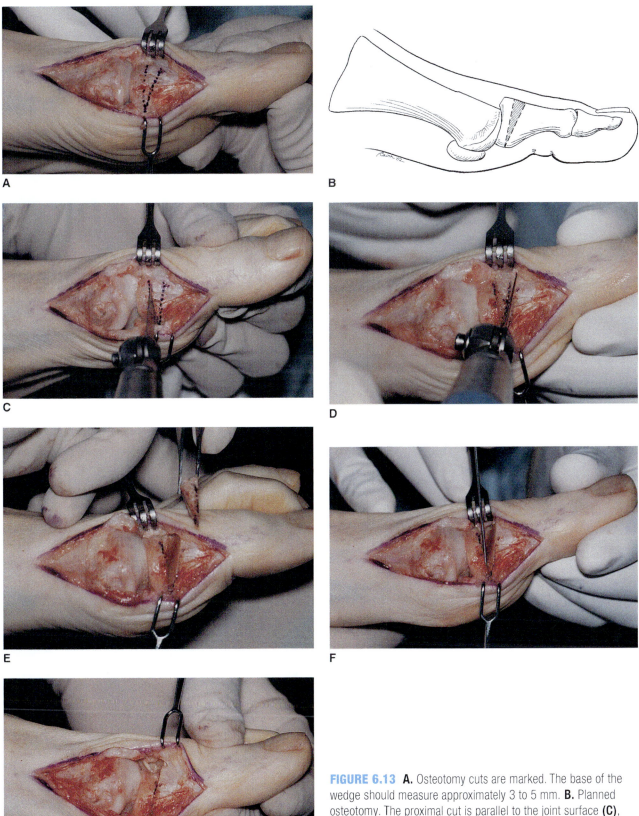

FIGURE 6.13 **A.** Osteotomy cuts are marked. The base of the wedge should measure approximately 3 to 5 mm. **B.** Planned osteotomy. The proximal cut is parallel to the joint surface **(C)**, and the distal cut is oblique **(D)**. **E.** The dorsal wedge is excised, ensuring that the plantar cortex and the periosteum remain intact. The plantar cortex is perforated with a K-wire **(F)** and then gently closed **(G)**.

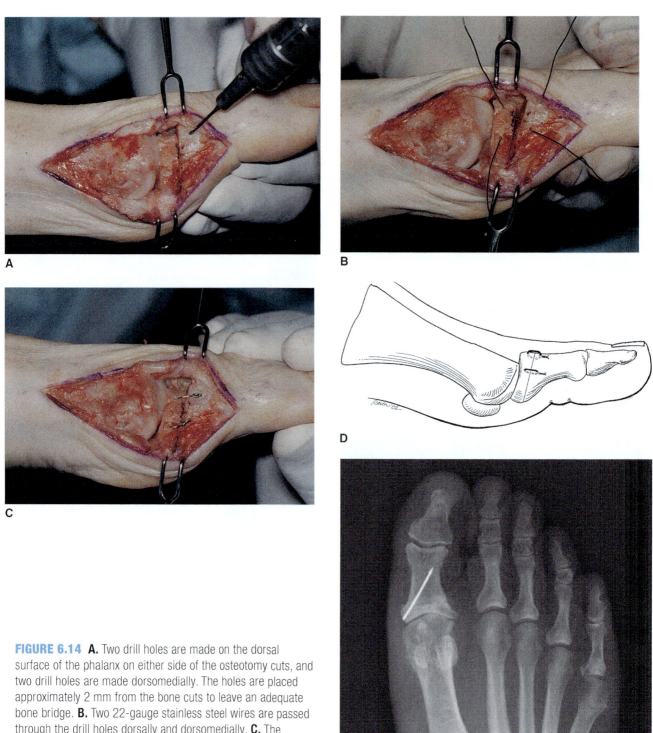

FIGURE 6.14 **A.** Two drill holes are made on the dorsal surface of the phalanx on either side of the osteotomy cuts, and two drill holes are made dorsomedially. The holes are placed approximately 2 mm from the bone cuts to leave an adequate bone bridge. **B.** Two 22-gauge stainless steel wires are passed through the drill holes dorsally and dorsomedially. **C.** The osteotomy is closed, the toe is supported, and the wires are tightened. The ends of the wires are buried in bone. **D.** Closing wedge osteotomy of the proximal phalanx with cheilectomy. **E.** Alternatively, the osteotomy site can be fixed with a 0.045 threaded K-wire that is cut flush and left in.

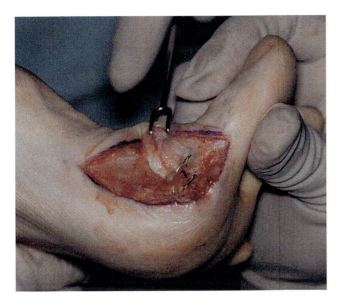

FIGURE 6.15 The toe is tested for range of motion and stability of the fixation. Approximately 70° to 75° of dorsiflexion is obtained at the end of the procedure in relation to the plantar foot.

- The tourniquet is released, the joint irrigated, and hemostasis obtained. We use 2-0 Vicryl suture to close the capsule.
- The skin is closed using 3-0 nylon sutures in interrupted horizontal mattress fashion. A sterile dressing and postoperative shoe are applied.
- Radiographs are obtained intraoperatively to assess bony apposition and fixation placement (Fig. 6.16).

PEARLS AND PITFALLS

- Avoid injury to the EHL and dorsal medial cutaneous nerve on approach.
- Preserve the collateral ligaments with medial and lateral exposure.

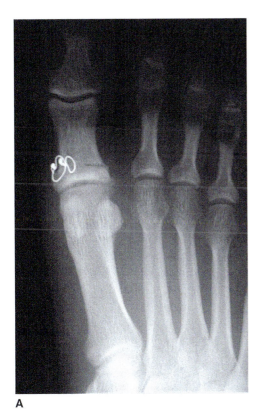
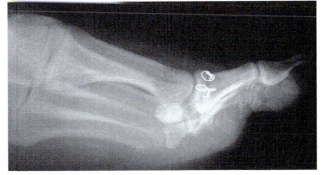

A B

FIGURE 6.16 Postoperative Anteroposterior **(A)** and lateral **(B)** radiographs.

- Resect enough bone (25% to 30%) to avoid residual impingement while avoiding destabilization of the joint with over resection of bone.

POSTOPERATIVE MANAGEMENT

- Following cheilectomy with phalangeal osteotomy, the patient is instructed to continue elevating the operated extremity. The foot is immobilized in a rigid postoperative shoe and the patient is allowed to heel weight bear. At 2 to 3 weeks postoperatively, the sutures are removed, and the patient is allowed to weight bear as tolerated in the postoperative shoe. Gentle passive ROM exercises are initiated 3 weeks postoperatively. Patients can elect to work on motion on their own or go to physical therapy. Starting at 4 weeks postoperatively, the patient is allowed to wean from the postoperative shoe into loose-fitting, closed-toe shoes as tolerated.
- This postoperative course is the same with or without the dorsiflexion osteotomy.

RESULTS AND COMPLICATIONS

Good results are reported following cheilectomy.[15-17] In a report of 68 feet following cheilectomy, AOFAS score improved from a preoperative average of 45 to 85 points at follow-up, average dorsiflexion improved from 19° to 39°, and the average ROM improved from 34° to 64°.[15] Overall, long-term studies following cheilectomy demonstrate that it is a reliable procedure with high satisfaction rates and moderately low recurrence rate with most recurrences in the first 2 years.[18] Results of combined cheilectomy and closing wedge osteotomy have been reported to be superior compared with cheilectomy alone.[19] An example of MTP dorsiflexion motion 3 years postoperatively is shown in Figure 6.17. Based on the review of 24 toes undergoing combined cheilectomy and closing wedge osteotomy, Thomas and Smith[19] concluded that addition of the dorsal-closing wedge osteotomy of the proximal phalanx increases patient satisfaction and functional outcome in patients with moderate hallux rigidus.

Other studies have confirmed satisfactory results after closing wedge osteotomy. Citron and Neil[20] reported the long-term results of dorsal wedge osteotomy in eight women (10 toes) with a mean age of 23 years. All the patients had relief from pain soon after the surgery. At 22 years of follow-up, five toes were completely symptom-free, four others had slight discomfort but were able to engage in all activities of daily living, and only one had required MTP fusion. Others have reported good functional outcome after closing wedge osteotomies.[5]

The osteotomy is technically more challenging than isolated cheilectomy and does carry potential of additional complications. However, there is concern regarding persistent pain and MTP joint stiffness in patients with hallux rigidus after cheilectomy. There are also reports confirming progression of the underlying degenerative disease process,[15,16,21] and abnormal MTP motion patterns have been noted following cheilectomy.[22] In a cadaveric model, the increase in dorsiflexion after cheilectomy was found to be caused by pivoting of the proximal phalanx on the metatarsal head at the level of the cheilectomy.[22] The abnormal MTP kinematics may account for the progression of the disease after cheilectomy. Mulier et al[21] observed that 7 of 13 of their young patients exhibited radiologic

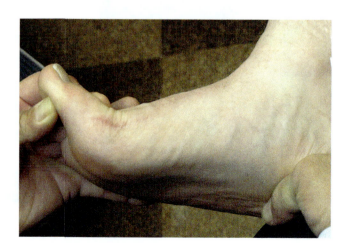

FIGURE 6.17 Clinical photograph (different patient) 3 years after surgery with improved dorsiflexion and a good clinical result.

progression of the disease within 4 years of their cheilectomies. Similarly, clinical and radiologic progression of the disease of at least one grade was seen in 32 of 68 feet in patients who underwent cheilectomy.[15] Fifteen (88%) of the 17 feet with grade I disease before surgery progressed one or two grades, and 24 (62%) of 39 feet with grade II hallux rigidus progressed to grade III.[15] Traditionally, the outcome of cheilectomy for hallux rigidus is thought to be more favorable in patients with milder disease.[4] However, Deland et al demonstrated satisfactory clinical outcomes in 81 patients with grade III disease who underwent cheilectomy and Moberg osteotomy indicating that select cases of advanced hallux rigidus can be treated with a joint-sparing procedure[11] (see ▶Video 6.1).

The complications of proximal phalangeal osteotomy with cheilectomy include nonunion, delayed union, or malunion. Avascular necrosis of the base of the phalanx and flexor hallucis longus tendon injury have been observed after other proximal phalangeal osteotomies, such as the akin osteotomy procedure, and are potential problems associated with the Moberg osteotomy. Persistent stiffness and limited increase in motion could result from an inadequate wedge resection. Inadvertent penetration of the phalangeal joint surface by the saw blade can also occur. This complication can be avoided by careful examination of the morphology of the phalanx and by placing a K-wire parallel to the joint surface to orient the first bone cut.

ACKNOWLEDGMENTS

We gratefully acknowledge the contribution of Dr. Harold Kitaoka for his work on this chapter.

REFERENCES

1. Davies-Colley N. Contraction of the metatarsophalangeal joint of the great toe (hallux flexus). *Br Med J.* 1887;1:728.
2. Hawkins BJ, Haddad RJ. Hallux rigidus. *Clin Sports Med.* 1988;7:37-49.
3. Canseco K, Long J, Marks R, et al. Quantitative motion analysis in patients with hallux rigidus before and after cheilectomy. *J Orthop Res.* 2009;27(1):128-134.
4. Hattrup SJ, Johnson KA. Subjective results of hallux rigidus following treatment with cheilectomy. *Clin Orthop Relat Res.* 1988;226:182-191.
5. Southgate JJ, Urry SR. Hallux rigidus: the long-term results of dorsal wedge osteotomy and arthrodesis in adults. *J Foot Ankle Surg.* 1997;36:136-140.
6. Yee G, Lau J. Current concepts review: hallux rigidus. *Foot Ankle Int.* 2008;29(6):637-646.
7. Seibert NR, Kadakia AR. Surgical management of hallux rigidus: cheilectomy and osteotomy (phalanx and metatarsal). *Foot Ankle Clin.* 2009;14(1):9-22.
8. Bonney G, Macnab I. Hallux valgus and hallux rigidus: a critical survey of operative results. *J Bone Joint Surg Br.* 1952;34:366.
9. Kessel L, Bonney G. Hallux rigidus in the adolescent. *J Bone Joint Surg Br.* 1958;40:668.
10. Moberg E. A simple operation for hallux rigidus. *Clin Orthop Relat Res.* 1979;142:55-56.
11. O'Malley MJ, Basran HS, Gu Y, Sayres S, Deland JT. Treatment of advanced stages of hallux rigidus with cheilectomy and phalangeal osteotomy. *J Bone Joint Surg Am.* 2013;95(7):606-610.
12. Karasick D, Wapner KN. Hallux rigidus deformity: radiologic assessment. *AJR Am J Radiol.* 1991;157:1029-1033.
13. Beeson P, Phillips C, Corr S, et al. Classification systems for hallux rigidus: a review of the literature. *Foot Ankle Int.* 2008;29(4):407-414.
14. Coughlin MJ, Shurnas PS. Hallux rigidus. Grading and long-term results of operative treatment. *J Bone Joint Surg Am.* 2003;85:2072-2088.
15. Easley ME, Davis WH, Anderson RB. Intermediate to long-term follow-up of medial approach dorsal cheilectomy for hallux rigidus. *Foot Ankle Int.* 1999;20:147-152.
16. Lin J, Murphy GA. Treatment of hallux rigidus with cheilectomy using a dorsolateral approach. *Foot Ankle Int.* 2009;30(2):115-119.
17. Mann RA, Clanton TO. Hallux rigidus: treatment by cheilectomy. *J Bone Joint Surg Am.* 1988;70:400-405.
18. Sidon E. Long-term follow-up of cheilectomy for treatment of hallux rigidus. *Foot Ankle Int.* 2019;40(10):1114-1121.
19. Thomas PJ, Smith RW. Proximal phalanx osteotomy for the surgical treatment of hallux rigidus. *Foot Ankle Int.* 1999;20(1):3-12.
20. Citron N, Neil M. Dorsal wedge osteotomy of the proximal phalanx for hallux rigidus: long-term results. *J Bone Joint Surg Br.* 1987;69:835-837.
21. Mulier T, Steenwerckx A, Thienpont E, et al. Results after cheilectomy in athletes with hallux rigidus. *Foot Ankle Int.* 1999;20:232-237.
22. Heller WA, Brage ME. The effects of cheilectomy on dorsiflexion of the first metatarsophalangeal joint. *Foot Ankle Int.* 1997;18:803-808.

7 Minimally Invasive Surgery (MIS) Cheilectomy With Moberg Osteotomy

Vandan D. Patel and Rebecca Cerrato

Hallux rigidus is a common degenerative condition of the first metatarsophalangeal (MTP) joint, characterized by osteophyte formation and pain with loss of motion. The classic osteophyte found involves the dorsal and central third of the articular surface of the first MTP joint, often involving both the metatarsal and proximal phalanx. This results in dorsal impingement with MTP joint dorsiflexion. Patients may also develop medial osteophytes and can present for evaluation of a painful bunion.[1] Dorsal impingement typically manifests as pain with push off during ambulation and dorsal skin irritation in shoe wear. It is classically found in patients older than 40 years of age and has a 2:1 female to male predominance.[1,2] Patients may also present with abnormal gait mechanics, increasing load onto the lateral aspect of the foot to minimize pain at the first MTP joint.[3]

Initial management consists of various nonoperative modalities, including rigid soled shoes or rigid inserts with Morton extension limiting the first MTP dorsiflexion. Anti-inflammatories and corticosteroid injection can provide symptomatic relief, while wider and deep toe boxes can reduce skin irritation over the dorsal joint.[1] Following failure of nonoperative management, surgical options can range from joint sparing procedures including cheilectomy and osteotomies to joint sacrificing procedures including arthroplasty and arthrodesis.[4]

Dorsal cheilectomy is indicated in early stages of the disease, where symptoms are predominantly related to the presence of dorsal osteophytes while joint space and motion is preserved. Coughlin and Shurnas demonstrated the 92% success rate with open cheilectomy in their series of 93 patients at a mean follow-up of 9.6 years.[5] More recent studies have also found good long-term results with open cheilectomy, with 69.3% of patients satisfied or very satisfied and 75.1% of patients who would repeat the operation at an average follow-up of 6.6 (5.0 to 10.9) years.[6] Cheilectomy is a viable option to improve pain, increase range of motion (ROM), maintain stability, and leave joint sacrificing procedures as secondary options.[1] In addition, the Kessel-Bonney osteotomy, which Moberg popularized, can be added. This dorsal closing wedge osteotomy of the proximal phalanx combined with dorsal cheilectomy moves the limited arc of motion of the joint to a more dorsiflexed position allowing better function and higher reported satisfaction.[7-9] O'Malley et al demonstrated success with open cheilectomy with Moberg osteotomy for Hattrup-Johnson grade 3 hallux rigidus in 69/81 satisfied patients with increased dorsiflexion from 32° to 60° and only four going onto arthrodesis at an average of 4.3 years.[10,11]

With the advent and popularization of minimally invasive surgery (MIS), cheilectomy is now possible through small stab incisions. The development of procedure-specific tools and instruments has advanced MIS techniques, and increasing literature is demonstrating comparable outcomes to classic open procedures. MIS procedures have the theoretical benefits of smaller incisions, better cosmesis, less soft tissue trauma, and faster recovery compared to their open counterparts. Small joint arthroscopy has also been introduced to supplement MIS procedures with direct visualization and examination of the joints.[12] MIS cheilectomy is an option for mild to moderate hallux rigidus with dorsal osteophytes causing impingement or irritation with shoe wear in patients who have failed nonoperative management.[13]

INDICATIONS AND CONTRAINDICATIONS

General indications for MIS cheilectomy are mild to moderate hallux rigidus with symptomatic dorsal osteophytes in those who have failed nonoperative management. In patients with severe joint degeneration, limited motion, and pain localized dorsally, MIS cheilectomy may be an alternative to fusion when the dorsal osteophyte is so prominent it limits shoe wear options and causes skin blisters or ulceration. Patients with greater than 6 months of pain, dorsal-based symptoms, pain at extremes of motion, greater than 50% joint space preservation, and radiographic dorsal osteophyte with minimal sagittal or axial plane deformity of the metatarsal are indicated. Experience with MIS and small joint arthroscopic instruments and techniques is a relative indication. Contraindications include advanced arthritis with positive grind test, greater than 50% joint space narrowing, midrange pain with passive MTP motion (grade 4), plantar or sesamoid pain, night or rest pain, lack of dorsal osteophyte, infection or compromised soft tissue, and joint malalignment necessitating corrective osteotomies.[13-16] While the literature describes success with up to grade 3 hallux rigidus and each patient should be evaluated individually, we recommend MIS cheilectomy in patients with grade 1 to 2 hallux rigidus with greater than 50% joint space preservation and dorsal osteophytes causing impingement pain at terminal dorsiflexion.

The indication for adding a Moberg osteotomy is based on intraoperative evaluation of dorsiflexion after cheilectomy procedure is completed. Limited dorsiflexion of less than 70° is a relative indication for addition of a Moberg osteotomy.[9] Patients should not only demonstrate limited dorsiflexion but also normal plantarflexion of the MTP so there is a sufficient arc of motion to essentially shift the functional ROM.[17] A Moberg-Akin biplanar osteotomy has been described for combined hallux rigidus and a hallux valgus interphalangeus angle 10° or greater.[18] Contraindications are similar to those cheilectomy previously described.

PREOPERATIVE PLANNING

A thorough and systematic history and physical should be performed. The ROM of the first MTP joint should be measured and documented. This can be measured using the axis of the proximal phalanx relative to the plantar surface of the foot or relative to the axis of the first metatarsal. The interphalangeal (IP) joint must be held in neutral to avoid overestimating motion. Careful examination of pain with passive motion of the MTP joint must be documented. Pain at terminal dorsiflexion indicates dorsal impingement, while pain at midarc motion and a positive MTP grind test indicates advanced degenerative changes. The soft tissue envelope and skin should be examined for signs of infection or compromise. Skin thickening or inflammation can also indicate shoe wear irritation at the prominence.

Weight-bearing radiographs should include anteroposterior (AP), oblique, and lateral views of the affected foot. The AP view can be used to evaluate the condition of the joint space, medial and lateral osteophytes, alignment of the MTP and IP joints, and condition of the surrounding joints. The oblique view can show additional osteophytes and joint space narrowing. The lateral view demonstrates the size and extent of the dorsal osteophytes on both sides of the MTP joint as well as further characterizes the joint space narrowing. Planned resection can be determined on this view, with up to 30% of the metatarsal head being acceptable. The Hattrup-Johnson classification is a simple radiographic grading system, which is helpful in characterizing the extent of disease. Grade 1 is mild to moderate osteophyte formation with good joint space preservation (Fig. 7.1A and B). Grade 2 is moderate osteophyte formation with joint space narrowing and subchondral sclerosis. Grade 3 is marked osteophyte formation and loss of visible joint space with or without subchondral cyst formation.[11] The Coughlin-Shurnas classification combines clinical and radiographic findings to grade the extent of disease (Table 7.1).[5] Advanced imaging is rarely indicated but can be helpful in assessing suspected intra-articular pathology.

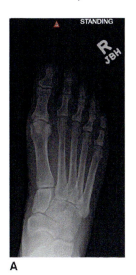
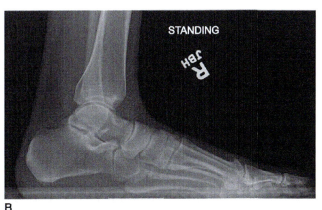

FIGURE 7.1 **A.** Anteroposterior weight-bearing foot radiograph with grade 1 (Hattrup-Johnson classification) hallux rigidus with preserved joint space. **B.** Lateral weight-bearing foot radiograph with grade 1 (Hattrup-Johnson classification) hallux rigidus with preserved joint space and dorsal metatarsal head spur.

SURGICAL TECHNIQUE

MIS Cheilectomy Technique

The procedure is an outpatient surgery. The appropriate MIS equipment should be available including a 3.1 × 13 mm wedge burr, MIS instruments (periosteal elevator, soft tissue rasp, beaver blade and handle), and high-speed power system specifically designed for MIS (Fig. 7.2A through C). Arthroscopic setup includes either a 1.9- or 2.7-mm 30° arthroscope, small joint shaver, saline irrigation on gravity, and small joint arthroscopic instruments (grasper, biter, and probe) (Fig. 7.3).

TABLE 7.1 Coughlin-Shurnas Grading for Hallux Rigidus

Grade	Dorsiflexion	Radiographic Findings	Clinical Findings
0	40°-60° and/or 10%-20% loss compared with normal side	Normal	No pain; only stiffness and loss of motion on examination
1	30°-40° and/or 20%-50% loss compared with normal side	Dorsal osteophyte is main finding, minimal joint space narrowing, minimal periarticular sclerosis, minimal flattening of metatarsal head	Mild or occasional pain and stiffness, pain at extremes of dorsiflexion and/or plantarflexion on examination
2	10°-30° and/or 50%-75% loss compared with normal side	Dorsal, lateral, and possibly medial osteophytes giving flattened appearance to metatarsal head, no more than 1/4 of dorsal joint space involved on lateral radiograph, mild to moderate joint space narrowing and sclerosis, sesamoids not usually involved	Moderate to severe pain and stiffness that may be constant; pain occurs just before maximum dorsiflexion and maximum plantarflexion on examination
3	≤10° and/or 75%-100% loss compared with normal side. There is notable loss of metatarsophalangeal plantarflexion as well (often ≤10° of plantarflexion)	Same as in grade 2 but with substantial narrowing, possibly periarticular cystic changes, more than 1/4 of dorsal joint space involved on lateral radiograph, sesamoids enlarged and/or cystic and/or irregular	Nearly constant pain and substantial stiffness at extremes of range of motion but not at midrange
4	Same as in grade 3	Same as in grade 3	Same criteria as grade 3, but there is definite pain at midrange of passive motion

Reprinted with permission from Coughlin MJ, Shurnas PS. Hallux rigidus grading and long-term results of operative treatment. *J Bone Joint Surg AM.* 2003;85(11):2072-2088. Copyright © 2003 by The Journal of Bone and Joint Surgery, Incorporated.

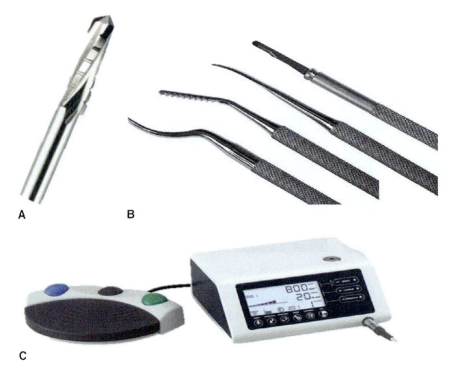

FIGURE 7.2 A. 3.1 × 13 mm wedge burr. **B.** MIS-specific instruments including beaver blade, periosteal elevators, and soft tissue rasps. **C.** MIS-specific power system with high torque and low speed that allows for adequate bone cutting/resection with less heat generation.

We prefer to place a nonsterile thigh tourniquet, though this is not inflated to allow additional cooling effect and debris extraction from the operative bleeding. General or regional anesthesia is used. We prefer light general anesthesia and perform an ankle block with a 50:50 mix of 0.5% Marcaine and 1% lidocaine.

The patient is positioned supine with the heels off at the end of the table (Fig. 7.4). An ipsilateral hip bump may be used to position the foot in a more vertical resting position. The operative heel will rest on and perpendicular to the image intensifier of the mini C-arm. We prefer the mini C-arm for ease of operation going back and forth between orthogonal views (Fig. 7.5). For a right-handed surgeon, the mini C-arm always comes in from the patient's right side regardless of the operative side (left side for left-handed surgeon). The limb is prepped and draped in usual sterile fashion, and appropriate surgical timeout is performed.

The bony landmarks are palpated and marked, including the metatarsal head, proximal phalanx, and extensor hallucis longus (EHL) tendon (Fig. 7.6). The dorsal medial cutaneous nerve (DMCN) should be marked if identifiable.

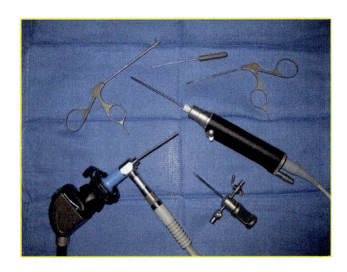

FIGURE 7.3 Small joint arthroscopy equipment including 1.9- or 2.7-mm 30° scope, small joint arthroscopy equipment (graspers, biters, and probe), and 2.5-mm shaver.

7 Minimally Invasive Surgery (MIS) Cheilectomy With Moberg Osteotomy

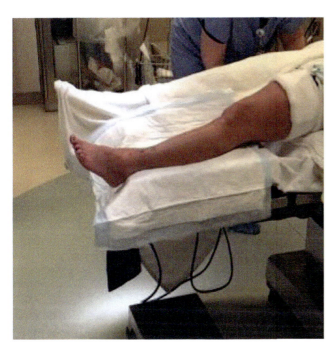

FIGURE 7.4 The patient is positioned with the foot over the end of the OR table to provide access for the mini C-arm to obtain orthogonal views.

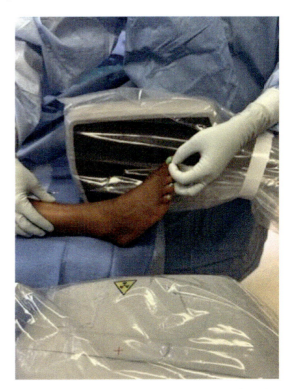

FIGURE 7.5 Mini C-arm is alternated between lateral view (shown) and anteroposterior view to assist surgeon in confirming correct position of burr and adequate bone resection.

A 3- to 5-mm dorsomedial stab incision is made using a beaver blade 2 cm proximal to the hallux MTP joint line (Fig. 7.7). When surgeons first start this procedure, a slightly larger incision will protect the skin from more excessive hand motions. The incision should be medial to the EHL tendon and plantar to the DMCN to avoid injuring either structure. Placing the portal too plantarly will create difficulty in reaching the entire osteophyte with the burr.

Blunt dissection is performed through the soft tissue to the bone with a curved hemostat. A curved periosteal elevator is then used to lift the capsule and dorsal soft tissues off the dorsal osteophyte and create a working pocket for the burr (Fig. 7.8).

The 3.1-mm wedge burr is introduced into this space. This is set to high torque and low speed (6,000 rpm) to minimize heat generation. Constant irrigation along the shaft of the burr, soft tissue, and bone is used to minimize thermal necrosis. The toe should not be held in plantarflexion to avoid tensioning and injuring the EHL tendon.

The burr begins at the base of the osteophyte and is advanced distally (Fig. 7.9A through C). Continue across the base until the osteophyte is removed. Engaging the osteophyte dorsally risks the EHL tendon and is avoided. Biplanar fluoroscopy is used to guide the burr and to assess resection. The burr is held in an agriculture grip position, and the burr is pulled toward the surgeons thumb (Fig. 7.10). Therefore, for a right-handed surgeon, the burr is moved medial to lateral for a left foot and lateral to medial for a right foot. The amount of resection desired is based on surgeon preference, similar to their open cheilectomies.

The burr will create a bony paste, which needs to be removed (Fig. 7.11). As the osteophyte is burred, intermittently pause to flush the debris with an angiocatheter and saline while applying manual pressure to express the debris. A soft tissue rasp can be used to remove soft tissue or capsular bone attachments. Careful fluoroscopic examination must be done to ensure proper debris removal. Any suspected opacity should warrant further débridement. For larger pieces, a small pituitary rongeur can be used. Saline irrigation should continue until the returned fluid is clear.

The burr can be advanced through the same portal dorsally over the base of the proximal phalanx to address any dorsal osteophytes at this level. This is done using a similar technique. Dorsiflexion of the toe can close down the MTP joint and bring the proximal phalanx to the burr.

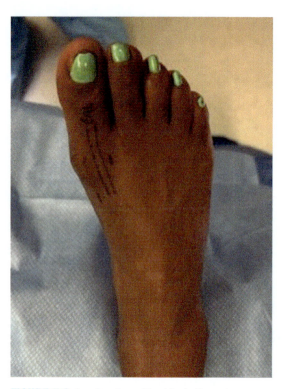

FIGURE 7.6 Landmarks outlined including extensor hallucis longus and joint line with the dorsomedial and dorsolateral portals marked out, as well as the proximal dorsomedial incision for the wedge burr.

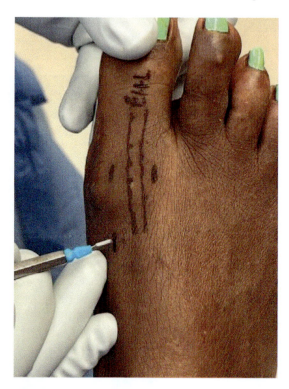

FIGURE 7.7 Beaver blade is used to make 2- to 3-mm incision at the dorsomedial incision marked approximately 2 cm proximal to metatarsophalangeal joint line and medial to extensor hallucis longus. After incision, hemostat used to spread subcutaneous tissue to minimize injury to dorsal medial cutaneous nerve.

Medial metatarsal or proximal phalanx osteophytes can be addressed through the dorsomedial portal. Lateral osteophytes may require an additional dorsolateral portal. This is made at the same level as the dorsomedial portal just lateral to the EHL tendon. Similar technique is used to create a soft tissue pocket and to insert the burr to remove lateral sided osteophytes.

At this point, we prefer to examine the MTP joint arthroscopically to assess for adequate resection, examine the articular surfaces, perform a synovectomy, and ensure removal of debris. Noninvasive distraction is applied to the toe using a 4 × 8 gauze in finger trap fashion (Fig. 7.12). A standard dorsomedial portal is made at the joint line. A small incision is made just through the skin medial to the EHL tendon at the level of the joint. Blunt dissection is done to the joint capsule, and the joint is bluntly entered with the straight hemostat.

A blunt trocar and cannula are placed through the prior dorsomedial cheilectomy portal, followed by a 2.7-mm arthroscope. Irrigation is to gravity. A small joint shaver is introduced through the additional dorsomedial portal at the joint and used to remove debris and synovitis (Fig. 7.13). The resection is carefully inspected, and the cuts can be smoothed down with the burr. An additional dorsolateral working portal can be made under direct visualization, just lateral to the EHL tendon at the level of the joint. This is done in similar technique with a small incision through the skin followed by blunt dissection and penetration into the joint. This portal can be used for additional débridement of bony fragments.

The joint is inspected for evaluation of the articular surfaces. An additional medial midaxial portal can be made for better visualization of the metatarsal head if needed. This is made at the distal portion of the MTP joint at the midaxial level using similar technique as prior portals. The arthroscope can be inserted to view the articular surface of the metatarsal head. The resection level is inspected by the arthroscope, and further removal or "touch-up" with the wedge burr can be performed with direct visualization using the arthroscope.

Once all debris and loose bodies are removed from the joint, the instruments are removed and the joint is again thoroughly irrigated. Fluoroscopy is used to confirm adequate resection and document ROM of the joint (Fig. 7.14).

7 Minimally Invasive Surgery (MIS) Cheilectomy With Moberg Osteotomy

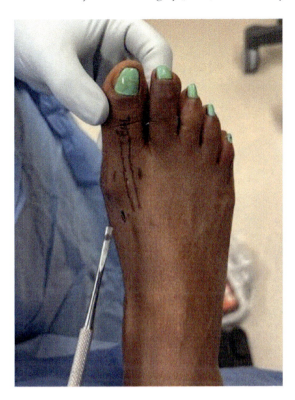

FIGURE 7.8 Following incision, soft tissue elevator introduced into incision and taken toward the joint on the dorsal metatarsal where it is used to enter capsule and elevate off dorsal metatarsal spur, moving carefully from medial to lateral.

Incisions may be closed with Steri-Strips or suture. We prefer placing No. 3-0 nylon interrupted stitches. Nonadherent gauze and a soft, compressive dressing are applied.

MIS Cheilectomy With Moberg Osteotomy Technique

The MIS cheilectomy is performed in the same fashion as described.

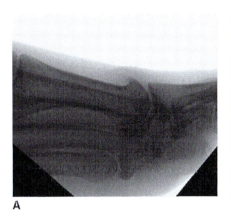

A

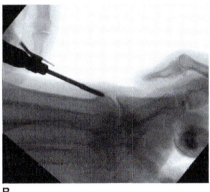

B

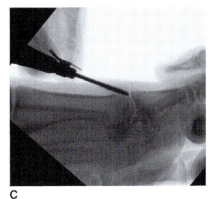

C

FIGURES 7.9 Lateral fluoroscopic views. **A.** Precheilectomy image showing dorsal metatarsal head osteophyte. **B.** Wedge burr initiated at the base of spur. **C.** Completion of resection with wedge burr. Note surgeon is not plantarflexing the hallux to reduce risk of injuring the extensor hallucis longus.

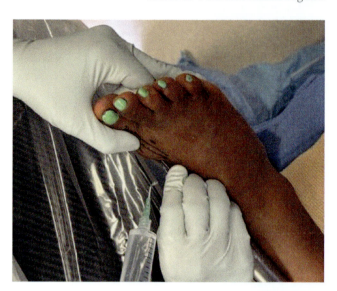

FIGURE 7.10 Pencil driver held with agricultural grip in order to control wedge burr across dorsal metatarsal head. Note additional irrigation at incision with angiocatheter and syringe.

After cheilectomy is completed, if dorsiflexion of the MTP joint is inadequate, an MIS Moberg osteotomy can be considered. Limited dorsiflexion of less than 70° is a relative indication for addition of a Moberg osteotomy.

A 2-mm longitudinal incision is made dorsally at the base of the proximal phalanx, medial to the EHL tendon. Fluoroscopic AP view can confirm the correct location for the incision. Blunt dissection is performed with a curved hemostat down to the bone. A periosteal elevator is used to create a working pocket from dorsal to plantar across the proximal phalanx base.

A 2 × 12 mm burr is placed onto the medial cortex of the proximal phalanx. Fluoroscopy is used to confirm the position and trajectory of the osteotomy distal to the joint and that the burr is not violating the plantar cortex (Fig. 7.15A). The toe is extended to protect the EHL tendon.

The osteotomy is performed perpendicular to the proximal phalanx base using the portal as a pivot point. The burr is advanced from medial to lateral, sparing the plantar cortex (Fig. 7.15B). Slight dorsal pressure on the toe can create the desired dorsal wedge size. Continuous irrigation is used to prevent thermal injury, and the portal is flushed to expel bone debris.

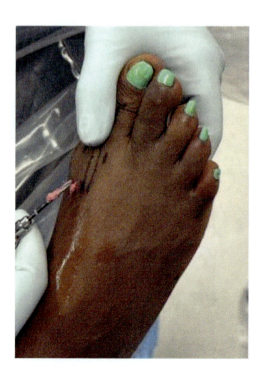

FIGURE 7.11 Resection of the dorsal spur creates bone paste seen on burr and at incision, which will require complete removal from joint to prevent inflammatory response and arthrofibrosis.

7 Minimally Invasive Surgery (MIS) Cheilectomy With Moberg Osteotomy

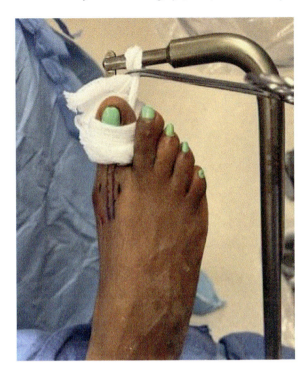

FIGURE 7.12 Noninvasive distraction is applied to the toe using a 4 × 8 gauze in finger trap fashion.

Closure of the dorsal wedge is confirmed on fluoroscopy. The osteotomy can be fixed with percutaneous placement of a screw or left to heal by osteoclasis[17,19] (Fig. 7.15C). Final fluoroscopy is used to document improved dorsiflexion arc of the toe.

PEARLS AND PITFALLS

Pearls

- A good physical examination, particularly assessment of ROM and pain, is critical in identifying patients who will benefit from cheilectomy alone.
- A thorough preoperative discussion is imperative to set the expectations regarding goals of the procedure, and risk of progressive arthritis should be discussed.
- Appropriate position of the dorsomedial portal is needed and should be planned with fluoroscopy if unsure to confirm appropriate trajectory and reach of the burr.
- Lateral osteophytes may require a dorsolateral portal to obtain thorough debridement.

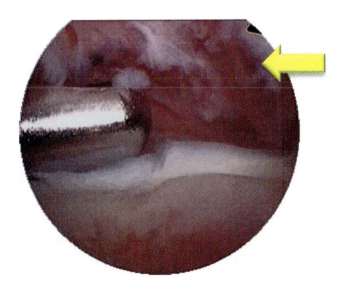

FIGURE 7.13 Arthroscopic view of the hallux MTP joint following cheilectomy with synovitis (*yellow arrow*).

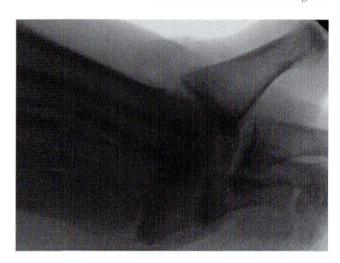

FIGURE 7.14 Final fluoroscopic evaluation is obtained to verify adequate and even resection, including maximum dorsiflexion view.

- Fluoroscopy should be used to guide and evaluate thoroughness of resection and to appropriately desired depth.
- Close examination of fluoroscopic opacities is needed to ensure that minimal bone debris remains.
- Confirm adequate dorsiflexion of the MTP joint under fluoroscopy and potential need for Moberg osteotomy.
- Arthroscopy is used for direct visualization of the bone cut, articular surface, synovitis, and to ensure through removal of bone debris.

Pitfalls

- Perform close preoperative radiographic evaluation to avoid operating on large angular or rotational deformities at the MTP joint.
- Identify and mark DMCN and avoid injury with careful placement of incision. Careful technique is used if the nerve is not identifiable.[20,21]

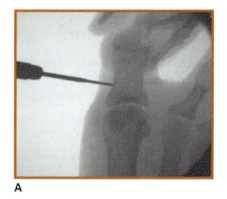
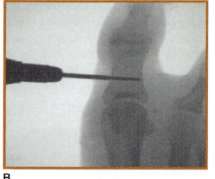

A

B

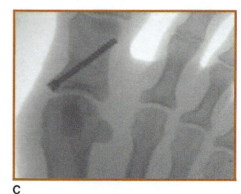

FIGURE 7.15 Percutaneous Moberg. **A.** Fluoroscopy is used to identify correct placement of a 2 × 12 mm cutting burr for osteotomy. **B.** The burr is taken across through the lateral cortex, leaving the plantar cortex intact. **C.** Optional fixation of the percutaneous Moberg osteotomy includes screw fixation.

C

- Excessively plantar placement of the initial dorsomedial portal will make lateral bone resection difficult.
- Thorough irrigation is necessary to avoid thermal injury and necrosis. Avoid high-speed burring and use short bursts with frequent cooling. Extend the skin incisions if needed.
- Left over bone debris can incite an inflammatory response leading to wound complications and joint stiffness.
- Plantarflexion of the toe during burring can increase risk of damage to the EHL tendon and dorsal soft tissues.
- Be prepared to convert to an open procedure at any point.
- Failure to begin early ROM and early weight bearing can lead to increased stiffness.

POSTOPERATIVE MANAGEMENT

The patient is placed in a soft dressing and allowed to weight bear as tolerated in a hard soled postoperative shoe. Any compressive wrap is taken down after 6 hours, but elevation is encouraged for the first 48 to 72 hours. Simple ROM is encouraged. The bandages are left in place until first follow-up in 10 to 14 days after surgery where sutures are removed if the portals are healed (Fig. 7.16). Other surgeons have their patients remove their dressing after several days to start early ROM. At this point, patients may return to normal shoe wear as their swelling allows and begin gentle advancement of activity. Gradual return to impact and sports may begin at 4 weeks. Physical therapy is not generally required.

RESULTS AND COMPLICATIONS

Although long-term results are lacking compared to classic open cheilectomy, the early to mid-term results of MIS cheilectomy have been promising.[5,6] Early adopters of the technique outside of the United States have begun to report their short- and mid-term results, with more data continuing to emerge.

Pastides et al prospectively followed the outcomes of their MIS cheilectomies in 47 feet, ranging from grade 1 to 3 hallux rigidus. At a mean of 17 months, they reported a mean AOFAS score of 87.1 and 32/35 patients recommended the procedure again. Two patients went on fusion, both with grade 3 disease.[22] Dawe et al compared open versus MIS cheilectomies reporting satisfaction scores of 9.1/10 and 8.6/10 for MIS and open groups, respectively. They only had a mean follow-up for 6 months for the MIS group and 35 months for the open group, and had one infection in each group. They concluded that both procedures had comparable early results.[23] Morgan et al completed an early prospective study comparing open and MIS cheilectomy, again showing comparable results.

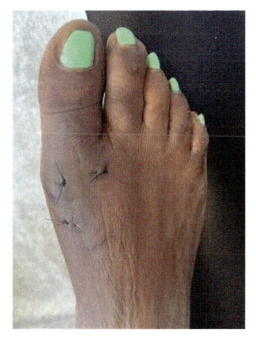

FIGURE 7.16 Clinical photo after patient returned 10 days s/p right hallux percutaneous metatarsophalangeal cheilectomy and arthroscopic synovectomy.

Manchester-Oxford Foot Questionnaire (MOXFQ) were completed pre- and postoperatively. The MIS group was followed to a median of 11 months and had an improvement in the MOXFQ score from 34/64 preoperatively to 19/64 postoperatively ($P < .02$). The open group also had a significant improvement in MOXFQ scores. Interestingly, the open group had three failures requiring conversion to fusion, while the MIS group had none. Their results showed effectiveness of MIS cheilectomy and similar improvements in pain, function, and social aspects with a potentially lower failure rate, though in a small cohort.[24]

Teoh et al followed 98 feet with MIS cheilectomy out to a mean of 50 months, demonstrating sustained improvement. Visual analogue scale (VAS) decreased from a mean of 8 to 3. Dorsiflexion was maintained at 69.1° compared to 11.3° preoperatively. MOXFQ scores were improved from 58.6 to 30.5. This score is worse than that reported by Morgan et al at 11 months, suggesting potential decline in results; however, this group started with a worse preoperative score and remained improved overall. They also reported a decrease in screening time and dosage of fluoroscopy at their center as they performed more MIS cheilectomies, suggesting a learning curve is present.[24,25] Similar outcomes were shown by Hickey et al who followed their group of 36 patients out to a mean of 4.69 years (2.0 to 7.3). Eighty-three percent recommended the procedure again, and 69% had mean postoperative pain improvement. In patients who still had pain, the mean pain score was 3.4/10. Eighty-one percent could wear fashionable shoes again. ROM was similarly improved.[26] The limited data of mid-term follow-up demonstrate comparable and sustained improvement for MIS cheilectomy.

Arthroscopy for dorsal impingement and cheilectomy can be used with MIS techniques. Arthroscopic-assisted spur resection is performed with visualization of the burr removing the dorsal spur. This is technically more difficult to perform with the limited joint space to perform the spur removal. Although early data showed mixed outcomes, Debnath et al found that their patients were 95% pain free after arthroscopic hallux rigidus treatment at 2 years. AOFAS scores improved from 43 to 97 and dorsiflexion from 8° to 30°. Two required joint sacrificing procedures at 2 years.[27-29] Glenn et al recently published their results of MIS cheilectomy supplemented with arthroscopy for examination of the joint, similar to our described technique. Unlike the arthroscopic-assisted approach, the MIS cheilectomy is performed first with the wedge burr using fluoroscopic guidance. The arthroscope is introduced into the joint following the dorsal bone resection, which now has a much larger work space to visualize and move around. At a mean follow-up of 16.5 months, they again demonstrated significantly improved VAS scores, dorsiflexion, and plantarflexion compared to preoperative measurements. They reported no revisions in that time period, and one patient who needed fusion at 3 years. On their reporting of arthroscopy findings, 100% of patients had bone debris despite thorough irrigation and 100% had synovitis. They attributed their lack of infection and wound issues as well as sustained outcomes to their more thorough débridement and inspection of the joint arthroscopically.[30] We agree with the authors regarding the benefits of arthroscopic evaluation; however, similar outcomes have been reported with and without arthroscopy after MIS cheilectomy.[25,26,30]

Kaplan et al has taken the procedure a step further by implementing it in the office setting. They describe a similar setup, using an intra-articular block of 5 mL 2% lidocaine and 0.5% bupivacaine 1:1 along with optional ankle or digital blocks. The procedure is then performed in a sterile, wide awake fashion in the office using a 1.9-mm, 0° needle arthroscope (NanoScope; Arthrex, Naples, Florida). They describe better cosmesis, reduced wound complications, reduced anesthesia complications, faster recovery, active patient participation, and health care cost savings as benefits of their technique.[16] Results and outcomes are yet to be reported.

The addition of the Moberg osteotomy remains an intraoperative decision by the surgeon. There is no direct comparison of MIS cheilectomy with and without Moberg osteotomy reported; however, the literature for open procedures can be extrapolated.[9,10] Mesa-Ramos et al performed cheilectomy with Moberg osteotomy in 26 feet and followed patients out to 18 months. They reported improvement in VAS scores from 7.44 to 1.69 and improvement in AOFAS scores from 58.45 to 92.36. All patients had improved ROM at 18 months.[31] De Prado added distal metatarsal plantarflexion osteotomy along with MIS cheilectomy and Moberg, finding 86% good or excellent results and improvement in AOFAS scores from 44 to 82 postoperatively.[19] De Arruda showed similar results in a series of seven patients with improved dorsiflexion, AOFAS scores, and VAS pain scores with no postoperative complications at a mean of 8 months postoperatively.[32] We do not routinely perform the MIS Moberg in conjunction with the MIS cheilectomy because we have not noticed a change in our patient's outcomes to warrant the increased recovery and delay in ROM. Ultimately, the addition of the Moberg osteotomy can be left to the surgeon's discretion.

The most common acute complications of MIS cheilectomy include thermal injury to soft tissue and bone, damage to tendons, nerve injury, and wound issues or infections.[33] Teoh et al reported two wound infections and two cases of delayed healing out of 98 patients. In all, 2/4 of these were smokers, and all were successfully treated with antibiotics. They had a 2% incidence of transient nerve palsy and two with permanent numbness in the DMCN. No patients had EHL tendon dysfunction.[25] In comparison, Hickey et al reported 1/36 with EHL tendon rupture 6 months postoperatively and 3/36 with numbness in the DMCN.[26] Two recent cadaveric studies measured the proximity of the DMCN to the dorsomedial incision. It was found an average of 3.8 mm from the incision and was cut in 2/13 specimens. They identified the danger zone to be at a third of the length of the metatarsal from the MTP joint. It was also suggested that the incisions be avoided between the 10 and 2 o'clock positions relative to the medial border of the EHL tendon to avoid the DMCN and the dorsolateral cutaneous nerve.[20,21] Glenn et al reported no nerve or EHL tendon injuries and no wound issues with their addition of arthroscopy to the procedure. Again they attribute this to a more thorough débridement of bone debris, which can be inflammatory and contribute to wound healing complications.[30] Stevens et al performed a retrospective comparison of MIS and open cheilectomy including 38 open and 138 MIS procedures. They reported no infections in the MIS group. They reported no difference in wound complications between the two groups (2.6% open vs 3.0% in MIS), and attributed the MIS wound issues to bone particles not being evacuated. The MIS group had one nerve injury and one EHL tendon rupture, similar to the findings in the other studies. Overall complication rates tended to be higher in the MIS group, though did not reach statistical significance (11.3% vs 2.6% RR 4.29, P = .076).[34]

A higher reoperation rate has been reported with MIS cheilectomy compared to open surgery. In a study by Stevens et al, at a mean of 3 years, one of the open group required fusion and 17 of the MIS group required reoperation (2.6% vs 12.8%, RR 4.86, P = 0.059). Within the MIS group, 10 (7.5%) patients had persistent stiffness and 9 went on to arthrodesis and 1 had interpositional arthroplasty. All of the reoperations were attributed to the MIS technique, mainly the residual bone debris. They felt that their operations and complications were not attributed to a learning curve with the MIS technique, as there was no decrease when comparing two yearly cohorts across 6 years.[34] In comparison, Teoh et al, who found a similar reoperation rate of 12% (n = 12, 7 arthrodesis, 4 repeat cheilectomy), attributed 42% of their reoperations directly to technique and a learning curve.[25] Interestingly, the groups who performed arthroscopy in conjunction with MIS cheilectomy reported no revision surgeries and one fusion at 3 years.[26,30]

There is some level of learning curve associated with all MIS foot and ankle procedures, and this may contribute to some complications and reoperations. Arthroscopy is helpful to augment especially if inexperienced with the burr and may provide a more thorough washout of bone debris, which can minimize wound complications.[12] Small joint arthroscopy has its own learning curve; however, following the cheilectomy, the working space for the arthroscope is much greater, and this can be the ideal scenario for surgeons to acquire skills for small joint arthroscopy.

REFERENCES

1. Walter R, Parera A. Open, arthroscopic, and percutaneous cheilectomy for hallux rigidus. *Foot Ankle Clin N Am.* 2015;20:421-431.
2. Coughlin MJ, Shurnas PS. Hallux rigidus: demographics, etiology, and radiographic assessment. *Foot Ankle Int.* 2003;24(10):731-743.
3. Canseco K, Long J, Marks R, et al. Quantitative motion analysis in patients with hallux rigidus before and after cheilectomy. *Orthop Res.* 2009;27(1):128-134.
4. Keiserman LS, Sammarco VJ, Sammarco GJ. Surgical treatment of the hallux rigidus. *Foot Ankle Clin.* 2005;10(1):75-96.
5. Coughlin MJ, Shurnas PS. Hallux rigidus grading and long-term results of operative treatment. *J Bone Joint Surg.* 2003;85(11):2072-2088.
6. Sidon E, Rogero R, Bell T, et al. Long-term follow-up of cheilectomy for treatment of hallux rigidus. *Foot Ankle Int.* 2019;40(10):1114-1121.
7. Kessel L, Bonney G. Hallux rigidus in the adolescent. *J Bone Joint Surg Br.* 1958;40:668.
8. Moberg E. A simple operation for hallux rigidus. *Clin Orthop Relat Res.* 1979;142:55-56.
9. Waizy H, Czardybon MA, Stukenborg-Colsman C, et al. Mid- and long-term results of the joint preserving therapy of hallux rigidus. *Arch Orthop Trauma Surg.* 2010;130:165-170.
10. O'Malley MJ, Basran HS, Gu Y, et al. Treatment of advanced stages of hallux rigidus with cheilectomy and phalangeal osteotomy. *J Bone Joint Surg.* 2013;95(7):606-610.
11. Hattrup SJ, Johnson KA. Subjective results of hallux rigidus following treatment with cheilectomy. *Clin Orthop Relat Res.* 1988;226:182-191.
12. Redfern D, Vernois J, Legre BP. Percutaneous surgery of the forefoot. *Clin Podiatr Med Surg.* 2015;32:291-332.
13. Schipper ON, Day J, Ray GS, et al. Percutaneous techniques in orthopedic foot and ankle surgery. *Orthop Clin N Am.* 2020;51:403-422.
14. Razik A, Sott AH. Cheilectomy for hallux rigidus. *Foot Ankle Clin N Am.* 2016;21:451-457.
15. Hunt KJ. Hallux metatarsophalangeal (MTP) joint arthroscopy for hallux rigidus. *Foot Ankle Int.* 2015;36(1):113-119.

16. Kaplan DJ, Chen JS, Colasanti CA, et al. Needle arthroscopy cheilectomy for hallux rigidus in the office setting. *Arthrosc Tech*. 2022;11(3):385-390.
17. De Prado M, Cuervas-Mons M, De Prado V, et al. Minimally invasive management of hallux rigidus. In: Scuderi GR, Tria AJ, eds. *Minimally Invasive Surgery in Orthopedics*. Springer International Publishing; 2016:783-801.
18. Hunt KJ, Anderson RB. Biplanar proximal phalanx closing wedge osteotomy for hallux rigidus. *Foot Ankle Int*. 2012;33(12):1043-1050.
19. De Prado M, Cuervas-Mons M. Minimal incision surgery in hallux rigidus. *J Foot Ankle*. 2022;16(1):9-11.
20. Teoh KH, Haanaes EK, Alshalawi A, et al. Minimally invasive dorsal cheilectomy of the first metatarsal: a cadaveric study. *Foot Ankle Int*. 2018;39(2):1497-1501.
21. Malagelada F, Dalmau-Pastor M, Fargues B, et al. Increasing the safety of minimally invasive hallux surgery—an anatomical study introducing the clock method. *Foot Ankle Surg*. 2018;24:40-44.
22. Pastides PS, El-Sallakh S, Charalambides C, et al. Minimally invasive cheilectomy for the treatment of grade I to III hallux rigidus: a prospective study reporting on early patient outcome. *Tech Foot Ankle Surg*. 2014;13(2):98-102.
23. Dawe ECJ, Ball T, Annamalai S, et al. Early results of minimally invasive cheilectomy for painful hallux rigidus. *Bone Joint J*. 2012;94(suppl XXII):33.
24. Morgan S, Jones C, Palmer S. Minimally invasive cheilectomy (MIS): functional outcome and comparison with open cheilectomy. *J Bone Joint Surg Br*. 2012;94:93.
25. Teoh KH, Tan WT, Atiyah Z, et al. Clinical outcomes following minimally invasive dorsal cheilectomy for hallux rigidus. *Foot Ankle Int*. 2019;40(2):195-201.
26. Hickey BA, Stew D, Namblar M, et al. Intermediate-term results of Isolated minimally invasive arthroscopic cheilectomy in the treatment of hallux rigidus. *Eur J Orthop Surg Traumatol*. 2020;30:1277-1283.
27. van Dijk CN, Veenstra KM, Nuesch BC. Arthroscopic surgery of the first metatarsophalangeal joint. *Arthroscopy*. 1998;14:851-855.
28. Iqbal M, Chana G. Arthroscopic cheilectomy for hallux rigidus. *Arthroscopy*. 1998;14(3):307-310.
29. Debnath U, Hemmady M, Hariharan K. Indications for and technique of first MTP arthroscopy. *Foot Ankle Int*. 2006;27(12):1049-1054.
30. Glenn RL, Gonzales TA, Peterson AB, et al. Minimally invasive dorsal cheilectomy and hallux metatarsophalangeal joint arthroscopy for the treatment of hallux rigidus. *Foot Ankle Orthop*. 2021;6(1):1-7.
31. Mesa-Ramos M, Mesa-Ramos F, Carpintero P. Evaluation of the treatment of hallux rigidus by percutaneous surgery. *Acta Orthop Belg*. 2008;74(2):222-226.
32. De Arruda JF, Baptista AD. Percutaneous cheilectomy combined with Waterman and Moberg osteotomies for the treatment of hallux rigidus. *Sci J Foot Ankle*. 2019;13(2):135-139.
33. Walther M, Chomej P, Kriegelstein S, et al. Minimal invasive cheilectomie. *Oper Orthop Traumatol*. 2018;30:161-170.
34. Stevens R, Bursnall M, Chadwick C, et al. Comparison of complication and reoperation rates for minimally invasive versus open cheilectomy of the first metatarsophalangeal joint. *Foot Ankle Int*. 2020;41(1):31-36.

PART THREE
TOTAL ANKLE REPLACEMENT

8 Salto Talaris Total Ankle Replacement

James S. Davitt

INTRODUCTION

The Salto Talaris (currently Smith-Nephew, Memphis, Tennessee) ankle replacement system was developed based on the Salto Mobile Version (Tornier N.V., Amsterdam, Netherlands). The original design was developed in France in the 1990s as a mobile-bearing ankle prosthesis.[1] The talar component was designed with dual radii of curvature for the talar component—with the lateral radius larger. The talar component is also broader anteriorly. This was done to replicate the talar dome morphology. However, there is controversy regarding this. A study based on three-dimensional computed tomography (CT) measurements of medial and lateral radii found that the medial radius was larger.[2] However, a CT study of 50 cadaveric tali found some variability.[3] By fitting circles to the anterior and posterior curves of the tali, these authors found that the anterior medial radius of curvature was smaller than the anterior lateral radius by a mean of 7.8 mm. Posteriorly, however, the medial radius was larger in 60% of the tali and smaller in 40% indicating more variability. Fluoroscopic studies done on 20 patients who underwent Salto total ankle replacement demonstrated approximately 1.5 mm of anterior to posterior translation of the mobile-bearing during gait.[4] The prosthesis was redesigned to take advantage of the mobile-bearing concept but build it into the implantation procedure. This led to the development and introduction of the fixed-bearing Salto Talaris design used in the United States in 2006.

IMPLANTS

The tibial implant initially came in three sizes (1, 2, and 3) with a smaller size 0 added in 2009 (Fig. 8.1A and B). The base plate is 4 mm thick. There is a 12-mm-long central keel with a hollow conical plug that is slightly tapered front to back to provide for compression and initial stability as it is inserted. Left and right sides are identical. It was redesigned in 2013 to add 1 mm of width and 2 mm of length to each size. In 2019, an extended version of sizes 1 to 3 was added for improved posterior coverage. The component is manufactured of cobalt-chrome coated with 200-μm plasma-sprayed titanium.

The talar component also comes in four sizes (0, 1, 2, and 3). The design is based on the dual radii of curvature of the talus with a biconvex surface to mimic a natural talus and improve stability over previous ankle implants (Fig. 8.2). Initial stability is achieved by three chamfer cut surfaces—posterior, anterior, and lateral along with a central hollow plug. In sizes 1, 2, and 3, the plug is a constant distance from the lateral chamfer allowing for the ability to change sizes. The size 0 has a slightly smaller distance between the plug and lateral chamfer as well as no fixed bone within the hollow plug. This may impact fixation of the size 0 talar component. The talar component is also cobalt-chrome coated with plasma-sprayed titanium and comes in left and right versions. As part of the redesign process, a flat cut talus is also available, which was initially part of the revision prosthesis.

Standard polyethylene inserts come in different thicknesses to achieve stability (8, 9, 10, 11, and 13 mm—combined thickness of poly and tibial base plate). The poly insert can be used to

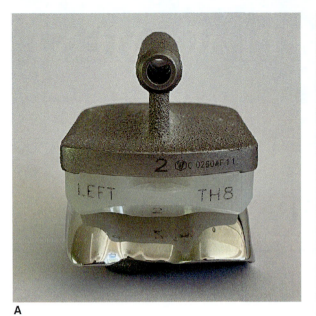 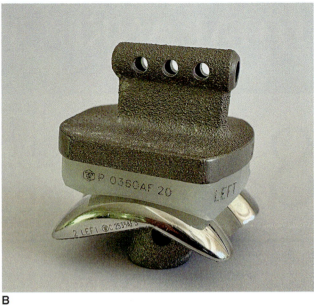

FIGURE 8.1 **A, B.** Salto Talaris ankle arthroplasty.

accommodate a one size smaller talar component for a better fit, that is, a size 3 tibia can function with a size 2 or size 3 talus. The poly insert is locked onto the tibial tray prior to implantation.

The basic procedure consists of measured resection—typically 9 mm from the tibia and 7 mm from the talus (or 5.5 mm for a size 0) using an extramedullary alignment guide. The tibial component cut is made with either 3° or 7° of posterior slope—most common is 3°. The initial talar cut is based off the same tibial extramedullary alignment. Once the cuts have been made, trial components are placed, which include a highly polished tibial base plate. This can rotate and translate above the talar trial and highly constrained trial liner. The ankle is taken through a range of motion as the tibial trial moves to find the "sweet spot." Once the ideal position is identified, the tibial keel cuts are made, which sets the final rotation and position of the tibial component. Essentially, this takes the mobile bearing out of the implant and into the implantation.

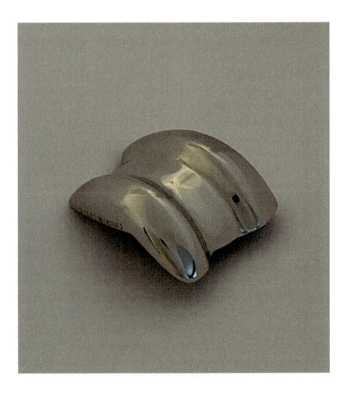

FIGURE 8.2 Note the biconvex superior surface for improved stability.

INDICATIONS AND CONTRAINDICATIONS

Standard indications for ankle arthroplasty are similar to arthroplasty in the hip and knee. End-stage osteoarthritis is the most common indication. Most ankle osteoarthritis is secondary to trauma and/or instability. Other indications include rheumatoid arthritis or other inflammatory arthropathies, pigmented villonodular synovitis, or similar erosive arthropathies. Contraindications include vascular insufficiency, neuropathy, active or potential for latent infection, severe uncorrectable deformity in or above the ankle, or significant osteoporosis/osteonecrosis. Of upmost importance is the ability to obtain a stable plantigrade foot under a balanced ankle. Often times that may require correction of the deformity or instability prior to contemplating an ankle arthroplasty.

PREOPERATIVE PLANNING

Weight-bearing radiographs of the ankle are essential in preoperative planning with a magnification marker. This allows for evaluation of alignment, deformity, and sizing of the implants. A hindfoot alignment view along with a full length long-standing view of the lower extremity (hip to ankle) have become standard in our institution to fully evaluate for potential additional corrections, that is, osteotomies, or manipulation of the extramedullary guide during the surgical procedure (Fig. 8.3A through E). Obviously, if there are foot deformities or muscle imbalance, weight-bearing radiographs of the foot are also warranted. CT scan can be helpful in identifying significant peritalar arthritis or larger periarticular cysts that may affect the surgical outcome.

SURGICAL TECHNIQUE

Positioning

The patient is positioned on the operative table supine with a bump under the ipsilateral hip to rotate the leg into a neutral position with the foot and toes pointing directly up. The knee is prepped into the field to help assess alignment in the coronal plane. The use of a thigh tourniquet is routine. The foot should be positioned near the end of the table to facilitate ease of surgery with the surgeon at the foot of the bed and the assistant usually on the lateral side of the operative ankle. This also facilitates performing a calcaneal osteotomy if necessary. Finally, a large C-arm is brought in from the opposite side. Often a bump under the knee is used to facilitate exposure. This can be moved under the ankle for fluoroscopy and talar preparation.

Approach

The Salto Talaris is inserted via the standard anterior approach beginning 7 to 8 cm above the ankle and extending distally to level of the talonavicular joint. The anterior compartment is incised over the extensor hallucis longus tendon to keep the anterior tibialis tendon completely covered within its sheath when possible. Distally, the superficial peroneal nerve should be swept or mobilized laterally and protected. Blunt dissection can then be used to develop the interval between the anterior tibialis and extensor hallucis longus tendons. The deep neurovascular bundle is retracted laterally. There are several crossing and sometimes larger veins that need to be coagulated.

The periosteum and capsule are then incised, and a Cobb elevator is used to create medial and lateral capsuloperiosteal flaps. It is important to maintain the integrity of this layer as it is used for closure. The medial and lateral gutters are completely exposed, and if the ankle joint is in varus, now is a good time to perform a medial release to help square the ankle joint. The medial release is done directly off the medial malleolus in a sleeve preserving the distal tibial periosteum with the deltoid. The release is complete when the posterior tibial tendon is visualized. The release can be completed after the distal tibial bone is removed as there will be more space to maneuver. Débride osteophytes to free up ankle joint paying particular attention to the medial and lateral gutters. Anything that prevents the joint from returning to a neutral alignment must be removed or it will affect the ability to identify the "sweet spot" during trialing.

An osteotome is used to remove the anterior osteophytes in order to visualize the tibial roof—the most superior surface of the articular surface as seen on the lateral radiograph (Fig. 8.4). Preoperative films are helpful to assess this level, which is the landmark for the tibial resection level. At this time,

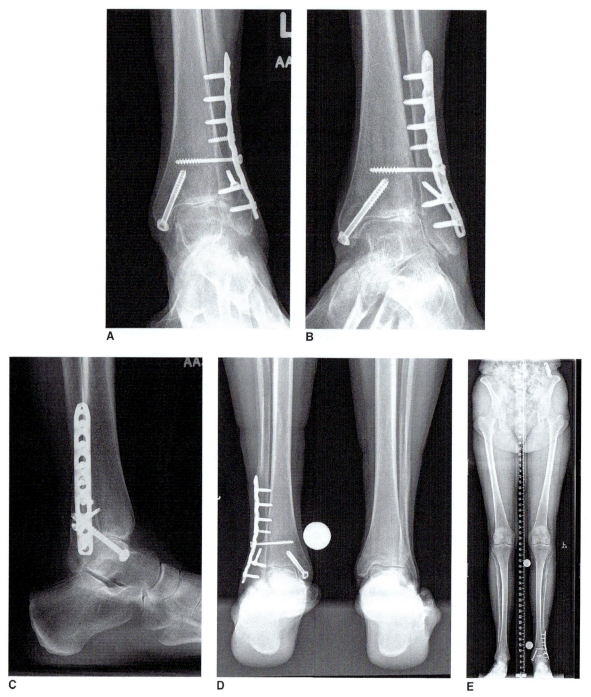

FIGURE 8.3 A-E. Standard preoperative views including anteroposterior, mortise, and lateral views of the ankle weight bearing. Also included are full length hip to ankle films and a hindfoot alignment view. Note the valgus on the arthritic left ankle.

it is helpful to remove the talar neck osteophytes. This will facilitate placement of the initial talar pin and simplify the process of performing the anterior chamfer cut on the talus.

Identify the tibial tubercle and place a 110-mm pin just through two cortices. Take care not to plunge. Oftentimes, this needs to be predrilled. This pin needs to be placed perpendicular to the tibia in all planes. An assistant is helpful here to gauge this. Full length lower extremity weight-bearing films preoperative are essential to assess for alignment. Frequently patients have arthritis at multiple joints, and any significant knee malalignment should be corrected prior to ankle replacement. The goal is to have the tibial base plate parallel to the surface of the floor when standing as visualized on an anteroposterior (AP) weight-bearing radiograph.

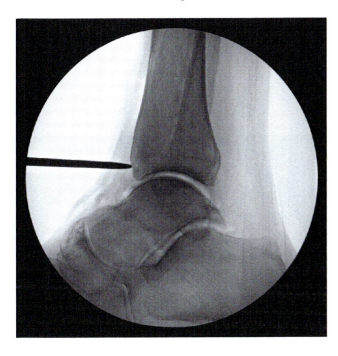

FIGURE 8.4 Osteotome at the level of the pilon roof.

Tibial Alignment

Varus/Valgus

The extramedullary alignment guide is applied with the 3° posterior slope block attached (7° available also). Knobs should all be loosely tightened. The guide should be set to the zero or center mark at the proximal end. Based on preoperative templating, this may need to be adjusted medially or laterally to correct for varus or valgus. Again, the goal is to obtain a neutral plafond on standing. This is typically aligned to the anatomic axis of the tibia when no proximal malalignment is present. However, if there is significant malalignment proximally, it should be identified and corrected prior to ankle replacement surgery. The alignment guide should run parallel to the tibial crest approximately two fingerbreadths anteriorly.

The center knob is loosened, and the distal portion of the guide translated to the level of the joint. Typically, the initial resection level is set to 0 mm. An osteotome in the joint (Fig. 8.5) can facilitate distal placement of the flange at the level of the pilon roof. The distal cut surface of the guide should

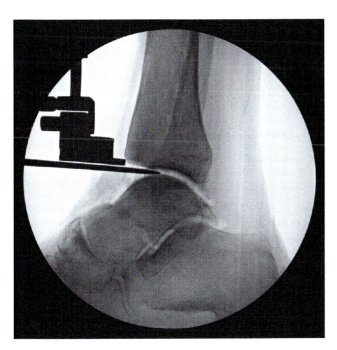

FIGURE 8.5 The pilon roof has been identified, and an osteotome defines the level of the distal tibia. The guide is set to 0 mm resection.

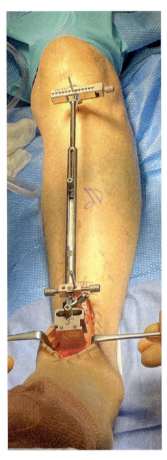

FIGURE 8.6 Extramedullary alignment guide pinned proximally and distally.

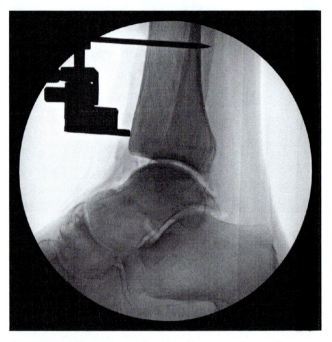

FIGURE 8.7 The resection level has been moved up to 9 mm, and the distal pin has been placed.

be parallel to a neutral plafond. The center knob is tightened. A second 110-mm pin is then placed. This can be placed through either the medial or lateral hole whichever will get the better purchase. Although the pins are self-drilling, a drill bit is preferred to minimize thermal necrosis. Pins should both be just bicortical. Fluoroscopy can be a helpful check to ensure a neutral plafond cut in the frontal plane. If necessary, the proximal guide can be shifted medially or laterally to correct any varus or valgus. The set screws on the pins are then tightened (Fig. 8.6). The other distal set screw should be loosened to allow the cut block to move.

The slope block is then translated proximally to the 9 mm level (Fig. 8.7) and the set screw tightened. One must ensure that the distal cut will remove enough bone to account for any significant abnormal wear. In a looser, oftentimes a valgus ankle, removing less tibia can help to minimize the thickness of the polyethylene and balance the soft tissues.

Rotational and Medial/Lateral Translation

Next, the rotational and medial to lateral translation adjustments are made with the tibial alignment jig.

It is first attached to the slope block. The gutters are identified to assess for rotation. This can be done by placing a medium pin in each gutter at the proximal corner of the joint or a thin malleable retractor can be used in each gutter. A long pin is then placed in the center hole of the adjustable arm, and the jig is rotated until the long pin bisects the angle created by the gutter pins/malleables. The rotational adjustment set screw is then secured. This ensures that the tibial cut matches the rotation of the native tibia.

Next, translation is assessed using medium pins in the holes on the side of the jig marked 0 to 3. The medial pin should be aligned with the medial corner of the ankle joint. The lateral pin should be at the lateral vertical joint space but not into the fibula (Fig. 8.8). Tighten the translation set screw. Remember you are not committed to a size yet.

8 Salto Talaris Total Ankle Replacement

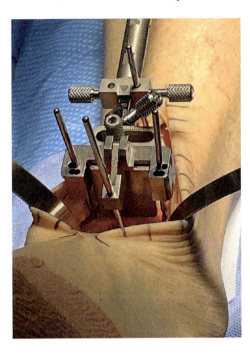

FIGURE 8.8 The rotational/translational guide has been applied with medium pins in the size 1 holes, and the central long pin remains from the rotational check.

Distal Tibial Cut

Apply the selected tibial cut guide after removing the alignment guide. There are two styles—the original with drill holes on the side and the newer version with cut slots. The author's preference is for the original style. The set screw is tightened. The middle hole on each side is drilled halfway through, and two medium pins are placed (Fig. 8.9). The cut guide can be removed, and fluoroscopy brought in to confirm appropriate medial to lateral positioning prior to final cut (Fig. 8.10). If the corners of the cut are incorrect, minor final adjustments can be made while preserving the proximal holes in the guide to protect the saw sweep. Once position is confirmed, drill all six holes bicortically starting with the proximal two and placing a medium pin in each of the proximal holes.

With the pins protecting the sweep of the saw, the distal tibial cut is made. Irrigation is used to cool the blade. The cut block is removed. A thin osteotome is used to connect the holes for the

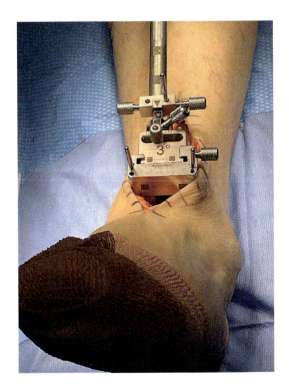

FIGURE 8.9 Tibial cutting block pinned through the middle holes. This allows a fluoroscopic check of the medial to lateral translation without burning the proximal hole.

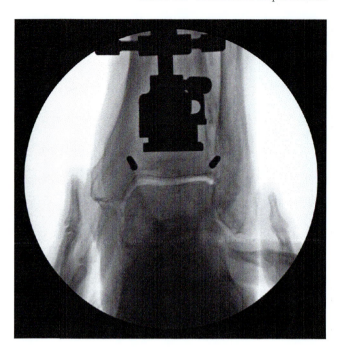

FIGURE 8.10 Now in the anteroposterior view, pins are marking the medial and lateral extent of the distal tibial cut. These have been placed in the middle holes of the guide so that if an adjustment needs to be made the proximal holes will be stable for the distal tibial cut.

vertical edges of the cut. The distal tibial bone is then removed piecemeal. At this time, all the bone is removed. This facilitates a size check at this time. The set screws on the two pins only are loosened so the whole alignment guide can be removed. The appropriate size tibial trial along with an 8-mm poly trial is assembled and inserted into the joint (Fig. 8.11). If it can be placed, then enough tibia has been resected, if not, now is a good time to recut the distal tibia.

If you have elected to make the size check, replace the tibial guide and retighten the set screws ensuring that the guide is in the same position as prior to removal. If the tibial cut was too distal, translate the cut block the appropriate amount proximally (usually 2 mm). Redrill the proximal screw holes and place medium pins and then recut the tibia.

Talar Alignment

The talar pin guide is then applied to the slope block. The ankle is positioned neutrally in terms of varus/valgus and dorsiflexion/plantarflexion. Ensure that the ankle is not translated anteriorly or

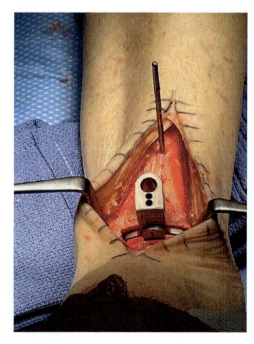

FIGURE 8.11 The guide has been removed to facilitate placement of the tibial trial and 8-mm poly. This is done to ensure that the tibial cut is proximal enough to accommodate the thinnest poly insert.

8 Salto Talaris Total Ankle Replacement

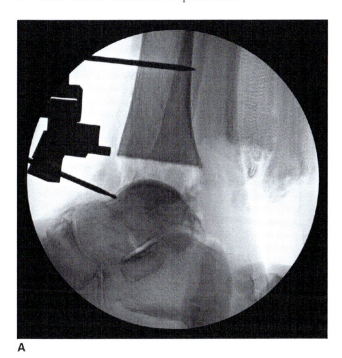
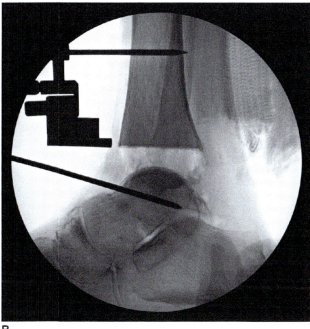

FIGURE 8.12 A, B. Talar alignment pin pointing toward the posterior third of the subtalar joint. The ankle is held in neutral position while the pin is drilled and placed. The posterior chamfer cut will parallel that pin.

posteriorly as well. A bump placed behind the distal tibia helps with this. Pin the talus through one of the holes in the pin guide (Fig. 8.12A). The pin guide is the angle of the posterior chamfer cut on the talus. The pin should point at the posterior third of the posterior subtalar joint (Fig. 8.12B). C-arm is quite helpful here. Usually, the center hole works best but adjust as needed. The alignment guide can be removed by loosening the set screws on the tibial pins, but leave all others snug in case the jig needs to be reapplied. Leave the talar pin in place.

Posterior Chamfer

Remove the cartilage from the talar dome if any remains. Check for uneven wear. Choose the talar pin guide based on the size of the talus. It is either a size 0 or size 1, 2, 3. Check for talar sizing with the talar gauge (lollipop). Remember that the talar component can be the same size as the tibia or one size smaller. If necessary to accommodate for uneven wear, a shim can be added to the worn side. Apply the posterior chamfer pin guide over the talar pin. The arms of the guide should parallel the talus. Lamina spreaders medially and laterally can help hold the guide in place (Fig. 8.13A and B). The set screw is tightened. The spreaders should rest on the highest point of the talus to avoid bending the pin. Next, the four pin holes are drilled and filled with medium pins. The pin pusher facilitates this. Typically, the central two are drilled and filled first followed by the peripheral ones as they require more soft tissue protection particularly laterally to avoid the superficial peroneal nerve. All pins need to be bicortical, and this should be confirmed with the fluoroscopy by swinging the C-arm into the lateral position (Fig. 8.14). The C-arm is left in the lateral position for the next several steps. The guide is removed, and the posterior chamfer cut made using the pins as a guide. Malleable retractors are placed in the gutters to protect the sweep of the saw blade. This is done under irrigation. The cut is complete when the dome moves. This is removed and the cut finished so that the entire top of all pins is visible, ensuring that the cut is flush with the guide pins (Fig. 8.15). In a smaller talus only three pins may be possible. In the newer 2.1 instrumentation, a talar cut through guide replaces the guide pins and is referenced off the initial talar alignment pin.

Anterior Chamfer

This cut can be made with either the standard guide or the 2.1 instrumentation. If osteophytes on the talar neck were not removed at the beginning, they should be removed now. This is critical as it affects the anterior positioning of the talar component. The standard instrumentation does not use

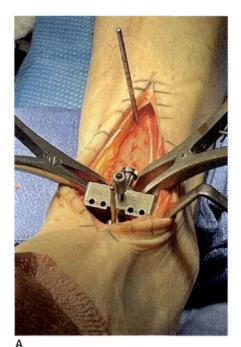 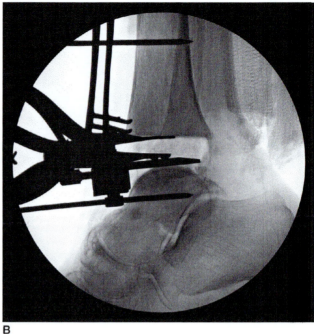

FIGURE 8.13 A, B. Posterior chamfer guide has been applied, and all cartilage has been removed from the talus. Lamina spreaders assist in holding the guide flush to the talar dome.

the talar pin, so it is removed. The anterior chamfer guide is inserted with the talar spacer in the oblong window. "ANT" should be in the front, and the guide should be flush on the posterior chamfer cut. With the foot held in neutral, the calibration line on the guide needs to be flush with the anterior cortex of the tibia (Fig. 8.16A and B). If it is anterior, more talar neck should be resected until it is flush. If it sits posterior, reposition the guide so that it sits flush. When positioning the guide, the handle should line up with the second or third toe. Once the position is set, lamina spreaders can be used to ensure that there is no movement of the jig. The surgeon holds the jig securely, while the

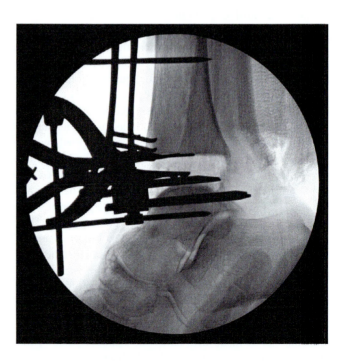

FIGURE 8.14 Pins have been placed. It is important that they extend beyond the posterior edge of the talus.

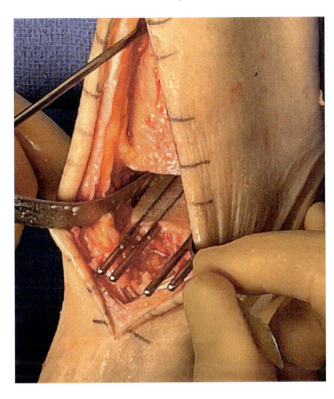

FIGURE 8.15 Posterior chamfer cut has been made flush with the top of the pins.

assist drills and fills the pin holes with two short pins (Fig. 8.17). These should not penetrate the far cortex. The reaming guide is exchanged with the talar spacer. The reamer is used to complete the cut in two steps, flipping the guide to complete. Ensure that the cut is flush. Remove the guide completely and finish the cut with a rongeur. The two chamfer cuts should meet at a sharp point. The apex of the cuts should be in line with the lateral process of the talus (Fig. 8.18). The 2.1 instrumentation is used in similar fashion over the talar alignment pin. However, it is often difficult to seat flush posteriorly. Therefore, the author has not used the newer guide in this step.

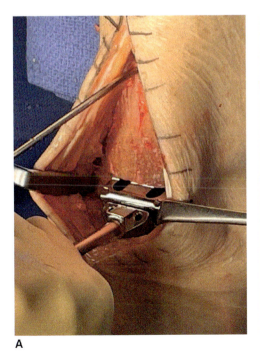
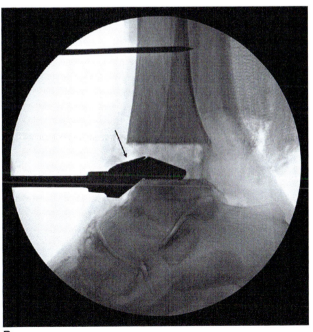

A B

FIGURE 8.16 A, B. The anterior chamfer guide has been applied. The groove marked by the *arrow* indicated that the anterior calibration line is in line with the anterior tibia.

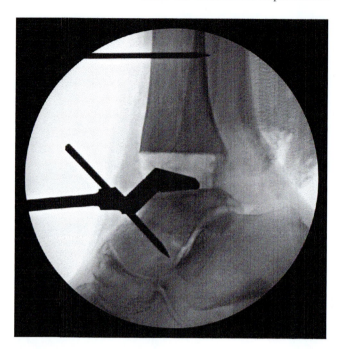

FIGURE 8.17 The anterior chamfer guide has been pinned in placed.

Lateral Chamfer and Plug Hole

The lateral chamfer cut guide is applied next. The 2.1 instrumentation has the advantage of also being a talar trial to help assess for sizing and positioning medial to lateral. When positioning, first ensure that the guide is positioned accurately medial to lateral with the handle in the same orientation as the previous guide. The guide should cover the talus as completely as possible but not extend past the cortical edges (Fig. 8.19A and B). Do not overstuff the joint. An option now is to also place the tibial and poly trials to assess for size and stability. The C-arm will need to be rotated into the anteroposterior view for complete examination. Now ensure that the lateral chamfer cut guide is positioned accurately over the previous chamfer cuts. Fluoroscopy in the lateral view is essential here. Once the position is felt to be optimal, a lamina spreader with the knob on the guide side can be placed to help with stabilizing the guide (Fig. 8.20). Often the guide is anterior, and a gentle tap on the handle of the guide can facilitate moving the guide posteriorly without altering the medial to lateral position. With the surgeon holding the guide, the drill bit is placed in the drill hole free hand and then drilled and filled with a short pin. The ankle is slightly plantarflexed while still holding the

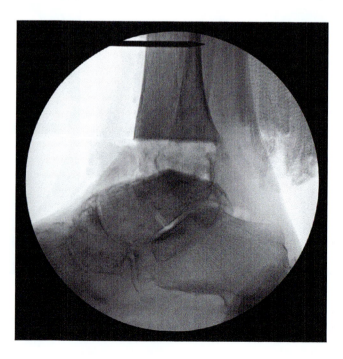

FIGURE 8.18 With the anterior chamfer completed, note how the peak of the talus is in line with the lateral talar process.

8 Salto Talaris Total Ankle Replacement

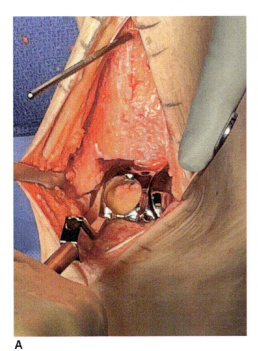
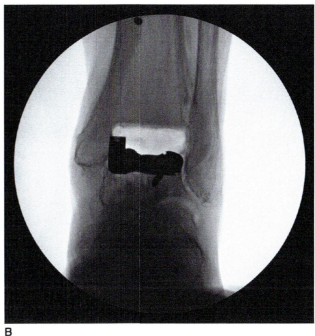

A.　　　　　　　　　　　　　　B.

FIGURE 8.19 **A.** The lateral chamfer guide using the 2.1 instrumentation. This is the author preferred guide. **B.** The lateral chamfer guide is applied and nicely covers the talus from medial to lateral on the anteroposterior view.

jig firmly in position, and the bell saw hole is drilled to a hard stop and either filler with the plug or detached from the drill and left for stability (Fig. 8.21). Now the lateral chamfer cut is made with a narrow oscillating saw taking care to protect neurovascular structures laterally. The guide is carefully removed so as not to crack through the bell saw hole. The cut piece of bone is usually small. Any remaining bone, particularly posterior, needs to be removed with rongeurs or a small saw. If left, malrotation of the talar component can occur. Important note, the size 0 talar component has a different plug size. In this case, after the guide is stabilized, the size 0 talar bushing is attached and the 7.9-mm drill is used to a positive stop. All guides can be removed.

If using the standard instrumentation, the guide is positioned with the lateral wing placed just inside the lateral cortex of the talus (Fig. 8.22). The guide still needs to be perfectly positioned at the apex of the chamfers on the lateral view. It can then be stabilized with the lamina spreader and pinned. The wing is removed, and the bell saw hole drilled to a hard stop and plugged. The lateral

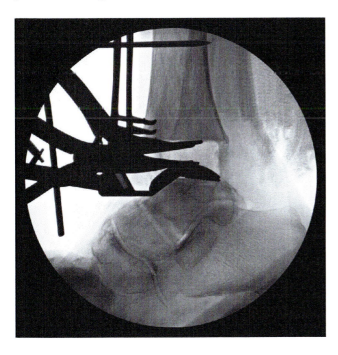

FIGURE 8.20 Now in the lateral position, the lateral chamfer guide is position and held with a lamina spreader. The guide can be used to accurately represent the talar trial.

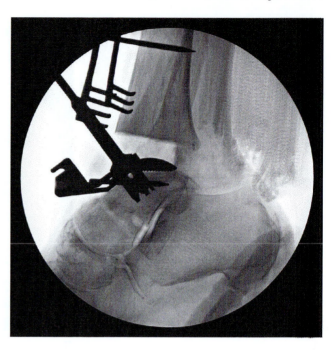

FIGURE 8.21 The guide has been pinned, and the plug hole drilled. The ankle must be plantarflexed to do this.

edge of the guide is used to make the lateral chamfer cut. If using a size 0 talus, the size 0 stem drill guide is placed and drilled with the drill left in place for stability for the lateral chamfer cut.

Trial Components—Finding the "Sweet Spot"

The joint is irrigated. The talar trial is placed first and impacted with the talar component impactor. The talar trials are side specific. The smooth tibial trial and appropriate poly insert are snapped together on the back table (Fig. 8.23). The tibial trials are universal, but the poly trials are side specific and should be oriented correctly anterior to posterior. The fit should be snug but not tight. Varus and valgus stability checks should be done in both dorsiflexion and plantarflexion. The smooth tibial trial will find its natural "sweet spot" particularly in rotation, and it is helpful to intentionally malrotate the tibial trial. This will allow it to reset itself, as the ankle is flexed and extended. The engraved anterior line on the smooth surface of the tibial trial should be flush with the anterior cortex of the tibia. If it is too anterior, it will need to be pushed back while drilling the keel. If it is slightly posterior, that position should be maintained with final component. This is also the position in which to decide if the XL base plate has

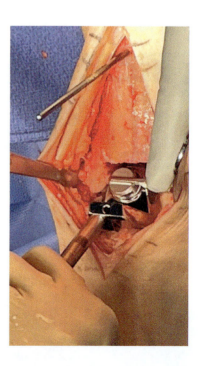

FIGURE 8.22 The original lateral chamfer guide.

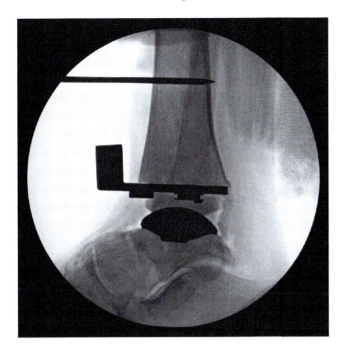

FIGURE 8.23 Trial components have been placed.

better posterior coverage. Fluoroscopy would be used here. Poly trials can be exchanged until stability is achieved. Medial releases, lateral ligament repairs, and Achilles lengthening or gastrocnemius recessions can all affect the stability of the ankle replacement. Final poly size should not be determined until those have been done. The joint should be stable with the ankle in dorsiflexion to both varus and valgus stresses. However, in plantarflexion, some mild (a few degrees) lateral instability is normal. At least 5 and preferably 10° to 15° of dorsiflexion should be achieved intraoperatively. If not, an Achilles lengthening or preferably a gastrocnemius recession should be done.

Once the sweet spot is identified and stability has been achieved, the ankle should be in neutral position for drilling the keel pins. The most distal hole is drilled and filled with a medium pin and then the next hole is drilled. Finally, the large proximal hole is drilled with the 7.9-mm drill to the positive stop. This all can be done with the C-arm in the lateral position to confirm that the base plate is securely flush with the tibia (Fig. 8.24). The keel is angled 4° proximal to provide for press fit as it is inserted.

Trial components are removed. The keel hole cut is completed with a small reciprocating saw, which also gently bevels the corners anteriorly. This is followed by the blue handled osteotome to

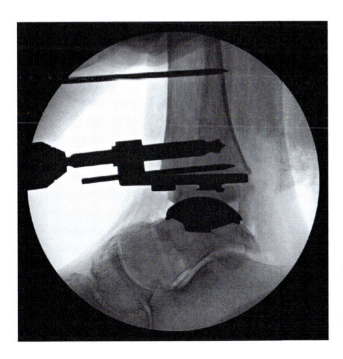

FIGURE 8.24 The keel hole has been initially prepared. Note how the drill holes angle proximally. As the keel follows this hole, the base plate is compressed against the tibial surface.

the appropriate depth corresponding to the tibial size. Finally, the blue handled rasp completes the keel hole preparation.

Final Components

All trial components are removed. The joint is irrigated. The talar component is inserted first with the talar impactor by lining up the plug hole with the drilled hole in the talus and then impacting it. In the case of a size 0 talus, plug hole is packed with autograft bone. The tibial base plate and polyethylene spacer are assembled on the back table with the insert assembler press. The posterior aspect of the keel hole is filled with graft after being attached to the inserter. Care should be taken to not allow the tibial component to fall off the insertion handle, as well as to orient the component correctly with the keel anterior. Under fluoroscopy, the tibial base plate is driven in after lining up the keel hole. Great care should be taken to not dorsiflex the tibial component during insertion (Fig. 8.25A). This can be avoided by going slowly and using C-arm to monitor. Bringing your

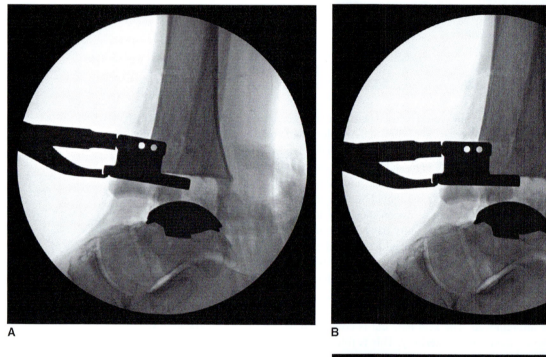

FIGURE 8.25 **A.** Insertion of the tibial component. Note how it is entering in a dorsiflexed position. **B.** By bringing the insertion handle distally, the position is corrected. **C.** Final position of the tibial component during insertion.

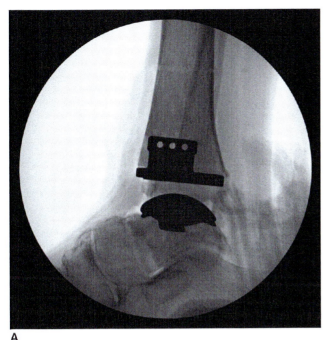 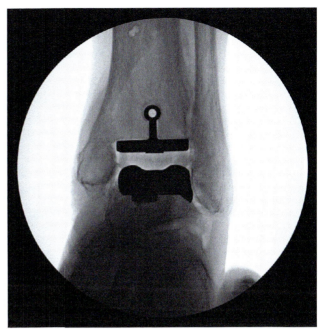

FIGURE 8.26 A, B. Final position of the implants.

hand distal as impaction occurs is helpful (Fig. 8.25B). This is of even more importance with the XL tibias due to the longer lever arm of the component. Impact the tibia until the trial position is achieved (Fig. 8.25C). Final stability checks are done again to ensure that nothing has changed and to ensure that the ankle joint is well balanced above a stable plantigrade foot (Fig. 8.26A and B).

Bone graft is impacted into the keel hole. The wound is copiously irrigated. The wound is closed in layers—capsuloperiosteal, extensor retinaculum, subcutaneous, and then skin. In our institution, the patient is then placed into a cast, which is split anteriorly with an added diamond anteriorly over the ankle joint to relieve pressure. The cotton padding is left in place (Fig. 8.27).

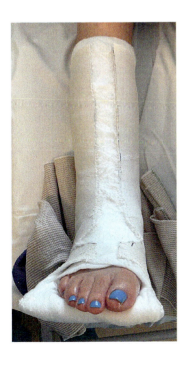

FIGURE 8.27 Standard postoperative cast. It has been spilt anteriorly to allow for swelling. It will be overwrapped with fiberglass on postoperative day 1 or 2 to allow static standing.

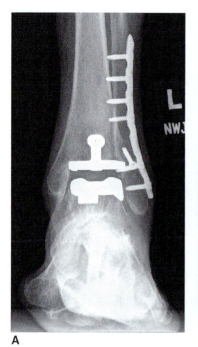 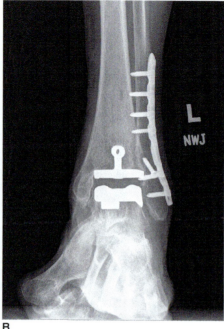 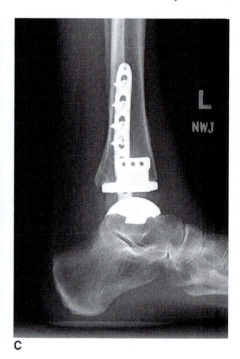

FIGURE 8.28 **A-C.** One-year follow-up radiographs of the patient in Figure 8.3.

PEARLS AND PITFALLS

- Maintain the integrity of the capsule-periosteal flap—important part of the closure.
- Examine the whole standing limb alignment—minor deviations between the tibial anatomic and mechanical axes can be accommodated by slight medial or lateral translation of the extramedullary guide proximally. However, significant proximal deformity should be corrected prior to ankle arthroplasty.
- Beware of the small ankle—particularly the size 0 tibia. This is where preoperative templating is essential. With the smaller implants, the spaces are tighter and fracture risk is increased by leveraging against a malleolus. Strongly consider preemptive malleolar screws placed percutaneously.
- Sometimes the tibial roof is more difficult to assess. In the author experience, it has been more common to resect too little distal tibia rather than too much. Using the trial tibial component with the 8-mm poly insert to check that there has been adequate resection has been helpful. If that is unable to be placed, a 2-mm recut is easily performed at that time rather than later in the case.
- When placing the talar alignment pin, holding the foot and ankle in neutral alignment is critical. The surgeon should hold the ankle while the assistant drills the hole and places the pin. Make sure that it points to the posterior third of the subtalar joint.
- The use of the lamina spreaders is helpful to maintain position of the talar jigs. Checking with fluoroscopy is a good idea, but this is also a two person job—one to hold the jig and one to pin it.
- The anterior chamfer guide must not be lined up too anteriorly. This will cause abnormal stresses and lead to early failure. Ensure that enough talar neck is removed. This can be done during the approach when removing the tibial spurs.
- Of all the 2.1 instrumentation, the lateral chamfer guide has been most helpful.
- In the varus ankle, an aggressive medial release is necessary for balancing the ankle. We begin anteriorly at the tip of the medial malleolus and subperiosteally release a sleeve of tissue off the medial malleolus from anterior to posterior all the way to the posterior tibial tendon. This includes both the deep and superficial fibers. Talar attachments of the deltoid are not released as this can injure blood supply.
- In the valgus ankle, consider resecting less tibia initially. These are often looser ankles and can require thicker poly inserts. Resecting less bone minimizes the risk of needing too thick a poly.
- For both varus and valgus ankle, hindfoot alignment views are imperative. A calcaneal osteotomy is usually easily done at the time of the arthroplasty and does not affect postoperative recovery much.

- When finding the "sweet spot" for the tibial component, take time and malposition it so rotation of the trial is necessary. Watch carefully to see that it sits flush prior to pinning. This can be achieved with compression axially through the heel.
- When driving in the larger tibial components, there is a tendency to dorsiflex the component during insertion due to larger moment arm. To ensure that this does not occur, use fluoroscopy and bring your hand distal.

POSTOPERATIVE MANAGEMENT

Approximately 50% of our patients are discharged home on the same day of surgery. The cast is overwrapped with fiberglass on postoperative day 1 (hospital) or 2 (outpatient done in office). At that point, the patient is allowed to stand statically with equal weight on both limbs for general daily activities as tolerated. However, no weight is allowed with ambulation. At 3 weeks, sutures are removed, and motion is initiated with a boot for protection. At 6 to 7 weeks, ambulation is initiated, and the patient is weaned from the boot as tolerated. Weight-bearing radiographs are obtained at the second follow-up visit and at 3 months, 6 months, and yearly thereafter (Fig. 8.28A through C).

RESULTS AND COMPLICATIONS

Ankle arthroplasty has been shown in prospective studies to provide significant improvement in overall function and ankle-specific function at 4 years postoperatively.[5] The Salto Talaris ankle arthroplasty demonstrates high levels of survivorship (greater than 95%) and improved function at mid-term follow-up (4 to 7 years).[6-9] Longer-term studies on ankle replacement are few. A recent large observation study on ankle replacements done in France had only 170 of 4,748 replacements that were followed for 10 years.[10] The original Salto cohort from France was followed from 7 to 11 years (mean of 8.9 years) and demonstrated 85% survivorship at 10 years with fusion or revision of a component as an end point.[11]

Complications of the Salto Talaris are similar to other ankle prostheses, and these include infection, neurovascular injury, wound healing problems, stiffness, subsidence or loosening of the prosthesis, and osteolysis. In one of the longer-term studies on the initial mobile-bearing Salto prosthesis, Bonnin et al[11] described reoperations as due primarily to bone cysts (11 of 85 patients) as well as fracture of the polyethylene (5) and other unexplained pain. There were six converted to a fusion and five revisions primarily for polyethylene fracture. Autogenous bone grafting of the cysts was completely successful in half of the cases. In the other half, residual cyst size was less than 5 mm. The authors discussed the higher incidence of osteolysis around the tibial keel. This was felt to be due to wear debris accessible from the joint. By modifying the technique and bone grafting, the tibial keel at the time of surgery, they have not had the need to secondarily bone graft tibial cysts. Interestingly, in a comparative study by some of the same authors involving the original Salto mobile-bearing design and the fixed-bearing Salto Talaris prosthesis, the fixed-bearing prosthesis developed significantly fewer radiolucent lines and subchondral cysts.[12] The main differences in the two designs are the mobile versus fixed bearing and the hydroxyapatite coating on the mobile-bearing metal components. In a separate comparative study between the Salto and Salto Talaris, the mobile-bearing prosthesis was reported as having a three times higher rate of revision at 3 years postoperatively.[13]

REFERENCES

1. Bonnin M, Judet T, Colombier JA, Buscayret F, Graveleau N, Piriou P. Midterm results of the Salto total ankle prosthesis. *Clin Orthop Relat Res.* 2004;424:6-18.
2. Siegler S, Toy J, Seale D, Pedowitz D. New observations on the morphology of the talar dome and its relationship to ankle kinematics. *Clin Biomech.* 2013;29:1-6.
3. Nozaki S, Watanabe K, Katayose M. Three-dimensional analysis of talar trochlea morphology: implications for subject-specific kinematics of the talocrural joint. *Clin Anat.* 2016;29(8):1066-1074.
4. Leszko F, Komistek RD, Mahfouz MR, et al. In vivo kinematics of the Salto total ankle prosthesis. *Foot Ankle Int.* 2008;29(11):1117-1125.
5. Sangeorzan BJ, Ledoux WR, Shofer JB, et al. Comparing 4-year changes in patient-reported outcomes following ankle arthroplasty and arthrodesis. *J Bone Joint Surg Am.* 2021;103(10):869-878.
6. Day J, Kim J, O'Malley MJ, et al. Radiographic and clinical outcomes of the Salto Talaris total ankle arthroplasty. *Foot Ankle Int.* 2020;41(12):1519-1528.

7. Hofmann KJ, Shabin ZM, Ferkel E, Jockel J, Slovenkai MP. Salto Talaris total ankle arthroplasty: clinical results at a mean of 5.2 years in 78 patients treated by a single surgeon. *J Bone Joint Surg Am.* 2016;98(24):2036-2046.
8. Marks RM. Mid-term prospective clinical and radiographic outcomes of a modern fixed-bearing total ankle arthroplasty. *J Foot Ankle Surg.* 2019;58(6):1163-1170.
9. Stewart MG, Green CL, Adams SB Jr, DeOrio JK, Easley ME, Nunley JA. Midterm results of the Salto Talaris total ankle arthroplasty. *Foot Ankle Int.* 2017;38(11):1215-1221.
10. Dagneaux L, Nogue E, Mathieu J, Demoulin D, Canovas F, Molinari N. Survivorship of 4,748 contemporary total ankle replacements from the French discharge records database. *J Bone Joint Surg Am.* 2022;104(8):684-692.
11. Bonnin M, Gaudot F, Laurent J-R, Ellis S, Colombier J-A, Judet T. The Salto total ankle arthroplasty: survivorship and analysis of failures at 7 to 11 years. *Clin Orthop Relat Res.* 2011;469(1):225-236.
12. Gaudot F, Columbier J-A, Bonnin M, Judet T. A controlled, comparative study of a fixed-bearing versus mobile-bearing ankle arthroplasty. *Foot Ankle Int.* 2014;35(2):131-140.
13. Assal M, Kutaish H, Acker A, et al. Three-year rates of reoperation and revision following mobile versus fixed-bearing total ankle arthroplasty: a cohort of 302 patients with 2 implants of similar design. *J Bone Joint Surg Am.* 2021;103(22):2080-2088.

9 Paragon 28 APEX 3D Fixed-Bearing Total Ankle Replacement

Christopher E. Gross and Daniel J. Scott

INTRODUCTION

Total ankle arthroplasty (TAA) has improved substantially over time, and the current generation of implants represent a new, incremental improvement over prior generations.[1] The newest, fourth generation implants have focused on lower profile tibial implants, which minimizes tibial bone resection. The fourth generation talar implants have tended to be curved implants that similarly try to minimize the amount of talar bone resection, while matching the normal contour of the talus. The APEX 3D total ankle (Paragon 28, Centennial, Colorado) is an example of one of these newest generation implants, which is a fixed bearing, semiconstrained total ankle. It was approved for use in July of 2020 by the U.S. Food and Drug Administration. The APEX offers the option of a flat tibial implant as well as a curved "arc" tibia. Theoretical benefits of the arc tibia include increased rotational stability from the curve shape of the tibial component.[2] Both tibial components include two press fit pegs in the posterior portion of the tibial component (into the strongest portion of tibial bone at that level), as well as a 3D-printed porous architecture on the tibia to maximize bony ingrowth. The APEX talar component offers the option of both a curved and flat cut option, both of which feature a biradial curvature on the talus to better recreate native talar motion. The curved talus features anterior and posterior chamfers, with the goal of increasing talar stability and minimizing bony resection. The polyethylene component is highly crosslinked and vitamin E infused, in an effort improve long-term wear characteristics and to reduce oxidation, respectively. Tibial component sizes range from 1 to 6, with all six sizes offering standard and long (increased anterior-posterior width) trays, as well as a short tray option on the size 1 for a total of 13 different tray options.[2] Talar components range from 1 to 5 in both curved and flat cut options. Finally, patient-specific custom cutting blocks are also available (MAVEN, Paragon 28, Centennial, Colorado), based on preoperative computed tomography (CT) scans, to help increase operative efficiency and accuracy of bony cuts.

INDICATIONS

- End-stage ankle arthrosis
- Ankle arthrodesis nonunion or malunion takedown, provided both medial and lateral malleoli are intact

CONTRAINDICATIONS

- Active infection surrounding the ankle or osteomyelitis
- Neuropathic arthropathy or Charcot arthropathy
- Skeletally immature patient
- Vascular insufficiency
- Inadequate soft tissue envelope
- Massive bone loss
- Loss of the medial or lateral malleolus

- Posterior ankle instability/subluxation.
- Motion is a not a limitation for us as even stiff ankles can benefit from an arthroplasty.

SPECIAL SITUATIONS

Age

- There is no consensus on what age is too young to consider TAA.
- The younger the patient, the increased amount of time the implant will be stressed, and the higher the patient will eventually need either a revision TAA or conversion to a fusion.
- Studies of newer-generation implants have shown promising results in younger (less than 50 years) patients.[3-5]
- Certainly, more long-term data are needed to determine the optimal age–related thresholds for total ankle replacement (TAR) versus arthrodesis.

Coronal Plane Deformity

- Historically, large coronal plane deformity has been a contraindication to TAA.[1,6]
- Over time, surgeons have become more facile with correcting larger and larger coronal plane deformities in the setting of TAA.[6,7]
- Currently, many surgeons are comfortable correcting coronal plane deformities as large as 30°.[1]
- Though there are not firm exclusion criteria in regard to coronal plane deformity, ultimately if the operative surgeon is not comfortable correcting large deformity or is not confident that they can successfully balance the ankle, a TAA should likely not be performed.

PREOPERATIVE ASSESSMENT

Preoperative assessment always begins with a through history and physical exam. Careful attention should be paid to the standing alignment of the limb in the coronal and sagittal planes. Any varus or valgus deformity of the limb should be noted. If there is any deformity of the hip, knee, or femur or tibia, long standing radiographs should be obtained, and consideration should be given to correcting a more proximal deformity prior to proceeding with TAA. The alignment of the foot should be noted, as any preoperative pes cavus or pes planus deformity will need to be corrected at the time of TAA or in a staged fashion. The surgeon should pay close attention to the soft tissues of the anterior ankle to ensure that the soft tissues will be robust enough to support healing. Any contracture of the Achilles tendon or gastrocnemius muscle should be noted, as this may also need to be addressed intraoperatively.

Weight-bearing ankle, and sometimes foot radiographs, will need to be obtained. As noted above, if any more proximal deformity exists in the limb, long-standing radiographs of the entire limb should be obtained. Surgeons should be prepared to address any coronal plane deformity noted on the ankle radiographs at the time of TAA. Varus ankle arthritis can require a multitude of procedures, including a deltoid ligament release, modified Broström, posterior tibial tendon lengthening or transfer to the middle cuneiform, peroneal tendon transfer (ie, peroneus longus to brevis), talonavicular and spring ligament capsulotomy, plantar fascia release, lateralizing calcaneal osteotomy, dorsiflexion first metatarsal osteotomy, or even hindfoot fusions in the setting of very rigid deformity. In contrast, valgus deformities can require a longus to brevis peroneal transfer medializing calcaneal osteotomies, medial column stabilizing procedures (Cotton osteotomy, first tarsometatarsal arthrodesis, and navicular-cuneiform arthrodesis), or hindfoot fusions. Often in the setting of large coronal plane deformity, bony resection will initially be minimized, to accommodate for the expected ligamentous balancing that will be needed to correct the deformity.

CT scans can be a useful adjunct preoperatively. CT allows for identification of bony cysts, which may need to be débrided and grafted. CT also helps surgeons better understand the existing tibial and talar bone stock. Weight-bearing CT can be useful to evaluate the alignment of the ankle and other hindfoot joints under physiologic load. CT is also required for custom cutting blocks to be created for the MAVEN APEX 3D TAA.

SURGICAL TECHNIQUE

Position

The patient is placed supine on radiolucent operating table with their heels at the edge of the bed. We then place a thigh tourniquet and oftentimes hold this in place with foam tape given that we traditionally have an indwelling nerve catheter that is inserted just above the knee. The operative ankle is then centered on the bed and then has enough padding placed underneath it such that the lateral fluoroscopic image can be taken without irradiating the contralateral leg. Typically, we use two blanket bumps under the operative legs. We place a nonsterile bump under the ipsilateral hip so the toes are pointing toward the ceiling. The leg is sterilely prepped and draped such that the tibial tubercle is exposed. Next, we drape the large intraoperative fluoroscopy, which will enter on the ipsilateral surgical ankle side with the monitor positioned over the contralateral upper extremity.

Approach

Before the anterior ankle approach, one must assess if a gastrocnemius recession or tendo-Achilles lengthening is needed with a Silfverskiold test. Once performed, a longitudinal incision is made on the anterior aspect of the ankle approximately 10 cm in length and 1 cm lateral to the anterior tibial crest (Fig. 9.1). Soft tissue dissection is undertaken, respecting that the superficial peroneal nerve oftentimes will travel in the distal one-half/one-third of the exposure. If identified, it must be protected throughout the procedure (Fig. 9.2). The extensor retinaculum is divided longitudinally. Next, the anterior tibial tendon is identified, and we sharply incise on the floor of the tibialis anterior to the tibia. The deep neurovascular bundle is retracted laterally. The anterior capsule is divided and reflected. One must ensure that the lateral and medial gutter are well exposed (Fig. 9.3). At this time, in a varus ankle, partial deltoid stripping is performed in order to balance the ankle and reduce the talus under the plafond. Once the joint is exposed, one must ensure that the ankle is not in varus or valgus before the alignment jig is placed.

Alignment Guide

A 3-mm stab incision is made in the proximal tibia. A 3 × 160 mm fluted Steinmann pin is aligned with an osteotome placed in the medial gutter and drilled into the tibial tubercle (Fig. 9.4). From this, an external tibial alignment guide (TAG) is suspended. It is important to make sure that the

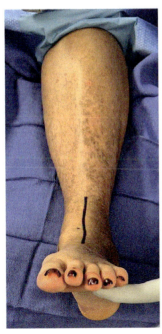

FIGURE 9.1 Use a 10-cm incision centered over the anterior ankle (roughly 60% over the tibia and 40% over the talus).

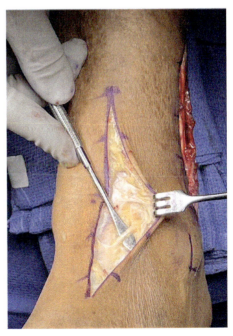

FIGURE 9.2 Avoid the superficial peroneal nerve as identified and protected here.

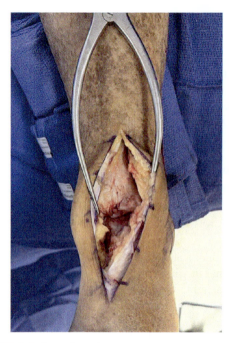

FIGURE 9.3 Once the ankle capsule is entered, carefully perform subperiosteal dissection.

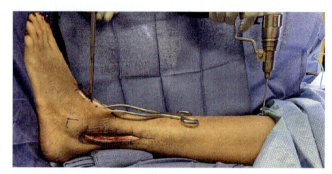

FIGURE 9.4 A Steinmann pin is drilled in the tibial tubercle in reference to an osteotome placed in the medial gutter to help establish rotation.

proximal portion of the tibial tubercle is utilized for the TAG to fit. The pin is placed perpendicular to the floor in the sagittal plane and pointing toward the ceiling in the coronal plane (Fig. 9.5A and B). The TAG is dropped until there are three finger breadths between it and the tibial crest. It is secured with proximal turn knob.

The TAG is telescoped distally until it approximates the tibiotalar joint line height. The joint line reference internal/external (I/E) pointer is attached and locked into the TAG's dovetail connection. Next, based on preference, the joint line reference I/E pointer is used visually guide I/E rotation against the second metatarsal, medial gutter, or gutter bisection. The most proximal gold screw is loosened and then tightened to adjust rotation. This position is secured by placing a 3 × 100 mm fluted Steinmann pin perpendicular and bicortically into one of the three distal TAG holes based on alignment requirements, targeting the flat region of metaphyseal bone.

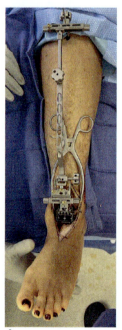

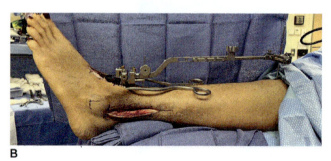

FIGURE 9.5 A, B. The tibial alignment guide is suspended from the proximal Steinmann pin.

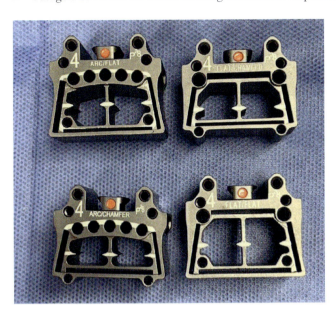

FIGURE 9.6 Four choices for tibia/talus resection (arc/flat, arc/chamfer, flat/chamfer, and flat/flat) that the APEX 3D offers. Typically we use one of the arc tibias given its unique geometry that may lead to improved tibial fixation.

The APEX system allows for flat/flat cuts (tibia/talus), flat/chamfer, arc/flat, and arc/chamfer. We will discuss the technique for the arc/chamfer first because discussing the three options is beyond the scope of this chapter (Fig. 9.6). The arc refers to the geometry of the tibia implant that optimizes the initial stability of the implants and allows for maximization of bone ongrowth. Furthermore, its cut is made with a drill to minimize bone necrosis that occur with a saw. We typically use the chamfer for the talus to minimize bone resection. We will also discuss the flat cut as well.

Next, the black metallic cutting block (arc/chamfer) is selected and attached into the dovetail connection based on preoperative estimations of tibial sizing. Under anteroposterior (AP) fluoroscopic guidance, we then rotate the proximal control knobs to adjust varus/valgus alignment. Once confirmed, the gold screw adjacent to the proximal control knobs is tightened. One must make sure that the holes are perfectly visible and that the gutters are clearly seen.

Medial/lateral (M/L) alignment is adjusted by rotating the distal control knobs. An AP fluoroscopic view is used to verify that the cutting block is aligned with the medial and lateral gutters. This is secured with a gold screw (Fig. 9.7A and B).

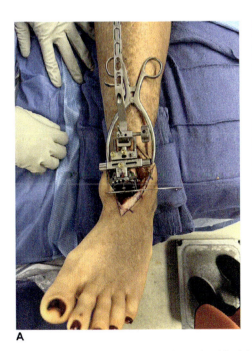
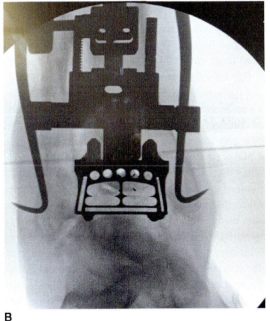

A   **B**

FIGURE 9.7 A. The black metallic cutting block is attached to the dovetail. **B.** Check for rotation, varus/valgus, and medial/lateral on anteroposterior radiograph.

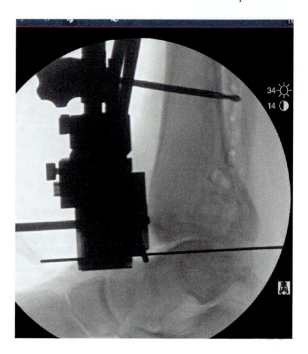

FIGURE 9.8 Ensure that the angel wing is a straight line. Then, check two things: resection height and slope. This line should be perpendicular to the tibial alignment to indication correct slope of cut. We typically cheat with "opening up the slope" pictured here to improve dorsiflexion range of motion. We place a pin in the lowermost tibia drill hole to check for resection of the tibial. The angel wing represents the resection height of the talus.

Next, the fluoroscopy is rotated to a lateral position. A joint line reference wing is placed in the talar resection guide. A top hat is placed into the lateral-most drill hole. The image is adjusted until the angel wing is one thin line (Fig. 9.8). The distal tibial slope is then checked based on the line created by the wing relative to the length of the tibia. If adjustments are needed, raise and lower the TAG on either the proximal or distal anterior tibial fixation pin locations, then retighten the locking turn knobs to secure position.

At this point, ensure that one is comfortable with the tibial resection height (as indicated by the top hat in one of the tibial drill holes) and the talar resection height (as indicated by the joint line reference wing). At this point, if one is happy with the tibial resection, but there is too little talus resection height, switch over to the metallic arc/flat guide, which will allow for 3 mm more of talar resection. This is oftentimes the standard for tight ankles. A chamfered talus would still be utilized later in the procedure.

Tibial Cut

Next, the plastic resection sizing block is placed (Fig. 9.9). Here, 2×2.4 mm Steinman pins are placed bicortically. Utilizing the 3.5-mm arc Tibia resection drill, drill bicortically into the medial most corner hole of the sizing resection block, ensuring the drill clears the posterior cortex, but does not penetrate beyond. The remaining holes are then sequentially drilled. The sizing block is then removed and replaced with the black metallic cutting block, sliding it over the 2×2.4 mm Steinmann pins and into the dovetail connection. The APEX 3D System offers both coupled and decoupled talar bone resection options. We will discuss the coupled technique given our philosophy that the entire ankle should have no deformity and be congruent when we are performing our cuts. In our hands, this minimizes the chance that we change the joint line height and ensures that we respect ligamentous balancing and osteotomies to correct our varus and valgus at the end of the case.

Once the metallic resection block is secured, two converging shoulder pins are placed into the guide, using the T handle to fully seat them such that there is no risk for torquing the assembly (Fig. 9.10). With the foot held in physiologic valgus, reducing the tibiotalar joint, the talus is secured by placing $2 \times 2.4 \times 110$ mm smooth Steinmann pins into the talus through the two distal most holes of the resection block. These pins are then cut flush to the cutting guide.

Next, the remainder of the arc drill holes are bicortically drilled. The 8×50 mm reciprocating saw blade is then used to perform the M/L gutter bone resection cuts, starting distally, then walking the saw blade up proximally. In order to ensure that the corner of the tibia is cut, we drop our hand within the assembly to direct our blade more superiorly (Fig. 9.11).

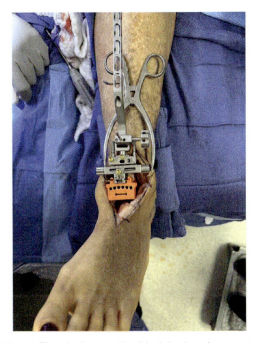

FIGURE 9.9 The plastic resection block is placed once rotation, slope, medial/lateral, height, and resection height are optimized.

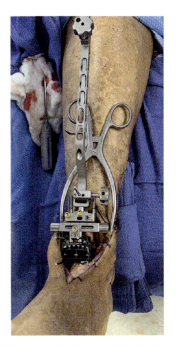

FIGURE 9.10 The assembly is secured to the talus while the ankle is held in physiologic valgus. This maneuver typically takes two people to perform.

Talar Cut, Preparation and Sizing: Chamfer

The dorsal talus is cut through the cutting slot with the 13 × 90 mm oscillating saw blade.

The two shoulder pins are removed and the entire TAG and cutting jig is removed. The 2 × 2.4 mm Steinmann pins remain. We then remove the cut superior talus (Fig. 9.12). Utilizing the arc Tibia osteotome, the resected tibial bone is freed away from the intact tibia, ensuring the osteotome is parallel to the cut surface. Using a variety of methods, the resected tibia is removed. Oftentimes, a small sliver of talus remains either medially or laterally, so we use the reciprocating saw blade to clean up the edges.

Once the bone is cleared from the ankle, in order to remove residual tibial ridges, we use the size-matched arc tibia rasp (Fig. 9.13A and B) in a push and pull fashion until we are pleased that the tibial surface is uniform. Next, we utilize the corresponding cut-style gap checker (Fig. 9.14) to evaluate that we have adequately removed enough bone. If one is not happy with the amount of talus resected, there is a 2-mm talar recut guide that can be used to carefully remove more bone.

Slide the size-matched arc tibia trial over the two smooth Steinmann pins already in place. Attach the modular tibial trial paddle and the talar distraction paddle to the parallel distractor (Fig. 9.15). To determine appropriate positioning, ensure that fluoroscopic markers are aligned. One should

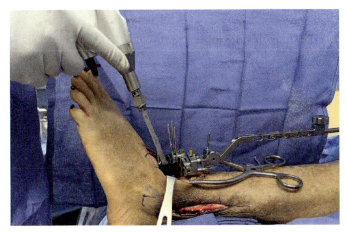

FIGURE 9.11 Drop one's hand to saw the corners.

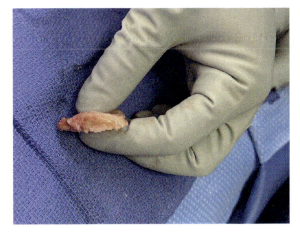

FIGURE 9.12 Surgeon holding the thin talus cut.

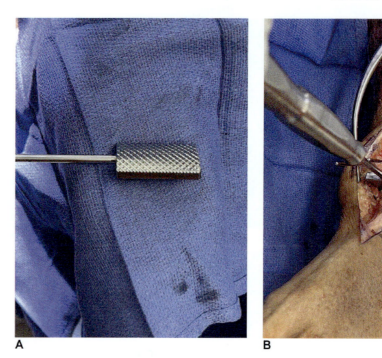

FIGURE 9.13 A. Arc tibia rasp. **B.** The arc tibial rasp is used to smooth out the drill holes. If this step is skipped or not vigorous enough, the trial will not sit flush.

see the punch outline just posterior to the midline on the lateral fluoroscopy view. The posterior lip indicates if the implant should be standard or long. Fine-tune the positioning of the tray using the AP positioning bolt. Distract the joint by squeezing the distractor handle. Two threaded shoulder pins are then placed to further secure the tibial trial (one pin must use the superior hole and one pin the inferior hole) (Fig. 9.16).

Next, insert the size-matched viper tip peg punch paddle by hand, sliding it until it drops into the corresponding punch guide. At this point, the talar paddle is connected to the distractor, and on the tibial side, the distractor connects to the viper tip paddle. The distractor is then distracted with suffi-

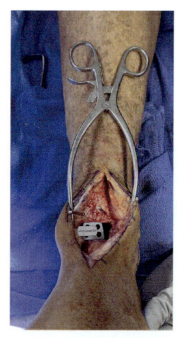

FIGURE 9.14 The surgeon uses the gap checker to ensure that enough bone on either side of the joint has been resected. If it does not fit, there is a talar recut guide available.

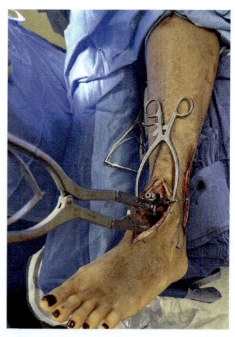

FIGURE 9.15 The tibial trial paddle and talar distraction paddle are used to open the joint to start tibia peg preparation.

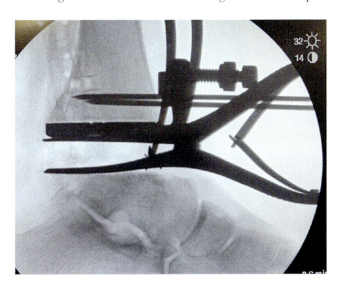

FIGURE 9.16 The tibial trial is placed over the Steinmann pins and held in place with a distractor.

cient pressure to engage the tibia bone. Utilizing the assembled tibia impaction tool construct, insert the impaction dimple underneath the viper tip peg punch paddle. This is impacted until the viper tip pegs are fully seated (Fig. 9.17).

The distractor and assembly are now removed. The appropriately sized talar trial sizing resection guide (Fig. 9.18) is placed into the joint to evaluate M/L talar coverage visually, ensuring that there is no impingement in the gutters. Attach the appropriately sized chamfer talar resection Guide and standard tibial trial paddle to the distractor. Under lateral fluoroscopy, ensure that the resection guide matches the curvature of the talus and the peak of the vertical position marker is aligned with the lateral process (Fig. 9.19). Gently distract, and then place two threaded shoulder pins into the medial and lateral converging pin holes in the talus guide. Remove the distractor. The 13 × 90 mm oscillating saw blade is then placed into the posterior cut slot to perform the posterior chamfer cut. The single-slotted resection insert is connected to the anterior chamfer cut and the corresponding-sized gold-tipped reamer is placed and reamed, holding it perpendicular to the resection insert (Fig. 9.20). The talar pins are removed and the guide is removed. Remove the posterior chamfer and clean up as needed. The medial and lateral anterior chamfer are cleaned with the provided square tip rongeur. At this point, we take extra care to débride the medial and lateral gutter of all soft tissue and bony debris to decrease the risk for impingement postoperatively.

The talar chamfer trial and poly trial are then inserted by hand into the joint (Fig. 9.21A and B). The ankle is ranged, allowing the talus to seat appropriately. The poly thickness is also checked at this stage. Next, the chamfer cuts are checked under lateral fluoroscopy. If there is any mismatch, there is an anterior and posterior chamfer checker. Once the talus is confirmed to be well positioned, we remove the tibial 2 × 2.4 mm Steinmann pins and then place these into the anterior most holes in the talus trial in order to secure its position (Fig. 9.21C).

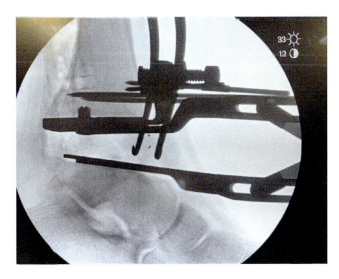

FIGURE 9.17 The viper tips are impacted until they are fully seated. While it can be confirmed by direct visualization, lateral fluoroscopy is ideal.

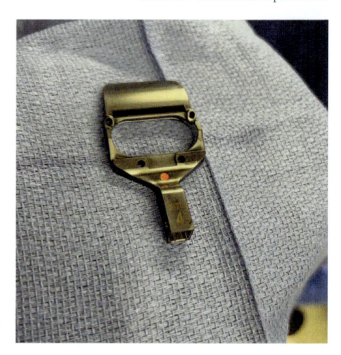

FIGURE 9.18 Tibial trial sizing guide. The surgeon places it on the talus, checking firstly that there is no impingement or over hang medially and laterally.

In plantar flexion, the talar reaming tower is locked into the trial using the provided hex driver. The talar fin reamer is used to drill superiorly and inferiorly (and then swept) to create room for the fin. The reaming tower and reamer are removed. Next, the trial components are removed.

Talar Cut, Preparation and Sizing: Flat Top

The flat-cut talus may be chosen if there is superior talar collapse or subchondral cystic changes or poor bone quality in the talar dome. The corresponding metallic resection guide is used (arc/flat) for bony resection. Attach the appropriately sized flat talar trial and standard tibial trial paddle to the distractor. Under lateral fluoroscopy, ensure that the flat talar trial is aligned with the vertical positioning marker on the tibial trial or the lateral process under lateral fluoroscopy. Under distraction, the flat talar trial position is secured by placing 2×2.4 mm threaded shoulder pins. Utilizing the talar peg drill, the medial and lateral talar trial peg holes are drilled until the positive stop. The poly trial is then placed and assessed.

Placement of Final Implant Through Closure

At this point, we irrigate the wound with 1 L of normal saline and switch top gloves. The tibial implant and plastic impact impactor are then placed into the tibia. A lamina spreader is needed to

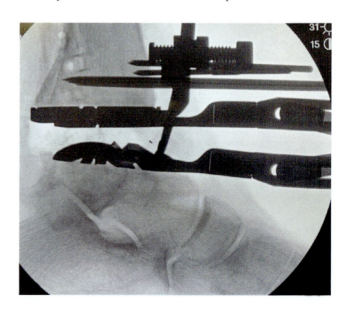

FIGURE 9.19 The surgeon ensures that resection guide matches the curvature of the talus. The dome of the guide should be contiguous with the posterior tibia. One knows it is a perfect lateral when the two peaks of the talar guide are seen.

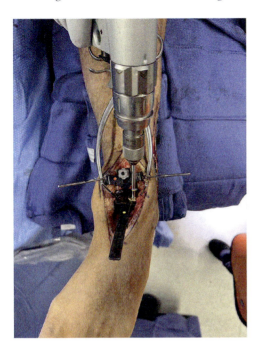

FIGURE 9.20 Next, the anterior chamfer is reamed.

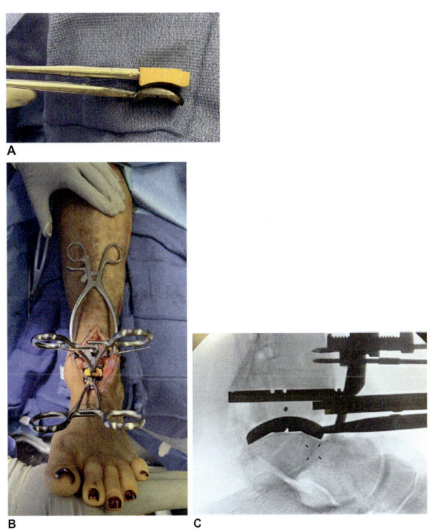

FIGURE 9.21 **A.** Talar chamfer trial and poly trial. **B.** The trial tibia, poly, and talus should fit and articulate with ease. **C.** The surgeon then checks a lateral fluoroscopic image to ensure that the chamfers have equal contact with the talus.

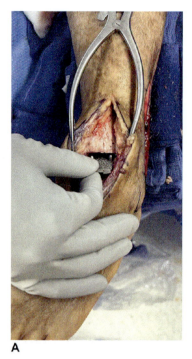
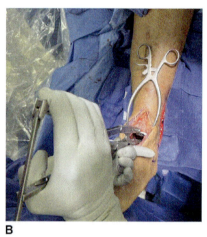
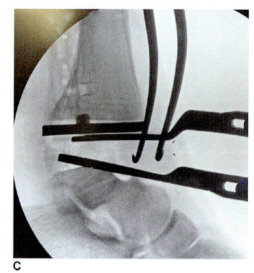

FIGURE 9.22 **A.** The first places the tibial tray by hand into the ankle. **B.** This is followed by using the distraction tool to open the joint and provide initial fixation. **C.** Here, the tibial tray is not yet flush with the tibia bone and needs to be impacted more.

push the implant pegs into the corresponding punched holes (Fig. 9.22A through C). The dimple is connected to the tibial impaction handle and under lateral fluoroscopy, the tibial implant is fully seated by striking the impaction handle with a mallet. The implant is confirmed as fully seated by both AP and lateral fluoroscopy. By hand, the talar implant is inserted such that the fin or pegs align with the reamed slot. The talar impactor is then struck with a mallet to press fit the talus (Fig. 9.23).

The poly implant should be inserted as far as possible by hand. The poly insertion tool is then attached to the tibial component and then locked, making sure to keep the alignment of the instrument parallel with the tibia component. The knob is then turned until the poly is fully engaged and then seated (a click is heard or felt) (Fig. 9.24A and B). Once the implant is in place, range the ankle. An anterior drawer test and varus stress test is performed to see if a Broström is needed. An AP fluoroscopic image is checked to see if a bony gutter débridement is needed (Fig. 9.25A through C).

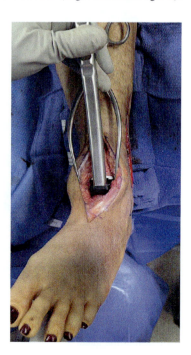

FIGURE 9.23 The surgeon then provides axial force with the talar impaction tool.

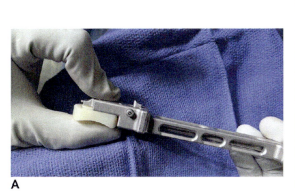
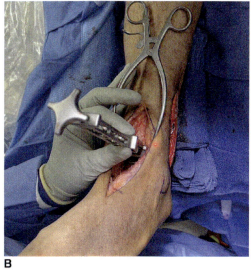

FIGURE 9.24 A, B. The poly is then placed into the joint by hand until it can no longer be pushed further. Poly insertion is completed using the device pictured above.

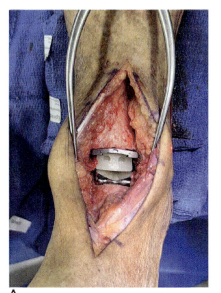
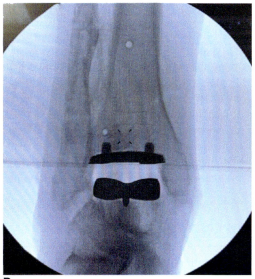
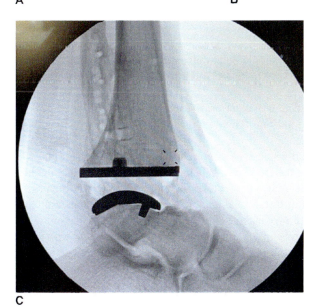

FIGURE 9.25 A. Final assembly. **B, C.** Final radiographs of assembly.

Patient-Specific Instrumentation

Preoperative planning case reports are generated using inputted CT and radiographic data. The standard anterior ankle approach is utilized; however, periosteum will need to be elevated where the tibial guide will contact the bone (in the metaphyseal cone of the tibia). The patient-specific instrumentation guide is placed over the anterior aspect of the tibia. It has a medial malleolus wrap that utilizes the notch of Harty as a reference point. No gapping between the guide and bone should be visible. A 2.4-mm Steinmann pin is placed into the medial converging sleeve, followed by the lateral fixation pin sleeve. Under an AP fluoroscopic view, the varus/valgus verification rod can be used to compare the position of the radiopaque markers against the position referenced in the surgical planning case reports.

The size-matched sizing resection block is placed and secured at this point. The above steps can now be performed.

POSTOPERATIVE MANAGEMENT

Before, we take down the tourniquet, we give 1 g of tranexamic acid unless it is contraindicated. Postoperatively, patients are routinely placed into a non–weight-bearing short leg cast. Drains are not used routinely, and there are emerging data suggesting that the use of drains in TAA is not routinely required.[8] Patients are often admitted overnight; however, some are discharged the same day, and there are emerging data to support same day discharges for uncomplicated primary TAAs.[9-13] Pain is managed postoperatively with the use of acetaminophen, nonsteroidal anti-inflammatories, and selective use of oral narcotics. Patients without risk factors for deep vein thrombosis or pulmonary emboli are routinely discharged on daily aspirin.

Patients are typically seen at 2 weeks after surgery, at which time the cast is removed, along with sutures assuming the wound is satisfactorily healed. Patients without concomitant osteotomies or hindfoot arthrodesis are routinely made weight bearing as tolerated in a controlled ankle motion (CAM) boot. Patients typically return at 6 weeks after surgery, at which time standing radiographs are obtained. They begin formal outpatient physical therapy focusing on ankle range of motion and strengthening and wean from their CAM boot.

Patients typically return at 3 months, 6 months, and 1 year postoperatively. After 1 year, the patient is seen annually for clinical and radiographic follow-up, to monitor implant stability as well as to evaluate for the development of ballooning periprosthetic cysts or heterotopic bone formation.

TECHNICAL TIPS

- Ideal patient positioning typically includes bringing the patient down to the end of the bed and placing a bump under the ipsilateral thigh to internally rotate the limb.
- A large C-arm is used and brought in from the ipsilateral (fibular) side, to allow the image intensifier to be closer to the ankle on lateral fluoroscopic images.
- During the approach, the superficial peroneal nerve is typically found crossing form lateral to medial in the distal third of the incision. This should be mobilized and retracted laterally. Sometimes, a small medial crossing branch may have to be sacrificed to allow for better mobilization of the nerve laterally.
- When using standard instrumentation, resection of anterior osteophytes on the tibia and talus can be helpful to more clearly visualize the joint line. This is typically accomplished with a small curved osteotome and double action rongeur.
- In patients with an ipsilateral total knee arthroplasty, the reference pin in the proximal tibia will often need to be placed distal to the end of the total knee. When there is a stemmed tibial implant in place, fluoroscopy can be utilized to offset the pin medial or laterally relative to the stem.
- When trying to gauge the proper amount of distal tibial and talar resection in the standard technique, the black metal cutting block can be very useful. This can be placed prior to beginning the tibial arc preparation. A free saw blade can be placed in the talar cutting guide, along with a free drill pin in the most superior hole for drilling the arc tibial holes. Obtaining a perfect lateral view, with the talar saw blade parallel, will best estimate combined tibial and talar resection.

- Removal of the distal tibial resected bone can be extremely challenging. Often, if the resected bone on the tibial side cannot be removed en bloc, this can be morselized with the help of a small reciprocating saw and a long, skinny rongeur. The resected talus can often be more easily removed, allowing for better visualization as the posterior portion of the resected tibia is removed.
- When impacting the tibial component, lift-off posteriorly is a common pitfall. A lateral fluoroscopic image is helpful to ensure that the implant and impactor are appropriately aligned. Lateral fluoroscopy can be very helpful both when punching the tibia during preparation and during final implant placement. If posterior tibial lift off is encountered, a helpful sequence of events includes the following:
  - Re-rasping the tibial arc cut
  - Re-punching the viper tip peg punch paddle
  - Impacting the tibial component first starting centrally, then posteriorly, then finishing impaction centrally
- Meticulous wound handling and closure is critical. The deep capsule should be completely closed and then the extensor retinaculum closed as an additional layer. Appropriate retinacular closures helps to prevent bow stringing, especially of the tibialis anterior tendon, which can cause pressure on the wound anteriorly.

COMPLICATIONS

Wound complications are one of the most feared complications of TAA and can have severe consequences if not managed appropriately.[14-16] As with other current generation TAAs, the APEX TAA should be monitored for early mechanical failure secondary to loosening and subsidence, especially tibial sided.[17,18] Patients should be monitored yearly for development of periprosthetic cysts, which may require débridement and grafting if they increase in size over time or threaten the stability of the implant. If we are suspicious for any radiographic irregularities, we reflexively order a CT scan to look for cysts or lucencies. Heterotopic bone can sometimes form in the medial or lateral gutter of the ankle, which can cause patients pain. Open or arthroscopic gutter débridement may be needed to remove the impinging bone. Both medium- and long-term data are needed to understand the longevity and function of this implant.

To date, there are no published studies on the results of the APEX 3D total ankle, likely owing to the fact that the implant has only been on the market a little over 2 years. Certainly short-, medium-, and long-term follow-up studies will be needed to demonstrate the function and longevity of the APEX 3D total ankle.

REFERENCES

1. Cody EA, Scott DJ, Easley ME. Total ankle arthroplasty: a critical analysis review. *JBJS Rev.* 2018;6(8):e8.
2. https://paragon28.com/wp-content/uploads/2022/10/P10-STG-0001-Rev-E_Apex-Total_Ankle_Replacement.pdf
3. Demetracopoulos CA, Adams SB Jr, Queen RM, DeOrio JK, Nunley JA II, Easley ME. Effect of age on outcomes in total ankle arthroplasty. *Foot Ankle Int.* 2015;36(8):871-880.
4. Gaugler M, Krahenbuhl N, Barg A, et al. Effect of age on outcome and revision in total ankle arthroplasty. *Bone Joint J.* 2020;102-B(7):925-932.
5. Pierce Ebaugh M, Alford T, Kutzarov K, Davis E, Greaser M, McGarvey WC. Patient-reported outcomes of primary total ankle arthroplasty in patients aged <50 years. *Foot Ankle Orthop.* 2022;7(1):24730114221082601.
6. Lee GW, Wang SH, Lee KB. Comparison of intermediate to long-term outcomes of total ankle arthroplasty in ankles with preoperative varus, valgus, and neutral alignment. *J Bone Joint Surg Am.* 2018;100(10):835-842.
7. de Keijzer DR, Joling BSH, Sierevelt IN, Hoornenborg D, Kerkhoffs G, Haverkamp D. Influence of preoperative tibiotalar alignment in the coronal plane on the survival of total ankle replacement: a systematic review. *Foot Ankle Int.* 2020;41(2):160-169.
8. Moncman TG, Fliegel B, Massaglia J, et al. Comparison between closed suction drainage and no drainage following total ankle arthroplasty. *Foot Ankle Int.* 2022;43(9):1227-1231.
9. Borenstein TR, Anand K, Li Q, Charlton TP, Thordarson DB. A review of perioperative complications of outpatient total ankle arthroplasty. *Foot Ankle Int.* 2018;39(2):143-148.
10. Gonzalez T, Fisk E, Chiodo C, Smith J, Bluman EM. Economic analysis and patient satisfaction associated with outpatient total ankle arthroplasty. *Foot Ankle Int.* 2017;38(5):507-513.
11. Kayum S, Kooner S, Khan RM, et al. Safety and effectiveness of outpatient total ankle arthroplasty. *Foot Ankle Orthop.* 2021;6(4):24730114211057888.
12. Langan TM, Rushing CJ, McKenna BJ, Berlet GC, Hyer CF. The safety profile of same-day outpatient total ankle arthroplasty. *J Foot Ankle Surg.* 2022;61(1):123-126.
13. Mulligan RP, Parekh SG. Safety of outpatient total ankle arthroplasty vs traditional inpatient admission or overnight observation. *Foot Ankle Int.* 2017;38(8):825-831.

14. Cody EA, Bejarano-Pineda L, Lachman JR, et al. Risk factors for failure of total ankle arthroplasty with a minimum five years of follow-up. *Foot Ankle Int.* 2019;40(3):249-258.
15. Gross CE, Hamid KS, Green C, Easley ME, DeOrio JK, Nunley JA. Operative wound complications following total ankle arthroplasty. *Foot Ankle Int.* 2017;38(4):360-366.
16. Reb CW, Watson BC, Fidler CM, et al. Anterior ankle incision wound complications between total ankle replacement and ankle arthrodesis: a matched cohort study. *J Foot Ankle Surg.* 2021;60(1):47-50.
17. Cody EA, Taylor MA, Nunley JA II, Parekh SG, DeOrio JK. Increased early revision rate with the INFINITY total ankle prosthesis. *Foot Ankle Int.* 2019;40(1):9-17.
18. Saito GH, Sanders AE, de Cesar Netto C, O'Malley MJ, Ellis SJ, Demetracopoulos CA. Short-term complications, reoperations, and radiographic outcomes of a new fixed-bearing total ankle arthroplasty. *Foot Ankle Int.* 2018;39(7):787-794.

10 Infinity Total Ankle Replacement

Brian M. Fisher and Jeremy J. McCormick

INDICATIONS AND CONTRAINDICATIONS

INFINITY total ankle arthroplasty (Stryker, Mahwah, NJ, United States) is indicated in patients with severe, end-stage ankle arthritis, which has failed to improve with conservative measures, such as activity modifications, oral anti-inflammatory medications, bracing, and corticosteroid injections. Contraindications for INFINITY total ankle arthroplasty include the presence of neuropathy, active infection, uncontrolled diabetes, or talus or tibia avascular necrosis. The authors consider utilizing a stemmed tibia implant named INBONE (Stryker, Mahwah, NJ, United States) rather than the minimal resection INFINITY tibial implant when there is concern about patient bone density, intra-articular deformity is greater than 15°, there is associated hindfoot deformity or prior hindfoot arthrodesis has been performed. In these situations there may be increased risk of failure of a low profile stemmed implant in these situations due to lack of adequate bone support or increased stress through the tibial implant. Further, INFINITY is not typically used in the setting of revision total ankle arthroplasty, where bone loss or concern for fixation may require the more robust tibia and talus fixation options of INBONE or INVISION total ankle arthroplasty systems (Stryker, Mahwah, NJ, United States).

PREOPERATIVE PLANNING

INFINITY total ankle arthroplasty may be performed utilizing standard instrumentation or via patient-specific cutting jigs. When utilizing standard instrumentation, the surgeon utilizes a rotational guide in the medial gutter of the ankle, a pin in the tibial tubercle, and then a guide arm, which overlies the tibial crest to create coronal and sagittal alignment for appropriate resection of both the tibial and talar articular surfaces. In order to utilize patient-specific instrumentation, a preoperative computed tomography (CT) scan is obtained with a specific protocol to include the ankle joint and the proximal tibia. The CT scan is then electronically submitted to Stryker, Inc and trained engineers, with the utilization of software and surgeon-driven individualized requests for alignment parameters, to create a surgical plan specific to that patient's anatomy (Fig. 10.1). These parameters include utilization of mechanical versus anatomic axis, location of the joint line, amount of bone resection, varus/valgus alignment, and rotation of the tibial implant. The preoperative plan is also able to estimate the tibia and talus implant sizes and can estimate whether previously placed hardware will interfere with planned surgical resections. The need for soft tissue balancing, additional osteotomies or arthrodesis in the hindfoot or forefoot, tendon lengthening or transfer, and other potential adjunct procedures should be planned preoperatively based on surgeon clinical evaluation of the patient and are not considered in the preoperative plan.

Once approved by the requesting surgeon, the software is then utilized to create 3D-printed guides for placement of the implant cutting jigs for both the tibia and talus. These guides use the bony contour of the anterior distal tibia and dorsal talar neck so that the planned resections and alignment seen on preoperative plan can be accurately executed intraoperatively. This is achieved by obtaining fluoroscopic images at specific points during the procedure and comparing the intraoperative images to the images predicted by the preoperative plan. If the fluoroscopic images do not match the preoperative plan, the surgeon may either make fine adjustments to the position of the jigs to match the preoperative plan or convert to using standard instrumentation. Preoperatively, surgeons should ensure familiarity with standard instrumentation should it be necessary.

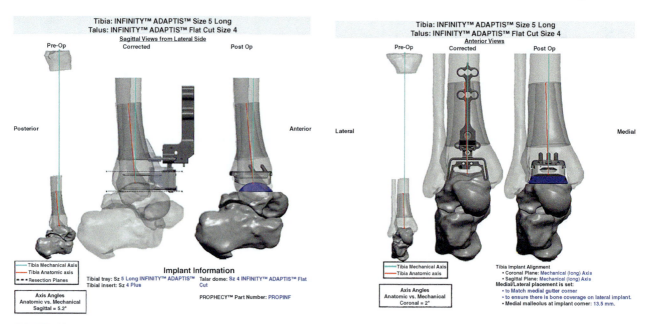

FIGURE 10.1 Initial pages of patient-specific total ankle arthroplasty report demonstrating anatomic and mechanical axis with proposed resection locations and final implant positioning.

It is the practice of the authors to utilize PROPHECY patient-specific instrumentation (Stryker, Mahwah, NJ, United States) for all INFINITY total ankle arthroplasty cases as it improves accuracy of implant alignment and decreases surgical time.[1,2] As such, the below surgical technique does not review the use of traditional external alignment guide.

SURGICAL TECHNIQUE

The patient is positioned in a supine position with a slight bump underneath the ipsilateral hip to allow the operative extremity to rest in neutral rotational position. The operative extremity is prepped and draped in the surgeon's preferred manner. A standard midline anterior ankle approach is undertaken using the interval between the tibialis anterior (TA) and extensor hallucis longus (EHL). The TA is retracted medially and the EHL and neurovascular bundle are retracted laterally. Once at the depth of the ankle joint capsule and periosteum, full-thickness flaps are developed. Some surgeons may choose not to dissect through the compartment contents and joint capsule as a single flap. The authors prefer to separate these layers to allow for capsular closure over the implant. It is essential while elevating the joint capsule and periosteum to completely elevate and remove all soft tissue from the underlying bone to allow the patient-specific guide to find the "perfect fit" on the tibia and talus bony surface (Fig. 10.2). This may be accomplished with Bovie electrocautery, curette, and/or periosteal elevator. Once the tibia surface is adequately cleared of soft tissue, attention is turned to use of the PROPHECY resect through guides.

The resect through guides come prepared with a patient-specific simulated 3D-printed tibia and talus based on the preoperative CT scan. It is recommended that the surgeon take the opportunity to evaluate the simulated surface of the tibia and compare it to the patient's anterior tibia to identify bony landmarks (Fig. 10.3A). Then, utilizing the resect through guide, the perfect fit is found on the simulated tibia surface to know where the guide will sit on the actual patient tibia. The surgeon should critically evaluate which osteophytes and bony undulations will guide a perfect "key" fit (Fig. 10.3B and C).

Once comfortable with the "perfect fit" of the resect-through guide on the printed model of the tibia, the guide is carefully placed on the anterior aspect of the patient's distal tibia until the same "perfect fit" is obtained (Fig 10.4A). At this time, bicortical pins are placed into the holes diagonally from each other in the proximal and distal aspect of the resect through guide for preliminary fixation (Fig. 10.4B). It is important that the surgeon continues to maintain pressure on the resect-through guide while wires are advanced to prevent small amounts of rotation or translation. In addition, the surgeon or assistant advancing the wire should do so slowly and perfectly in line with the hole in the resect through guide to avoid skiving or pushing the guide (and resultant implant) into an undesired

10 Infinity Total Ankle Replacement

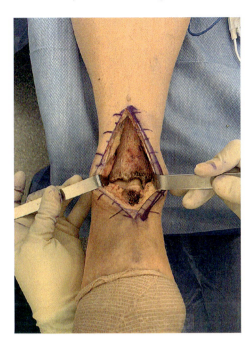

FIGURE 10.2 Anterior approach to the ankle. Note complete elevation of periosteum and soft tissue from the anterior surface of the tibia.

position. An AP radiograph is obtained under fluoroscopy at this time, adjusting the position of the ankle until a perfect bullseye is obtained (Fig. 10.5A and B). If the surgeon prefers, they can place unicortical pins initially, advancing them to bicortical fixation once the alignment has been verified radiographically.

It is only once this perfect AP fluoroscopic shot is obtained that it should be compared to the preoperative report. The overlay of the rings on the distal tibia from the resect-through guide should be critically evaluated on fluoroscopy and compared to the preoperative report to ensure correct orientation of the distal tibia cut (Fig. 10.5B and C). If the two are a match, with the targeting bullseye lined up, the surgeon may proceed. However, if the radiographs do not match the PROPHECY report, adjustments may be made to the PROPHECY guide position. This can be accomplished by

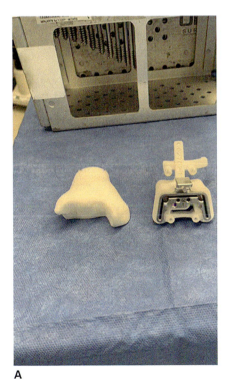
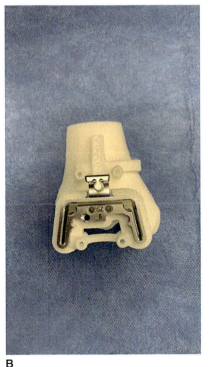
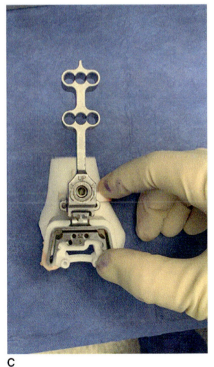

A B C

FIGURE 10.3 A. The 3D-printed replica of the anterior tibia surface and resect-through tibia guides. **B, C.** Assessing "perfect fit" of the tibia PROPHECY guide.

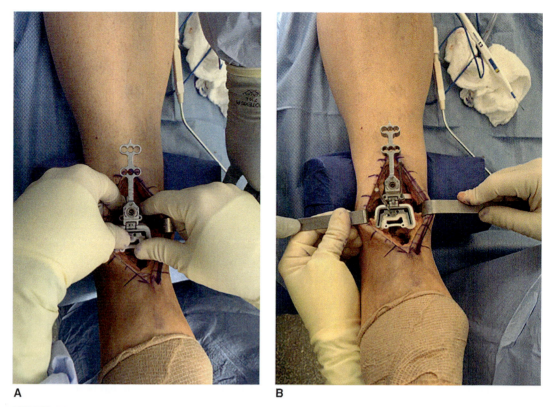

FIGURE 10.4 A. Obtaining fit on a patient's anterior tibia similar to the perfect fit on the 3D-printed replica. **B.** Pins are placed bicortically in holes diagonal from one another.

completely removing the pins securing the guide, repositioning the guide, and placing pins into opposite pin sites. Alternatively, a single pin could be removed, and the guide slightly rotated to allow the fluoroscopy to match the preoperative report. The removed pin is then placed into a different pin site to avoid placing the guide into the prior incorrect position.

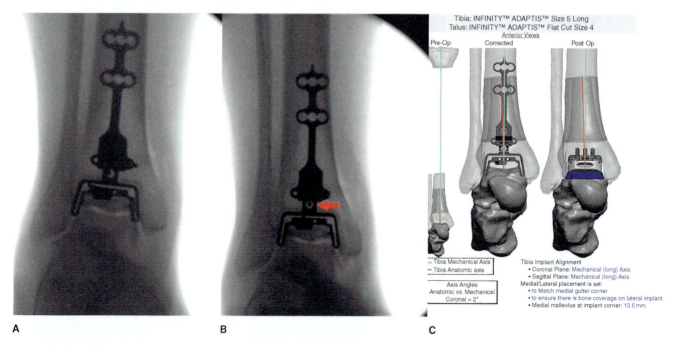

FIGURE 10.5 A, B. Fluoroscopy is obtained and position of the ankle is adjusted until the perfect bullseye is seen (*red arrow*). **C.** Fluoroscopy is compared to the preoperative report to ensure that position of the resect-through guide on the distal tibia is a match ("Olympic rings," cut guide projection).

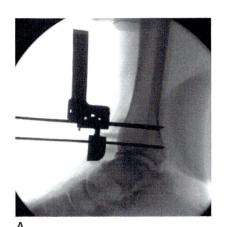
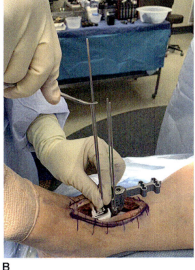
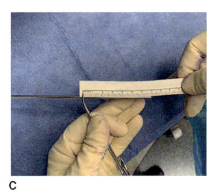

FIGURE 10.6 **A.** Fluoroscopy demonstrating pin position with distal medial pin depth up to, but not protruding through, the posterior cortex. **B, C.** An additional wire of the same length is placed on the anterior aspect of guide, marked at the end of secured wire, and measured for accurate depth of cut with the sagittal saw.

Once the guide is confirmed to be in the correct position, it is fully secured with two additional bicortical pins, being careful to ensure the pins do not plunge posteriorly and damage posterior anatomic structures, such as the medial neurovascular bundle or flexor hallucis longus tendon. A lateral fluoroscopic radiograph is obtained to ensure that the resection level is also appropriate as compared to the preoperative report. The authors make a point at this step to ensure that the length of the pins are just beyond the posterior tibial cortex, particularly the distal, medial pin as it is closest to the posteromedial structures of the ankle (Fig. 10.6A). An additional wire of the same length is then placed on the anterior aspect of guide against the fixed wire. The additional wire is then marked at the proximal end of the fixed wire (Fig. 10.6B). The length of the remaining portion of the free wire is then measured to estimate the depth of expected tibia resection from the top of the resection guide (Fig. 10.6C). This step helps avoid excessive excursion of the saw blade posteriorly and the potential of resultant damage to the posterior neurovascular and tendinous structures when making the tibia bone cut. The fixed pins are then trimmed flush to the PROPHECY guide so they do not interfere with the saw blade during distal tibia resection (Fig. 10.7A and B). An additional wire is placed

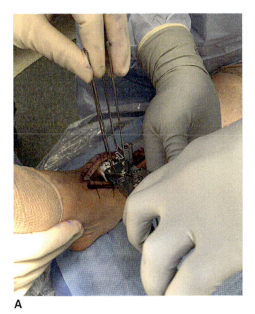
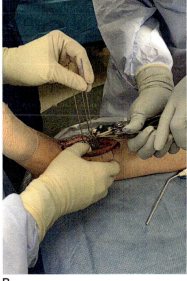
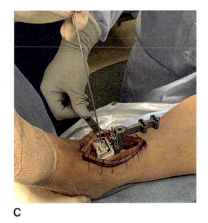

FIGURE 10.7 **A, B.** Wires are trimmed close to the guide to not interfere with the saw. **C.** A diagonal pin is placed to further stabilize the guide. It is also trimmed although not flush to the guide to allow for easier removal at the completion of the distal tibia resection.

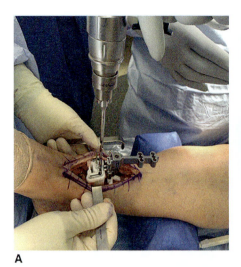 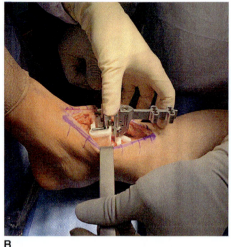 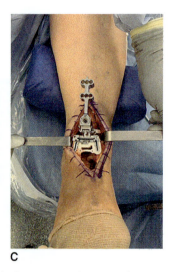

FIGURE 10.8 **A.** The corner drill is utilized through the resect through guide in each corner bicortically to ensure the corner is resected well to allow for proper implant seating. **B.** Corner protectors are then placed. **C.** Final setup including all pins and corner protectors prior to completing the distal tibia cut.

through an oblique hole in the patient-specific guide for further stability (Fig. 10.7C). The pin is then trimmed to be out of the way of the saw but not flush with the cutting guide. If this oblique pin is cut flush to the guide, it will be difficult to remove the pin or guide after tibial resection. A corner drill is then utilized bicortically, ensuring the drill stays in line with the corner guide holes in the cutting jig (Fig. 10.8A). Each corner is then filled with a corner protector peg that both stabilizes the cut guide and avoids inadvertent excursion of the saw blade when making the tibial cuts (Fig. 10.8B and C).

An oscillating saw is utilized to make the bone cuts through the tibia resect-through guides. When performing tibia cuts, the surgeon should use a blade that is narrow enough to oscillate without

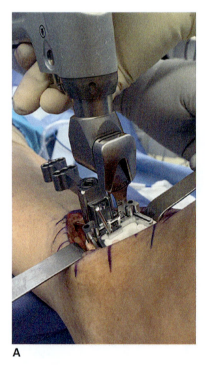 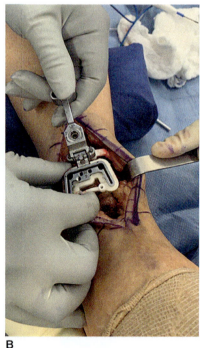 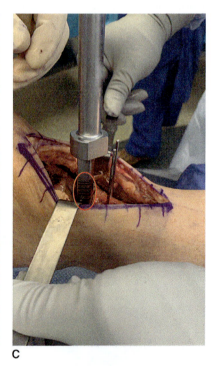

FIGURE 10.9 **A.** An oscillating saw is utilized to perform the tibial cut through the guide, with care taken not to plunge posteriorly. The depth measurement on the saw should be utilized to correlate with the previously measured anticipated depth of the distal tibia cut. **B.** Cross pin is removed and the distal tibia cutting guide is removed from the distal tibia surface. **C.** The corner chisel is utilized with a mallet to complete the corner cut. The chisel is sunk to the depth of the anticipated tibial size based on the preoperative report (*red circle*).

causing displacement of the jig. Often, utilization of a Kocher clamp on at least one of the wires can further stabilize the jig. Typically, the authors make the proximal transverse cut followed by the medial and lateral cuts. If the surgeon elected to use the depth measurement technique described previously, they should pay close attention to the depth of resection that was measured (Fig. 10.9A). If doubt remains whether the posterior cortex has been cut, fluoroscopy may be used to check the depth of cut. The authors typically err on the side of a more conservative depth so as not to injure the posterior ankle structures.

Once the tibia cuts have been completed, the surgeon has the option to complete the talus cut through the same cut guide. This technique, known as "coupling" the cuts, works well in the situation where the ankle does not have significant deformity. When the cuts are "coupled," the talus cut is mated exactly to the tibia cut. Some surgeons believe that this offers an advantage to placement and subsequent stability of the implants. In the case of ankle deformity, it is critical that the surgeon corrects all deformity and temporarily pins the ankle in a straight position before considering coupling the cuts. This will help assure the result of the cuts is a well-aligned total ankle replacement. While this "coupled" technique is a viable option for total ankle replacement surgery, the author's preference is to perform the procedure with "uncoupled" cuts, independently cutting the tibia with the cut guide described above and the talus with a separate cut guide as described later in this chapter. Particularly with the use of the PROPHECY guides, the authors believe that "uncoupled" cuts allow for more reproducible deformity correction and, therefore, use this technique as their standard.

Once tibia cuts have been completed, the tibial cut guide is then removed (Fig. 10.9B). The proximal row of K-wires should be left in place as these will be necessary for placement of the tibial trial component. The corner chisel is then used to ensure that the corner cuts have been completed and any remaining posterior cortex is no longer intact. The corner osteotome has markings for each size of tibial implant; thus, the surgeon should seat the osteotome to the marked depth for the anticipated implant size as projected on the PROPHECY report (Fig. 10.9C). A threaded bone retrieval pin is then placed within the resected segment of the distal tibia. The bone retrieval pin can be premarked to match the depth of the planned tibia implant and advanced to that marking to ensure that the pin is well seated (Fig. 10.10A). A handle is then attached to the pin and traction is applied with gentle manipulation of the bone segment until the bone of the distal tibia resection can be completely removed (Fig. 10.10B and C). Care should be taken to avoid moving in a medial or lateral direction with the retrieval instrument once it is inserted into the tibia bone resection to avoid causing a

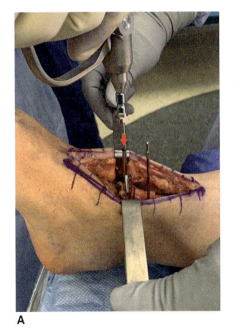
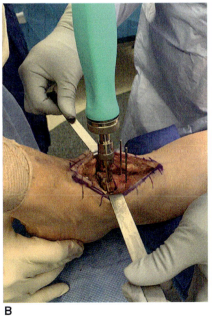
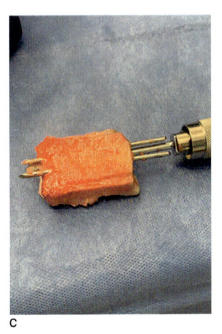

A   **B**   **C**

FIGURE 10.10 **A.** A bone retrieval instrument is then placed within the resected segment of the distal tibia, ensuring the pin is well seated as measured to the depth of the predicted implant as identified on the report. The depth is marked with a purple marker on the back table (*red arrow*). **B.** A handle is then applied to the pin, and traction is applied to manipulate the tibia bone out of the wound. **C.** The goal is to remove the distal tibia resection in one piece.

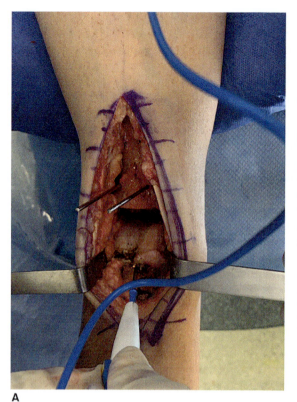 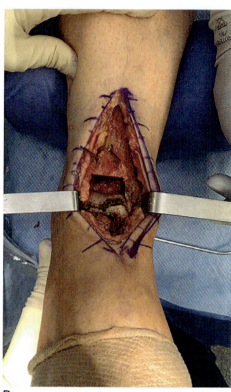

FIGURE 10.11 A. Talus with intact cartilage and soft tissue prior to removal. **B.** Talus following cartilage removal with Bovie and curette.

medial malleolus fracture. If the surgeon is unable to remove the tibial bone resection en bloc, one can use an osteotome to remove the anterior half of the tibia bone block and subsequently remove the posterior half once the talus resection is completed.

Attention is now turned to the talus. A combination of Bovie electrocautery and curette is used to remove remaining soft tissue from the dorsal head and neck of the talus. Cartilage is also removed from the anterior half of the talar body to allow for positioning of the PROPHECY talar guide, ensuring the underlying bone, including osteophytes, is not disrupted (Fig. 10.11). It is recommended that the surgeon take the opportunity to evaluate the simulated surface of the talus that is generated as part of the patient-specific guide system and compare it to the patient's dorsal talus to identify bony landmarks. The talar block is then used to find the perfect fit on the model talus surface to know generally where the guide will sit *in vivo*. The surgeon should critically evaluate which osteophytes and bony undulations that "key" into the guide (Fig. 10.12).

Once comfortable with the "perfect fit" of the talus guide on the model, it is carefully placed on the dorsal aspect of the patient's talar neck and body until the perfect fit is achieved (Fig. 10.13A). Two wires are then placed dorsal to plantar through the talus guide to secure it to the talus while the surgeon maintains pressure on the block to keep it in position (Fig. 10.13B). Two additional wires are then placed from anterior to posterior (AP) through the guide and into the talus bicortically, again while the surgeon is maintaining pressure on the block to maintain appropriate position (Fig. 10.13C). Fluoroscopy is used to obtain a perfect lateral of the talus and the position of the AP wires is observed. The two AP wires should perfectly overlap to judge the plane of the proposed talar resection. The location of this resection is modeled in relation to the position of these wires on the patient-specific report. For a minimal resection, or chamfer cut talus, the resection will be above the wires. For a flat-cut talus, the resection will be below the wires. The plane of the proposed talar resection is compared to the preoperative report. If pleased with the position of the talus resection, the surgeon may proceed. If not, adjustment to the position of the talus PROPHECY block is required (Fig. 10.14).

The INFINITY total ankle system (Stryker, Mahwah, NJ, United States) has the option of utilizing a chamfer cut or flat cut talus. The chamfer cut is used in situations where there has not been

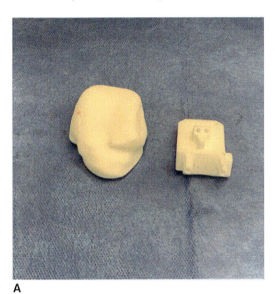 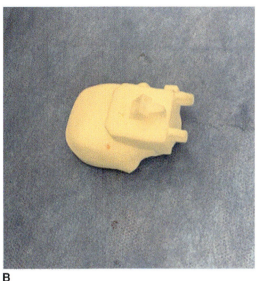

FIGURE 10.12 **A.** Patient-specific talus 3D model and associated guide. **B.** Simulated perfect fit on the talus with the block prior to placing it on the patient's talus to understand where perfect fit will occur.

talar bone loss or flattening and the surgeon is interested in preserving as much talar bone as possible at the time of ankle replacement. In theory, this allows the patient to retain bone stock in the talus that could be helpful if the patient ever requires revision total ankle replacement. This chamfer cut method does require a few additional steps to accomplish the multiplane talar cut. The flat cut should be utilized when there has been talus bone loss, and the chamfer cut implant would not appropriately fit on the native talus after bone resection. The bone resection for the flat cut implant is in a single plane and, for some surgeons, is preferred. Ultimately, selection of the talus implant is left to the surgeon's discretion, considering both patient factors and technical factors. The Stryker continuum of total ankle implants does allow for an INBONE or INVISION talus to mate with an INFINITY tibia if necessary. For this case example, a flat-cut talus resection was performed.

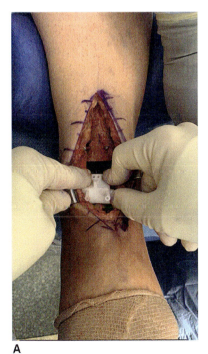 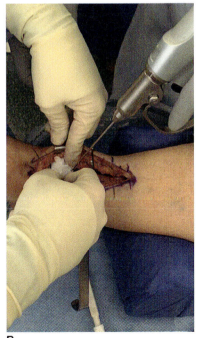 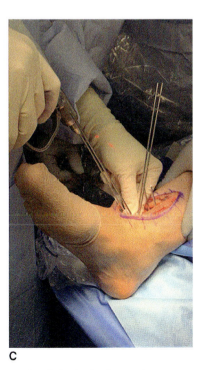

FIGURE 10.13 **A.** Perfect fit is found with the talus jig on the patient's talus. **B.** Once perfect fit is obtained, two pins are placed through the guide in a proximal to distal fashion to hold the jig in place. **C.** Anterior-posterior wires are placed through the PROPHECY guide.

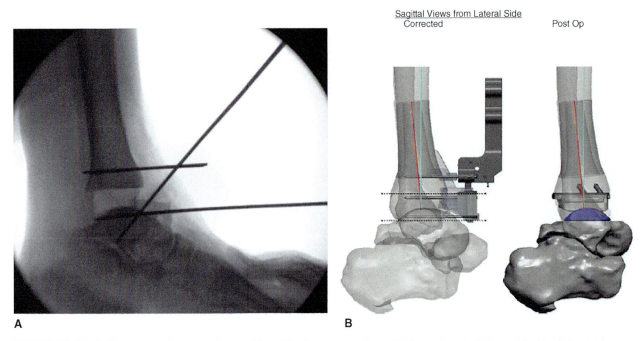

FIGURE 10.14 A. Fluoroscopy demonstrating position of the transverse wires with the anticipated talar cut for the flat-cut talus being 2 mm distal to the pin location. **B.** Position of the wires on fluoroscopic view compared to the PROPHECY report to ensure appropriate alignment.

Once the desired position of the talus component is obtained, the dorsal-plantar wires are removed and the patient-specific block is removed, leaving the AP wires in place. The talus cutting jig is then placed over the AP wires. For this example, with the flat-cut talus, the word "FLAT" will be upright and legible (if it was a chamfer cut talus, the talus cutting jig would be flipped with "CHMF" visualized) (Fig. 10.15A and B). Gutter pins are placed through the cut guide to protect the medial and lateral malleoli in positions suggested in the preoperative report. An additional oblique pin is also placed through the cut guide for additional stability (Fig. 10.15C). The AP pins are cut flush to the

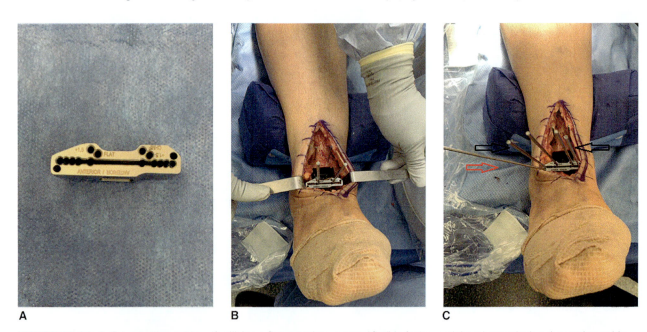

FIGURE 10.15 A. Talus cutting guide—if utilizing a flat-cut talus, ensure "flat" is facing upright prior to placing the cutting guide on the wires in the talus. **B.** For the flat-cut talus, slide the cutting guide onto the anterior-posterior wires through the holes just on top of the cutting slot. **C.** Place the oblique wire (*red arrow*) into the cutting guide for improved stability. Also place gutter wires (*black arrows*) to protect the medial and lateral malleoli during talar resection.

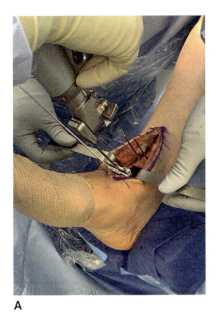 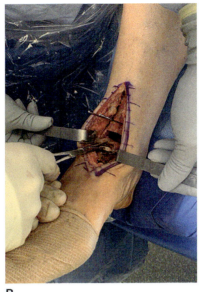 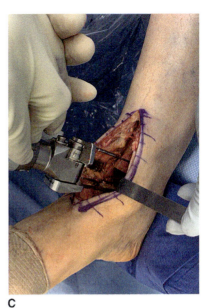

FIGURE 10.16 **A.** Resection of the talar dome is undertaken with an oscillating saw. The surgeon can look over the guide into the ankle joint to observe the depth of the talar cut. **B.** Once the talus resection is completed, the resected talar dome is removed from the ankle and gutter pins are removed. **C.** If any bone remains, particularly on the periphery of the talus, this is removed free-hand with the oscillating saw to ensure the blade stays flush in plane with the prior resection.

cut guide and the oblique pin is left with some length to ease later pin retrieval. An oscillating saw is then utilized to make the talar bone cut through the talus cut guide (Fig. 10.16A). Like the tibia cut, a blade that is narrow enough to oscillate without causing displacement of the jig should be used while performing the talus resection. Often utilization of a Kocher clamp on at least one of the wires can further stabilize the jig. The surgeon should again pay close attention to the depth of cut; with the talus resection guide, the posterior aspect of the talus can be visualized in the joint as the resection is being performed. The resected talus is removed from the ankle (Fig. 10.16B). The surgeon should then utilize the oscillating saw or a reciprocating saw to ensure that the talus resection level is smooth and flat, particularly paying attention to the medial and lateral aspects of the talus (Fig. 10.16C).

At this point, the ankle is prepared for trialing. The tibia trial is placed over the two remaining tibia K-wires (Fig. 10.17A). Position of the tibial implant in an anterior-posterior plane as visualized clinically and on lateral fluoroscopy is adjusted with a screwdriver in the screw mechanism on the anterior aspect of the trial, which can bring the trial anteriorly. The trial implant is positioned to ensure adequate anterior-posterior cortical coverage, biasing toward anterior coverage of the distal tibial cortex (Fig. 10.17B). Fluoroscopy and clinical evaluation are undertaken to ensure that the anterior portion of the implant is flush with the anterior tibia surface without significant overhang (Fig. 10.18A). Lateral fluoroscopy is used to determine if the component would need to be a "long" or "standard" version. The standard length of the actual implant ends at the V notch in the trial visualized on a lateral fluoroscopic image of the trial implant. The long length is the entirety of the trial implant (Fig. 10.18B). Typically, the authors err toward a larger implant to optimize the cortical coverage of the implant. Once the tibial trial is in the desired position, an awl is used to create a path for the central tibial peg while being impacted with a mallet (Fig. 10.19A). The awl for the central peg should be left in place and sequentially the second awl should be utilized with a mallet to impact bone in both the anteromedial and anterolateral holes. It is important to ensure that the awls are completely seated to impact the appropriate amount of bone to avoid malposition of the tibial implant during implantation.

The talus and polyethylene trial are then placed within the ankle while keeping the tibial trial in place (Fig. 10.19B and C). Initial selection of talus size in the author's hands is usually based on the preoperative report. In the INFINITY system, the talus size can be the same numerical size or one numerical size smaller than the tibial implant (size 4 tibia can mate with a size 4 or size 3 talus). Typically, the smallest thickness polyethylene trial is utilized initially but may be increased

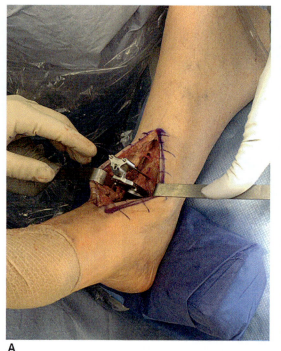
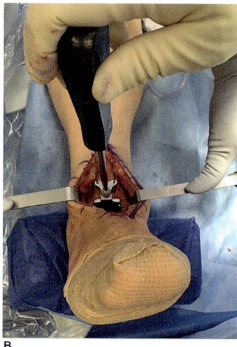

FIGURE 10.17 **A.** The tibial trial is placed over the retained wires in the distal tibia until there is contact between trial and anterior tibia. **B.** Position of the tibia trial in an anterior-posterior direction may be adjusted for optimal cortical coverage by turning the position screw in the trial.

depending on the stability of the ankle. Before the final position of the talus is set, the ankle is ranged in dorsiflexion and plantarflexion to allow for appropriate rotational positioning of the talus component, the so-called sweet spot. The talus component is then pinned into place with dorsal to plantar directed pins through the talus trial (Fig. 10.20A). Fluoroscopy is obtained in both AP and lateral views to ensure correct sizing and positioning of the talus component. On lateral view, the posterior

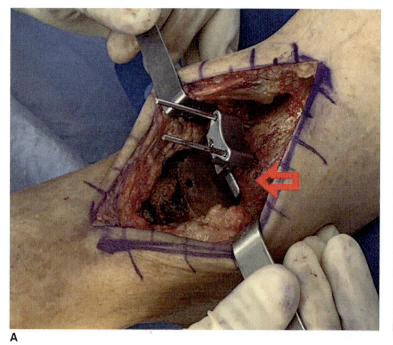
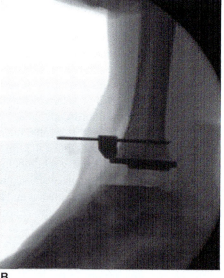

FIGURE 10.18 **A.** Appropriate position of the tibial trial with the anterior portion of the trial being flush with the anterior distal tibia (*red arrow*). **B.** Position of the tibial trial seen on lateral fluoroscopy.

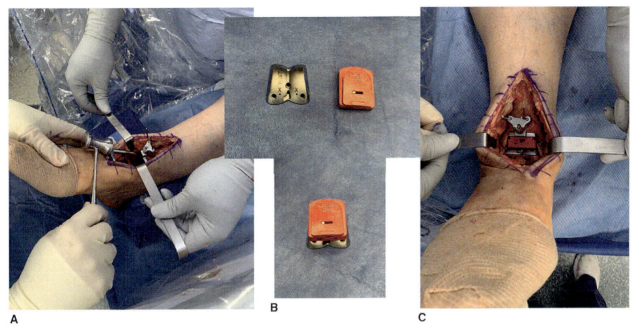

FIGURE 10.19 A. Awls are used to broach a path for the tibial implant pegs. This figure shows the #1 awl being driven into the central position. Once the #1 awl is inserted completely, it is left in place to stabilize the tibial trial while the #2 awl is used to broach the medial and lateral peg holes. Once this is completed, the #1 awl is removed. **B, C.** The talus and polyethylene trials are assembled and subsequently placed in the ankle joint with the polyethylene mating with the tibial component.

aspect of the talus trial should replicate the position identified on the preoperative PROPHECY report. On the AP view, there should be no overhang of the talus trial component medial or lateral into the gutters (Fig. 10.20B and C), as this can lead to postoperative impingement and pain. In addition to the fluoroscopic evaluation, the surgeon should carefully examine the medial and lateral gutters clinically to determine if there is any overhang of the implant or gutter impingement. This is done by carefully examining the medial and lateral gutters with the talus trial in place and observing

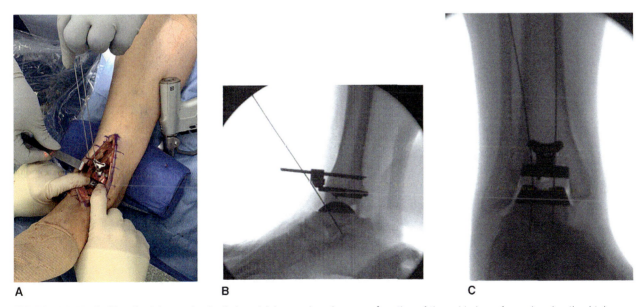

FIGURE 10.20 A. After the talus and polyethylene trials are placed, range of motion of the ankle is performed and optimal talar rotation is identified by allowing the talus to rotate into optimal position while dorsiflexing and plantarflexing through the trial articulating surface. Once satisfied with the position of the talus both in the coronal and sagittal plane, the trial talus component is secured with two K-wires. **B, C.** Fluoroscopy in both AP and lateral planes is obtained to ensure proper position of the talus component. On the AP view, there is no overhang of the talus medially or laterally into the gutters.

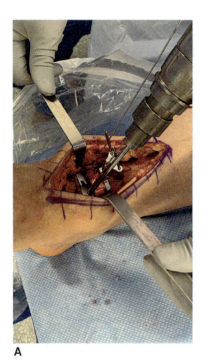 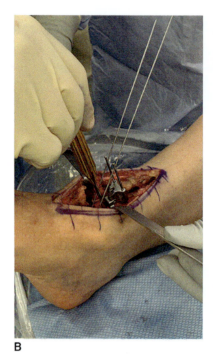 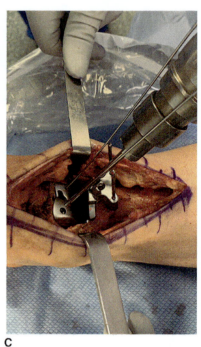

FIGURE 10.21 **A.** Once the position of talus is appropriate and it is pinned in position, a drill is utilized to ream the medial and lateral talus pegs through the talus trial, being careful to stay in line with the trajectory of the holes in the trial. **B.** The polyethylene trial is removed. **C.** The drill is used to ream the central talus peg through the talus trial.

the gutters through range of motion. If there is any gutter impingement, the talus trial implant can be recentered on the talus by backing out the fixation wires, making fine adjustments, and then replacing the wires. If the talus is felt to be in its most central position, then the surgeon should consider downsizing the implant. If the talus is already one size number less than the tibia, then the trial component should be centered in the best position possible, minimizing medial and/or lateral overhang. For the authors, it is more common to have a talus component that is one size smaller than the tibia component. If there is any doubt, the authors will typically choose the smaller size talus implant to avoid gutter impingement.

Once the talus is deemed to be in satisfactory position and pinned into position with two K-wires, the ankle is plantarflexed and a reamer is used to create three peg holes through the talus trial. The surgeon should be careful to ensure the reamer is directly in line with the talus trial holes and seats fully to ensure the final talar component will sit flush against the bone (Fig. 10.21A). The anteromedial and anterolateral holes can be created with the polyethylene component still in place. For the central hole to be reamed, the polyethylene typically must be removed (Fig. 10.21B and C). At this point, once all three peg holes have been drilled, the wires, talus trial, and tibia trial are removed and the surgical site is thoroughly irrigated to remove any residual bone or debris prior to final implant placement.

Final implants are then opened and prepared on the back table. The insertion handle is placed on the tibial implant (Fig. 10.22A and C). The tibial pegs are then aligned with the previously created peg holes in the distal tibia and preliminarily pushed manually with the surgeon's thumbs into position (Fig. 10.23A and B). The tibial impactor is placed into position against the implant and impacted gently with a mallet (Fig. 10.24A). The tibia implant is inspected grossly and under fluoroscopy to ensure it is completely seated (Fig. 10.24B). A small plastic phalange is then placed into the tibia component to protect it while the talar implant is inserted. The insertion handle is threaded in the talus component. The talar implant is then placed by plantar flexing the ankle and giving slight distraction (Fig. 10.25A and B). The talar pegs are aligned with the previously reamed holes, and the implant is pushed into the holes manually to engage the pegs. The talus impactor and a mallet are then used to impact the talar component into position (Fig. 10.25C). The talus implant is inspected grossly and under fluoroscopy to ensure it is completely seated (Fig. 10.25D).

10 Infinity Total Ankle Replacement

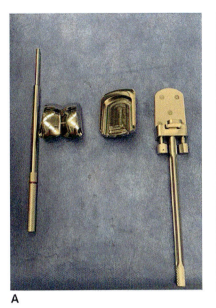 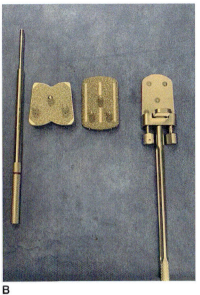 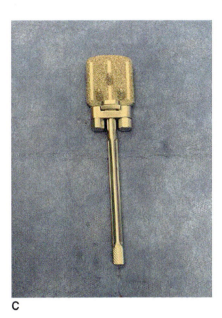

FIGURE 10.22 **A.** Infinity components with associated insertion handles. **B.** A 3D-printed porous ingrowth surface is appreciated on the undersurface of the talus (*left*) and tibial (*right*) components. **C.** The tibial component is attached to the inserter by engaging the screws of the insertion handle into the associated holes on the anterior aspect of the implant.

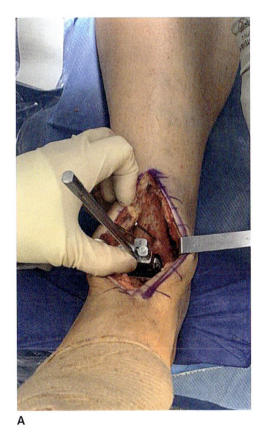 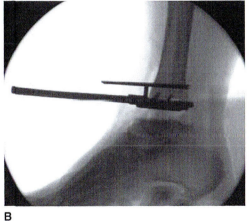

FIGURE 10.23 **A.** The tibial component is placed into the ankle and the pegs are engaged into the previously broached holes with manual pressure. **B.** Fluoroscopy demonstrates initial engagement of the pegs into the tibia. There is a small gap that remains between the tibia implant and the tibia bone making clear that the implant will need further impaction.

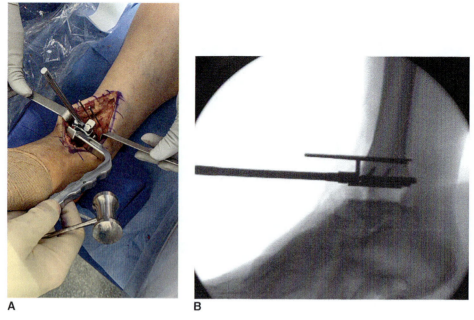

FIGURE 10.24 A. The tibial impactor is placed onto the tibial tray and a mallet is used to impact the tibial component in line with the trajectory of the pegs on the implant. **B.** Fluoroscopy demonstrating the complete seating of the tibial component.

The polyethylene trial is then placed, and the medial and lateral gutters of the ankle are débrided with a combination of an oscillating micro sagittal saw and pituitary rongeur (Fig. 10.26). It is essential to perform bony resection of overhanging bone and osteophytes and remove impinging soft tissue within the medial and lateral gutters of the ankle. In doing so, the surgeon will reduce the risk of postoperative pain from gutter impingement. Next, ankle stability and range of motion is evaluated. If symmetric instability is present, the polyethylene thickness may be increased. If there is asymmetric instability to varus, consideration is given to medial release and increase in polyethylene thickness or adding a lateral ligament stabilization procedure. If there is asymmetric instability

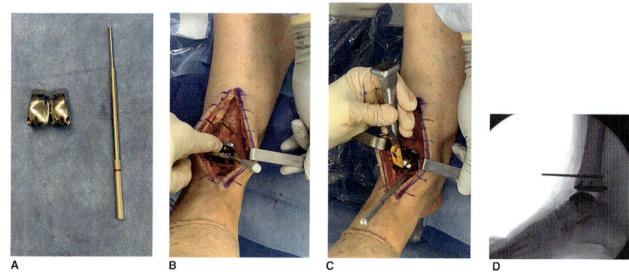

FIGURE 10.25 A. The talus insertion handle is screwed into either the medial or lateral aspect of the anterior aspect of the talus component. **B.** The talus component is placed by plantarflexing the ankle and engaging the pegs manually into the previously broached holes. **C.** The talus impactor is placed superior to the component and a mallet is used to impact the talar component into the talus until it is flush. **D.** Fluoroscopy demonstrates complete seating of the talus component.

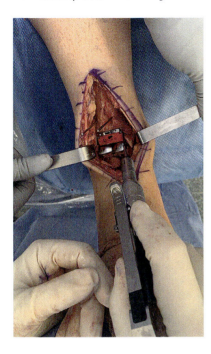

FIGURE 10.26 Polyethylene size is trialed until coronal stability is achieved with adequate range of motion. Gutter débridement is then performed with an oscillating saw to remove residual talar bone impinging in the medial and/or lateral gutter.

to valgus, consideration is given to increase in the thickness of polyethylene or adding a medial deltoid stabilization procedure. If the ankle has limited range of motion to dorsiflexion, the surgeon may perform an Achilles tendon or gastrocnemius fascia lengthening. In addition to ankle stability and range of motion, it is important that the patient's foot posture be well aligned beneath the ankle replacement. Discussion of techniques for ligament stabilization and balancing, assessment of ankle range of motion, and deformity correction at the time of total ankle arthroplasty is outside the scope of this chapter, but it is critically important to the success of the implant. In this case example, the patient did not have significant deformity; therefore, we did not need to perform specific ligament balancing procedures.

Once the surgeon is pleased with gutter débridement, stability, and range of motion, the final polyethylene size is selected. The INFINITY total ankle replacement utilizes a fixed bearing, ultra-high molecular weight polyethylene. Fully engaging the polyethylene into the tibial component is essential for optimal function of the implant and a specific polyethylene insertion device is utilized (Fig. 10.27A). Two posts are screwed into small holes on the anterior aspect of the tibial component (Fig. 10.27B). The polyethylene is loaded into the insertion device while the plunger is pulled back completely and locked. The insertion device is then slid over the posts that were threaded into the tibial component and the inserter is then secured with a nut over each post (Fig. 10.27B). The plunger is used to initially engage the polyethylene into the tibial component (Fig. 10.28A). Once the threads of the plunger contact the housing, the plunger is turned clockwise to advance the polyethylene into the tibial component in a controlled manner (Fig. 10.28B). The inserter and guide rods are then removed, and the polyethylene is inspected to ensure it is fully seated. If it is not fully seated, there will be a small gap between the polyethylene and the tibial component. In this case, an impactor can be used to carefully complete insertion of the polyethylene (Fig. 10.28C). Caution is advised to not impact too forcefully as this may result in tibial component loosening.

Fluoroscopic AP, lateral, and mortise views are utilized to inspect the final total ankle arthroplasty to ensure complete seating of implants, appropriate alignment of implants, and adequate débridement of medial and lateral gutters (Fig. 10.29). The ankle is then irrigated and a layered closure is performed of the joint capsule/periosteum, extensor retinaculum, subcutaneous tissue, and skin. This closure is typically performed with the tourniquet still inflated unless the tourniquet had been previously deflated after appropriate duration of time as dictated by the surgeon. Most commonly, this occurs in a situation where adjunctive procedures are necessary for deformity correction driving the case to a longer duration of operative time.

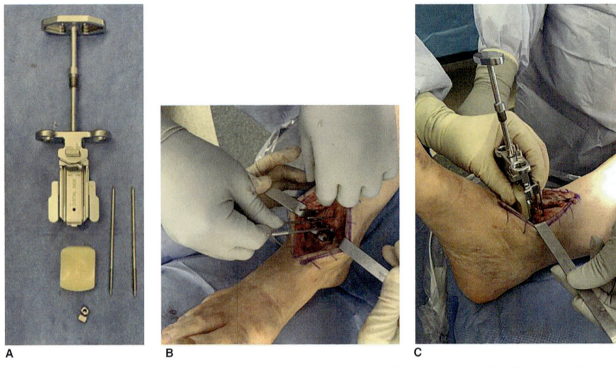

FIGURE 10.27 **A.** Polyethylene with inserter including guide rods and nuts. **B.** Guide rods are screwed into the holes on the anterior aspect of the tibial component. **C.** The polyethylene inserter is slid over the guide rods and nuts are used to secure the inserter to the rods and the tibial implant.

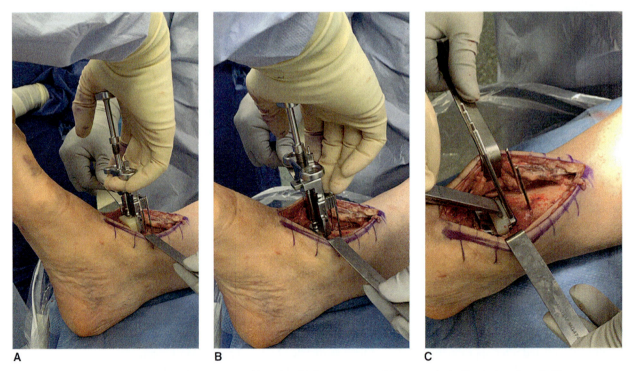

FIGURE 10.28 **A.** Polyethylene is initially engaged into the tibial component with a posteriorly directed motion. **B.** The polyethylene is further advanced into the tibial component by turning the handle clockwise once the threads on the plunger engage the housing. This is done until the plunger bottoms out. **C.** If there is still space between polyethylene and tibia component, the polyethylene is manually impacted with light mallet taps using a finishing tool.

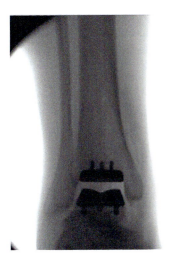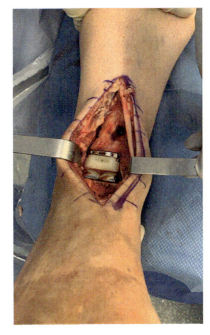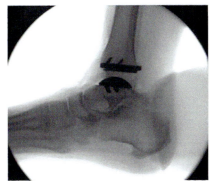

FIGURE 10.29 Final clinical and radiographic appearance of the Infinity total ankle arthroplasty with polyethylene fully inserted into the tibia component.

PEARLS AND PITFALLS

- Utilize the 3D-printed simulated tibia and talus to obtain a feel for where the perfect fit of the patient-specific guide will occur prior to placing the guides on the patient's anatomy.
- Ensure that all soft tissue including the periosteum and joint capsule is removed from the bony surface of the tibia and talus prior to utilizing patient-specific guides to allow for "perfect fit."
- The patient-specific report should be critically evaluated and compared to fluoroscopic images throughout the surgical case to ensure that bony resection matches the preoperative plan and subsequently matches the planned alignment of the total ankle arthroplasty.
- Utilize the described technique to measure the depth of tibial resection to avoid lacerating posterior tendinous and neurovascular structures.
- The corner drill and subsequently the corner osteotome should be utilized to allow for a flush corner cut to create optimal stability of the tibial implant and reduce the risk of a stress riser at the medial shoulder of the ankle resection that can lead to fracture of the medial malleolus.
- Optimize tibial component cortical contact by adjusting the anterior/posterior position of the tibial implant.
- To improve longevity of the total ankle implant, the surgeon should balance soft tissues and correct foot alignment to avoid asymmetric contact pressure within the total ankle, which could lead to polyethylene wear and implant loosening.

POSTOPERATIVE MANAGEMENT

Following total ankle arthroplasty, the operative ankle is placed in a well-padded splint. This is important to control postoperative edema, which can contribute to postoperative wound complications. The patient is instructed to strictly elevate the extremity for the first 2 weeks postoperative while maintaining non–weight-bearing (NWB) status on the operative side. After 2 to 3 weeks, sutures are removed, and the patient is placed into a short leg fiberglass cast with the ankle at neutral dorsiflexion for an additional 3 to 4 weeks for a total of 6 weeks of immobilization and NWB. If the patient has not had adjunctive procedures that require 6 weeks of postoperative casting, and the surgical incision appears completely healed, the patient can be placed in a controlled ankle motion (CAM) boot at the time the sutures are removed. This is at the discretion of the surgeon.

At 6 weeks postoperative, the patient is placed in a tall CAM boot, allowed gradual weight bearing, and begins physical therapy focusing on edema control and range of motion. As range of motion is restored, the patient begins working on ankle strengthening outside of the boot.

At 10 to 12 weeks postoperative, the patient is weaned out of the CAM boot and into an ankle stabilizing orthosis (ASO) brace. Physical therapy is advanced to include closed and open chain strengthening, gait retraining, and proprioceptive training. At approximately 4 months after surgery, the patient can wean out of the ASO brace. As the patient's symptoms and function improve, they can begin resuming lower impact activities such as walking, golf, and hiking but are encouraged to wait until 6 months postoperative to resume medium impact activities, such as tennis and pickleball.

RESULTS AND COMPLICATIONS

Early reports from the designers of the INFINITY implant showed promising data with a 97% implant survival rate at mean 35.4 months.[3] Other data have been published demonstrating a 90% implant retention at a mean 13 months follow-up. In this series, 4% of revisions were performed for infection rather than aseptic implant loosening.[4] More recent studies demonstrate 95.3% implant survival[5] and the largest study performed to date by nondesign surgeons was published out of the United Kingdom demonstrating 99% 2-year survival of implants.[6] In addition, all patient-reported outcome measures demonstrated significant improvement when compared to preoperative values. Further studies are required to evaluate mid- and long-term outcomes and complication rates and how they compare with other currently available implants.

Complications following total ankle arthroplasty include implant loosening, gutter impingement, peri-implant cysts, intraoperative or postoperative fracture, wound healing complications, and deep periprosthetic infection. Unfortunately, like other lower extremity procedures, significant complication with total ankle arthroplasty can occur, leading to outcomes including amputation.[7]

REFERENCES

1. Daigre J, Berlet G, Van Dyke B, Peterson KS, Santrock R. Accuracy and reproducibility using patient-specific instrumentation in total ankle arthroplasty. *Foot Ankle Int.* 2017;38(4):412-418.
2. Saito GH, Sanders AE, O'Malley MJ, Deland JT, Ellis SJ, Demetracopoulos CA. Accuracy of patient-specific instrumentation in total ankle arthroplasty: a comparative study. *Foot Ankle Surg.* 2019;25(3):383-389.
3. Penner M, Davis WH, Wing K, Bemenderfer T, Waly F, Anderson RB. The infinity total ankle system: early clinical results with 2- to 4-year follow-up. *Foot Ankle Spec.* 2019;12(2):159-166.
4. Cody EA, Taylor MA, Nunley JA 2nd, Parekh SG, DeOrio JK. Increased early revision rate with the INFINITY total ankle prosthesis. *Foot Ankle Int.* 2019;40(1):9-17.
5. Saito GH, Sanders AE, Cesar Netto C, O'Malley MJ, Ellis SJ, Demetracopoulos CA. Short-term complications, reoperations, and radiographic outcomes of a new fixed-bearing total ankle arthroplasty. *Foot Ankle Int.* 2018;39(7):787-794.
6. Townshend DN, Bing AJF, Clough TM, Sharpe IT, Goldberg A. Early experience and patient-reported outcomes of 503 INFINITY total ankle arthroplasties. *Bone Joint J.* 2021;103-B(7):1270-1276.
7. Randsborg PH, Jiang H, Mao J, et al. Two-year revision rates in total ankle replacement versus ankle arthrodesis. *JBJS Open Access.* 2022;7(2):e21.00136.

11 Lateral Approach Total Ankle Arthroplasty

Kevin A. Schafer and Lew C. Schon

INTRODUCTION

While nearly a dozen implants are available for anterior approach total ankle arthroplasty, only one, The Zimmer Trabecular Metal, exists for use via a lateral, transfibular approach. This implant has been Food and Drug Administration cleared since 2012 and is a semi-constrained implant with a highly cross-linked polythylene liner snap fitted into the tibial component (fixed bearing). Although this implant is Food and Drug Administration cleared only for use with cemented fixation, many surgeons worldwide choose to implant the prosthesis without cement.[1-3]

There are several unique material properties of this implant. The implant interface is constructed from porous tantalum (Trabecular Metal), which has a similar microstructure and porosity to cancellous bone. It has a low modulus of elasticity similar to subchondral bone, and a high coefficient of friction.[4,5] Together, these properties are intended to promote bone ingrowth, enhance implant stability, and minimize implant stress shielding that can result in marginal bone loss.[4,5] This tantalum interface is distinctive, as other arthroplasty implants have a titanium alloy bone interface that is either 3D printed (porous) or plasma spray coated. The biomechanical properties of tantalum more closely resemble those of bone,[6] and tantalum may have superior osseointegration compared to titanium.[7]

Additionally, there are several unique advantages afforded by arthroplasty through a lateral approach:

1. Curved tibial and talar bone resection can be performed. Compared to flat or chamfered cuts from an anterior approach, curved cuts increase the contact area between the implant and bone, allow for minimal bone resection, and position the components against denser bone at the anterior and posterior tibia.[8] Together, these properties may enhance implant stability and may decrease the likelihood of implant subsidence.
2. The stabilizing implant rails can be placed perpendicular to the flexion-extension plane, improving stability against anterior to posterior shear stress.
3. A fibular osteotomy facilitates easier correction of varus and valgus deformity and can correct fibular deformity or malunion.
4. A lateral approach involves dissection between two perforating branches of the peroneal artery (terminal calcaneal branch and anterior perforating branch) and is associated with a low rate of wound complications (less than 4%).[1,2]

While the use of a rigid alignment frame is not unique to this implant, it is a powerful component of the surgical technique. This frame allows for careful, controlled correction of most multiplanar deformities, with the tibia and talus then rigidly fixed to the frame. Arthroplasty can then be performed relative to this corrected alignment. Although supplemental bony and soft tissue procedures may still be needed to maintain corrected ankle alignment after frame removal, our experience has been that mild to severe deformity corrections are maintained. This phenomenon is not well defined and is likely multifactorial: (1) inherent gap balancing of the technique by correcting the deformity under traction in the frame with medial collateral release as needed, making a curved coupled talotibial cut with a router, filling the arthroplasty gap with the appropriately sized components as assessed with stability testing, and then repairing the lateral ligament sleeve at a corrected tension while the ankle remains fixed in the frame in the desired alignment, (2) sagittal plane conformity of the opposed, truncated conical arthroplasty surfaces, and (3) the anatomic coronal constraint of the malleoli (not unique to this system, although fibular length and alignment adjustments likely provide additional stability in severe deformity).

In the following sections, we will detail the critical steps in indicating, evaluating, and performing this arthroplasty. The authors' surgical tips and preferred techniques can be used together with manufacturer's surgical technique guide for a comprehensive reference to lateral total ankle arthroplasty.

INDICATIONS AND CONTRAINDICATIONS

Primary total ankle arthroplasty is indicated in patients with tibiotalar arthritis secondary to degenerative, posttraumatic, or inflammatory etiologies. Revision arthroplasty of a non-Zimmer total ankle or an ankle fusion take-down to a Zimmer total ankle can also be performed through the lateral approach. However, templating should be performed preoperatively to confirm adequate bone stock, as stemmed or thicker revision components are not yet available for the Zimmer total ankle.

Arthroplasty specifically through a lateral approach may be advantageous in several clinical scenarios. Patients with a traumatized anterior soft tissue envelope can undergo arthroplasty without a repeat insult to the anterior blood supply. Also, a fibular malunion or deformity is straightforward to address with the fibular osteotomy that is necessary for this approach. Additionally, patients with large sagittal and coronal plane deformity can benefit from the versatility of the rigid frame, which enables controlled deformity correction followed by implantation of well-positioned components in a single stage procedure. Next, performing curved bone resections from the lateral approach may be preferable in patients with a flat or flatter talar dome when a curved or chamfered talar cut is desired, as talar resection can be minimized. In the setting where the ankle joint is distal to the talonavicular joint, a lateral approach also facilitates easier bony resection, as the midfoot does not block access to the ankle joint. Lastly, a lateral approach is particularly advantageous during a takedown of an existing arthrodesis, as the recreation of the flexion extension axis is directly visualized.

Ankle arthroplasty is contraindicated when there is inadequate bone stock to support the implant at either the talus or tibia. This can occur in severe cases of avascular necrosis, or with large periarticular cyst formation secondary to arthritis. Similarly, fibular bone loss, either form prior trauma, congenital deformity, or from removal during ankle arthrodesis, presents a challenge to reconstruct a joint with an adequate stabilizing lateral buttress. However, rotational fibular transfers during arthroplasty have been described with encouraging early results.[9] Arthroplasty is also contraindicated in patients with neuroarthropathy and advanced peripheral vascular disease given the high risk of perioperative complications and concerns regarding implant longevity. Similarly, an active local or systemic infection also precludes arthroplasty. Arthroplasty specifically through a lateral approach is also contraindicated if there is an inadequate lateral soft tissue envelope.

Relative contraindications to ankle replacement should also be considered. A history of prior infection poses an increased risk of a periprosthetic infection, and many surgeons prefer arthrodesis in this setting. However, the authors have successfully performed arthroplasty in such patients when clinical evidence (examination, inflammatory labs, bone biopsy, intraoperative evaluation) suggests infection has been eradicated. Performing arthroplasty in younger (less than 50 years old), active patients is also controversial given concerns for accelerated wear in more active patients, and given the likelihood of future revision procedures. However, the authors discuss the risk and benefits of arthrodesis versus arthroplasty with younger patients on a case-by-case basis given the potential for sustained functional improvement with arthroplasty.[10,11]

Final relative contraindications to consider are significant joint instability (deltoid insufficiency, lateral ligament instability), global limb malalignment, and a nonreconstructable nonplantigrade foot. If these issues can be addressed during arthroplasty or in a staged fashion, then ankle replacement may still be a viable option. If these issues cannot be addressed, arthroplasty will result in eccentric implant loading and likely early failure, and arthrodesis is preferred. Lastly, severe coronal or sagittal plane deformities may be better treated with arthrodesis. The authors have treated varus/valgus deformities up to 40° and translational deformities of 3 cm, but long-term follow-up of similar cases is required to better define arthroplasty limitations.

PREOPERATIVE PLANNING

Preoperative planning begins with a detailed history. Any modifiable risk factors that can contribute to perioperative complications are identified and addressed. Patients on disease modifying antirheumatic drugs may need to either hold or coordinate medication dosing to minimize wound complications. Patients with diabetes must have their hemoglobin A1c controlled, with the authors preferring a 7.5 mg/dL cutoff.[12] Additionally, patients diagnosed with osteoporosis should have an endocrine evaluation to determine whether biologics are indicated. Lastly, smoking cessation for at least 4 weeks preoperatively is important given the well-documented increase in perioperative complications following joint arthroplasty.[13,14]

We next proceed with a thorough physical examination. With the patient standing, the overall alignment of the lower extremity and foot are carefully assessed, as creating a neutrally aligned ankle and plantigrade foot are prerequisites to a successful outcome. The patient is then observed while ambulating, allowing for dynamic deformities to be identified. On seated examination, the soft tissues are inspected for any preexisting incisions or soft tissue trauma to confirm an adequate lateral soft tissue envelope. A neurovascular examination is then conducted to assess for weakness, neuropathy, or inadequate vascularity. If there are any concerns regarding vascularity, we routinely obtain arterial duplex studies. Next, an assessment of tendon and joint function is performed with active and passive ankle, subtalar, and transverse tarsal motion. Any deficits are characterized as rigid or passively correctable. Tendon deficits are noted. Lastly, the stability of the collateral ligaments is assessed. Collectively, this comprehensive examination identifies any coexisting pathology that may need to be addressed so that arthroplasty results in a stable, well-aligned prosthesis above a plantigrade foot.

Standing plain radiographs of the foot and ankle are next routinely obtained. If there is more global deformity on examination, tibia and fibula or full length standing radiographs may be necessary. Radiographs are carefully examined for the severity of arthritis at the ankle and adjacent joints. The alignment of the ankle, hindfoot, and midfoot are also studied. Additionally, images can characterize bone loss (particularly a flat top talus or erosions of the tibial plafond), existing hardware, cysts, and malunions or nonunions (typically at the medial or lateral malleoli).

Advanced imaging can be helpful in several instances. If bone cysts or voids are visualized, a computed tomography (CT) describes these lesions in detail. We prefer using a weight-bearing CT scan so that ankle and hindfoot alignment can simultaneously be studied in additional detail. This is particularly useful in patients with additional pathology including subtalar arthritis or lateral impingement. If there are concerns regarding tendon or ligament integrity, an ankle magnetic resonance imaging (MRI) offers a detailed evaluation of these structures. An MRI can also be helpful in evaluating the hindfoot in patients with both ankle and subtalar joint pain.

Prior to proceeding with surgical management of ankle arthritis, nonoperative treatments are recommended for attempted symptomatic relief. These include activity modification, shoe modifications or orthotics in the setting of flexible deformity, ankle braces, icing, anti-inflammatories, vitamin D augmentation, and steroid or viscosupplementation injections. When patients fail these interventions, the risks and benefits of surgical management are discussed.

SURGICAL TECHNIQUE

Anesthesia, Positioning, and Room Setup

Upon arrival to the operating room, popliteal and adductor canal blocks guided by ultrasound are performed for perioperative analgesia. The patient is then positioned supine on a bean bag positioner, and anesthesia is administered. However, spinal anesthesia is an alternative if preferred by the surgeon or anesthesia provider. A pneumatic thigh tourniquet is applied, although rarely inflated by the authors. The patient is then positioned with their heels 6 inches from the end of the table to provide enough room for the frame. A 4.5 tall × 8 wide × 25 long foam positioner is then inserted under the operative extremity to provide a stable working platform above the contralateral extremity that is wide enough to support the frame (Fig. 11.1A). The authors use a custom foam positioner with adequate stiffness to support the frame and the leg without collapsing. Alternatively, stacked blankets can be used if a foam positioner is not available. Importantly, this foam or blanket platform facilitates obtaining a lateral fluoroscopic image without the nonoperative leg interfering. An arm board is placed by the contralateral leg to move it away from the working surface and help support it

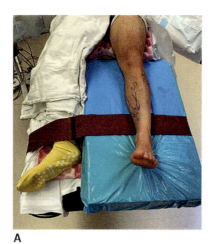 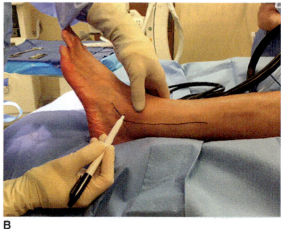

FIGURE 11.1 Preoperative positioning and incision. **A.** The operative extremity is elevated above the nonoperative extremity on a wide foam platform. An arm board is placed along the nonoperative extremity for extended support given the width of this platform. The operative extremity is then internally rotated using a beanbag positioner so that the toes point straight up and down. Both the foam platform and the nonoperative leg are then secured to the table. **B.** A longitudinal incision is made along the posterior border of the fibula, beginning 10 to 12 cm proximal to the ankle joint. Distally, the incision is curved around the tip of the fibula toward the sinus tarsi for 3 cm.

during the procedure. Finally, the beanbag is adjusted at the pelvis to internally rotate the extremity 15° to 20°, until the toes are pointing straight up and down (see Fig. 11.1A). A large C-arm is then positioned opposite to the operative extremity, perpendicular to the long axis of the table.

Prior to surgical incision, 1 g of tranexamic acid is administered in patients who are not at an increased risk of thrombosis.[15] We also position the operating table in a 10° to 15° Trendelenburg position. In our experience, these interventions have allowed us to complete almost all procedures without inflating the tourniquet.

Surgical Approach

Step 1. Lateral Dissection and Fibular Osteotomy

A longitudinal incision is made along the posterior border of the fibula, beginning 10 to 12 cm proximal to the ankle joint. Distally, the incision is curved around the tip of the fibula toward the sinus tarsi for 3 cm (Fig. 11.1B). If a prior incision is in close proximity, it is generally utilized to minimize wound complications. During superficial dissection, care is taken to identify any crossing branches of the superficial peroneal nerve. About 1.5 cm proximal to the ankle joint line, the peroneal retinaculum is released off of the posterior fibula to facilitate reflection of the distal fibula. This dissection is carried distally until reaching the superior peroneal retinaculum, which is left intact (Fig. 11.2A). Distally, a blunt object is inserted into the sinus tarsi (Fig. 11.2B). The blunt tip of a surgical forceps or a freer are commonly used, with a blunt object preferred to avoid damage to adjacent subtalar cartilage and crossing nerve branches. Sharp longitudinal dissection is then performed between this point and the fibular tip and is continued along the distal fibular periosteum slightly posterior to the midline. A single soft tissue sleeve is then elevated anteriorly containing fibular periosteum, the anterior talofibular ligament, and distal extent of the anterior inferior tibiofibular ligament (AITFL) (Fig. 11.2B and C). With superior traction on this elevated soft tissue sleeve, subperiosteal dissection continues across the lower 1.5 cm of the anterior tibia, allowing full visualization of the anterior joint line (Fig. 11.2C and D). Care is taken not to dissect too proximally along the lateral distal tibia, as a perforating branch of the peroneal artery can be transected.

With the necessary releases performed, a lateral fibula plate is then provisionally placed to facilitate future reduction and fixation. In cases of fibular malunion or severe deformity, this step can be skipped given the anticipated change in fibular alignment. We routinely place a proximal bicortical nonlocking screw and drill for three distal locking screws (Fig. 11.3A). The hardware is then removed and the holes marked with surgical ink in preparation for the osteotomy (Fig. 11.3B).

11 Lateral Approach Total Ankle Arthroplasty

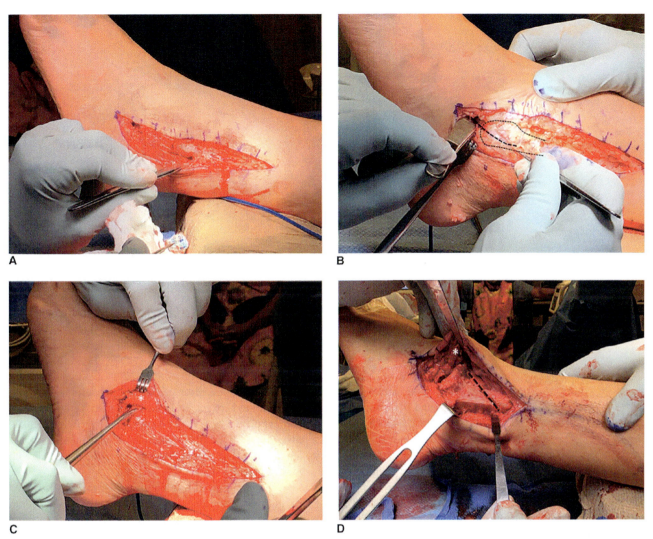

FIGURE 11.2 Lateral dissection to facilitate fibular reflection. **A.** 1.5 cm proximal to the joint line, the peroneal retinaculum is released off of the posterior fibula to facilitate upcoming reflection of the distal fibula inferiorly. This dissection is carried distally until reaching the superior peroneal retinaculum, which is left intact. **B.** Distally, a blunt object is inserted into the sinus tarsi. Sharp dissection is then carried out longitudinally between this point and the distal fibula (*dashed line* along silhouette of distal fibula). **C.** This entire soft tissue sleeve is elevated anteriorly as one flap off of the fibula (*asterisk* in **C** and **D**), containing fibular periosteum, the anterior talofibular ligament, and distal extent of the anterior inferior tibiofibular ligament. **D.** This dissection plane is carried anteriorly across the anterior tibia, elevating the anterior ankle capsule until a blunt object can be inserted all the way across the anterior tibia. This graphic also nicely demonstrates the posterior release of the peroneals from the distal fibula, distal to the planned osteotomy site (*dashed line*).

A K-wire is placed in the fibula 1.5 cm above the ankle joint and checked on imaging (Fig. 11.4). A microsagittal saw is then used to osteotomize the fibula perpendicular to the coronal plane of the ankle, angled 45° from proximal posterior to anterior superior. This osteotomy orientation allows for fibular shortening, lengthening, and coronal plane correction as needed.

The distal fibula is then mobilized by first placing a Cobb elevator into the incisura distally, roughly parallel with the long axis of the fibula (Fig. 11.5A). The Cobb is then gently rotated externally to place tension on the remaining anterior AITFL fibers not released during elevation of the soft tissue sleeve from the distal fibula as described above. These remaining AITFL fibers are then sharply released from the tibia. The Cobb is then inserted into the incisura from proximal to distal or distal to proximal and similarly rotated to place tension on the posterior inferior tibiofibular ligament fibers that can be sharply released from the tibia (Fig. 11.5B). Dissection of posterior inferior tibiofibular ligament fibers directly off bone will minimize risk of injury to the nearby peroneal artery. The fibula is then reflected inferiorly with traction from a towel clip. Any inhibiting

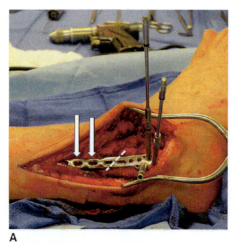 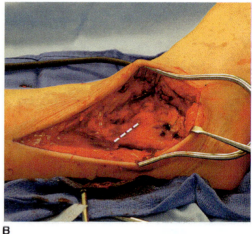

FIGURE 11.3 Provisional fibular plating. **A.** An anatomic lateral fibular plate is applied to the fibula, with plate positioned assessed fluoroscopically. A bicortical nonlocking screw is then drilled for and inserted proximal to the planned osteotomy (*white arrows* identifying potential plate holes for this screw, *dashed line* indicating planned osteotomy), securing the plate down to bone. Locking towers are then attached to the plate distally, and three unicortical holes are drilled and measured. **B.** Hardware is then removed, and the drill holes are marked with a surgical marker to facilitate identification during future fibular reduction and fixation.

remaining syndesmotic attachments are released, but the superior peroneal retinaculum, calcaneofibular ligament, and posterior talofibular ligament are kept intact. In cases of severe contracture, a partial release of the posterior talofibular ligament off the talus may be necessary to obtain adequate talar exposure. A 1.6-mm K-wire is then passed through the fibula and into the calcaneus to secure the reflected fibula against the lateral skin (Fig. 11.5C). The wire is then cut, bent, and protected with a pin cap. The tibiotalar joint should now be well visualized.

The ankle joint capsule is then released. A Cobb is inserted into the tibiotalar joint and twisted repeatedly to release the capsule. These twisting motions are continued anteriorly and posteriorly, as the Cobb is rolled from inside to outside the joint. After exiting just above and below the tibial plafond, the Cobb is gently pulled proximally to further release the capsule from the tibia. Next, a talar sizing depth gauge is inserted from lateral to medial, and a fluoroscopic image is obtained to confirm adequate placement (Fig. 11.5D). When the gauge measures in between sizes, the smaller size is chosen to preserve medial malleolar bone stock.

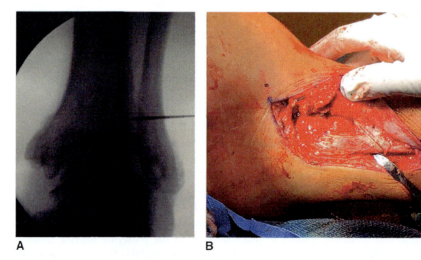

FIGURE 11.4 Fibular osteotomy. **A.** A K-wire is placed between 1.5 and 2 cm proximal to the tibiotalar joint line. **B.** The wire serves as a guide during the oblique osteotomy.

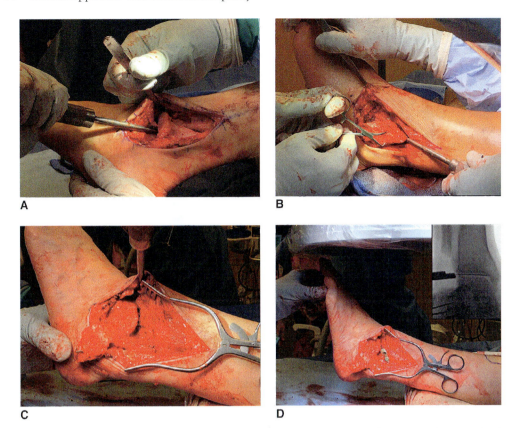

FIGURE 11.5 Fibular reflection and talar sizing. **A.** A Cobb is inserted into the incisura to place rotational tension on the anterior syndesmosis to facilitate sharp release. **B.** This is repeated to place tension on the posterior syndesmosis, and a towel clip is used to provide distal traction. **C.** The fibula is pinned to the lateral calcaneus. **D.** The talar sizer is inserted after capsular release, and fluoroscopy is used to check proper positioning.

In a fair number of cases, the distal and lateral edge of the tibia impairs direct visualization of the joint line. Removing a small wedge of bone may be required to facilitate milling and implant placement (Fig. 11.6).

In the case of a severe or rigid varus deformity, or when there is significant bony impingement at the medial ankle gutter, a medial arthrotomy can be performed. In many cases, this medial approach is not required, as milling from the lateral incision allows for visualization and débridement of the medial gutter. When necessary, however, a longitudinal incision is made in line with the saphenous

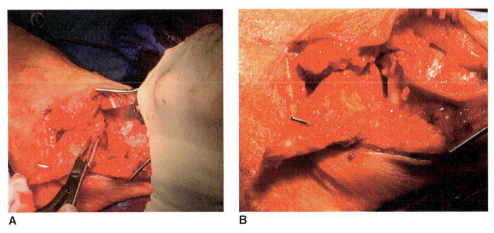

FIGURE 11.6 Removal of lateral tibial overhang. **A.** The lateral tibia frequently extends over the edge of the tibiotalar joint line, impairing visualization of the talar dome. **B.** With this small wedge of bone removed (which will be removed during upcoming milling anyway), the joint line is now fully visualized.

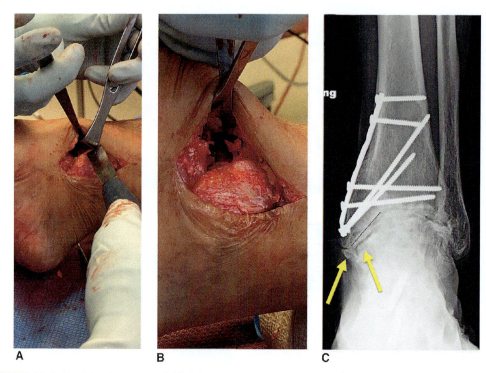

FIGURE 11.7 Medial arthrotomy and débridement. **A.** After medial exposure in line with the saphenous neurovascular bundle, the anterior edge of the medial malleolus is removed (*dashed line* in **C**). **B.** Removal of this anterior edge of the medial malleolus facilitates visualization across the anterior tibiotalar joint. **C.** Additional sources of impingement at the tip of the medial malleolus and medial talus (*yellow arrows*) are also addressed. While debris in the medial gutter may be visible from the lateral approach, a medial approach is utilized to address significant medial impingement and perform a thorough gutter débridement (as indicated by the pathology).

bundle at the joint line, and subperiosteal dissection off of the medial malleolus is carried anteriorly until an arthrotomy is made. An osteotome is then used to remove the anterior edge of the medial malleolus (Fig. 11.7A and B), as this bone is often a source of impingement. There may be additional impingement at the body-neck junction at the medial talus or at the tip of the medial malleolus (Fig. 11.7C). With a rigid varus deformity, the superficial deltoid ligament can be released off the tibia. This is performed by carrying the subperiosteal dissection posteriorly from the site of the arthrotomy in the prior step, peeling the ligament off the medial malleolus rather than cutting it transversely. In working from anterior to posterior, care is taken to protect the posterior tibial tendon. The deep deltoid fibers are left intact to function as a restraint against lateral talar translation in the following steps as the deformity is corrected with traction in the frame.

Step 2. Frame Application and Deformity Correction

The operative extremity is then positioned in the frame. The heel is placed on the heel cup with 2 to 3 cm between the heel and the footplate to provide room for distraction. The height of resting supports under the gastrocnemius can be adjusted until the tibial crest is parallel with the rods of the frame (Fig. 11.8A). The extremity should be rotated internally approximately 10° to 15° until the medial border of the foot parallels the medial aspect of the footplate (Fig. 11.8B). The rotation of the foot can then be secured with sliding clamps on the footplate at the metatarsal heads. The rotation of the talus is then assessed by attaching a router guide to the frame and inserting the probe through the "position" slot of the router guide. If rotation is correct, the backside of the probe should rest flush against the anterolateral talus (Fig. 11.8C).

The first of four partially threaded Schanz pins is then inserted. The first pin is placed through the calcaneus from medial to lateral and allows for the traction to correct coronal hindfoot alignment relative to the foot plate and frame. The pin is inserted just above the medial edge of the heel cup (Fig. 11.8A) and is oriented parallel to the footplate if there is no coronal plane deformity. If there is a varus deformity, the pin is angled to exit more distally laterally (parallel to the deformity) so

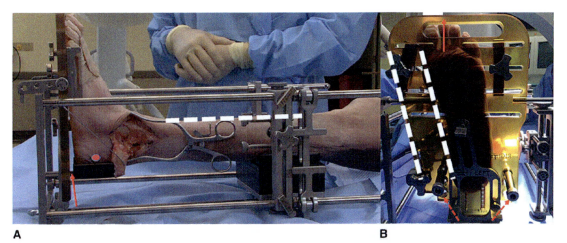

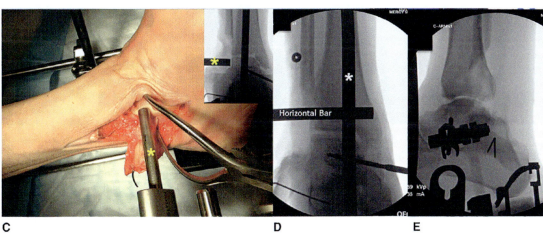

FIGURE 11.8 Frame positioning and talar alignment. **A.** Leg height is adjusted until the tibia is parallel to the bars on the frame. A space is left between the heel and the footplate (*red arrow*) to allow room for distraction. The *red dot* marks the planned location of calcaneal pin insertion, just above the heel cup. **B.** The extremity is rotated internally until the medial border of the foot parallels the medial surface of the footplate. The second toe should point straight up and down (*solid red arrow*). The *dashed red arrows* identify the calcaneal pin clamps that are used to bring the foot down to the plate. **C.** The back end of the probe (probe marked by *yellow asterisk*) is placed against the lateral talus to assess rotation, with rotation adjusted until the probe is flush. **D.** The probe is inserted across the ankle to serve as a horizontal bar and reference for talar and tibial alignment. A tibial alignment rod (*white asterisk*) can also be inserted to assess tibial alignment more proximally. **E.** A talar pin is inserted through a clamp on the frame, with the clamp positioned below the talar dome to prevent interference with lateral fluoroscopy of the talus.

that correction of the pin parallel to the footplate corrects hindfoot alignment. The opposite angular correction is made for a valgus deformity.

The calcaneal pin is then secured to the footplate via medial and lateral pin holders. These pin holders are fastened to bring the heel down to the footplate and can be tightened asymmetrically to help correct deformity (ie, tighten more medially in varus deformity). The probe is then inserted through the router guide and placed anterior to the skin at the distal tibia to serve as a horizontal alignment guide (Fig. 11.8D). The router guide needs to be tightened to ensure the probe rests in a perfectly horizontal position. The surgeon then fine-tunes the alignment until the talar dome is parallel to the horizontal bar. This can be performed by additional manipulation of the calcaneal pin or by applying distal traction on the frame itself. A laminar spreader can also be inserted at the joint line to help correct more severe deformity.

With talar alignment corrected relative to the frame, it is secured to the frame with a second pin. This pin is placed medially at the junction of the lower and middle thirds of the talus at the junction of the talar neck and body. The starting point is usually 1 cm distal and anterior to the tip of the medial malleolus. The talar pin is inserted through an external fixator clamp on a talar pin post on the frame (Fig. 11.8E) and is angled from distal to proximal so that the clamp does not block

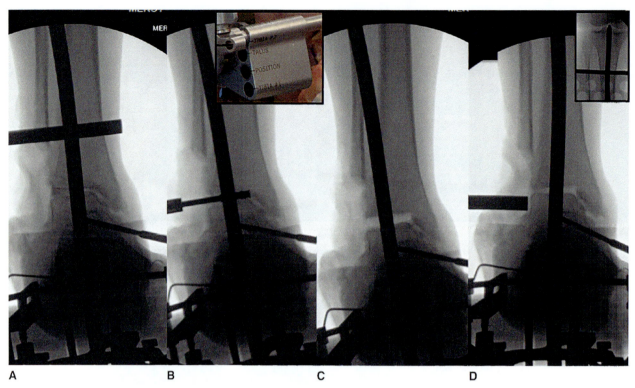

FIGURE 11.9 Correcting varus deformity. **A.** The talus is parallel to the horizontal alignment bar, but the varus joint alignment and lack of joint space prohibit a correction of the tibial plafond. **B, C.** The distal most aspect of the tibia is removed with the router to create a space for the foot plate and talus to move relative to the tibia. The *inset* in item **(B)** depicts the four slots in the router guide, with the "tibia 2" slot located at the top of the guide. **D.** The hindfoot is then rotated clockwise (for a right ankle) while applying traction until both the tibia and talus are aligned neutrally to the mechanical axis.

fluoroscopic views of the talar dome. Prior to tightening the talar pin to the frame, it can be used as a joystick to further correct talus alignment if the above steps were not sufficient. We advise against excessive bending of this pin as this is a sign that further medial gutter débridement, superficial deltoid release, or intra-articular bony resection is needed.

The alignment of the tibia is next adjusted so that the mechanical axis of the tibia is perpendicular to the footplate and corrected talus. On fluoroscopy, the tibial plafond should be parallel to the horizontal bar, and the tibial alignment bar should intersect the medial tibial spine on an AP knee image (Fig. 11.9D, inset image). Tibial position can be adjusted by pulling directional traction on the frame. If there is no room at the joint line to adjust residual tibial malalignment (such as in rigid varus), the distal most aspect of the tibial plafond can be removed with the router to create a working space for a reduction. This is performed by inserting the router through the "tibia 2" slot in the router guide (Fig. 11.9B, inset image). Subsequent manipulation of the frame can then allow for residual deformity correction (Fig. 11.9). An intact deep deltoid ligament, now slightly less taught after distal tibial bone resection, prevents excessive lateral talar translation during this alignment correction. The tibia is then secured in place with two Schanz pins (Fig. 11.10, items 3 and 4). The distal most pin is inserted first, and in most nondeformity cases, it can be inserted from medial to lateral (Fig. 11.10, item 3). In the case of sagittal deformity, this pin is placed from anterior to posterior (Figs. 11.10, item 3* and Fig. 11.11). To correct sagittal deformity, a horizontal radiolucent crossing rod is attached to the frame, and the Schanz pin is inserted off this crossing bar, just medial to tibialis anterior (Fig. 11.11C). This pin is then manipulated with compression or distraction to correct sagittal deformity (Fig. 11.11A and B). A laminar spreader inserted between the pin to bar clamp and the T-handle chuck is helpful to apply additional anterior distractive force in a controlled fashion (Fig. 11.11C). A final coronal assessment is made clinically and radiographically at the ankle and the knee, and the proximal tibial pin is inserted from medial to lateral (Fig. 11.10, item 4).

Once a distal tibial Schanz pin is placed, we feel it is crucial to place a small carbon bar connecting the talar pin to the distal tibial pin (Fig. 11.10, white asterisk). This dramatically improves construct rigidity and prevents micromotion of the tibia and talus during milling.

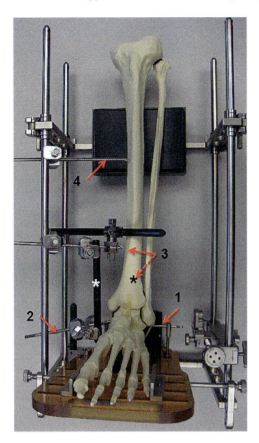

FIGURE 11.10 Complete frame assembly. Four Schanz pins are placed. The calcaneal pin is placed first, followed by the talus pin. The distal tibial pin can then be placed either medial to lateral or anterior to posterior (*black asterisk*), as indicated by the deformity. A short carbon bar is then attached to both the distal tibial pin and talar pin (*white asterisk*) to enhance rigidity. A fourth pin is then inserted at the proximal tibia from medial to lateral. Aside from the calcaneal pin, all pins should be placed through the clamps attached to the frame to minimize secondary malalignment.

Step 3. Milling and Implant Insertion

In preparation for bone milling, the router guide is aligned. This router guide is first locked in the neutral position, and the probe is placed through the "position" slot. The position of the router guide is then adjusted until the tip of the probe is at the apex of the joint line. Next, the router guide is unlocked, and the talar dome is traced with the probe. The height of the router guide is further adjusted to improve tracing of the talar arc. The probe is then removed, and the router (bur with a router bit, hereafter referred to as the router) is inserted through the guide into the "talus" slot. The amount of talar resection is then visualized by tracing the arc of the talus. The router guide (Fig. 11.9B, inset image) can be translated proximally so that minimal talus is resected (target is two-thirds the width of the router, or 4 mm). If there is inadequate (poor quality or quantity) tibial bone stock, it may be advisable to lower the joint line and resect more talus to preserve more tibia.

Finally, tibial slope is assessed. The router is inserted in the "tibia 1" slot of the guide, and the most anterior and posterior points of contact between the router and the tibia are noted. A straight line connecting these points is then compared to the foot plate (neutral slope). An anterior distal tibial angle of the final implant as low as 75° ("opening" anteriorly 15°) is acceptable (Fig. 11.12B). An excess slope in either direction correlates to the router guide being translated too far in that direction (ie, anterior translation of the router creates an anterior opening of the tibia, Fig. 11.12C). The three clamps securing the router guide position are then firmly tightened when the desired path has been traced.

In the case of severe deformity, bone loss, or a takedown fusion, tracing the joint line can be challenging. In these cases, we attach a silhouette guide to the routing bracket. These size-specific guides project the exact implant position on a lateral fluoroscopic image (Fig. 11.13).

The final step before milling is to set the depth of the router. The router is placed against the talus, and a trial talus implant is positioned between the router guide and the bur guard stop on the bur guard sleeve (Fig. 11.14A). The sleeve is then adjusted to the width of the trial, with a bur guard stop creating a positive lateral to medial stop during milling. The router is then inserted into the "tibia 2" slot and advanced through the central tibia. A fluoroscopic image is obtained to ensure appropriate depth. The bur guard stop is now tightened to prevent inadvertent migration medially.

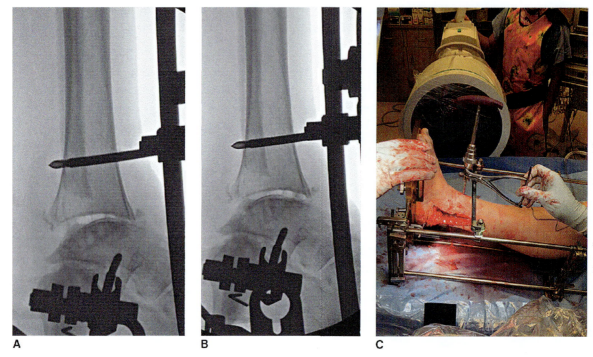

FIGURE 11.11 Sagittal deformity correction. **A.** The distal tibial pin is placed from anterior to posterior. **B, C.** The pin is then pulled anteriorly with manual traction and a laminar spreader, allowing for controlled anterior translation.

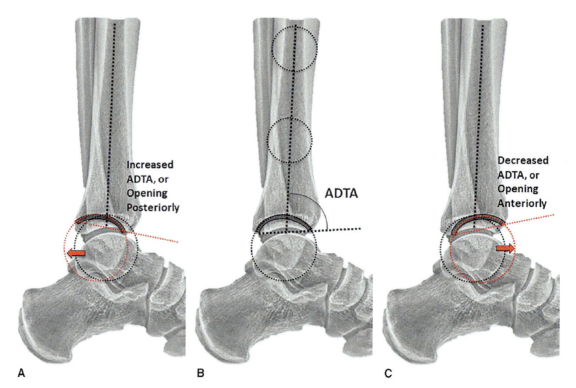

FIGURE 11.12 Milling arc relation to implant position. **A.** When the milling arc is translated posteriorly, as depicted the *red circle*, the intersection of this arc with the bone will create a posteriorly tilted tibial implant or "opening" posteriorly. This can also be described as an increased anterior distal tibial angle (ADTA). **B.** A well-centered milling path will recreate an anatomic ADTA, which on average is between 80° and 84°. **C.** Similarly, if the milling arc is translated anteriorly, as depicted by the *red circle*, the ADTA will decrease and the implant will be "opening" anteriorly.

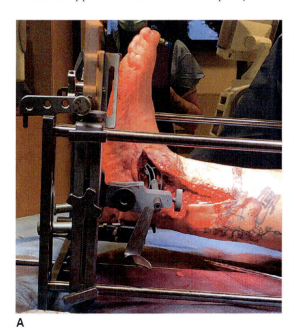
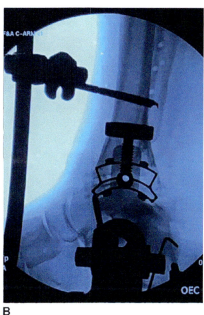

FIGURE 11.13 Silhouette guide placement. **A.** When anatomic landmarks are altered or absent (bone voids, take down fusion procedure), tracing the arc of the joint line arc can be challenging. In these cases, we attach a silhouette guide of the appropriate size to the frame, which attaches to the same component as the router guide. **B.** Lateral fluoroscopy is then obtained, and the guide can be adjusted until the desired implant position is obtained. The router is then attached to mill this exact path for the implant.

Prior to milling, retractors are placed anteriorly and posteriorly to protect the capsule and adjacent neurovascular structures. A Z-retractor is inserted posteriorly between the capsule and tibia to retract the flexor hallucis longus and neurovascular bundle from the path of the router (Fig. 11.15). During anterior milling, this retractor is similarly placed between the capsule and anterior tibia.

Milling is then performed with a peck and sweep technique. We start by milling centrally and in the talus (the hardest bone), pecking through bone until at the desired depth. We then sweep anteriorly and posteriorly while continuously pecking, which uses all surfaces of the router to cut bone. During initial milling, we do not remove the final 1 cm depth of bone at the anterior and posterior margins of the tibia and talus, as adjacent neurovascular structures are at risk. Instead, we first mill the central portions of the tibia and talus and remove this bone with a rongeur (Fig. 11.15A). With

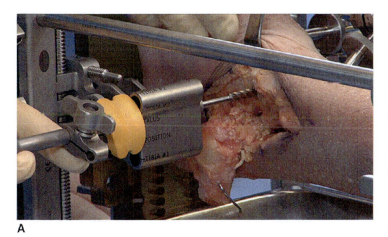
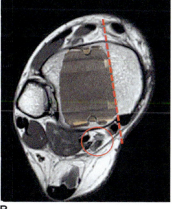

FIGURE 11.14 Anatomical considerations for milling. **A.** The talar trial is used to set the depth for milling. **B.** An axial MRI with a superimposed implant demonstrates that the router can come into contact with the neurovascular bundle at the posterior and medial tibia (*red circle*) within the depth of milling (marked by the *dashed red line*). As a result, we do not mill the final 1 cm depth of bone at the anterior and posterior margins until the central bone is removed. With this bone removed, the remaining bone can carefully be removed under direct visualization.

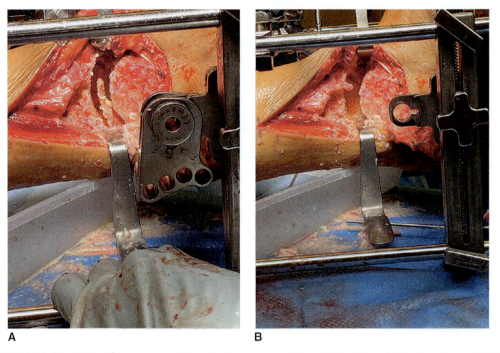

FIGURE 11.15 Milling of the talus and tibia. **A.** The central portions of the tibia and talus have been milled, leaving a central wafer of bone that can be removed with a rongeur. **B.** After removal of this central bone, the remaining bone anteriorly and posteriorly at the tibia can now be directly visualized, allowing for safe milling adjacent to neurovascular structures.

this bone removed, the surgeon can then directly visualize the remaining anterior and posterior bone for safer removal (Fig. 11.15B). The final step is to mill the central shelf of bone at the joint line using the "tibia 2" slot. During all milling, we continuously irrigate the router and bone to prevent thermal necrosis. Our preference is to attach a Frazier suction tip to cystoscopy tubing to facilitate continuous deep irrigation.

The router guide is then removed, and the rail guides are placed into the resection slot. A spreader pin is inserted in the appropriate slot between the guides to push the guides flush against the resection

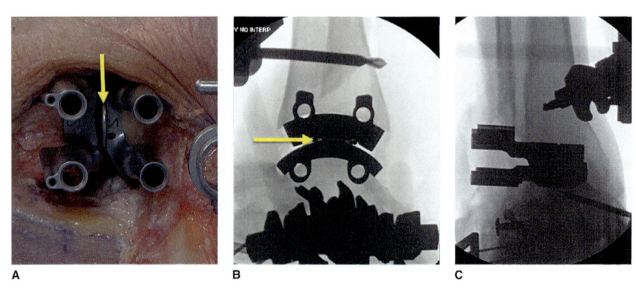

FIGURE 11.16 Rail guide placement. **A.** Rail guides are positioned at the talus and tibia. A spreader pin is inserted between the rail guides to create good apposition between the guides and the bone (*yellow arrow*). **B.** A lateral fluoroscopic image shows both an excellent profile of the guides (round shape to rail guide holes) and excellent positioning at both the tibia and talus (no tibial overhang, no talar notching). The spreader pin is again visualized (*yellow arrow*). **C.** An AP image shows excellent depth of rail guide placement (no lateral overhang) and neutral alignment.

surfaces (Fig. 11.16). A wiggle of the guides ensures that they are flush to the surface of the bone. AP and lateral fluoroscopic images are then obtained to assess rail guide position. A spreader pin is placed between the tibial and talar guides to rigidly compress the metal surfaces against the bone. When in the correct position, the rail guides are pinned in place, and the rail guide holes are drilled. The guides are then removed, and trial implants are inserted (Fig. 11.17).

The stability of the trial implants is then assessed. The tibiotalar carbon bar is removed, and the footplate is released from the frame. Stability during dorsiflexion and plantarflexion is then assessed (Fig. 11.17A). At maximum dorsiflexion, we apply a gentle valgus stress (Fig. 11.17B), assessing laxity with tactile feedback and with fluoroscopic imaging (Fig. 11.17C and D). A varus stress is not applied given risk of a medial malleolus fracture. If there is too much laxity, a +2- or +4-mm tibial trial is placed. Once implant size is selected, the polyethylene liner is attached to the tibial implant, and the implants are attached to the corresponding insertion handles. In preparation for final implant insertion, we thoroughly irrigate the joint with a sterile iodine suspension (BD Surgiphor™) followed by saline.

The tibial trial is replaced, and the talar component is then inserted orthogonally to the frame with direct visualization of the rail guides. While one team member is inserting the implant the final 2 cm, the other provides a dorsiflexion stress to keep the implant rails seated as the implant is advanced. The tibial trial is then removed, and the tibial implant is similarly inserted. A plastic tipped impactor is used for final placement under image guidance (Fig. 11.17E and F).

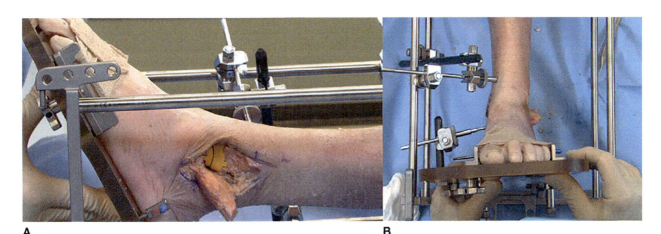

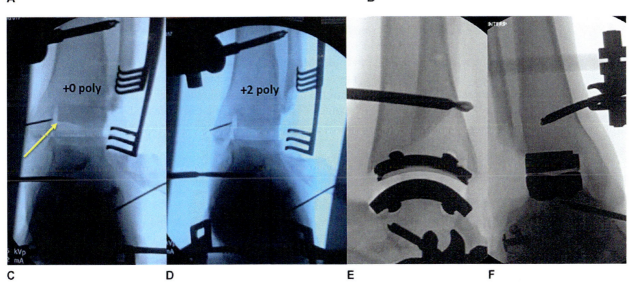

FIGURE 11.17 Trial implant placement and stability testing. **A.** With the trial implants inserted, the foot plate is released from the frame to assess plantarflexion-dorsiflexion stability. **B.** A valgus stress is then applied in maximum dorsiflexion to assess stability. **C.** Fluoroscopic image during valgus stability test with a +0 polyethylene liner. The *arrow* points to medial gapping at the trial implant interface, indicating instability. **D.** Repeat valgus stress examination with a +2 polyethylene liner, with medial lift off now eliminated. **E.** Lateral fluoroscopic image after final implants inserted. **F.** Anteroposterior fluoroscopic image with final implants inserted.

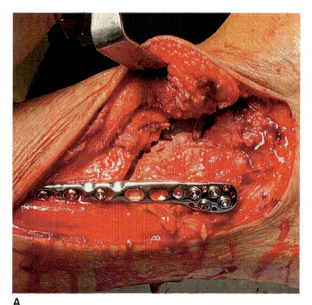
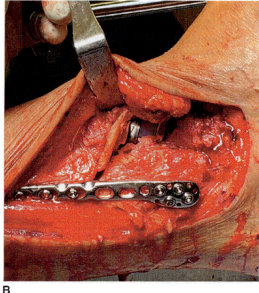

FIGURE 11.18 Fibular plating and bone grafting. **A.** The fibular plate has been applied with three bicortical nonlocking screws proximally and four locking screws distally. In this case, the fibula had to be lengthened after correction of deformity. **B.** The fibular gap is bone grafted; using a wedge of bone, we routinely remove with a rongeur during milling (such a wedge depicted in Fig. 11.15A).

Step 4. Fibular Reduction and Adjunct Procedures

The distal fibula is then repositioned anatomically. If a lateral plate was placed during the approach, the existing distal locking screws and proximal cortical screw are placed to guide the reduction. At least three bicortical screws are placed into the proximal segment (Fig. 11.18). Based upon the degree of preoperative deformity, the distal fibula may need to be fixated in a new position. In this setting, additional bone cuts or bone grafting can be performed to restore normal fibular length and alignment (Fig. 11.18A). Bone is routinely put aside during milling in the event bone graft is needed to fill any gaps at the fibular osteotomy (Fig. 11.18B).

The integrity of the syndesmosis is then assessed with a cotton test. We place a towel clip on the fibula and apply lateral traction. If there is excessive motion, flexible syndesmotic fixation is placed (Fig. 11.19). We prefer to test syndesmotic stability prior to lateral ligament and partial AITFL repair. We routinely begin weight-bearing knee bending exercises (discussed below) at 2 weeks postoperatively, a time at which repaired ligaments are still healing. Testing for stability prior to ligament repair reassures us that we will have adequate stability for these exercises in the acute postoperative period without compromising the healing repaired ligaments.

Additionally, we assess the size of the medial malleolus at the level of the plafond. If the medial to lateral width is less than 8 to 10 mm, we routinely place a fully threaded 4.0-mm screw to stabilize the malleolus. If there is valgus instability, a deltoid reconstruction can be performed. Our preferred technique is to begin with an synthetic augment—InternalBrace™ (Arthrex)—reconstruction between the talus and medial malleolus, drilling horizontally above the tibial implant. If residual instability exists, a semitendinosus deltoid reconstruction is then performed.

Step 5. Closure

Prior to closure, we routinely place vancomycin powder anterior and posterior to the joint. The previously elevated soft tissue sleeve containing fibular periosteum and the lateral ligaments is then repaired (Fig. 11.20). If there is not sufficient fibular periosteum or remnant ligament for repair, a suture anchor is placed in the fibula to facilitate anatomic repair. Deep fascia and periosteum are repaired over the fibula plate while protecting the superficial peroneal nerve (see Fig. 11.20).

Once the lateral wound has been closed, the extremity is removed from the frame and the flexion-extension arc is then assessed. If there is less than 15° of dorsiflexion, a percutaneous tendoachilles hemisection is performed with three cuts 2.5 cm apart from one another. Lastly, we routinely recommend a bone marrow aspirate concentrate injection to patients to enhance implant ingrowth and

11 Lateral Approach Total Ankle Arthroplasty

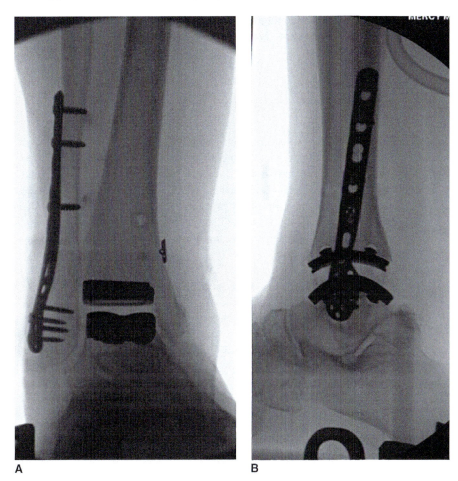

FIGURE 11.19 Final implant placement. **A.** Mortise fluoroscopic image at the conclusion of implant placement, fibular reduction, and syndesmotic fixation. **B.** Lateral fluoroscopic image demonstrating excellent implant alignment.

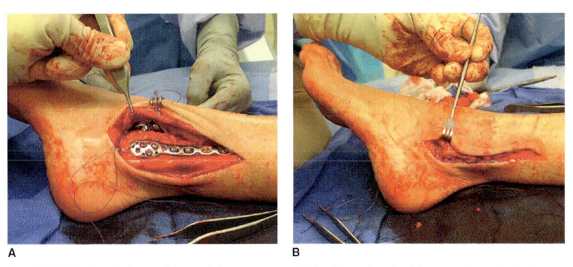

FIGURE 11.20 Lateral closure. **A.** The soft tissue sleeve containing the ATFL, anterolateral capsule, and part of the AITFL is repaired. The forceps are holding this sleeve. **B.** The fascia over the fibular plate proximally and the lateral ligament repair distally has been completed. Of note, these pictures show a repair with the ankle removed from the frame. We now routinely perform this closure with the ankle in the frame, as explained in the text.

healing of the fibular osteotomy,[16] injecting around the joint and fibular osteotomy. The extremity is then placed into a bulky, well-padded short leg U and posterior splint with the ankle resting in neutral dorsiflexion.

PEARLS AND PITFALLS

Pearls

Step 1: In the case of an equinus contracture, the footplate may need to be adjusted to an equinus position to bring the foot flat onto the plate. Bone milling can be completed with the foot in equinus. We prefer to adjust the footplate to match the equinus rather than begin with a tendoachilles lengthening, as the restricted motion is partly attributable to osteophytes and adherent capsule that are removed/released as part of the arthroplasty procedure. We prefer to address residual equinus as the last step in our case after all soft tissue and bony work has been completed.

Step 2: When inserting the distal tibial Schanz pin, apply a counter force on the tibia to avoid inadvertent posterior translation.

Step 3: During tibial implant insertion, it may be difficult to initially seat the implant in the rail slots. We first gently plantarflex the ankle to seat the edge of the implant, and then apply dorsiflexion to maintain rail guide alignment as the implant is advanced.

Step 4: We now routinely repair the lateral ligament complex with the ankle in the frame. This allows for less tension on the ligament repair, periosteal repair, and fascial closure. This also allows us to repair the ligament in a position of a well-aligned arthroplasty, improving our soft tissue balancing.

Pitfalls

Step 1: Incomplete releases of the tibial capsule will make it more challenging to correct deformity in the frame and to retract the capsule and adjacent neurovascular structures during milling.

Step 2: The surgeon can place the calcaneal pin, parallel to the talar joint surface, prior to placement in the frame or once in the frame. However, drilling the talar pin before the leg is in the frame is not recommended. When the talar pin is drilled independent from the clamp on the frame, the angle of pin insertion may not allow for a smooth attachment to the pin-to-rod clamp. As a result, forcing the off-axis pin into the clamp on the frame alters talar alignment.

Step 3: Over impacting the talus medially may require a medial approach to adjust position.

Step 4: Failure to recognize and remove lateral talar osteophytes can impair fibula reduction and may result in postoperative lateral gutter pain.

POSTOPERATIVE MANAGEMENT

Patients remain splinted for 10 to 14 days, when sutures are then removed and patients are transitioned to a boot brace and a posterior splint (typically used for plantar fasciitis). At this first postoperative visit, we begin a deep knee bending protocol that we feel is crucial for maintaining motion without introducing excessive stress at the bone-implant interface. While barefoot, patients are instructed to squat down by bending their knees, creating a dorsiflexion ankle stretch that is held for approximately 10 seconds. Slow repetitions are continued for 20 minutes and repeated 5 times a day until 3 months postoperatively. Straight knee, Achilles stretching can be also used to improve dorsiflexion. When not performing knee bends, patients are strictly non–weight bearing for 6 weeks. At the first visit, we also institute splinting in neutral dorsiflexion using a posterior night splint typically used for plantar fasciitis while patients rest or sleep. We discourage the use of the boot unless the patient is ambulating because use of the boot may put pressure on the incisions. The night splint, the boot and avoiding plantarflexion beyond 20° is crucial to protect the ligament repair(s) and is continued for 3 months postoperatively.

At 6 weeks postoperatively, we begin progressive weight bearing in the boot brace. Patients begin with 20 lbs and add 20 lbs every other day until full weight bearing. Although weight bearing is permitted, twisting exercises are strictly prohibited to protect the fibular and lateral ligament repair.

At 12 weeks postoperatively, patients wean from the boot brace to a shoe, using a cloth brace to support the ankle during longer periods of walking or exercise. While walking and biking are encouraged, we recommend against regular impact activities such as running to minimize polyethylene wear and maximize implant longevity. We next see the patients back at 6 months, 12 months, and then annually. During the postoperative period, we obtain standing radiographs of the ankle from the 6-week visit onward.

In our practice, patients are generally advised that the healing process is 75% complete at 3 months and 90% complete at 6 months. We continually remind patients preoperatively and postoperatively that it takes a full year to maximize their clinical outcome.

RESULTS AND COMPLICATIONS

Several clinical series have documented excellent short-term and midterm outcomes after lateral approach total ankle arthroplasty. This procedure reliably improves patient pain (Visual Analog Scale pain scores) at 1-, 2-, and 5-year follow-up.[1-3,17] A clinical series demonstrated a 2.5-fold improvement in American Orthopaedic Foot and Ankle Society scores at 2- and 5-year follow-up,[1,17] although this metric has poor validity despite being one of the most widely reported outcome scores.[18] SF-12 physical function and mental component tests have also shown significant improvement at 2 and 5 years.[1,17]

Excellent recovery of motion has been described in multiple series. At 2-year follow-up, Usuelli et al documented an improvement of preoperative plantarflexion and dorsiflexion by almost two- and fourfold, respectively. Follow-up of 86 of 89 of these patients at 5 years demonstrated sustained motion improvement.[17] Similarly, Barg et al found the total arc of motion doubled when comparing preoperative and postoperative goniometer measurements,[2] which is a significantly greater increase in motion compared to many existing series analyzing alternative implants.[19] However, most of these existing studies have measured motion clinically with a goniometer, which does not isolate tibiotalar motion from combined ankle and midfoot motion. To our knowledge, a comparison of radiographically measured motion between lateral and anterior approach arthroplasty has not yet been performed. Potential greater gains in motion with lateral arthroplasty may be secondary to less anterior scarring with the transfibular approach but may also be attributable to more anatomic implant contours.

Radiographic outcomes with this implant have also been encouraging. Multiple series have documented excellent correction of sagittal and coronal plane deformity between 12-month and 5-year follow-up.[1-3,17] At 5-year follow-up in 86 patients, Usuelli et al also reported no cases of implant subsidence.[17] In this series, 9% of patients had visible peri-implant lucencies, but no patients had cysts. This is in contrast to Barg et al, who documented 34.5% of patients had radiolucent lines about the tibial prosthesis, although these findings were not progressive out to 24 months and not associated with pain or function.[2] Kormi et al evaluated the rate of osteolytic lesion formation with CT scans at 5-year follow-up and found only 10% of patients had detectable lesions.[20] This is in contrast to Lintz et al, who performed a similar CT analysis on several popular anteriorly placed implants at shorter follow up (44 months) and found at least one cyst in 81% of patients.[21]

Reports of implant survivorship have also been excellent. At 12 months, two surgeons publishing their first clinical experience with this implant recorded 100% survivorship.[2,3] At 24 months, three series reported between 93% and 100% survivorship.[1,2,22] At 5 years, Usuelli et al found 97.7% of patients were free from revision or implant removal, with two patients requiring explanation for septic loosening. There were no periprosthetic fractures or polyethylene dissociations in this series.

Variable rates of secondary reoperations have been reported, ranging between 11% and 20% at 12- to 24-month follow-up.[1-3] The most frequent reason for secondary reoperation is for symptomatic lateral hardware, accounting for 70% of all secondary procedures in one series. The rate of secondary procedures may be partially attributable to the learning curve of this approach,[23] as many series describe a surgeons first experiences with the lateral approach. Our rate of secondary symptomatic lateral hardware is 5% to 10%.

Other potential complications include delayed wound healing, nonunion or delayed union of the fibular osteotomy, medial malleolus fractures, and gutter impingement. Reported rates of delayed wound healing have been low, ranging from 2.3% to 3.6%.[2,17] Rates of fibular nonunion have also been extremely low. Three studies documenting surgeries performed by fellowship-trained orthopedic foot and ankle surgeons found no fibular delayed unions or nonunions in a total of 164 procedures.[1-3] Secondary surgery for gutter débridement is also infrequent (1.9%).[20] Lastly, intraoperative or postoperative medial malleolus fracture are rare (1.8% to 1.9%).[2,20]

In summary, lateral approach total ankle arthroplasty is a reliable procedure for treating ankle arthritis, with patients reporting significant improvement in pain, function, and motion. Short-term and midterm follow-up has demonstrated excellent survivorship with low rates of cyst formation, implant subsidence, or aseptic loosening. Like all total ankle arthroplasty systems, a successful patient outcome requires careful surgical technique. The authors' preferred technique detailed in this chapter has been refined over the past 10 years and has led to excellent clinical outcomes.

REFERENCES

1. Usuelli FG, Maccario C, Granata F, Indino C, Vakhshori V, Tan EW. Clinical and radiological outcomes of transfibular total ankle arthroplasty. *Foot Ankle Int.* 2019;40(1):24-33.
2. Barg A, Bettin CC, Burstein AH, Saltzman CL, Gililland J. Early clinical and radiographic outcomes of trabecular metal total ankle replacement using a transfibular approach. *J Bone Joint Surg Am.* 2018;100(6):505-515.
3. Tan EW, Maccario C, Talusan PG, Schon LC. Early complications and secondary procedures in transfibular total ankle replacement. *Foot Ankle Int.* 2016;37(8):835-841.
4. Aubret S, Merlini L, Fessy M, Besse JL. Poor outcomes of fusion with trabecular metal implants after failed total ankle replacement: early results in 11 patients. *Orthop Traumatol Surg Res.* 2018;104(2):231-237.
5. Huang G, Pan ST, Qiu JX. The clinical application of porous tantalum and its new development for bone tissue engineering. *Materials (Basel).* 2021;14(10):2647.
6. Fan H, Deng S, Tang W, et al. Highly porous 3D printed tantalum scaffolds have better biomechanical and microstructural properties than titanium scaffolds. *Biomed Res Int.* 2021;2021:2899043.
7. Piglionico S, Bousquet J, Fatima N, Renaud M, Collart-Dutilleul PY, Bousquet P. Porous tantalum vs. titanium implants: enhanced mineralized matrix formation after stem cells proliferation and differentiation. *J Clin Med.* 2020;9(11):3657.
8. Bischoff JE, Schon L, Saltzman CL. Influence of geometry and depth of resections on bone support for total ankle replacement. *Foot Ankle Int.* 2017;38(9):1026-1034.
9. Usuelli FG, de Cesar NC, Maccario C, Paoli T, D'Ambrosi R, Indino C. Reconstruction of a missing or insufficient distal fibula in the setting of a total ankle replacement: the Milanese technique. *Foot Ankle Surg.* 2022;28(2):186-192.
10. Brodsky JW, Scott DJ, Ford S, Coleman S, Daoud Y. Functional outcomes of total ankle arthroplasty at a mean follow-up of 7.6 years: a prospective, 3-dimensional gait analysis. *J Bone Joint Surg Am.* 2021;103(6):477-482.
11. Consul DW, Chu A, Langan TM, Hyer CF, Berlet G. Total ankle arthroplasty survivorship, complication, and revision rates in patients younger than 55 years. *Foot Ankle Spec.* 2022;15(3):283-290.
12. Cancienne JM, Cooper MT, Laroche KA, Verheul DW, Werner BC. Hemoglobin A1c as a predictor of postoperative infection following elective forefoot surgery. *Foot Ankle Int.* 2017;38(8):832-837.
13. McConaghy K, Kunze KN, Murray T, Molloy R, Piuzzi NS. Smoking cessation initiatives in total joint arthroplasty: an evidence-based review. *JBJS Rev.* 2021;9(8).
14. Sahota S, Lovecchio F, Harold RE, Beal MD, Manning DW. The effect of smoking on thirty-day postoperative complications after total joint arthroplasty: a propensity score-matched analysis. *J Arthroplasty.* 2018;33(1):30-35.
15. Nodzo SR, Pavlesen S, Ritter C, Boyle KK. Tranexamic acid reduces perioperative blood loss and hemarthrosis in total ankle arthroplasty. *Am J Orthop (Belle Mead NJ).* 2018;47(8).
16. Hernigou P, Guissou I, Homma Y, et al. Percutaneous injection of bone marrow mesenchymal stem cells for ankle nonunions decreases complications in patients with diabetes. *Int Orthop.* 2015;39(8):1639-1643.
17. Maccario C, Paoli T, Romano F, D'Ambrosi R, Indino C, Usuelli FG. Transfibular total ankle arthroplasty: a new reliable procedure at five-year follow-up. *Bone Joint J.* 2022;104-B(4):472-478.
18. Hunt KJ, Hurwit D. Use of patient-reported outcome measures in foot and ankle research. *J Bone Joint Surg Am.* 2013;95(16):e118(1-9).
19. Zaidi R, Cro S, Gurusamy K, et al. The outcome of total ankle replacement: a systematic review and meta-analysis. *Bone Joint J.* 2013;95-B(11):1500-1507.
20. Tiusanen H, Kormi S, Kohonen I, Saltychev M. Results of trabecular-metal total ankle arthroplasties with transfibular approach. *Foot Ankle Int.* 2020;41(4):411-418.
21. Lintz F, Mast J, Bernasconi A, et al. 3D, weightbearing topographical study of periprosthetic cysts and alignment in total ankle replacement. *Foot Ankle Int.* 2020;41(1):1-9.
22. DeVries JG, Derksen TA, Scharer BM, Limoni R. Perioperative complications and initial alignment of lateral approach total ankle arthroplasty. *J Foot Ankle Surg.* 2017;56(5):996-1000.
23. Maccario C, Tan EW, Di Silvestri CA, Indino C, Kang HP, Usuelli FG. Learning curve assessment for total ankle replacement using the transfibular approach. *Foot Ankle Surg.* 2021;27(2):129-137.

12 The Stryker INBONE II Total Ankle Arthroplasty System

M. Pierce Ebaugh and William C. McGarvey

INTRODUCTION

The continued advancement of total ankle arthroplasty combined with a posttraumatic population has resulted in increased numbers of total ankle replacements being performed for the treatment of end-stage tibiotalar arthritis.[1-5] The INBONE II prosthesis (Stryker Orthopedics, Mahwah, NJ) replaced the INBONE I in 2010 as one of the most frequently utilized total ankle replacements. It has an intramedullary tibial component and has presented excellent midterm outcomes and survivorship.[1,3,6] The introduction of PROPHECY technology (Stryker Orthopedics, Mahwah, NJ) in 2012 advanced the prosthesis, adding patient specific instrumentation (PSI) to allow for proper component positioning in all cases.[7] The following chapter outlines the authors technique for employing the PSI of INBONE II in ankle arthroplasty.

CONTRAINDICATIONS

- Complete avascular necrosis of the talus
- Nonachievable plantigrade foot
- Prior osteomyelitis with elevated laboratory markers or evidence of ongoing infection
- Poor soft tissue envelope without ability for proper plastic surgery intervention
- Severe neuromuscular disorder
- Neuropathic ankle joint

Relative Contraindications

- Severe osteoporosis
- Partial avascular necrosis of the talus
- Inadequate tibial or talar bone stock

PREOPERATIVE EVALUATION

We routinely perform standard clinical evaluation and thorough physical exam including standing and gait analysis in shorts to evaluate proximal deformity. Medications including anticoagulants, immunosuppressants, and other potential complicating pharmacologics are vetted. Bilateral comparison weight-bearing radiographs are performed of both the ankle and foot. Additionally, we employ hip knee ankle full leg length films for patients with objective proximal deformity and/or leg length evaluation. Saltzman hindfoot alignment views are often obtained for reference. For ankles with deformity, stress views to evaluate deformity flexibility are performed. A thorough outpatient laboratory and imaging evaluation then occurs. We routinely use the computed tomography (CT) PSI protocol in addition to a weight-bearing (or mimicked via neutral dorsiflexion radiolucent platform) CT of the entire foot and ankle in the standard axial, sagittal, and coronal views.[7] The surgeon should specify when ordering the CT, that all views be included, as the PSI protocol only requires axial views. An arterial/venous ultrasound is also routinely performed to identify chronic venous thrombosis or arterial occlusion that may result in significant postoperative edema or wound concerns. Hemoglobin A1C, erythrocyte sedimentation rate, and C-reactive protein levels are obtained to ensure proper blood glucose control in diabetics, lack of underlying infections in cases of prior surgery or open injury, and/or poorly controlled inflammatory disorders. All modifiable risk factors identified by the above data are addressed to the fullest possible extent and any remaining risk factors presented as patient education to ensure willingness to proceed. We employ liberal use of plastic and/or vascular surgery consultations to ensure optimization of all modifiable risk factors.

Preoperative Deformity

In general, proximal and severe compensatory foot deformities are addressed prior to ankle arthroplasty. Mild to moderate foot deformities are addressed at the time of arthroplasty. Depending on the degree of preoperative deformity and origination, foot and/or ankle balancing procedures may be required prior to arthroplasty. If these are performed, we routinely wait 12 to 24 weeks following index procedure prior to arthroplasty to allow for union and timely weight bearing to reduce disuse osteopenia. The discussion of the particular corrections is outside of the scope of this chapter.

SURGICAL TECHNIQUE

Operating Room Set Up

The patient is positioned at the end of the table with a radiolucent end board. The ankle is placed on top of a platform of blankets to elevate it out of the way of the opposite extremity for lateral/sagittal views. Fluoroscopy is directed to be brought in ipsilateral to the operative side. A skin marker is utilized to outline the PSI jig on the 3D printed patient ankle model for intraoperative reference (Fig. 12.1A through C).

Approach

For the INBONE II total ankle system, a standard direct anterior approach to the ankle is undertaken. Other similar approaches have been described with excellent results, and it is up to the surgeon's discretion as to whether to employ these depending on circumstances surrounding prior surgical incisions, free flaps, tobacco use, or other comorbidities.[8] Prior to beginning the approach, we place wires in a vertical orientation into the medial malleolus to combat intraoperative fracture; screws are then placed over the wires at the end of the case. This is based off of whether the authors deem the medial malleolus to be at risk for fracture in the early postoperative period. To reserve tourniquet time, these are done prior to exsanguination of the limb.

It is our preference to carefully dissect and free the superficial peroneal nerve, particularly at the distal aspect of the approach to avoid potential iatrogenic injury. In some cases, a vessel loop can be useful in both nerve retraction and identification during closure. Careful incision of the extensor retinaculum in between the extensor hallucis longus and tibialis anterior is performed, with special attention paid to anterior neurovascular bundle identification and cautery of associated vasculature by placing an additional vessel loop here. At this point, we recommend cautery to complete the dissection, as the PSI guides are manufactured to exact bony anatomy and any residual soft tissue on the tibia and talus may induce guide malalignment. Additionally, cautery allows for preservation of periosteal and capsular tissue, which we include in our closure as we believe it aids in stabilization of medial/lateral ankle ligaments, prevention of hematoma formation directly under the incision, along with prevention of contamination should superficial infection occur. The dissection of capsular tissue continues distally until the talonavicular capsule is opened. This allows for proper seating of the PSI guide, but should be repaired at the end of the case. In cases of varus deformity through the mid/hindfoot, this capsule does not require repair as it assists in deformity correction.

Instrumentation

Prior to fitting the PSI guides, a Ray-Tec type sponge is used to débride the anterior tibia and talus of any residual cauterized tissue and the wound is thoroughly irrigated. Special attention at this point should be paid to any loose anterior tibial osteophytes as noted by the prophecy report. These should

12 The Stryker INBONE II Total Ankle Arthroplasty System

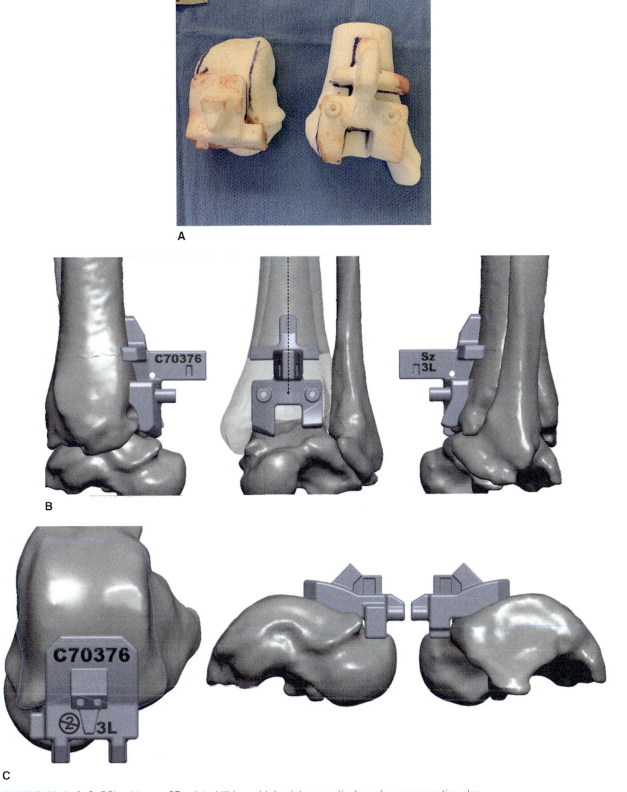

FIGURE 12.1 A-C. PSI guides on 3D printed tibia and talus intraoperatively and on preoperative plan.

be removed. A bump is placed behind the ankle, allowing the calcaneus to translate posteriorly, protecting the posteromedial neurovascular bundle, and allowing the talus to fall out of the way preventing abutment of guide. The tibial prophecy guide is then placed securely on the tibia matching

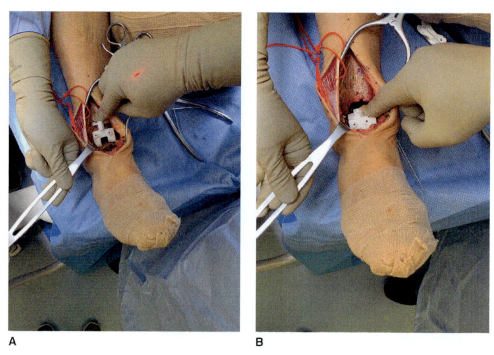

FIGURE 12.2 A, B. PSI guide placement on tibia and talus, respectively.

its counterpart position on the 3D-printed model (we find it helpful to outline this position prior to the case with a marking pen) (Figs. 12.1 and 12.2).

Notes regarding the prophecy tibial guide: Often the report will display a medial arm to be built onto the guide. We find this to hinder position as it requires additional dissection medially to properly fit and does not easily allow for guide adjustment. The authors request that their prophecy guides do not include this arm, as we feel it can create malalignment. Additionally, the pin placed through the center of the guide for coronal plane alignment has a tendency to have motion associated with it. This can be mitigated by ensuring enough of the pin is pulled distally through the guide to balance the proximal portion without it running into the talar neck. Fluoroscopy with a larger image intensifier is useful for the alignment portions of the case to moderate parallax.

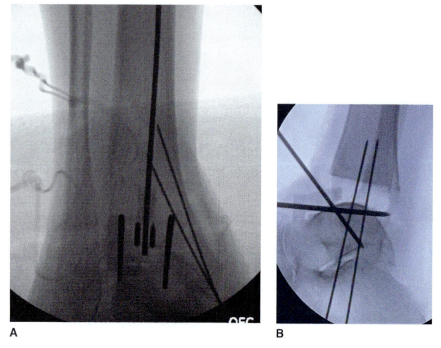

FIGURE 12.3 A, B. PSI guides have been pinned into place, note the prophylactic medial malleolus fixation.

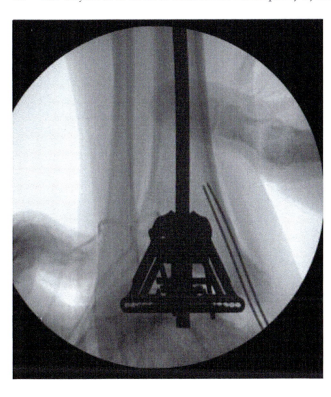

FIGURE 12.4 The cut block is placed and the intramedullary reamer shaft is laid inside the anterior fins of the antirotation notch to match with the tubercle and represent stem alignment.

Once radiographic coronal plane alignment is confirmed, pins are placed through the guide. This alignment should be rechecked for accuracy once all pins are placed (Fig. 12.3). Sagittal radiographic alignment is then checked for accuracy against the prophecy report. The prophecy guide is removed and the cut guide placed.

Note: In rare situations, the authors choose to couple the cuts; however, the majority of patients that require INBONE systems have degrees of deformity or instability that make accuracy of coupling difficult. If the surgeon wishes to couple their cuts, we suggest doing so in manually correctable deformities of less than 4° in the coronal plane.

Prior to performing the cuts, we perform an additional check of the coronal plane with the cut guide on by applying the intramedullary reamer shaft to sit within the two anterior fins of the tibial cut block (Fig. 12.4). This provides additional reference via length, acting to confirm the relationship to the tibial tubercle for rotational referencing. The antirotation notch is drilled and the cuts performed. While the cuts are performed, we focus on collinear blade work to avoid binding and potential skiving. The cuts are also repeated to ensure all residual bone is removed; we feel this is a crucial step in sclerotic patients. The surgeon should focus particularly in saw blade excursion at the corners. In cases of poor bone quality, a reciprocating saw may be employed to allow better tactile feedback toward the posterior portion of the cuts. Additionally, in cases of hypertrophic osteophyte formation or long-standing arthritis, the osteophytes will exceed the length of the capture guide slot requiring continuation of the cut after guide removal to ensure that the remnant does not create a fracture in an undesirable plane during final bone resection. Once the tibial cutting block guide is removed, the corner cutter is introduced carefully into the medial and then later corners of the tibial cut and advanced carefully with a mallet to the appropriate depth posteriorly as determined by the preoperative plan. The anterior to posterior sizes are marked off in the cutting guide itself. Care must be taken to follow the cuts made by the saw in order not to create a new path. The bone is then irrigated. It is important to note that the INBONE system design lends itself toward residual bone often being left in the medial and lateral corners/shoulders. This can create both tibial base plate malalignment and stem placement inaccuracy when the prophecy stem CT guide is inserted following the talar cut. We typically utilize a reciprocating saw or power rasp to remove this bone. In addition, it is particularly important to note that the tibial bone block removal is not insignificant and is at times a rate-limiting step to the surgical procedure. Often the screw-tipped bone removal joystick will allow for en bloc bone excision. If this fails, the remaining bone may require an osteotomy to aid in piecemeal removal. Further access may be obtained by removing the talar cut remnant to get better access to the tibial remnant. Special bone removal tools are available and the authors will incorporate angled curettes, long narrow rongeurs, and pituitary rongeurs to assist in this step (Fig. 12.5A through C).

We then turn our attention to the talus. All residual cartilage should be removed from the dome to ensure accurate placement of the prophecy guide. The guide is held in place manually and the

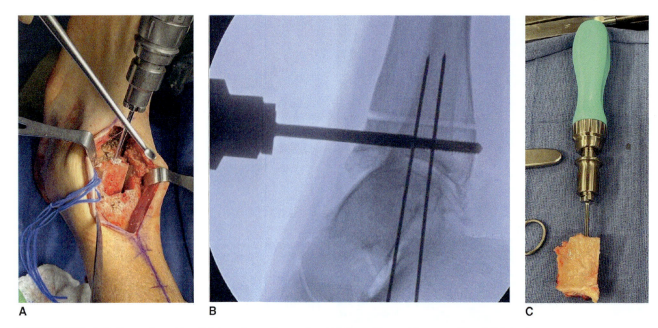

FIGURE 12.5 **A-C.** Screw tipped joystick insertion with curette aid followed by en bloc resection of tibial cut.

wires passed. The cut is checked for accuracy on a perfect lateral radiograph of the talus. The cut is performed, block removed, and wound thoroughly irrigated with pulsatile irrigation. Of note, often the medial and lateral edges of the talus have residual bone. We typical use a reciprocating saw run flush/flat against the talar cut to gently remove this bone.

Next, the prophecy stem guide block is inserted. It should be noted that it needs to sit flush against the tibia and the accuracy of the corners should be checked. Prior to placing wires, we utilize the purple-colored extraction handle (M4 attachment screw used to remove center block after peck drilling) inserted at the top of the prophecy guide (Fig. 12.6). This is used to confirm the coronal alignment and the stem medial/lateral translation. If this shows inaccuracy, we recommend rechecking

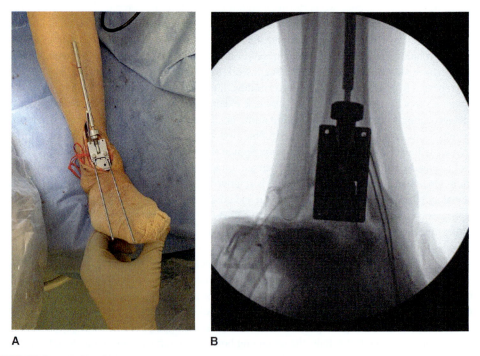

FIGURE 12.6 **A, B.** The M4 purple ring extraction handle is placed into the top of the prophecy peck drill guide block. The alignment guide block can then be confirmed on fluoroscopy to ensure accurate stem placement.

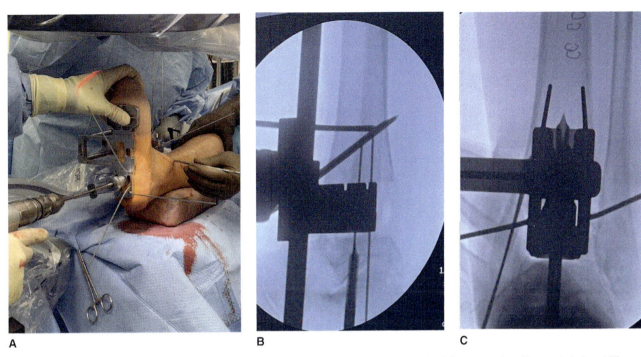

FIGURE 12.7 A-C. Peck drill advancement with control of INBONE PSI jig, ensuring to check intraoperative alignment during drilling.

the corner cuts. The stem guide is secured into place, and the purple stick step is rechecked followed by anterior to posterior translation on the lateral radiograph. We continue by assembling the peck drill bracket. The entry point of the peck drill is marked through the drill sleeve and then a small incision made on the plantar foot. This incision is deepened to bone by spreading with a long narrow hemostat to ensure that the bone-drill interface is unencumbered by soft tissue that could cause the drill tip to skive on the sloped plantar medial calcaneal wall. The initiation of this step is critical to maintain drill trajectory accuracy. When beginning the peck drill, go slowly as the bracket has play in it which can throw off the drill trajectory (Fig. 12.7). If you find yourself slightly malaligned, know that varus/valgus and dorsi/plantarflexion stress placed on the bracket can correct this, but we caution attempting to correct large degrees of malalignment (Fig. 12.8). If this is the case, the stem guide should be removed and the bone cuts checked for accuracy.

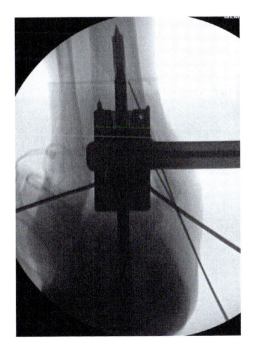

FIGURE 12.8 The peck drill is advanced into the tibial shaft. Note the foot being held in alignment during drilling to guide accuracy.

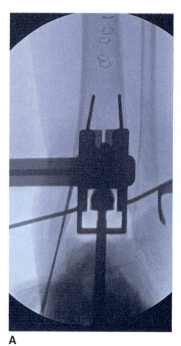 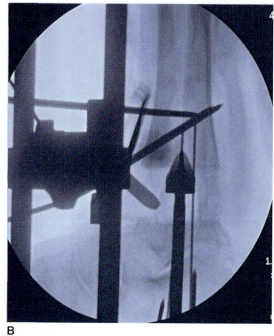

FIGURE 12.9 A, B. Reaming the tibia.

Next, the reamer attachment is assembled and the step performed. We generally recommend utilizing the sharp reamer. The posttraumatic nature of ankle arthritis often creates sclerotic densities that persist proximally; the dull reamer can skive on this dense bone-altering alignment. Additionally, we recommend reaming slightly proximal to the extent of the stem, to ensure capability of stem modularity or proximal cement insertion if the stem fixation floats in the medullary canal. Line to line reaming of the stem and under reaming of the base stem is also recommended to ensure a solid press fit if bone quality allows (Fig. 12.9).

Thoroughly irrigate the canal and remove all instruments for stem insertion. Tibia sizing is then confirmed. This step is crucial for checking how the baseplate will insert/sit and for making any final adjustments. Trial components are available and assist in determining soft tissue balance and necessary polyethylene thickness at this stage (Fig. 12.10). Unless significant bone loss or bony compromise is present, we often utilize a three-part stem construct, which can be assembled on

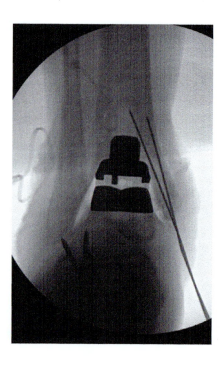

FIGURE 12.10 Trials are placed and ligamentous balance assessed.

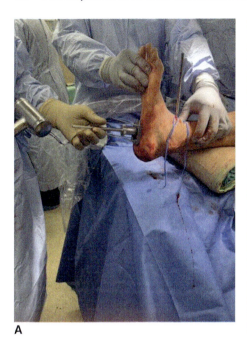 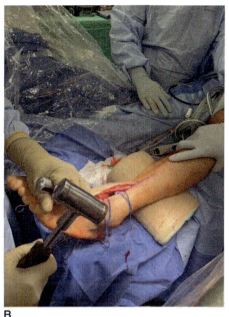 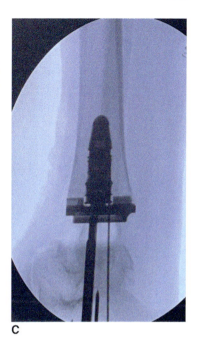

FIGURE 12.11 A-C. Stem insertion using a straight tamp through the jig and a curved tamp via the wound.

the back table and inserted as one piece in most cases. When significant cystic disease of the distal tibia is present, we suggest increasing the stem length to four-part or greater. The baseplate is then connected by seating the Morse taper. The stem is malleted into the canal in a controlled fashion. A curved bone tamp can be helpful here for guiding the stem properly. Liberal use of biplanar fluoroscopy is critical to ensure appropriate stem travel (Fig. 12.11). Any deviations in stem position should be addressed before a false tract or canal enlargement are created, which can lead to loosening or malposition.

The talus can now be trialed, sized, drilled, and placed. Recent trends have shown that some surgeons have been using the INIFINITY system flat cut talus implant with ADAPTIS porous coated technology in place of the INBONE II grit blasted talus with larger posterior stem. While it is noted that this may leave create a mismatch between the previous peck drill hole and posterior ADAPTIS stem, this is minimal overall and can be supplemented with bone cement. We believe the bone INgrowth versus ONgrowth offered is the important focus.[9] It should be noted that ADAPTIS flat cut talus component use is off label for INBONE; this intriguing concept warrants longer term data to determine the value of this exchange.

Next, we trial the polyethylene component again. Of note, we look for maintenance of range of motion (ROM) while creating the greatest amount of tension in the medial and lateral ankle collateral ligaments. Ligamentous balancing is on a per case basis, and need is evidenced by tension of one ligament with significant laxity of another. This is outside of the scope of this chapter. The polyethylene component is then inserted (Fig. 12.12).

Finally, medial malleolus screws are inserted over previously placed wires as needed. Final fluoroscopy is performed. We then begin a meticulous layered closure. We typically place vancomycin powder into the wound. We then close the tibial periosteum, ankle capsule, and talonavicular joint capsule with a running absorbable braided suture. We feel this lends to joint stability and hematoma control. We then perform the same stitch on the extensor retinaculum. Subcutaneous tissue and epidermis are then managed.

PEARLS AND PITFALLS

- Complete tissue removal from the anterior tibia is essential for fitting of the prophecy guide
- Distal translation of the center prophecy guide wire to avoid micromotion in the guide
- Incomplete removal of residual bone in the medial and lateral shoulders/corners of the tibial cut
- Inaccurate placement of the prophecy peck drill block resulting in translation or coronal/sagittal plane malalignment

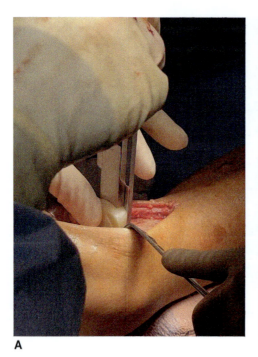 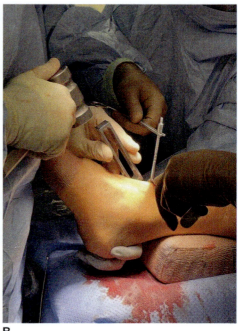

FIGURE 12.12 A, B. The polyethylene component is first inserted most of the way using the jig. It is seated into place using an impactor. In cases of poor bone quality, we leave the jig connector in place with a nut attached **(B)**. We hold this while impacting to avoid dorsiflexion of the tibial component.

POSTOPERATIVE CARE

The patient is placed into a posterior splint and returns for a wound check at 4 days, often a compression wrap technique is performed.[10] At this point they are transitioned into a controlled ankle motion (CAM) boot to begin ROM. Weight bearing and boot transition is dependent upon wound healing, bone quality, and associated procedures but rarely occurs prior to 4 weeks. Physical therapy is often employed for gait training and balance. Total CAM boot weight bearing occurs for 8 weeks, and then the patient is transitioned to a ankle stabilizing orthosis (ASO) style ankle brace.

COMPLICATIONS

Glazebrook et al defined total ankle complications that are most often seen following arthroplasty.[11] For the purposes of this chapter, we have reduced the discussion to two categories seen more often in the acute peri/postoperative period: intra/postoperative fracture and wound healing/deep infection.

Fracture of the medial or lateral malleolus in ankle arthroplasty can be a devastating complication leading to implant loosening and failure postoperatively. Prior studies have noted rates in other total ankle systems as high as 20%.[12] Despite the intramedullary fixation of the INBONE II, we routinely prophylactically fixate the medial malleolus prior to beginning the arthroplasty portion of our case. We often note a thin medial shoulder at the point of implant and medial malleolus transition into the tibial metaphysis. We employ two K-wires to fixate the medial malleolus at the beginning of the case, and then place fully threaded screws over these wires at the end of the case.[12] As previously stated, this is dictated by the quality of the bone and other risk factors to suggest fracture. One such concern is the proximity of the PSI guide pin holes to the tibial metaphyseal cortex, which can be quite close in cases involving smaller statured patients. In the authors' opinion, this can provide a significant stress riser, which can precipitate malleolar fracture in the early postoperative phase. In cases where medial malleolus stress fracture occurs, if the diagnosis is made prior to fracture completion and displacement, the patient can often be treated nonoperatively with non–weight bearing and CAM boot placement owing the stability from the medial malleolus screws. If the fracture completes or displaces, we suggest returning to the operating room for plate fixation in addition.

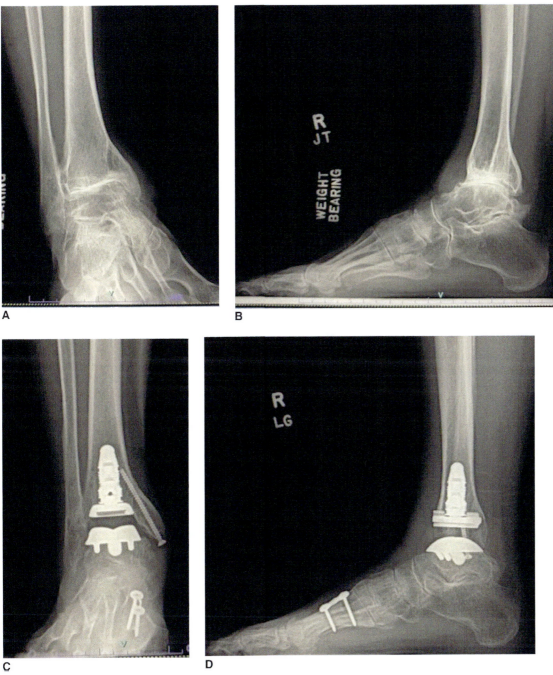

FIGURE 12.13 A-D. Displays case of 66-year-old man with prior skiing trauma **(A, B)**. Upon evaluation, deformity was found to be limited to the ankle joint. He underwent INBONE II total ankle arthroplasty with a gastroc recession. He is successfully weight bearing without assistance and pain free at 10 weeks postoperatively **(C, D)**.

Incisional healing issues are frequently found in total ankle arthroplasty with rates of 6.6% in one literature review.[11] The authors prefer a proactive approach to avoiding wound healing complications. Preoperatively patients are screened for diabetes, tobacco use, and vascular issues. For patients with inflammatory arthritis, we work with the patient's rheumatologist to safely transition medications that are associated with increased risk of wound complications. Significant prior surgical incisions in trauma patients often warrant a plastic surgery referral for suggestions and follow-up. Intraoperatively, we monitor soft tissue handling technique and tourniquet times, specifically trying to reduce time utilizing self-retaining retractors, which can lead to unrecognized soft tissue ischemia and necrosis. For those with prior free or rotational flap coverage, we utilize our plastic surgery col-

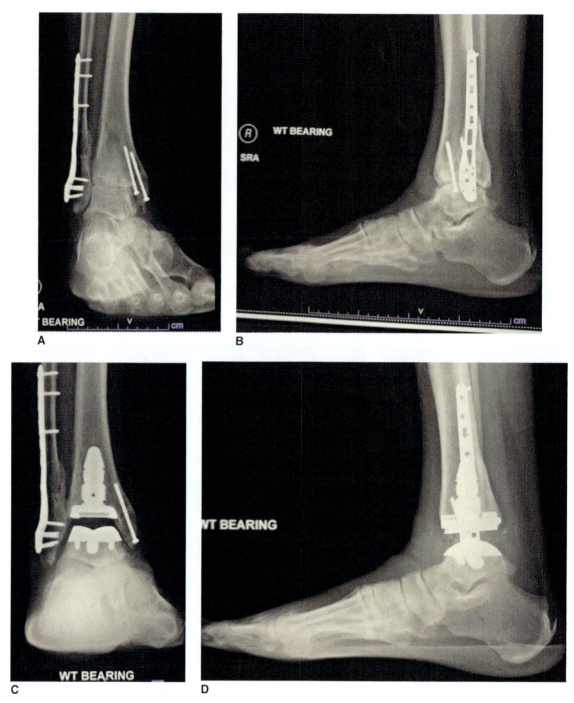

FIGURE 12.14 A-D. A 71-year-old gentleman involved in an motor vehicle accident 4 years prior to ankle replacement surgery. He sustained an ankle fracture and was treated with open reduction internal fixation. He developed progressive onset of pain and limitation of motion. Conservative treatments including injections gave him transient or little relief. The foot achieved neutral but he was somewhat stiff. He had pain with weight-bearing and reasonable plantar flexion.

leagues for access and closure. Surgeons should give thoughts to their choice of approach. Despite this, the authors continue to utilize a direct anterior approach to the ankle. However, a recent study suggests an anteromedial approach trends toward reduced wound complications.[8]

Deep infection is an infrequent complication found in ankle arthroplasty with rates of 1.7% in one literature review.[11] Aggressive surgical management follows confirmation of infection, with algorithms consistent with hip and knee arthroplasty literature, the discussion of which is out the scope of this chapter.

Impingement is often a concern in total ankle arthroplasty. The authors find anecdotally that is an uncommon occurrence when utilizing INBONE secondary to PSI guiding component sizing as well as the trapezoidal design tapering cuts into the gutters.

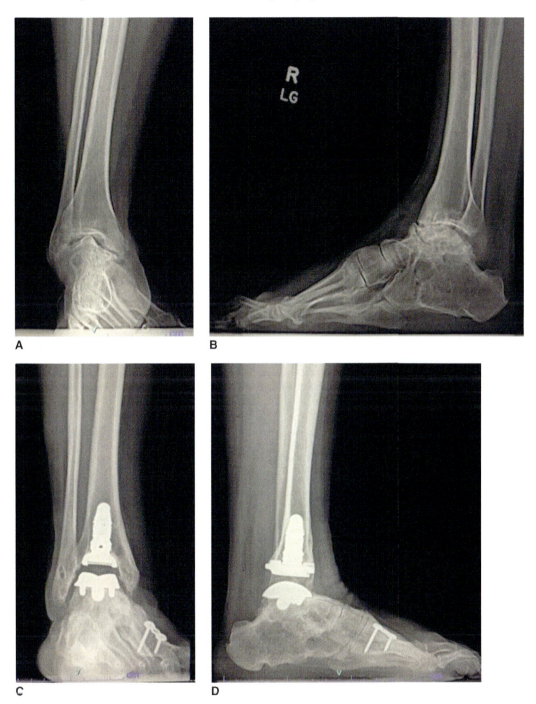

FIGURE 12.15 **A-D.** A 41-year-old female with congenital foot and ankle deformities. She underwent multiple surgeries to correct her foot but developed a significant degenerative ankle on top of the previously reconstructed foot. At the time of surgery, she's a mother of two but had increasing pain that was limiting her ability to function and also care for her family and children. Her exam demonstrated that she walked on the outside of her foot, had a callus on her lateral midfoot, and lacked the ability to get to neutral by about 10°.

RESULTS

The INBONE II prosthesis has enjoyed successful mid-term outcomes as both a primary and a revision component. Hsu and Haddad evaluated INBONE II for radiographic and clinical outcomes, with a 3-year survival rate of 97%. The single patient of the cohort who underwent revision of the talar component for subsidence did not require any further operations. Visual analog scale pain, American Orthopedic Foot and Ankle Society (AOFAS) hindfoot score, and ROM all significantly increased. Rushing et al produced results at a mean follow-up 7 years (range 5 to 9 years) of 15 INBONE II total ankle arthroplasties with survivorship of 93.7%. Only one ankle required revision during that time period and all maintained their initial coronal and sagittal alignments. These findings were reinforced by Gagne et al who displayed 51 ankles with a mean follow-up of 6.4 years (range, 5 to 9) with a survivorship of 98% and an overall reoperation rate of 7.8%.

Prior to the advent of INVISION total ankle revision componentry, INBONE II was often utilized to revise failed ankle prostheses. In a retrospective review of revision total ankle replacement that utilize INBONE II componentry, the survivorship was nearly 80% at 4 years with improvement in Foot Function Index as well as AOFAS hindfoot score.

The most common mechanism of failure in the aforementioned studies is aseptic loosening/subsidence of the talar componentry. Prior criticisms of the INBONE II system centered around the peck drilling through the hindfoot for stem reaming access and its affect on the vascular supply of the talus. Dyke et al challenged this theory, demonstrating with ^{18}F linked positron emission tomography CT that talus vascular perfusion persists following index total ankle arthroplasty with the INBONE II.[13]

In conclusion, we find that INBONE II total ankle replacement utilizing PSI provides the surgeon with the stability, modularity, and survivability to address the ever increasing number of patients with end stage ankle arthritis (Figs. 12.13 through 12.15).

REFERENCES

1. Gagne OJ, Day J, Kim J, et al. Midterm survivorship of the INBONE II total ankle arthroplasty. *Foot Ankle Int.* 2022;43(5):628-636.
2. Raikin SM, Rasouli MR, Espandar R, Maltenfort MG. Trends in treatment of advanced ankle arthropathy by total ankle replacement or ankle fusion. *Foot Ankle Int.* 2014;35(3):216-224.
3. Rushing CJ, Mckenna BJ, Zulauf EA, Hyer CF, Berlet GC. Intermediate-term outcomes of a third-generation, 2-component total ankle prosthesis. *Foot Ankle Int.* 2021;42(7):935-943.
4. Saltzman CL, Salamon ML, Blanchard GM, et al. Epidemiology of ankle arthritis: report of a consecutive series of 639 patients from a tertiary orthopaedic center. *Iowa Orthop J.* 2005;25:44-46.
5. SooHoo NF, Zingmond DS, Ko CY. Comparison of reoperation rates following ankle arthrodesis and total ankle arthroplasty. *J Bone Joint Surg Am.* 2007;89(10):2143-2149.
6. Hsu AR, Haddad SL. Early clinical and radiographic outcomes of intramedullary-fixation total ankle arthroplasty. *J Bone Joint Surg Am.* 2015;97(3):194-200.
7. Bernasconi A, Najefi AA, Goldberg AJ. Comparison of mechanical axis of the limb versus anatomical axis of the tibia for assessment of tibiotalar alignment in end-stage ankle arthritis. *Foot Ankle Int.* 2021;42(5):616-623.
8. Halai MM, Pinsker E, Daniels TR. Effect of novel anteromedial approach on wound complications following ankle arthroplasty. *Foot Ankle Int.* 2020;41(10):1198-1205.
9. Overgaard S, Lind M, Glerup H, Bünger C, Søballe K. Porous-coated versus grit-blasted surface texture of hydroxyapatite-coated implants during controlled micromotion: mechanical and histomorphometric results. *J Arthroplasty.* 1998;13(4):449-458.
10. Schipper ON, Hsu AR, Haddad SL. Reduction in wound complications after total ankle arthroplasty using a compression wrap protocol. *Foot Ankle Int.* 2015;36(12):1448-1454.
11. Glazebrook MA, Arsenault K, Dunbar M. Evidence-based classification of complications in total ankle arthroplasty. *Foot Ankle Int.* 2009;30(10):945-949.
12. McGarvey WC, Clanton TO, Lunz D. Malleolar fracture after total ankle arthroplasty: a comparison of two designs. *Clin Orthop Relat Res.* 2004;424:104-110.
13. Dyke JP, Garfinkel JH, Volpert L, et al. Imaging of bone perfusion and metabolism in subjects undergoing total ankle arthroplasty using 18F-fluoride positron emission tomography. *Foot Ankle Int.* 2019;40(12):1351-1357.

13 Exactech Vantage Fixed-Bearing Total Ankle Replacement

Jensen K. Henry and Constantine A. Demetracopoulos

INTRODUCTION

The current generation of total ankle replacement (TAR) has evolved dramatically from prior iterations. The majority of implants on the market today feature low-profile designs that minimize bony resection, more closely replicate native anatomy, and rely on osseous integration.[1] One of these low-profile implants is the Vantage TAR (Exactech, Gainesville, Florida), which is a fixed-bearing, semiconstrained two-component total ankle implant that was approved for use in 2016 (Fig. 13.1).[2] There is also a mobile-bearing version of this implant approved for use outside of the United States. Features of the Vantage include a tibial component with a central press-fit cage and three pegs that are perpendicular to the tibial axis, and a biconcave talar component with a larger medial than lateral radius of curvature to better reproduce talar morphology.[3,4] The Vantage talus has both flat-cut and curved options, the latter of which is created from four chamfered sides that are rasped smooth. The curved surface is theorized to increase stability and decrease shear stress at the bone-implant interface of the talar component.[5] Tibial and talar sizes both range from 1 to 4; a unique feature of the Vantage is that any size the tibia may be matched with any size of the talus. There is also a patient-specific instrumentation (PSI) feature, which provides 3D-printed cutting guides to align the tibial and talar cuts to a preoperative plan based on computed tomography (CT) imaging.

INDICATIONS AND CONTRAINDICATIONS

Indications

- End-stage arthritis of the ankle,[6] which may be secondary to:
  - Posttraumatic (prior ankle fracture)
  - Chronic ankle instability
  - Primary osteoarthritis
  - Underlying progressive collapsing foot deformity (PCFD), E1
  - Inflammatory arthritis (ie, rheumatoid arthritis, gout)
  - Other: including hemochromatosis, adjacent joint arthritis

Absolute Contraindications[6]

- Active infection of the ankle, osteomyelitis, or sepsis
- Excessive bone loss/bony defect
- Neuropathic arthropathy or Charcot arthropathy
- Inadequate soft tissue envelope around the ankle
- Skeletally immature patient
- Confirmed metal allergy
- Vascular deficiency of the limb
- Dementia or other neurological, psychological, or mental barrier that would limit the patient's ability to comply with recovery and precautions
- Avascular necrosis of the entire talus

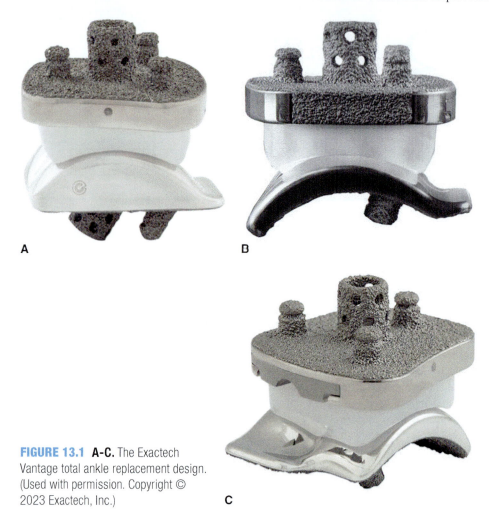

FIGURE 13.1 A-C. The Exactech Vantage total ankle replacement design. (Used with permission. Copyright © 2023 Exactech, Inc.)

Special Indications/Relative Contraindications

- Previous ankle arthrodesis
  - Although takedown of an ankle arthrodesis and conversion to TAR has been described, the procedure is challenging and has a substantial risk of intraoperative and postoperative complications.[7,8]
  - TAR can be beneficial in a patient with a symptomatic ankle arthrodesis nonunion or malunion. It may be considered in a patient with a well-healed ankle arthrodesis, who presents with end-stage associated hindfoot arthritis.[7]
  - Both medial and lateral malleoli are required to convert an ankle arthrodesis to TAR.[8]
  - Moreover, in our experience, these patients have a higher rate of TAR failure.[9]
- Significant deformity
  - Coronal plane deformity has long been discussed as a potential risk factor for TAR failure.[10-12]
  - Recent studies have shown that TAR success is contingent upon surgical correction of preoperative deformity.[10-12]
  - Therefore, deformity that cannot be reconstructed is a contraindication to TAR.
- Severe osteoporosis
  - Currently, there is no threshold or cutoff for bone density prior to TAR.
  - However, surgeons should be cautious in patients with systemic or local osteoporosis because poor bone density may increase the risk of TAR failure or complications.[13,14]
- Age
  - Young age, with associated higher demand and increased patient life expectancy, was traditionally a contraindication for TAR.[15]
  - However, as implants and techniques have improved, there is increased interest in utility of TAR for younger patients.

- Studies of newer-generation implants have shown promising results in younger (less than 50 years) patients.[15,16]
- Further, long-term data are needed to determine if there should be age-related thresholds for TAR versus arthrodesis, or age-based guidelines for what type of TAR implant is the best for a patient.
- Revision
  - The low-profile design of the Vantage TAR means that it is best suited for primary replacement procedures.
  - The use of the Vantage implant in revision TAR is limited to cases where there is ample remaining bone stock to allow for osseous integration to the implant.
  - Cases with severe bone loss or tibial and talar loosening from micromotion of a low-profile implant may benefit from revision with a stemmed implant.

PREOPERATIVE PLANNING

Preoperative planning is a key element of successful TAR surgery. Preoperative planning consists of thorough physical examination, weight-bearing radiographs, and CT of the ankle. In the examination, surgeons should identify prior incisions or soft tissue abnormalities that would affect the approach or benefit from a consultation with a plastic surgeon. The surgeon should also comprehensively assess alignment of the proximal limb, ankle, and foot. Malalignment of the limb more proximally (eg, from severe knee arthritis or a prior tibial shaft fracture) must be identified prior to the TAR and may need to be corrected prior to addressing the ankle. Associated deformity of the foot may be corrected at the time of TAR or may be addressed in staged fashion. Contracture of the gastrocnemius muscle and/or Achilles tendon should also be noted.

From weight-bearing radiographs, the surgeon should assess coronal angulation (varus or valgus), sagittal deformity (dorsiflexion or plantarflexion of the distal tibial plafond). Translation of the talus in the mortise should also be noted. For example, medial translation of the talus in a varus ankle must be corrected intraoperatively. Anterior or posterior translation of the talus on the lateral radiograph may reflect chronic instability, which may need to be addressed intraoperatively to adequately balance the ankle. The hindfoot, midfoot, and forefoot should also be assessed for additional procedures that may be needed to properly balance the ankle and foot (Table 13.1).

CT is the most useful tool to assess bone quality and cysts, which may require bone grafting at the time of surgery. Weight-bearing CT (WBCT) is a novel modality that can be valuable for preoperative planning. WBCT allows for accurate and precise evaluation of alignment at each joint, particularly allowing rotational assessment that is challenging with plain radiographs. CT or WBCT is required if the surgeon uses the PSI feature using 3D-printed custom cutting guides.

TABLE 13.1 Additional Procedures that May Be Required to Balance the Ankle and Foot

Varus Ankle Potential Procedures	Valgus Ankle Potential Procedures
• Deltoid ligament release	• Lateral ligament repair (Broström)
• Medial release—TN joint capsule, PTT	• Achilles lengthening/gastrocnemius recession
• Lateral ligament repair (Broström)	• Medializing calcaneal osteotomy
• Achilles lengthening/gastrocnemius recession	• Medial column stabilization—Cotton osteotomy vs first TMT fusion vs NC fusion
• Lateralizing calcaneal osteotomy	• Peroneus brevis to longus transfer
• First metatarsal dorsiflexion osteotomy	• Deltoid/spring ligament reconstruction
• Peroneus longus to brevis transfer	• Fibular lengthening osteotomy
• Tibialis anterior transfer to centralize	• Hindfoot fusions for rigid/large deformity
• PTT (or FHL) transfer to peroneus brevis	
• Hindfoot fusions for rigid deformity	

TN, talonavicular joint; PTT, posterior tibial tendon; FHL, flexor hallucis longus; Cotton osteotomy, dorsal opening wedge osteotomy of the medial cuneiform; TMT, tarsometatarsal; NC, naviculocuneiform.

SURGICAL TECHNIQUE

Position

The patient is placed supine on an operating table that is radiolucent at the legs. The feet are positioned at the end of the table, with the operative ankle centered on the bed. If the surgeon uses a tourniquet, a well-padded nonsterile tourniquet is placed on the operative thigh. A nonsterile bump is placed under the ipsilateral hip so that the ankle joint is facing up. The leg is prepped and draped in a sterile fashion. We recommend that large intraoperative fluoroscopy is used, with the monitor at the contralateral shoulder of the patient, with the beam entering from the ipsilateral side.

Approach

The anterior approach to the ankle is used. The skin incision is linear and made approximately 1 cm lateral to the tibial crest over the ankle joint, extending 6 cm above and below the level of the ankle joint (Fig. 13.2). Dissection is carried out through the subcutaneous tissues, and the superficial peroneal nerve (SPN) is identified laterally in the wound and mobilized laterally. A small nick in the extensor retinaculum is made at the level of the joint over the extensor hallucis longus (EHL) tendon, and the surgeon can visually confirm that the tendon visualized is the EHL rather than the tibialis anterior (TA) (see Fig. 13.2). The extensor retinaculum is then opened longitudinally. It is important to maintain the integrity of this later for eventual closure to prevent bowstringing and wound breakdown.

Once the extensor retinaculum has been opened, the neurovascular bundle is identified deep to the EHL in the wound. Crossing vessels are coagulated so that the bundle can be mobilized laterally. A longitudinal capsulotomy is then performed, and the capsule is elevated off the bone medially and laterally to visualize the ankle joint. Take care to protect the bundle throughout this step. A large Gelpi retractor is placed deeply in the wound, below the bundle, at the level of the joint (see Fig. 13.2).

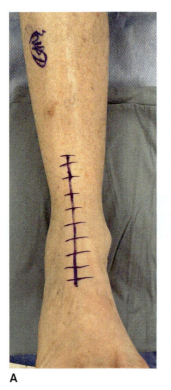
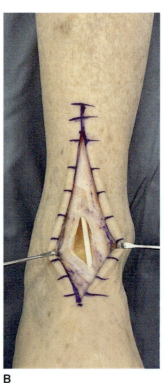
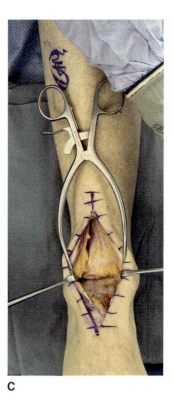

FIGURE 13.2 The anterior approach to the ankle joint is used. **A.** The anterior incision used for the Vantage total ankle replacement. **B.** Incision through the extensor retinaculum with the extensor hallucis longus tendon visible. **C.** After capsulotomy, the ankle joint is visualized.

Alignment Guide

Once the ankle joint is exposed, a shim is placed in the medial gutter to help target the external alignment guide. A small (subcentimeter) incision is made over the tibial tubercle, and the tibial tubercle pin is inserted parallel in the axial plane to the medial shim (Fig. 13.3). The proximal portion of the guide is attached over the tubercle pin and secured at approximately two fingerbreadths from the skin; this can be adjusted later to fine-tune the slope. The distal portion of the alignment guide is grossly centered over the distal tibia. A pin is placed in the most proximal hole of the guide to provisionally secure the guide—after this pin, smaller adjustments can still be made (up to 10°).

First, adjust rotation of the alignment guide. Place the rotation alignment rod ("the flag") in the tibial cutting block, and adjust the alignment guide rotation so that the flag is parallel with the second/third ray of the foot as well as with the orientation of the medial gutter shim. Lock the rotation using the hex screwdriver in the central locking screw. Next, coronal alignment is addressed under fluoroscopic guidance. Varus/valgus position is adjusted at the proximal portion of the alignment guide by sliding the entire longitudinal arm of the guide medially or laterally. The implant should be placed neutral to the axis of the tibia. Medial/lateral position is adjusted over the guide at the level of the ankle joint using the hex screwdriver. The vertical portion of the tibial cutting guide should align with the medial gutter; avoid excessive resection of the medial malleolus. Appropriate position is confirmed with the mortise view of the anteroposterior (AP) fluoroscopy (Fig. 13.4).

Once the position of the alignment guide is appropriate on the AP image, the resection level and slope can be addressed. Insert the angel wing into the tibial cutting block (Fig. 13.5), and obtain a perfect lateral fluoroscopic image with the angel wing appearing at its peak thinness (see Fig. 13.4). Once this lateral image is obtained, adjust the slope by sliding the proximal portion of the guide closer or further from the skin. Next, the resection height is set via the hex screwdriver; this is typically 7 mm proximal to the tibial plafond (see Fig. 13.4) but may vary based on the surgical plan. Once satisfied with the slope and resection level on the lateral view, the surgeon should return to the AP (mortise) view and confirm the coronal alignment is still adequate. Then, the guide can be pinned in the block and the tibial cutting guide.

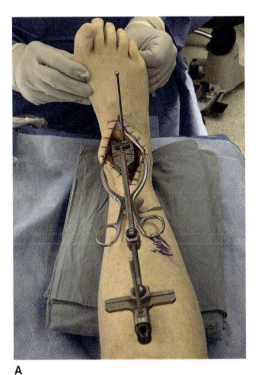
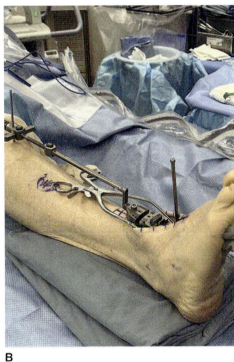

FIGURE 13.3 A, B. The external alignment guide positioned over the tibia. The axial alignment of the tibial tubercle pin is parallel to the medial shim in order to guide adequate rotational position of the cuts and the implant.

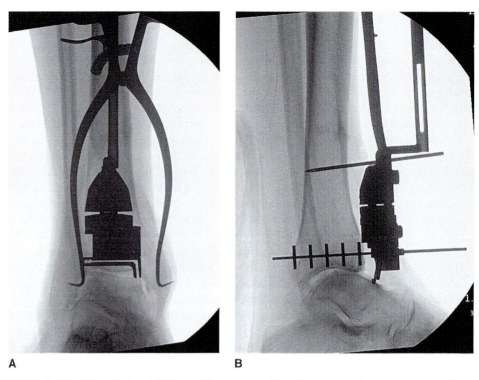

FIGURE 13.4 **(A)** AP (mortise) and **(B)** lateral C-arm view of the alignment guide in adequate position.

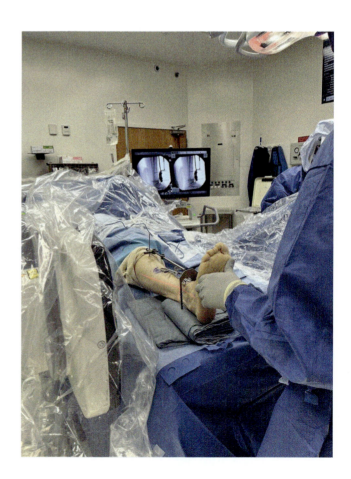

FIGURE 13.5 The angel wing is placed in the tibial cutting block. A perfect lateral fluoroscopic image is obtained.

Tibial Cut

After the alignment guide and cutting guide are securely pinned, the distal tibia is cut using an oscillating saw. The large reciprocating saw is then used through the medial aspect of the cutting block. The distal tibial cutting block is removed. An osteotome can be used to complete the cuts if needed. Remove the resected tibial bone. Any small step-offs or irregularities in the tibial cut can be smoothed with a small reciprocating saw. If a rounded talus is desired, follow the subsequent steps (pictured); if a flat-cut talus is used, proceed to the flat-cut talus section (not pictured).

Rounded Talus: Talar Cut, Preparation, and Sizing

If there is residual cartilage on the talus, this should be removed so that the talar cutting block can sit flush on the bone. The talar cutting block has two options for the amount of talar resection, 2 and 4 mm. The standard 4-mm cutting block is typically used, especially in the cases of tight ankles. The 2-mm cut can be used if there is substantial loss of talar height and the curved talar option is still desired. The length of the alignment guide is adjusted to ensure that the talar cutting block is sitting flush on the talar dome. Hold the foot in neutral dorsiflexion with slight heel valgus and pin the talar cutting block. Place the angel wing in the talar cutting block, and obtain a lateral fluoroscopic image to confirm that the slope of the cut is appropriate (Fig. 13.6); at this point, the resection level has been determined. Next, the talus is cut using the oscillating saw. Since the talar cutting block is not a capture guide, attention should be paid to the direction and depth of the saw cut to avoid inadvertently injuring the malleoli, the posterior neurovascular bundle, or the flexor hallucis longus (FHL) tendon. Remove the talar capture pins and the guide, and then, remove the talar bone. Insert the gap check tool to ensure that an adequate amount of bone has been resected (Fig. 13.7). Once satisfactory, the alignment guide can be removed.

Use the talar lollipop on the cut talar dome to choose the best talar size and guide the talar rotation. The objective is to have adequate talar medial-lateral coverage without overhang and rotational alignment with the second metatarsal. Insert the distraction tool to tension the soft tissues and hold the talar lollipop in place (Fig. 13.8). Obtain a lateral fluoroscopic image to confirm the adequate anterior-posterior position of the talar lollipop (see Fig. 13.8). Pin the talar lollipop anteriorly, and then, remove the tensioner and the lollipop.

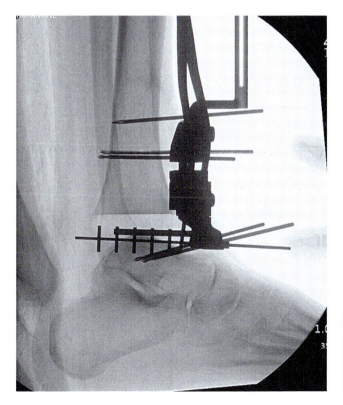

FIGURE 13.6 The angel wing is placed in the talar cutting block and a lateral fluoroscopic image is obtained to confirm that the slope of the cut is appropriate.

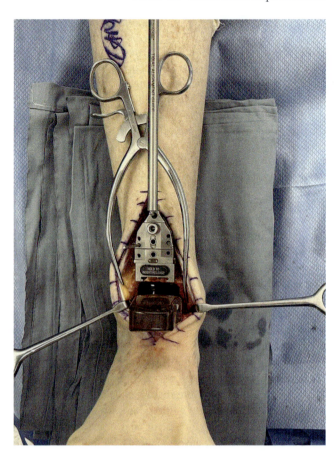

FIGURE 13.7 The gap check tool confirms that enough bone has been resected to accommodate the implant and that there will not be impingement from the fibula.

Then, place the size-specific talar cutting block over the pins (Fig. 13.9) and fix with two additional pins medially and laterally. Confirm that it is flush to the bone; this can be performed using the lateral fluoroscopic image and by visually checking that the posterior chamfer slot is directly in contact with bone. Make the first chamfer cut through the posterior slot using the oscillating saw; do not plunge into the back of the ankle. Then, use the anterior mill tool in the two anterior slots. Remove the anterior pins before the next cut, and then, use the oscillating saw for the final chamfer cut (through two slots of the cut guide). At this point, the pins and the talar cutting guide can be removed, and all resected bone can be removed. Ensure that osteophytes on the talar neck are removed but stay anterior to the milling slots. Use the curved rasp to smooth the cut talus into a rounded surface.

Insert the talar trial onto the cut talar surface, ensuring adequate medial-lateral position. Hold the talar trial in place with the tensioner, and provisionally fix with the central screw (Fig. 13.10). Confirm with a lateral fluoroscopic image that the talar trial sits flush to the bone and is in adequate anterior-posterior position (see Fig. 13.10). The anterior talar peg holes can be drilled now, or after the tibial trial is placed.

Flat-Cut Talus: Talar Cut and Sizing

The flat-cut talus may be chosen if there is significant talar collapse, cystic changes or poor bone quality in the talar dome, or due to surgeon preference due to reproducibility and simplicity. If the flat-cut talus is used, place the adjustable talar cutting block onto the alignment guide and shift the block as distal as possible to adequately tension the soft tissues. The paddle should sit flush and centered on the talar bone. Insert the angel wing into the talar cutting block. As in the steps for the rounded talus, hold the foot in neutral dorsiflexion with slight heel valgus and pin the cutting block. A lateral fluoroscopic image is obtained to confirm the slope of the talar cut. The adjustable talar cutting block is then pinned proximally.

The resection height of the talar flat cut is then set using the adjustable talar cutting block. The typically used resection height is 8 mm, but this may be adjusted from 2 to 12 mm based on the

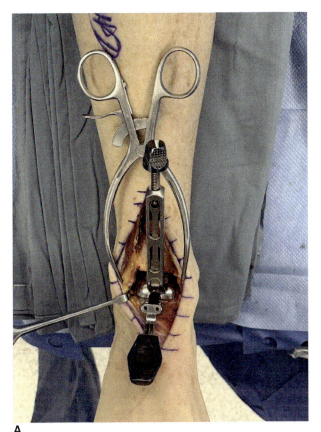
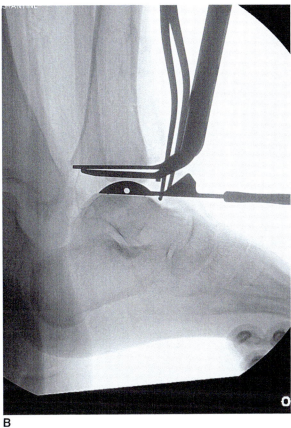

FIGURE 13.8 A. The talar lollipop and the distraction tool in place. The black paddle on the talar lollipop can be used to assess rotation, which should line up with the second ray. **B.** On the lateral fluoroscopic image, the radiolucent circle should align with the lateral process of the talus.

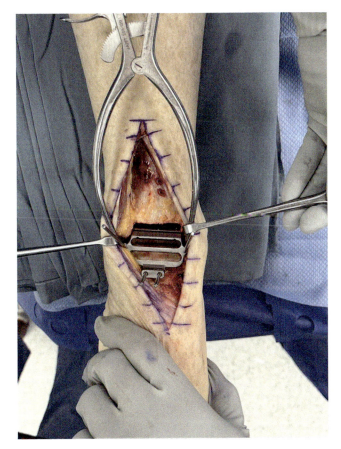

FIGURE 13.9 The size-specific talar cutting block is placed over the pins and fixed with two additional pins medially and laterally. Confirm that it is flush to the bone using fluoroscopy and visually checking that the posterior chamfer slot is directly in contact with bone.

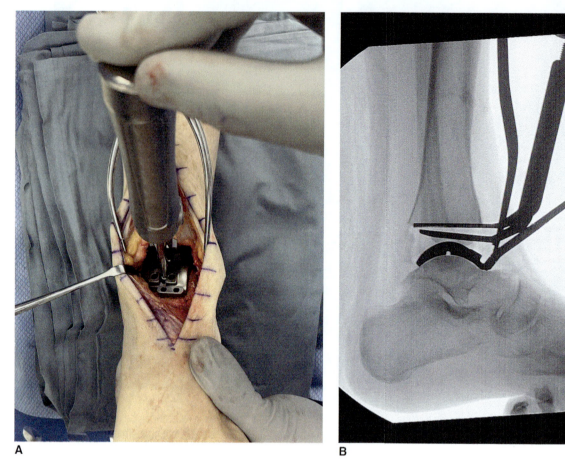

FIGURE 13.10 **A.** The talar trial is inserted along with the tensioner, and held in place with the central screw. **B.** The lateral fluoroscopic image is obtained to confirm that there is excellent contact between the trial and the cut talar bone.

extent of talar dome collapse and desired resection amount. If there is severe talar collapse, resection height may be reduced to 2 to 4 mm. The talar cutting block is then pinned more distally in the talus. The talus is cut with the oscillating saw, and the resected bone is removed.

Insert the flat-cut talus trial, confirming adequate size and rotation. Then, insert the flat-cut fixed-bearing gap check tool to ensure that adequate bony resection was achieved. A lateral fluoroscopic image is used to confirm talar trial position. Once the talus has been sized and the gap is confirmed satisfactory, remove the alignment guide, pin the flat cut talus trial in place, and remove the gap check tool. The anterior peg holes in the trial are drilled with the talus drill, followed by the center cage hole using the coring drill. Intraoperative fluoroscopy images for the flat-cut talus sequence are shown in Figure 13.11.

Tibial Sizing and Preparation

Size the tibia using the tibial sizing guide. Ensure adequate anterior-to-posterior coverage using the lateral fluoroscopic image. Insert the size-specific tibial trial (tibial punch guide) and the punch liner (Fig. 13.12). Confirm adequate position on both AP and lateral fluoroscopy (see Fig. 13.12). Then, pin the tibial punch guide with bicortical cross pins, and repeat the fluoroscopic images to ensure that the guide did not move and there is no lift-off posteriorly. If the talar pegs were not drilled before because the surgeon wanted to confirm tibial position first, complete that step now. Then, remove the punch liner, the central talar screw, and the talar trial.

Ensure that the anterior screw on the tibial trial is tightened to rest against the anterior tibial cortex (Fig. 13.13). This will prevent the tibial trial from translating posteriorly. The pegs and cage for the tibial implant are then punched (see Fig. 13.13). Remove the punch guide and the tibial pins and trial.

13 Exactech Vantage Fixed-Bearing Total Ankle Replacement

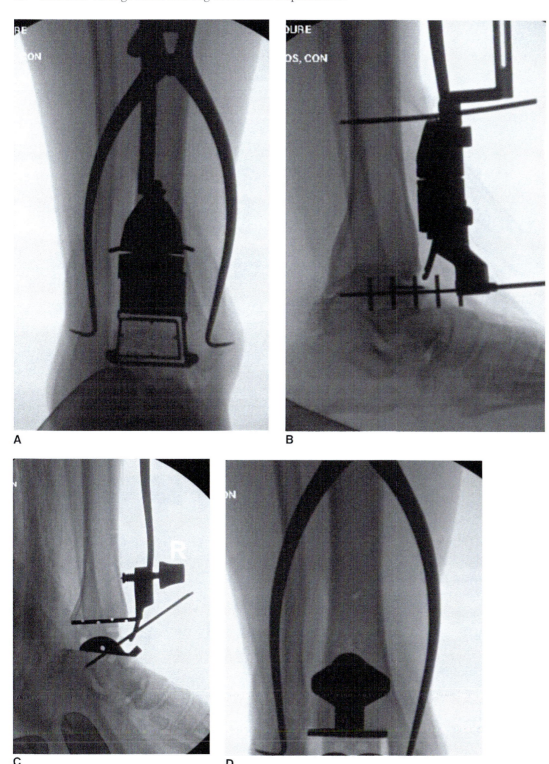

FIGURE 13.11 Intraoperative fluoroscopy images **(A-F)** for the flat cut talus.

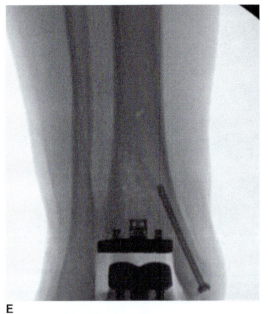
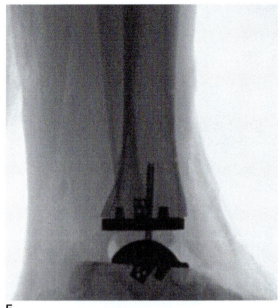

FIGURE 13.11 *(Continued)*

Implant Insertion

Manually insert the tibial component into the joint and align it with the punched holes, starting with the central cage followed by the anterior pegs. Insert the tibial impactor and align it with the implant. Mallet to impact the tibia, ensuring that the impactor is aligned with the limb

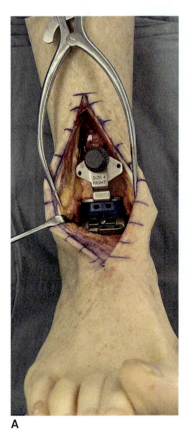
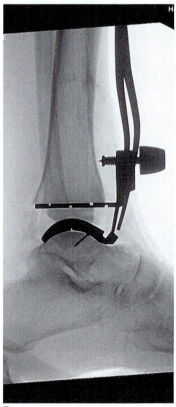
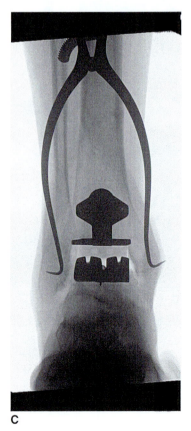

FIGURE 13.12 A. Intraoperative photo and anteroposterior **(B)** and lateral **(C)** fluoroscopy of the tibial punch guide. On the lateral fluoroscopic image, notches in the tibial trial indicate the implant length as well as the location of the pegs and the central cage.

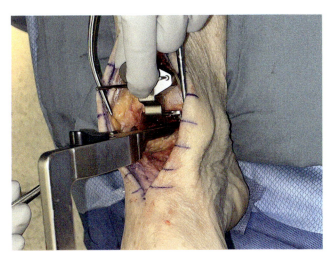

FIGURE 13.13 Prior to punching the tibia, ensure that the anterior screw on the tibial trial is tightened to apply pressure to the anterior tibial cortex. Take extreme caution during punching the tibia. The force during this step can lead to intraoperative fracture (often anterolaterally at the tibia, which should be recognized and plated immediately). Moreover, off-axis or inadequate punching can lead to inadequate space/orientation for the pegs/cage, which can lead to the implant not seating correctly to the bone.

(Fig. 13.14). Impact the tibia so that it is flush to bone without radiographic evidence of lift-off posteriorly. Then, insert the talar implant by manually lining the pegs to the peg holes and impacting. Insert the trial polyethylene (tibial liner trial) and manually test the balance of the ankle. The ankle should have supple dorsiflexion/plantarflexion with 1- to 2-mm joint opening between the polyethylene insert and the talus symmetrically on the medial and lateral sides. Once the adequate liner size is selected, insert the final polyethylene. Push the polyethylene fully into the tibial tray, and then, insert the size-specific locking clip until it is fully seated and flush with the tibial tray (Fig. 13.15).

Patient-Specific Instrumentation

There is a PSI option available for the Vantage total ankle system. This option utilizes a preoperative CT scan to generate custom cutting guides for use in surgery. The surgeon may elect to use PSI for multiple reasons: elimination of intraoperative use of the alignment guide, which may reduce operative time and intraoperative fluoroscopy use; planning implant placement for cases with existing hardware in the distal tibia; and the benefit of preoperative alignment planning. However, surgeons may choose to proceed with standard instrumentation based on expertise and comfort with the alignment guide; cases in which they want to perform soft tissue and/or bony alignment corrections prior to TAR implantation; or cases of severe deformity that may not be completely accounted for in the PSI planning guides.

If PSI is to be used, osteophytes should not be removed at the original approach, as these are used as a reference for the cutting guide. Take care to ensure that the soft tissue and periosteum are removed from the distal tibia and the talus to facilitate adequate contact between the cutting guide and bone. The tibial guide is then placed, and fluoroscopy is used to confirm adequate alignment and verify that the position of the guide reflects the presurgical plan. Once satisfied, the guide is pinned,

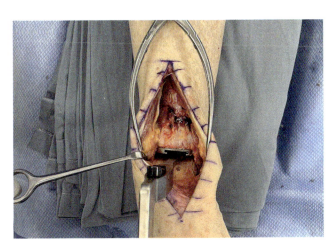

FIGURE 13.14 The tibial component is impacted carefully. When impacting the tibial component, lift-off posteriorly is a common pitfall. A lateral fluoroscopic image is helpful to ensure that the implant and impactor are appropriately aligned. Start with the tibial impactor on the posterior lip of the tibial tray, and then, move it more centrally on the implant to seat it down. However, too much back-and-forth with the tibial impactor will just the implant to toggle and rock in the sagittal plane.

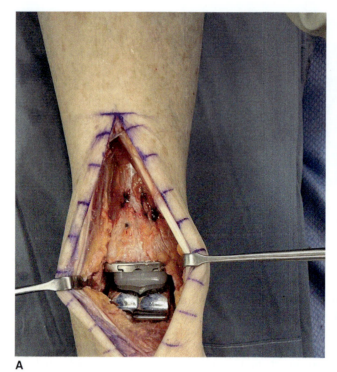
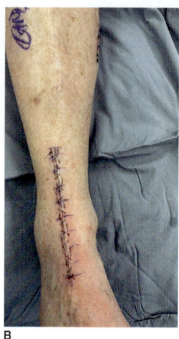

FIGURE 13.15 A. The final implants inserted. The locking clip is flush with the tibial tray to hold the polyethylene liner in place. **B.** The wound is closed in layers with a horizontal mattress or running horizontal mattress for the skin. There should be minimal soft tissue tension to minimize wound complications and soft tissue breakdown in this vulnerable area.

and the distal tibia is cut through the guide. This is repeated for the talar cut. After completion of the appropriate cuts, the PSI cutting guide is removed and the tibial and talar bone is removed. The surgeon can then follow the standard technique to prepare the tibial and talar bone cuts for placement of the implants as noted above.

Final Steps and Closure

Final radiographs are taken to confirm adequate implant alignment and contact to the bone (Fig. 13.16). Ensure that there are no periprosthetic fractures that occurred during the procedure. The gutters are thoroughly débrided using a combination of the small reciprocating saw, osteotomes, and rongeurs. The wound is copiously irrigated; surgeon or institution practice may dictate the use of a povidone-iodine wash for arthroplasty cases. Additional procedures are performed based on the preoperative plan to balance the foot and ankle.

If a tourniquet is used, it is deflated at this step and hemostasis is achieved. Closure of the anterior wound is performed in layers. The ankle capsule is closed using absorbable braided sutures in a figure-of-8 fashion. The extensor retinaculum is similarly closed over the neurovascular bundle and extensor tendons. Subcutaneous tissue is closed with a buried monofilament layer, and the skin is closed with nonabsorbable sutures in a horizontal mattress or running horizontal mattress fashion (see Fig. 13.15). Sterile dressings and a short-leg splint are placed.

PEARLS AND PITFALLS

- In positioning the patient, ensure that the feet are at the end of the bed and there is a large bump under the ipsilateral hip. If the bump is too small, the leg/ankle rotates externally away from the surgeon's natural field of view, which makes visualization and accurate assessment of limb rotation more challenging.
- The C-arm should enter on the ipsilateral side, so the surgeon can achieve the best resolution and field of view of the foot. This is beneficial for accurate positioning of the angel wing on the lateral radiograph.

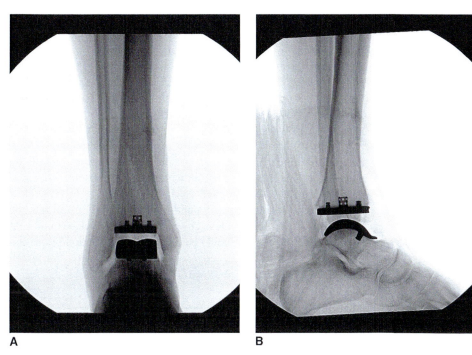

FIGURE 13.16 Final AP **(A)** and lateral **(B)** fluoroscopy images of the Vantage implant.

- The SPN is lateral in the wound, but there is often a crossing branch that runs centrally over the ankle joint. It is typically better to sacrifice this branch rather than unintentionally injure it with traction or during other steps of the case, which can lead to a painful neuroma/neuritis.
- In cases where standard instrumentation is used, it may be necessary to address osteophytes and deformity at the joint prior to placement of the jig. If the standard instrumentation is used, large osteophytes at the tibial plafond and anterior talar neck should be removed using an osteotome, rongeur, and/or the small reciprocating saw. In the case of PSI, these osteophytes should be preserved in order to facilitate accurate placement of the PSI guide. In a varus ankle deformity, it may be necessary to perform a release of the deltoid ligament off its tibial insertion.
- If the patient has a total knee replacement or other implant at the knee, the tubercle pin should be inserted under fluoroscopic guidance, typically more distal or medial/lateral to the stem to avoid contact.
- There may be cases where due to prior trauma, deformity, or anatomic variation, there is a discrepancy between the rotational alignment of the medial gutter and the second/third ray of the foot. Moreover, there will be cases in which the anatomic axis and the mechanical axis of the tibia differ (ie, a malunited tibial diaphyseal fracture). In these cases, the surgeon will need to use clinical judgment to determine the ideal axial alignment of the alignment guide.
- In order to accurately gauge the position of the angel wing, a perfect lateral image is needed. It is often helpful to "wag" the C-arm machine and adduct/abduct the limb to achieve this.
- In posttraumatic cases, the posterior neurovascular bundle and FHL tendon may be adherent to the posterior capsule and ankle. The surgeon should take extreme caution in these cases to not injure these structures with the anterior-to-posterior motion of the saw blade. The surgeon may also elect to cut perform cuts with the ankle in plantarflexion to relieve tension off the posterior structures.
- Removal of the distal tibial resected bone can be challenging. If possible, lever a curved Lambotte osteotome off the alignment guide to "walk" the resected bone out in one piece. Do not lever off the tibial bone. Alternately, tibial bone removal can be done piecemeal using a reciprocating saw and a rongeur.
- The talar cutting guide must be pinned flush to the talus. A laminar spreader or the tensioner can be used to provide adequate tension during this step to ensure that the guide is sufficiently seated to the bone without gapping or malalignment and is pinned appropriately.
- When milling the anterior talus, it is better to push, rather than drag, the milling tool. This provides more thorough milling of the anterior talus. It can help to first go straight down and make a pilot hole with the milling tool, then orient the tool obliquely and push across the anterior talus.

- Do not overuse the rasp, which can lead to blunting of the rounded talar dome and poor bone-implant contact. Moreover, ensure that the rasp is in contact with the bone through the entire arc of movement; lift-off at any point can lead to irregularities of the talus.
- Take extreme caution during punching the tibia. The force during this step can lead to intraoperative fracture (often anterolaterally at the tibia, which should be recognized and plated after insertion of the tibial component). Moreover, off-axis or inadequate punching can lead to inadequate space/orientation for the pegs/cage, which can lead to the implant not seating correctly to the bone.
- When impacting the tibial component, lift-off posteriorly is a common pitfall. A lateral fluoroscopic image is helpful to ensure that the implant and impactor are appropriately aligned. Start with the tibial impactor on the posterior lip of the tibial tray, and then, move it more centrally on the implant to seat it down. However, too much back-and-forth with the tibial impactor will cause the implant to toggle and rock in the sagittal plane.
- Meticulous closure of the wound is critical to minimize wound complications. Ensure that the extensor retinaculum layer is completely and securely closed over the extensor tendons to prevent bowstringing and pressure on the wound. Suture tails should be short to avoid irritation/projection through the skin.

POSTOPERATIVE MANAGEMENT

Postoperatively, patients are initially placed in a short-leg plaster splint and kept non–weight bearing. We no longer routinely use suction drains for primary TARs; recent literature has actually shown that use of a suction drain may be associated with increased risk of wound infections.[17] Depending on the patient's comorbidities and the extent of additional procedures performed, the patient may be discharged home either the day of surgery or the following day. Pain management is multimodal and consists of acetaminophen, nonsteroidal anti-inflammatory drugs (NSAIDs), and judicious use of oral opioids. Patients are discharged with medication to prevent venous thromboembolism per hospitalist or medical doctor recommendations.

Patients return for the first postoperative visit at 2 weeks after surgery. The splint is removed and sutures are removed if there is adequate wound healing. The patient is typically placed in a controlled ankle motion (CAM) boot unless there are soft tissue or other concerns, in which case a non–weight-bearing plaster cast is utilized. The patient then returns at 4 weeks or 6 weeks postoperatively, depending on the additional procedures performed. At this visit, the postoperative radiographs are obtained and the patient begins to advance weight bearing in the CAM boot.

Once the patient is fully weight bearing in the CAM boot (typically at 8 to 10 weeks postoperatively), they can progress out of the CAM boot into supportive footwear. They are seen at 2 months postoperatively for another clinical check and radiographs. They continue to progress activity as tolerated with the direction of a physical therapist. The patient is seen again at 4 months, 6 months, and 1 year postoperatively. After 1 year, the patient is seen annually for clinical and radiographic follow-up to assess component position and peri-implant lucency.

RESULTS AND COMPLICATIONS

Early results of the Vantage implant are limited due to its relative short time on the market. To date, there is one study of the fixed-bearing implant in the United States: in 22 patients with minimum 2-year follow-up, there was 100% survivorship.[18] In this series, one patient sustained an intraoperative medial malleolus fracture and delayed wound healing. There were two European studies of the mobile-bearing version of the implant. In the first, which included 39 patients with a minimum 1-year follow-up, there were no complications requiring revision or reoperation.[19] In the second, there were no reoperations or revisions in 50 TARs, although 6% of patients had peri-implant lucency or cyst formation at 1 year postoperatively. All studies reported significant improvements in patient-reported outcomes scores and radiographic alignment.[18-20]

Intraoperative complications are rare. The anterolateral tibia is at risk for fracture from the anterolateral peg, particularly in posttraumatic sclerotic bone. If the fracture is noted intraoperatively and treated with open reduction internal fixation, this does not portend a worse outcome. Wound complications are uncommon but can have severe consequences if not appropriately managed.[21] Like most current generation, low-profile implants, the Vantage TAR should be monitored for early mechanical failure secondary to loosening and subsidence, especially at the tibial component.[22,23] Although often asymptomatic, peri-implant cysts and lucencies should be monitored radiographically and may require operative treatment before they become symptomatic or progress to implant loosening.[23] Long-term data are still required, however, to determine ultimate survivorship and complication rates of this implant.

ACKNOWLEDGMENTS

The authors acknowledge Isabel Shaffrey, BS, for her tremendous effort and help in preparation of this manuscript.

REFERENCES

1. Gross CE, Palanca AA, DeOrio JK. Design rationale for total ankle arthroplasty systems. *J Am Acad Orthop Surg.* 2018;26:353-359.
2. Department of Health and Human Services. *FDA/HHS approval of vantage total ankle. 510(k) Premarket Notification.* 2016. Accessed April 11, 2023. https://www.accessdata.fda.gov/scripts/cdrh/cfdocs/cfpmn/pmn.cfm?ID=K152217
3. Siegler S, Toy J, Seale D, Pedowitz D. The Clinical Biomechanics Award 2013—Presented by the International Society of Biomechanics: New observations on the morphology of the talar dome and its relationship to ankle kinematics. *Clin Biomech (Bristol, Avon).* 2014;29(1):1-6.
4. Wiewiorski M, Hoechel S, Anderson AE, et al. Computed tomographic evaluation of joint geometry in patients with end-stage ankle osteoarthritis. *Foot Ankle Int.* 2016;37(6):644-651.
5. Exactech. *Exactech Vantage Design Rationale.* https://www.exac.com/product/vantage-ankle-fixed-bearing-design-rationale/
6. Exactech. *Vantage Total Ankle Operative Technique.* 2022. https://www.exac.com/wp-content/uploads/2019/04/721-00-30_RevA_Vantage_Ankle_Fixed_Bearing_Operative_Technique_Web_1350376.pdf
7. Coetzee JC, Raduan F, McGaver RS. Converting ankle arthrodesis to a total ankle arthroplasty. *Orthop Clin North Am.* 2021;52:181-190.
8. Greisberg J, Assal M, Flueckiger G, Hansen ST. Takedown of ankle fusion and conversion to total ankle replacement. *Clin Orthop Relat Res.* 2004;424:80-88.
9. Chu AK, Wilson MD, Houng B, Thompson J, So E. Outcomes of ankle arthrodesis conversion to total ankle arthroplasty: a systematic review. *J Foot Ankle Surg.* 2021;60:362-367.
10. Queen RM, Adams SB, Viens NA, et al. Differences in outcomes following total ankle replacement in patients with neutral alignment compared with tibiotalar joint malalignment. *J Bone Joint Surg Am.* 2013;95:1927-1934.
11. Lee GW, Wang SH, Lee KB. Comparison of intermediate to long-term outcomes of total ankle arthroplasty in ankles with preoperative varus, valgus, and neutral alignment. *J Bone Joint Surg Am.* 2018;100:835-842.
12. de Keijzer DR, Joling BSH, Sierevelt IN, Hoornenborg D, Kerkhoffs GMMJ, Haverkamp D. Influence of preoperative tibiotalar alignment in the coronal plane on the survival of total ankle replacement: a systematic review. *Foot Ankle Int* 2020;41:160–169.
13. So E, Rushing CJ, Prissel MA, Berlet GC. Bone mineral density testing in patients undergoing total ankle arthroplasty: should we pay more attention to the bone quality? *J Foot Ankle Surg.* 2021;60:224-227.
14. Cody EA, Lachman JR, Gausden EB, Nunley JA, Easley ME. Lower bone density on preoperative computed tomography predicts periprosthetic fracture risk in total ankle arthroplasty. *Foot Ankle Int.* 2019;40:1-8.
15. Samaila EM, Bissoli A, Argentini E, Negri S, Colò G, Magnan B. Total ankle replacement in young patients. *Acta Biomed.* 2020;91:31-35.
16. Demetracopoulos CA, Adams SB, Queen RM, Deorio JK, Nunley JA, Easley ME. Effect of age on outcomes in total ankle arthroplasty. *Foot Ankle Int.* 2015;36:871-880.
17. Moncman TG, Fliegel B, Massaglia J, et al. Comparison between closed suction drainage and no drainage following total ankle arthroplasty. *Foot Ankle Int.* 2022;43(9):1227-1231.
18. King MA, Vesely BD, Scott AT. Early outcomes with the vantage total ankle prosthesis. *Foot Ankle Surg Tech Rep Cases.* 2022;2:100121.
19. Mosca M, Caravelli S, Vocale E, et al. Clinical radiographical outcomes and complications after a brand-new total ankle replacement design through an anterior approach: a retrospective at a short-term follow up. *J Clin Med.* 2021;10:4-11.
20. Alsayel F, Alttahir M, Mosca M, Barg A, Herrera-pérez M, Valderrabano V. Mobile anatomical total ankle arthroplasty improvement of talus recentralization. *J Clin Med.* 2021;10:1-12.
21. Gross CE, Hamid KS, Green C, Easley ME, DeOrio JK, Nunley JA. Operative wound complications following total ankle arthroplasty. *Foot Ankle Int.* 2017;38:360-366.
22. Cody EA, Bejarano-Pineda L, Lachman JR, et al. Risk factors for failure of total ankle arthroplasty with a minimum five years of follow-up. *Foot Ankle Int.* 2019;40:249-258.
23. Henry JK, Rider C, Cody E, Ellis SJ, Demetracopoulos C. Evaluating and managing the painful total ankle replacement. *Foot Ankle Int.* 2021;42(10):1347-1361.

14 Cadence Total Ankle Replacement

Justin Tsai, Daniel Fuchs, and David Pedowitz

INDICATIONS AND CONTRAINDICATIONS

Total ankle arthroplasty (TAA) is a procedure performed to address symptomatic end-stage ankle arthritis that has failed to improve with nonoperative management. Ankle arthritis usually develops secondary to prior trauma to the ankle. It can also develop secondary to a systemic inflammatory condition such as rheumatoid arthritis or following septic arthritis. Unlike hip or knee arthritis, primary/idiopathic ankle arthritis is rare.[1] Nonoperative treatment of ankle arthritis includes anti-inflammatory medication, corticosteroid injections, physical therapy, bracing, and activity modifications. For the symptomatic patient in which the above measures have failed, surgical treatment is indicated.

Surgical treatment traditionally involved ankle arthrodesis. Although successful ankle arthrodesis does address the pain associated with ankle arthritis, the impact on the patient's ability to return to presurgical activity level and the increase in rate of adjacent joint arthritis are concerning sequelae, especially in the younger, more active patient with relatively preserved preoperative range of motion.[2]

It is, therefore, no surprise that TAA has emerged as a desirable alternative to ankle arthrodesis over the past several decades. Initial prostheses demonstrated poor survivability secondary to design flaws, which have been improved on with each successive generation of implants.[3] The combination of advancements in survivorship and more ubiquitous exposure during fellowship training have led to an increase in the percentage of ankle replacements performed versus ankle fusions performed for the treatment of symptomatic ankle arthritis.[4]

The Cadence© total ankle (Smith + Nephew Inc., Memphis, Tennessee) is a fourth-generation, three component, fixed bearing implant, which was first introduced for clinical use in 2016. It shares some features with the other implants in its generation, including minimal bone resection, porous metal-backed surfaced to promote ongrowth, and streamlined instrumentation to allow for reproducible technique.[5]

Some unique features of the Cadence implant:

- Side (left or right) specific tibial, talar, and polyethylene components
- Tibial incisura on the tibial implant to accommodate the fibula
- Anterior and posterior biased polyethylene inserts to help correct residual anterior and posterior subluxation of the talus on the tibia
- Highly cross linked (HXL) ultra-high molecular weight polyethylene (UHMWPE) insert

There are both absolute and relative contraindications to use of TAA.[6] Absolute contraindications include active infection, compromised peripheral vascular flow, Charcot arthropathy, and poor overlying soft tissue envelope. In the past, factors such as younger age and/or moderate to severe preoperative coronal plane deformity have been described as relative contraindications, although recent studies have demonstrated that these patients can have similar outcomes to those without these underlying factors.[7,8] Septic arthritis or osteomyelitis of the ankle, preexisting ankle fusion, or poor preoperative range of motion also do not necessarily preclude successful TAA.[9-11]

PREOPERATIVE PLANNING

The preoperative evaluation for a Cadence total ankle replacement (TAR) requires weight-bearing ankle radiographs (Fig. 14.1A through C). Additional radiographs such as weight-bearing foot radiographs, a hindfoot alignment view and tibia-fibula or standing leg radiographs which include knee alignment, should be obtained if there is suspected deformity proximal or distal to the ankle joint. computed tomography (CT) scan is useful to prepare for bone grafting of cysts, resection of osteophytes, and to assess for arthritis of the subtalar joint. Weight-bearing CT scan, if available, may provide additional useful information regarding alignment, deformity, and adjacent joint arthritic changes. A comprehensive understanding of any lower extremity deformities and adjacent joint arthritis is mandatory to plan for staged or concomitant osteotomies or fusions.

Preoperative templating with physical or digital templates is recommended. This will improve intraoperative efficiency by identifying the anticipated implant size for the talus and tibia. The surgeon should be familiar with compatibility between tibia and talus sizes. Understandably, given the congruency of the bearing surface, the talar size dictates the polyethylene size (not thickness) as only same sizes match the exact articular congruity of the talar component. Specifically, for the Cadence, a given size for the talus component is compatible with the same size tibia component or

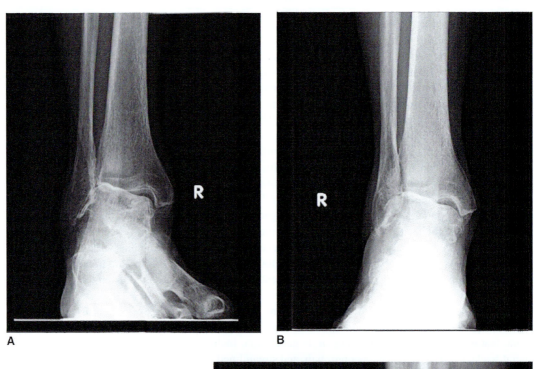

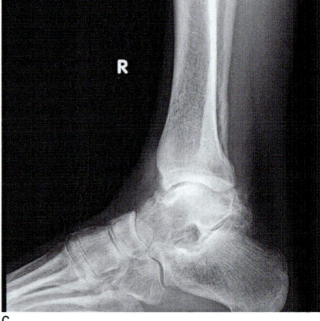

FIGURES 14.1 A-C. Weight-bearing radiographs are obtained during initial evaluation and consideration of total ankle arthroplasty.

a tibia component one size larger. For example, a size 2 talus is compatible with a size 2 or 3 tibia. Similarly, one could not use a tibial component smaller than the talar component. In this example, using a size 3 talus, requiring a size 3 polyethylene liner, could not fit on a size 2 tibia as the tibial component would be too small to cover the entire liner.

For the Cadence system, tibial components are also available with extended length (XL) sizes to help achieve additional posterior coverage when needed. The XL tibial component for a given size provides the same medial to lateral coverage as the non-XL. The additional length of the XL implant for a given size is the same anterior to posterior length as the standard tibia component one size larger. For example, a size 2 XL and 3 XL tibia component each have the same anterior to posterior length but different medial to lateral coverage.

The Cadence total ankle provides options for a bone preserving chamfer cut talus component as well as a flat cut talus component. The flat cut talus is particularly useful in cases where the talar dome has significant bone wear, mild collapse or erosion, and in the setting of prior ankle arthroplasty resulting in decreased bone stock at the talar dome. In most cases, the need for a flat cut talus component should be identified preoperatively and the surgeon should specify that these implants are to be made available for the procedure.

Additionally, the Cadence system provides an option to use an anteriorly or posteriorly biased polyethylene insert to correct anterior or posterior subluxation. The anterior biased inserts have 2-mm increased thickness of the polyethylene at the anterior aspect of the insert to prevent anterior subluxation. The converse is true for the posterior biased inserts. The decision to use a biased polyethylene insert can be made intraoperatively based on trialing; however, the potential need for the biased implants should be identified preoperatively to assure that the appropriate equipment and implants are available for the procedure.

SURGICAL TECHNIQUE

A midline incision is made over the anterior ankle and a standard anterior approach is performed. Full-thickness flaps are developed, and the superficial peroneal nerve is protected at the distal aspect of the incision (Fig. 14.2). The extensor retinaculum is divided, the tibialis anterior tendon sheath opened, and the floor of the tendon sheath is incised along with the capsule (Fig. 14.3). Full-thickness flaps are then utilized to expose the tibiotalar joint medially and laterally (Fig. 14.4).

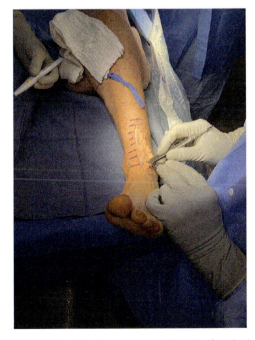

FIGURE 14.2 Anterior exposure with back of scalpel indicating the superficial peroneal nerve at the distal aspect of the incision.

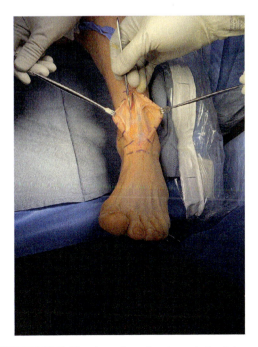

FIGURE 14.3 The deep dissection is carried out deep to the tibialis anterior tendon.

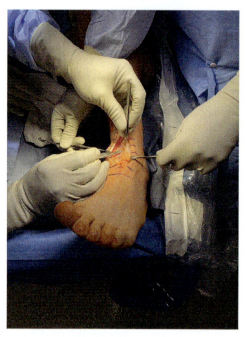 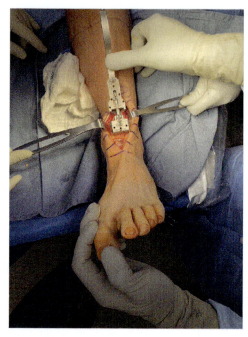

FIGURE 14.4 Capsule incised and full-thickness elevation of all structures lateral to the tibialis anterior tendon.

FIGURE 14.5 Tibial alignment guide in place, centered over anatomic and mechanical axis of tibia and with medial corner of ankle joint.

Osteophytes are carefully removed and the medial and lateral gutters are débrided in order to gain full exposure and prevent impingement. Care should be taken not to remove the distal tibia anterior cortex, which provides important structural support to the tibial component. Laminar spreaders can be placed and tensioned to place the ligaments on stretch and then releases are performed to balance the joint. The tibial alignment guide is then placed after it has been assembled on the back table. Its clamp is applied around the proximal tibia, with the proximal translation block sitting at the level of the tibial tubercle and the tibial rod in line with the tibial crest. The appropriate size tibial cut guide can be placed onto the distal alignment block based on preoperative templating. Most patients are sizes 1 to 3. While preoperative templating is useful, the smaller cut guide is generally applied as a rule and for larger sizes, the larger guide can be used based on intraoperative radiographs. In general, if one aligns the most proximal hole on the medial side of the guide with the medial corner of the ankle joint, the guide is in the general vicinity of where it will finally be placed (Fig. 14.5).

The alignment block and cut guide should be perpendicular to the axis of the tibia in the coronal and sagittal plane. Sagittal plane alignment is estimated by positioning the tibial rod approximately three finger breaths from the anterior aspect of the tibia. A long shouldered bone pin is placed through the proximal portion of the distal alignment block (Fig. 14.6).

Fluoroscopy is then used to fine-tune alignment with sequential images taken along the course of the tibia. Adjustments are first made in the coronal plane at the level of the proximal tibial clamp to achieve neutral varus-valgus alignment such that the tibia rod is in line with the tibia on a full length radiograph. If the tibial anatomical axis is not in line with the mechanical axis, this must be accounted and adjusted for. Once varus-valgus alignment has been achieved, attention is directed at the height of the tibial cut. Because raising the cut level of the tibia necessarily takes more medial malleolus due to the medial slope of the distal tibia, determining the height of the tibial cut first then allows one to ensure an adequate medial malleolar bridge without having to go back and forth between lateral and anteroposterior (AP) radiographs.

Lateral projection fluoroscopy is then performed. The sagittal rod is used and aligned with the axis of the tibia by making adjustments at the articulation between the tibial rod and the proximal tibia clamp. Once the coronal and sagittal alignment have been confirmed, a second long shoulder pin is placed through the distal tibia alignment block.

While still using lateral fluoroscopy, the distal tibia resection height should be set. The tibial resection template should be placed through the slot of the distal tibia cut guide (Fig. 14.7).

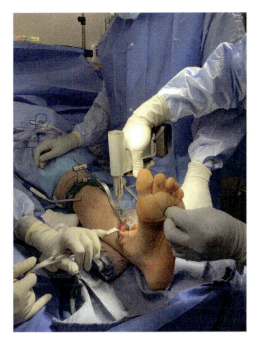

FIGURE 14.6 After rough alignment of the tibial alignment guide has been established, pin in place with a long shouldered pin.

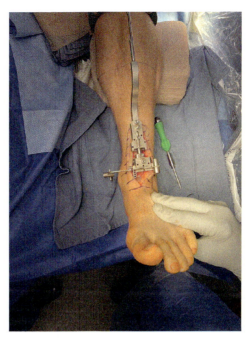

FIGURE 14.7 The tibial resection template should be placed through the slot of the distal tibia cut guide.

A perfect lateral view should be obtained, which is confirmed by a perfect circle appearance at the anterior aspect of the tibial resection template. Then the distal/proximal location of the distal tibia cut guide is adjusted such that the inferior tips of the posts are aligned with the most superior aspect of the tibial plafond. This resection level will allow for placement of the thinnest (6 mm) polyethylene insert in a relatively stiff ankle. The authors have found that often this resection level can be brought distal, to take less bone. To assess this, we obtain a lateral radiograph with the resection wing in place, and then pull on the ankle in an axial fashion to see what flexibility the ankle has. If there is significant distraction between the tibia and talus, the resection height of the tibial cut is brought distally. We have found that in these cases, the sagittal alignment tabs on the resection wing can be brought to the apex of the talar dome (Fig. 14.8).

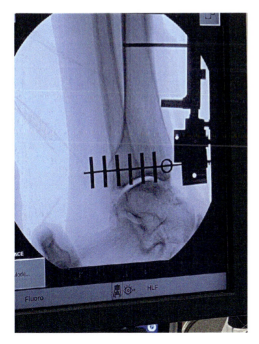

FIGURE 14.8 The distal/proximal location of the distal tibia cut guide is adjusted such that the inferior tips of the posts are aligned with the most superior aspect of the tibial plafond. In some cases, the inferior tips can be placed at the superior aspect of the talar dome to take less bone.

Next, rotational alignment is established. The provided gutter indicators are placed within the medial and lateral gutters for reference. The angle bisector is placed into the distal tibia alignment block. The set screw for rotational alignment is loosened and adjusted such that the bisector is perfectly between the gutter indicators (Fig. 14.9). Typically, this will also align with the second ray or between the second and third rays. The set screw is tightened to lock in rotation. Lastly, the medial to lateral position of the distal tibia cut guide is set using anterior to posterior fluoroscopy views with perfect circles of the pin holes. The guide is adjusted such that the fibula will not be violated and enough medial malleolus is spared to limit risk of malleolar fracture. Once this is set, the cut guide is compressed to the anterior surface of the distal tibia and tighten the set screw.

The tibia resection is then performed. A straight bone pin with trocar tip is placed into the most lateral hole that will allow the pin to remain medial to the fibula. Next a straight bone pin with drill bit is used to sequentially drill from distal to proximal along the three medial holes to establish the vertical cut of the medial malleolus. A straight bone pin with trocar is then placed into the most proximal medial hole to protect the medial malleolus during the saw cut. The saw is then used through the cut guide to perform the distal tibia cut. This can be done under lateral fluoroscopic guidance to avoid plunging and neurovascular injury. The cut guide is then removed and the corner osteotome is used to complete the vertical component of the medial malleolus cut (Fig. 14.10). An osteotome can also be used to complete the lateral cut at the Chaput tubercle anterolaterally.

The bone fragment is then removed. This can be one of the most time-consuming parts of TAR as this bone is often excessively scarred posteriorly due to prior trauma. The use of the corner osteotome on both the medial and lateral sides of the tibial cut can greatly assist in freeing up this bone anteriorly. Care should be taken not to lever on the osteotome as a great deal of force can be transmitted to the bone and fracture of the malleoli could occur. A reciprocating saw can be used to complete the posteromedial cut if necessary. A 5-mm Shanz pin can be utilized to help remove the fragment. Sometimes, a large osteotome levered anteriorly on the anterior tibia can achieve removal of the distal tibial resection as a single piece of bone. This technique, however, is not without the hazards of malleolar fracture and forcible impaction and deformation of the anterior distal tibia and is, therefore, not used by the authors. Rather, a quarter inch osteotome is then used to break up the distal tibial bone into two or three pieces, which can subsequently be removed using a large toothed

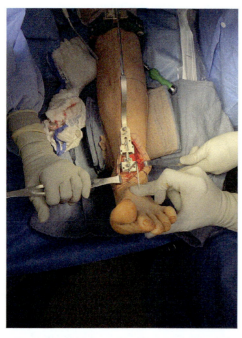

FIGURE 14.9 The angle bisector is placed into the distal tibia alignment block. The set screw for rotational alignment is loosened and adjusted such that the bisector is perfectly between the gutter indicator or in line with the second ray.

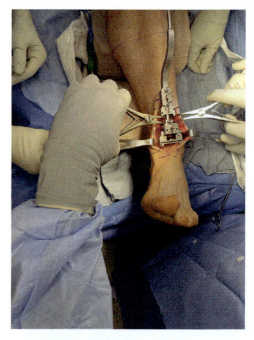

FIGURE 14.10 Corner osteotome used to complete the vertical component of the medial malleolar cut.

pituitary rongeur. Smaller pituitary rongeurs, often used for neurosurgery and head and neck surgery, should not be used as they are fragile and often cannot withstand the forces necessary for bone removal in this area.

The small versus large talar cut guide is then selected based on preoperative templating and is placed into position. The small guide should be trialed first. If the lateral most hole sits medial to the lateral gutter, then the cut will not cover the entire medial to lateral width of the talus and the larger guide should be used. The guide is placed such that it sits flush with the talar neck and just anterior to the talar body. The locking screw for the proximal/distal adjustment of the distal tibia alignment block is then loosened. Laminar spreaders are placed and tensioned to place the collateral ligaments on stretch and compress the talar cut guide to the talus (Fig. 14.11). The proximal/distal locking screw is tightened and the laminar spreaders can be removed. One or two long shouldered bone pins are then inserted to secure the cut guide for the chamfer talus. The foot must be held in plantigrade position while these pins are placed. Straight bone pins with trocar tips are placed into the holes along the cut guide to protect the malleoli. The talus cut is then performed with the saw blade.

All pins and guides are then removed. The gap sizer is used to confirm adequate resection to allow for placement of implants and the thinnest polyethylene insert (6 mm). The authors then obtain a single AP radiograph with the green joint space evaluator in place to ensure proper alignment has been achieved. It is at this point that additional modifications of the cuts can still be made before impacting the final implants. If there is not adequate room for the spacer, a 2-mm tibial cut guide can be used to remove an additional 2 mm of bone.

There is the option for a flat cut talus in addition to the option for the chamfer cut. For use in the case of revision or talus deformity/bone loss, the flat cut provides a clear advantage to ensure adequate bony coverage and to limit the chance of subsidence. When using the flat cut implant, the guide is a simple flat cut guide that attaches to the alignment jig and is adjustable for various heights of a talar resection.

Next, the talus is sized by aligning the appropriate guide along the cut surface of the talus. Medial/lateral and anterior/posterior fit are assessed and, if between sizes, the smaller size is selected. Once the correct size is established, rotation is set clinically by aligning the handle of the guide with the second ray. Medial to lateral position is set by direct visualization. Anterior to posterior position is confirmed with lateral fluoroscopy. A direct lateral is confirmed by achieving a perfect circle within the guide's proximal paddle and within the posterior corner of the corresponding to the cut slot. The curvature of the talar sizer should align with the contour of the remaining talus anteriorly and posteriorly. The more posterior triangle on the sizer silhouette seen on the lateral radiograph has a hole in it and should correspond with the center of both the tibia and the lateral process of the talus. Once position is confirmed, the guide is compressed to the bone by tensioning against the distal tibia, and

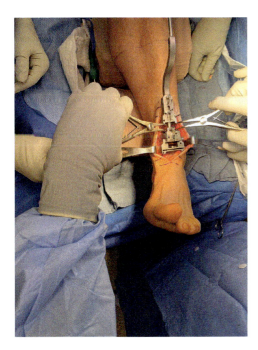

FIGURE 14.11 Laminar spreaders utilized to evenly compress the talar cut guide evenly to the talus with tension on the collateral ligaments.

short-shouldered pins are used to secure the guide. The holder for the talar sizer is removed and the posterior chamfer cut is performed with a saw blade.

The talar sizer holder is replaced and the guide is again compressed to the talus by tensioning against the tibia. The shouldered bone pins are replaced with straight bone pins and the talar sizer is removed, leaving the straight bone pins in place. The talar chamfer cut guide is placed over the straight bone pins and secured with medium shoulder bone pins. Care is taken not to breach the subtalar joint with these pins, but if there is poor quality bone, the authors will occasionally use long pins to ensure stability of the guide. The straight bone pins are removed, and the talar chamfer reamer guide is placed. Each hole is reamed to a hard stop, though any holes that align with the medial or lateral malleolus should be skipped. The reamer guide is then flipped and the holes are again reamed. The reamer guide is then replaced with the talar chamfer drill guide and the two implant post holes are drilled to a hard stop. All guides are then removed.

The talar trial is impacted into place and appropriate position confirmed with lateral fluoroscopy. Tibial size is then determined based on preoperative templating, a tibial sizer depth gauge, and as indicated by the tibial cut guide used during tibial preparation. The appropriate tibial trial is then placed with a trial polyethylene insert. Different thickness trial inserts can be trialed, as well as anterior versus posterior biased inserts, until good stability and range of motion is achieved. The ankle is taken through a range of motion to allow the tibial trial component to find its optimal position. Appropriate implant size and alignment is confirmed with lateral fluoroscopy (Fig. 14.12). The position is then maintained by pinning the trial to the tibia with two short shouldered bone pins. The post drill is then used to drill for the two tibial implant posts through the trial to a hard stop. All pins and trial implants are then removed.

The wound is thorough irrigated and all debris is removed. The final implants are then placed. The tibial tray is placed using an insertion handle and mallet. This is done under lateral fluoroscopic guidance to assure that the implant remains parallel to the cut surface of the tibia throughout insertion and that the posterior wedge of the tibial implant engages the bone. Care is taken not to be too aggressive with this step as this can potentially lead to posterior subluxation of the implant. The anterior border of the implant should always sit flush with the anterior surface of the tibia since when the distal tibia was prepared, the guide was held against the anterior tibial cortex. It is for this reason that the properly placed implant will never be countersunk posterior to the anterior cortex. The insertion handle is removed and a plastic insert is placed into the tibial component for protection during talus implantation. The talus is then impacted into place followed by the polyethylene insert. The insert can be placed by hand or using an insertion device. The ankle is once again evaluated for range of motion and stability and final fluoroscopic images are obtained.

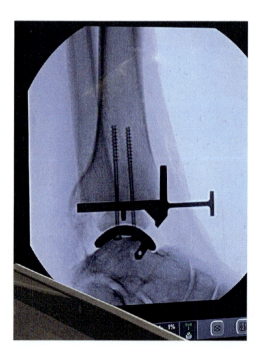

FIGURE 14.12 Lateral fluoroscopy with trial components in place.

After final irrigation, closure is performed of the capsule, extensor retinaculum, and skin. A well-padded splint is applied with the ankle placed in neutral position. The authors find that placement of a closed suction drain is typically not required.

POSTOPERATIVE MANAGEMENT

Postoperatively, the patient is placed into a well-padded splint and non–weight-bearing precautions are maintained for the first 2 weeks. One week postoperatively, patients are placed in an Unna boot compression type bandage for edema control, which we find helps the skin and suture line heal (Fig. 14.13). After 2 weeks, sutures are removed and a removable fracture boot is applied. Patients are made weight bearing as tolerated and wear a contralateral shoe even-up to make sure the pelvis is well balanced to the boot. The boot may be removed for sleep and bathing. Active range of motion is started at that time. Physical therapy is started at 6 weeks, and the patient is able to transition out of the fracture boot as they feel comfortable. Weight-bearing radiographs are obtained according to surgeon protocol, including dorsiflexion and plantarflexion views (Fig. 14.14A through E). For right-sided surgery, driving is delayed until the sixth postoperative week. Adjustments are made as needed if concomitant procedures are performed with the TAA.

PEARLS AND PITFALLS

- Consider utilizing a Z-type incision of the retinaculum, particularly in cases in which there is a longer anticipated surgical time which might normally preclude adequate closure of the retinaculum.
- To avoid damage to the deep neurovascular bundle, deep dissection is performed directly under the tibialis anterior with the tendon retracted. The tibialis anterior sheath is incised anteriorly, the tendon retracted, and the floor of the tibialis anterior tendon sheath incised deeply. The lateral tissues are then reflected and retracted as a single sleeve so that the neurovascular bundle is not dissected, avoiding additional postsurgical scarring. With this technique, the extensor hallucis longus tendon is not dissected and the bundle underneath safely protected throughout the entirety of the procedure.
- Subperiosteal dissection of the deltoid ligament is often employed in the setting of chronic varus deformity. This is done sharply, anteriorly, and bluntly with a Cobb elevator more posteriorly until the posterior tibial tendon is encountered.

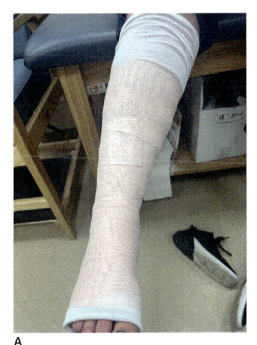
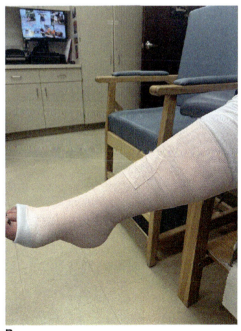

FIGURE 14.13 A, B. Unna boot utilized at week 2 to control edema and minimize wound complications.

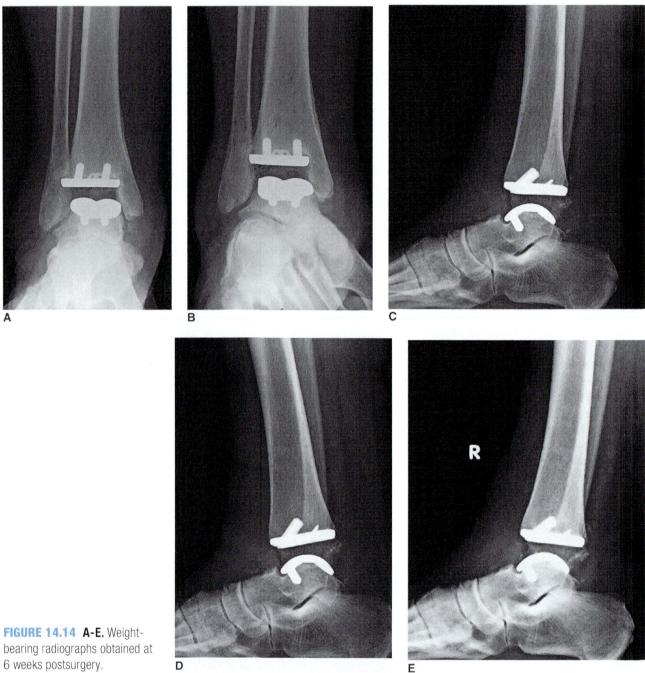

FIGURE 14.14 A-E. Weight-bearing radiographs obtained at 6 weeks postsurgery.

- Ensuring neutral coronal and sagittal alignment is paramount to implanting a durable implant. C-arm machines with a larger field of view, as those typically used for vascular surgery, can be helpful in getting full length tibial radiographs. Medial-lateral calibration to decrease the imaged area can be used to minimize patient and surgeon radiation exposure with such a machine.
- The authors have found the following to be the most efficient order in setting the tibial cut:
  - Varus/valgus alignment (AP view)
  - Tibial sagittal alignment (lateral view)
  - Tibial resection height (lateral view)
  - Rotation alignment
  - Medial/lateral alignment (AP view)
- Emphasis should be made to all involved in the operation that although tempting to do so, once bony cuts have been made, the ankle should not be brought through a range of motion. This will erroneously put the malleoli at risk for fracture as the larger talus engages the unprotected malleoli

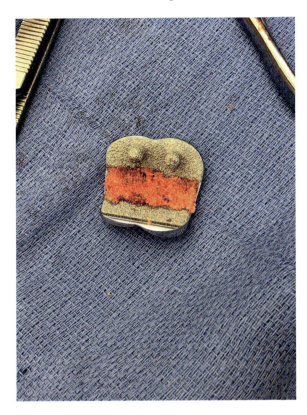

FIGURE 14.15 Bone graft from drill reamings spread onto the undersurface of the talar implant.

in dorsiflexion. For this reason, range of motion and stability should only be assessed with trial implants in place.
- The talar component trial should not have any overhang on the medial or lateral aspects of the resected talus. This will result in impingement. This should be confirmed both visually and radiographically as it can be difficult to see the posterior coverage of the talus.
- When using the flat cut guide, the authors generally set the cut guide to a 3-mm cut. A free saw blade is then placed in the guide and a lateral radiograph is obtained to estimate the cut. Regardless of which talar implant has been selected, the ankle should be held in neutral when pinning it in place. Residual plantar flexion or dorsiflexion will result in the final implant being placed too posterior or anterior, respectively.
- Occasionally, when using a chamfer talar implant, there can be a small gap between the trial and the proximal talar cut. This is thought to be due to plantar flexion of the guide for anterior chamfer reaming. In this scenario, the authors save the bone from the drill used in the reaming of the tibial and talar posts and spread it over the proximal flat portion of the final implant before impaction (Fig. 14.15). Regardless of the implant choice, final implantation should result in clear bony contact between the tibial and talar surfaces on AP and lateral radiographs.

RESULTS AND COMPLICATIONS

Although a thorough discussion of the clinical, functional, and radiographic results of TAA is beyond the scope of this chapter, in general TAA as a procedure demonstrates excellent improvement in pain, function, and radiographic parameters at a minimum of 2 years.[12] Complications that have been described acutely following total ankle include iatrogenic medial malleolar fracture, nerve injury, delayed wound healing, and infection.[6] Once out of the acute perioperative phase, common sequelae include impingement, osteolysis, loosening/subsidence, and heterotopic ossification. Of these, impingement is the most common reason for reoperation.[13] As is the case with any complex procedure, a learning curve has been described in which complications rates are higher in surgeons and institutions with less experience/volume performing TAA.[14] As the surgeon becomes more comfortable with the procedure, complication rates fall.[15,16]

Several studies have demonstrated favorable intermediate clinical and radiographical outcomes of TAA performed using the Cadence implant exclusively. Rushing et al described their clinical and radiographic results in 32 patients, all with at least 1-year follow-up. Their cohort demonstrated implant survivorship of 93.7% and significantly improved coronal and sagittal plane alignment. There was an overall complication rate of 28.1%, with the most common being an intraoperative medial malleolar fracture.[17] Kooner et al included functional results in their prospective case series involving 69 patients and found following surgery patients demonstrated a significant decrease in ankle osteoarthritis score as well as significant increase in SF-36 physical component score.[18] All surgeries were performed by a single surgeon, who was part of the design team for the implant. Implant survivorship in their case series was 100% at 2 years. Interestingly, even though fibrous union of the tibial component was present in just over a quarter of their cases (26.1%), this had no impact on functional scores. Finally, in a similar study involving a single surgeon who was part of the design team, Fram et al demonstrated a significant increase in functional scores, decrease in pain score, and improvement in coronal plan alignment.[19] Mean arc of motion following surgery was 36.5°. Kim et al also reported excellent outcomes in their single center retrospective study, demonstrating survivorship of 93.7% and reoperation rate of 6.3% with minimum follow up of 2 years. Greater than a third (35.8%) of their patients demonstrated tibial-sided periprosthetic lucencies, with those patients demonstrating worse patient reported outcome measurement information system physical function scores than those without lucencies.[20] In summary, the Cadence TAA implant demonstrates excellent survivorship, significant improvements in functional score and radiographic alignment, and low major complication rate at a minimum of 2-year follow-up. Future work needs to be done on the long-term outcomes using not only this implant but also its fourth generation competitors.

REFERENCES

1. Saltzman CL, Salamon ML, Blanchard GM, et al. Epidemiology of ankle arthritis: report of a consecutive series of 639 patients from a tertiary orthopaedic center. *Iowa Orthop J.* 2005;25:44-46.
2. Coester LM, Saltzman CL, Leupold J, Pontarelli W. Long-term results following ankle arthrodesis for post-traumatic arthritis. *J Bone Joint Surg Am.* 2001;83(2):219-228.
3. Gougoulias NE, Khanna A, Maffulli N. History and evolution in total ankle arthroplasty. *Br Med Bull.* 2009;89:111-151.
4. Paracha N, Idrizi A, Gordon AM, Lam AW, Abdelgawad AA, Razi AE. Utilization trends of total ankle arthroplasty and ankle fusion for tibiotalar osteoarthritis: a nationwide analysis of the United States population. *Foot Ankle Spec.* 2022;19386400221110132.
5. Gross CE, Palanca AA, DeOrio JK. Design rationale for total ankle arthroplasty systems: an update. *J Am Acad Orthop Surg.* 2018;26(10):353-359.
6. Cody EA, Scott DJ, Easley ME. Total ankle arthroplasty: a critical analysis review. *JBJS Rev.* 2018;6(8):e8.
7. Gaugler M, Krähenbühl N, Barg A, et al. Effect of age on outcome and revision in total ankle arthroplasty. *Bone Joint J.* 2020;102-B(7):925-932.
8. Hobson SA, Karantana A, Dhar S. Total ankle replacement in patients with significant pre-operative deformity of the hindfoot. *J Bone Joint Surg Br.* 2009;91-B(4):481-486.
9. Shi GG, Huh J, Gross CE, et al. Total ankle arthroplasty following prior infection about the ankle. *Foot Ankle Int.* 2015;36(12):1425-1429. Accessed July 27, 2022. https://pubmed.ncbi.nlm.nih.gov/26231198/
10. Greisberg J, Assal M, Flueckiger G, Hansen ST. Takedown of ankle fusion and conversion to total ankle replacement. *Clin Orthop Relat Res.* 2004;424:80-88.
11. Brodsky JW, Kane JM, Taniguchi A, Coleman S, Daoud Y. Role of total ankle arthroplasty in stiff ankles. *Foot Ankle Int.* 2017;38(10):1070-1077.
12. Syed F, Ugwuoke A. Ankle arthroplasty: a review and summary of results from joint registries and recent studies. *EFORT Open Rev.* 2018;3(6):391-397.
13. Stewart MG, Green CL, Adams SB, DeOrio JK, Easley ME, Nunley JA. Midterm results of the Salto Talaris total ankle arthroplasty. *Foot Ankle Int.* 2017;38(11):1215-1221.
14. Matsumoto T, Yasunaga H, Matsui H, et al. Time trends and risk factors for perioperative complications in total ankle arthroplasty: retrospective analysis using a national database in Japan. *BMC Musculoskelet Disord.* 2016;17(1):450.
15. Usuelli FG, Maccario C, Pantalone A, Serra N, Tan EW. Identifying the learning curve for total ankle replacement using a mobile bearing prosthesis. *Foot Ankle Surg.* 2017;23(2):76-83.
16. Clement RC, Krynetskiy E, Parekh SG. The total ankle arthroplasty learning curve with third-generation implants: a single surgeon's experience. *Foot Ankle Spec.* 2013;6(4):263-270.
17. Rushing CJ, Berlet GC, Hyer CF. Early outcomes with the CADENCE total ankle prosthesis. *Foot Ankle Orthop.* 2020;5(4):2473011420S00419.
18. Kooner S, Kayum S, Pinsker EB, et al. Two-year outcomes after total ankle replacement with a novel fixed-bearing implant. *Foot Ankle Int.* 2021;42(8):1002-1010.
19. Fram B, Corr DO, Rogero RG, Pedowitz DI, Tsai J. Short-term complications and outcomes of the cadence total ankle arthroplasty. *Foot Ankle Int.* 2022;43(3):371-377.
20. Kim J, Rajan L, Bitar R, et al. Early radiographic and clinical outcomes of a novel, fixed-bearing fourth-generation total ankle replacement system. *Foot Ankle Int.* 2022;43(11):1424-1433.

15 The Kinos Axiom Total Ankle System

Eitan M. Ingall and J. Kent Ellington

INTRODUCTION

The Kinos Axiom Total Ankle System is designed to preserve normal ankle joint kinematics. The trochlear surface of the normal talus is a skewed truncated conic saddle shape with an apex lateral orientation, facilitating triplanar motion through the normal gait cycle.[1,2] Biomechanical studies have also shown that the ankle does not have a fixed axis of rotation but rather is a sliding and rolling joint with the highest contact points moving from posterior to anterior as the foot moves from plantar to dorsiflexion.[3] Further cadaveric testing of 3D printed, customized surfaces designed to replicate this complex joint motion have shown promising mobility and stability behavior that closely mimic that of a normal ankle joint.[4-6] As such, the Axiom is designed to mimic these features of normal joint kinematics during gait (Fig. 15.1).

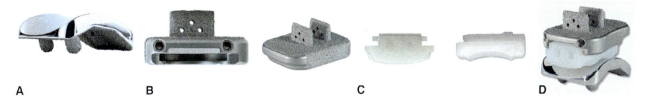

FIGURE 15.1 The talar (A), tibial (B), polyethylene bearing surface (C), and fully assembled (D) Kinos Axiom total ankle prosthesis.

INDICATIONS AND CONTRAINDICATIONS

The indications and contraindications for the Kinos Axiom Total Ankle System are the same as most other ankle arthroplasty systems. These generally include the following:

Indications

- The primary indication for total ankle arthroplasty is symptomatic, end-stage arthritis of the tibiotalar joint.
- Degenerative, rheumatic or other inflammatory arthritis, posttraumatic or postinfectious arthritis.

Contraindications

- Active infection/osteomyelitis
- Neuropathy
- Extensive cystic changes of the talus or evidence of avascular necrosis and/or collapse

PREOPERATIVE PLANNING

- Patients with end-stage ankle arthritis typically present with deep anterior ankle pain, worse with weight bearing, and may describe crepitus or other mechanical symptoms.
- Conservative measures including physical therapy and bracing should be undertaken prior to surgical management. Furthermore, corticosteroid injection to the ankle can be both diagnostic and therapeutic.
- Careful physical examination must be performed and include a detailed neurovascular examination to identify neuropathy or vascular pathology. Range of motion (ROM) at the ankle and subtalar joint should be carefully examined, and ankle stability should be assessed. Any concomitant deformities of the foot should also be noted.
- Weight-bearing three-view radiographs of the foot and the ankle should be obtained and evaluated for any deformity. The subtalar joint should be carefully evaluated for any evidence of arthrosis.
- We recommend that weight-bearing computed tomography (CT) scan of the foot ankle be performed, if available. A 3D rendering of this weight-bearing CT is then used to create a preoperative plan to template tibial and talar resection and determine implant rotation and sizing (Fig. 15.2). If weight-bearing CT is not available, the same preoperative plan can be developed from a standard CT image series. We routinely review this plan prior to surgery for guidance on our cut guide placement and amount of resection. Furthermore, in the operating room, this preoperative plan can be easily referenced to ensure proper placement of cut guides in situ.
- Beginning in 2023, this preoperative CT scan can also be used for the manufacturing of patient specific cut guides. A plan similar to the one shown in Figure 15.7 can be generated that allows the surgeon to use an additively manufactured titanium cut guide to plan bony resection. These cut guides are designed to perfectly mate with the bony landscape of the patient's distal tibia and talus, respectively, allowing for precise cuts without the use of an extramedullary guide.

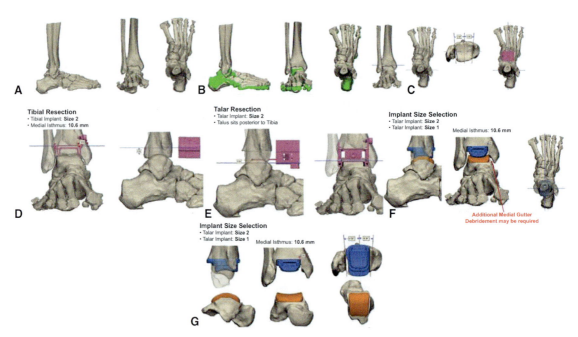

FIGURE 15.2 Kinos Axiom preoperative plan based upon 3D rendering of weight-bearing CT. **A, B.** The *green outline* demonstrates the new position of the foot and ankle after arthroplasty. **C.** Shows templated implant rotation. **D, E.** Templated tibial and talar resection and **(F, G)** show implant sizing.

SURGICAL TECHNIQUE

Positioning and Approach

- The patient is positioned supine on a radiolucent table with a thigh tourniquet applied to the operative extremity.
- The incision is planned just lateral to the tibial crest and in line with the second webspace.
- Incision is made through skin and subcutaneous tissue and the superficial peroneal nerve is identified, mobilized, and retracted laterally (Fig. 15.3).
- The extensor retinaculum is encountered, and the extensor hallucis longus (EHL) and tibialis anterior (TA) are identified. We prefer to incise the extensor retinaculum lateral to the TA, almost directly over the EHL so as to keep the TA tendon within its independent tendon sheath.
- The deep neurovascular bundle is isolated and retracted laterally. Crossing vessels are meticulously coagulated.
- Medial and lateral flaps are created in a periosteal sparing fashion so as to expose the gutters medially and laterally and the talonavicular (TN) joint distally. Many patients have a contracture of the TN joint with or without osteophyte formation. If present, we will release the TN capsule and débride any osteophytes in order to decompress the joint.
- Any large osteophytes are removed with a rongeur and osteotome (unless patient specific cutting guides are to be used, discussed below).

Alignment Guide Placement

- The tibial tubercle is identified and a pin is inserted into the tibia approximately in line with the second webspace.
- Assemble the guide for the appropriate foot (right/left) and place it onto the tubercle pin (Fig. 15.4).
- At this point, the guide should be placed in approximately the correct position, to be later microadjusted based on fluoroscopy. The tibial cut guide should be approximately one finger breadth proximal to the distal tibial plafond. The height is then locked at about two finger breadths off the crest. This puts the guide in an approximate position that can later be fine-tuned under fluoroscopy.
- The rotation shim is placed into the tibial cut guide and aligned with the second webspace. The rotation screw is then locked and a K-wire can be placed to further secure the guide.
- Once the jig is provisionally secured, fluoroscopic fine-tuning is performed (Fig. 15.5).

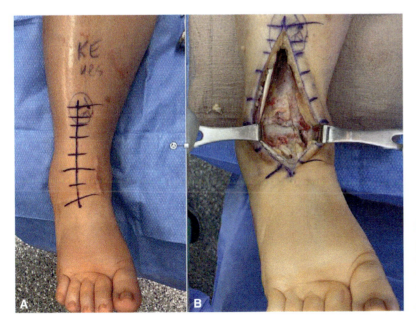

FIGURE 15.3 A. Direct anterior approach is planned. **B.** Completed surgical exposure with extensor hallucis longus retracted laterally and tibialis anterior still in its sheath retracted medially. The talonavicular joint is exposed at the distal aspect of the wound.

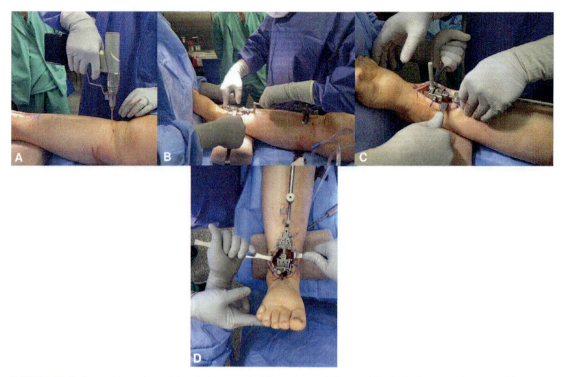

FIGURE 15.4 Assembly and provisional placement of the extramedullary guide. A pin is placed into the tibial tubercle **(A)**, the extramedullary guide is positioned **(B, C)**, and the rotation is grossly set to be in line with the second webspace **(D)**.

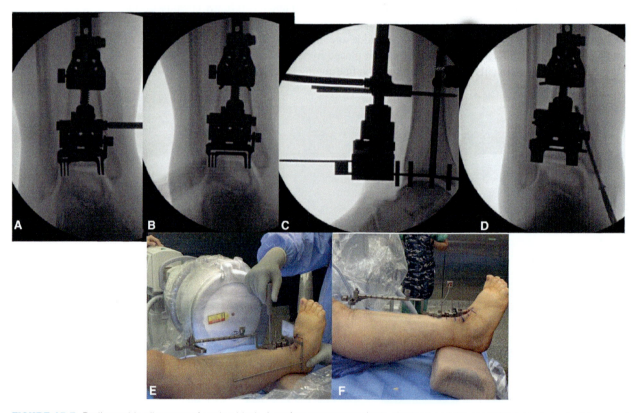

FIGURE 15.5 Radiographic alignment of cutting block. A perfect anteroposterior is obtained and the medial to lateral size is determined. In **(A)**, the jig is felt to be slightly too medial, with too much valgus. This is adjusted and confirmed to be in better position **(B)**. A perfect lateral is obtained with the angle wing in a "razor's edge" profile and can be adjusted as appropriate **(C, E)**. A prophylactic medial malleolar screw is routinely placed at this point **(D)**. The guide is secured with pins once final position is confirmed **(F)**.

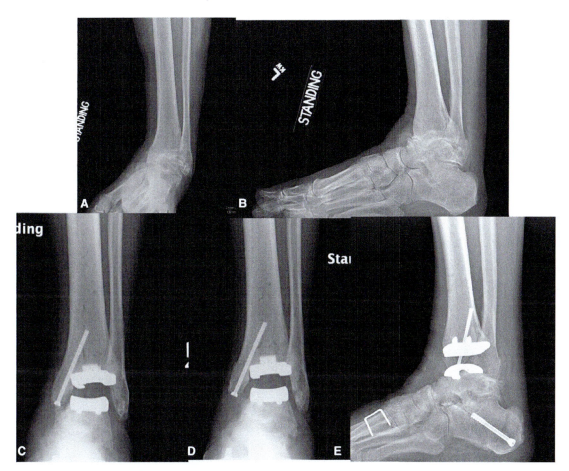

FIGURE 15.6 Preoperative standing ankle radiographs of a severe varus ankle arthritis in a 62-year-old male **(A, B)**. He underwent a single stage total ankle arthroplasty with adjunctive foot procedures including a dorsiflexion first ray, Dwyer osteotomies, medial release, and Brostrom lateral ligament repair. Three-month weight-bearing anteroposterior, oblique, and lateral radiographs are pictured **(C-E)**.

- A perfect anteroposterior radiograph is obtained, and the medial to lateral implant size is determined. The medial to lateral position is adjusted so that the medial cut exits into the medial gutter and the lateral cut does not extend into the incisura.
- A true lateral radiograph is obtained with the angel wing in place. It is critical to obtain a "razor's edge" profile of the angel wing to evaluate templated cut. The tibial cut will be at the proximal aspect of the bars and the talar cut will be at the distal end of the bars. The Axiom is designed for an 8-mm bony resection off the tibia. As mentioned previously, this is around one finger breadth above the plafond.
- The slope of the cut can be adjusted. It should be noted that the tibial plafond declinates at a 7° to 9° angle from anterior to posterior (ie, the tibial lateral surface angle)[7] to facilitate ankle dorsiflexion. It is the authors' preference to plan the cut with this anatomic feature in mind.
- One study suggested that a narrow medial malleolus may increase the risk for fracture and/or medial sided pain postoperatively.[8] Due to its anatomic design, Axiom tibial cuts often leave the medial malleolus at 10 to 11 mm or slightly narrower. We, therefore, frequently place a prophylactic screw. We place the screw slightly more medial and more vertical than we would for a medial malleolar fracture so as to not interfere with later implant placement.
- For patients with varus or valgus arthritis (Fig. 15.6), the cuts can be planned to correct significant deformity. Adjunctive foot realignment procedures (calcaneal osteotomy, plantar/dorsiflexion osteotomies of the first ray, etc.) may also be necessary.
- *Custom implants and patient-specific resection guides:* In patients with unusual talar or tibial plafond morphology, custom implants can be made along with patient-specific resection guides (Figs. 15.7 and 15.8). Patient-specific resection guides can also be used with standard implants. The Axiom patient-specific cut guides are additively manufactured to match the specific anatomy

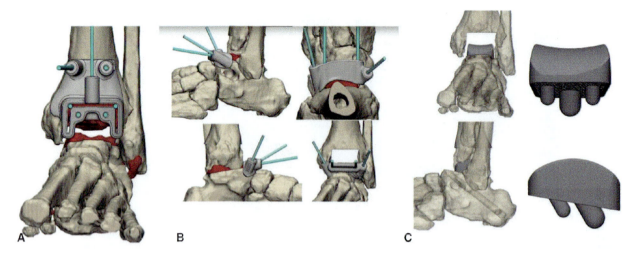

FIGURE 15.7 An example of a preoperative plan using patient-specific instrumentation and a custom implant. A plan for placement of the tibial guide **(A)** and talus guide **(B)** is shown. In this case, a custom implant was used **(C)** due to the unusual talar morphology in this patient. Small, medium, and large implants are provided for the surgeon to choose from at the time of surgery.

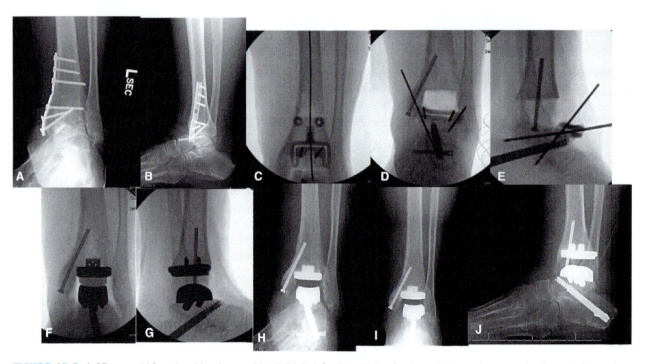

FIGURE 15.8 A 67-year-old female with prior combined tibial plafond and talus fracture status post open reduction and internal fixation who went on to develop tibiotalar and subtalar arthritis with partial talar collapse **(A, B)**. Her preoperative plan was shown in Figure 15.7. Because of the morphology of her talus, a custom implant was designed and printed. Intraoperatively, patient-specific cut guides were used to make the tibial and talar cuts, respectively **(C-E)**. A custom talus was implanted **(F, G)**. Two-month weight-bearing radiographs are shown **(H-J)**.

15 The Kinos Axiom Total Ankle System

of the patients' tibial plafond and talus. The cut guides are 3D printed in titanium alloy instead of plastic to facilitate easy on-lay onto the topography of the bone in situ. These patient-specific resection guides are available for noncustom cases as well.

Tibial and Talar Cuts

- The horizontal tibial cut is made with an oscillating saw, and the tibial cut is made with a reciprocating saw. The corner chisel is then used to complete the tibial cut.
- The cut tibia is removed en bloc with a removal screw.
- With the foot dorsiflexed to neutral, the standard or flat top talar guide is placed into the manifold. The gear is then extended until it rests just on top of the talus (see Fig. 15.8E). The angel wing is again used to template the talar cut. The Axiom system is designed to preserve as much talus bone as possible. The standard cut removes 3.5 mm of bone and the flat top cut removes 8.5 mm of bone.
- The talar cut is made with an oscillating saw, and the cut talus is removed.
- Adequate bony resection is confirmed with a gap sizing tool (15 mm) to ensure that the minimum necessary bone is removed in order to fit the final implants. If it is too tight, it is recommended that a second cut is made to take more bone (Fig. 15.9).

Tibial and Talar Sizing, Final Bony Preparation

- Once the cut bone is removed, the alignment guide is removed and the tibial pin site closed with a 2-0 monocryl suture.
- Figures 15.10 and 15.11 describe the step by step clinical and radiographic, respectively, trialing and final bony preparation.
- On the tibial side, the screw can be adjusted to make micro adjustments in the plafond slope.
- The back of the trial corresponds to the "long" tibial tray, and the notch corresponds to the standard size.

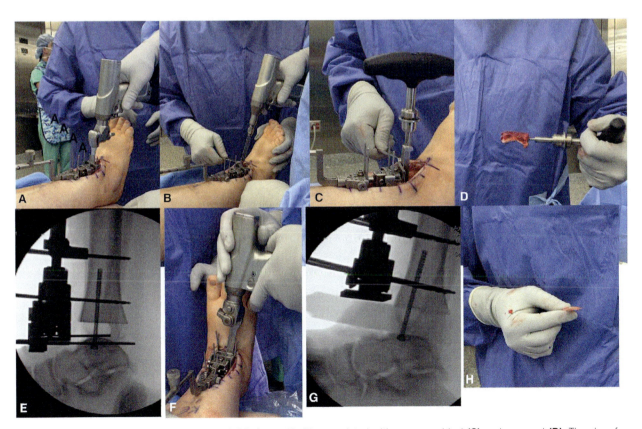

FIGURE 15.9 Tibial and talar cuts. The distal tibia is cut **(A, B)**, completed with a corner chisel **(C)** and removed **(D)**. The chamfer talar cut is then planned on the lateral view **(E)**, cut **(F, G)**, and removed **(H)**.

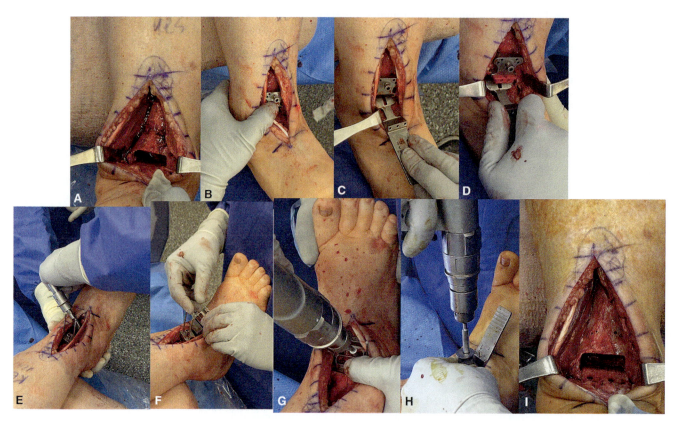

FIGURE 15.10 Tibial and talar sizing and final preparation. The tibial and talar sizing guides are placed into the ankle **(A-C)** and sizing is confirmed on fluoroscopy. These are pinned in place. A trial poly is inserted **(D)**. Once sizing is deemed satisfactory, the plafond is broached for the tibial component fin **(E)**. The talus rail and peg guide is placed **(F)**, chamfer cuts are made **(G)**, and the rail drill guide is placed **(H)**. **I.** Final cuts in situ.

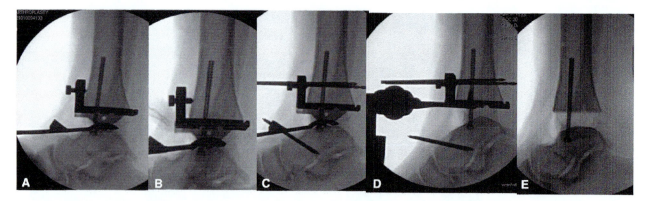

FIGURE 15.11 Confirmation of tibial and talar sizing under fluoroscopy. The tibial sizing guide is placed and felt to be too posterior **(A)**, so the screw is adjusted to bring the tibial trial more anterior **(B)**. The talar chamfer cut guide is introduced **(C)** and pinned in place. The chamfer cuts will be at the level of the clear space in the guide. The chamfer guide is removed and the broach is introduced to broach the fins for the tibial component **(D)**. Final cuts are evaluated **(E)**.

15 The Kinos Axiom Total Ankle System

- The talus can be prepared with chamfer cut or flat top cut, as described earlier. The final preparation varies slightly, with the chamfer cut described in detail below.
- The chamfer cut guide should be placed directly in line with the lateral process of the talus on lateral fluoroscopy.
- The Axiom system has no limitation on pairing the size of the tibia with the size of the talus. In other words, any size tibia can be paired with any size talus (ie, a size 4 tibia with a size 1 talus), to best match the patients' anatomy. This prevents issues with tibial-talar component mismatch that leads to overhang into the gutters or undercoverage of the cut talus surface.

Final Implant Insertion

- The Axiom total ankle can be cemented on both the tibial and talar components. We often use cement, particularly in the cases of osteoporotic bone or significant cystic changes. We also will often add bone marrow aspirate in both cemented and press-fit implants as shown in Figure 15.12A. The goal of this is to improve the biologic environment of the bone-implant surface to promote ingrowth.
- The tibial component is inserted into the wound and the fins are placed into the previously broached slots. The tibial tray can be aligned into position with use of a retractor as shown in Figure 15.12C and is then impacted into its final position. A smooth lamina spreader can aid in final seating of the implant, taking care not to damage the talus.
- The talar component is then placed and impacted and the polyethylene liner is placed and final position and ROM is evaluated (Fig. 15.13).

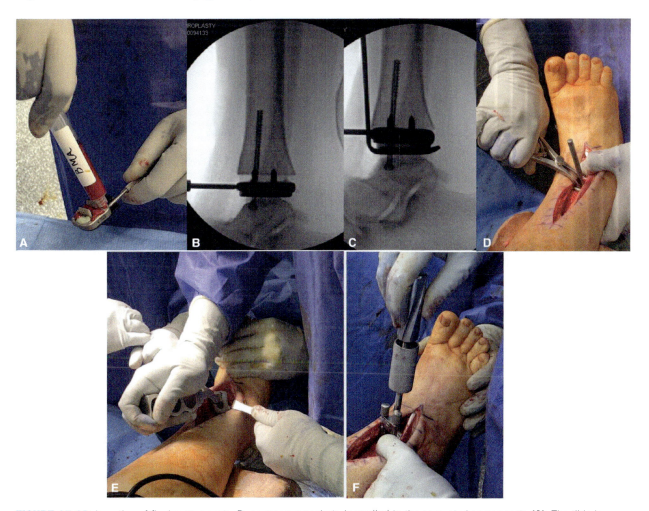

FIGURE 15.12 Insertion of final components. Bone marrow aspirate is applied to the cemented components **(A)**. The tibia is seated first and aligned **(B-D)**. The talus is then placed and impacted into final position **(E)**. Finally, the polyethylene is seated using the inserter **(F)**.

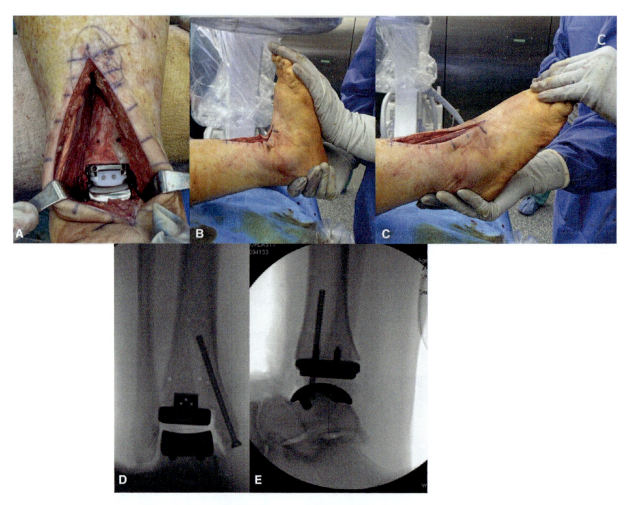

FIGURE 15.13 Final implants in situ **(A)** and demonstration of range of motion **(B, C)**. Final anteroposterior **(D)** and lateral **(E)** fluoroscopy.

POSTOPERATIVE PROTOCOL

- Patients are placed in a well-padded AO splint and instructed to remain non–weight bearing.
- At 2 weeks, sutures are removed if deemed appropriate, patient is transitioned to a boot, and ROM is encouraged.
- Full weight bearing is permitted at 4 weeks.
- Physical therapy is initiated at 2 to 3 weeks and continued for a total of 10 to 12 weeks to assist with ROM, gait mechanics, and edema control.

DISCUSSION: DESIGN RATIONALE AND IMPLANT FEATURES

As mentioned in the introduction, the Kinos Axiom Total Ankle System is designed to closely mimic natural triplanar joint kinematics. Early biomechanical literature described the ankle joint as a cylindrical hinge,[9,10] and many current prosthetic designs mimic this anatomy. All other widely used total ankle replacement (TAR) devices were designed with articulating surfaces shaped as either a cylinder or a truncated cone with its apex oriented medially. These designs followed morphological concepts established several decades ago and have been. Consequently, they afford limited side-to-side and rotational motion of the ankle. In contrast to this prior anatomical understanding, recent studies using CT imaging and 3D computer modeling have shown that that the surfaces of the tibiotalar joint resemble a truncated saddle-shaped cone with its apex oriented laterally. This new understanding of ankle morphology led to the development of a TAR device that attempts to mimic plafond anatomy and intends to restore more normal ankle kinematics and ROM. One study directly compared ankle and foot movements of 10 cadaveric, intact ankles to (1) those of 3D printed copies of the natural articulating surfaces and to (2) a 3D printed Axiom type saddle-shaped truncated cone with apex lateral orientation.[4] Their results demonstrated that the Axiom TAR kinematics very closely approximate that of the natural ankle joint.

This Axiom talar implant is made of cobalt chromium alloy, has left and right specific implants, and is available in five sizes. As mentioned above, newer studies suggest that the dorsal surface of the talus functions as a laterally based cone. The shape of the Axiom talar dome is a hyperbolic paraboloid that follows this morphology. This facilitates flexion/extension coupled with internal external rotation and independent inversion/eversion. As a result, there is broad, stable contact throughout gait, maintaining contact over larger ROM. This minimizes lift off, point loading, and edge loading.

The tibial component is made of titanium alloy. It is available in long and standard lengths and is anatomically contoured for left and right tibias, respectively. The tibial component is unique in that there are two fins aligned perpendicular to the plane of motion. Tibial loosening has been a long-standing and well-documented problem in total ankle arthroplasty. The vertical buttresses are designed to maximally resist clinical loading. Stemmed tibial implant designs are underway and will be available soon.

The surface of the Axiom tibial and talar components is a proprietary porous surface architecture designed for maximal osseointegration (TIDAL Technology). It is a 3D-printed synthetic porous biomaterial.[11] Multiple preclinical small and large animal model studies have suggested a very high strength and fatigue resistance compared with other surface architectures. These studies have shown TIDAL implants approach the shear strength of intact bone.[12,13] Finally, the polyethylene bearing is a biomechanically accurate articulating surface with left and right specific implants. It is made of vitamin E treated highly cross-linked polyethylene. It is available in heights from 6 to 12 mm, with larger options soon available up to 20 mm.

To date, there are no published clinical outcomes studies on the Axiom TAR. The implant is just reaching 2-year clinical follow-up (end of 2022), and a rigorous data collection effort on clinical and radiographs outcomes is underway. Reports on short- and mid-term outcomes will soon follow.

REFERENCES

1. Siegler S, Chen J, Schneck CD. The three-dimensional kinematics and flexibility characteristics of the human ankle and subtalar joints—part 1: kinematics. *J Biomech Eng.* 1988;110:364-373.
2. Siegler S, Toy J, Seale D, Pedowitz D. The clinical biomechanics award 2013—presented by the international society of biomechanics: new observations on the morphology of the talar dome and its relationship to ankle kinematics. *Clin Biomech.* 2014;29(1):1-6.
3. Siegler S, Konow T, Belvedere C, Ensini A, Kulkarni R, Leardini A. Analysis of surface-to-surface distance mapping during three-dimensional motion at the ankle and subtalar joints. *J. Biomech.* 2018;76:204-211.
4. Belvedere C, Siegler S, Ensini A, et al. Experimental evaluation of a new morphological approximation of the articular surfaces of the ankle joint. *J Biomech.* 2017;53:97-104.
5. Siegler S, Belvedere C, Ensini A, et al. Effect of variation in ankle morphology on replaced joint kinematics and load transfer. *Foot Ankle Surg.* 2016;22(2):54.
6. Belvedere C, Siegler S, Ensini A, et al. Experimental evaluation of current and novel approximations of articular surfaces of the ankle joint. *J. Biomech.* 2018;75:159-163.
7. Guo C, Zhu Y, Hu M, Deng L, Xu X. Reliability of measurements on lateral ankle radiographs. *BMC Musculoskelet Disord.* 2016;17(1):1-8.
8. Lundeen GA, Dunaway LJ. Etiology and treatment of delayed-onset medial malleolar pain following total ankle arthroplasty. *Foot Ankle Int.* 2016;37(8):822-828.
9. Inman VT. *The Joints of the Ankle.* The Williams and Wilkins Co; 1976.
10. Scott SH, Winter DA. Talocrural and talocalcaneal joint kinematics and kinetics during the stance phase of walking. *J Biomech.* 1991;24(8):743-752.
11. Kelly CN, Miller AT, Hollister SJ, Guldberg RE, Gall K. Design and structure–function characterization of 3D printed synthetic porous biomaterials for tissue engineering. *Adv Healthc Mater.* 2018;7(7):1-16.
12. Mcgilvray KC, Easley J, Seim HB, et al. Bony ingrowth potential of 3D-printed porous titanium alloy: a direct comparison of interbody cage materials in an in vivo ovine lumbar fusion model. *Spine J.* 2019;18(7):1250-1260.
13. Kelly CN, Francovich J, Julmi S, et al. Fatigue behavior of As-built selective laser melted titanium scaffolds with sheet-based gyroid microarchitecture for bone tissue engineering. *Acta Biomater.* 2019;94:610-626.

PART FOUR
SPORTS

16 Hamstring Peroneals

Mark Drakos

INTRODUCTION

Peroneal tendon disorders comprise a significant proportion of lateral ankle injuries and are often associated with chronic ankle pain, ankle instability, or preexisting anatomical abnormalities such as cavovarus foot type. Although the incidence of peroneal tendon injuries in the general population remains unknown, peroneal tendon pathology was observed in 23% to 77% of patients with lateral ankle instability.[1] Moreover, cadaveric studies suggest a prevalence of 11% to 37% in specimens with longitudinal split tears or attritional tears to the peroneus brevis[2] and a 2016 retrospective magnetic resonance imaging (MRI) study observed peroneal pathology in 35% of asymptomatic cases.[2] While more common than typically realized, peroneal tendon injuries represent a misunderstood and overlooked source of chronic lateral ankle pain and instability. Similarities in clinical presentation and the vague nature of pain following ankle trauma contribute to a large percentage of peroneal tendon injuries, more specifically tendon tears, being misdiagnosed as lateral ligamentous injuries.[3,4] Furthermore, most peroneal tendon pathology exists within the spectrum of tendinopathy and represents degenerative changes rather than acute ruptures. Clinicians, therefore, must carefully consider patients with lateral ankle injuries or with a history of lateral ankle pain, as pain and disability can persist without proper diagnosis and treatment.

The peroneal muscles form the peroneus longus and peroneus brevis tendons in the distal two-thirds of the fibula. The peroneus longus and brevis provide active and passive ankle stabilization predominantly in the eversion and plantarflexion motion.[5,6] The peroneus brevis originates 2 to 3 cm proximal to the tip of the fibula and courses distally down the posterior lateral malleolus toward its insertion on the fifth metatarsal base. Around 4 cm proximal to the lateral malleolus, the peroneus brevis is observed anterior and medial to the peroneus longus, both secured in a protective synovial sheath.[7] The tendons are stabilized within the sheath by a fibro osseous tunnel formed by the retromalleolar groove within the fibula anteriorly, the superior peroneal retinaculum posterolaterally, and the calcaneofibular and posterior talofibular ligaments medially.[7,8] The superior peroneal retinaculum, in particular, is crucial in maintaining tendon stability within the retromalleolar groove and has been considered the most important factor in preventing tendon subluxation or dislocation.[8]

While there is no standard of treatment for peroneus brevis tendon tears, current treatment options include conservative treatment, peroneal tendoscopy,[9] débridement and tubularization of the remaining tendon, tenodesis,[10,11] transfer of the flexor hallucis longus (FHL) or flexor digitorum longus (FDL) tendons,[12] and reconstruction with an autograft or allograft.[13] Since nonoperative treatment has been shown to produce poor clinical outcomes with a failure rate of up to 83% for chronic tears, surgical intervention is advised for most patients with symptomatic peroneal pathology.[14] Tenodesis of the brevis to the longus has traditionally been performed for severe tears, but Pellegrini et al recently demonstrated this procedure to be biomechanically ineffective in restoring tendon tension while also sacrificing the integrity of the muscle-tendon unit.[15] Transfer of the FHL or FDL has also been advocated for but likewise has been associated with biomechanical limitations.

Peroneus brevis reconstruction using a semitendinosus allograft has shown to produce good clinical and patient outcomes.[16] Furthermore, Pellegrini et al found that the measured tension following allograft reconstruction significantly exceeded that of tenodesis under all tested loading conditions ($p < .022$).[15] However, concerns over the high cost and availability of the graft, the potential for disease transmission, delayed incorporation and stretching of the graft, the risk of potential immune response, and long-term graft strength question the viability of such a procedure.[24,25] In light of these shortcomings, we instead recommend a reconstruction using a hamstring autograft to treat a severe peroneus brevis tear. This article will describe our indications for surgery, demonstrate the steps of hamstring tendon harvest in the supine position, and illustrate the operative technique to reconstruct the peroneus brevis.

INDICATIONS AND CONTRAINDICATIONS

Patients presenting with persistent ankle pain, instability, and decreased function are indicated for surgical management. Traditionally, operative treatment for peroneal tendon tears has been based on a 50% cross-sectional area threshold of the native tendon; autograft reconstruction is indicated when less than 50% of the native tendon's cross-sectional area remains after débridement and excision or if the native tendon is beyond repair.[16] Contraindications include severe peripheral vascular disease, fatty infiltration, and fibrosis of the peroneus brevis.

PREOPERATIVE PLANNING

Several factors should be considered when developing an operative strategy for a peroneus brevis reconstruction with hamstring autograft. A thorough analysis of patient history, clinical examination, and radiographic evaluation should first be conducted for each patient. Patients should also be evaluated for symptoms and risk factors of chronic conditions such as lateral ankle instability, cavovarus malalignment, low-lying peroneus brevis muscle belly, and a peroneus quartus tendon. Malalignment can be identified using weight-bearing anteroposterior and lateral radiographs as well as the hindfoot alignment view to assess varus heel alignment. Stress radiographs of the ankle and anterior drawer tests should also be performed to rule out concomitant lateral ankle instability. Additionally, MRI and ultrasound are important to determine the extent of the tear and the presence of any other pathology that may necessitate the need for concomitant procedures such as lateral ligament reconstruction, peroneus brevis low-lying muscle belly resection, peroneus quartus tendon resection, lateral sliding calcaneal osteotomy for cavovarus, and ankle arthroscopy to address intra-articular pathology. We do not routinely use arthroscopy unless indicated preoperatively based on MRI findings. Moreover, the addition of concomitant procedures depends on the degree of deformity as well as rigidity. These preoperative findings should then be confirmed with direct visualization at the time of surgery. Once the patient is deemed an appropriate candidate for autograft reconstruction, the surgeon must decide which approach to take regarding incision placement and tendon harvest.

In our opinion, the historical débridement, tubularization, and repair procedures can have satisfactory outcomes. However, many patients will still have pain due to the persistent presence of underlying tendinopathy. Therefore, when split tears are present within the setting of tendinopathy as evidenced by MRI or visual and tactile evaluation of the tendon, we have chosen to use autograft reconstruction with gracilis as our procedure of choice.[17] If it is an acute tear associated with a dislocation, we will simply do a débridement and repair as these are often in young people and without any underlying tendinopathy. In the setting of a cavovarus, we will often incorporate a longus to brevis tendon transfer to minimize some of the deforming forces.

SURGICAL TECHNIQUE

First, the hamstring graft is harvested. The patient is placed in the supine position and a thigh tourniquet is applied. An oblique 3-cm longitudinal incision is made over the proximal medial tibia. A knife is used to dissect sharply through the skin and subcutaneous tissue, and then blunt dissection is carried out to the level of the sartorial fascia. The sartorial fascia is then incised in line with its fibers (Fig. 16.1). Both the gracilis and semitendinosus are visualized on the deep aspect of the sartorial fascia. Based on surgeon discretion, one or both tendons, in cases where one tendon alone was not feasible, are removed from all adhesins using a Metzenbaum scissor and harvested with a

16 Hamstring Peroneals

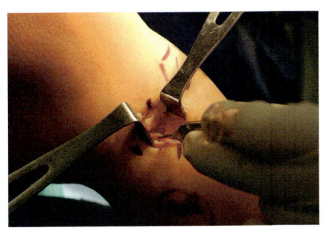

FIGURE 16.1 The incision of sartorial fascia in line with fibers is demonstrated.

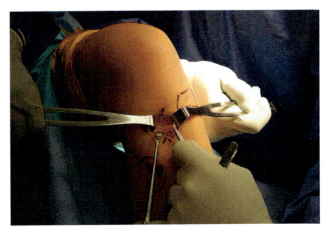

FIGURE 16.2 The gracilis hamstring tendon is harvested with a tendon stripper.

tendon stripper (Fig. 16.2). Once the tendon is harvested, it is stripped of all muscle adhesions with a large curette. The graft is then tubularized on a GRAFTMASTER with 2-0 Vicryl with two sutures coming out of each end (Fig. 16.3).

Once the hamstring graft is harvested, attention is turned to the ankle joint. An approximately 7-cm curvilinear incision is made over the course of the peroneal tendons (Fig. 16.4). Sharp dissection is carried through the peroneal retinaculum and is then incised both proximally and distally. Scar tissue and tenosynovium surrounding the peroneal tendons are removed and the tendons are

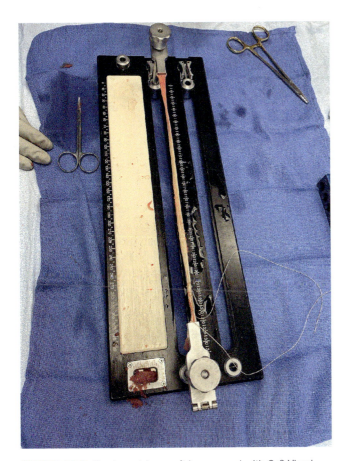

FIGURE 16.3 The hamstring graft is prepared with 2-0 Vicryl suture.

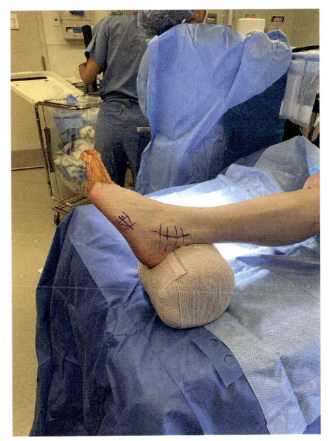

FIGURE 16.4 The curvilinear incision over the peroneal tendons as well as the additional incision over the fifth metatarsal base are prepared via a window technique incision.

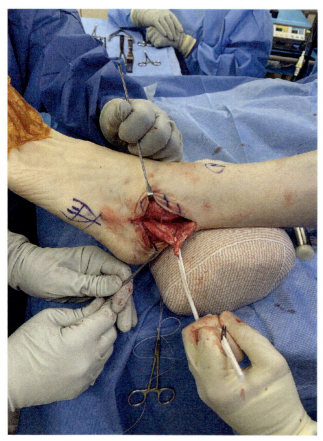

FIGURE 16.5 The torn peroneus brevis tendon is visualized after scar tissue and tenosynovium surrounding the peroneal tendons are removed.

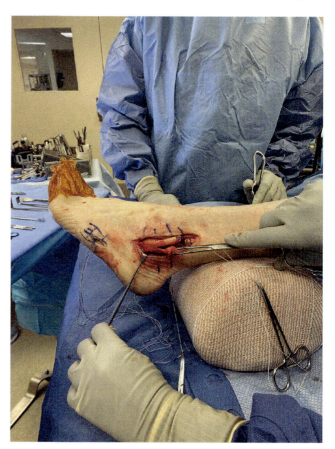

FIGURE 16.6 Example of resection of the brevis and longus in a case of significant tendinopathy.

then assessed and débrided (Fig. 16.5). Any diseased tissue is excised. In cases with significant tendinopathy, the whole peroneus brevis is resected. If the longus is involved, the diseased tendon is resected until only the healthy tendon remains (Figs. 16.6 and 16.7). A side to side tenodesis of longus to brevis is then completed proximally.

After the peroneal tendon is exposed, an anchor is placed in the fifth metatarsal base to secure the graft distally with fluoroscopic guidance (Fig. 16.8). If the metatarsal base is exposed after the incision over the peroneal tendons, the anchor can be placed onto the bone without any additional incisions. In cases where the metatarsal base is not exposed during the initial incision, a separate 3-cm incision can be made over the fifth metatarsal base to decrease the length of the incision when placing the anchor (Fig. 16.9). There should be a skin bridge between the incisions to avoid violating the sural nerve.

Once prepared, the graft is secured to the bone and proximally shuttled under the skin bridge within the peroneal retinaculum (Figs. 16.10 and 16.11). A Pulvertaft maneuver is performed to secure the graft to the distal stump of the native tendon, where it is then sutured in a figure-of-8 fashion with a #2 suture tape, doubled back, and tied onto the original anchor to create what is known as a "double-loaded anchor" (Figs. 16.12 through 16.14). The tension is set with the foot in slight eversion and dorsiflexion. The suture is performed 3 cm above the lateral malleolus to prevent any volume effect of increased pressure within the retromalleolar groove.[18] By doing this, the surgeon creates a double-bundle effect to achieve excellent tension and increase the width of the graft to model the dimensions of the native tendon. The graft is then tubularized and tensioned in dorsiflexion and slight eversion of the ankle (Fig. 16.15). Afterward, the peroneal retinaculum is repaired over the peroneal tendons, and the wounds were irrigated and closed (Fig. 16.16).

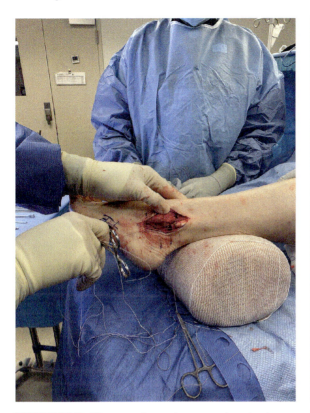

FIGURE 16.7 After resection, sutures are placed onto the distal stump of the remaining tendon in preparation of autograft insertion.

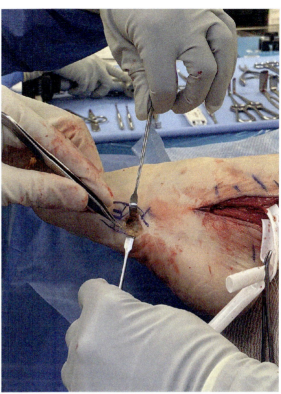

FIGURE 16.8 A 3-cm incision is made over fifth metatarsal base in preparation for anchor placement.

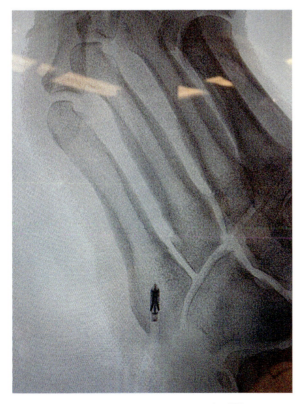

FIGURE 16.9 The anchor is placed onto the fifth metatarsal base. The skin bridge.

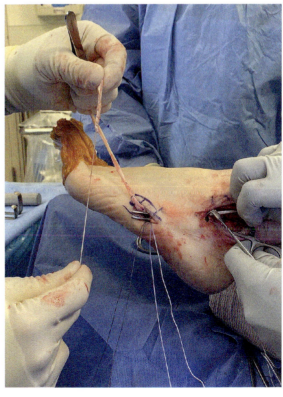

FIGURE 16.10 The gracilis graft is shown after being secured onto the fifth metatarsal base after suture anchor fixation.

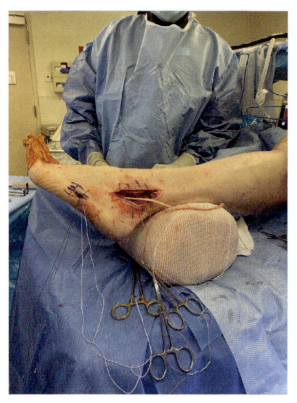

FIGURE 16.11 The graft is shuttled underneath skin bridge, thereby decreasing the incision length.

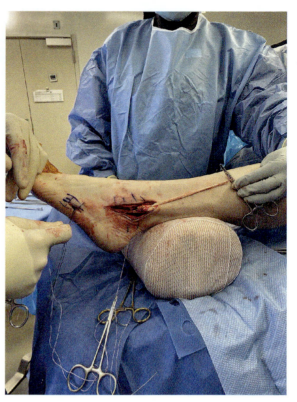

FIGURE 16.12 The graft is secured to the distal stump of the native tendon and tensioned using the Pulvertaft maneuver.

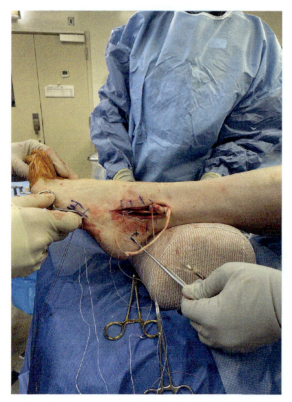

FIGURE 16.13 Any excess graft tendon is swung back down distally to create a double-bundle effect.

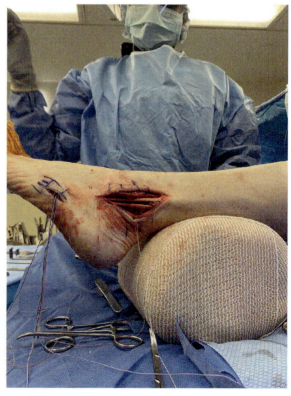

FIGURE 16.14 Distal bone to tendon fixation of excess graft onto fifth metatarsal via a second set of sutures, otherwise known as a "double-loaded anchor."

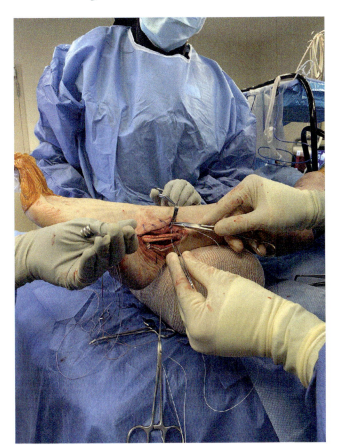

FIGURE 16.15 The final tubularization of hamstring graft is shown.

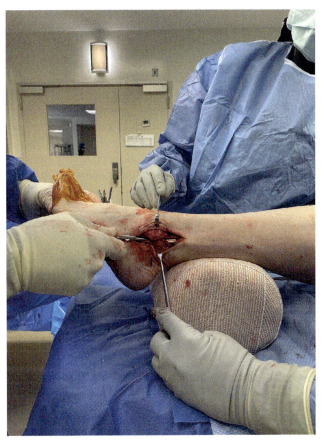

FIGURE 16.16 Repair of retinaculum over the peroneal tendon is shown.

POSTOPERATIVE MANAGEMENT

After the wounds are closed and the dressings are applied, the patient is placed in a splint with the foot in a neutral ankle position, where they remain non–weight bearing for 2 weeks. At 2 weeks postoperative, the patient is transitioned into a controlled ankle motion boot where they remain non–weight bearing for an additional 4 weeks but start both active and passive range of motion (ROM). At 6 weeks postoperative, the patient can begin weight bearing and physical therapy. At this point, the patient can begin dorsiflexion and plantarflexion exercises, as well as inversion and eversion exercises. At 10 to 12 weeks postoperative, they are transitioned into an ankle stabilizing orthosis brace that they slowly progress out of for up to 6 months postoperative. According to Kumar et al, 3 months following this procedure, patients were able to resume pain-free physical activity in both the foot and donor site and return to sports by 5 to 6 months postoperative.[19] With adequate recovery and physical therapy, many patients can return to sports and activities within 6 months.

RESULTS AND COMPLICATIONS

Complications of this procedure include postoperative wound infection, sural nerve damage, graft failure, and failure of graft incorporation. We believe the potential risk for donor site morbidity associated with autografts to be outweighed by their biological superiority to allogenic tissue in terms of its better healing potential and faster reincorporation.[18-20] The graft can also be undertensioned, leading to decreased strength and excursion. Thus, careful attention must be paid to not under or overtension the graft as both may result in poorer outcomes. Due to the excursion of the native peroneal tendon and musculature, we again recommend tensioning in dorsiflexion and 5° to 10° of eversion. Postoperatively, the more common phenomenon is stretching out of the repair rather than stiffness due to over-restraint. Wound complications and damage to the saphenous nerve can occur at the donor site and lead to numbness in the area of the skin surrounding the knee.[21] While there are few studies on the use of hamstring autografts for the treatment of irreparable peroneal tendon ruptures, those that do show relatively low complication rates.[3,21,22] Chrea et al reported complications in 3 out of 31 patients who underwent reconstruction. One out of the three was involved in a postoperative motor vehicle accident that required reoperation and another presented with a history of chronic peroneal and lateral ligament pathology. Nishikawa et al described a case report of three patients who underwent peroneal tendon reconstruction with a semitendinosus autograft.[18] The authors reported no complications along with no ankle inversion or eversion strength deficits at 6 months postoperatively based on isokinetic strength testing results. Regarding complications at the harvest site, Cody et al performed a study of 37 patients who underwent hamstring harvest for a variety of different foot and ankle procedures.[23] In their study, 32 patients (86%) reported no pain at the site of the hamstring harvest while the remaining 5 patients (14%) reported mild to moderate pain symptoms. Furthermore, patient strength at an average of 38 months postoperatively was evaluated with isokinetic strength testing and was found to have minimal strength deficits in the involved knee.

Published outcomes of peroneal tendon reconstruction with a hamstring autograft are likewise positive. Chrea et al reported that patients demonstrated pre- to postoperative improvement in every Patient Reported Outcomes Measurement Information Score domain evaluated, with significant improvement in physical function, pain interference, pain intensity, and global physical health. As a general rule, if there is good muscle excursion and contraction, re-establishing the connection to the insertion with a normal tendon has a very successful impact on pain and a significant improvement on eversion strength.

PEARLS AND PITFALLS

Pearls

- Gracilis tendon autograft is preferred in situations where one hamstring tendon is needed, as it has minimal to no effect on the functional/strength capacity of the hamstring.
- Examining the peroneal tendon first before autograft can lead to a better diagnosis of which/how many hamstring tendons should be used for autograft.
- Early ROM to avoid scarring.
- Using a skin bridge to avoid wound problems and sural nerve injury.

Pitfalls

- Carefully diagnose between lateral ligamentous injury and peroneus brevis tear.
- Infection.
- Sural nerve injury.
- Scar of the tendon reconstruction which would prevent healing.
- Undertension.
- Overtension.

ACKNOWLEDGMENTS

We gratefully acknowledge the contributions of Mr. David Cho and Ms. Saanchi Kukadia for their work on this chapter.

REFERENCES

1. DiGiovanni BF, Fraga CJ, Cohen BE, Shereff MJ. Associated injuries found in chronic lateral ankle instability. *Foot Ankle Int.* 2000;21(10):809-815.
2. O'Neil JT, Pedowitz DI, Kerbel YE, Codding JL, Zoga AC, Raikin SM. Peroneal tendon abnormalities on routine magnetic resonance imaging of the foot and ankle. *Foot Ankle Int.* 2016;37(7):743-747.
3. Chrea B, Eble SK, Day J, et al. Clinical and patient-reported outcomes following peroneus brevis reconstruction with hamstring tendon autograft. *Foot Ankle Int.* 2021;42(11):1391-1398.
4. Dombek MF, Lamm BM, Saltrick K, Mendicino RW, Catanzariti AR. Peroneal tendon tears: a retrospective review. *J Foot Ankle Surg.* 2003;42(5):250-258.
5. Konradsen L, Voigt M, Højsgaard C. Ankle inversion injuries. The role of the dynamic defense mechanism. *Am J Sports Med.* 1997;25(1):54-58.

6. Ziai P, Benca E, von Skrbensky G, et al. The role of the peroneal tendons in passive stabilisation of the ankle joint: an in vitro study. *Knee Surg Sports Traumatol Arthrosc.* 2013;21(6):1404-1408.
7. Davda K, Malhotra K, O'Donnell P, Singh D, Cullen N. Peroneal tendon disorders. *EFORT Open Rev.* 2017;2(6): 281-292.
8. van Dijk PAD, Kerkhoffs GMMJ, Chiodo C, DiGiovanni CW. Chronic disorders of the peroneal tendons: current concepts review of the literature. *J Am Acad Orthop Surg.* 2019;27(16):590-598.
9. Bojanić I, Dimnjaković D, Bohaček I, Smoljanović T. Peroneal tendoscopy—more than just a solitary procedure: case-series. *Croat Med J.* 2015;56(1):57-62.
10. Heckman DS, Reddy S, Pedowitz D, Wapner KL, Parekh SG. Operative treatment for peroneal tendon disorders. *J Bone Joint Surg Am.* 2008;90(2):404-418. https://journals.lww.com/jbjsjournal/Fulltext/2008/02000/Operative_Treatment_for_Peroneal_Tendon_Disorders.28.aspx
11. Demetracopoulos CA, Vineyard JC, Kiesau CD, Nunley JA. Long-term results of debridement and primary repair of peroneal tendon tears. *Foot Ankle Int.* 2013;35(3):252-257.
12. Seybold JD, Campbell JT, Jeng CL, Short KW, Myerson MS. Outcome of lateral transfer of the FHL or FDL for concomitant peroneal tendon tears. *Foot Ankle Int.* 2016;37(6):576-581.
13. Nishikawa DRC, Duarte FA, de Cesar Netto C, Monteiro AC, Albino RB, Fonseca FCP. Internal fixation of displaced intra-articular fractures of the hallux through a dorsomedial approach: a technical tip. *Foot Ankle Spec.* 2018;11(1):77-81.
14. Krause JO, Brodsky JW. Peroneus brevis tendon tears: pathophysiology, surgical reconstruction, and clinical results. *Foot Ankle Int.* 1998;19(5):271-279.
15. Pellegrini MJ, Glisson RR, Matsumoto T, et al. Effectiveness of allograft reconstruction vs tenodesis for irreparable peroneus brevis tears: a cadaveric model. *Foot Ankle Int.* 2016;37(8):803-808.
16. Redfern D, Myerson M. The management of concomitant tears of the peroneus longus and brevis tendons. *Foot Ankle Int.* 2004;25(10):695-707.
17. Rider CM, Hansen OB, Drakos MC. Hamstring autograft applications for treatment of achilles tendon pathology. *Foot Ankle Orthop.* 2021;6(1):2473011421993458.
18. Nishikawa DRC, Duarte FA, Saito GH, et al. Reconstruction of the peroneus brevis tendon tears with semitendinosus tendon autograft. Mayr J, ed. *Case Rep Orthop.* 2019;2019:5014687.
19. Kumar G, Simon R, Jose DP, Ravi S, Punnoose DJ. Repair of peroneus brevis tear with autologous gracilis: a case report. *J Foot Ankle Surg Asia Pac.* 2021;9(1):25-29.
20. Eble SK, Hansen OB, Patel K, Drakos MC. Lateral ligament reconstruction with hamstring graft for ankle instability: outcomes for primary and revision cases. *Am J Sports Med.* 2021;49(10):2697-2706.
21. Ellis SJ, Rosenbaum AJ. Hamstring autograft reconstruction of the peroneus brevis. *Tech Foot Ankle Surg.* 2018;17(1): 3-7.
22. Mook WR, Parekh SG, Nunley JA. Allograft reconstruction of peroneal tendons: operative technique and clinical outcomes. *Foot Ankle Int.* 2013;34(9):1212-1220.
23. Cody EA, Karnovsky SC, DeSandis B, Tychanski Papson A, Deland JT, Drakos MC. Hamstring autograft for foot and ankle applications. *Foot Ankle Int.* 2017;39(2):189-195.

17 Lateral Ankle Ligament Repair and Reconstruction

L. Daniel Latt

INDICATIONS AND CONTRAINDICATIONS

History: Recurrent Ankle Sprains

Lateral ankle sprains are one of the most common musculoskeletal injuries in both athletes and nonathletic individuals. The vast majority of ankle sprains will heal without sequelae; thus, most patients who suffer an ankle sprain should be treated with a short period of immobilization followed by bracing and physical therapy. A patient whose symptoms have not resolved despite 3 months of nonoperative treatment after an initial ankle sprain or who has had recurrent ankle sprains should undergo a workup and be considered a possible candidate for operative intervention.

Mechanical Instability

Mechanical instability or laxity is present when the lateral ankle ligaments (LALs) do not provide adequate constraint to the relative motion between the fibula and the talus. Laxity can be the result of either chronically torn, attenuated, or healed but elongated LALs. The anterior talofibular ligament (ATFL) is the most commonly torn, followed by the calcaneofibular ligament (CFL) (Fig. 17.1).

Functional Instability and Pain

Functional instability is present when the patient reports the feeling of giving way of the ankle during activities of daily living or athletic pursuits. Instability symptoms can be the result of insufficient active or passive restraints to ankle motion. While the majority of patients with chronic LAL injuries report instability symptoms, there is a small percentage that report only pain without instability. Despite the lack of laxity or instability, it is the author's experience that these patients still benefit from LAL repair or reconstruction.

Contraindications

Lateral ankle ligament repair or reconstruction is contraindicated in patients with chronic infection or poorly controlled diabetes. It is relatively contraindicated in patients with hindfoot arthritis or hindfoot malalignment unless these conditions are treated concomitantly or in a staged fashion.

PREOPERATIVE PLANNING

Physical Examination

A focused physical examination is important to confirm the diagnosis, rule out other causes of the symptoms, and determine if any of the commonly associated conditions are present. The

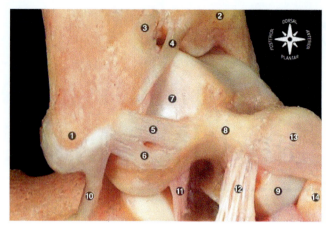

FIGURE 17.1 The anterior talofibular ligament consists of a superior and an inferior band that originate from the center of the anterior face of the distal fibula and insert on the lateral process of the talus at the junction of the dome and neck (5 and 6). The calcaneofibular ligament originated distally on the anterior face of the distal fibula and inserts on the calcaneus just proximal to the peroneal tubercle (10). (Reprinted with permission from Springer: Golanó P, Vega J, de Leeuw PA, et al. Anatomy of the ankle ligaments: a pictorial essay. *Knee Surg Sports Traumatol Arthrosc,* 2010;18(5):557-5369.)

physical examination should include inspection for swelling or prominence of the lateral malleolus as well as the determination of standing alignment. Varus malalignment is strongly associated with chronic ankle instability (CAI) as the lateral ligaments are constantly resisting the external rotation moment created by the hindfoot varus. The peek-a-boo heel (the ability to see the medial aspect of the heel when viewing the foot from directly anterior) is a reliable sign of subtle hindfoot varus. Palpation is used to determine the precise location of the symptoms in relation to the distal fibula (anterior or posterior as well as supramalleolar, retromalleolar, or inframalleolar). The range of motion (ROM) of the subtalar joint should be compared to the contralateral side. Normal ROM is 10° eversion and 30° inversion but is quite variable. Eversion strength should be assessed with manual muscle testing both to assess hey ability of the active ankle stabilizers and to aid in the diagnosis of peroneal tendonitis or tear. Special tests include anterior drawer to evaluate for laxity of the ATFL (Fig. 17.2A), talar tilt to evaluate for laxity of the CFL (Fig. 17.2B), and syndesmotic testing (squeeze test and external rotation stress test) to rule out high ankle sprain.

Weight-Bearing Foot and Ankle Radiographs

Three weight-bearing radiographic views of the ankle should be obtained to look for avulsion fractures, arthritis, and malalignment. If hindfoot varus is noted on physical examination, three views weight bearing of the foot should also be obtained. When malalignment is suspected, comparison views of the contralateral extremity can be helpful. Additionally, equivocal physical exam findings can be confirmed using stress radiographs (anterior drawer on lateral radiograph and talar tilt on mortice radiograph).

MRI

Noncontrasted MRI of the ankle should be obtained to confirm the chronic tearing, absence, or attenuation of the LALs and to search for concomitant injuries such as peroneal tendonitis, peroneal tendon tear, peroneal subluxation, deltoid ligament injury, syndesmotic injury, and osteochondral lesion of the talus.

Diagnostic Ultrasound

Dynamic ultrasound examination of the peroneal tendons and lateral ligaments may be added when there is suspicion of peroneal tendon or peroneal retinacular injury as ultrasound has been shown to be more sensitive for peroneal tendon subluxation.[1]

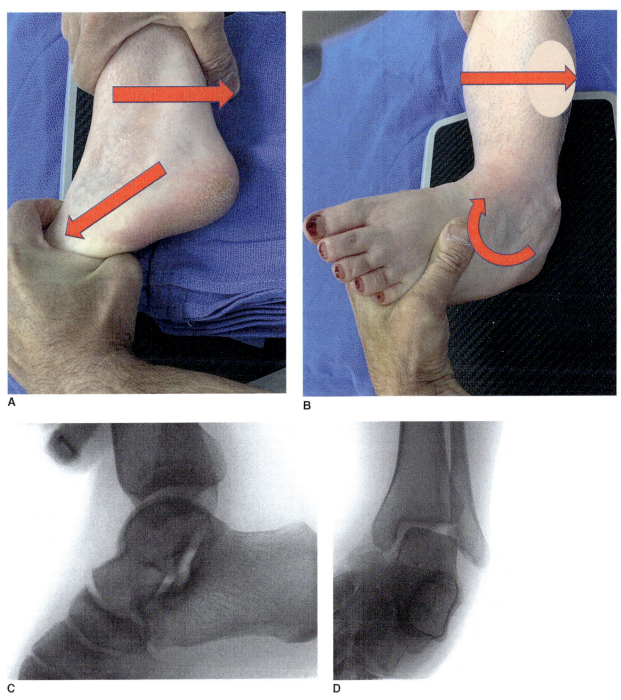

FIGURE 17.2 Physical exam tests for laxity of the lateral ankle ligaments include **(A)** anterior drawer test for anterior talofibular ligament laxity, which is performed with the ankle in 20° plantarflexion by applying an anteromedially directed force on the calcaneus (along the line from the tip of the fibula to the great toe), and **(B)** talar tilt for calcaneofibular ligament laxity, which is performed with the ankle in neutral flexion by applying and inversion moment. The sensitivity of these tests is improved by comparing to the contralateral extremity or by performing with fluoroscopy (shown here). Positive anterior drawer test **(C)** under fluoroscopy and **(D)** positive talar tilt test.

SURGICAL TECHNIQUE (▶ VIDEO 17.1)

Historical Overview

Anatomic repair of the ankle ligaments was first described by Broström over 50 years ago[2] and has undergone many modifications during this time including those by Gould[3] and Karlsson,[4] and more recently through an arthroscopic approach. Nonanatomic reconstructions were popular for the treatment of instability that either was not amenable to repair or for revision of failed repair, but have largely been supplanted by anatomic graft–based reconstruction. A thorough description of the current and historic treatments for CAI is beyond the scope of this chapter and can be found elsewhere.[5] The remainder of this chapter will cover anatomic repair and reconstruction of the LALs through an open approach. These two surgeries are more similar than they are different and thus the anatomic repair will be covered in detail first followed by the modifications to the technique that are used when performing graft-augmented repair (reconstruction).

Repair

Equipment/Implants and Positioning

Lateral ankle ligament repair does not require any special equipment. The classic Broström[2] is a suture-based mid-substance imbrication of the ligaments and the technique described by Karlsson[4] is a insertional repair using bone tunnels. Most modern techniques rely on suture anchors for fixation of the ligaments at their insertion onto the fibula. There are a myriad of suture anchors including metal, plastic, bioabsorbable, and suture only anchors in the 2 to 3 mm range. The author's preferred anchor is a double-loaded suture only 2 mm anchor. These anchors give acceptable fixation in this application because the cortex of the distal fibula is quite robust in most patients.

The patient is positioned in the lateral decubitus position with a tourniquet around the thigh. The preferred anesthetic is the combination of a general anesthetic combined with a popliteal nerve block as this both improves the patient tolerance to lateral positioning and provides optimal intraoperative and postoperative pain relief.

Ankle arthroscopy can be performed prior to ligament repair or reconstruction. Arthroscopy can be used evaluate/treat an osteochondral lesions of the talus (OLTs), loose bodies, and anterolateral impingement. OLT is present in approximately 25% patients with chronic ankle instablity.[6] The author's preference is to perform ankle arthroscopy in conjunction with ankle ligament repair only when an OLT is symptomatic, as the majority of OLTs are asymptomatic and do not cause significant morbidity. On the other hand, the ease and precision of surgical dissection is adversely affected by the tissue edema following arthroscopy.

Fluoroscopic Exam

A mini C-arm is used to perform a fluoroscopic evaluation under anesthesia of ankle laxity either before or after sterile prep. Performance of the exam prior to sterile prep allows for a comparison to the contralateral ankle, which can be helpful when the presence of laxity is uncertain. Both anterior drawer and talar tilt should be evaluated. To maximize the sensitivity of the exam, the anterior drawer should be performed on a properly aligned lateral image (Fig. 17.2C) and the talar tilt on a properly aligned mortise (Fig. 17.2D). Anterior translation of 2.3 mm or greater is generally accepted as representing laxity on anterior drawer,[7] but the specificity of any particular value is poor.[8] Moreover, the decision of whether to perform ligament repair should not be based solely on the evaluation of laxity as there is a subset of patients that have functional instability due to LAL injury but lack demonstrable laxity.[9] The author prefers to fluoroscopically evaluate both anterior drawer and talar tilt and then use this information to determine whether to perform isolated repair of the ATFL or combined repair of ATFL and CFL.

Approach

Isolated LAL repair or reconstruction can be performed through the classic J-shaped incision just slightly anterior and distal to the distal fibula (Fig. 17.3A), whereas an extensile lateral incision over the midline of the fibula should be used when the procedure is combined with peroneal tendon or peroneal retinacular procedures (Fig. 17.3B). The J-shaped incision has a cosmetic advantage because it nearly follows the skinfolds leading to minimal scarring. This incision also provides improved access to the structures needed for the repair without the need for extensive dissection. The subcutaneous tissues are then bluntly dissected. However, in patients with a large anterior fibular fat pad, it is preferable to sharply transect the fat pad with a scalpel so that it can be repaired at the end of the procedure. The extensor retinaculum should be identified between the layers of the fat pad and its edge should be created directly adjacent and parallel to the anterior face of the fibula (Fig. 17.3C). Subperiosteal dissection is then sharply performed parallel to the anterior face and tip of the fibula (Fig. 17.3D). This subperiosteal dissection elevates the ATFL and CFL in conjunction with the ankle joint capsule. The dissection is complete when the lateral articular surface of the talus is completely visualized.

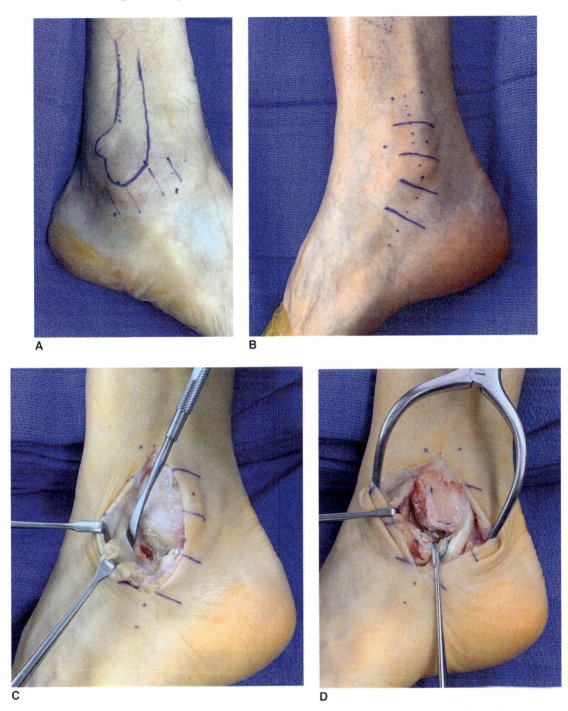

FIGURE 17.3 A. The classic transverse or hockey stick incision for lateral ankle ligament repair is made parallel and just slightly distal to the anterior face of the distal fibula. **B.** The lateral extensile incision is made parallel to the course of the peroneal tendons but centered over the distal fibula. **C.** The inferior extensor retinaculum is located within the fat pad just anterior to the fibula. **D.** The periosteum of the distal fibula is incised at the lateral border of the anterior face of the fibula.

Fixation

The anterior face and tip of the fibula should then be cleared of fibrous tissue using a curette to create the footprints for the ATFL and CFL. One anchor is then placed at the center of each of the ATFL and CFL footprints (Fig. 17.4A). The anchors should be pulled to test the fixation or set the knot against the cortex. The sutures are then sewn through the ATFL and CFL using a horizontal

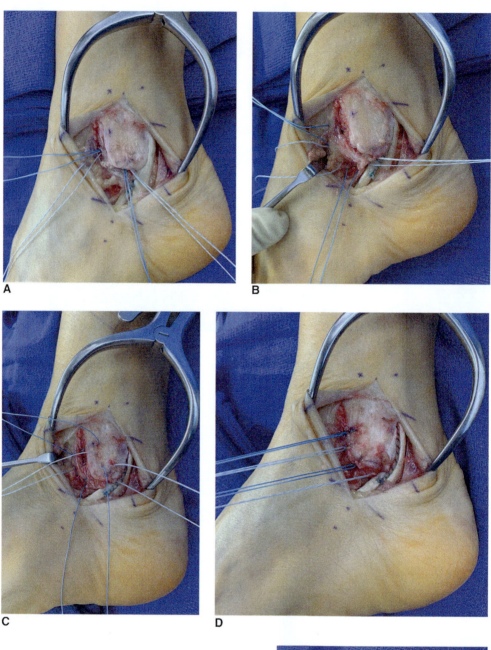
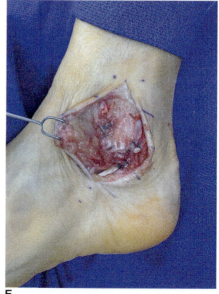

FIGURE 17.4 A. Anchors placed at the anterior talofibular ligament (ATFL) and calcaneofibular ligament (CFL) footprints. **B.** Sutures passed through the ATFL and CFL approximately 1 cm distal to the fibula. **C.** Sutures are tied and one. limb of each suture is then passed back through the periosteum of the fibula to create a vest over pants. **D.** Vest over pants created by tying the two limbs of each suture together. **E.** Extensor retinaculum brought up and tied to the periosteum of the fibula with running absorbable suture.

mattress suture where the horizontal limbs of the suture nearly completely cover the area of the LALs (Fig. 17.4B). The ankle is then held in slight eversion with care taken to ensure that the talus is reduced under the tibia (posterior translation) while the sutures are tied. One of each of the pair of sutures can then be bought back through the proximal end of the ligament and pulled under the periosteum of the distal fibula (Fig. 17.4C), which when tied both increases the area of fixation and creates a vest over pants repair (Fig. 17.4D). The extensor retinaculum is then pulled up and sutured to the cut edge of the distal fibula. Tying the extensor retinaculum to the distal fibula in this way has the effect of adding an additional 50% of initial pullout strength to the repair,[10] acts as a checkrein that limits hindfoot inversion to approximately 10° that prevents the ankle from getting into the position where injury could occur, and covers over the sutures to decrease the prominence of the knots (Fig. 17.4E).

Closure

The tourniquet is then let down. Hemostasis is obtained with direct pressure and electrocautery. The fat pad can then be repaired with absorbable suture. The skin is then closed with inverted deep dermal absorbable suture and 3-0 nylon vertical mattress sutures. Local anesthetic is instilled into the wound. A sterile dressing is applied. A well-padded short leg fiberglass cast in neutral position is then placed.

Graft-Augmented Repair

Graft-augmented repair (reconstruction) differs from primary repair in that the allograft, autograft, or synthetic graft is used to replace or augment the torn or attenuated native ligament tissue instead of fixing the native tissues at their attachments. The author's preference is to perform graft augmentation or reconstruction in the setting of (1) revision surgery, (2) for patients with inadequate tissues (hypermobility disorders, chronic malalignment), and (3) when the tissues are found to be absent or attenuated during surgery. Reconstruction can be performed through either the classic anterior transverse incision or an extensile lateral incision (Fig. 17.5A).

Graft Choices

Lateral ankle ligament reconstruction can be performed using either allograft or autograft tendon (eg, graciliis or semitendinosis, Fig. 17.5A) or synthetic material (eg, Flexband, Artelon Inc, Marietta, Georgia) to replace the absent or attenuated ligaments. The author's preference is to use synthetic graft when performing augmentation of mildly attenuated tissues in the setting of neutral alignment (Fig. 17.6) or when correcting mild malalignment and to use allograft when the native ligament tissues are absent or the malalignment is severe. When using allograft, a 4- to 5-mm diameter graft is sufficient (Fig. 17.5B). The grafts are fixed into each of the tunnels with small (5 × 15 mm) interference screws.

Graft Placement and Fixation

The placement of the tunnels or sockets into which the grafts are fixed should correspond to the anatomic footprint of the native ligaments. For the ATFL, this is from the anterior face of the distal fibula to a point on the neck of the talus just anterior to the articular surface of the lateral talus. The insertion points of the CFL are the tip of the fibula and adjacent to the peroneal tubercle of the calcaneus. These landmarks should be identified fluoroscopically with short 0.062-inch K-wires (Fig. 17.5C). The author's preferred technique is to first locate the distal insertion of the ATFL using the tip of a K-wire on a lateral of the ankle. It is crucial that the spot chosen is in the middle of the talar neck from superior to inferior and immediately adjacent to the articular surface of the talar dome. This spot is not easily located by direct visualization or palpation but can be reliably found on fluoroscopy if properly aligned lateral images are obtained. The center of ATFL footprint on the anterior face of the distal fibula is then located with direct visualization. If using a synthetic graft, only a single socket is placed into the distal fibula, whereas for allograft or autograft, two tunnels are made, which are joined at the back of the fibula. The CFL footprint is then located on the calcaneus by palpation of the peroneal tubercle and confirmed on fluoroscopy to be posterior and inferior to the crucial angle of Gissane. Once the three or four tunnel positions

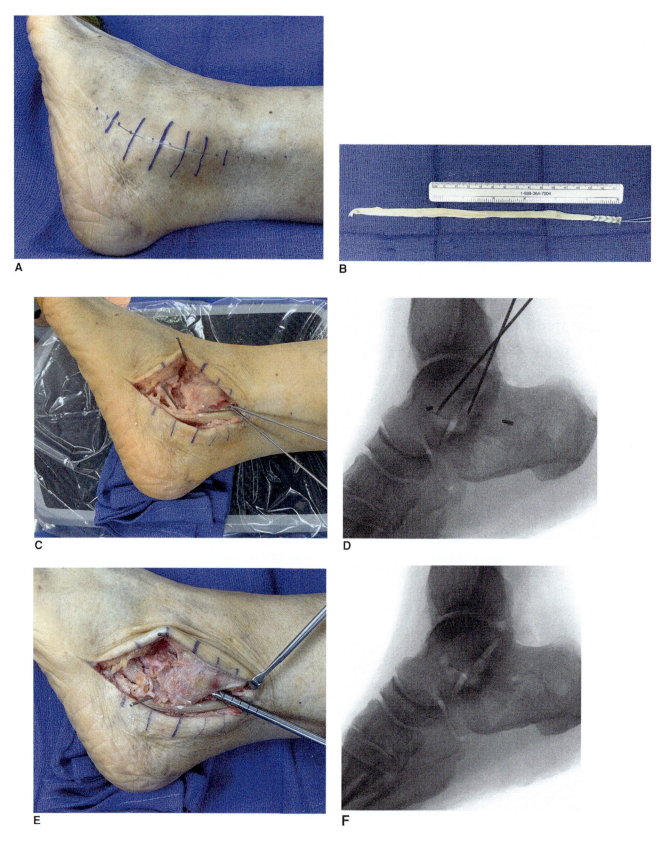

FIGURE 17.5 Lateral ankle ligament reconstruction with allograft. **A.** Extensile lateral approach to the distal fibula. **B.** Tendon allograft with one end whipstitched to aid in passing graft, **(C, D)** locating tunnels with guidewires using fluoroscopy. **E, F.** Drilling of tunnels/sockets with 5-mm cannulated drill.

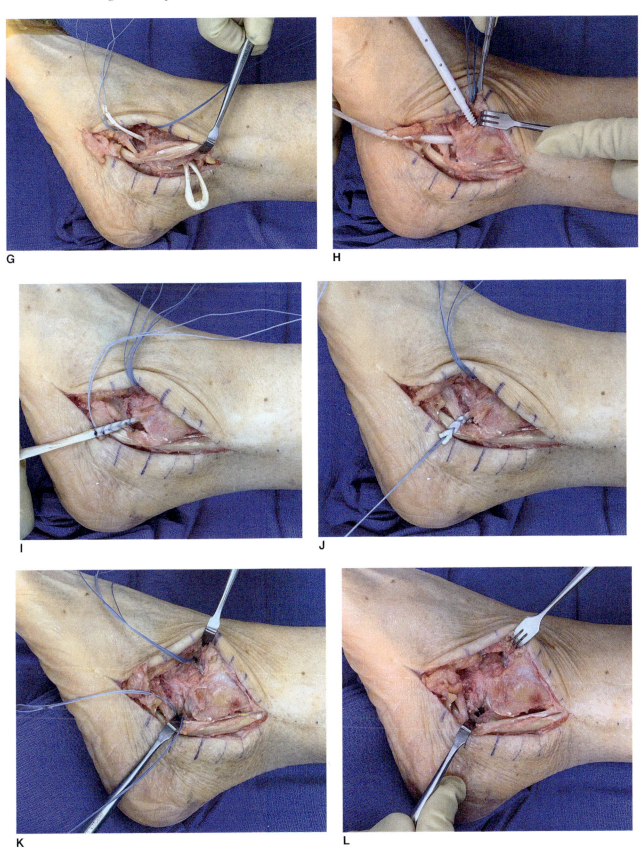

FIGURE 17.5 *(Continued)* **G.** Passing the graft. **H.** Fixing the proximal portion of the graft with an interference screw. **I.** Whipstitching the calcaneofibular ligament (CFL) portion of the graft. **J.** The CFL portion of the graft is trimmed to the correct length. **K.** The CFL graft is then fixed in its tunnel deep to the peroneal tendons. **L.** Completed reconstruction.

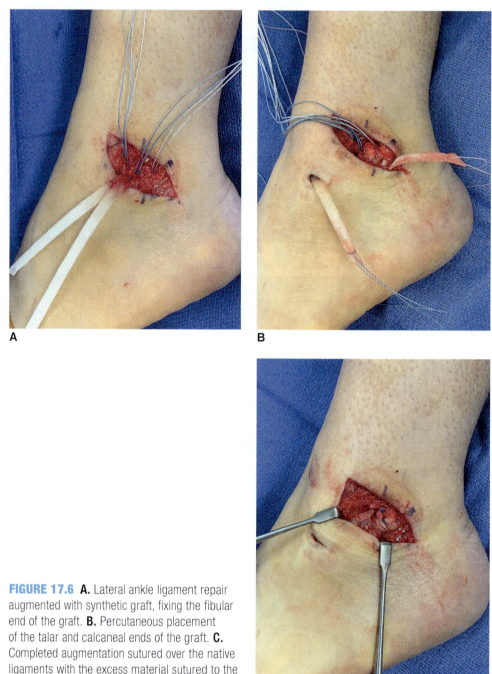

FIGURE 17.6 A. Lateral ankle ligament repair augmented with synthetic graft, fixing the fibular end of the graft. **B.** Percutaneous placement of the talar and calcaneal ends of the graft. **C.** Completed augmentation sutured over the native ligaments with the excess material sutured to the periosteum of the distal fibula.

have been confirmed on fluoroscopy (Fig. 17.5C and D), they are drilled with a 4.5- or 5-mm cannulated drill (Fig. 17.5E and F) and the grafts can be passed (Fig. 17.5G). When the native tissues are present, the author's preference is to pass the grafts superficial to the imbricated native tissues and then suture the grafts to the native tissues. This maintains the physiologic relationship of the synovial joint capsule to the cartilage and avoids exposure of the grafts to the intra-articular environment, which retards healing. The grafts should be tensioned with the ankle and subtalar joints held in neutral position then trimmed to appropriate length and fixed with interference screws (Fig. 17.5H through L).

PEARLS AND PITFALLS

While LAL repair and reconstruction are not especially technically demanding, there are a number of pearls that can make the procedure proceed more efficiently and a number of pitfalls that should be avoided to improve the chances of success.

Pearls

Fluoroscopic Exam
Anterior drawer and talar tilt should be evaluated after the induction of anesthesia but before starting surgery to confirm the laxity that was assessed preoperatively.

Gould Modification
The addition of the Gould modification (advancement of the extensor retinaculum to the distal fibula) to the ligament repair augments the strength of the repair by 50%[10] and provides a way to cover over the knots from the anchors. It also functions to limit inversion of the hindfoot (to ~10°), which helps to prevent reinjury.

Tunnel Placement
The use short K-wires allows for more precise tunnel localization, as shorter wires can more easily be aligned on fluoroscopic imaging to confirm tunnel position and direction. This is especially important in the case of the talar neck socket for the ATFL in which it is easy to drill out the inferior cortex and break through into the sinus tarsi.

Pitfalls

Correction of Malalignment
Failure to address varus malalignment either prior to or concomitant with LAL repair will lead to a high chance of failure, either in the form of mechanical failure of the construct or persistent pain after surgery. The type of procedure used for the correction of the varus hindfoot depends on the particular deformity, a complete discussion of which is outside the scope of this chapter. In general, mild to moderate deformities can be treated with a single procedure. First metatarsal dorsiflexion is preferred when there is forefoot driven hindfoot varus, which corrects with Coleman block testing. Calcaneal osteotomies (Dwyer closing wedge, lateral translation, or Malerba Z osteotomies) are preferred when the hindfoot varus is not forefoot driven or when hindfoot stiffness prevents correction with Coleman block testing. More severe deformities require a cavovarus foot reconstruction consisting of a combination of procedures such as calcaneus osteotomy, first metatarsal osteotomy, plantar fascia release, peroneus longus to brevis tenodesis, posterior tibial tendon lengthening or transfer, and talonavicular capsulotomy. Whichever procedure or combination of procedures is chosen, it should result in the restoration of the physiologic slight valgus of the hindfoot. The author's preference is to not rely on the use of orthoses for the correction of hindfoot varus in patients undergoing operative treatment of lateral ankle instability as the hindfoot varus is the underlying cause of the ligament disorder and undercorrection of alignment or noncompliance can lead to failure of the ligament reconstruction.

Bulky Knots
Suture bulk should be kept to a minimum and knots should be placed distally as bulky knots over the distal fibula can cause irritation with shoe wear. The author's preferred technique is to place the knots as distal as possible and then to cover them with the extensor retinaculum, which is sutured to the periosteum of the distal fibula.

Failure to Recognize or Treat Concomitant Disorders
Peroneal tendon injuries (tendonitis, tears, subluxation) often coexist with LAL injuries[6] because the peroneals act as an active stabilizer of the ankle. Therefore, they are often injured when they forcibly contract in an attempt to prevent the excessive inversion during an instability event. Failure to diagnose and treat concomitant peroneal tendon injury can lead to persistent pain and dissatisfaction after ankle ligament repair.

Intra-articular derangements such as OLT, loose bodies, and anterolateral impingement also occur in association with CAI.[6] The failure to diagnose and treat these lesions can cause persistent pain despite ankle ligament repair. The author's preferred method of addressing intra-articular disorders is to utilize diagnostic ankle injection in patients complaining of anterior ankle joint line pain and to perform arthroscopy in those who report temporary relief of symptoms.

Sural Neuritis

Care must be taken to avoid injury to both the sural nerve proper (which runs posterior and then inferior to the fibula) and the anastomotic branch from the sural to the superficial peroneal nerve (which can run over the distal fibula). Gentle blunt dissection through the fat pad anterior and distal to the tip of the fibula can serve to avoid nerve injury while preserving as much of the fat pad as possible. The fat pad can be reapproximated during closure as long as the dissection has not been overly aggressive.

POSTOPERATIVE MANAGEMENT

Postoperative protocols and determination of readiness for return to sport vary widely among studies.[11] The author's preferred postoperative protocol is listed in Table 17.1. The same protocol can be used after either repair or reconstruction. A well-padded short leg fiberglass cast is preferred as the initial immobilization because it prevents inversion (which would stress the repair/reconstruction), partially offloads the extremity, and ensures compliance.

RESULTS AND COMPLICATIONS

Anatomic repair and reconstruction of the LALs are highly successful procedures with excellent clinical outcomes, low rates of recurrent instability, and high levels of return to sport. The mid to long-term success of modified Broström (including all variations of ATFL/CFL repair) has been examined in a number of studies.[12-16] In these studies, the recurrence rate varies from 0% to 6% and return to sport at preinjury level is reported to range from 58% to 94%.[13-15] One study in 30 high-level athletes[12] found excellent results in 12 patients and good results in 16 at average of 10.4 years after surgery with 28 of the 30 returning to preinjury activity levels.

Anatomic reconstruction with tunneled allograft, autograft, or synthetic graft is a newer procedure. The outcomes are similar to those for repair[17-20] with one study reporting 84% excellent patient satisfaction.[21] Another study compared activity level, function, and return to sport between repair and reconstruction and did not find significant differences.[19] However, return to sport varies substantially across studies with a range of 64% to 97%[18] (average 80%), but some patients only returned at a lower level.[22]

Complications are an infrequent occurrence after LAL repair or reconstruction, the most common complications are wound problems (approximately 2%), sural or superficial peroneal nerve injury (4% to 6%), and recurrent instability.[6] Complex regional pain syndrome occurs rarely (0.3%).[6] Tunnel fracture is a rare but devastating complication that can occur with anatomic reconstruction[5] as the tunnels represent a stress concentrator in the distal fibula.[23]

TABLE 17.1 Post Operative Protocol After Lateral Ankle Ligament Repair or Reconstruction

Weeks Postsurgery	Immobilization	Activity
0-3	Well-padded short leg cast	WBAT
3-6	CAM boot	WBAT, pf/df ROM 5 times per day
6-12	Ankle stirrup splint (eg, Aircast Air Stirrup)	PT eversion strengthening, modalities, ROM ankle, NO inversion stretching till 3 mo after surgery
12-24	Soft ankle brace (eg, ASO, Breg Wraptor, Bioskin Trilock)	Resume athletic activities in brace
>24	None	Full activity, no restrictions

pf, plantar flexion; df, dorsiflexion; WBAT, weight bearing as tolerated; ROM, range of motion; PT, physical therapy; CAM, controlled active motion; ASO, ankle stabilizing orthosis.

REFERENCES

1. Taljanovic MS, Alcala JN, Gimber LH, Rieke JD, Chilvers MM, Latt LD. High-resolution US and MR imaging of peroneal tendon injuries. *Radiographics*. 2015;35(1):179-199.
2. Broström L. Sprained ankles. VI. Surgical treatment of "chronic" ligament ruptures. *Acta Chir Scand*. 1966;132(5):551-565.
3. Gould N, Seligson D, Gassman J. Early and late repair of lateral ligament of the ankle. *Foot Ankle*. 1980;1(2):84-89.
4. Karlsson J, Bergsten T, Lansinger O, Peterson L. Surgical treatment of chronic lateral instability of the ankle joint. A new procedure. *Am J Sports Med*. 1989;17(2):268-273. discussion 273-4
5. Roward Z, Latt LD. Fracture through a distal fibular tunnel used for an anatomic lateral ankle ligament reconstruction. *Foot Ankle Orthopaed*. 2018;3(2):
6. DiGiovanni BF, Fraga CJ, Cohen BE, Shereff MJ. Associated injuries found in chronic lateral ankle instability. *Foot Ankle Int*. 2000;21(10):809-815.
7. Nyska M, Amir H, Porath A, Dekel S. Radiological assessment of a modified anterior drawer test of the ankle. *Foot Ankle*. 1992;13(7):400-403.
8. Netterström-Wedin F, Matthews M, Bleakley C. Diagnostic accuracy of clinical tests assessing ligamentous injury of the talocrural and subtalar joints: a systematic review with meta-analysis. *Sports Health*. 2022;14(3):336-347.
9. Takao M, Innami K, Matsushita T, Uchio Y, Ochi M. Arthroscopic and magnetic resonance image appearance and reconstruction of the anterior talofibular ligament in cases of apparent functional ankle instability. *Am J Sports Med*. 2008;36(8):1542-1547.
10. Aydogan U, Glisson RR, Nunley JA. Extensor retinaculum augmentation reinforces anterior talofibular ligament repair. *Clin Orthop Relat Res*. 2006;442:210-215.
11. Camacho LD, Roward ZT, Deng Y, Latt LD. Surgical management of lateral ankle instability in athletes. *J Athl Train*. 2019;54(6):639-649.
12. Lee KT, Park YU, Kim JS, Kim JB, Kim KC, Kang SK. Long-term results after modified Broström procedure without calcaneofibular ligament reconstruction. *Foot Ankle Int*. 2011;32(2):153-157.
13. Li X, Killie H, Guerrero P, Busconi BD. Anatomical reconstruction for chronic lateral ankle instability in the high-demand athlete: functional outcomes after the modified Broström repair using suture anchors. *Am J Sports Med*. 2009;37(3):488-494.
14. Maffulli N, Del Buono A, Maffulli GD, et al. Isolated anterior talofibular ligament Broström repair for chronic lateral ankle instability: 9-year follow-up. *Am J Sports Med*. 2013;41(4):858-864.
15. Petrera M, Dwyer T, Theodoropoulos JS, Ogilvie-Harris DJ. Short- to medium-term outcomes after a modified brostrom repair for lateral ankle instability with immediate postoperative weightbearing. *Am J Sports Med*. 2014;42(7):1542-1548.
16. So E, Preston N, Holmes T. Intermediate- to long-term longevity and incidence of revision of the modified brostrom-gould procedure for lateral ankle ligament repair: a systematic review. *J Foot Ankle Surg*. 2017;56(5):1076-1080.
17. Ellis SJ, Williams BR, Pavlov H, Deland J. Results of anatomic lateral ankle ligament reconstruction with tendon allograft. *HSS J*. 2011;7(2):134-140.
18. Li H, Song Y, Li H, Hua Y. Outcomes after anatomic lateral ankle ligament reconstruction using allograft tendon for chronic ankle instability: a systematic review and meta-analysis. *J Foot Ankle Surg*. 2020;59(1):117-124.
19. Matheny LM, Johnson NS, Liechti DJ, Clanton TO. Activity level and function after lateral ankle ligament repair versus reconstruction. *Am J Sports Med*. 2016;44(5):1301-1308.
20. Wang W, Xu GH. Allograft tendon reconstruction of the anterior talofibular ligament and calcaneofibular Ligament in the treatment of chronic ankle instability. *BMC Musculoskelet Disord*. 2017;18(1):150
21. Coughlin MJ, Schenck RC Jr, Grebing BR, Treme G. Comprehensive reconstruction of the lateral ankle for chronic instability using a free gracilis graft. *Foot Ankle Int*. 2004;25(4):231-241.
22. Dierckman BD, Ferkel RD. Anatomic reconstruction with a semitendinosus allograft for chronic lateral ankle instability. *Am J Sports Med*. 2015;43(8):1941-1950.
23. Sammarco VJ. Complications of lateral ankle ligament reconstruction. *Clin Orthop Relat Res*. 2001;391:123-132.

18 Débridement, Repair, and Regeneration of Osteochondral Lesions of the Talus

John M. Rawlings and Richard D. Ferkel

INTRODUCTION

Articular cartilage lesions continue to be a challenging problem for the orthopedic community. The growth of athletic participation and an increase in active individuals across all age groups have necessitated the development of improved strategies to treat symptomatic osteochondral defects.[1] For example, osteochondral lesions of the talus (OLTs) can occur in up to 40% of patients with chronic ankle instability[2] and in up to 70% of patients with ankle fractures,[3] both of which are quite common in the active population.[4,5] With increasing prevalence and recognition of these injuries, surgeons need to improve both nonoperative and operative treatment of these injuries. This chapter will discuss strategies and treatments for OLTs.

INDICATIONS AND CONTRAINDICATIONS

The first step to evaluating any patient with ankle pain is obtaining a comprehensive history and physical examination, followed by weight-bearing radiographs (when possible) to include anteroposterior, lateral, and mortise views. In cases of known lesions of the talus, a computed tomography (CT) scan should be obtained to further evaluate the size and characteristics of the lesion. Magnetic resonance imaging (MRI) is appropriate for patients with acute or chronic ankle pain of unknown etiology or when an OLT is known but may not explain all the patient's symptoms or signs.

The decision to treat OLTs surgically is not always clear cut. Berndt and Harty[6] and others have advocated surgical treatment in stage III lateral lesions and all stage IV lesions. They recommended nonoperative treatment for stage III medial lesions, unless symptoms persisted. Several other authors have had difficulty distinguishing between stage II (a partially detached osteochondral fracture remains in its native bed) and stage III (completely detached but nondisplaced osteochondral lesion) lesions according to the Berndt and Harty classification. More recently, Flick and Gould reported superior results with surgical treatment, even with a number of stage II lesions.[7]

We currently use the Ferkel-Sgaglione CT classification[8] (Table 18.1, Fig. 18.1) and/or the Anderson MRI classification[9] (Table 18.2, Fig. 18.2) to preoperatively stage OLTs. All symptomatic stage I and II lesions—and stage III lesions in children with open physes—are treated conservatively in a weight-bearing, short-leg cast or boot. To date, there is no evidence to suggest that a non–weight-bearing cast improves clinical outcomes, and thus, it is not advocated. Initial conservative treatment is recommended for 6 to 12 weeks, with the length of time determined by size and extent of the lesion. In adults, operative intervention is indicated in all symptomatic stage III and IV lesions that fail conservative treatment or in stage I and II lesions that fail nonoperative management.

TABLE 18.1 Computed Tomography Classification

Stage	
Stage I	Cystic lesion within dome of talus, intact roof on all views
Stage IIA	Cystic lesion with communication to talar dome surface
Stage IIB	Open articular surface lesion with overlying nondisplaced fragment
Stage III	Undisplaced lesion with lucency
Stage IV	Displaced fragment

Reprinted with permission from Ferkel RD, Sgaglione NA. Arthroscopic treatment of osteochondral lesions of the talus: long-term results. *Orthop Trans*. 1993-1994;17:1011.

PREOPERATIVE PLANNING

Once it has been determined that surgical treatment is the correct course of action, it must then be determined which surgical technique will be utilized to achieve the best result. Fortunately, surgical advances and improving technology have generated considerable research in cartilage restoration.

Resurfacing techniques designed to produce hyaline-like repair tissue, such as autologous chondrocyte implantation, or transfer hyaline tissue, such as osteochondral allografts and autografts, may have improved outcomes, particularly on large (greater than 10 to 15 mm diameter) lesions. However, allograft options are sometimes prohibitively expensive and difficult to obtain, and autograft options

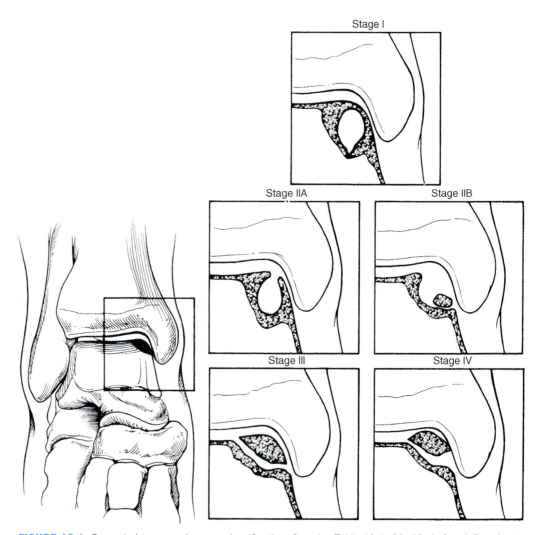

FIGURE 18.1 Computed tomography scan classification. See also Table 18.1. (Modified after J. Daugherty and Richard Ferkel. Reprinted with permission from Kerker J, Ferkel RD. Articular cartilage defects of the ankle. In: Ferkel RD, ed. *Foot and Ankle Arthroscopy*. 2nd ed. Wolters Kluwer; 2017:192. Illustration by Susan Brust.)

18 Débridement, Repair, and Regeneration of Osteochondral Lesions of the Talus

TABLE 18.2 Magnetic Resonance Imaging (MRI) Classification	
Stage I	Subchondral trabecular compression
	Plain radiograph normal, positive bone scan
	Marrow edema on MRI
Stage IIA	Formation of subchondral cyst
Stage II	Incomplete separation of fragment
Stage III	Unattached, undisplaced fragment with the presence of synovial fluid around fragment
Stage IV	Displaced fragment

Reprinted with permission from Anderson IF, Crichton KJ, Grattan-Smith T, et al. Osteochondral fractures of the dome of the talus. *J Bone Joint Surg Am.* 1989;71(8):1143-1152. Copyright © 1989 by The Journal of Bone and Joint Surgery, Incorporated.

result in donor site morbidity with or without a staged procedure. As a result, interest in scaffolding-type procedures has increased as the grafts used are cheaper than osteochondral allografts. These grafts also result in hyaline-like cartilage that more closely matches native cartilage compared to bone marrow stimulation (BMS) alone. These techniques may also better fill the defect than BMS alone.[10,11]

SURGICAL TECHNIQUE

Various arthroscopic setups and approaches are available to treat OLTs. These include the supine position with an ankle and thigh holder, the supine position with a thigh holder and the table bent to allow the knee to flex to 90°, the lateral decubitus position, and the prone position. Regardless of the method used, the therapeutic alternatives are the same. The senior author's preferred position is the supine position with an ankle and thigh holder (Fig. 18.3).

Small joint 2.7-mm 30° and 70° arthroscopes and small joint instrumentation are particularly useful in treating these lesions because they enable the arthroscopist to see a wide angle of vision

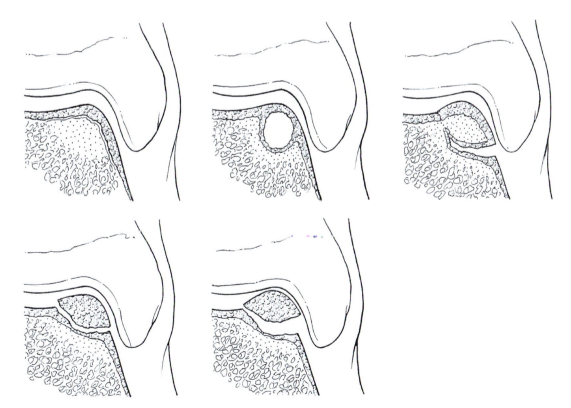

FIGURE 18.2 Anderson magnetic resonance imaging classification. See also Table 18.2. (Reprinted with permission from Kerker J, Ferkel RD. Articular cartilage defects of the ankle. In: Ferkel RD, ed. *Foot and Ankle Arthroscopy.* 2nd ed. Wolters Kluwer; 2017:193. Illustration by Susan Brust.)

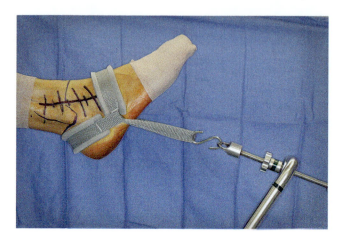

FIGURE 18.3 Intraoperative picture of a right ankle with soft tissue distraction with the patient in the supine position with a thigh holder. The relevant anatomy, including the superficial peroneal nerve, is marked.

with minimal distraction and to work in small spaces. Occasionally, a 1.9-mm 30° arthroscope is necessary in tight joints.

Arthroscopic evaluation of osteochondral lesions starts with a complete 21-point examination utilizing anteromedial, anterolateral, and posterolateral portals.[12,13] Care is taken to examine not only the talus but also the tibial articular surfaces because some patients will either have isolated or associated tibial plafond lesions that are symptomatic and require treatment. The arthroscope must be placed in all three portals (anteromedial, anterolateral, posterolateral) so that no area is left uninspected.

Technique 1: Arthroscopic Débridement and Bone Marrow Stimulation of Small Talar Chondral Lesions

For noncystic lesions that are less than 10 to 15 mm in diameter, all loose articular cartilage is removed down to healthy, bleeding bone (Fig. 18.4A through D). The edges of the cystic lesion should be cut at 90° to promote blood pooling, and the base of the lesion is drilled with a 1.1-mm (0.045-in) Kirschner wire (K-wire). Arthroscopic awls may also be used, but we prefer drilling as some literature has shown improved biological features compared with BMS.[14] The drilling can be performed directly through available portals or percutaneously if the location of the lesion allows, or alternatively retrograde drilling can be performed with a guide. We prefer to avoid transmalleolar drilling through the medial or lateral malleolus to avoid iatrogenic damage to otherwise healthy cartilage. However, occasionally, it is necessary to use the transmalleolar portal for access to the osteochondral lesion (Figs. 18.5A and B).

Traction is removed, and the portals are closed with 4-0 nylon suture in a vertical mattress fashion.

Technique 2: Arthroscopic Repair of Acute Talar Osteochondral Lesions

Acute anterolateral lesions are usually displaced and may be upside-down in the joint and is called a LIFT lesion (lateral, inverted, osteochondral fracture of the talus).[15] Anterolateral lesions are best approached with the arthroscope in the anteromedial portal, inflow posterolaterally, and instrumentation anterolaterally. Loose lesions can be reduced and fixated or excised through the anterolateral portal (Figs. 18.6A and B). A small joint cannula can then be used to stabilize the K-wire while drilling into the base of the lesion to assist in fixation of the loose osteochondral fragment. Fixation can be maintained with K-wires, screws, or absorbable pins (Fig. 18.7A and B). It is rare to use a K-wire for fixation unless it is drilled from a transtalar approach. Usually, two or three pins are necessary for stable fixation. Prior to fixating the fracture, the bed needs to be curetted to good bleeding bone and all fibrous material removed. The fracture is then reduced and stabilized.

Acute anterolateral OLTs are often not amenable to "arthroscopic fixation." If necessary, a longitudinal Broström-type approach is performed. The talus is then plantar flexed, inverted, and displaced anteriorly. The lesion and bed can be débrided and bone grafted, if necessary. The acute OLT is then reduced and pinned. Rarely, a lateral malleolus osteotomy is necessary to access these lesions. Once the lesion is exposed, preparation and fixation of the lesion is performed in the same manner as described above.

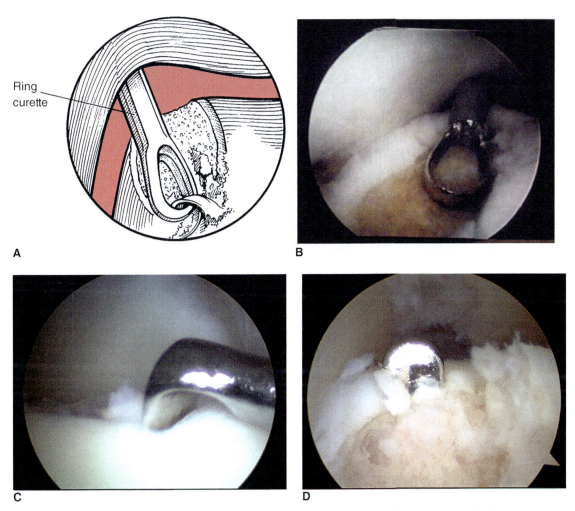

FIGURE 18.4 **A.** Use of a ring curette to remove any fibrous tissue or unstable cartilage from the underlying bony bed of a right ankle. The visualization is from a posterolateral portal, and the curette is introduced through the anteromedial portal. (Reprinted with permission from Kerker J, Ferkel RD. Articular cartilage defects of the ankle. In: Ferkel RD, ed. *Foot and Ankle Arthroscopy*. 2nd ed. Wolters Kluwer; 2017:203. Illustration by Susan Brust.) **B.** Arthroscopic view showing use of a ring curette in a right ankle. Visualization is through a posterolateral portal, and the curette is in an anteromedial portal. (Reprinted with permission from Kerker J, Ferkel RD. Articular cartilage defects of the ankle. In: Ferkel RD, ed. *Foot and Ankle Arthroscopy*. 2nd ed. Wolters Kluwer; 2017:203.) **C.** Use of an arthroscopic "hoe" in a right ankle to create stable vertical walls around the medial lesion anteriorly, as seen from the anterolateral portal. (Reprinted with permission from Kerker J, Ferkel RD. Articular cartilage defects of the ankle. In: Ferkel RD, ed. *Foot and Ankle Arthroscopy*. 2nd ed. Wolters Kluwer; 2017:204.) **D.** Use of an arthroscopic "hoe" in a right ankle to create stable vertical walls around the medial lesion anteriorly, as seen from the posterolateral portal. (Reprinted with permission from Kerker J, Ferkel RD. Articular cartilage defects of the ankle. In: Ferkel RD, ed. *Foot and Ankle Arthroscopy*. 2nd ed. Wolters Kluwer; 2017:204.)

Technique 3: Arthroscopic Bone Grafting of Cystic Talar Osteochondral Lesions With an Intact Cartilage Cap

In the unusual occasion when a large cyst is present with the overlying cartilage intact, a bone graft should be performed. One method advocated in the past was to ream a large enough hole through a transmalleolar approach to create a small window on the medial dome of the talus. Bone graft from the distal tibia or calcaneus can then be inserted and impacted through the transmalleolar approach. This is not recommended because of the morbidity associated with the large hole and the possible development of arthritic change. A preferred method is to insert a guide pin percutaneously near the sinus tarsi at the junction of the talar neck and body. Once the guide pin is verified to be in the posteromedial osteochondral defect, the hole is cored or drilled out and the bone graft is inserted through a cannula and impacted with a plunger (Figs. 18.8A through C). Bone graft substitute can also be inserted through a drilled hole in the sinus tarsi. As an alternative to using bone graft, Kennedy

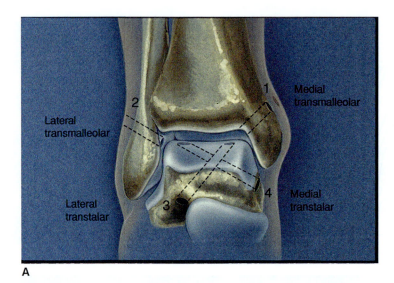

FIGURE 18.5 A. Transmalleolar and transtalar drilling, both laterally and medially. (From Kerker J, Ferkel RD. Articular cartilage defects of the ankle. In: Ferkel RD, ed. *Foot and Ankle Arthroscopy*. 2nd ed. Wolters Kluwer; 2017:196. Copyright © Richard D. Ferkel.). **B.** Transmalleolar drilling technique. (*A*) Dorsiflexion and plantarflexion of the ankle allows multiple drill holes to be made in the talus with limited holes through the tibia. (*B*) Initial drill hole made in the talus. (*C*) Plantarflexion allows the same pin to drill a hole more posteromedially in the talus. (*D*) Extreme dorsiflexion allows the same pin to drill a hole more anteromedially into the talus. (Reprinted with permission from Kerker J, Ferkel RD. Articular cartilage defects of the ankle. In: Ferkel RD, ed. *Foot and Ankle Arthroscopy*. 2nd ed. Wolters Kluwer; 2017:207. Illustrations by Susan Brust.)

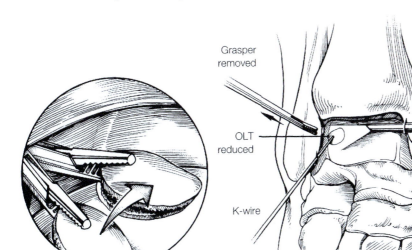

FIGURE 18.6 Acute osteochondral lesion of the talus. **A.** Loose body is located centrally in the joint and reduced back into the bleeding talar bed. **B.** Once the loose lesion is reduced, it is held in place with a probe or grasper temporarily until it is secured with fixation or temporarily with pins. (Reprinted with permission from Kerker J, Ferkel RD. articular cartilage defects of the ankle. In: Ferkel RD, ed. *Foot and Ankle Arthroscopy*. 2nd ed. Wolters Kluwer; 2017:197. Illustration by Susan Brust.)

et al described their technique of injecting a surgical-grade calcium sulfate bone graft through the sinus tarsi to fill osteochondral lesions of the talar dome[16] (Fig. 18.9). Other people have injected an allograft paste.

Another alternative for bone grafting these lesions is to make a small window in the medial wall of the talus below the medial malleolus and to remove the cystic lesion using curved curettes. The bone graft can then be obtained from the distal or proximal tibial and inserted up into the cystic defect of the talus. This can usually be done only when the lesions are quite large and extend below

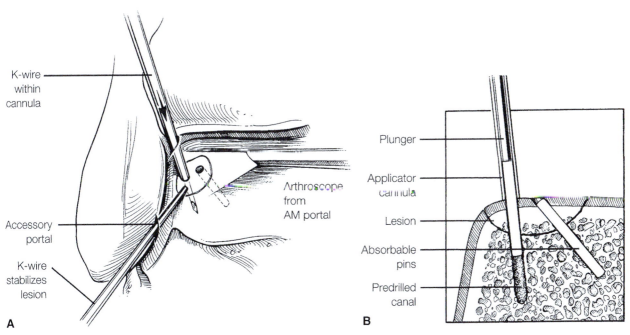

FIGURE 18.7 Acute osteochondral lesion of the talus. **A.** The acute lesion is stabilized so that absorbable pins can be inserted. **B.** Insertion of absorbable pins is done arthroscopically using a plunger after measuring the appropriate length of the pin and predrilling the hole. (Reprinted with permission from Kerker J, Ferkel RD. Articular cartilage defects of the ankle. In: Ferkel RD, ed. *Foot and Ankle Arthroscopy*. 2nd ed. Wolters Kluwer; 2017:195. Illustration by Susan Brust.)

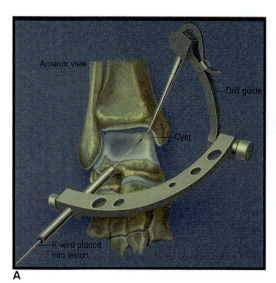
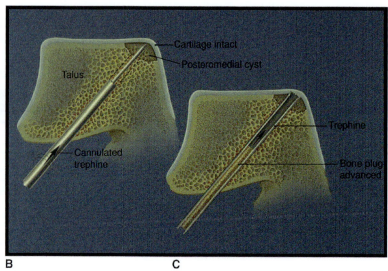

FIGURE 18.8 Transtalar drilling of an osteochondral lesion of the medial dome of the talus. **A.** A K-wire is inserted using a drill guide by drilling from the sinus tarsi posteromedially. **B.** A cannulated trephine is used to core out the bone from the lateral aspect of the talus into the area of the osteochondral defect. (Reprinted with permission from Kerker J, Ferkel RD. Articular cartilage defects of the ankle. In: Ferkel RD, ed. *Foot and Ankle Arthroscopy*. 2nd ed. Wolters Kluwer; 2017:209.) **C.** Using a plunger, the bone plug is advanced into the area of the osteochondral lesion. (From Kerker J, Ferkel RD. Articular cartilage defects of the ankle. In: Ferkel RD, ed. *Foot and Ankle Arthroscopy*. 2nd ed. Wolters Kluwer; 2017:209. Copyright © Richard D. Ferkel, Illustrations by Susan Brust.)

the tip of the medial malleolus. Sometimes an arthroscopic approach to bone grafting is not feasible and an open approach should be used with bone grafting using the distal tibia or iliac crest.

Technique 4: Arthroscopic Treatment of Large Cystic Talar Osteochondral Lesions With Bone Autograft, Bone Marrow Aspirate Concentrate (BMAC), and Extracellular Matrix Cartilage Allograft (Also Referred to as Micronized Cartilage) (See ▶Video 18.1)

For large unstable cystic OLTs, the lesion is identified, and all loose articular cartilage and cystic membrane are removed down to healthy, bleeding bone (Fig. 18.10). The edges of the cystic lesion should be cut at 90° to promote blood pooling, and the base of the lesion is drilled with a 1.1-mm

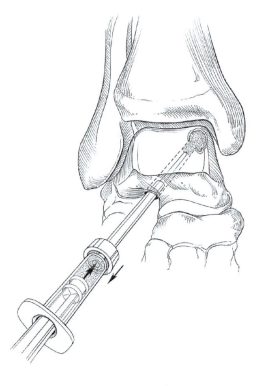

FIGURE 18.9 Injectable bone graft inserted through the sinus tarsi up into the cystic osteochondral lesion. (Reprinted with permission from Kerker J, Ferkel RD. Articular cartilage defects of the ankle. In: Ferkel RD, ed. *Foot and Ankle Arthroscopy*. 2nd ed. Wolters Kluwer; 2017:210. Illustration by Susan Brust.)

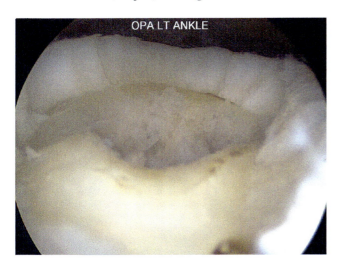

FIGURE 18.10 All loose articular cartilage and cystic membrane are removed down to healthy, bleeding bone. Be sure to remove all of the cystic membrane or at least as much as is possible.

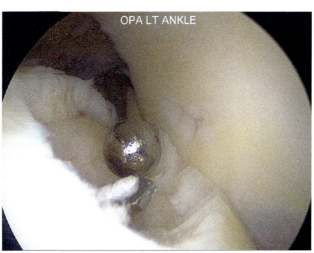

FIGURE 18.11 Retrograde drilling can be performed with a Micro Vector drill guide, typically starting percutaneously at the sinus tarsi for osteochondral lesions of the talus of the medial dome. Visualization is from the posterolateral portal, and the drill guide is inserted through the anteromedial portal.

(0.045-in) K-wire to promote healing. The drilling can be performed directly through available portals or percutaneously if the location of the lesion allows, or alternatively retrograde drilling can be performed with a guide, typically starting percutaneously at the sinus tarsi for OLTs of the medial dome (Fig. 18.11, see Fig. 18.5A). We prefer to avoid drilling through the medial or lateral malleolus to avoid iatrogenic damage to otherwise healthy cartilage, but this is another option, when necessary (see Fig. 18.5B).

The removed loose articular cartilage is morselized on the back table to later be mixed with extracellular matrix cartilage allograft (EMCA) (also referred to as micronized cartilage). Alternatively, the loose articular cartilage may be removed with a shaver that has an attached filtration system to catch the cartilage for later use.

Typically performed prior to the arthroscopy, bone marrow aspirate (Fig. 18.12) and bone graft are harvested from the iliac crest with a percutaneous bone graft harvester to obtain adequate bone graft to fill the defect (Fig. 18.13). At least 60 mL of bone marrow aspirate is obtained and spun down to get about 4 to 5 mL of bone marrow aspirate concentrate (BMAC). Bone grafting cystic osteochondral lesions is done when the depth of the cyst is greater than 6 mm.

A dry arthroscopy is then performed, and sterile swabs or suction swabs are utilized to completely dry out the osteochondral lesion. A delivery cannula is placed directly into the lesion through the portal that provides the most unobstructed route to the lesion, and an obturator advances the bone graft through the portal until the defect is filled (Fig. 18.14A and B). A freer elevator is additionally utilized to impact the bone graft to create a flush border with the surrounding intact bone while keeping the bone graft from filling beyond the bone-cartilage border.

On the back table, the morselized autologous cartilage is mixed with the EMCA and BMAC. This mixture is made to provide enough fluid to make a paste without making the final product runny. After the paste is well mixed, a delivery system is utilized to carefully and slowly push the mixture on top of the packed bone graft (Fig. 18.15A through D). A freer elevator is additionally utilized to smooth the mixture to create a flush border with the surrounding intact cartilage. Fibrin glue is then placed and allowed to dry for 6 minutes.

Once the fibrin glue is dried, the stability is checked and traction is removed. The portals are closed with 4-0 nylon suture in a vertical mattress fashion.

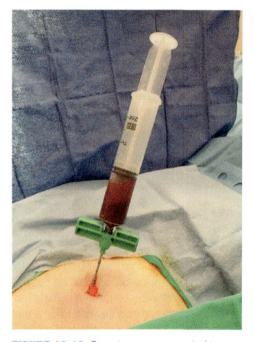

FIGURE 18.12 Percutaneous removal of bone marrow aspirate from a left anterior iliac crest using a Jamshidi needle.

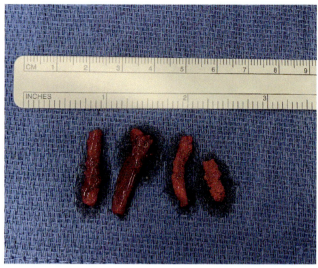

FIGURE 18.13 Bone graft has been taken from the iliac crest using a percutaneous harvester.

Technique 5: Arthroscopic Treatment of Large Talar Chondral Lesions With Matrix-Induced Autologous Chondrocyte Implantation

Another option for large chondral lesions is to use a staged procedure with matrix-induced autologous chondrocyte implantation (MACI). The first phase of the procedure includes a diagnostic ankle arthroscopy using previously described techniques to evaluate the lesion and confirm that MACI treatment is appropriate. Débridement of noninvolved parts of the ankle can then be performed, but the lesion should be left alone until the second stage. At the same time, the cartilage biopsy is removed from the ipsilateral knee at the intercondylar notch. From standard knee arthroscopy

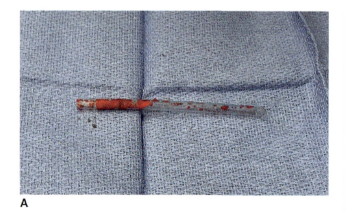

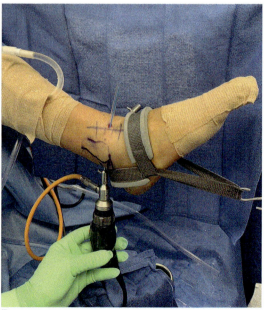

FIGURE 18.14 A. Shuttle with bone graft placed inside the tube. In this case, a shuttle was made by utilizing plastic tubing from sterile packaging and cutting one end at a 45° angle. **B.** The bone graft shuttle has been placed through the anterolateral portal while viewing from the posterolateral portal in a right ankle.

18 Débridement, Repair, and Regeneration of Osteochondral Lesions of the Talus

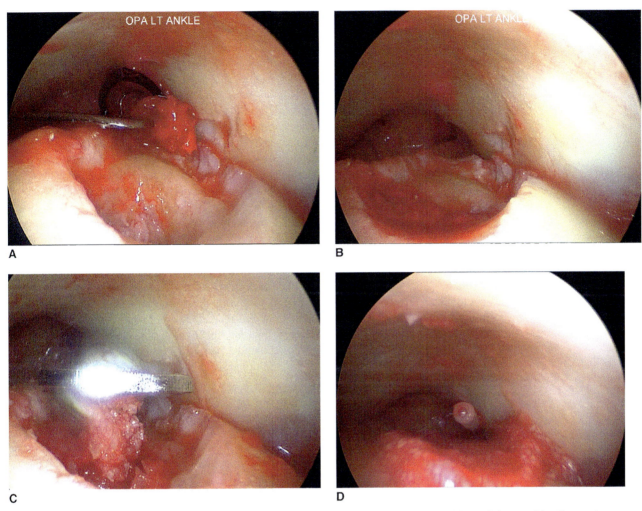

FIGURE 18.15 **A.** A delivery cannula is placed directly into the lesion through the anteromedial portal that provides the most unobstructed route to the lesion, and an obturator advances the bone graft through the portal until the defect is filled. In this case, plastic tubing was utilized by cutting the end at a 45° angle, and the blunt side of a large Steinmann pin was used as a plunger. Visualization is through a posterolateral portal. **B.** The bony cystic defect has been filled with bone graft and compressed down with a freer elevator. Visualization is through a posterolateral portal. **C.** The mixture of morselized autologous cartilage and extracellular matrix cartilage allograft mixed with bone marrow aspirate concentrate is delivered into the cartilage defect. Visualization is through a posterolateral portal. **D.** The cartilage defect is filled with the mixture, the surface is smoothed, and fibrin glue is placed on top. Visualization is through a posterolateral portal.

portals, cartilage is harvested from the lateral aspect of the intercondylar notch by a sharp ring curette (a 200- to 300-mg sample is necessary). Care is taken to avoid detaching the cartilage completely so that it does not float free in the knee joint. A tissue grasper is then used to remove the cartilage piece with a gentle twisting motion, and the piece is removed through a cannula to prevent its entrapment in the anterior soft tissue. The tissue is then stored in packaging provided by the Vericel Corporation (Vericel, Cambridge, Massachusetts). The cartilage biopsy can be obtained from the ankle instead of the knee, but we do not feel that the ankle should be used for the biopsy site since it creates another osteochondral lesion, even in a non–weight-bearing area.

The second phase of the procedure is the implantation phase. This is typically performed at a minimum 6 to 12 weeks after the cells have been cultured and placed onto the membrane. In most cases, the implant is available for 5 years after biopsy. Implantation can be performed by open surgery or occasionally by arthroscopy. The size and location of the lesion will often dictate which approach is optimal. Bone graft can be inserted into cystic osteochondral lesions prior to inserting the MACI membrane using a sandwich technique to place two membranes over the bone graft site. However, if there is significant bone loss, a different procedure such as an allograft needs to be considered.

TRADITIONAL OPEN SURGERY

A tourniquet is placed to ensure that the surgical field remains bloodless. The location of the lesion determines the positioning of the patient. Medial lesions are positioned supine, and a bump is placed under the contralateral hip. A medial malleolar osteotomy is performed to gain access to the lesion. First, the medial malleolus is predrilled for two 4.0-mm cancellous lag screws or a medial malleolar hook plate (Fig. 18.16). Then, under fluoroscopy, guide pins are used as a cutting guide for the saw to assist in making the osteotomy in the correct plane (Fig. 18.17). Imaging should confirm that the saw will exit lateral to the extent of the OLT so that the entire lesion can be accessed.[17]

If the lesion is lateral, it can be accessed by predrilling the fibula for two interfragmentary lag screws and then making an oblique fibular osteotomy. Releasing the anterior talofibular ligament and the anterior capsule allows for the fibula to be rotated posteriorly. A cuff of tissue is left on the fibula for later Broström-type repair of the lateral ligaments.[17]

After adequate exposure is obtained, the OLT can then be débrided to stable vertical margins. A no. 15 blade can be used to obtain sharp vertical borders. The subchondral bone must be left intact in order to prevent osseous bleeding. After deflating the tourniquet, the lesion is dried with thrombin-soaked pledgets. The lesion is then measured to determine the exact size of the defect (Fig. 18.18). A sterile suture foil package is then pressed into the defect to form a template. The MACI membrane is then cut to match this template. After further drying with thrombin, the membrane is placed onto the lesion and pressed gently into place, ensuring that the cell side is facing down into the lesion (Fig. 18.19). Fibrin glue is then applied to the membrane, sealing it in place. After the fibrin has set (5 to 7 minutes), range of motion testing should then be performed to ensure that the MACI graft is stable. 6-0 Vicryl sutures can be applied for additional security but are rarely needed because the membrane is self-adherent.

The osteotomy is then reduced and repaired with two screws. An additional transverse screw at the proximal portion of the medial malleolar osteotomy is used for additional fixation due to the oblique nature of the osteotomy. If a hook plate is utilized, it is secured with compression across the medial malleolar osteotomy (Fig. 18.20A and B). Lateral osteotomies can be fixed with a neutralization one-third tubular plate after placing the interfragmentary lag screws. The Broström repair is

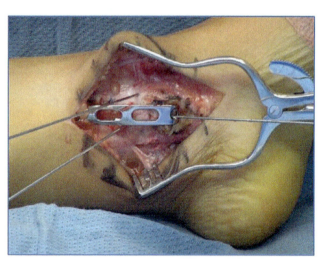

FIGURE 18.16 In this case, a hook plate was applied and predrilled prior to performing the medial malleolar osteotomy, making the anatomic reduction go much more smoothly at the end of the case. (Reprinted by permission from Springer: Berkowitz JJ, Ferkel RD. New and emerging techniques in cartilage repair: matrix-induced autologous chondrocyte implantation (MACI). In: Canata G, d'Hooghe P, Hunt K, et al., eds. *Sports Injuries of the Foot and Ankle. A Focus on Advanced Surgical Techniques.* Springer; 2019:125-131. Copyright © 2019 ISAKOS.)

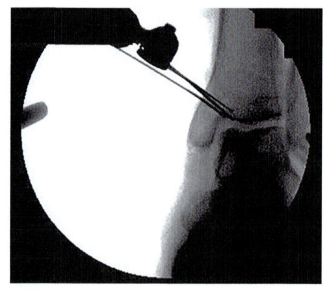

FIGURE 18.17 Under fluoroscopy, guide pins are placed as cutting guides to perform an osteotomy in the precise plane desired. (Reprinted by permission from Springer: Berkowitz JJ, Ferkel RD. New and emerging techniques in cartilage repair: matrix-induced autologous chondrocyte implantation (MACI). In: Canata G, d'Hooghe P, Hunt K, et al., eds. *Sports Injuries of the Foot and Ankle. A Focus on Advanced Surgical Techniques.* Springer; 2019:125-131. Copyright © 2019 ISAKOS.)

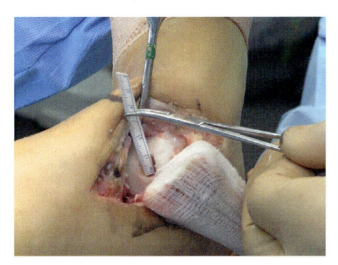 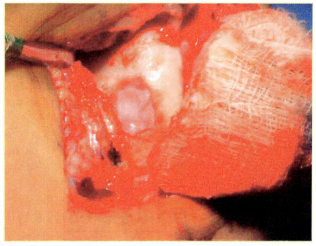

FIGURE 18.18 The osteochondral lesion of the talus is measured with a sterile ruler. (Reprinted by with permission from Springer: Berkowitz JJ, Ferkel RD. New and emerging techniques in cartilage repair: matrix-induced autologous chondrocyte implantation (MACI). In: Canata G, d'Hooghe P, Hunt K, et al., eds. *Sports Injuries of the Foot and Ankle. A Focus on Advanced Surgical Techniques.* Springer; 2019:125-131. Copyright © 2019 ISAKOS.)

FIGURE 18.19 The matrix-induced autologous chondrocyte implantation membrane is applied to the lesion with gentle pressure, followed by the application of fibrin glue. (Reprinted by with permission from Springer: Berkowitz JJ, Ferkel RD. *New and emerging techniques in cartilage repair: matrix-induced autologous chondrocyte implantation* (MACI). In: Canata G, d'Hooghe P, Hunt K, et al., eds. *Sports Injuries of the Foot and Ankle. A Focus on Advanced Surgical Techniques.* Springer; 2019:125-131. Copyright © 2019 ISAKOS.)

then performed. The incisions are then closed with 3-0 Vicryl sutures, followed by 4-0 nylon vertical mattress sutures.

ARTHROSCOPIC TECHNIQUE

Due to the less technically demanding nature of the MACI procedure, it is reasonable to perform the procedure entirely arthroscopically, thereby avoiding the morbidity of an osteotomy. It has been suggested that rolling the graft into the cannula delivery system in the arthroscopic technique may damage the cells,[18] but better studies need to be performed to determine whether this is clinically correct.

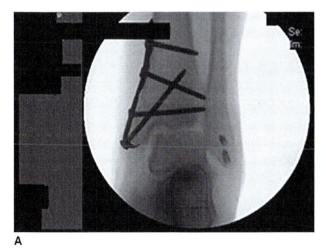 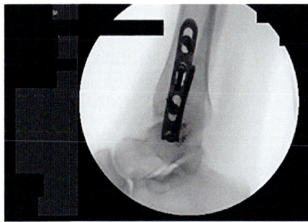

A B

FIGURE 18.20 A, B. Anteroposterior and lateral radiographs of the ankle after fixation of the medial malleolar osteotomy. (Part **A:** Reprinted by permission from Springer: Berkowitz JJ, Ferkel RD. New and emerging techniques in cartilage repair: matrix-induced autologous chondrocyte implantation (MACI). In: Canata G, d'Hooghe P, Hunt K, et al., eds. *Sports Injuries of the Foot and Ankle. A Focus on Advanced Surgical Techniques.* Springer; 2019:125-131. Copyright © 2019 ISAKOS.; Part **B:** Reprinted by permission from Springer: Berkowitz JJ, Ferkel RD. New and emerging techniques in cartilage repair: matrix-induced autologous chondrocyte implantation (MACI). In: Canata G, d'Hooghe P, Hunt K, et al., eds. *Sports Injuries of the Foot and Ankle. A Focus on Advanced Surgical Techniques.* Springer; 2019:125-131. Copyright © 2019 ISAKOS.)

The all arthroscopic second stage procedure is performed with the same setup and through the same portals as the first stage. After débridement of any loose cartilage fragments and synovitis, débridement of the lesion should occur at this time, using different angled curettes to obtain stable vertical borders. The lesion is then accurately measured, and the MACI graft is cut to size. Next, the arthroscopic fluid flow is stopped, and all fluid is drained from the ankle joint. Thrombin-soaked pledgets are inserted from the portal closest to the lesion and used to dry the lesion.

Arthroscopic forceps, or a specialized cannula delivery system, can be used to deliver the matrix into the ankle joint.[19] A probe and a freer elevator can then be used to precisely fit the matrix into the lesion. Fibrin glue should then be placed over the matrix with a commercially available applicator. Once the fibrin is set (5 to 7 minutes), the ankle is taken through extension and flexion to ensure that the matrix is stable. All instruments should then be removed, and the portals closed with 4-0 nylon vertical mattress sutures.

PEARLS AND PITFALLS

- To avoid injury to the superficial peroneal nerve, premark the location of the nerve prior to prepping and draping and use the nick and spread technique prior to placing the arthroscopic cannula into the joint.
- Regularly utilizing the posterolateral portal improves comfort with the placement of the portal and greatly enhances visualization and treatment of more challenging posterolateral and posteromedial OLTs. This portal is located in the "soft spot" directly adjacent to the lateral edge of the Achilles tendon, approximately 1.2 cm above the tip of the fibula; the exact level of the portal varies depending on the patient's anatomy. The portal is established by placing an 18-gauge spinal needle through the posterolateral portal just medial (under) to the transverse tibiofibular ligament.
- Posteromedial OLTs can be challenging, but careful arthroscopic setup and placement of anteromedial, anterolateral, and posterolateral portals facilitate complete arthroscopic management of these challenging lesions without requiring a medial malleolar osteotomy (Table 18.3).
- A thorough débridement of all diseased tissue (including the entire cystic membrane, if present) from the lesion is necessary, and stable vertical walls should be obtained.
- For both transtalar and transmalleolar drilling, a drill guide system with articulating arms allows for consistently accurate placement of K-wires for drilling.
- When placing bioabsorbable pins for acute osteochondral lesion repairs, placing the pins at slightly divergent angles will help keep the fragment from moving after placement of the pins.
- Prior to placing bone graft and EMCA/morselized cartilage, it is critical to develop a dry bone bed to avoid having the products float away from the prepared bed. We have found this is best performed by utilizing multiple suction swabs.
- When planning an MACI procedure, be prepared to perform an open procedure with or without an osteotomy if the lesion proves to not be amenable to arthroscopic MACI graft placement.

POSTOPERATIVE MANAGEMENT

Postoperatively, a bulky compression dressing is applied, as well as a posterior splint with the ankle at 90° to the tibia. Alternatively, a cast may be applied and split with a cast saw in the recovery room. The leg is elevated, and toe range of motion is encouraged immediately. Our patients are kept on non–weight-bearing status for at least 2 weeks. Home range of motion exercises are initiated at this time. The period of non–weight bearing is determined by the type of procedure and the size of the lesion.

TABLE 18.3 Tips for Improved Access to Posteromedial Osteochondral Lesions of the Talus

1. Keep anteromedial portal close to anterior tibial tendon
2. Move anterolateral portal more centrally
3. Good separation of ankle from table
4. Angle posterolateral portal toward lesion
5. Correct equipment availability: 30 and 70 scopes, curettes, hoe

Our rehabilitation protocol involves four phases: early phase (less than 8 weeks), transition phase (8 to 12 weeks), midphase (3 to 5 months), and final phase (6 to 12 months). The goal during the first phase is to achieve full range of motion by 8 weeks. Stationary bike activities without resistance can be initiated during this phase. The transition phase involves proprioceptive exercises, isometric and then eccentric strengthening, and closed kinetic chain presses. The midphase increases walking distance and speed on a progressive basis. Load training is also increased with cycling, skating, and light jogging. The final phase is the initiation of sport-specific training based on the patient's needs. The Tegner activity level score improved from 1.3 preoperatively to 4.0 postoperatively, which is statistically significant. The average time to return to sports was not calculated in this paper.

RESULTS

Dekker et al[20] recently performed a critical analysis review of treatment strategies for OLTs. Although many of the studies referenced are level IV retrospective studies, BMS has had overwhelmingly positive results and has been associated with clinical improvements in 65% to 90% of cases in appropriately sized lesions. In a recent long-term (minimum 10-year follow-up) study of 45 patients who underwent BMS for OLTs, there was a 93.3% survival rate and an 85.7% return to sport, which strongly supports the long-term durability of this procedure.[21] However, in slight contrast to these results, Ferkel et al found that 35% of patients had deterioration of their results over time.[22] Arthroscopic repair of acute osteochondral fractures has been shown to have even better results than BMS for chronic injuries.[23]

Despite good results in small OLTs, BMS has been shown to have increased rates of unsuccessful results in large OLTs. Chuckpaiwong et al[24] had a large series of over one hundred patients, and they found no failures if the lesion was less than 15 mm in diameter in contrast to only one patient who met criteria for success in the group of patients (32 patients in this group) with lesions greater than 15 mm in diameter. Choi et al[25] confirmed these findings by showing that lesions less than 150 mm^2 had significantly better results. Guo et al found a strong correlation in good to excellent results in patients with lesions less than 10 mm in diameter.[26] A more recent systematic review suggested that BMS may be best reserved for OLTs measuring less than 107.4 mm^2 in area and/or less than 10.2 mm in diameter.[27]

Of particular interest are large lesions with subchondral cysts and uncontained (shoulder) lesions. Lesions with subchondral cysts have demonstrated outcomes with failure rates as high as 53%,[28] and uncontained lesions have shown significantly worse clinical outcome scores when treated with BMS techniques when compared to contained lesions.[29] Unfortunately, there are very few studies that have compared surgical techniques in large, cystic, and/or uncontained lesions, but more advanced techniques continue to be employed in the hopes of obtaining superior results in these more challenging scenarios.

In patients with OLTs associated with subchondral cysts but intact overlying cartilage that were treated with retrograde drilling and autologous bone grafting, one study of 41 osteochondral lesions revealed good outcomes with results better than patients with similar injuries but *without* an intact cartilage cap, which advocates for preserving an intact cartilage cap when possible.[30]

Cartilage regenerative techniques have much fewer studies but have also shown promising results. In a study of EMCA use versus BMS alone in equine models, EMCA use was found to have improved histologic scores for repair-host integration and better formation of collagen type II compared to BMS alone.[10] Shimozono et al[11] recently performed a retrospective cohort study of EMCA with BMS versus BMS alone and found that EMCA with BMS provides better cartilage infill in the defect on MRI.

We have reported two papers on the use of ACI for OLTs after failed BMS surgery. The long-term results with a mean follow-up of 70 months revealed 79% of patient with good to excellent results.[31,32] In a meta-analysis of ACI/MACI for the treatment of OLTs, data for 213 patients with nearly 3 years of follow-up and a mean lesion size of 2.3 cm^2 reported a mean success rate of 89.9%.[33] However, there have also been studies that show no significant difference in functional outcomes when comparing MACI and BMS even when diffusion-weighted imaging suggested more normalized tissue repair in the MACI group.[34,35]

COMPLICATIONS

Complications of BMS techniques are very rare but include infection, deep vein thrombosis, stiffness, complex regional pain syndrome, plantar fasciitis, and possible damage to neurovascular structures in association with arthroscopic portal placement.[36] Graft and patch hypertrophy are specific complications of ACI but were decreased in second- and third-generation ACI and MACI techniques.[37] If an osteotomy is performed, nonunion and hardware-related pain are also possible complications.

REFERENCES

1. Wodicka R, Ferkel E, Ferkel R. Osteochondral lesions of the ankle. *Foot Ankle Int.* 2016;37(9):1023-1034.
2. Okuda R, Kinoshita M, Morikawa J, et al. Arthroscopic findings in chronic lateral ankle instability: do focal chondral lesions influence the results of ligament reconstruction? *Am J Sports Med.* 2005;33(1):35-42.
3. Hintermann B, Regazzoni P, Lampert C, et al. Arthroscopic findings in acute fractures of the ankle. *J Bone Joint Surg Br.* 2000;82(3):345-351.
4. Hootman JM, Dick R, Agel J. Epidemiology of collegiate injuries for 15 sports: summary and recommendations for injury prevention initiatives. *J Athl Train.* 2007;42(2):311-319.
5. Scheer RC, Newman JM, Zhou JJ, et al. Ankle fracture epidemiology in the united states: patient-related trends and mechanisms of injury. *J Foot Ankle Surg.* 2020;59(3):479-483.
6. Berndt AL, Harty M. Transchondral fractures (osteochondritis dissecans) of the talus. *J Bone Joint Surg Am.* 1959;41:988.
7. Flick AB, Gould N. Osteochondritis dissecans of the talus (transchondral fractures of the talus): review of the literature and new surgical approach for medial talar dome lesions. *Foot Ankle.* 1985;5:165.
8. Ferkel RD, Sgaglione NA. Arthroscopic treatment of osteochondral lesions of the talus: long term results. *Orthop Trans.* 1993-1994;17:1011.
9. Anderson IF, Crichton KG, Grattan-Smith T, et al. Osteochondral fractures of the dome of the talus. *J Bone Joint Surg Am.* 1987;71:1143.
10. Fortier LA, Chapman HS, Pownder SL, et al. BioCartilage improves cartilage repair compared with microfracture alone in an equine model of full-thickness cartilage loss. *Am J Sports Med.* 2016;44(9):2366-2374.
11. Shimozono Y, Williamson ERC, Mercer NP, et al. Use of extracellular matrix cartilage allograft may improve infill of the defects in bone marrow stimulation for osteochondral lesions of the talus. *Arthroscopy.* 2021;37(7):2262-2269.
12. Ferkel RD. *Ankle and Foot Arthroscopy: Contemporary Approach to Diagnosis and Treatment.* Smith & Nephew Inc.; 2009.
13. Ferkel RD, Fischer SP. Progress in ankle arthroscopy. *Clin Orthop.* 1989;240:210.
14. Kraeutler MJ, Aliberti GM, Scillia AJ, et al. Microfracture versus drilling of articular cartilage defects: a systematic review of the basic science evidence. *Orthop J Sports Med.* 2020;8(8):2325967120945313.
15. Dunlap BJ, Ferkel RD, Applegate GR. The "LIFT" lesion: lateral inverted osteochondral fracture of the talus. *Arthroscopy.* 2013;29(11):1826-1833.
16. Kennedy JG, Suero EM, O'Loughlin PF, et al. Clinical tips: retrograde drilling of talar osteochondral defects. *Foot Ankle Int.* 2008;29:616-619.
17. Arroyo W, Ferkel RD. Distal fibular oblique osteotomy for lateral talus exposure. *Tech Foot Ankle Surg.* accepted for publication. 2023.
18. Biant LC, Simons M, Gillespie T, et al. Cell viability in arthroscopic versus open autologous chondrocyte implantation. *Am J Sports Med.* 2017;45(1):77-81.
19. Giannini S, Buda R, Ruffilli A, et al. Arthroscopic autologous chondrocyte implantation in the ankle joint. *Knee Surg Sports Traumatol Arthrosc.* 2014;22:1311-1319.
20. Dekker TJ, Dekker PK, Tainter DM, et al. A treatment of osteochondral lesions of the talus. *JBJS Rev.* 2017;5(3):e4
21. Corr D, Raikin J, O'Neil J, et al. Long-term outcomes of microfracture for treatment of osteochondral lesions of the talus. *Foot Ankle Int.* 2021;42(7):833-840.
22. Ferkel RD, Zanotti RM, Komenda GA, et al. Arthroscopic treatment of chronic osteochondral lesions of the talus: long-term results. *Am J Sports Med.* 2008;36(9):1750-1762.
23. Kelbérine F, Frank A. Arthroscopic treatment of osteochondral lesions of the talar dome: a retrospective study of 48 cases. *Arthroscopy.* 1999;15(1):77-84.
24. Chuckpaiwong B, Berkson EM, Theodore GH. Microfracture for osteochondral lesions of the ankle: outcome analysis and outcome predictors of 105 cases. *Arthroscopy.* 2008;24(1):106-112.
25. Choi WJ, Park KK, Kim BS, et al. Osteochondral lesion of the talus: is there a critical defect size for poor outcome? *Am J Sports Med.* 2009;37(10):1974-1980.
26. Guo QW, Hu YL, Jiao C, et al. Arthroscopic treatment for osteochondral lesions of the talus: analysis of outcome predictors. *Chin Med J (Engl).* 2010;123(3):296-300.
27. Ramponi L, Yasui Y, Murawski CD, et al. Lesion size is a predictor of clinical outcomes after bone marrow stimulation for osteochondral lesions of the talus: a systematic review. *Am J Sports Med.* 2017;45(7):1698-1705.
28. Robinson DE, Winson IG, Harries WJ, et al. Arthroscopic treatment of osteochondral lesions of the talus. *J Bone Joint Surg Br.* 2003;85(7):989-993.
29. Choi WJ, Choi GW, Kim JS, et al. Prognostic significance of the containment and location of osteochondral lesions of the talus: independent adverse outcomes associated with uncontained lesions of the talar shoulder. *Am J Sports Med.* 2013;41(1):126-133.
30. Anders S, Lechler P, Rackl W, et al. Fluoroscopy-guided retrograde core drilling and cancellous bone grafting in osteochondral defects of the talus. *Int Orthop.* 2012;36(8):1635-1640.
31. Nam EK, Ferkel RD, Applegate GR. Autologous chondrocyte implantation of the ankle: a 2- to 5-year follow-up. *Am J Sports Med.* 2009;37(2):274-284.
32. Kwak SK, Kern BS, Ferkel RD, Chan KW, Kasraeian S, Applegate GR. Autologous chondrocyte implantation of the ankle: 2- to 10-year results. *Am J Sports Med.* 2014;42(9):2156-2164.

33. Niemeyer P, Salzmann G, Schmal H, et al. Autologous chondrocyte implantation for the treatment of chondral and osteochondral defects of the talus: a meta-analysis of available evidence. *Knee Surg Sports Traumatol Arthrosc.* 2012;20(9):1696-1703.
34. Magnan B, Samaila E, Bondi M, et al. Three-dimensional matrix-induced autologous chondrocytes implantation for osteochondral lesions of the talus: midterm results. *Adv Orthop.* 2012;2012:942174.
35. Apprich S, Trattnig S, Welsch GH, et al. Assessment of articular cartilage repair tissue after matrix-associated autologous chondrocyte transplantation or the microfracture technique in the ankle joint using diffusion-weighted imaging at 3 Tesla. *Osteoarthritis Cartilage.* 2012;20(7):703-711.
36. McGahan PJ, Pinney SJ. Current concept review: osteochondral lesions of the talus. *Foot Ankle Int.* 2010;31(1):90-101.
37. Gomoll AH, Probst C, Farr J, et al. Use of a type I/III bilayer collagen membrane decreases reoperation rates for symptomatic hypertrophy after autologous chondrocyte implantation. *Am J Sports Med.* 2009;37(Suppl 1):20S-23S.

19 Osteochondral Autologous Transfer Systems (OATS) for the Treatment of Talar Osteochondral Lesions: The OATS Procedure

Ahmed Khalil Attia and McCalus V. Hogan

INTRODUCTION

Management for symptomatic osteochondral lesions of the talus (OLTs) is challenging given the poor healing potential of articular cartilage and limited access to the ankle joint. While OLTs may occur in any location on the talar dome, they are more common on the centromedial aspect of the talar dome[1] and are frequently associated with inversion ankle sprains and lateral ankle instability. In addition to trauma, ossification defects, abnormal vasculature, emboli, or endocrine disorders may account for focal pathological subchondral fractures of the talus.[2,3] It is not uncommon for acute OLTs to go undetected and end up being treated as chronic lesions.

Arthroscopic débridement and microfracture/drilling of the OLTs has been the standard of care for first-time management of subacute and chronic lesions, especially those under 10 mm.[2-4] The goal of this strategy is to recruit mesenchymal stem cells that differentiate within the defect.[2,3] It is straightforward, is inexpensive, and does not preclude a cartilage repair procedure at a later time. Moreover, it does not include donor site morbidity or osteotomy site nonunion. It is done arthroscopically, minimizing the risk for soft tissue complications. Although favorable intermediate to long-term results have been reported,[5] débridement and drilling/microfracture provides fibrocartilage to fill the defect rather than restoring the physiological hyaline cartilage surface. Due to inferior durability of fibrocartilage in comparison to native hyaline cartilage, débridement and drilling/microfracture is as durable as the adjacent hyaline cartilage. In other words, a contained OLT with intact hyaline cartilage border is necessary for a successful outcome. This can be challenging in edge lesions and large OLTs. Osteochondral autograft transfer systems (OATS) on the other hand restores native hyaline cartilage.

One of the most important variables that guide the management strategy of OLTs is the size of the lesion. As noted above, débridement and drilling/microfracture procedures are effective in the vast majority of smaller diameter lesions under 10.2 mm in diameter but may be less successful in the treatment of many larger diameter OLTs.[4] In smaller defects, the fibrocartilage relieves mechanical symptoms and the surrounding hyaline cartilage provides an adequate mechanical support. With larger defects, however, the natural viscoelastic properties and mechanical support of the talar dome articular surface are compromised. Long-term results point to deterioration of results over time in up to 35% of patients.[3] However, microfracture is a technically simple procedure, and thus it remains an attractive first line in smaller lesions greater than 10 mm and even in larger OLTs due to the many advantages mentioned earlier.

While OATS procedure can be done using allografts, we prefer using autografts whenever possible. Autografts are biologically superior and have been shown to provide superior results while avoiding the risk of disease transmission associated with allografts. On the other hand, allografts are not associated with donor site morbidity, especially if multiple grafts are needed, and are technically easier to use.

INDICATIONS AND CONTRAINDICATIONS

Indications

- Symptomatic OLTs smaller than 10 mm that:
  - Failed débridement and microfracture
  - Are stage V lesions with extensive subchondral cyst that needs bone grafting
- Symptomatic OLTs 10 mm or larger:
  - Failed conservative management
  - Displaced fragments

Contraindications

- Skeletal immaturity as there is high potential for healing with an open physis
- Infection
- Medical comorbidities that preclude surgical intervention
- Diffuse ankle arthritis that requires a more aggressive strategy such as ankle fusion, or replacement
- Large talar shoulder lesions without a stable rim, which is requirement for a successful outcome
- Ankle and hindfoot malalignments unless concomitantly corrected
- Ankle instability unless concomitantly corrected
- Asymptomatic OLTs
- Kissing lesions (talar dome and tibial plafond)
- Diffuse AVN of the talus

PREOPERATIVE PLANNING

While not necessary, it is recommended that the first step in preoperative planning is to determine whether the OLT is the cause of the ankle pain using a local anesthetic and steroid intraarticular ankle injection. Pain relief following the injection confirms that the OLT is the source of the pain and surgical planning can proceed. The injection also provides pain relief while the patient waits for the surgery to be scheduled. If the injection fails to provide substantial pain relief, alternative or additional diagnosis should be sought to explain the source of pain.

Obtain three weight-bearing radiographic views of the ankle (Fig. 19.1). While small OLTs may be missed, it may identify large OLTs and bone cysts. The main advantage of plain radiographs is that of showing any lower extremity malalignment. These may need to be addressed at the time of an OATS procedure. They also show open physis in younger patients, which would preclude an OATS procedure. There is a high potential for healing with an open physis and violating it should be avoided.[6] Plain radiographs can also be used for OLT staging based on Brendt and Harty's radiographic classification:[7] (I) small subchondral compression, (II) partial fragment detachment, (III) complete fragment detachment without displacement, and (IV) complete fragment detachment with displacement.

At least one advanced imaging modality such as computed tomography (CT) scans, preferably weight-bearing computed tomography (WBCT), or magenetic resonance imaging (MRI) is always required (Fig. 19.2). We routinely obtain both CT scans and MRI for all our patients who are to receive an OATS procedure. MRIs are often the first advanced imaging requested for patients with traumatic ankle events that fail to respond to nonoperative management such as ankle sprains. MRI provides valuable information on the state of lateral ankle ligaments, peroneal tendons, and other soft tissues around the ankle that would potentially require concomitant procedures at the time of OATS to optimize outcomes.

19 Osteochondral Autologous Transfer Systems

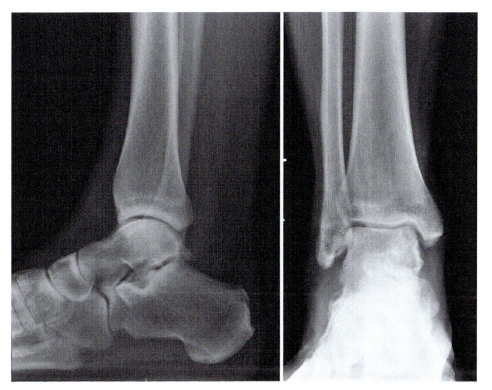

FIGURE 19.1 Plain weight-bearing ankle films of a 37-year-old male who had ankle pain for several months after twisting his ankle while skating. They show a large medial osteochondral lesions of the talus.

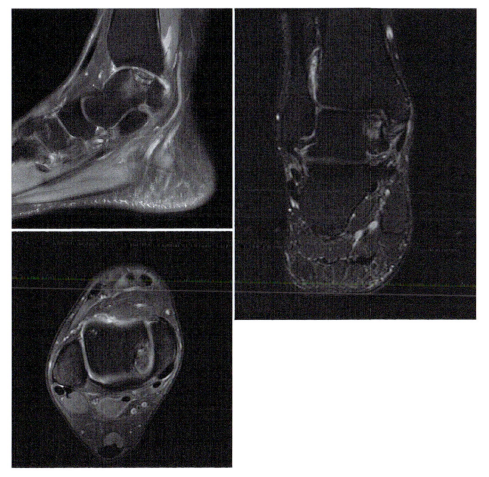

FIGURE 19.2 T2-weighted sagittal, coronal, and axial magnetic resonance imaging images of the same patient showing a large posteromedial talar shoulder osteochondral lesions of the talus that measures 15 × 8 mm.

Advances in MRI technology have allowed detailed characterization of the articular cartilage thickness and defects. The downside to MRI is that it detects bone marrow edema associated with OLTs, which often leads to overestimation of the lesion size and extent. Additionally, MRI is not the best modality to delineate subchondral cysts. Hence, we believe a CT scan should be obtained if an OATS procedure is planned. Not affected by bone marrow edema, CT scans are the most accurate in determining the exact size and characteristics of the OLTs as well as the extent of talar dome involvement. OLTs can be staged based on their CT appearance according to the Ferkel et al classification[3] into: (I) cystic lesion in talar dome with intact roof, (IIA) cystic lesion with communication to talar dome surface, (IIB) open articular surface lesion with overlying nondisplaced fracture, (III) nondisplaced lesion with lucency, (IV) displaced fragment, and (V) subchondral cyst. WBCT can also provide a 3D image of the overall ankle alignment.

In revision cases, we review the arthroscopic images and videos of the previous surgeries and compare those with the findings of diagnostic arthroscopy at the time of OATS procedure.

SURGICAL TECHNIQUE

Medial Malleolar Osteotomy

Several different patterns of medial malleolar osteotomy have been described. Regardless of the chosen technique, the osteotomy must allow perpendicular access to the medial talar dome. We use the oblique medial malleolar osteotomy.[8]

- Perform a curved incision centered over the medial malleolus similar to that performed for open reduction internal fixation of the medial malleolar fracture (Fig. 19.3A).
- Identify and retract the tibialis anterior tendon.
- Create an anterior arthrotomy to identify the junction between the medial malleolar and tibial plafond articular surfaces. Identify the joint line and visualize the anterior talus and the anterior aspect of the OLT (Fig. 19.3B).
- Open the flexor retinaculum to identify and protect the posterior tibial tendon (PTT) (Fig. 19.3C). The PTT runs along the groove in the posterior aspect of the medial tibia in its own sheath. With the PTT properly retracted, the posterior medial neurovascular bundle will also be protected.
- Leave as much of the periosteum as possible on the medial malleolar fragment to preserve the blood supply.
- Predrill the medial malleolus. This helps anatomical reduction of the medial malleolar osteotomy at the end of the OATS procedure.
- Create two parallel drill holes across the desired osteotomy position as perpendicular as possible to the osteotomy plane. The orientation of these drill holes would be the same as screws placed for conventional open reduction and internal fixation for medial malleolar fractures (Fig. 19.4A).
- It is crucial to confirm the proper course for these drill holes fluoroscopically, in orthogonal anteroposterior and lateral planes.
- Plan for the osteotomy to enter the tibial plafond just lateral to the OLT even if that violates the weight-bearing surface of the plafond.
- Under fluoroscopic control, introduce a K-wire obliquely to mark the desired plane and position of the osteotomy (Fig. 19.4B). Start slightly proximal and aim slightly more laterally than the intended osteotomy plane. This allows access for the saw blade and osteotome without having to remove the guide pin.
- Mark the osteotomy across the periosteum using diathermy or a marker perpendicular to the tibial shaft axis.
- Perform the osteotomy using a micro sagittal saw obliquely to the level of the tibial plafond subchondral bone parallel to the guide pin (Fig. 19.5A). Use fluoroscopic guidance periodically to confirm proper saw blade orientation.
- Use cold saline irrigation to reduce the risk of heat osteonecrosis.
- Stop the saw at the subchondral bone level and then carefully penetrate the joint with an osteotome or chisel in a controlled manner to avoid injury to the talar dome.
- Release the PTT sheath from the medial malleolus and reflect the medial malleolus on the deltoid ligament (Fig. 19.5B).

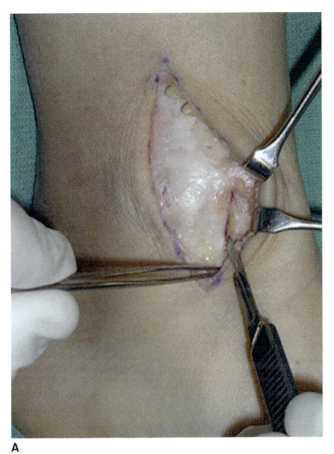
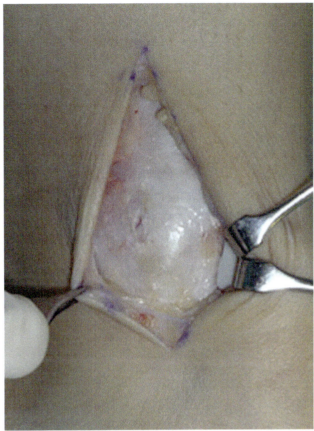
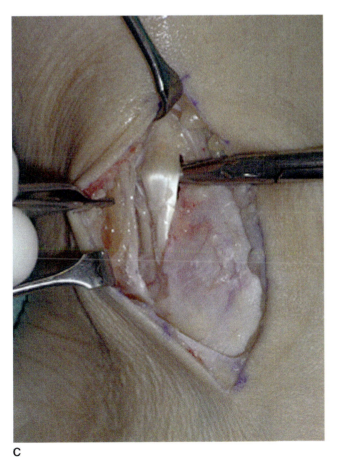

FIGURE 19.3 **A.** Medial incision for malleolar osteotomy. Locate joint and perform medial capsulotomy. **B.** Medial talar dome is visible through the arthrotomy with capsule retracted, which defines the anterior margin of the osteotomy. Osteochondral lesion of the talus may be accessed by arthrotomy alone, but this is more common for lateral lesions. **C.** The posterior tibial tendon is identified and protected during the osteotomy.

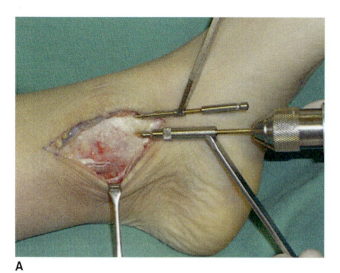
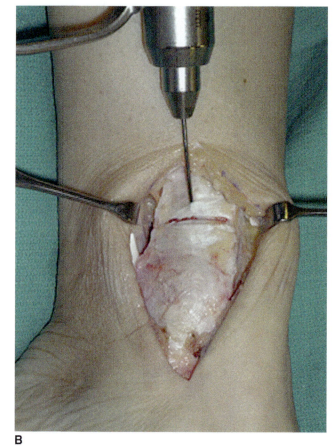

FIGURE 19.4 A. Predrilling for later placement of medial malleolar screws. **B.** K-wire defines the trajectory of the osteotomy and is inserted more proximal and lateral than the intended osteotomy.

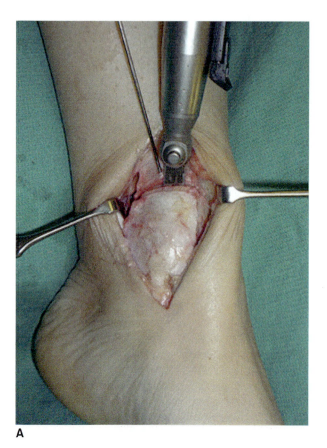
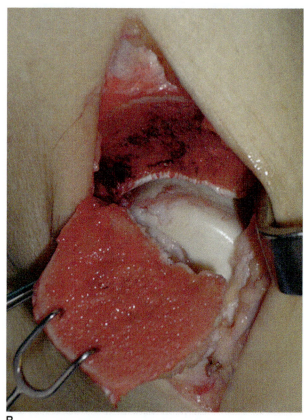

FIGURE 19.5 A. Microsagittal saw is used to perform the osteotomy, parallel with K-wire. **B.** The medial malleolus is reflected, exposing the osteochondral lesion of the talus.

Lateral Malleolar Osteotomy

Lateral molecular osteotomy is performed for access to lateral lesions of the talus. Commonly, a modified Broström lateral ankle ligaments repair is needed for lateral ankle instability. Releasing the lateral ankle ligaments (anterior talofibular ligament [ATFL] and calcaneofibular ligament [CFL]) and the capsule off the fibula as done in a Broström procedure in addition to inversion, plantar flexion, and anterior subluxation of the talus are usually sufficient to expose lateral osteochondral lesions without requiring a lateral malleolar osteotomy.

- Create a curvilinear incision extending from the posterior aspect of the fibula tip to the sinus tarsi. Careful dissection is then carried out to avoid injury to the branches of the superficial peroneal nerve anteriorly, and the sural nerve and peroneal tendons posteriorly. The incision can be extended proximally if a fibular osteotomy is needed.
- Release the joint capsule with the ATFL and CFL from the fibula similar to a modified Broström release.
- After ligament release, plantar flex, invert, and anteriorly sublux the talus. If the exposure is not sufficient with soft tissue release alone, a fibular osteotomy is added.
- Plan for a short oblique fibular osteotomy similar to the pattern created by a Weber B ankle fracture to avoid disrupting the syndesmosis ligaments.
- Mark the osteotomy starting site using cautery or a marking pen perpendicular to the long axis of the fibula. Keep periosteal stripping of the distal fibula to a minimum.
- Provisionally position a distal fibula plate on the lateral aspect of the intact fibula spanning the proposed osteotomy site.
- Predrill the fibula through the provisionally positioned plate and remove the plate.
- Identify, retract, and protect the peroneal tendons while performing the osteotomy.
- Fibular osteotomy is performed with a microsurgical saw making sure the osteotomy exits below the syndesmosis ligamentous (anterior inferior tibiofibular ligament [AITFL] and posterior inferior tibiofibular ligament) attachment (Fig. 19.6A through C).
- Use cold saline irrigation at the osteotomy site to limit osseous heat necrosis.
- Alternatively, Chaput osteotomy can be performed for centrolateral OLTs that cannot be accessed through fibular osteotomy alone. Two osteotomies are performed. The fibula is cut parallel to the tibial plafond proximal to the AITFL attachment (about 10 cm proximal to the tibial plafond). The tibial plafond is then cut at 45° in the coronal plane, aiming posterolaterally. Note that if this approach is used, care must be taken to protect the AITFL attachment. The tibial plafond is fixed with two screws, one parallel to the plafond and another one perpendicular to the osteotomy.

Recipient Site Preparation

- Débride the OLT sharply using a blade to achieve a stable circumferential rim of articular cartilage if possible (Fig. 19.7A). Ensure that the defect is contained with a bony rim all around the bone defect. The press fit will be compromised if the medial talar dome at the bone defect lacks medial wall structural integrity (Fig. 19.8). Lack of medial wall structural support such as seen in a talar shoulder legion should be identified on preoperative CT scans. Since the talus is wider at the base on the medial side, adequate bony support can be achievable in some lesions despite lack of medial cartilage rim at the top. If the OLT lacks medial bony support, structural allograft reconstruction should be considered instead of OATS.
- Assess the defect size and orientation with the sizing guide and with reference to preoperative CT (Fig. 19.7B). Larger defects may warrant two or even three graft cylinders (Fig. 19.8B).
- The assistant positions the foot and ankle in maximal eversion for medial OLTs (Fig. 19.9A). Conversely, for lateral OLTs, the foot and ankle are positioned in maximal inversion.
- Advance that chisel 11 to 12 mm into the talus (Fig. 19.9B).
- Maintain the proper recipient reamer orientation to the desired depth. Avoid changing the orientation of the reamer once it has been advanced into the subchondral bone.
- Once the reamer has been advanced to the desired depth, twist the reamer handle forcefully 90° and then 90° again (Fig. 19.9C).
- Gently toggle the reamer to separate the defective cartilage from the surrounding healthy cartilage.
- Extract the diseased osteochondral cylinder with the chisel (Fig. 19.9D).
- Alternatively, a reamer on power of corresponding size can be used to create the recipient site in sclerotic subchondral bone. Predrill the reamer guide pin to maintain desire orientation.
- If a powered reamer is used, make sure to avoid thermal osteonecrosis by irrigating with cold saline.

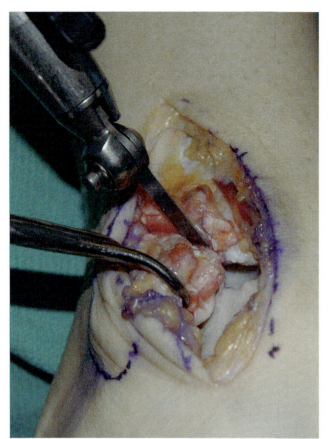
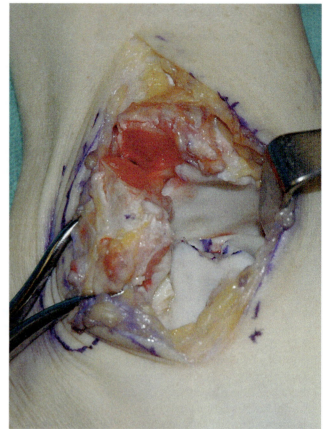
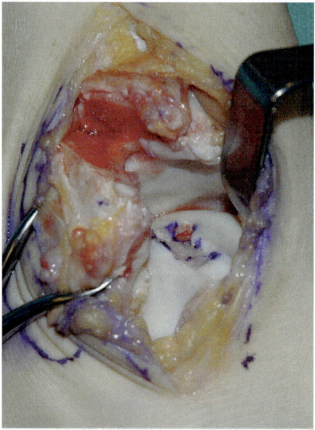

FIGURE 19.6 **A.** Lateral malleolar osteotomy performed obliquely with a microsagittal saw at the joint line for improved access, similar to creating a Weber B type ankle fracture. The syndesmotic ligaments remain intact. **B.** Towel clip applied to externally rotate malleolus. In this view, the lesion is contained laterally. **C.** Osteochondral lesion in the lateral talus exposed. In this more dorsal view, the extent of the lesion is appreciated.

19 Osteochondral Autologous Transfer Systems

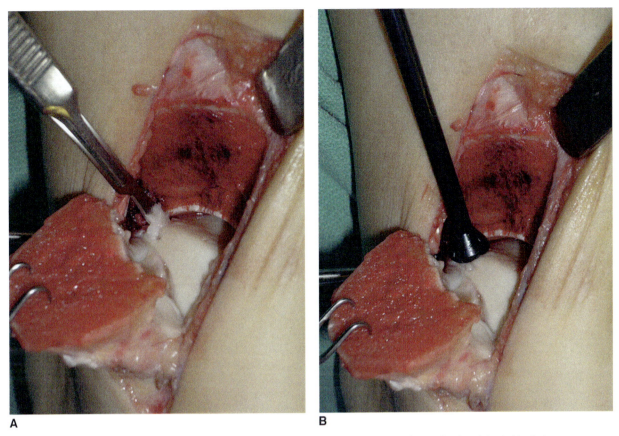

FIGURE 19.7 **A.** Débride the osteochondral lesion. **B.** The defect is sized to determine optimal recipient chisel size.

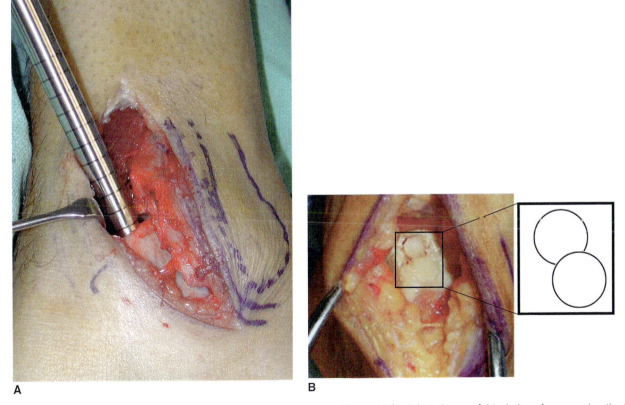

FIGURE 19.8 **A.** In addition to ligament releases, anterior tibial notching or plafondplasty is a useful technique for accessing the talar dome without an osteotomy to access a relatively posterior lateral osteochondral lesions of the talus. **B.** If the talar defect is large, multiple overlapping plugs are inserted, as in a Venn diagram.

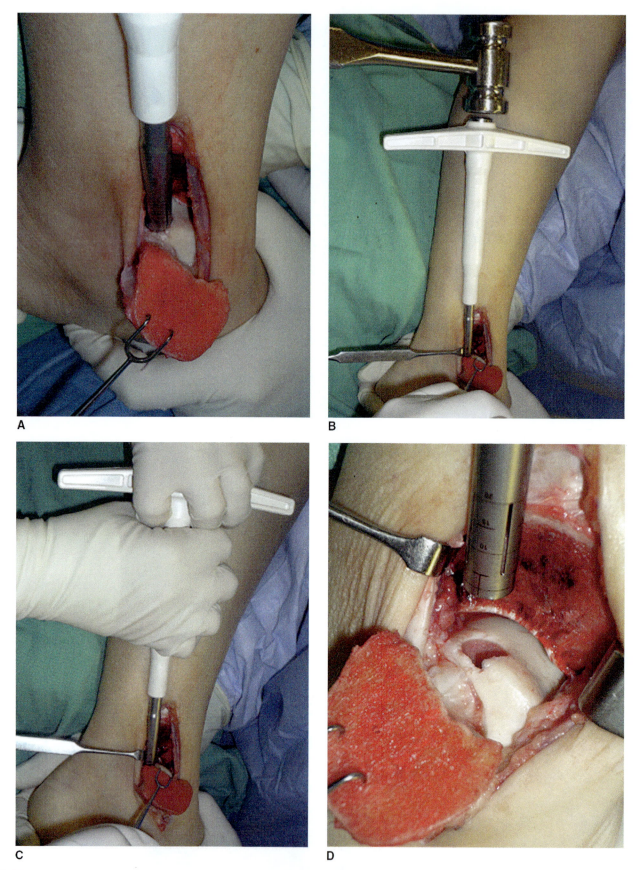

FIGURE 19.9 **A.** Evert the ankle to permit vertical access of the recipient chisel. **B.** Recipient chisel oriented properly on the osteochondral lesion, without violating the medial talar dome subchondral bone, keeping the defect contained. Mallet used to advance chisel. **C.** Once fully seated, chisel is twisted to free the diseased cartilage cylinder. **D.** Recipient site is prepared. A slight medial cartilage defect is seen, but the recipient site is still contained.

Osteochondral Graft Harvesting From Ipsilateral Superior Lateral Femoral Condyle

- Perform a superolateral arthrotomy with the knee extended, immediately lateral to the patella (Fig. 19.10A through C).
- Choose the optimal site for graft harvesting. Use the same sizing guide as was used for the recipient site to determine the proper trajectory for the harvesting reamer.
- Select the corresponding donor reamer. The diameter of this reamer is 1 mm larger than the recipient's reamer to allow for press fit of the graft into the recipient site (Fig. 19.11A).
- Be extra careful not to contact the cartilage surface with the reamer until proper reamer position and trajectory has been confirmed. The tip of the donor reamer is sharp and will cut the cartilage with the slightest pressure.
- Perpendicular to the harvest side, impact the reamer to a depth of 10 mm (1 to 2 mm less than the depth of the recipient hole). Make sure you do not change the orientation of the reamer once it has been advanced (Fig. 19.11B).
- Use the depth markings on the reamer to judge the depth and importantly to maintain perpendicular alignment by keeping the cartilage perpendicular to the markings.
- Once depth has been achieved, rotate the reamer handle 90° and then 90° again (Fig. 19.11C).
- Gently toggle the reamer to release the graft and remove the reamer from the knee.
- Note that the graft is not to be removed from the reamer at any time until it is delivered into the recipient site.

Osteochondral Graft Transfer

- Before the graft is transferred into the recipient site, the base of the recipient site should be carefully smoothed out using rongeurs, curettes, or a power reamer if the base is sclerotic. Cysts should be packed with calcaneal bone graft. Then inject 1 to 2 mL of bone marrow aspirate concentrate into the recipient hole. Properly orient the donor reamer over the recipient site and maintain contact with the reamer directly over the defect (Fig. 19.12A).

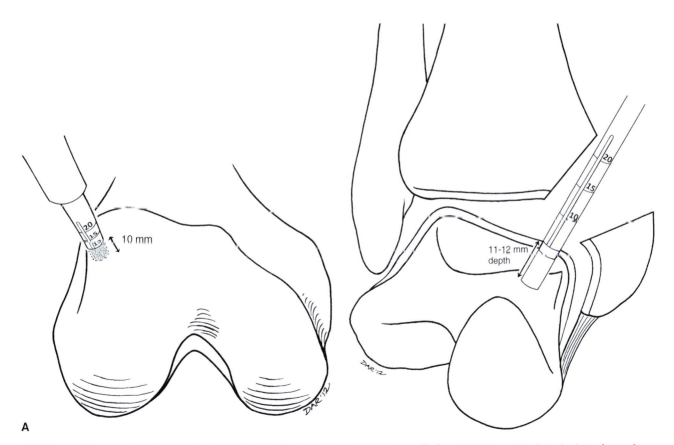

FIGURE 19.10 A. Drawing of osteochondral autograft transfer systems procedure. **B.** Superolateral approach to the knee for graft harvesting. **C.** Lateral knee arthrotomy performed.

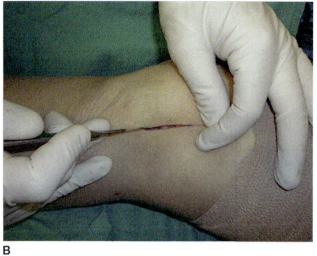
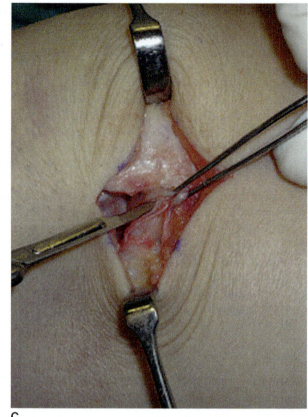

FIGURE 19.10 (Continued)

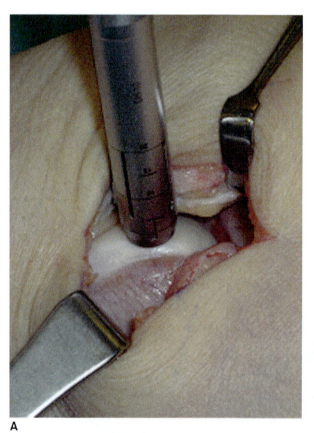
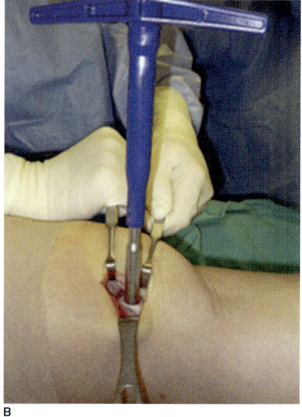

FIGURE 19.11 **A.** Superolateral femoral condyle exposed with patella retracted medially. Donor chisel oriented to allow optimal graft harvesting. **B.** Harvesting chisel impacted without changing trajectory once chisel is introduced. **C.** Chisel is fully seated, then twisted to free the cylindrical graft.

19 Osteochondral Autologous Transfer Systems

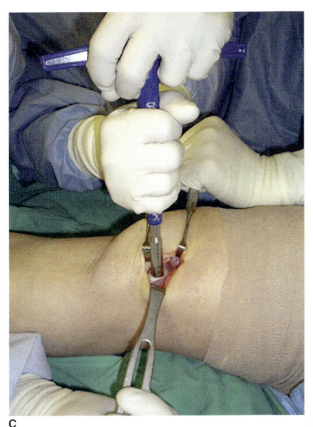

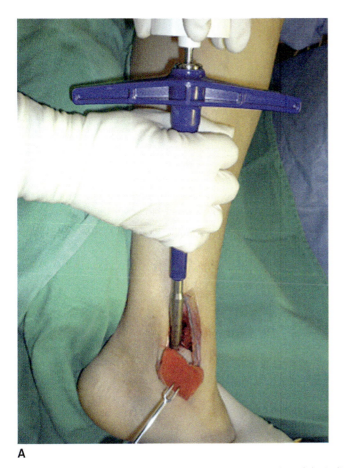

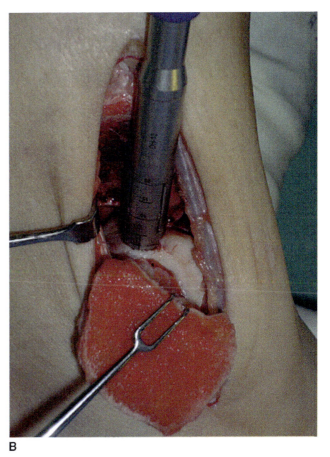

FIGURE 19.11 *(Continued)*

FIGURE 19.12 **A.** Donor chisel with graft oriented with recipient site. Tamp within the chisel advances the graft into the recipient site. **B.** Fenestrations in chisel confirm that graft is advancing. Chisel typically releases graft before it is fully seated. **C.** Graft is sitting slightly high relative to the adjacent cartilage and should be adjusted.

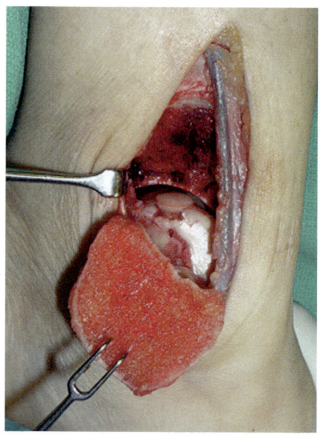

FIGURE 19.12 *(Continued)* **C**

- Advance the graft into the recipient site by advancing the tamp within the donor reamer (Fig. 19.12B).
- Through the fenestrations in the reamer, visualize that the graft is being advanced (Fig. 19.12C).
- A corresponding tamp or sizing guide can be used to carefully achieve optimal final graft position by gently tapping the graft into position (Fig. 19.13A through C). Be careful when manipulating the graft as the cartilage may shear off of the bone or the bone may fragment. If there is minimal defect around the graft cartilage cap, micronized allogenic cartilage extracellular matrix can be used around the cartilage rim of the graft to achieve a better seal with improved outcomes.[9]
- Not all OTLs are circular in shape, and multiple grafts may be needed based on the size and geometry of the defect. Grafts can be inserted side by side, or in a snowman configuration. In the latter, two grafts of similar or different diameters overlap one another to cover the entirety of the OTL. Regardless of the technique used, space between grafts should be avoided.

Closure

Medial Malleolus Osteotomy Closure

- Reduce the medial malleolus using a pointed reduction clamp. Temporarily place a drill bit into one of the predrilled holes on the medial malleolus to orient the reduction used as a joystick to find the hole on the tibia and advance that drill bit into position.
- Use a partially threaded long cancellous compression screw to fix the medial malleolus while keeping the drill bit in place to prevent rotations. Remove the drill bit and insert the second screw (Fig. 19.14).
- If there is concern about shortening, fully threaded screws can be used while avoiding overcompression.
- Confirm anatomical reduction by lining up the medial malleolus with the tibial plafond anteriorly and using intraoperative fluoroscopy to obtain standard three ankle views. Fluoroscopy should confirm anatomical reduction and extraarticular screw position (Fig. 19.15).
- A medial buttress plate can also be added, depending on the stability of the osteotomy.
- Approximate the flexor retinaculum with the PTT in its anatomical position and close the anterior ankle arthrotomy. Close the knee arthrotomy and approximate the subcutaneous layers and skin for the knee and ankle.

19 Osteochondral Autologous Transfer Systems

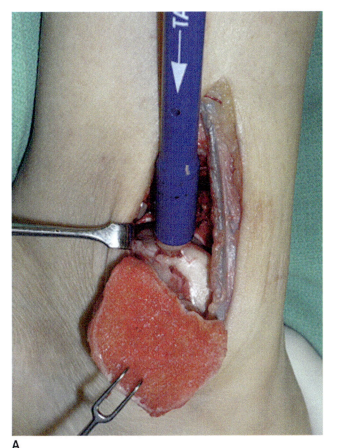

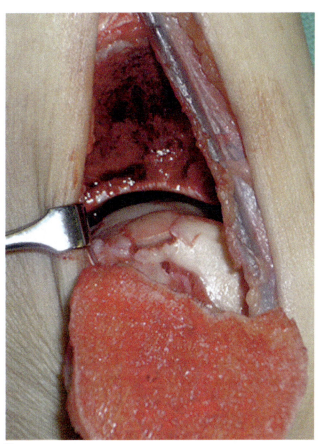

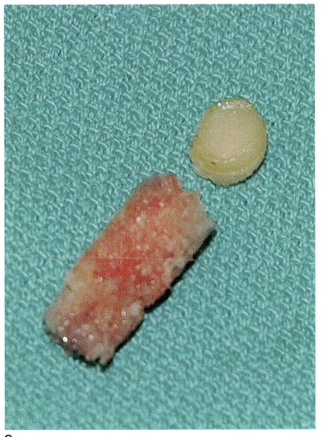

FIGURE 19.13 **A.** Smooth tamp used to perform final seating of graft. The tamp is tapped lightly to advance graft in a graduated manner. **B.** Graft seated flush with surrounding native cartilage. Medial articular defect is not fully resurfaced, but the majority of osteochondral lesion is resurfaced with stable graft. **C.** This harvested osteochondral cylinder was manipulated after being removed from the harvesting chisel, resulting in the cartilage cap being sheared from the bone. We recommend leaving the osteochondral cylinder in the chisel during graft transfer.

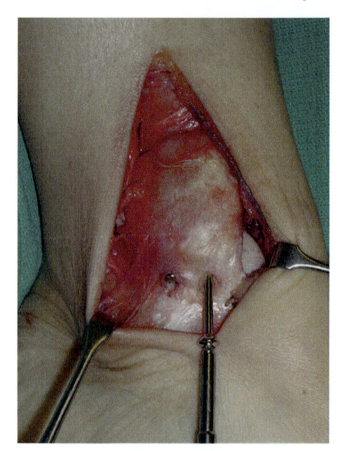

FIGURE 19.14 Osteotomy reduced and secured with two malleolar screws placed in the predrilled holes. View through arthrotomy confirms reduction of anterior tibial plafond.

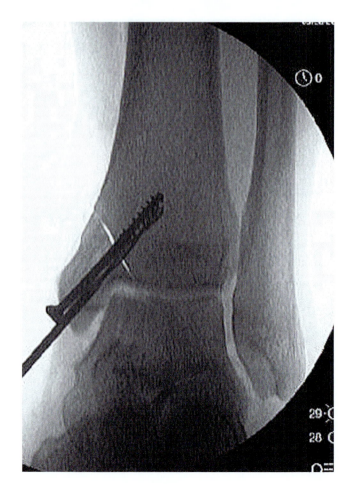

FIGURE 19.15 Anteroposterior radiograph shows a small gap in the medial malleolar osteotomy after fixation, despite anatomic reduction. This is anticipated and due to the thickness of the saw blade.

Lateral Malleolus Osteotomy

- At the conclusion of the cartilage repair procedure, reduce the fibula and secure the osteotomy with the predrilled lateral fibular plate.
- Confirm the reduction clinically and with intraoperative fluoroscopy.
- Proceed with Broström Gould lateral ligament repair using two suture anchors. We routinely use knotless anchors to avoid leaving prominent knots that can cause local irritation especially in thin individuals. Incorporate the inferior extensor retinaculum into the repair (Gould modification) in pants over vest fashion.
- We add an InternalBrace (Arthrex, Naples, FL) if the quality of the lateral tissues is questionable, in the setting of revision lateral ankle ligament repair, and in individuals with hindfoot varus and heavy professional athletes. Confirm the position of the internal brace at the talar neck to avoid penetration into the subtalar joint.
- Closure in layers of the arthrotomy, subcutaneous tissues, and skin of the ankle and knee.

PEARLS AND PITFALLS

Medial Malleolar Osteotomy

- The flexor digitorum longus tendon lies directly posterior to PTT and must not be mistaken for the PTT to avoid injuries to the latter while performing the osteotomy.
- Releasing the PTT sheath and inverting the foot allows for easier retraction of the PTT before performing the medial malleolar osteotomy. It also facilitates reflection of the medial malleolus after completion of the osteotomy.
- Creating a more conservative osteotomy that avoids the weight-bearing tibial plafond may not allow perpendicular access of the OLT and hinders successful OATS procedure. While an ideal osteotomy may violate the weight-bearing surface of the tibial plafond, this rarely leads to any complications if done carefully.
- Even with careful controlled osteotomy technique, the medial malleolus fragment rarely separates in a uniform plane. These minor irregularities often provide greater stability at the time of reduction.
- When reducing the osteotomy, use the drill bit inserted into the medial malleolus hole as a joystick, hole finder, temporary fixation, and antirotation device.
- Marking the drill holes with a marking pen right after drilling makes them easier to find later as you reduce the osteotomy.

Lateral Malleolar Osteotomy

- When treating lateral OLTs with lateral ankle instability, avoid using the curved J approach described by Broström. Use the lateral extensile incision instead to allow performing a lateral malleolar osteotomy and addressing peroneal tendons pathologies if needed.
- When performing lateral fibular osteotomy, the syndesmosis ligaments must not be violated.

Graft Transfer

- Never change the orientation of the donor or the recipient reamer once it has been advanced.
- Once the donor graft has been extracted it is not to be removed from the reamer at any time until it is delivered into the recipient site.
- The tip of the donor reamer is sharp and will cut the cartilage with the slightest pressure. Do not touch the cartilage until you are sure of the orientation and location.
- Grafts harvested from the ipsilateral lateral knee need to be rotated 180° before being inserted into the medial OLTs recipient site to match the talar contour.
- Knee cartilage is thicker than ankle cartilage; thus, despite having anatomic congruency of the graft and adjacent native cartilage, the graft may appear countersunk on fluoroscopy or postoperative radiographs.

POSTOPERATIVE MANAGEMENT

The postoperative plan is discussed with the patient at the preoperative visits and again on the day of surgery. The patients are instructed to remain non–weight bearing using crutches or a knee scooter (once their knee incision heals) for 6 weeks. The operative ankle remains in a short three-sided splint until their first postoperative appointment at 2 to 3 weeks postoperatively. The splint is removed, and wounds are inspected. Sutures are removed if the wounds have healed. A short leg cast is applied, which remains for 3 more weeks. At the 6 week postoperative appointment, the cast is removed, and the patients are allowed touchdown weight bearing for balance in a long boot for an additional 6 weeks. Based on their progress, patients are gradually transitioned out of the boot and ankle range of motion exercises, proprioception, strengthening, pain and swelling control modalities, and sports-specific conditioning protocols are employed by the physical therapists. We prescribe aspirin or enoxaparin based on each patient's individual risk factors for deep vein thrombosis until full mobility has been restored.

RESULTS AND COMPLICATIONS

A recently published systematic review of mid-term outcomes (mean 62.8 months) of 500 ankles that underwent OATS procedure showed good to excellent outcomes and a low complications rate.[10] The mean American Orthopaedic Foot and Ankle Society (AOFAS) score improved from 55.1 ± 6.1 preoperatively to 86.2 ± 4.5 postoperatively, with 87.4% of patients being reported as having excellent or good results.[10] They reported a 10% overall complication rate, with donor site morbidity being the most common (5%).[10] In a prospective multicenter study, Hangody et al reported 92% good to excellent results at a mean of 9.6 years' follow-up.[11] Larger prospective studies with long-term follow-up are still needed to provide superior evidence to support the encouraging findings of many smaller series with short to immediate follow-up.[8]

In a prospective study of 43 patients, Baltzer et al suggested that best results were obtained in patients with smaller defects, amenable to treatment with a single osteochondral transfer.[12] For management of type V lesions, Scranton et al demonstrated 90% good to excellent results at intermediate follow-up in 50 patients and all medial molecular osteotomies healed uneventfully.[13] Al-Shaikh et al reported an average AOFAS score of 88 points for primary cases and 91 points for those failing prior surgical treatment at intermediate follow up.[14] Imhoff et al in a long-term follow-up of OATS procedures, reported on 26 OATS procedures at an average follow-up of 12 years.[15] They reported significant improvement in AOFAS scores, Tegner scores, and VAS pain scores. Follow-up MRI scans suggested normal integration or minimal incongruity at the transplant–native cartilage interface were predictive of best AOFAS scores. They also suggested that patients undergoing OATS as a primary procedure had better function and less pain than did those undergoing OATS procedure as a revision surgery.[15]

REFERENCES

1. Elias I, Zoga AC, Morrison WB, Besser MP, Schweitzer ME, Raikin SM. Osteochondral lesions of the talus: localization and morphologic data from 424 patients using a novel anatomical grid scheme. *Foot Ankle Int.* 2007;28(2):154-161.
2. Easley ME, Latt LD, Santangelo JR, Merian-Genast M, Nunley JA II. Osteochondral lesions of the talus. *J Am Acad Orthop Surg.* 2010;18(10):616-630.
3. Ferkel RD, Zanotti RM, Komenda GA, et al. Arthroscopic treatment of chronic osteochondral lesions of the talus: long-term results. *Am J Sports Med.* 2008;36(9):1750-1762.
4. Ramponi L, Yasui Y, Murawski CD, et al. Lesion size is a predictor of clinical outcomes after bone marrow stimulation for osteochondral lesions of the talus: a systematic review. *Am J Sports Med.* 2017;45(7):1698-1705.
5. Rikken QGH, Dahmen J, Stufkens SAS, Kerkhoffs GMMJ. Satisfactory long-term clinical outcomes after bone marrow stimulation of osteochondral lesions of the talus. *Knee Surg Sports Traumatol Arthrosc.* 2021;29(11):3525-3533.
6. Bauer M, Jonsson K, Lindén B. Osteochondritis dissecans of the ankle. A 20-year follow-up study. *J Bone Joint Surg Br.* 1987;69(1):93-96.
7. Berndt AL, Harty M. Transchondral fractures (osteochondritis dissecans) of the talus. *J Bone Joint Surg Am.* 1959;41-A:988-1020.
8. Easley ME, Orr JD, Nunley JA. Osteochondral transfer procedure autologous defects in the articular cartilage for repairing talus: OATS procedure. In: Kitaoka HB, ed. *Master Techniques in Orthopaedic Surgery: Foot and Ankle.* Wolters Kluwer; 2013.
9. Drakos MC, Hansen OB, Eble SK, et al. Augmenting osteochondral autograft transplantation and bone marrow aspirate concentrate with particulate cartilage extracellular matrix is associated with improved outcomes. *Foot Ankle Int.* 2022;43(9):1131-1142.

10. Shimozono Y, Hurley ET, Myerson CL, Kennedy JG. Good clinical and functional outcomes at mid-term following autologous osteochondral transplantation for osteochondral lesions of the talus. *Knee Surg Sports Traumatol Arthrosc.* 2018;26(10):3055-3062.
11. Hangody L, Dobos J, Baló E, Pánics G, Hangody LR, Berkes I. Clinical experiences with autologous osteochondral mosaicplasty in an athletic population: a 17-year prospective multicenter study. *Am J Sports Med.* 2010;38(6):1125-1133.
12. Baltzer AW, Arnold JP. Bone-cartilage transplantation from the ipsilateral knee for chondral lesions of the talus. *Arthroscopy.* 2005;21(2):159-166.
13. Scranton PE Jr, McDermott JE. Treatment of type V osteochondral lesions of the talus with ipsilateral knee osteochondral autografts. *Foot Ankle Int.* 2001;22(5):380-384.
14. Al-Shaikh RA, Chou LB, Mann JA, Dreeben SM, Prieskorn D. Autologous osteochondral grafting for talar cartilage defects. *Foot Ankle Int.* 2002;23(5):381-389.
15. Imhoff AB, Paul J, Ottinger B, et al. Osteochondral transplantation of the talus: long-term clinical and magnetic resonance imaging evaluation. *Am J Sports Med.* 2011;39(7):1487-1493.

20 Open Reduction and Internal Fixation Fifth Metatarsal

Kenneth J. Hunt and Benjamin Ebben

INTRODUCTION

The fifth metatarsal is the most fractured metatarsal in adults.[1] Fractures involving the proximal aspect of this bone carry an incidence of 21 to 46 per 100,000 person-years.[2] The mechanism of injury is multifactorial involving a combination of foot posture, repetitive loading of the lateral foot, and the pull from the peroneus brevis and lateral band of the plantar fascia.[3] Fractures occur at multiple locations within this region and are often indiscriminately combined under the heading of a Jones fracture, named for the original describing author.[4] In order to completely understand the approach to managing these injuries, it is important to have a clear understanding of fracture location and contributing factors, including sport, foot posture, and radiographic features of the injury.

There is, at minimum, inconsistency and ambiguity surrounding the term Jones fracture in the literature. Michalski et al[1] recently revealed that there is poor interrater observer reliability among American Orthopedic Foot and Ankle Society surgeons both in defining where a Jones fracture is located along the proximal fifth metatarsal as well as the preferred management strategy for fractures in this location.[1] Multiple anatomic classification schemes have been developed that separate the base of the metatarsal into three zones based on the relationship of the fracture line to the proximal fourth and fifth intermetatarsal articulation.[5,6] Others have suggested that the classification be simplified to a 2-part anatomical system, using only metaphyseal and metadiaphyseal, to guide therapeutic approach.[7,8] Where the accepted classification of these injuries will end up is unclear and beyond the scope of this chapter. In this chapter, we will focus on the surgical treatment of fractures of the proximal metadiaphysis of the fifth metatarsal, which includes zones 2 and 3. We will refer to these injuries as Jones fractures.

INDICATIONS AND CONTRAINDICATIONS

Jones fractures do not always require surgical management, even in good surgical candidates. Historically, Jones fractures have been thought to occur in a vascular watershed area that puts these fractures at risk for nonunion or refracture when treated nonoperatively.[9] Most proximal fifth metatarsal fractures heal with nonoperative treatment, regardless of anatomic fracture classification. This was supported in a very recent large retrospective study of over 834 proximal fifth metatarsal fractures with minimum 5-year follow-up.[2] Using the classification system described by Lawrence and Botte,[6] the authors reported union rates for nonoperatively treated fractures as 97.3% with average time to union of 7.5 weeks for zone 1 fractures, 96.8% with average time to union of 7.7 weeks for zone 2, and 92.4% with average time to union of 9.2 weeks for zone 3.[2] Union can be defined clinically as pain-free ambulation and the absence of pain on palpation, as was the situation for many cases in the above study. For these particular injuries, it is recognized that radiographic union often trails clinical union or fails to occur altogether with stable asymptomatic fibrous union instead.

Based on published healing and complication rates, a decision analysis model demonstrated a preference for surgical intervention for Jones fractures.[10] In general, elderly, sedentary, and patients with significant comorbidities that might preclude healing should be offered conservative treatment for fifth metatarsal fractures. Surgery for a primary Jones fracture is typically indicated for patients with higher activity demands, and athletes with incentives that prioritize an accelerated recovery, return to play, and lower risk of refracture. In these patients, the evidence supports primary surgical management to circumvent the risk of nonunion and the associated delay in training and competition.[11,12]

Foot Morphology and Radiographic Alignment

There is a known association between foot morphology and risk of Jones fractures. However, it is not always the classic cavovarus posture commonly thought to contribute to Jones fracture risk. Hunt et al[13] demonstrated an increase in peak and mean forces at the fifth metatarsal base during sports activities in athletes with a history of Jones fractures. O'Malley et al described a 30% nonunion rate in National Basketball Association (NBA) athletes with Jones fractures, citing forefoot metatarsus adductus and a curved fifth metatarsal with a prominent base as an associated foot type.[14] Similarly, data from the National Football League (NFL) combine suggest that differences in coronal plane alignment, rather than sagittal plane alignment, were associated with Jones fractures.[15] A recent systematic review similarly indicates that it is metatarsus adductus, rather than pes cavus or hindfoot varus that correlates with Jones fracture risk.[16] Consideration should be given to foot posture in the treatment of Jones fracture. This should include supportive orthoses and braces to offload the base of the fifth metatarsal during postoperative rehabilitation. Surgical correction of foot alignment or deformity should be considered in the revision setting if a fracture recurs or does not heal despite excellent surgical technique and healing factors.

Torg's classification is useful in guiding treatment, and it must not be confused with the fracture location-based classifications mentioned earlier. The Torg classification is used to describe radiographic fracture line characteristics and serves as a surrogate for chronicity and propensity for fracture healing.[17] Type 1 fracture lines are narrow with minimal cortical hypertrophy and no intramedullary sclerosis. Type 2 and 3 fractures display increasing degrees of fracture widening, periosteal thickening, and obliteration of the medullary canal with sclerotic bone. Type 2 and 3 fractures are typically associated with higher chronic loads to the fifth metatarsal base leading up to fracture formation.

PREOPERATIVE PLANNING

The radiographic workup of Jones fracture should reveal the nature and location of the fracture and identify risk factors that might be mitigated during treatment. For a suspected Jones fracture, a weight-bearing anterior-posterior (AP), oblique, and lateral radiograph series should suffice for diagnosis, fracture classification, and surgical planning (Fig. 20.1A through C). Computed tomography (CT) is typically reserved for later in the recovery, regardless of management strategy, to confirm the presence or absence of osseous trabeculae spanning the fracture site. CT can be helpful but is not typically necessary in the diagnosis of delayed union or nonunion in the nonoperatively treated fracture setting. Persistent pain implies incomplete healing and redirecting to surgical management should be considered regardless of imaging findings. We will routinely use CT at 6 to 8 weeks postoperatively in elite-level athletes and again prior to clearance to unrestricted play. Magnetic resonance imaging (MRI) can be utilized as a diagnostic tool if there is no fracture line present on plain radiographs but bone stress injury or fracture is suspected on exam. MRI is most frequently considered in the setting of acute or chronic pain at the base of the fifth metatarsal with negative radiographs to diagnose stress fracture and stress reaction (Fig. 20.2A and B).

Other radiographic views and imaging studies may be necessary when considering deformity as a contributor to fracture nonunion or refracture. A hindfoot alignment view can quantify hindfoot varus in the cavovarus foot. Weight-bearing CT has become increasingly more available and utilized in the workup of alignment and deformity (Fig. 20.3).

SURGICAL TECHNIQUES

Intramedullary Screw Fixation

For first-time, acute fractures with Torg type 1 radiographic findings, we prefer primary treatment with a solid intramedullary screw after cannulated ream and tap. We will employ this technique first line even in patients with underlying foot posture that predispose a risk of proximal fifth metatarsal injury, such as cavovarus deformity, metatarsus adductus, and chronic lateral ankle instability. For this situation, we will also routinely incorporate orthobiologic augmentation. For acute fractures, bone marrow aspirate (BMA) or bone marrow aspirate concentrate (BMAC) is utilized because it

20 Open Reduction and Internal Fixation Fifth Metatarsal

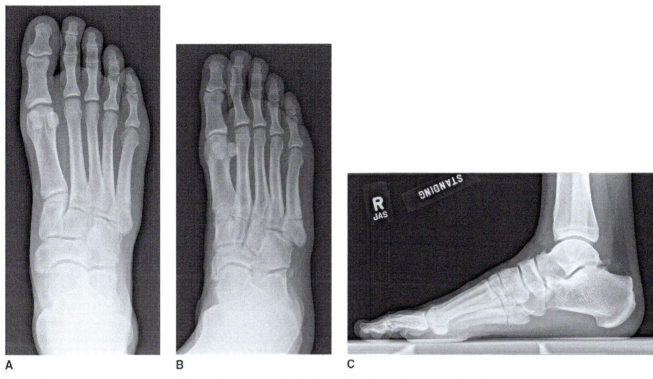

FIGURE 20.1 Anteroposterior **(A)**, oblique **(B)**, and lateral **(C)** radiographs of elite athlete with Jones fracture.

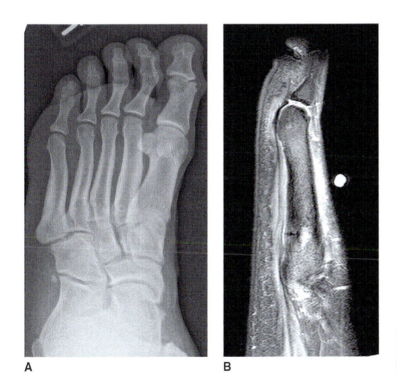

FIGURE 20.2 Oblique radiograph **(A)** and T2-weighted magnetic resonance imaging image **(B)** of fifth metatarsal stress fracture with mild bone edema.

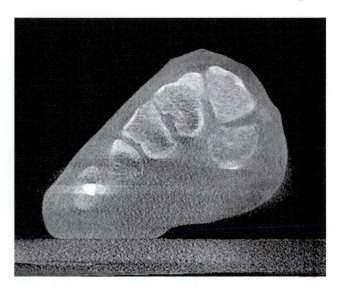

FIGURE 20.3 Coronal weight-bearing computed tomography scan showing loading on lateral foot at the base of the fifth metatarsal due to cavovarus alignment.

can be injected into the nonsclerotic fracture site percutaneously, eliminating soft tissue dissection and potential vascular disruption associated with alternative open augmentation options. We reserve open grafting for cases that already obligate direct open access to the fracture site such as in a sclerotic Torg 3 fracture or revision setting.

For the intramedullary screw technique, optimization of patient positioning and fluoroscopy setup is paramount and meticulous attention here will facilitate the establishment of an optimal guidewire start point and trajectory prior to cannulated drilling. It is helpful to use the large C-arm image intensifier platform as an extension of the operating room table (Fig. 20.4). For this, we position the patient semilateral with a large bump beneath the ipsilateral hip. It is surgeon preference whether or not to use tourniquet, but it does not typically need to be inflated for percutaneous screw placement. The C-arm image intensifier can be sterilely draped with the operative extremity and included in the sterile

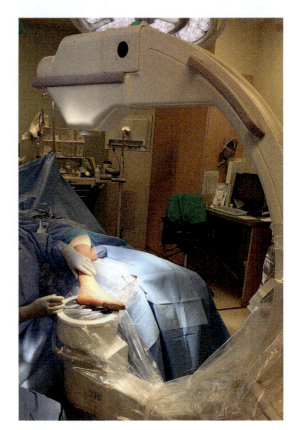

FIGURE 20.4 Intraoperative photograph depicting image intensifier within the sterile field. This allows easy imaging of the foot during pin and screw placement.

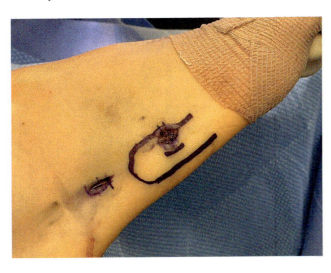

FIGURE 20.5 Clinical photograph depicting location of skin incision, centered approximately 2 cm proximal to the fifth metatarsal base.

field. In order to obtain an AP fluoroscopic image, the operative hip is slightly flexed and externally rotated. The operative knee is flexed and this enables placement of the foot plantigrade on the image intensifier. In order to obtain a lateral image, the hip is internally rotated back to neutral and the knee is extended. The hip can then be abducted and the foot elevated off the image intensifier toward the fluoroscopy transducer. This setup eliminates the need for back and forth C-arm maneuvering, which can be time-consuming at the beginning of the case when trying to establish the optimal start point.

Palpate and draw out the anatomic landmarks, specifically the base of the fifth metatarsal and the peroneus brevis insertion. The peroneus brevis tendon will be dorsal to the percutaneous incision used for guidewire placement. It is standard to place this incision roughly 1 to 2 cm posterior to the proximal fifth metatarsal tuberosity. This will also be influenced by patient body habitus and foot size. Fluoroscopy can be used to plan the skin incision with a guidewire placed on top of the skin directed down the center of the intramedullary canal. Then place a mark in line with the guidewire about 2 cm proximal to the base of the fifth metatarsal. This is the location of the longitudinal incision (Fig. 20.5).

After incision, the soft tissues should always be spread with a hemostat, in-line with the eventual guidewire placement, down to bone. This technique is recommended to avoid injuring the peroneus brevis tendon or the sural nerve, which typically resides within a few millimeters dorsally. Use of cannulated guides for all drilling and canal preparation is critical to avoid soft tissue injury.

Guidewire positioning dictates the success of the case. Use a pin guide to protect surrounding soft tissues as you place the pin against the base of the fifth metatarsal. It is important to remain

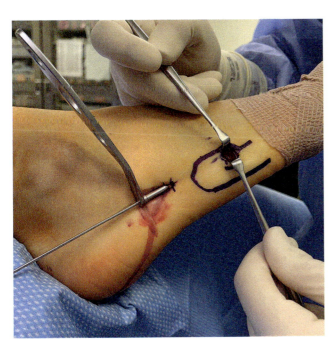

FIGURE 20.6 Clinical image depicting placement of pin guide to allow pin placement without risk to surrounding soft tissues.

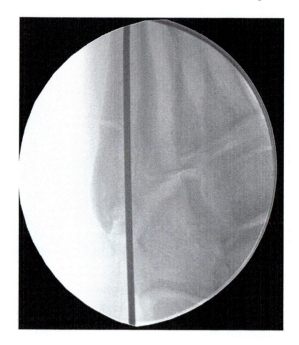

FIGURE 20.7 Intraoperative fluoroscopic image demonstrating placement of pin as medial as possible.

against the cuboid and as superior as possible while remaining in line with the fifth metatarsal canal (Fig. 20.6). The phrase "high and inside" can aide in remembering the ideal start point relative to the proximal fifth metatarsal tuberosity (Fig. 20.7). The goal is to position the entry point of the guidewire dorsal and medial to the tip of the tuberosity.[18] The start point determines the final screw head position and correct placement can avoid potential complications like impingement on the cuboid and cuboid edema syndrome.[19]

Once the pin is confirmed in the correct position on orthogonal fluoroscopic images, a 3.2-mm cannulated drill is advanced over the pin to create a start point in the metatarsal. Once the intramedullary canal is penetrated, the drill is advanced on reverse along the wire across the fracture site and just past the anticipated end point of the screw (Fig. 20.8). The drill is then removed and sequential cannulated taps are applied to provide a path for the screw. It is important to hold the fracture manually reduced during the tap to avoid distraction across the fracture site during screw placement (Fig. 20.9). It is important to ensure that the tap advances

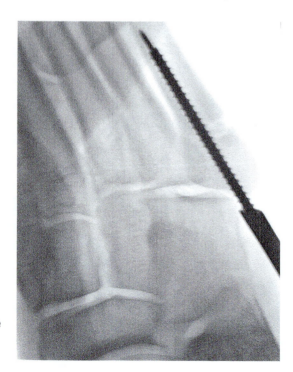

FIGURE 20.8 Intraoperative fluoroscopic oblique image demonstrating a cannulated 3.2-mm drill to initiate the screw tract past the fracture site.

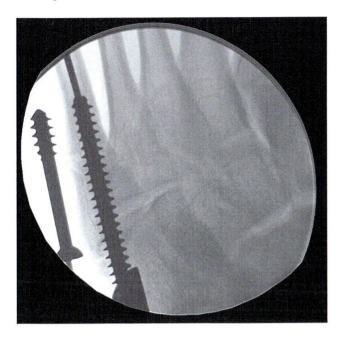

FIGURE 20.9 Intraoperative fluoroscopic image depicting placement of a 6.5-mm tap over the intramedullary pin. Note the selected screw placed within the fluoroscopy field to confirm sufficient tap length to accommodate the screw.

just beyond the tip of the screw once inserted. The goal is to get all threads of the screw across the fracture site to maximize compression, while keeping the screw length just short of the apex of curvature of the fifth metatarsal. The authors will place the screw against the foot and obtain a fluoroscopic image to confirm appropriate tap and screw length before insertion (Fig. 20.9). The diameter of the screw is determined based on the torque noted during the tap process. Once there is enough torque to cause movement of the metatarsal, slow down the pace of the tap, allowing the bone to acclimate. That is the correct diameter. The vast majority of cases call for a 5.5- or 6.5-mm diameter screw.

Finally, the pin is removed and the selected solid screw is placed through the same incision. Ensure adequate tension on the screw and compression of the fracture on fluoroscopy before disengaging the screw driver from the screw head to avoid the challenge of re-engaging percutaneously. Biplanar fluoroscopic images should be obtained to confirm screw placement (Fig. 20.10). The wounds are then irrigated with sterile saline and repaired with nonabsorbable suture.

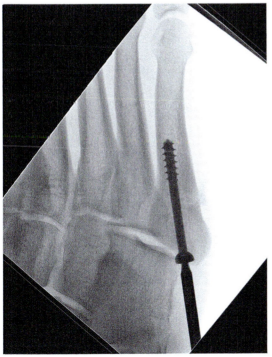

A

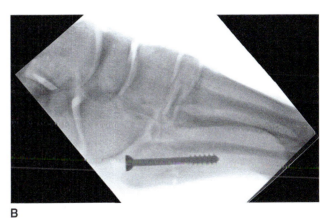

B

FIGURE 20.10 Anteroposterior **(A)** and lateral **(B)** fluoroscopic images confirming placement of screw and compression of fracture.

HARVESTING BMA AND CANCELLOUS AUTOGRAFT

Even in primary cases, it can be helpful to supplement with orthobiologics. Biologic augmentation can result in higher union rates.[20] There are a number of factors to consider in deciding whether and which biologics to incorporate, including cost, added risk, invasiveness, fracture displacement, and outcomes data. The injection of BMAC, with or without demineralized bone matrix (DBM), is a safe and inexpensive means of adding growth factors to the fracture site during surgery with high associated union rates.[21] Prior to injecting any biologic, it is helpful to prepare the fracture site unless the fracture is truly nondisplaced. Through a percutaneous technique, a small curette can be used to débride cancellous bone at the fracture site (Fig. 20.11A). The periosteum is gently elevated on both sides of the fracture to prepare space for graft material. Bone marrow is aspirated from the iliac crest as this is the site with the highest concentration of growth factors and progenitor cells.[22] BMAC is then mixed with DBM to form a paste, and this paste is injected into the intramedullary canal and subperiosteal area of the fracture through a percutaneous incision (Fig. 20.11B). The material should be injected just before screw placement while the fracture is more mobile and

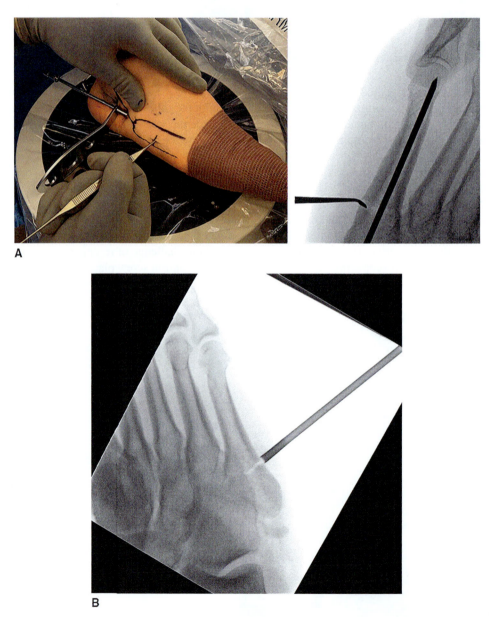

FIGURE 20.11 **A.** A small curette is used to débride fracture margins percutaneously. **B.** Intraoperative fluoroscopic image demonstrating placement of bone marrow aspirate/demineralized bone matrix into and around the fracture site.

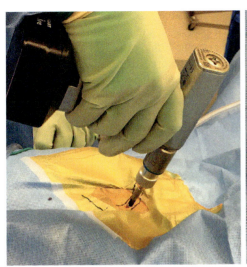
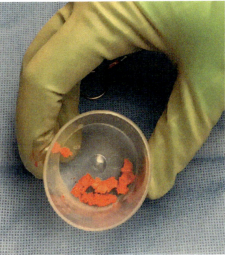

FIGURE 20.12 Clinical photographs depicting harvest of iliac crest cancellous autograft using a 7-mm trephine through a small incision over the iliac crest. Sufficient bone is typically harvested in one to two passes with the trephine.

fracture cleft access is easier. Ideally, the BMAC/DBM is injected after the screw has been started, but before it crosses the fracture site in order to prevent proximal extravasation from the intramedullary canal.

A recent systematic review of 26 studies and 718 surgically treated Jones fractures found an increased union rate (98.5% versus 93.8%) in fractures fixed with biologic augmentation.[20] No differences were found in pooled time to union, return to play rate, time to return to play, or refracture risk. Another study of revision cases described a 100% union rate with biologic augmentation using iliac crest cancellous autograft or BMAC combined with DBM.[21]

In cases where there is sclerosis along the fracture margin, or in cases of nonunion or refracture, the authors prefer to apply cancellous autograft from the iliac crest. This is performed by making a small incision over the fracture site on the lateral/plantar border of the bone. The periosteum is incised, exposing the bone and fracture site. It is important to preserve the periosteum and close this as a separate layer after the graft is placed. A small curette or burr can then be introduced and the fracture edges aggressively débrided to disrupt sclerotic bone formation and facilitate the unimpeded flux of blood and growth factors across the fracture. We prefer harvesting of cancellous autograft from the ipsilateral iliac crest using a cannulated trephine (Fig. 20.12). The graft is then packed into the prepared fracture site. It is important to pack in the bone graft before compressing the fracture with screw or plate. The periosteum is then closed followed by skin.

PEARLS AND PITFALLS OF INTRAMEDULLARY SCREW

- A start point that is relatively plantar will create a screw trajectory that is plantar to dorsal and risks perforation of the dorsal cortex in the distal segment. This trajectory will also limit screw length.
- There is a natural lateral bowing to most fifth metatarsal shafts. The degree of bowing varies from none to a type 2 bunionette deformity. On the AP radiographic view, the planned screw length should not extend into the area of bowing as the placement of a stiff intramedullary screw will induce a medial deviation of the distal fragment and cause lateral gapping at the fracture site. In the author's experience, screw lengths from 36 to 50 mm achieve this goal.

SURGICAL TECHNIQUE: PLANTAR PLATING

Plantar or plantar lateral plating is an increasingly accepted technique for Jones fractures. Conceptually, a plantar plate will provide compression on the tension side of the bone, thus reducing the risk of fracture gapping with weight-bearing activities. Plating has been shown to have biomechanical superiority to intramedullary screw fixation.[23] The plating technique has been associated with excellent results in the elite athlete population.[24] The authors prefer plantar plating for the setting of nonunions, particularly in cases where foot posture increases tension forces on the fifth metatarsal base.

The plating technique entails a single incision over the fracture site, providing enough space to fit a plate on the plantar lateral cortex of the bone (Fig. 20.13). Cancellous autograft is applied to the fracture site and the compression holes in the plate are utilized to maximize bone contact and compression. Postoperative rehabilitation is similar to the screw technique with careful monitoring of the surgical incision for healing before allowing weight bearing. If there is concern about fracture stability and/or osteopenia, a dual plating technique can be used to allow early weight bearing without risk of hardware failure (Fig. 20.14).

PEARLS AND PITFALLS OF PLANTAR PLATING

- For all open approaches in the treatment of proximal fifth metatarsal fractures, we recommend meticulous development of dorsal and plantar periosteal flaps (see Fig. 20.6). Closure of this layer helps ensure containment of bone graft and other biological augments. This is readily achievable in cases of intramedullary fixation but can be difficult with plantar plating as the added bulk of the plate may limit excursion of the plantar periosteal flap. In this situation, it is okay to incorporate fascia from the abductor digiti minimi.

POSTOPERATIVE MANAGEMENT

Postoperatively, the authors place the patient into a non–weight-bearing, well-padded splint for 10 to 14 days. Then sutures are removed and the patient is allowed to weight bear as tolerated in a short controlled ankle motion (CAM) boot. We prefer a CAM boot to a sandal since this has been shown to create a better loading environment than a sandal or athletic shoe.[25] The boot is discontinued at 6 weeks postoperatively if the fracture appears healed on radiographs. We will obtain a CT scan to confirm healing in athletes at 8 weeks postsurgery. If healing is present, the athlete is allowed to advance into shoes and begin a return to sport program, carefully monitoring for foot symptoms. Nonimpact and light load activities can be initiated at 2 weeks postoperatively once the incision has healed. Return to play is allowed when an athlete is able to participate in full speed training sessions without pain. In the author's experience, this is typically around 10 to 12 weeks.

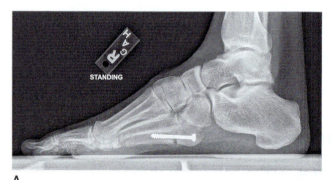
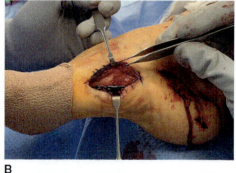
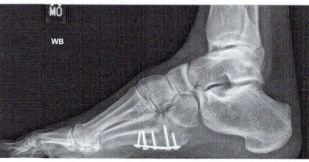

FIGURE 20.13 Preoperative lateral radiograph **(A)** demonstrating cavus foot with nonunion of Jones fracture. Intraoperative photograph **(B)** demonstrating placement of plantar compression plate with iliac crest autograft at nonunion site, and postoperative lateral radiograph **(C)** demonstrating a healed fracture.

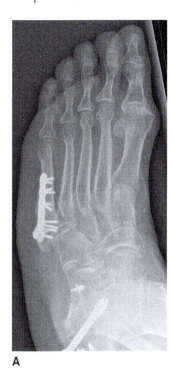
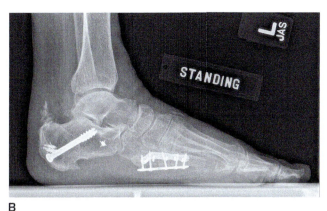

FIGURE 20.14 Oblique **(A)** and lateral **(B)** radiographs demonstrating a dual plating technique in patient with an unstable fracture and osteopenia.

RESULTS AND COMPLICATIONS

Published outcomes following Jones fracture surgery are, for the most part, excellent.[11,12,14,21,26] Most athletes are able to return to sport and it is exceedingly rare that a Jones fracture would end an athletic career, even if a revision surgery is required. Still, the reported complication rate following surgery for Jones fractures is as high as 19%.[27] The most common complication following operative treatment of Jones fractures is refracture or nonunion, representing half of all complications. It can be difficult to differentiate between these two results. While the overall nonunion rate has been reported as only 4% when taking into account the published literature,[12] certain populations of athletes have demonstrated a higher nonunion rate. O'Malley et al described a 30% nonunion rate in NBA athletes treated surgically for Jones fractures.[14] Anderson et al[26] described a 12% refracture rate in NFL athletes with Jones fractures treated with intramedullary screws, requiring reoperation in the refracture group. All athletes ultimately returned to sport and there was an association between timing of return to sport and refracture risk.[26] Early return to sport may delay fracture healing in soccer but may not impact the long-term union rate.[28]

Other complications include symptoms related to the screw and rarely wound healing complications.[27] More serious complications, including thermal necrosis and osteomyelitis, have been described in the Japanese literature,[29] underscoring the critical importance of careful technique and counseling patients with regard to surgical risks prior to Jones fracture surgery.

CONCLUSION

Jones fractures are a very common injury in the active population. While there is a role for nonoperative management for these injuries in some patients, there remains a tendency to treat Jones fractures surgically due to accelerated return to sport and reduced refracture risk associated with operative treatment. Surgical techniques and implants have evolved, but the gold standard treatment for acute Jones fractures remains a percutaneously placed intramedullary screw, with or without biologic augmentation. Revision techniques are effective in cases of nonunion or refracture. In a revision setting, for cases of nonunion or refracture after primary surgical fixation, predisposing foot posture factors may need to be addressed. This is considered on a case by case basis and may involve osteotomies to correct metatarsus adductus and/or hindfoot varus.

REFERENCES

1. Michalski MP, Ingall EM, Kwon JY, Chiodo CP. Reliability of fifth metatarsal base fracture classifications and current management. *Foot Ankle Int.* 2022;43(8):1034-1040.
2. Pettersen PM, Radojicic N, Grun W, Andresen TKM, Molund M. Proximal fifth metatarsal fractures: a retrospective study of 834 fractures with a minimum follow-up of 5 years. *Foot Ankle Int.* 2022;43:602-608.
3. DeVries JG, Taefi E, Bussewitz BW, Hyer CF, Lee TH. The fifth metatarsal base: anatomic evaluation regarding fracture mechanism and treatment algorithms. *J Foot Ankle Surg.* 2015;54:94-98.
4. Jones RI. Fracture of the base of the fifth metatarsal bone by indirect violence. *Ann Surg.* 1902;35(6):697-700.
5. Dameron TB Jr. Fractures of the proximal fifth metatarsal: selecting the best treatment option. *J Am Acad Orthop Surg.* 1995;3:110-114.
6. Lawrence SJ, Botte MJ. Jones' fractures and related fractures of the proximal fifth metatarsal. *Foot Ankle.* 1993;14:358-365.
7. Chuckpaiwong B, Queen RM, Easley ME, Nunley JA. Distinguishing Jones and proximal diaphyseal fractures of the fifth metatarsal. *Clin Orthop Relat Res.* 2008;466:1966-1970.
8. Polzer H, Polzer S, Mutschler W, Prall WC. Acute fractures to the proximal fifth metatarsal bone: development of classification and treatment recommendations based on the current evidence. *Injury.* 2012;43:1626-1632.
9. Smith JW, Arnoczky SP, Hersh A. The intraosseous blood supply of the fifth metatarsal: implications for proximal fracture healing. *Foot Ankle.* 1992;13:143-152.
10. Bishop JA, Braun HJ, Hunt KJ. Operative versus nonoperative treatment of jones fractures: a decision analysis model. *Am J Orthop (Belle Mead NJ).* 2016;45:E69-E76.
11. Attia AK, Taha T, Kong G, Alhammoud A, Mahmoud K, Myerson M. Return to play and fracture union after the surgical management of jones fractures in athletes: a systematic review and meta-analysis. *Am J Sports Med.* 2021;49:3422-3436.
12. Roche AJ, Calder JD. Treatment and return to sport following a Jones fracture of the fifth metatarsal: a systematic review. *Knee Surg Sports Traumatol Arthrosc.* 2013;21:1307-1315.
13. Hunt KJ, Goeb Y, Bartolomei J. Dynamic loading assessment at the fifth metatarsal in elite athletes with a history of jones fracture. *Clin J Sport Med.* 2021;31:e321-e326.
14. O'Malley M, DeSandis B, Allen A, Levitsky M, O'Malley Q, Williams R. Operative treatment of fifth metatarsal jones fractures (zones II and III) in the NBA. *Foot Ankle Int.* 2016;37:488-500.
15. Carreira DS, Sandilands SM. Radiographic factors and effect of fifth metatarsal Jones and diaphyseal stress fractures on participation in the NFL. *Foot Ankle Int.* 2013;34:518-522.
16. Riegger M, Muller J, Giampietro A, et al. Forefoot adduction, hindfoot varus or pes cavus: risk factors for fifth metatarsal fractures and jones fractures? A systematic review and meta-analysis. *J Foot Ankle Surg.* 2022;61:641-647.
17. Torg JS, Balduini FC, Zelko RR, Pavlov H, Peff TC, Das M. Fractures of the base of the fifth metatarsal distal to the tuberosity. Classification and guidelines for non-surgical and surgical management. *J Bone Joint Surg Am.* 1984;66:209-214.
18. Watson GI, Karnovsky SC, Konin G, Drakos MC. Optimal starting point for fifth metatarsal zone II fractures: a cadaveric study. *Foot Ankle Int.* 2017;38:802-807.
19. Roberts L, Bernasconi A, Netto CC, Elliott A, Hamilton W, O'Malley M. Cuboid edema syndrome following fixation of proximal fifth metatarsal fractures in professional athletes. *Foot Ankle Spec.* 2019;12:373-379.
20. Attia AK, Robertson GAJ, McKinley J, d'Hooghe PP, Maffulli N. Surgical management of jones fractures in athletes: orthobiologic augmentation: a systematic review and meta-analysis of 718 fractures. *Am J Sports Med.* 2022;3635465221094014.
21. Hunt KJ, Anderson RB. Treatment of Jones fracture nonunions and refractures in the elite athlete: outcomes of intramedullary screw fixation with bone grafting. *Am J Sports Med.* 2011;39:1948-1954.
22. Hyer CF, Berlet GC, Bussewitz BW, Hankins T, Ziegler HL, Philbin TM. Quantitative assessment of the yield of osteoblastic connective tissue progenitors in bone marrow aspirate from the iliac crest, tibia, and calcaneus. *J Bone Joint Surg Am.* 2013;95:1312-1316.
23. Duplantier NL, Mitchell RJ, Zambrano S, et al. A biomechanical comparison of fifth metatarsal jones fracture fixation methods. *Am J Sports Med.* 2018;46:1220-1227.
24. Bernstein DT, Mitchell RJ, McCulloch PC, Harris JD, Varner KE. Treatment of proximal fifth metatarsal fractures and refractures with plantar plating in elite athletes. *Foot Ankle Int.* 2018;39:1410-1415.
25. Hunt KJ, Goeb Y, Esparza R, Malone M, Shultz R, Matheson G. Site-specific loading at the fifth metatarsal base in rehabilitative devices: implications for Jones fracture treatment. *PM R.* 2014;6:1022-1029. quiz 9
26. Lareau CR, Hsu AR, Anderson RB. Return to play in national football league players after operative jones fracture treatment. *Foot Ankle Int.* 2016;37:8-16.
27. Dean BJ, Kothari A, Uppal H, Kankate R. The jones fracture classification, management, outcome, and complications: a systematic review. *Foot Ankle Spec.* 2012;5:256-259.
28. Miller D, Marsland D, Jones M, Calder J. Early return to playing professional football following fixation of 5th metatarsal stress fractures may lead to delayed union but does not increase the risk of long-term non-union. *Knee Surg Sports Traumatol Arthrosc.* 2019;27:2796-2801.
29. Morimoto Y, Komatsu T, Tokuhashi Y. Four cases with rare complications of intramedullary screw fixation for jones fracture. *Acta Med Okayama.* 2020;74:537-544.

21 Open Reduction and Internal Fixation of Navicular Stress Fractures

Andrew J. Rosenbaum and Martin O'Malley

INTRODUCTION

Navicular stress fractures were first described by Towne et al in 1970.[1] Although fairly uncommon, they are becomingly increasingly more recognized in the athletic population with up to 35% of all stress fractures of the foot and ankle occurring in the navicular.[2,3] The highest incidence of this fracture is seen in running and jumping athletes. Additionally, navicular stress fractures are rarely seen in nonathletes. In a systematic review by Mallee et al, 98.5% of stress fractures were in athletes.[4] Men in their mid-20s are most at risk.

The pathogenesis of navicular stress fractures remains incompletely understood. They are thought to be due to chronic overuse and repetitive loading of the bone, which predisposes individuals to microfractures, and then stress fractures. The navicular also has a relatively poor blood supply, which increases the risk for stress fractures and nonunion. The dorsalis pedis and posterior tibial arteries are responsible for the majority of the blood supply to the navicular. However, an avascular zone in the central one-third of the bone exists, rendering this region susceptible to damage.[5] Although this area of limited blood flow has traditionally been hypothesized as to why the navicular is so vulnerable to stress fractures, this theory has been refuted. In a cadaveric study by McKeon et al, 58.8% of naviculars had no avascular zones, and only 11.8% of naviculars had the classic dorsal and central hypovascular zones. For this reason, it is now felt that other factors also contribute to the development of stress fractures. Regardless of the underlying etiology, most navicular stress fractures occur at the junction between the central and lateral one-third of the bone.

Multiple intrinsic and extrinsic variables also contribute to the development of navicular stress fractures. Navicular stress fractures are most common in males, with young male athletes the most at-risk population. However, female sex is also an independent risk factor for stress fractures. Other intrinsic factors include a history of previous stress fracture, underlying metabolic bone disease, abnormal foot biomechanics, and genetics.[6] In a recent study by Becker et al, foot kinematics were evaluated between runners with and without a history of navicular stress fractures.[7] Decreased plantar flexion range of motion, greater hindfoot eversion, and reduced forefoot abduction excursion were associated with fracture.[7]

Extrinsic factors associated with navicular stress fractures include rigorous training, poor nutrition, and improper footwear. In a randomized control trial, custom orthoses were found to significantly reduce the incidence of lower extremity stress fractures.[8] Regardless of the underlying etiology, the management of navicular stress fractures is challenging and influenced by multiple variables, including fracture pattern, displacement, comorbidities, and level of activity. While no consensus exists on the optimal treatment of navicular stress fractures, the literature strongly suggests an aggressive approach with surgical intervention.[9]

CLASSIFICATION

Saxena et al developed a tarsal navicular stress fracture classification system based on computed tomography (CT) findings (Table 21.1). This classification system is important, as it helps with clinical decision-making. Type 0.5 is a stress reaction, in which findings are negative on CT and only evident on magnetic resonance imaging (MRI) (Fig. 21.1). Type I fractures are those involving the dorsal cortex (Fig. 21.2). Type II fractures extend from the dorsal cortex into the navicular body (Fig. 21.3). Type III fractures are complete fractures through both cortices (Fig. 21.4).[10]

INDICATIONS AND CONTRAINDICATIONS

Nonsurgical management of navicular stress fractures is indicated in sedentary individuals and those at high risk for complications following surgery. This includes active nicotine users and those with significant medical comorbidities, such as poorly controlled diabetes mellitus and vascular compromise. Avascular necrosis of the navicular, bipartite navicular, large intraosseous cysts, and advanced talonavicular arthritis are also contraindications for primary open reduction and internal fixation (ORIF). In patients where concern exists for compliance with postoperative weight-bearing restrictions, conservative treatment is offered. Further, stress reactions and dorsal navicular capsular avulsion fractures (type 0.5 and type 1, respectively) are initially treated nonsurgically in the absence of a concurrent stress fracture.

Torg et al published a meta-analysis of 250 cases treated nonsurgically and noted 96% success.[11] However, strict non–weight-bearing protocols for a minimum of 6 weeks are paramount to success. In a review of 86 patients with navicular stress fractures, Khan et al found an 86% healing in those made non–weight-bearing for a minimum of 6 weeks versus 20% success in those treated with

TABLE 21.1 The Saxena Classification

Type 0.5	Normal CT, evidence of stress reaction on MRI	Figure 21.1
Type 1	Dorsal cortex fracture	Figure 21.2
Type 2	Fracture extends to midpoint of navicular	Figure 21.3
Type 3	Both cortices affected	Figure 21.4

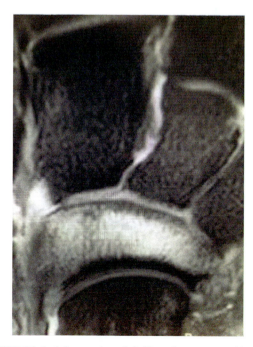

FIGURE 21.1 A Saxena type 0.5. There is pronounced bone marrow edema throughout the navicular, consistent with a stress reaction.

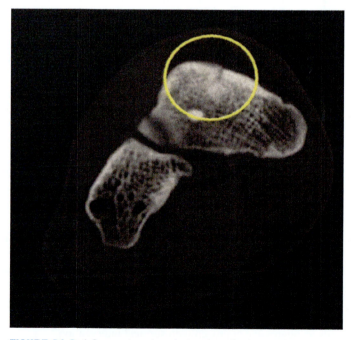

FIGURE 21.2 A Saxena type 1 navicular stress fracture.

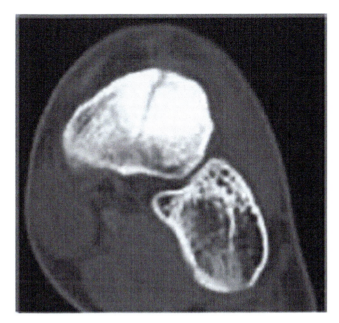

FIGURE 21.3 A Saxena type 2 navicular stress fracture.

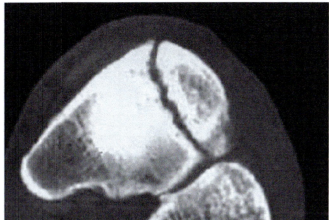

FIGURE 21.4 A Saxena type 3 navicular stress fracture.

weight-bearing casts or less than 6 weeks non–weight-bearing.[12] Other studies are less supportive of nonsurgical treatment. Fitch and colleagues found that 51% of navicular stress fractures failed conservative treatment and underwent bone grafting with subsequent good results.[13]

Open reduction and internal fixation of navicular stress fractures is warranted for type II and III fractures in athletic individuals and those with type 1 stress fractures concerned about the possibility of nonsurgical treatment failing (Table 21.2). Type 0.5 fractures are initially treated conservatively. Other indications for surgical intervention include all nonunions, failed prior nonsurgical treatment, and refracture. Although excellent outcomes have been observed in surgically treated navicular stress fractures, we let all patients know that the optimal treatment remains somewhat unclear and that nonsurgical treatments can be successfully employed at times. We, therefore, recommend surgical intervention for navicular stress fractures to professional, collegiate, and highly competitive athletes and very active individuals.

PREOPERATIVE PLANNING

The initial diagnosis of a navicular stress fracture can be challenging. Many patients present with vague discomfort that can lead to a delay in diagnosis. Initially, patients may describe medial midfoot pain and discomfort only with weight bearing or sports. Over time, the pain becomes more constant and may also be present at night. Tenderness at the "N-spot" is often seen on physical exam (Fig. 21.5). This is the area of maximal discomfort and is described as the prominence over the proximal and dorsal navicular.[14]

TABLE 21.2 Treatment Algorithm for Navicular Stress Fractures

Type 0.5 fractures	Non–weight bearing in short leg cast × 4 weeks, with transition into non–weight-bearing controlled ankle motion boot × 2 additional weeks
Type 1 fractures	Non–weight bearing versus percutaneous screw placement
Type 2 fractures	• Open reduction and internal fixation (ORIF) with bone marrow aspirate concentrate (BMAC) and graft • 1 and possibly 2 screws
Type 3 fractures	• ORIF with BMAC and graft • 1 and possibly 2 screws
Postoperative protocol	• Non–weight bearing × 6 weeks • Computed tomography (CT) scan at 6 and 10 weeks to assess healing • Return to play when evidence of healing on CT

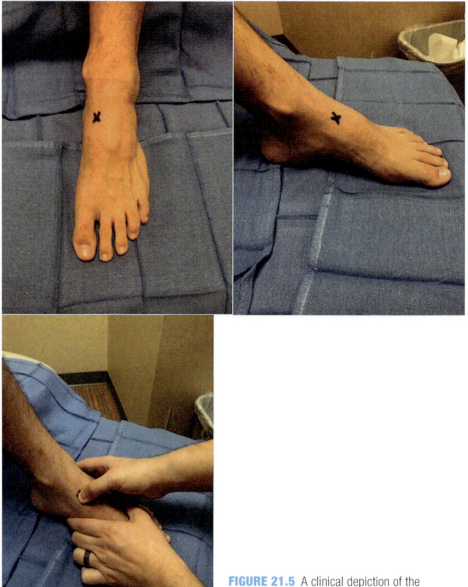

FIGURE 21.5 A clinical depiction of the "N" spot.

Weight-bearing radiographs of the foot and ankle are critical but may be normal. Khan et al found that plain radiographs were only positive in 18% of patients with CT confirmed stress fractures.[11] Despite this, plain radiographs are useful to look for concurrent pathology and foot alignment. When radiographs demonstrate a navicular stress fracture, a CT scan is obtained next (Fig. 21.6). The CT plays an important role in preoperative planning, as it provides optimal visualization of the fracture line (Fig. 21.7). This test may also aide in identifying sclerosis at the fracture margins, which is indicative of a possible nonunion. Further, CT is effective postoperatively in assessing fracture healing. Dorsal cortical proliferation can be seen as soon as 6 weeks following ORIF or initiation of nonsurgical treatment and is typically the first radiologic sign of healing.[15]

A subtle radiographic clue that a stress fracture may be present is dorsal sclerosis of the navicular. When this is present on plain films, bone scan or MRI is warranted. Even if radiographs are completely normal, an MRI or bone scan is ordered if clinical suspicion remains high. MRI is our preferred test when there are negative radiographs but high suspicion, as bone scans lack anatomic resolution and fail to depict the fracture pattern. Additionally, while a negative bone scan can rule out a navicular fracture, a positive bone scan requires CT imaging to confirm and more specifically classify the fracture (nonunion versus acute, complete versus incomplete, presence of cysts or other degenerative changes). Although MRI often provides adequate detail of the fracture, CT may be obtained as well to provide additional insight.

21 Open Reduction and Internal Fixation of Navicular Stress Fractures

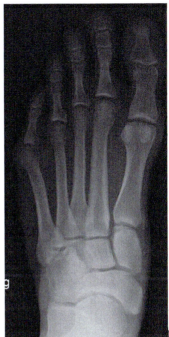

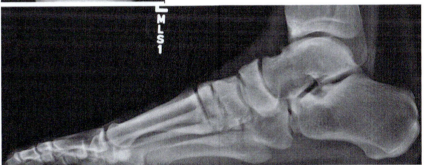

FIGURE 21.6 Anteroposterior and lateral radiographs of an 18-year-old division 1 basketball player who presented with pain in the dorsal hindfoot following an ankle sprain. Radiographs demonstrate a navicular stress fracture.

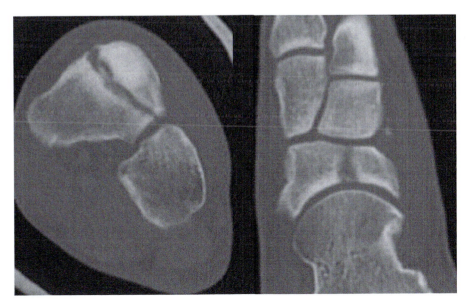

FIGURE 21.7 Coronal and axial computed tomography (CT) images of the navicular fracture seen in Figure 21.6. Note the sclerotic margins seen on the CT, consistent with a chronic process.

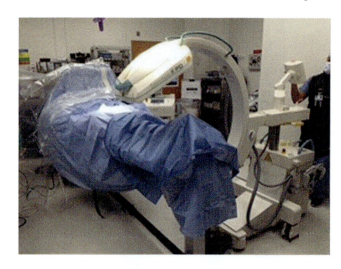

FIGURE 21.8 Photograph demonstrating the operating room setup with intraoperative three-dimensional imaging to aid in placement of fixation.

A navicular stress fracture ORIF is usually performed under regional anesthesia as outpatient surgery. If allograft or other biologics are going to be used during surgery, this is discussed with the patient prior to surgery.

SURGICAL TECHNIQUE

Regional anesthesia is administered and a thigh tourniquet is used. The patient is positioned supine with a bump under the ipsilateral hip to maintain the foot in a neutral position (Fig. 21.8). If iliac crest bone marrow aspirate concentrate (BMAC) is going to be harvested, it is done so from the ipsilateral iliac crest under sterile technique with local anesthetic (Fig. 21.9). Additionally, six dowels of bone graft are also harvested from the same entry site with the Jamshidi needle. If anterior ankle impingement symptoms are present, both bony and soft tissue causes of impingement should be addressed at the time of surgery. This can be done through arthroscopic techniques or via an anteromedial ankle arthrotomy. Patients may also have underlying foot deformity (eg, cavovarus or pes planovalgus alignment) when presenting with a navicular stress fracture. Concurrent reconstruction is rarely indicated, and such deformity is managed with custom orthoses postoperatively.

When imaging fails to demonstrate characteristics of a more chronic fracture or nonunion, a smooth Kirschner wire is placed under fluoroscopic guidance from medial to lateral in the navicular. If the

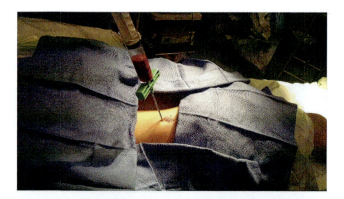

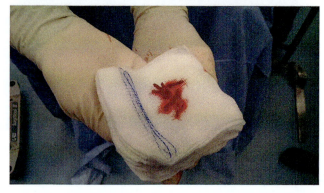

FIGURE 21.9 Iliac crest bone marrow and bone graft harvest technique.

fracture involves the lateral one-third of the bone, a lateral to medial screw is placed instead. In such instances, a small stab incision is made over the lateral aspect of the navicular to facilitate wire placement. It is important to remain as perpendicular as possible to the fracture. A 2.7-mm cannulated drill bit is then used over the wire, and a 3.5-mm drill bit is then used to overdrill the near cortex. Iliac crest BMAC is then placed into the fracture site under fluoroscopic guidance. The K-wire is then removed and the iliac crest autograft is packed into the drilled hole. A solid 3.5-mm cortical screw is than placed, achieving compression by technique across the fracture. Through an additional stab incision, a second 3.5 screw can be placed if the patient's anatomy permits or if the fracture is rotationally unstable.

For navicular fracture nonunions, or displaced fractures, a dorsal approach is used to expose the fracture. Fluoroscopy is used to identify the fracture site and a dorsal incision is made. For more medial fractures, the dissection is between the tibialis anterior and extensor hallucis longus tendons. For more lateral fractures, one dissects between the extensor hallucis longus and extensor digitorum longus tendons. It is imperative to identify and protect the superficial peroneal nerve and deep neurovascular bundle during the approach. An 18-gauge needle is helpful to identify the fracture site, and the fibrous material interposed is débrided with a dental pick and small rongeur. If the fracture is difficult to identify with fluoroscopy, intraoperative CT can be used if available. The sclerotic fracture edges are then drilled with a 1.6-mm K-wire to fenestrate the surfaces of the fracture and expose healthy cancellous tissue. Autograft and BMAC are placed at the fracture site (Fig. 21.10). One or two 3.5-mm cortical screws are then placed in a lag by technique fashion to stabilize and compress the fracture, as described above (Fig. 21.11). Separate stab incisions are often required for screw placement, which should start at either the most medial or lateral aspect of the navicular, depending on fracture location. Optimal screw position should be as close as possible to perpendicular to the fracture in all planes. This typically requires a gradual dorsal to plantar trajectory in the sagittal plane. A layered closure is then performed and the patient is immobilized in a splint and made non–weight bearing.

PEARLS AND PITFALLS

- Navicular stress fractures are uncommon injuries that predominantly occur in running or jumping athletes.
- The diagnosis of a navicular stress fracture can be challenging. If radiographs appear normal, obtain an MRI.
- If radiographs demonstrate a fracture, a CT should be performed next to better understand the fracture characteristics.
- For type 0.5 and type 1 fractures, immobilization and nonweighting for 6 weeks is crucial for healing; surgery can be considered for type 1 fractures in patients concerned about the possibility of nonsurgical treatment failing.

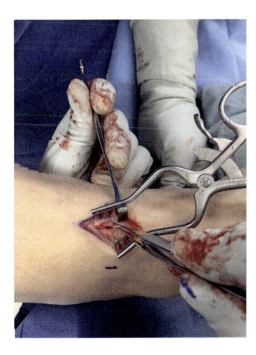

FIGURE 21.10 Placement of iliac crest autograft at the fracture site.

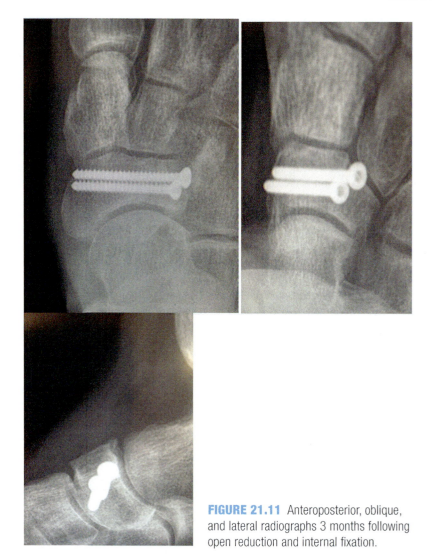

FIGURE 21.11 Anteroposterior, oblique, and lateral radiographs 3 months following open reduction and internal fixation.

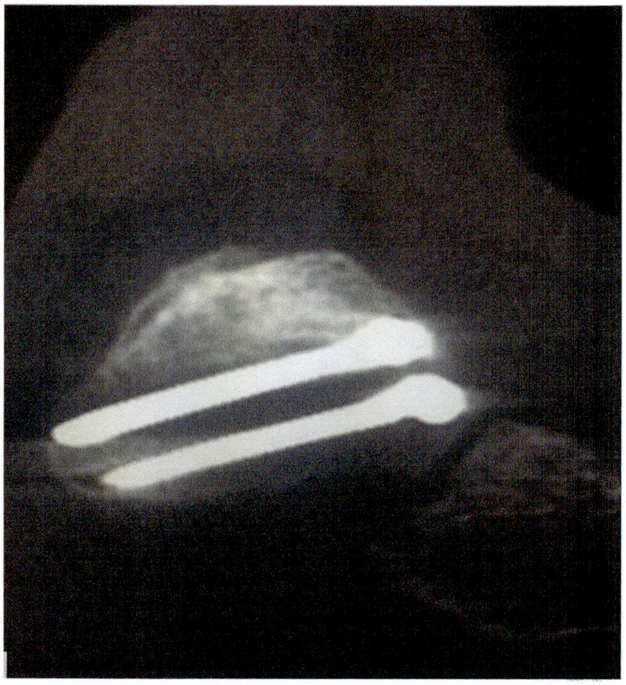

FIGURE 21.12 CT imaging confirming healing of the navicular stress fracture seen in Figure 21.11.

- Athletes benefit from early ORIF in type 2 or 3 fractures and in the setting of nonunion or refracture.
- A 3.5-mm cortical screw should be placed in a lag by technique fashion. If the initial screw has inadequate purchase, or the fracture remains rotationally unstable, a second screw should be placed.
- Screw placement should be perpendicular to the fracture for optimal compression.
- Proper screw trajectory is critical to healing and a common pitfall is screw placement perpendicular to the fracture in only one plane. Fluoroscopy or intraoperative CT should be used to ensure appropriate screw placement in all planes.
- Biologic augmentation should be performed at the time of ORIF with BMAC and/or iliac crest bone graft.
- Pack bone graft and BMAC into the fracture site both before and after screw placement (types 1, 2, and 3)
- Keep a soft tissue sleeve over navicular to protect the bone graft as the fracture is compressed during screw placement.
- Sources of anterior ankle impingement should also be addressed at time of surgery.
- Following ORIF, non–weight bearing for 6 weeks is pivotal.
- At 2 weeks postoperative, patients transitioned into non–weight-bearing controlled ankle motion boot with initiation of active range of motion exercises.
- Vitamin D and calcium supplementation may be beneficial to enhance healing.
- CT scan is performed at 6 and between 10 and 12 weeks following ORIF or the initiation of nonoperative treatment.
- Once the CT scan demonstrates healing, athletes can return to sports. This ultimately takes approximately 4 to 5 months.

POSTOPERATIVE MANAGEMENT

Patients are immobilized in a well-padded splint for the first 2 weeks after surgery. At that time, sutures are removed and they are transitioned into a boot for early range of motion. Patients are strictly non–weight-bearing for the first 6 weeks following surgery and are then permitted to gradually weight bear in the boot for another 6 weeks. CT is performed at 6 weeks and between weeks 10 and 12 to assess healing (Fig. 21.12). Once a CT scan demonstrates definitive fracture healing, activities are progressed accordingly and a return to sports is allowed. Sport-specific training usually begins at approximately 12 weeks, pending evidence of healing on imaging. We counsel elite athletes that return to in game competition is often 6 to 12 months. Vitamin D supplementation is prescribed at a dose of 50,000 IU/weekly for the first 6 weeks following surgery. Orthotics are used postoperatively if an underlying foot deformity is present and felt to have contributed to the development of the navicular stress fracture.

RESULTS AND COMPLICATIONS

The outcomes following treatment of navicular stress fractures correlate with fracture severity.[10] McCormick et al found that 100% of partial navicular stress fractures healed uneventfully, whereas nonunions arose from complete and displaced fractures.[16] In cases that heal after surgery, American Orthopaedic Foot & Ankle Society and SF-36 scores are approximately 92. However, they are in the low 70s in cases that develop a nonunion.[16] Nonunion may occur in up to 20% of surgically treated fractures.[16] However, the use of autologous bone grafting at the fracture site may help to decrease the likelihood of a nonunion.[16]

Other complications of navicular stress fractures include pain, stiffness, delayed union, arthritis, osteonecrosis, and navicular collapse leading to shortening of the foot's medial column and deformity. Such complications are associated with significant morbidity and can impede return to sports.

REFERENCES

1. Towne L, Blazina M, Cozen L. Fatigue fracture of the tarsal navicular. *J Bone Joint Surg.* 1970;52:376-378.
2. Bennell KL, Malcolm SA, Thomas SA, et al. Risk factors for stress fractures in track and field athletes. A twelve-month prospective study. *Am J Sports Med.* 1996;24:810-818.
3. Brukner P, Bradshaw C, Khan KM, White S, Crossley K. Stress fractures: a review of 180 cases. *Clin J Sport Med.* 1996;6:85-89.

4. Mallee WH, Weel H, van Dijk CN, et al. Surgical versus conservative treatment for high-risk stress fractures of the lower leg (anterior tibial cortex, navicular and fifth metatarsal base): a systematic review. *Br J Sports Med.* 2015;49:370-376.
5. Waugh W. The ossification and vascularisation of the tarsal navicular and their relation to Köhler's disease. *J Bone Joint Surg Br.* 1958;40-B:765-777.
6. Wright AA, Taylor JB, Ford KR, Siska L, Smoliga JM. Risk factors associated with lower extremity stress fractures in runners: a systematic review with meta-analysis. *Br J Sports Med.* 2015;49:1517-1523.
7. Becker J, James S, Osternig L, Chou LS. Foot kinematics differ between runners with and without a history of navicular stress fractures. *Orthop J Sports Med.* 2018;6:2325967118767363.
8. Franklyn-Miller A, Wilson C, Bilzon J, McCrory P. Foot orthoses in the prevention of injury in initial military training: a randomized controlled trial. *Am J Sports Med.* 2011;39:30-37.
9. Jones MH, Amendola AS. Navicular stress fractures. *Clin Sports Med.* 2006;25:151Y158.
10. Saxena A, Fullem B, Hannaford D. Results of treatment of 22 navicular stress fractures and a new proposed radiographic classification system. *J Foot Ankle Surg.* 2000;39(2):96-103.
11. Torg JS, Pavlov H, Roberts MM, Eremus J, Drakos MC, Arnoczky SP. The tarsal navicular stress fracture revisited: the unequivocal case for conservative, non-surgical management. *Foot Ankle Orthop.* 2016;1:2473011416S00018.
12. Khan KM, Fuller PJ, Brukner PD, Kearney C, Burry HC. Outcome of conservative and surgical management of navicular stress fracture in athletes: eighty-six cases proven with computerized tomography. *Am J Sports Med.* 1992;20:657-666.
13. Fitch KD, Blackwell JB, Gilmour WN. Operation for non-union of stress fracture of the tarsal navicular. *J Bone Joint Surg Br.* 1989;71(1):105-110
14. Burne SG, Mahoney CM, Forster BB, Koehle MS, Taunton JE, Khan KM. Tarsal navicular stress injury: long-term outcome and clinicoradiological correlation using both computed tomography and magnetic resonance imaging. *Am J Sports Med.* 2005;33:1875-1881.
15. Hossain M, Clutton J, Ridgewell M, Lyons K, Perera A. Stress fractures of the foot. *Clin Sports Med.* 2015;34(4):769-790.
16. McCormick JJ, Bray CC, Davis WH, Cohen BE, Jones CP III, Anderson RB. Clinical and computed tomography evaluation of surgical outcomes in tarsal navicular stress fractures. *Am J Sports Med.* 2011;39(8):1741-1748. Case series of 10 operatively treated navicular stress fractures with functional and radiologic outcomes at 42 months.

22 Os Trigonum Resection

J. Chris Coetzee

INTRODUCTION

Posterior ankle impingement syndrome (PAIS) is fairly common in dancers and athletes that require repetitive hyper plantarflexion of their ankles. Most common problem is an os trigonum or Stieda process, but secondary soft tissue hypertrophy and scarring can also contribute to pain and disability. Nonsurgical care includes physical therapy (PT), short-term rest, and activity modification and anti-inflammation medication. Only when these measures fail to provide relief over a minimum of 3 months should surgery be considered.

INDICATIONS AND CONTRAINDICATIONS

Sports that require regular and repetitive hyper plantarflexion of the ankle can cause posterior ankle pain and impingement, especially in people born with an os trigonum or Stieda process. Dancers, specifically ballerinas, are most often affected as they spent a lot of time in the relevé position. Kicking sports like soccer can be a factor as well.

Posterior ankle impingement syndrome can be caused by both osseous and soft tissue structures, but most cases needing surgery will have bony impingement as well.[1-4] An os trigonum is present in 13% of the population[5] and is usually asymptomatic.

Indications for Surgical Management
- Symptomatic PAIS with an os trigonum
- Failure of conservative management for at least 3 months
- Diagnosis confirmed with imaging studies including radiographs and an magnetic resonance imaging (MRI)

Contraindications for Surgical Management
- Pain of unknown origin
- Presence of an os trigonum on radiograph, but an MRI with no sign of posterior impingement, soft tissue inflammation, or marrow edema

Nonoperative treatment is initiated in the early stage of PAIS. However, because of the osseous etiology of acquired os trigonum syndrome, surgical intervention is often required because of recalcitrant posterior ankle pain and a bony end point in plantarflexion. The traditional open surgical excision of the os trigonum through a posteromedial has good results, relatively few complications and provides the advantage of performing flexor hallicis longus (FHL) tenolysis.[6,7]

An arthroscopic technique could be used by an experienced arthroscopic surgeon and has shown comparable clinical outcomes regarding pain, function, and satisfaction.[8] There is evidence in the literature that there is no difference in the outcome and return to dance with an open versus an arthroscopic approach and the surgeon should use the technique he/she is most comfortable with.[9]

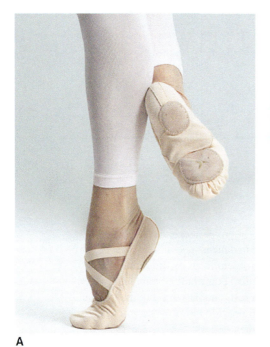
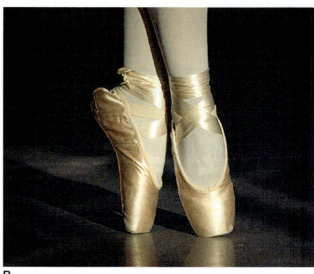

FIGURE 22.1 **A.** Relevé position. **B.** Pointe position. Both can cause posterior impingement syndrome. Lateral standing radiograph confirms a large os trigonum posterior to the ankle.

DIAGNOSIS AND PREOPERATIVE PLANNING

Radiographs

Standard anteroposterior, lateral, and oblique radiographs should be done as well as a weight-bearing lateral with the foot in maximum plantarflexion. These studies will show the presence of an os trigonum or Stieda process, as well as the likelihood of posterior impingement caused by it (Figs. 22.1 and 22.2).

Magnetic Resonance Imaging

An MRI is more valuable than a computed tomography (CT) scan in PAIS.[10] It will help to determine whether the posterior pain is from soft tissue or osseous origin. Also, a symptomatic os trigonum or Stieda process should show marrow edema and signal change in the os trigonum and often the posterior distal tibia (Figs. 22.3 and 22.4).[11,12]

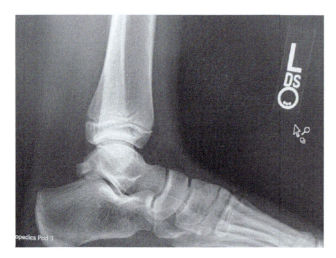

FIGURE 22.2 Lateral standing radiograph confirms a large os trigonum posterior to the ankle.

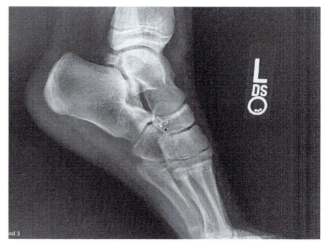

FIGURE 22.3 A relevé lateral confirms impingement between the os trigonum, between the calcaneus, and posterior tibia.

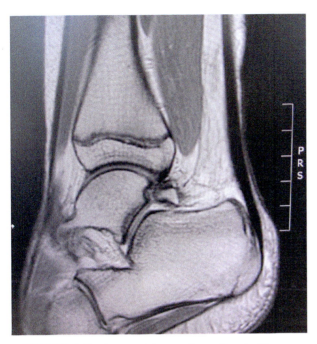

FIGURE 22.4 The large os trigonum is confirmed with an magnetic resonance imaging.

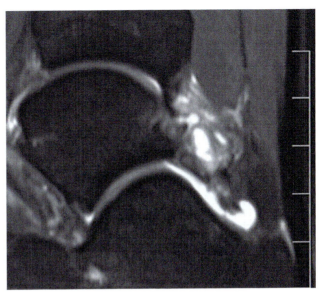

FIGURE 22.5 T2 sequence shoes significant posterior inflammation and marrow edema.

Physical Examination

Pain and tenderness in the posterior and posterolateral ankle in maximum plantarflexion. There could be restricted active and/or passive plantarflexion. If there is secondary flexor hallucis tenosynovitis (fairly common in ballerinas), pain will be exacerbated with dorsiflexion of the great toe. FHL tendinosis is present in about 70% of cases with PAIS secondary to an os trigonum.[1,13]

SURGICAL TECHNIQUE

An os trigonum excision could be done arthroscopically or with a mini-open technique. There is no difference in outcome in open versus arthroscopic os trigonum excision and a mini-open technique is easier to accomplish for the inexperienced ankle arthroscopist.[9]

With an open technique, either a lateral or medial approach could be used. The os trigonum is closer to the lateral side of the ankle, but it is difficult to access the FHL tendon from lateral. It is not uncommon to have an FHL tenosynovitis or stenosing tenosynovitis especially in ballerinas with PAIS. With that in mind, a medial approach is preferred.

The patient is placed supine with a sandbag under the opposite buttock. A 3-cm incision is made posteromedial over the ankle (Fig. 22.5).

The interval between the flexor digitorum longus (FDL) anterior and the neurovascular bundle posterior is used to access the posterior ankle (Figs. 22.6 and 22.7).

Careful dissection is used with the ankle in a neutral position to expose the FHL tendon. A tenosynovectomy is done to release any stenosis of the tendon, especially around the posterior aspect of the talus.

The FHL is then retracted medially to expose the os trigonum. The os starts at the lateral tubercle of the FHL groove, but the interval can be obscured by fairly dense soft tissue. A Freer elevator or small osteotome is used to find the interval between the os and the posterior aspect of the talus (see ▶Video 22.1). Careful sharp dissection is then used to mobilize and remove the os trigonum.

There is often significant soft tissue hypertrophy posterior to the ankle in chronic PAIS. This tissue should also be excised either with sharp dissection or and arthroscopic shaver could be used through the open approach. Both the tibiotalar and subtalar joints should be inspected to ensure no articular cartilage issues which could be débrided if present.

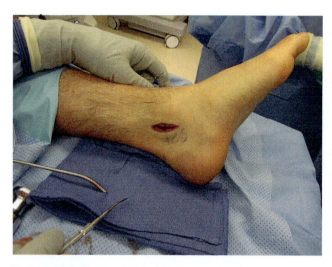

FIGURE 22.6 The surgical incision is between posteromedial in the interval between flexor digitorum longus and the neurovascular bundle.

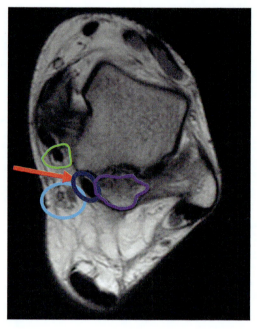

FIGURE 22.7 MRI with the anatomic structures marked. This gives a schematic visualization of the posteromedial surgical approach (*red arrow*). The plane is between the flexor digitorum longus (*green circle*) and the neurovascular bundle (*light blue circle*). The next structure that is exposed is the flexor hallucis longus (*dark blue circle*) and the os trigonum (*purple circle*).

An intraoperative lateral and plantarflexion lateral radiograph is done to confirm resection of the os and no further posterior impingement (see Fig. 22.8).

A short leg cast or controlled ankle motion (CAM) boot is used for 10 to 14 days to allow soft tissue healing before PT is started.

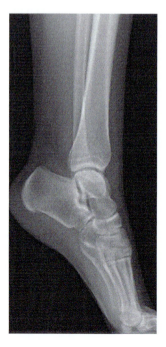

FIGURE 22.8 Postoperative simulated relevé to confirm complete resection of the os trigonum.

22 Os Trigonum Resection

PEARLS

- A headlamp is invaluable due to the small workspace with a mini-open approach.
- A medial approach is preferable over a lateral as it allows débridement and release of the FHL.
- Place a sandbag under the opposite buttock to externally rotate the leg for easier access of the posteromedial ankle.
- If a posterolateral approach is used, it might be easier to do the procedure prone.
- Identify and protect the neurovascular bundle.
- Once the FHL is identified and retracted, use a Freer elevator or small osteotome to find the cleavage between the os trigonum and posterior talus.
- The rehabilitation program is as important, if not more, as the surgery.

PITFALLS

- Don't attempt an arthroscopic excision if not very comfortable with posterior ankle scope techniques.
- Don't proceed with deep dissection until the neurovascular bundle is identified and protected.
- Do an intraoperative radiograph to confirm complete resection of the os and débridement of the posterior ankle.

POSTOPERATIVE MANAGEMENT

A short leg cast, or CAM boot, is used for 2 weeks to allow the soft tissue to heal. Patient can be partial to weight bearing as tolerated with or without crutches. At 2 weeks, the sutures are removed and PT starts. PT is of utmost important to ensure full range of motion and equal balance and proprioception prior to return to sports. This is especially important in ballerinas as any deficit could lead to compensatory injuries.

Phase I: Weeks 0 to 2
- Week 1: CAM boot and partial weight bearing with crutches
- Week 2: Weight bearing as tolerated and work into shoe as able
  - Start PT

Phase II: Weeks 2 to 6 (1 to 2× week PT)
- Weight bearing as tolerated
- Exercises 2 to 4 weeks:
  - Gait training
  - Active range of motion (AROM) plantarflexion without maximal contraction
  - AROM dorsiflexion to neutral
  - Gentle FHL stretching in non–weight-bearing
  - Intrinsic activation in sitting (short foot/dome exercise)
  - Toe yoga: active toe flexion, extension, spreads
  - Balance progressions with short foot/dome
  - Proximal neuromuscular reeducation and strengthening (hip, lumbopelvic, core)
- Exercises 4 to 6 weeks:
  - Dynamic balance progressions
  - Band-resisted plantarflexion high rep/low load
  - Dance specific progressions**
  - Closed chain plié and relevé (progressive weight bearing to standing)
  - Balance progressions en relevé supported with ball under heel
  - Plantarflexion progressions without gripping through Achilles tendon
  - Plantarflexion with lateral or medial theraband focusing on neutral ankle alignment
  - Plantarflexion with toe flexion/extension for intrinsic activation

Phase III: Weeks 6 to 12 (1× week PT)
- Exercises 6 to 8 weeks:
  - Progress dorsiflexion stretching

- Cardio/fitness—bicycling, elliptical
  - Standing calf strengthening gastroc (knee extended) and soleus (knee flexed)

**Modified return to dance class at 6 weeks

- Exercises 9 to 12 weeks:
  - Progressive weight-bearing plyometrics
  - Functional performance criteria: able to perform 25 single leg calf raises gastroc (knee extended) and soleus (knee flexed)
  - Initiate sports-specific training
  - Pass functional tests for general sport (dance**)

**Dance specific concepts to consider:

1. Balance exercises with small to medium size ball under the heel. This can help with control at different levels of relevé.
2. Pointing the ankle and learning to relax the Achilles tendon. Dancers are often able to figure this out. Have the patient maximally plantar flex, place their fingers on the Achilles, and try to relax it while maintaining the ankle motion and intrinsic contraction needed for midfoot. Dancers often overcontract with their gastroc to maximally plantar flex the ankle which in turn "jams" the posterior ankle. Pointe shoe dancers use intrinsics to "pull up" out of a pointe shoe while relaxing their gastroc when en pointe.
3. Theraband plantarflexion focusing on neutral ankle. The theraband will either have inversion or eversion pull during plantarflexion AROM.
4. Return to dance considerations to be made with therapist and patient based on style, age, experience, pain, edema, strength, and neuromuscular control.
5. Dance functional tests: (a) airplane test, (b) topple test, (c) sauté test, and (d) pass on the pencil test for return to pointe
   a. "Airplane test: The dancer assumes single-leg stance, with the trunk and nonsupport lower extremity extended parallel to the ground. The patient then performs five controlled single-leg squats in this position, as the arms horizontally adduct toward the ground. A 'pass' is indicated by successful completion of four out of five repetitions, without lower extremity alignment deviations or loss of trunk control."[14]
   b. "Topple test is an assessment of total body control during a pirouette, a 360° rotation of the entire body while in single-leg balance. A 'pass' is indicated by successful performance of the pirouette with the balance leg in full knee extension, gesture leg in passé position, maintenance of vertical trunk position during the descent from the skill, and proper control of the supporting leg during deceleration."[14]
   c. "Single-leg sauté test is an assessment of dynamic trunk control and lower extremity alignment as the dancer performs 16 consecutive single-leg jumps. A 'pass' is defined as at least 8 of the 16 jumps executed with a neutral pelvis, upright and stable trunk, proper lower extremity alignment, appropriate toe-heel landing, and a fully pointed foot in the air."[14]
   d. "Pencil test: The pencil is placed on the dorsal talar neck. When the straight edge of the pencil can clear the distal-most part of the tibia just proximal to the malleoli, it is considered a 'pass,' as this represents that there is greater than or equal to 90° of ankle plantarflexion."[14]

RESULTS AND COMPLICATIONS

There are multiple papers on arthroscopic and open os trigonum excisions. In general, the results are very good with either procedure, with no clear preference for one. The average return to dance is between 8 and 10 weeks, but it could be longer to be fully pain free.[4,6,7]

Most common complication is sural nerve injury with the arthroscopic or lateral open approach. Due to the small incisions, wound issues are minimal. Posterior scar tissue can delay return to dance until full relevé is possible.

Several Recent Articles Show Results as Highlighted Below

Heyer et al reported their results of an open medial approach to os trigonum excisions in dancers. A total of 95% were able to return to their preoperative level of dance at an average time of 7.9 weeks, but it could take up to 18 weeks to be completely pain free. They reported no major complications.[6]

Morelli reported on 12 dancers treated with an endoscopic os trigonum excision. Average return to dance was 8.7 weeks and they also had no major complications.[8]

Walsh et al reported on 54 ankles in dancers with open medial os trigonum excisions. There was statistically significant improvement in outcomes scores and all patients return to their previous level of dance. Only 83% were completely pain free.[7]

REFERENCES

1. Hamilton WG. Stenosing tenosynovitis of the flexor hallucis longus tendon and posterior impingement upon the os trigonum in ballet dancers. *Foot Ankle*. 1982;3(2):74-80.
2. Nault M, Kocher MS, Micheli IJ. Os trigonum syndrome. *J AAOS*. 2014;22(9):545-553.
3. Giannini S, Buda R, Mosca M, Parma A, Di Caprio F. Posterior ankle impingement. *Foot Ankle Int*. 2013;34(3):459-465.
4. Coetzee JC, Seybold JD, Moser BR, et al. Management of posterior impingement in the ankle in athletes and dancers. *Foot Ankle Int*. 2015;36(8):988-994.
5. Tsuruta T, Shiokawa Y, Kato A, et al. Radiological study of the accessory skeletal elements in the foot and ankle. *Nihon Seikeigeka Gakkai Zasshi*. 1981;55(4):357-370.
6. Heyer JH, Rose DJ. Os trigonum excision in dancers via an open posteromedial approach. *Foot Ankle Int*. 2017;38(1):27-35.
7. Walsh K, Durante E, Moser BR, et al. Surgical outcomes of os trigonum syndrome in dancers: a case series. *Orthop J Sports Med*. 2020;8(7): 2325967120938767.
8. Morelli F, Mazza D, Serlorenzi P, et al. Endoscopic excision of symptomatic os trigonum in professional dancers. *J Foot Ankle Surg*. 2017;56(1):22-25.
9. Guo QW, Hu YL, Jiao C, Ao YF, Tian de X. Open versus endoscopic excision of a symptomatic os trigonum: a comparative study of 41 cases. *Arthroscopy*. 2010;26(3):384-390.
10. Gursoy M, Dag F, Mete BD, Bulut T, Uluc ME. The anatomic variations of the posterior talofibular ligament associated with os trigonum and pathologies of related structures. *Surg Radiol Anat*. 2015;37(8):955-962.
11. Hillier JC, Peace K, Hulme A, Healy JC. Pictorial review: MRI features of foot and ankle injuries in ballet dancers. *Br J Radiol*. 2004;77(918):532-537.
12. Russell JA, Shave RM, Yoshioka H, Kruse DW, Koutedakis Y, Wyon MA. Magnetic resonance imaging of the ankle in female ballet dancers en pointe. *Acta Radiol*. 2010;51(6):655-661.
13. Hamilton WG. Posterior ankle pain in dancers. *Clin Sports Med*. 2008;27(2):263-277.
14. Filipa A, Barton K. Physical therapy rehabilitation of an adolescent preprofessional dancer following os trigonum excision: a case report. *J Orthop Sports Phys Ther*. 2018;48(3):194-203.

PART FIVE
ACHILLES

23 Graft Reconstruction for Treatment of Chronic Achilles Tendon Ruptures

Carson Rider, Drew Murphy, Stephanie S. Gardner, and John Z. Zhao

Chronic Achilles tendon ruptures can present after a misdiagnosed acute rupture, delay in presentation, or as a failure of previous treatment. Clinically, patients are noted to have increased resting dorsiflexion compared to the uninjured side, decreased plantarflexion strength, often a palpable gap along the Achilles tendon, and an abnormal Thompson test. It should be noted that while the Thompson test is very reliable in the setting of an acute Achilles rupture, once there is significant atrophy of the gastrocsoleus complex in the setting of chronic Achilles pathology, a squeeze on the calf can cause the tibialis posterior muscle to exert a similar plantarflexion of the ankle, which can be confused for an intact Achilles. It is important in the chronic injury to compare the amount of plantarflexion of the ankle with the contralateral side. There still may be plantarflexion of the ankle with calf squeeze, but usually less than the uninjured side. Patients report difficulty due to weakness with certain activities that require push off, including ambulation, running, and climbing.

Management of chronic Achilles tendon ruptures is challenging and controversial. Previous discussions on tendon gap excision and shortening, V-Y lengthening, fascial turndown, and flexor hallucis longus (FHL) transfer have been well described[1-5] and are options for surgical treatment for chronic Achilles rupture. However, portions of the tendon are frequently fibrotic in the chronic setting, requiring resection of the diseased tissue. This can result in large gaps of missing tendon tissue, thus making repair difficult with V-Y lengthening or fascial turndown alone. Achilles tendon graft reconstruction, with either autograft or allograft, can serve as an option to help bridge these large tissue gaps during surgical repair.

INDICATIONS AND CONTRAINDICATIONS

Graft reconstruction is indicated when the patient has failed nonoperative or previous operative treatment, desires an increase in push off strength, and has a tendon defect greater than 5 cm. Ability to place the ankle at neutral on the table after reconstruction is ideal, and the inability to accomplish this should be a consideration for this graft technique. Residual equinus contracture is rare regardless of technique chosen. This procedure capitalizes on restoring function of the gastrocsoleus complex in cases where there is not significant fatty atrophy of either muscle belly. Either allograft or autograft can be used. As for autograft, hamstring is more commonly used due to ease of harvest and the ability to harvest multiple tendons if needed.[6] Autograft is cheaper and minimizes risk of disease transmission or graft rejection. However, there is a risk of donor site morbidity.[6-8] An FHL muscle/tendon transfer may be concomitantly performed to augment plantarflexion strength.

PREOPERATIVE PLANNING

A thorough history and physical exam should be carefully performed for each patient. Preinjury activity level should be assessed, and appropriate patient expectations should be established prior to surgery. Surgical risk factors for wound complications must be assessed, such as vasculopathy, uncontrolled diabetes mellitus, smoking, malnutrition, and history of wound healing complications. The potential surgical site should be evaluated for prior incisions or scarring, and preoperative plastic surgery consultation may be considered if soft tissue coverage is expected to be a concern for the procedure. In high-risk patients, smaller windowed incisions may be considered. Active ongoing infection at the site of surgical repair is an absolute contraindication for the procedure; however, a staged procedure can be considered, initially with débridement of infected tissue and resolution of the infection.

A bilateral Thompson test should be performed to compare baseline function of the Achilles tendon unit. Passive ankle dorsiflexion can also be evaluated, as increased passive ankle dorsiflexion could indicate Achilles tendon attenuation. A focused component of the examination is the resting equinus of the ankle in the prone position, both with the knee flexed and extended. In chronic cases, scar and fibrotic tissue may sometimes have filled in at the prior rupture site, making it difficult to palpate a gap in the tendon.

In addition to standard ankle films for radiographic evaluation, magnetic resonance imaging (MRI) advanced imaging should be obtained to better characterize the injury. MRI technique should include the gastrocsoleus muscle belly for assessment of the condition of the muscle. Extensive fibrosis or fatty changes may indicate less flexibility of the muscle for primary repair and suggest the need for grafting technique. The site of rupture should be localized, and tendon tissue quality should be evaluated on fluid-sensitive sequences. In this fashion, length of diseased tissue resection can be preoperatively measured, as well as lengths of the remaining distal stump and final gap length (Fig. 23.1). If the distal stump has at least 2 to 3 cm of healthy tissue, the graft can be docked into the remaining native tissue stump. However, if the remaining healthy stump is shorter than 2 cm, or if it is avulsed off the bone, osseous fixation of the graft into the calcaneal tuberosity is recommended.

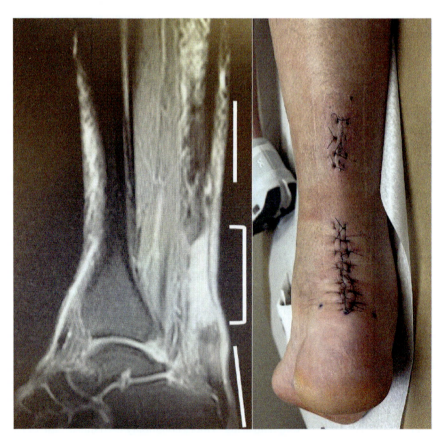

FIGURE 23.1 Preoperative magnetic resonance imaging and incision placement. The tendon defect (5 cm) is measured (*bracket*) to help plan the incisions and graft requirements during the reconstruction procedure. In this case, "windowed" incisions (*heavy lines*) were used to minimize the risk of wound complication. The incisions made during the case are demonstrated.

Measurement of the residual gap length can aid preoperative planning for autograft harvesting. The average diameter of the gracilis tendon is 3.5 to 4.3 mm and the average diameter of the semitendinosus tendon is 4 to 5 mm. The lengths of each tendon vary from 22 to 30 cm. In our experience, if the residual gap length is less than 5 cm, harvesting the gracilis alone is usually sufficient to reconstruct the gap with multiple Pulvertaft passes. However, in cases where the residual gap is greater than 5 cm, we recommend harvesting both the gracilis and semitendinosus tendons for adequate reconstruction.

SURGICAL TECHNIQUE

Harvesting Hamstring Autograft

We harvest the hamstring tendons with the patient in the prone position to decrease operating room time, but this can also be performed with the patient in the supine position for graft harvest and then transition to the prone position for the tendon reconstruction. A sports surgeon partner can be asked to help with the harvest for those foot and ankle surgeons who are not well versed in harvesting the hamstrings. We drape out both lower extremities to be able to compare the resting Achilles tension to the noninjured side. The incision for the hamstring harvest should be parallel to the medial face of the tibia, centered between the tibial tubercle and posteromedial aspect of the tibia (Fig. 23.2). The proximal aspect of the incision should be in line with the top of the tibial tubercle. The incision is typically 3 to 4 cm in length.

The skin is incised and blunt dissection is carried down to the sartorial fascia. The saphenous nerve should be preserved and protected. Clean off the sartorial fascia with an elevator until the fascia can be fully visualized. Sharply incise the fascia in line with its fibers just a few millimeters medial to the tibia. The hamstring tendons can be palpated between layers 1 and 2 of the knee by sweeping from anterior to posterior with your finger. Flexing and extending the knee can facilitate the palpation of the tendons as needed. If adhesions are present, remove them.

A right-angle clamp is placed around the gracilis tendon and a Penrose drain is placed around the tendon for countertraction. A Langenbeck retractor can also be used for countertraction. Metzenbaum scissors are used to remove any remaining adhesion from the medial head of the gastrocnemius muscle. After the tendon is completely mobilized, a tendon stripper is placed over the tendon. Flex the knee and guide the tendon stripper toward the ischial tuberosity (Fig. 23.3). Sharply transect the distal insertion of the gracilis tendon and remove any muscle fibers with a metal ruler. The semitendinosus tendon will be deep and insert inferior to the gracilis tendon insertion. Harvest the semitendinosus tendon in the same way as above if needed for reconstruction. When done

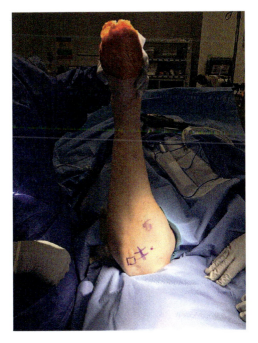

FIGURE 23.2 Incision location for hamstring harvest. The tibial tubercle is marked with a square. A dot is placed on the posteromedial border of the proximal tibia. An oblique incision is then made halfway between these palpable bony landmarks, with the proximal extent of the incision starting at the proximal-most aspect of the tibial tubercle. The incision is oriented proximal-medial to distal-lateral.

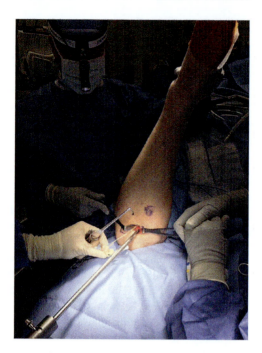

FIGURE 23.3 Hamstring autograft harvest. The tendon stripper is placed around the tendon, counterpressure is applied, and the stripper is pushed toward the ischial tuberosity to harvest the hamstring tendon(s) required to reconstruct the Achilles tendon defect. In this figure, the gracilis tendon has already been harvested. The semitendinosus tendon is visible and was also harvested in this case.

harvesting the hamstring tendons, irrigate the wound and close the sartorial fascia with a running 3-0 Vicryl stitch. The rest of the wound is closed in layers.

The graft is prepared on the back table using a locking 0-Vicryl suture on the ends of the graft. Make sure to leave the suture ends long so the graft can be easily shuttled during the reconstruction (Fig. 23.4). If using both the gracilis and semitendinosus grafts, they can be bundled together to make one graft.[5]

GRAFT RECONSTRUCTION TECHNIQUE

Various incision locations have been described in the literature, but we prefer a direct midline incision when reconstructing chronic Achilles pathology. A previous study showed that there is less blood supply to the central portion of the Achilles tendon,[9] so this should be considered when planning skin incisions. Regardless of the incision location, a skilled plastic surgeon should be avail-

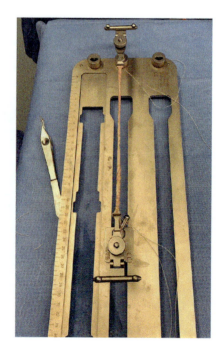

FIGURE 23.4 Graft preparation. The graft is prepared on the back table using tubularizing 0-Vicryl locking sutures. The suture tails are left long to facilitate passing the graft during the reconstruction.

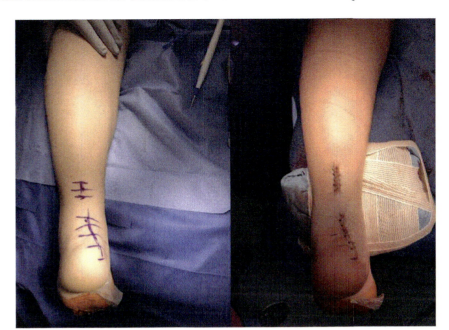

FIGURE 23.5 "Windowed" incisions. Note the lateral-based distal incision, which has been shown in a previous study[10] to have lower rates of infection and wound complication during treatment of chronic Achilles pathology.

able to help with surgical planning, especially in the setting of revision cases utilizing larger skin incisions. A 4- to 5-cm incision is used and is placed slightly proximal to the center of the tear. If the injury is more than 3 months out, a larger incision is made to allow for adequate scar removal. Smaller "windowed" incisions can be used when the patient is at risk for wound complications (Fig. 23.5).

If there is a true fascia layer over the tendon, isolate and preserve it for closure at the end of the case. The sural nerve and saphenous vein should be protected during the approach. Aggressive débridement of scar tissue is performed to free up the native Achilles tendon. A Cobb elevator helps to create a plane circumferentially around the tendon. Avoid aggressive dissection in the deep posterior compartment unless an FHL transfer is planned or if it is needed to maximally mobilize the tendon. Once the tendon has been freed, we completely excise the abnormal portion of the Achilles until healthy looking tendon is presented both proximal and distal (Fig. 23.6). At this point, the existing gap should ideally match the preoperative templated gap.

A locking 0-Vicryl suture is used to tag both ends of the existing Achilles tendon. Attention is then turned to distal docking of the graft. In patients with 2 to 3 cm of healthy distal stump remaining, we prefer to use this portion of the native stump to dock our graft using a curved tissue passer to anchor

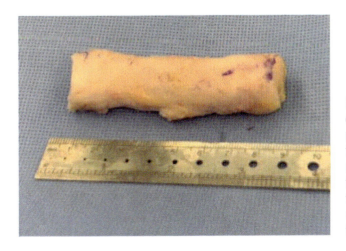

FIGURE 23.6 Complete excision of diseased Achilles tendon. The resected portion of the Achilles tendon is thickened and scarred due to chronic rupture. The diseased portion of the tendon is often visibly unhealthy and the tendon is thicker and harder than native tendon upon palpation during the case.

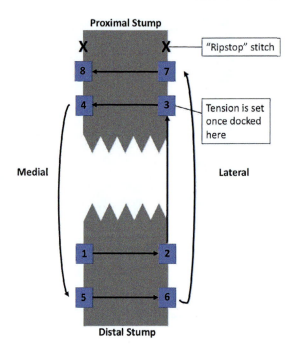

FIGURE 23.7 Schematic of graft passage and docking steps. Note the use of a "ripstop" stitch just proximal to the docking site in the proximal stump. This stitch serves as a barrier within the native stump to prevent graft migration and proximal pullout of the graft.

the graft via a Pulvertaft weave. When using the curved tissue passer, be sure to firmly spread the tips after penetrating the far side of the tendon to help generate a path for the graft. The tissue passer is inserted into the medial aspect of the Achilles stump, pushed through the lateral tendon edge, and one limb of the graft 0-Vicryl tagging suture is pulled from the lateral to medial direction. Stop pulling once the edge of the graft is resting flush with the medial aspect of the native distal stump. The graft is then docked with a buried figure-of-8 braided nonabsorbable tape on the medial and lateral aspects of the distal Achilles stump. Since only one limb of the suture tail was initially pulled through the distal Achilles stump, the remaining limb should be passed from lateral to medial with a free needle and then tied to the previously shuttled 0-Vicryl limb to add an additional point of graft fixation. The graft is now secured into the distal portion of the healthy, native tendon.

If there is minimal or no residual healthy distal stump, anchor the graft into the calcaneal tuberosity using an osseous fixation device (ie, tenodesis screw). If direct anchoring to the bone is chosen, a rasp or saw should be used to roughen the bone just anterior to the normal attachment of the Achilles tendon. Any remaining diseased Achilles stump can be resected to make room for the osseous fixation device. A free suture can be passed through the eyelet of the tenodesis screw prior to its insertion, which allows the tenodesis screw to serve as an anchor for reinforcing the construct at the conclusion of the reconstruction. Dock the graft into the calcaneus using the osseous fixation device and maintain the free limbs of the suture to be used later during the case.

After securing the graft distally, attention is turned to connecting the graft to the proximal portion of the healthy tendon. It is crucial to dock the graft proximally under an appropriate amount of tension, ensuring that adequate dorsiflexion to neutral can be obtained without jeopardizing the integrity of the construct. The contralateral limb can be used intraoperatively to help guide the amount of tension within the construct. The proximal 0-Vicryl limbs of the graft are then pulled from lateral to medial through the proximal edge of the healthy tendon with the curved tissue passer (Fig. 23.7). With the foot positioned under appropriate tension—so that resting tension is similar to the contralateral side—the graft is secured to the medial and lateral aspects of the proximal native Achilles stump with buried figure-of-8 sutures. The tension of the construct is now set.

If there is additional graft length remaining, the graft can be shuttled back down distally. To avoid damaging the graft in the original distal stump docking site, locate an area within the distal Achilles stump that is distal to the original graft docking site. The graft is then shuttled once more into this location in the distal Achilles stump from a medial to lateral direction using the tissue passer, and it is secured again with buried figure-of-8 sutures. This technique creates a cerclage of autograft between the distal insertion site and healthy, proximal native tendon. If a tenodesis screw was utilized for distal fixation, the graft can also be anchored down to the screw with the limbs of the free

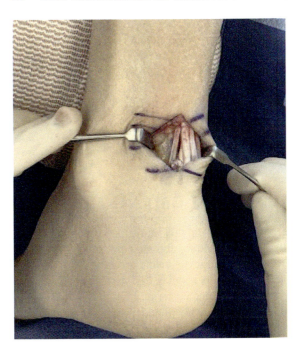

FIGURE 23.8 Multiple passes with graft. If residual graft length is available, multiple passes into the native tendon can be made using a Pulvertaft weave until the graft length has been exhausted.

suture within the screw eyelet using a free needle. At this point, there should be continuity of the graft between the proximal and distal aspects of the defect. However, if there is remaining length on the graft, it can be passed proximally again and secured in a similar "box-weave" fashion. Continue to make passes with the tissue weaver until the graft length has been exhausted, securing the graft after each pass with buried suture. Again, take care to avoid penetrating the previous weave locations to maintain graft integrity. We can typically make multiple autograft passes between the distal and proximal stumps for defect sizes measuring 2 to 3 cm in length (Fig. 23.8). It is important to note that the resting equinus position of the repaired limb should be equal or slightly greater than the uninjured limb.

Once all the graft length has been exhausted, the medial and lateral limbs of the construct should be tubularized together with a running suture. This will bring the limbs of the construct together to form a single, centralized unit (Fig. 23.9). A 3-0 Vicryl suture can be used to fill in residual gaps

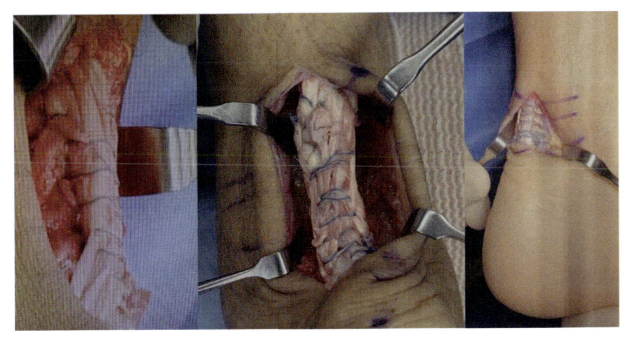

FIGURE 23.9 Examples of final graft constructs.

between the constructed limbs and to bury any knots that are present on the posterior surface of the tendon so that the tendon surface is smooth. A suture "ripstop" stitch should be placed proximal to the docking site in the proximal tendon stump to prevent proximal suture migration.

A Thompson test is performed to verify continuity of the constructed Achilles. Satisfactory tension restoration should allow dorsiflexion to neutral. The wound is irrigated and the fascial layer is repaired with a running 3-0 Vicryl suture if present. The rest of the wound is closed in layers. We use two strips of folded 4 × 8 gauze to make "goalposts" on either side of the incision to minimize direct pressure on the wound. A short leg splint is applied with the foot resting in resting equinus. If using allograft reconstruction, the graft is passed and secured in a similar way as described above.[5]

OPTIONAL FHL TENDON TRANSFER AUGMENTATION

We will add an FHL tendon transfer to the reconstruction in highly active patients with significant muscle atrophy noted on MRI. Additionally, in long-standing chronic cases greater than 3 to 6 months, infection where large segments were affected, large segments greater than 10 cm, or any case where the surgeon feels that more muscle would be beneficial, FHL transfer will improve strength during recovery. The FHL is harvested through the same posterior incision as stated above. Dissection should remain lateral to the FHL tendon to decrease likelihood of neurovascular injury. We harvest around 4 cm of the FHL tendon from within the tarsal canal. After harvest, the distal end is tagged with a locking 0-Vicryl suture.

In patients with a healthy distal Achilles stump, we use a Pulvertaft weave of the FHL tendon into the distal tendon using the curved tissue passer after the auto or allograft was passed. For cases without a healthy distal stump or in cases with significant suture traffic in the distal stump, we use the osseous fixation device technique as mentioned previously, incorporating both the graft and FHL tendon into the distal insertion site. The FHL tendon is tensioned by placing the foot in 10° to 15° of plantarflexion. Care should be taken to not overly plantarflex the ankle with this technique and ensure that the ankle can be brought to just past neutral on the table after final tensioning. Based on the technique of distal fixation, the FHL tendon is either secured to the distal Achilles stump using a buried figure-of-8 suture or brought down to the osseous fixation device using the free suture tape in the eyelet. The tagging 0-Vicryl suture limbs from the FHL graft are then tied to any remaining suture tails to add an additional point of distal fixation to the construct (Fig. 23.10).

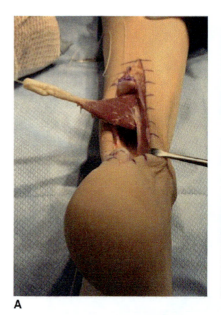
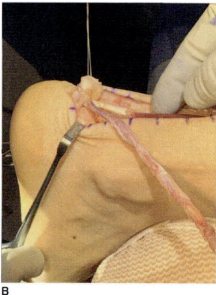
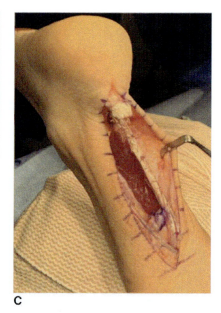

FIGURE 23.10 Flexor hallucis longus (FHL) augmentation. **A.** The FHL tendon is harvested through the posterior incision. **B.** The FHL tendon and graft are docked into the calcaneus just anterior to the native distal stump. **C.** Final construct with autograft spanning the Achilles defect with FHL tendon augmentation.

PEARLS AND PITFALLS

Pearls

- Graft reconstruction can be used to address large (greater than 5 cm) tendon defects in the setting of chronic tissue attenuation to provide a healthier collagen unit in continuity.
- If more than 2 to 3 cm of healthy native tendon stump remains distally, dock the graft into the native stump using a Pulvertaft weave.
- If the native distal stump is not healthy, dock the graft into the bone using osseous fixation.
- Factors that might indicate augmentation with a FHL transfer: delayed treatment more than 3 to 6 months, advanced MRI changes of muscle fibrosis or fatty atrophy, lack of intraoperative flexibility of the proximal muscle, and delayed staged reconstruction in the setting of infection.
- Windowed incisions can be used to minimize the risk of wound complications.
- At the completion of the procedure, the limb should be in the same or slightly greater resting equinus as the contralateral limb.

Pitfalls

- Larger incisions increase the risk of wound complications. Utilizing smaller bridge incisions may mitigate this risk.
- Extreme caution should be exercised with this procedure in active smokers or other patients at risk for wound healing problems.
- Donor site morbidity in the setting of hamstring autograft harvest, which is overall fairly low,[11] should be discussed with patients preoperatively.

POSTOPERATIVE MANAGEMENT

- Strict non–weight bearing for 4 weeks.
- Splinted initially in the operative room in resting equinus (around 10° of plantarflexion). A fiberglass roll should be used as a bolster under the heel so that accidental weight bearing by the patient does not endanger the repair.
- The splint is removed at the 2-week postoperative visit and the wound is inspected. We typically place the patient into another splint for an additional 2 weeks to allow for undisturbed wound healing, since complete wound healing is critical for success with this operation.
- Sutures are removed at 4 weeks and patients are then placed into a controlled ankle motion walking boot with two heel wedges (each ¾ inch) to keep the ankle in plantarflexion.
- Weight bearing in the boot with wedges (three for taller patients, two for shorter patients [under 5 feet 6 inches]) and formal physical therapy is started at 4 weeks postoperatively. A functional rehabilitation handout is also provided to patients at this time.
- One wedge is removed per week, not removing the last wedge, after therapy is initiated until placement back into a regular shoe with a heel lift around the 8 to 10 postoperative week (this is guided primarily by resolution of postoperative swelling and wound healing).
- Light exercise is started around 3 to 4 months and full activity 6 to 9 months after surgery.

RESULTS AND COMPLICATIONS

High-quality studies that report long-term outcomes of graft reconstruction for management of chronic Achilles ruptures are lacking. Perhaps the most devastating complications that can occur after graft reconstruction are wound breakdown and infection. Graft reconstruction techniques utilizing larger incisions are associated with increased wound complication rates. A recent study showed that graft reconstruction for large Achilles defects had an infection rate of 8.96%.[10] The risk of infection and wound breakdown can be minimized by utilizing windowed incisions and the lateral-based distal incision as described above.[10] The relatively high infection and wound complication rate should be discussed with patients prior to surgery to help manage patient expectations. Donor site morbidity from hamstring autograft harvest is overall low,[11] and this complication may be avoided by utilizing allograft tendon during the reconstruction. Allografts can be expensive and difficult to obtain in some surgical settings, and the risk of infection transmission and immunogenic reactions, which is overall low, should again be discussed with patients preoperatively.

REFERENCES

1. Deese JG, Gratto-Cox G, Clements FD, Brown K. Achilles allograft reconstruction for chronic Achilles tendinopathy. *J Surg Orthop Adv.* 2015;24(1):75. Accessed March 22, 2021.
2. Guclu B, Basat HC, Yildirim T, Bozduman O, Us AK. Long-term results of chronic Achilles tendon ruptures repaired with V-Y tendon plasty and fascia turndown. *Foot Ankle Int.* 2016;37(7):737-742.
3. Hahn F, Meyer P, Maiwald C, Zanetti M, Vienne P. Treatment of chronic Achilles tendinopathy and ruptures with flexor hallucis tendon transfer: clinical outcome and MRI findings. *Foot Ankle Int.* 2008;29(8):794-802.
4. Wegrzyn J, Luciani JF, Philippot R, Brunet-Guedj E, Moyen B, Besse JL. Chronic Achilles tendon rupture reconstruction using a modified flexor hallucis longus transfer. *Int Orthop.* 2010;34(8):1187-1192.
5. Rider CM, Hansen OB, Drakos MC. Hamstring autograft applications for treatment of Achilles tendon pathology. *Foot Ankle Orthop.* 2021;6(1):1-9.
6. Beer AJ, Tauro TM, Redondo ML, Christian DR, Cole BJ, Frank RM. Use of allografts in orthopaedic surgery: safety, procurement, storage, and outcomes. *Orthop J Sports Med.* 2019;7(12):1-10.
7. Hinsenkamp M, Muylle L, Eastlund T, Fehily D, Noël L, Strong DM. Adverse reactions and events related to musculoskeletal allografts: reviewed by the World Health Organisation Project NOTIFY. *Int Orthop.* 2012;36(3):633-641.
8. Yasuda K, Tsujino J, Yasumitsu Ohkoshi YT, Kaneda K. Graft site morbidity with autogenous semitendinosus and gracilis tendons. *Am J Sports Med.* 1994;23(6):706-714.
9. Yepes H, Tang M, Geddes C, Glazebrook M, Morris SF, Stanish WD. Digital vascular mapping of the integument about the Achilles tendon. *J Bone Joint Surg Am.* 2010;92(5):1215-1220.
10. Rider CM, Hansen OB, Drakos MC. Achilles pathology and surgical approach determine post-operative infection rate. *Foot Ankle Orthop.* 2022;7(1).
11. von Essen C, McCallum S, Eriksson K, Barenius B. Minimal graft site morbidity using autogenous semitendinosus graft from the uninjured leg: a randomised controlled trial. *Knee Surg Sports Traumatol Arthrosc.* 2022;30(5):1639-1645.

24 Haglund Deformity With Flexor Hallucis Longus Tendon Transfer

Kelly K. Hynes

INTRODUCTION

Insertional tendinopathy makes up about 30% of all causes of Achilles tendon pain.[1] Haglund deformity is a prominent posterior superior border of the calcaneus and is considered part of the spectrum of calcific insertional tendinopathy. Patients present with painful swelling in the posterior aspect of the heel and ensuing problems with rubbing and discomfort from the posterior part of the shoe occurs. True Haglund syndrome is caused by a mechanically induced irritation of the Achilles tendon and associated retrocalcaneal bursa. Patients may present at a younger age with calcific insertional tendinopathy, sometimes bilateral, which should alert the clinician to the possibility of a more generalized inflammatory arthropathy.

The terms "tendinopathy" and "tendinosis" are now widely accepted in the literature as histopathologic studies of débrided tendon have shown a lack of inflammatory response; mucoid degeneration and collagen disorganization, fatty infiltration, and increased thickness are the more common findings.[2]

Conservative treatments include reducing pressure on the affected area with soft heel counters, open back shoes, and heel lifts. Night splints may be used in the setting of an equinus contracture; however, their efficacy has not been shown in the literature.[3] Repetitive weight-bearing activities should be limited and eccentric Achilles stretching with formal physical therapy is encouraged. We do not advocate the use of steroid injections around the Achilles tendon due to concerns regarding rupture. Studies of extracorporeal shockwave therapy have revealed varying results, but some benefit has been shown when combined with a physical therapy program.[4] The majority, around 80%, of patients can be reassured regarding the success of nonoperative treatments.[5]

Surgical treatment of insertional Achilles tendinopathy in the form of Achilles tendon débridement, tendon detachment, Haglund excision, and tendon reattachment with or without flexor hallucis longus (FHL) tendon transfer augmentation has been the mainstay of operative treatment of this condition with generally good outcomes. An FHL tendon transfer may also be used in other presentations of Achilles tendon deficiency such as a delayed presentation of an Achilles tendon rupture.

INDICATIONS AND CONTRAINDICATIONS

The decision to operate will ultimately depend on the duration of symptoms, the level of discomfort, and the disability that this causes.

- Stiffness/pain especially after a period of rest
- Disability limiting daily or recreational activities
- Failure of conservative treatments (greater than 3 to 6 months)
- Difficulty with comfort in shoe wear
- Degenerative rupture of the Achilles tendon

Surgery should be avoided in the presence of

- Skin breakdown
- Active or chronic infection
- Poorly controlled diabetes
- Peripheral vascular disease
- Peripheral neuropathy
- Tobacco use

PREOPERATIVE PLANNING

Lateral radiographs of the heel (Fig. 24.1) are useful in quantifying the degree of calcification within the tendon insertion, which can help to predict the degree of degeneration present, the likelihood of disrupting the Achilles insertion, and, therefore, the need for surgical augmentation and postoperative protocol implications. In patients with insertional Achilles tendinopathy, 65% to 80% will have an enthesophyte seen on the lateral radiograph while in people without foot pain, 25% to 35% will have an enthesophyte present.[6] Retrocalcaneal bursitis can be seen as a loss of the normal soft tissue shadowing in the space anterior to the Achilles tendon (Kager triangle) and in long-standing cases may lead to erosion of the cortex of the posterosuperior prominence. Various measurements have been described in attempting to quantify the size of the Haglund deformity.

In some cases, magnetic resonance imaging (MRI) assessment of the Achilles insertion and Haglund deformity may be helpful in preoperative planning. Assessment of the thickness of the tendon and intrasubstance degeneration has been found to have implications for the success of nonsurgical management. One study found that patients who have greater than 8-mm tendon thickness required surgical treatment 70% to 90% of the time (Fig. 24.2).[7] The specific indications for MRI in insertional Achilles tendinopathy are not well established. In the author's experience, patients who have a large Haglund deformity radiographically and clinically are not imaged with MRI preoperatively as an open approach with more significant detachment will be required to sufficiently access the entire area of pathology; therefore, no change in surgical management would occur based on MRI findings. In patients with less clinically apparent disease or where the pathology may be in question, an MRI may be helpful both to confirm the diagnosis as well as to assess the extent of the tendinopathy. In a small number of cases with primarily ventral changes of the tendon, endoscopic calcaneoplasty and tendon débridement may be an option for treatment. This option is also more likely to be considered in patients for who a prolonged weight-bearing time and recovery may not be well tolerated.

There have been descriptions of some alternative procedures to standard open débridement, detachment, Haglund excision, and reattachment, which will not be explored in detail here. Consideration should be made based on physical exam if an adjunctive procedure to improve dorsiflexion range of motion, such as a gastrocnemius recession, is indicated. Minimally invasive techniques for Haglund

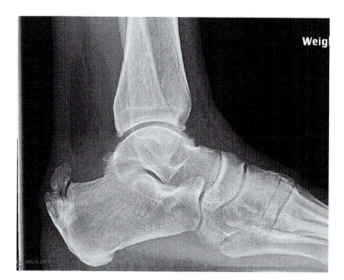

FIGURE 24.1 Lateral view of heel with a calcaneal prominence. The retrocalcaneal bursa is just posterior to the calcaneus and anterior to tendon attachment.

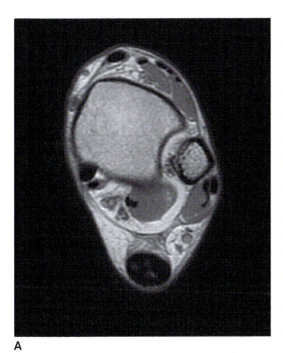 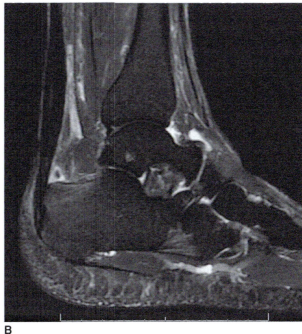

FIGURE 24.2 A. Axial cut of magnetic resonance imaging (MRI) showing intrasubstance degeneration. **B.** Sagittal MRI image of Achilles tendon insertion showing thickening of the tendon at the insertion and large calcaneal prominence.

deformity débridement have been described but thus far have been limited from widespread use for cases when significant tendon detachment may be necessary due to limitations of percutaneous reattachment and/or FHL transfer. Minimally invasive techniques are rapidly evolving, and there may be accepted such alternatives to the presently described technique in the not too distant future.

SURGICAL TECHNIQUE

Technique 1: Haglund Excision Through Tendon-Splitting Approach

- The patient is placed in a prone position, with the foot elevated with a bolster or blankets under the leg (Fig. 24.3A).
- The approach is through a posterior midline incision (Fig. 24.3B). Care should be taken to avoid injury to the sural nerve, which may be seen lying along the tendon's lateral border in the subcutaneous tissue.
- Alternatives to the posterior midline approach have been described, although they are less commonly used. J-Shaped, transverse, medial, and lateral approached have all been reported.
- A tendon-splitting approach (Fig. 24.4A) is used, and the tendon carefully dissected to expose degenerative tissue, intrasubstance tears, and intrasubstance calcifications (Fig. 24.4B). A primary goal of this procedure is to perform a thorough débridement of the degenerative areas of tendon and calcifications. This tendon-splitting approach provides excellent access to FHL should augmentation be required.
- Varying degrees of tendon detachment may be required in order to gain sufficient exposure of the degenerative areas of tendon insertion and Haglund deformity. By some reports, 70% to 80% tendon detachment is usually needed to gain sufficient exposure.[8] Where possible, leaving the most medial and lateral extents of the tendon attachment intact is very helpful to maintain resting tendon tension and is feasible in all but the most severe cases.
- Abnormal tendon is excised (Fig. 24.5A). While it may be challenging to distinguish normal from abnormal tendon, uniform tissue that has lost the natural tendon striations and is much thicker in texture than normal tendon should be excised. One way of describing the abnormal tendon has been like the texture of "crab meat," which is meant to describe disorganization of the fibers and

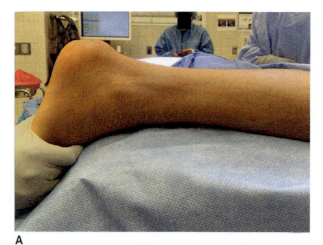
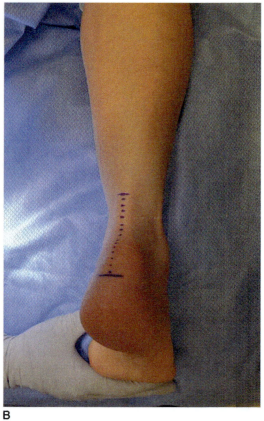

FIGURE 24.3 **A.** Prone positioning with blankets under the leg. **B.** Incision marked for posterior approach.

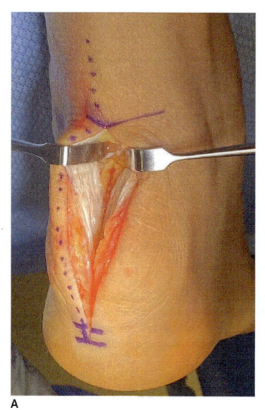
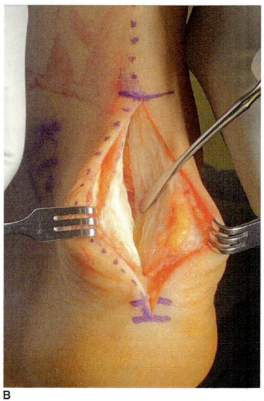

FIGURE 24.4 **A.** The Achilles tendon is split in the midline. **B.** The Achilles is dissected sharply to reveal the intratendinous tearing and degeneration.

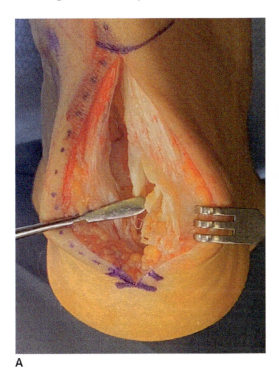 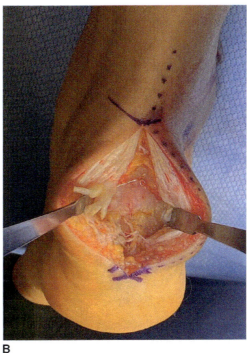

FIGURE 24.5 A. The Achilles is partially detached from the calcaneal tuberosity to expose further degeneration and bursal thickening. **B.** The inflamed bursa and fibrosed fat are removed to reveal the posterior-superior calcaneal prominence or Haglund deformity.

may provide some guidance for the surgeon in débridement. If it is still difficult to determine normal from abnormal tissue, the primary goal of the procedure is to debulk the tendon to a more normal thickness. Inflamed bursa and scarred or fibrosed fat are removed from above the retrocalcaneal space to define the Haglund deformity (Fig. 24.5B).
- Once all abnormal tissue from the tendon, and retrocalcaneal space are removed, there is a clear view of the Haglund deformity, calcaneal tuberosity, and posterior subtalar joint (Fig. 24.6).
- The Haglund deformity is resected with an oscillating saw with a typical excised fragment being 2 cm wide × 3 cm tall × 1 cm deep exposing a large insertion footprint for the Achilles tendon repair (Fig. 24.7).
- At this point, the remaining Achilles tendon insertion is assessed, and it is determined if augmentation with FHL tendon transfer is required—often if only poor-quality tendon tissue remains or a significant portion of the tendon insertion was débrided, the author typically considers greater than 50% of the tendon having been débrided as an indication to proceed with FHL transfer; however, the evidence for exact indications for augmentation is lacking.
- If no FHL transfer is performed, the tendon is repaired to the insertion with suture anchors. Both single row (two suture anchors) and double row (four suture anchor) techniques have been described.[9] It is at the surgeon's discretion as to whether a single or double row technique is chosen. This should be determined taking into consideration the degree of detachment that has been required to be performed. If a robust tendon attachment remains, consideration of less fixation should be given since suture anchors may cause patients pain as well as add unnecessary foreign material burden. If the majority of the tendon or complete detachment is performed, the added fixation of four anchors may be necessary. In the double-row technique, four holes are drilled for suture anchors into the exposed calcaneal footprint (Fig. 24.8A). These holes are spaced approximately 15 mm apart.
- The two proximal suture anchors preloaded with nonabsorbable suture tape are inserted (Fig. 24.8B). The suture from each anchor is then passed through each side of the Achilles tendon approximately 15 mm from the distal tendon insertion (Fig. 24.8C).

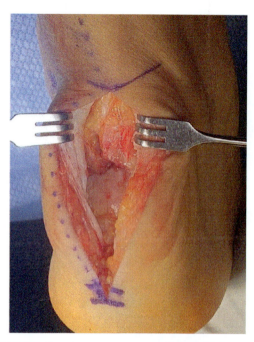

FIGURE 24.6 The abnormal tendon is débrided as there are areas of thickening, calcification within the tendon, and tendon degeneration giving a clear view of the Haglund deformity. If significant tendon is detached, repair with suture anchors with or without flexor hallucis longus tendon transfer (described below) is performed.

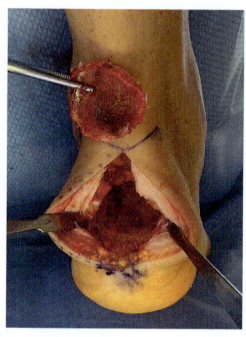

FIGURE 24.7 The calcaneal prominence is resected with a saw showing the fragment of bone removed from the incision approximately 2 × 3 cm in diameter.

- Once suture form each side is passed to the other, creating a suture bridge type pattern over the repair site (Fig. 24.9). Each pair of sutures is then loaded onto a suture anchor, tensioned, and inserted into the predrilled distal holes while maintaining appropriate plantar flexion of the foot to restore appropriate repair tension (Fig. 24.10).
- The tendon split is repaired with a running suture (see Fig. 24.8A), and the wound is closed with a 4-0 subcuticular monocryl suture (see Fig. 24.8B).

Technique 2: FHL Tendon Transfer (Augmentation)

- If it is determined that a significant portion of the tendon attachment was dissected, augmentation may be required with FHL tendon. The literature usually describes a number of this being indicated when less than 50% of the insertion remains and this is the guidance used by this author.
- Any fat overlying the FHL is excised, and then the deep fascia between the superficial and deep compartments is released.
- The hallux is flexed and extended to help identify the muscle belly of FHL (Fig. 24.11A).
- Great care should be taken while dissecting around the tendon of the FHL because the tibial nerve is immediately to the medial side (Fig. 24.11B).
- A tendon hook or curved clamp is placed around the tendon, and the ankle and hallux are plantarflexed to deliver maximal tendon from the fibro-osseous tunnel (Fig. 24.12A). The tendon is followed as it travels between the medial and lateral tubercles of the posterior talus, and the FHL tendon is released from its sheath (fibro-osseous tunnel). The tendon is cut as distally as possible; a small tendon stripper may help. Great care must be taken to avoid injury to the tibial nerve (Fig. 24.12B). A whip stitch is inserted into the FHL tendon. The tendon size is measured using a standard tendon sizer. The reamer size selected is typically 1 mm greater than the tendon diameter.
- A threaded guide wire is passed plantarly through the prepared calcaneus approximately 1 cm anterior to the posterior border of the calcaneus. This increases the mechanical advantage by maximizing the lever arm of the transferred tendon (Fig. 24.11A and B).

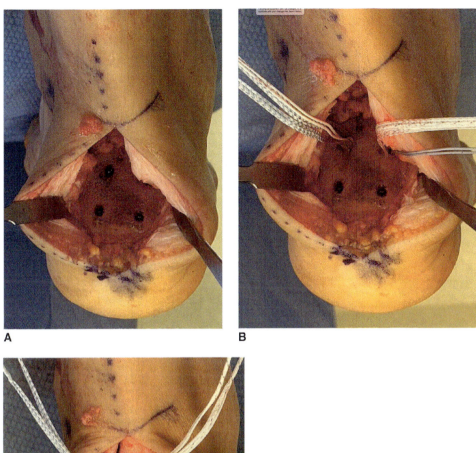
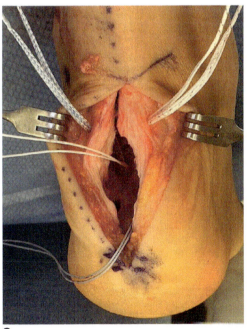

FIGURE 24.8 A. Drill holes for the placement of four suture anchors are made approximately 1.5 cm away from each other on the repair footprint. **B.** Preloaded suture anchors are inserted into the proximal holes. **C.** The suture tape is passed through the tendon on either side of the split approximately 1.5 cm from the distal insertion.

- Reaming is done over the guidewire with selected drill based on the size determined by the tendon size (Fig. 24.11C).
- The suture and attached tendon are pulled through the prepared drill hole using the guidewire (Fig. 24.12A), and the tendon is secured with an interference screw that is the size of the reamer used in preparing the hole once appropriate tension and foot position are achieved (Fig. 24.12B).
- With the tendon transfer securely fixed, the Achilles tendon is repaired to its insertion and the tendon split is closed (Fig. 24.12C).

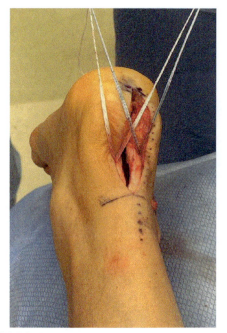

FIGURE 24.9 The suture pairs are separated and one limb from each side is brought together.

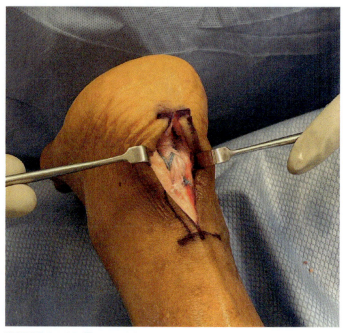

FIGURE 24.10 The repair is completed with insertion of the loaded distal anchors into the prepared drill holes.

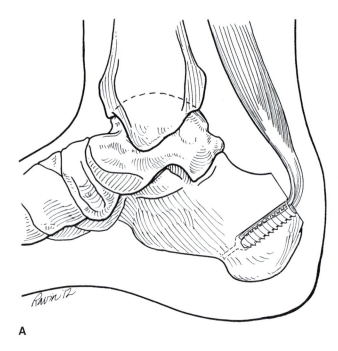

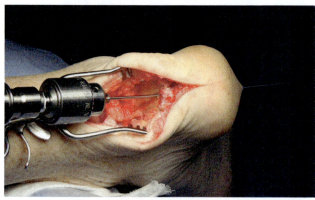

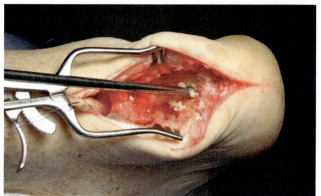

FIGURE 24.11 A. Tunnel placement for the flexor hallucis longus tendon. **B.** Threaded guidewire passed through calcaneus. **C.** Tunnel is prepared.

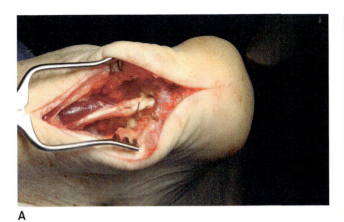
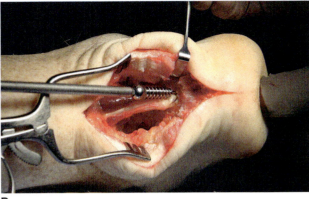
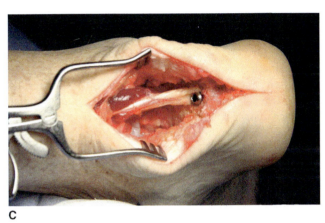

FIGURE 24.12 **A.** The tendon is pulled through into the tunnel. **B.** Tendon secured with 7 × 25 mm interference screw. **C.** Completed flexor hallucis longus tendon augmentation. Closure is routine.

PEARLS AND PITFALLS

- Avoid lateral position if considering a tendon-splitting approach
- Gentle skin handling
- Flexing the knee and plantarflexing the foot relieves tension on the Achilles tendon if required
- Adequate bony resection must be achieved to ensure decompression of the retrocalcaneal space
- Cautious dissection around the FHL tendon to protect the tibial nerve
- Adequate débridement is important in achieving symptomatic relief

POSTOPERATIVE MANAGEMENT

- Consider thromboprophylaxis, especially for high-risk patients
- Splint in plantar flexion with posterior (+/− anterior) slab of plaster of Paris
- Wound check 10 days
- Immobilization in an orthopedic walking boot with heel lift for 6 weeks if greater than 50% of the tendon insertion is detached or an augmentation procedure is performed
- Physiotherapy to regain gastrocnemius-soleus strength

RESULTS AND COMPLICATIONS

We have found that a significant improvement in pain and function can be expected after this surgery, which is also supported in the literature.[10] Patient satisfaction for this procedure is typically reported as between 85% and 95% satisfied. The complication rate in the literature is between 15% and 35% with most of those complications being considered "minor" such as scar hypertrophy and hypersensitivity. While these issues may be considered minor, they do contribute to patient dissatisfaction.[11]

There are also some potential serious problems that the patient should also be aware of including infection,[12,13] Achilles tendon rupture or avulsion, nerve injury, and persistent pain. Wound problems are a source of worry around the Achilles tendon, and great care should be taken when handling the soft tissues and posterior skin. Maintaining full-thickness skin flaps is recommended. Possible nerve damage includes injury to the sural nerve laterally or the posterior tibial nerve or its branches medially. This can be avoided by incision placement, using careful dissection technique, and controlling the position of the saw blade.

Removing too much bone at the insertion of the Achilles tendon may result in avulsion of the tendon (if no concurrent repair is performed). Removing insufficient bone from the posterior-superior aspect of the calcaneus may result in inadequate decompression of the retrocalcaneal bursa and persistent pain. In an effort to provide guidelines for how much tendon may be detached without risking rupture, Kolodziej et al[14] performed a cadaver study and concluded that as much as 50% of the Achilles tendon may be resected safely. Wagner et al reported on 75 patients and found equivalent satisfaction between those patients who had partial and complete detachment of the tendon.[15] It should be noted, however, that with complete detachment, postoperative restrictions are typically more prolonged. The protracted recovery period may be a source of dissatisfaction with many studies indicated that recovery may take up to 12 months. Patients should be advised preoperatively.

Sammarco and Taylor reported results of 39 feet that underwent excision of the posterior calcaneal tuberosity and reattachment of the Achilles tendon with bone anchors. The investigators reported a rate of 97% excellent or good results with an average of 3-year follow-up. Complications included one recurrence of painful prominence, one wound infection, and one incisional neuroma.[16] After 2 years of follow-up, Jarde et al reported the results of resection in 74 feet, with excellent or good results in 73%, fair in 16%, and poor in 11%.[17] Schneider et al found that complete relief of symptoms after resection was achieved in 34 (69%) of 49 feet and that the course of rehabilitation averaged 6 months. Nunley et al reported results of resection for insertional Achilles tendinopathy utilizing the central approach. Average recovery time was 6 months, and a 96% (22 of 23) satisfaction rate at 7-year follow-up with minimal to no loss of strength. Brunner et al described results of 36 patients (39 feet) who underwent calcaneal ostectomy for Haglund deformity with mean follow-up of 51 months. The mean American Orthopaedic Foot and Ankle Society score following surgery was 86/100 points; the mean SF-36v2 health survey score following surgery was 144/152. Six of the 36 patients interviewed, however, would not recommend the procedure to others, citing mainly prolonged recovery time, between 6 months and 2 years.

The determination of when to augment with the FHL tendon has been a topic of debate. It has often been recommended when greater than 50% of the insertion is excised. A recent randomized control trial found no difference in functional outcomes between patients who did and did not undergo FHL augmentation.[18] It is a safe means of augmentation and with modern techniques and implants does not require additional incisions for a more distal harvest.[19] Schon et al[20,21] studied the results of FHL transfer with Achilles tendon débridement surgery in older, sedentary patients and found that 57% of patients reported no hallux weakness and 76% reported no loss of balance due to hallux weakness and overall pain and function were significantly improved. In another retrospective study looking at FHL transfer with Achilles débridement, 92% of patients could perform a single leg heel rise at final follow-up and the rate of complications was low. In summary, FHL tendon transfer is a safe means of augmentation and with modern techniques and implants does not require additional incisions for a more distal harvest.[19]

REFERENCES

1. Chimenti RL, Cychosz CC, Hall MM, Phisitkul P. Current concepts review update: insertional Achilles tendinopathy. *Foot Ankle Int.* 2017;38(10):1160-1169.
2. Li HY, Hua YH. Achilles tendinopathy: current concepts about the basic science and clinical treatments. *Biomed Res Int.* 2016;2016:6492597.
3. de Vos RJ, Weir A, Visser RJ, de Winter T, Tol JL. The additional value of a night splint to eccentric exercises in chronic midportion Achilles tendinopathy: a randomised controlled trial. *Br J Sports Med.* 2007;41(7):e5.
4. Mansur NSB, Matsunaga FT, Carrazzone OL, et al. Shockwave therapy plus eccentric exercises versus isolated eccentric exercises for Achilles insertional tendinopathy: a double-blinded randomized clinical trial. *J Bone Joint Surg Am.* 2021;103(14):1295-1302.
5. Kunkle BF, Baxter NA, Hoch CP, et al. Success rate of non-operative treatment of insertional Achilles tendinitis. *Foot & Ankle Orthopaedics.* 2022;7(2).
6. Kang S, Thordarson DB, Charlton TP. Insertional Achilles tendinitis and Haglund's deformity. *Foot Ankle Int.* 2012;33(6):487-491.
7. Nicholson CW, Berlet GC, Lee TH. Prediction of the success of nonoperative treatment of insertional Achilles tendinosis based on MRI. *Foot Ankle Int.* 2007;28(4):472-477.
8. Barg A, Ludwig T. Surgical strategies for the treatment of insertional Achilles tendinopathy. *Foot Ankle Clin.* 2019;24(3):533-559.

9. Lakey E, Kumparatana P, Moon DK, et al. Biomechanical comparison of all-soft suture anchor single-row vs double-row bridging construct for insertional Achilles tendinopathy. *Foot Ankle Int*. 2021;42(2):215-223.
10. Nunley JA, Ruskin G, Horst F. Long-term clinical outcomes following the central incision technique for insertional Achilles tendinopathy. *Foot Ankle Int*. 2011;32(9):850-855.
11. Hörterer H, Baumbach SF, Oppelt S, et al. Complications associated with midline incision for insertional Achilles tendinopathy. *Foot Ankle Int*. 2020;41(12):1502-1509.
12. Brunner J, Anderson J, O'Malley M, et al. Physician and patient based outcomes following surgical resection of Haglund's deformity. *Acta Orthop Belg*. 2005;71(6):718-723.
13. Schneider W, Niehus W, Knahr W. Haglund's syndrome: disappointing results following surgery–a clinical and radiographic analysis. *Foot Ankle Int*. 2000;21:26-30.
14. Kolodziej P, Glisson R, Nunley JA. Risk of avulsion of the Achilles tendon after partial excision for treatment of insertional tendonitis and Haglund's deformity: a biomechanical study. *Foot Ankle Int*. 1999;20(7):433-437.
15. Wagner E, Gould JS, Kneidel M, Fleisig GS, Fowler R. Technique and results of Achilles tendon detachment and reconstruction for insertional Achilles tendinosis. *Foot Ankle Int*. 2006;27(9):677-684.
16. Sammarco GJ, Taylor AL. Operative management of Haglund's deformity in the nonathlete: a retrospective study. *Foot Ankle Int*. 1998;19(11):724-729.
17. Jardé O, Quenot P, Trinquier-Lautard JL, Tran-Van F, Vives P. Maladie de Haglund traitée par résection tubérositaire simple. Etude angulaire et thérapeutique. A propos de 74 cas avec deux ans de recul [Haglund disease treated by simple resection of calcaneus tuberosity. An angular and therapeutic study. Apropos of 74 cases with 2 years follow-up]. *Rev Chir Orthop Reparatrice Appar Mot*. 1997;83(6):566-573.
18. Hunt KJ, Cohen BE, Davis WH, Anderson RB, Jones CP. Surgical treatment of insertional Achilles tendinopathy with or without flexor hallucis longus tendon transfer: a prospective randomized study. *Foot Ankle Int*. 2015;36(9):998-1005.
19. Yassin M, Gupta V, Martins A, Mahadevan D, Bhatia M. Patient reported outcomes and satisfaction following single incision Flexor Hallucis Longus (FHL) augmentation for chronic Achilles tendon pathologies. *J Clin Orthop Trauma*. 2021;23:101650.
20. Schon LC, Shores JL, Faro FD, Vora AM, Camire LM, Guyton GP. Flexor hallucis longus tendon transfer in treatment of Achilles tendinosis. *J Bone Joint Surg Am*. 2013;95(1):54-60.
21. de Cesar NC, Chinanuvathana A, Fonseca LFD, Dein EJ, Tan EW, Schon LC. Outcomes of flexor digitorum longus (FDL) tendon transfer in the treatment of Achilles tendon disorders. *Foot Ankle Surg*. 2019;25(3):303-309.

25 Endoscopic Treatment of Insertional Achilles Deformity

Jordi Vega, Matteo Guelfi, and Miki Dalmau-Pastor

INTRODUCTION

Insertional Achilles tendinopathy is usually related to a deformity of the posterosuperior part of the calcaneal tuberosity, which is referred to as Haglund syndrome. It is a common cause of posterior heel pain characterized by painful swelling of an inflamed retrocalcaneal bursa, Achilles insertional tendinopathy, and enlarged calcaneal tuberosity.[1,2] It is considered an overuse injury of the insertion of the Achilles tendon that may be due to an excessive contact during dorsiflexion of the ankle between the Achilles tendon and a prominent posterosuperior part of the calcaneal tuberosity or Haglund deformity. Both intratendinous calcification and partial tears of the Achilles tendon insertion are common components associated to Achilles tendinopathy.[1,2]

Treatment is initially conservative, including nonsteroidal anti-inflammatory drugs, activity modification and/or rest, plantar orthoses and shoe modification, physiotherapy including eccentric training and stretching exercises, and/or shockwave therapy.[2,3] If conservative treatment fails, surgical treatment should be proposed.

Surgical procedures on insertional Achilles tendinopathy can be open or minimally invasive (percutaneous or endoscopic).[4-6] Open surgical procedures treating Haglund syndrome are characterized by a higher risk of wound healing complications and the need for detachment with subsequent reattachment of the Achilles tendon.[4,7] In contrast, endoscopic techniques have the advantage of addressing the pathology without the need for complete Achilles detachment with a low risk of soft tissue complications.[4,8,9] For these reasons, endoscopy has gained further popularity in the surgical management of Achilles insertional tendinopathy.[4,6]

INDICATIONS AND CONTRAINDICATIONS

As mentioned above, complications related to skin incisions after Achilles tendon open surgical procedure (up to 21%)[10] have favored the use of endoscopic techniques. Endoscopy allows for a minimally invasive management of insertional Achilles tendinopathy. The small skin incisions reduce the risk of complications related to the healing of surgical wounds. This makes endoscopic procedures highly recommended in patients with such risk, which includes obesity, smokers, or patients with vascular problems in lower extremities.

In addition to a lower risk of wound complications, endoscopy allows for a more accurate surgery and less soft tissue aggression. As a result, postoperative pain is reduced, and early weight bearing and physiotherapy can be performed, which presents advantages especially in young and active patients.

Classically, endoscopic procedures for insertional Achilles tendinopathy included calcaneoplasty, retrocalcaneal bursa excision, and Achilles tendon débridement. Other endoscopic procedures have been described, such as endoscopic Achilles tendon reinforcement or augmentation with anchors or biological augmentation with endoscopic flexor hallucis longus (FHL) tendon transfer.[7,11,12] Recently, an endoscopic Achilles tendon detachment and reattachment using a double-row suture bridge has been described.[12] In the authors' experience, Achilles tendon reinforcement with anchors is required in about 10% of cases after endoscopic calcaneoplasty, particularly in young and high demanding patients who have a high risk of postoperative tendon detachment.

In cases of severe insertional Achilles tendinopathy on magnetic resonance imaging (MRI)/ultrasound (US), or with a tear of more than 50% of the tendon, the calcaneoplasty could be biologically augmented with a FHL tendon transfer.[13-15] The endoscopic FHL tendon transfer provides a mechanical and biological support to the injured Achilles tendon. As a result, the transferred FHL tendon would help the Achilles tendon during healing process.

Given the above, endoscopic treatment of insertional Achilles tendinopathy does not have any specific contraindication. However, as endoscopic techniques treating insertional Achilles tendon pathology are highly demanding procedures, they are not ideal for novice surgeons or surgeons without experience in other foot and ankle endoscopic procedures.

PREOPERATIVE PLANNING

A general evaluation of the patient will help to determine compliance for the surgical procedure, including the postoperative treatment or rehabilitation process. Before the surgery, the patient needs to understand the procedure and its risks along with the nonsurgical alternatives. Patients need to be aware of potential complications, such as a prolonged recovery time, swelling, range of motion restriction, neurovascular injury, tendon entrapment, Achilles tendon rupture, or recurrent symptoms. The step-by-step rehabilitation program should be explained before surgery.

Alteration of lower extremity axis or any foot deformity should be detected during the preoperative work up in order to decide if any previous treatment is required, or if any kind of postoperative aid such as insoles or specific physiotherapy exercises will be needed.

A Silfverskiold test should be performed in every patient. In case of a gastrocnemius contracture, some authors advocate for a gastrocnemius lengthening as an adjunct procedure combined with the Achilles insertional treatment.[16]

Imaging studies are routinely obtained to evaluate insertional Achilles tendinopathy. On lateral weight-bearing radiographs of the ankle, several findings should be detected. A Haglund deformity and the presence of posterior calcaneal bone spur and/or intratendinous calcifications are common signs of insertional Achilles tendinopathy. US and MRI are useful to observe Achilles tendon characteristics, bursitis, intratendinous calcifications, or calcaneal bone spurs.[17] However, MRI is recommended as it has a highest diagnostic accuracy when compared to US.[18] Although both can be obtained, our recommendation is to obtain just a US only when MRI is not possible.

SURGICAL TECHNIQUE

- The procedure can be performed under spinal or general anesthesia. Alternatively, and in order to obtain better postoperative pain control, a popliteal block may be used in addition to general anesthesia.
- Patient is placed in a prone position. To have free ankle movement, the foot and ankle must be placed at the edge of the table. A soft support is placed to flex the knee 10° to 15°. The pelvis is rotated to obtain a neutral position of the affected limb. The contralateral lower extremity is separated from the surgical leg (Fig. 25.1).
- Bilateral procedures are rarely performed simultaneously.
- A thigh tourniquet is recommended.
- Hindfoot endoscopy is performed with a standard arthroscope (4.0 mm and 30° scope), a 4.0-mm arthroscopic motorized shaver, and basic and large arthroscopic instruments. Both gravity or pump flow can be used at the surgeon's discretion.
- Cutaneous landmarks—the distal tip of the lateral malleolus, the Achilles tendon, and the calcaneal tuberosity—should be highlighted before starting the surgery.
- Hindfoot endoscopic portals or portals placed between the Achilles tendon and the Haglund deformity, originally described by van Dijk, can be used.[8,19] With the aim to better visualize the area and with instruments to access the insertional area of the Achilles tendon, Vega et al[20] modified the classic hindfoot endoscopy portals. Modified portals are placed slightly distal and anterior to the classic. The posterolateral portal (0.5-cm skin longitudinal incision) is performed first and is used

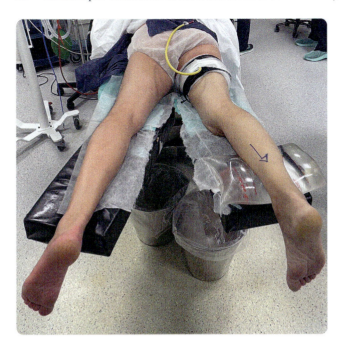

FIGURE 25.1 Patient positioning.

for scope introduction. The arthroscopic instruments are introduced through the posteromedial portal (0.5-cm skin longitudinal incision) (Fig. 25.2).

- A distal midline Achilles portal has been described and used for Haglund resection and bone anchor introduction.[20] The distal midline Achilles portal is located at the midline of the Achilles tendon and close to its insertional area. Proper location of this portal is checked under endoscopic or even radiological aid with the help of a needle. Both, the skin and tendon incisions are performed longitudinally in order to minimize Achilles tendon damage (Fig. 25.3).

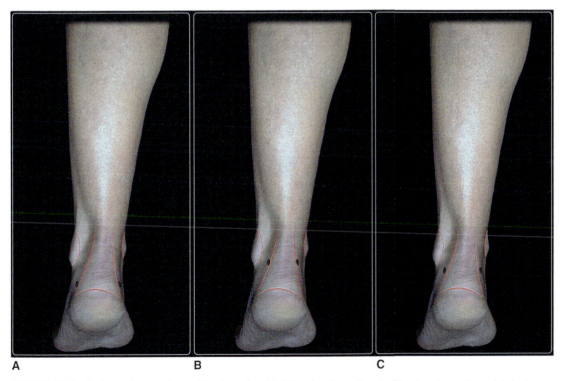

FIGURE 25.2 Endoscopic portals used for insertional Achilles tendinopathy. **A.** Direct endoscopic portals between the Achilles tendon and the Haglund deformity. **B.** Classic hindfoot endoscopic portals. **C.** Modified endoscopic portals.

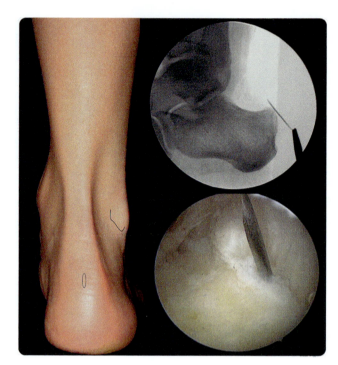

FIGURE 25.3 Distal midline Achilles portal. A needle is introduced through the portal and in a proximal direction. Radiological and endoscopic control of the needle placement.

- A protocolized endoscopic technique is performed to create a working area. Posterior ankle soft tissue between the Achilles tendon and the tibiotalar and subtalar joint is débrided with an arthroscopic shaver as described by van Dijk.[8] Anatomical structures of the posterior ankle should be identified. The posterolateral aspect of the subtalar joint is first identified. Next, the arthroscopic shaver is directed medially and proximal to the subtalar joint, to locate the FHL tendon. The FHL tendon is an important landmark, as the neurovascular tibial bundle is located medial to it.
- Once the working area is created, the scope and instruments are redirected to the posterior area. With the arthroscopic shaver in contact with the superior surface of the calcaneus, removal of the soft tissue and bursectomy is performed until the posterior part of the calcaneal tuberosity is visualized. After calcaneal bursectomy, and with the ankle in plantarflexion, the anterior surface of the Achilles tendon and its insertional area can be observed (Fig. 25.4).

Endoscopic Calcaneoplasty

- The Haglund deformity can be resected with the instruments inserted through the posterolateral and posteromedial hindfoot endoscopic portals or its modification as previously described

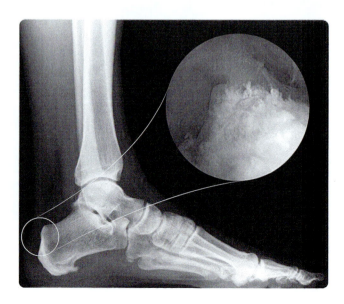

FIGURE 25.4 Endoscopic view of the calcaneal tuberosity with the scope introduced through the modified posterolateral portal. Arthroscope and visualization directed posteriorly.

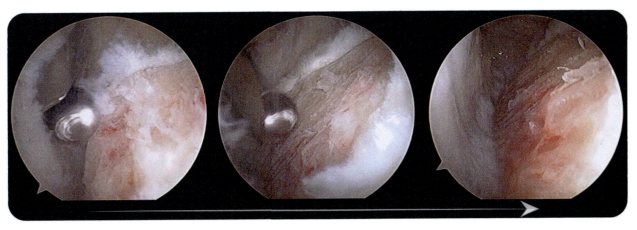

FIGURE 25.5 Endoscopic resection of Haglund deformity with arthroscope and instruments inserted through the posterolateral and posteromedial modified hindfoot endoscopic portals.

(Fig. 25.5). The authors' preference is to perform the calcaneal ostectomy with an arthroscopic burr inserted through a distal midline Achilles portal (Fig. 25.6).
- Care should be taken to protect the Achilles tendon during calcaneoplasty. The cutting end of the instrument should be directed toward the bone and away from the tendon.
- Bone resection could be underestimated when endoscopically performed. Radiological control is recommended to observe the calcaneal ostectomy. A Kirschner wire (K-wire) placed under radiological control can be used as a guide for the bone resection.
- If any pathology of the tendon, such as intratendinous calcification or insertional partial tendon tear is observed in imaging studies or during endoscopic procedure, débridement of the pathological tissue can be performed with an arthroscopic shaver.
- In the case of calcaneal spur, it can be removed under endoscopic view with the help of an arthroscopic burr introduced through an accessory portal performed close to the bony spur, and the arthroscope placed between the tendon and the skin. However, this is a difficult endoscopic procedure because usually the spur is not easy to visualize endoscopically, and a radiological view is required in most of the cases. For this reason, the authors' preference is to remove the calcaneal spurs under radiological control and the use of a minimally invasive surgery burr.

Endoscopic Single Row Achilles Tendon Reinforcement or Augmentation

- In order to avoid the risk of Achilles tendon detachment after calcaneoplasty, endoscopic Achilles tendon reinforcement or augmentation with anchors in a single row has been described.[20]

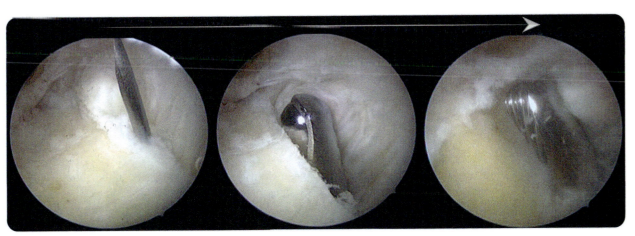

FIGURE 25.6 Endoscopic resection of Haglund deformity with arthroscope introduced through a modified hindfoot endoscopic portal, and arthroscopic shaver and burr inserted through the distal midline Achilles portal.

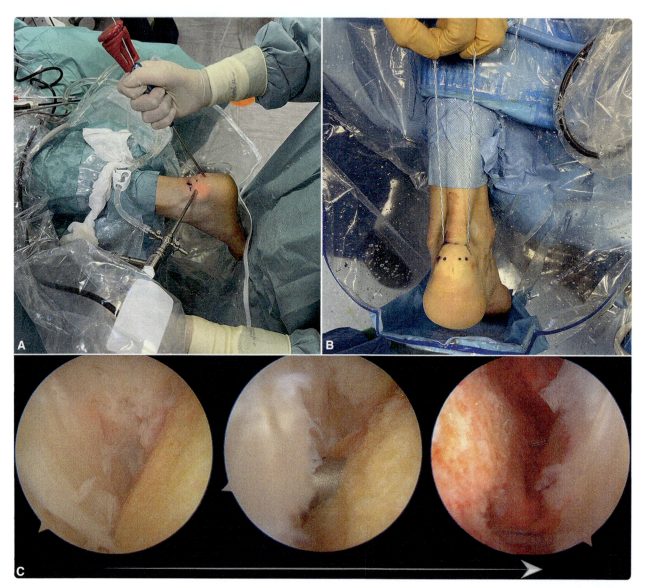

FIGURE 25.7 Endoscopic single row Achilles tendon reinforcement. **A.** Introduction of bone anchors through the distal midline Achilles portal. **B.** Sutures are taken out through the posterolateral and posteromedial endoscopic portals prior to penetrating the Achilles tendon. **C.** Endoscopic view of bone anchors insertion.

- After calcaneoplasty, one or two bone anchors are inserted to the calcaneus and introduced through the distal midline Achilles tendon portal (Fig. 25.7).
- The authors' preferred anchor is a nonmetallic bone anchor, 3.5 to 4 mm diameter, with one or two high resistance sutures. The anchor should be placed at the insertional area or 0.5 cm proximal to it. The tunnel for the anchor should be drilled parallel to the plantar sole. If only one anchor is placed, it will be located in the midline of the calcaneus. On the other hand, if two anchors are needed, one will be placed medial and the other lateral to the midline of the calcaneus, at a minimum distance of 1 cm between anchors.
- With a straight suture passer, the Achilles tendon is percutaneously penetrated 0.5 cm proximal to the anchor and under endoscopic control (Fig. 25.8).
- Sutures are retrieved with an arthroscopic grasper introduced through one of the portals. Through the same portal, the nitinol wire is pulled out with the help of the arthroscopic grasper.
- Next, one of the suture limbs of the bone anchor is introduced inside the nitinol wire loop. The nitinol is pulled and the suture penetrates the tendon and the skin. The same steps are performed for each suture limb until all sutures penetrate the tendon.

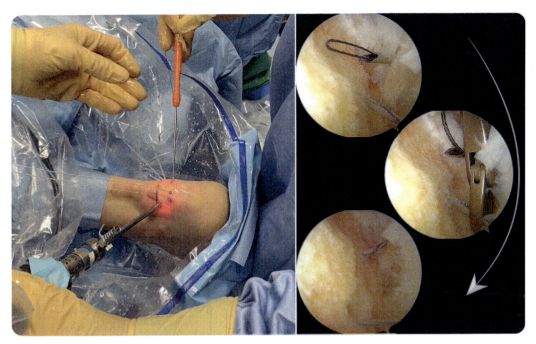

FIGURE 25.8 External and endoscopic view showing Achilles tendon penetration with a straight suture passer for a single row augmentation.

- With a mosquito clamp, the tendon is separated from the subcutaneous layer and the suture limbs retrieved subcutaneously from the posteromedial portal or posterolateral portal. The arthroscope is not required for this step.
- Running knots are performed with the ankle plantarflexed in order to relax the Achilles tendon and make easy contact with the calcaneus.

Endoscopic Suture Bridge Achilles Tendon Reinforcement or Augmentation

- Following the same philosophy of the endoscopic single row Achilles tendon reinforcement, a second and distal row can be performed. In order to increase the strength of the Achilles tendon augmentation, a suture bridge configuration can be performed (Fig. 25.9).
- When performing the suture bridge reattachment, anchors with tape-like sutures are suggested for the proximal row in order to provide a low-profile construct, while knotless anchors are used for the distal row providing a tendon reinforcement without risk of knot impingement. The authors prefer to use soft anchors with high resistance and flat suture for the proximal row (1.6- to 2-mm soft anchor) and knotless anchors for the distal row (3.5- to 4-mm knotless anchor).
- Once the calcaneoplasty is completed, the first row of anchors is placed and sutures passed through the Achilles tendon as previously described. Although the sutures can be knotted to fix the first row, it is not mandatory as they will be fixed in the second row.
- Next, two distal approaches are performed for the placement of the distal row anchors. These are located at both sides of the posterior and distal calcaneal bone.
- With a mosquito clamp, the tendon is separated from the subcutaneous layer, from the distal to the proximal portals.
- With the help of an arthroscopic grasper introduced from the distal portals, the sutures are retrieved subcutaneously in a suture bridge configuration—one limb from the same side anchor and one limb from the opposite side anchor.
- Finally, a tunnel for the anchors is drilled, and knotless anchors are loaded with sutures and introduced with the ankle in plantarflexion.

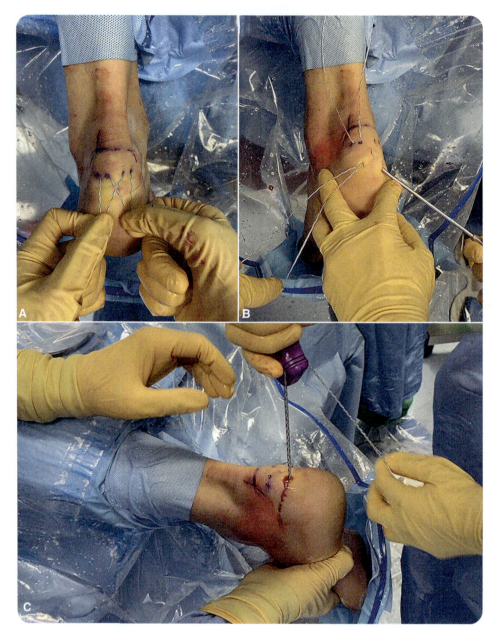

FIGURE 25.9 Suture bridge Achilles tendon reinforcement **(A)**. After the proximal row, sutures are subcutaneously retrieved in a bridge configuration **(B)** and from two distal approaches created at both sides of the posterior and distal calcaneal bone **(C)**.

- The authors use this suture bridge reinforcement without detachment of the healthy Achilles tendon. However, endoscopic Achilles tendon detachment and reattachment has been recently described.[12]

Endoscopic FHL Tendon Transfer

- The endoscopic FHL tendon transfer is usually performed with the scope introduced through the posterolateral portal and instruments through the posteromedial portal. When the FHL tendon transfer is planned, the FHL tendon must be identified during the creation of the endoscopic working.
- If a calcaneoplasty is being performed, it must be completed before the FHL tendon transfer.
- When the working area has been created and the FHL tendon is visible, the posterior fibulotalocalcaneal ligament, or Rouvière and Canela ligament,[21] is cut as proximal as possible in order to allow free movement of the FHL tendon. This allows a straight FHL tendon trajectory to the most posterior aspect of the calcaneal bone.

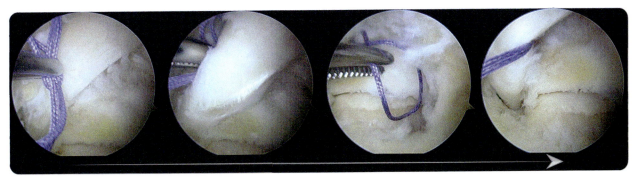

FIGURE 25.10 FHL tendon looping with a suture and with the help of a mosquito clamp.

- Next, the FHL tendon retinaculum is released with the help of an arthroscopic shaver or scissors.
- With the help of a mosquito clamp introduced through the posteromedial portal, the tendon is looped with a suture (Fig. 25.10). By pulling the suture, the tendon is subluxated from its calcaneal groove between the posterolateral and posteromedial talar tubercles.
- Next, the FHL tendon is harvested. According to FHL tendon zones previously described,[20,22] the tendon can be cut at zone 1 or 2. In order to have a longer tendon to be transferred, the authors' preference is to cut the tendon at zone 2, when the tendon courses under the sustentaculum tali.
- In order to harvest the FHL tendon at zone 2, the scope is introduced inside the fibro-osseous FHL tendon sheath after pulling the sutures grasping the tendon.
- Under direct endoscopic vision, and with the help of a needle, the right point to cut the tendon is identified at the level of the sustentaculum tali. With a beaver blade (number 64), the tendon is percutaneously cut at that point while the assistant is pushing the suture to visualize and transect the tendon as distal as possible to obtain the longest tendon to transfer (Fig. 25.11).
- Once the tendon is cut, it is pulled out through the posteromedial portal.
- The tendon is grasped with a Krackow suture or similar. A high-resistance suture (#0 or #2) is recommended.
- Next, the FHL tendon is introduced into a calcaneal tunnel and secured with a screw. A blind tunnel is drilled in the most posterior and superior part of the calcaneus, as close as possible to the Achilles tendon.
- A K-wire with an eyelet introduced through the posteromedial portal is used as guide for the drill. The drilling direction should be from dorsal to plantar and centered at midpoint between medial to lateral. It is recommended to drill same diameter tunnel as the tendon diameter. The aimed blind-tunnel length is 25 to 30 mm (Fig. 25.12).
- Once the tunnel is drilled, sutures are introduced into the eyelet of the K-wire. By pushing out the K-wire from the plantar aspect, the sutures are passed through the tunnel, and by pulling the

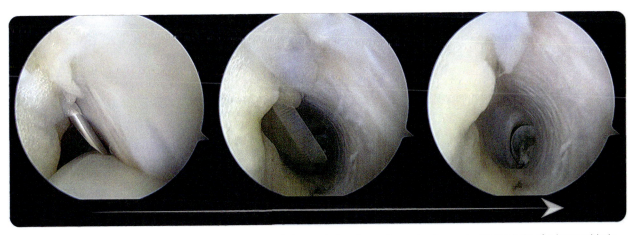

FIGURE 25.11 FHL tendon cut at its zone 2. The tendon is harvested under endoscopic view and with the help of a beaver blade introduced percutaneously.

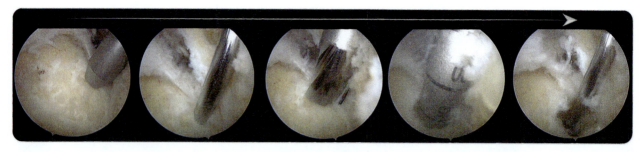

FIGURE 25.12 Endoscopic view of tunnel placement and drilling. The ideal blind-tunnel length is 25 to 30 mm.

sutures, the tendon is introduced into the tunnel (Fig. 25.13). It is recommended that a minimum of 15 mm tendon is introduced into the tunnel.
- Under direct endoscopic vision, a nitinol wire is introduced into the tunnel through the posteromedial portal. Using the nitinol wire as a guide, the biotenodesis or interference screw is introduced to secure the tendon into the tunnel. In order to have a strong transferred tendon secure into the tunnel, the ideal screw size should be with the same tunnel diameter, and a minimum of 15 mm length (Fig. 25.14).
- The tendon is secured with the ankle in plantarflexion. Tension of the transferred FHL tendon is performed by pulling the sutures before introducing the screw. Advancement of the screw and a final endoscopic control is performed (Fig. 25.15).

Closure and Dressing

- Incisions are closed and a soft bandage applied.
- If the procedure performed was an isolated calcaneoplasty, immobilization is not mandatory. Weight bearing is encouraged according to the patient's tolerance. The patient can start physiotherapy in the next days after surgery.
- After an Achilles tendon reattachment or FHL tendon transfer, a controlled ankle motion walker boot is used for 4 weeks. The boot is plantarflexed at about 15° to 20° for the first 2 weeks. The third week the boot is changed to 0° and weight bearing is allowed. After the fourth week the boot is removed, and the patient can start physiotherapy.

POSTOPERATIVE MANAGEMENT

- Once the portals are healed, the sutures are removed.
- Weight bearing with the aid of crutches is used until the patient is comfortable to mobilize without aid.
- Postoperative physiotherapy includes passive and active ankle motion and muscle strengthening with elastic bands. In the case of FHL tendon transfer, exercises to stimulate flexor hallucis brevis muscle are recommended.
- Progressive increases in muscle strength and activity are encouraged. Daily activity and return to sports activities are expected according to Achilles tendon healing.

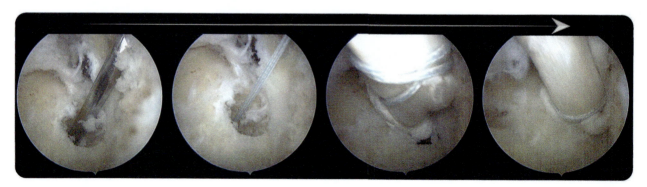

FIGURE 25.13 Endoscopic view of FHL tendon introduction into the calcaneal tunnel.

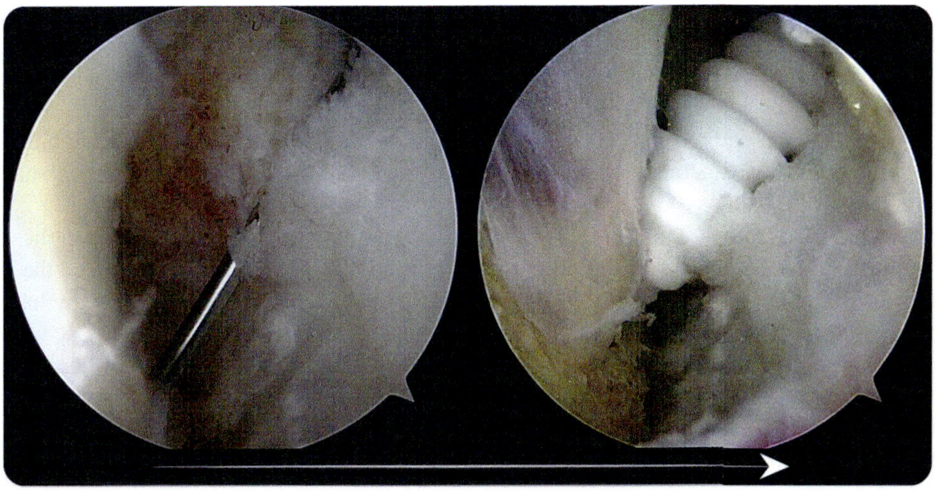

FIGURE 25.14 Endoscopic view of FHL tendon fixation with a biotenodesis screw used as an interference screw.

RESULTS AND COMPLICATIONS

The first favorable outcomes of endoscopic calcaneoplasty were reported by van Dijk in 2001.[8] Since then, several studies regarding endoscopic techniques to address insertional Achilles tendinopathy have been published over the years with excellent results. A recent systematic review based on 35 studies reported better clinical functional outcomes, lower complication rate, and shorter recovery time for the endoscopic technique compared to an open calcaneoplasty procedure.[23]

In the last 10 years, a new generation of techniques has been proposed to extend the endoscopic indications treating insertional Achilles tendinopathy. The insertional Achilles tendon augmentation with a single- or double-row anchors and the use of the FHL tendon transfer in the insertional Achilles tendinopathy are the most popular, with promising results shown despite a limited number of clinical studies available.

Excellent clinical results for the endoscopic calcaneoplasty associated with tendon augmentation with a single-row anchor have been reported.[20] In this study, no major complications were observed, and all the patients returned to their daily activities without limitations, except for two patients who described complaints with sports activity.

Another recent study reported an overall success rate of 93.3% when performing endoscopic FHL tendon transfer to augment Achilles tendon disorders.[24] Despite this, a high rate of minor complications (20%) was observed, with only one patient requiring revision surgery. However, this study was not specific to insertional Achilles tendinopathy. In our experience, the FHL tendon transfer provides a faster return to daily and sports activities of the patients.

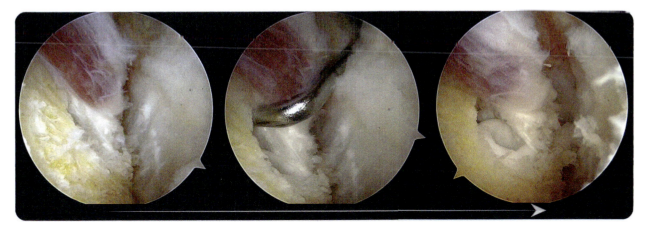

FIGURE 25.15 Endoscopic final view of the FHL tendon transferred to the calcaneal bone near to the Achilles tendon insertion.

Although no clinical data are available, advantages of the double row anchor technique are the absence of prominent knots and the reduced surgical time related to not tying the knots. In addition, this insertional area augmentation allows for a shorter time of immobilization and a faster postoperative rehabilitation.

To the best of our knowledge, no case series studies regarding the endoscopic Achilles tendon detachment and reattachment with anchors have been published in the English international literature.

Endoscopic procedures treating insertional Achilles tendinopathy are not free of complications. The main risk of the technique is in relation to the endoscopic working area creation and the injury of the neurovascular tibial bundle. Injury of the tibial nerve during hindfoot endoscopy has been reported in 3% of patients.[25-29] However, the incidence of tibial nerve injury may increase when the surgeon is not experienced in endoscopic foot and ankle techniques. Attention must be paid when creating the working area as the neurovascular tibial bundle is located close, and in some cases in contact[30] with the FHL tendon, which is the main endoscopic landmark.[31]

Endoscopic portals are safe as skin incisions are far from neurovascular structures.

The risk of Achilles tendon detachment after calcaneoplasty exists, especially after excessive bony resection or in patients with a high level of activity.[32,33] Postoperative immobilization, and/or Achilles tendon augmentation with anchors, as described here, can reduce the risk of Achilles tendon detachment after calcaneoplasty.

PEARLS AND PITFALLS

- Both gravity and pump flow can be used at the surgeon's discretion. When pump, low pressure is recommended to avoid soft tissue edema that could potentially make difficult an eventual open procedure in the area.
- It is recommended to debride the soft tissue near the portals to obtain an adequate arthroscopic view of the Achilles tendon insertional area.
- When endoscopic FHL tendon transfer, place the modified posteromedial slightly anterior in order to obtain as easier access to the more posterior aspect of the calcaneal bone.
- The distal midline Achilles portal can be used to perform the calcaneal tunnel, transferred the FHL tendon and to secure it with screw. In order to avoid tendon damage at the insertional area and during every surgical step, introduction of an arthroscopic cannula through the portal will protect the Achilles tendon.
- A common problem when FHL tendon is fixed in the calcaneal tunnel is to introduce the screw in the wrong direction. Introduction of the nitinol wire guide into the tunnel before the FHL tendon is a simple way to ensure that the screw will progress in the correct direction and secure the transferred tendon.
- In order to increase the tendon contact with the bone when tendon augmentation after calcaneoplasty, the ankle must be plantarflexed and the tendon pushed against the bone with the surgeon or assistant fingers while single row suture knots are performed, or sutures fixed in the double row.

REFERENCES

1. van Dijk CN, van Sterkenburg MN, Wiergerinck JI, Karlsson J, Maffulli N. Terminology for Achilles tendon related disorders. *Knee Surg Sports Traumatol Arthrosc*. 2011;19:835-841.
2. Maffulli N, Kader D. Tendinopathy of tendon Achillis. *J Bone Joint Surg Br*. 2002;84:1-8.
3. Johnston E, Scranton P, Pfeffer GB. Chronic disorders of the Achilles tendon: results of conservative and surgical treatments. *Foot Ankle Int*. 1997;18:570-574.
4. Wiegerinck JI, Kerkhoffs GM, van Sterkenburg MN, Sierevelt IN, van Dijk CN. Treatment for insertional Achilles tendinopathy: a systematic review. *Knee Surg Sports Traumatol Arthrosc*. 2013;21:1345-1355.
5. Lalond KA. The surgical treatment of Achilles tendinopathy: a treatment algorithm. *Tech Foot Ankle Surg*. 2012;11:113-117.
6. Guelfi M, Vega J, Salini V. Trattamento endoscopico delle patologie del tendine d'Achille: tecniche chirurgiche e indicazioni. *G Ital Ortop Traumatol*. 2020;46:62-73.
7. Maffulli N, Tesla V, Capasso G, Sullo A. Calcific insertional Achilles tendinopathy: reattachment with bone anchors. *Am J Sports Med*. 2004;32:174-182.
8. van Dijk CN, Van Dyk GE, Scholten PE, Kort NP. Endoscopic calcaneoplasty. *Am J Sports Med*. 2001;29:185-189.
9. Ortmann FW, McBryde AM. Endoscopic bony and soft-tissue decompression of the retrocalcaneal space for the treatment of Haglund deformity and retrocalcaneal bursitis. *Foot Ankle Int*. 2007;28:149-153.
10. Yang B, Liu Y, Kan S, et al. Outcomes and complications of percutaneous versus open repair of acute Achilles tendon rupture: a meta-analysis. *Int J Surg*. 2017;40:178-186.

11. Hunt KJ, Cohen BE, Davis WH, Anderson RB, Jones CP. Surgical treatment of insertional Achilles tendinopathy with or without flexor hallucis longus tendon transfer: a prospective, randomized study. *Foot Ankle Int.* 2015;36:998-1005.
12. Lopes R, Ngbilo C, Padiolleau G, Boniface O. Endoscopic speed bridge: a new treatment for insertional Achilles tendinopathy. *Orthop Traumatol Surg Res.* 2021;107(6):102854.
13. Elias I, Raikin SM, Besser MP, Nazarian LN. Outcomes of chronic insertional Achilles tendinosis using FHL autograft through single incision. *Foot Ankle Int.* 2009;30:197-204.
14. Wilcox DK, Bohay DR, Anderson JG. Treatment of chronic Achilles tendon disorders with flexor hallucis longus tendon transfer/augmentation. *Foot Ankle Int.* 2000;21:1004-1010.
15. Den Hartog B. Flexor hallucis longus transfer for chronic Achilles tendinosis. *Foot Ankle Int.* 2003;24:233-237.
16. Chimenti RL, Cychosz CC, Hall MM, Phisitkul P. Current concepts review update: insertional Achilles tendinopathy. *Foot Ankle Int.* 2017;38(10):1160-1169.
17. Chimenti RL, Chimenti PC, Buckley MR, Houck JR, Flemister AS. Utility of ultrasound for imaging osteophytes in patients with insertional Achilles tendinopathy. *Arch Phys Med Rehabil.* 2016;97(7):1206-1209.
18. Gatz M, Bode D, Betsch M, et al. Multimodal ultrasound versus MRI for the diagnosis and monitoring of Achilles tendinopathy. A prospective longitudinal study. *Orthop J Sports Med.* 2021;9(4):23259671211006826.
19. van Dijk CN, Scholten PE, Krips R. A 2-portal endoscopic approach for diagnosis and treatment of posterior ankle pathology. *Arthroscopy.* 2000;16:871-876.
20. Vega J, Baduell A, Malagelada F, Allmendinger J, Dalmau-Pastor M. Endoscopic Achilles tendon augmentation with suture anchors after calcaneal exostectomy in Haglund syndrome. *Foot Ankle Int.* 2018;39:551-559.
21. De Leeuw PAJ, Vega J, Karlsson J, Dalmau-Pastor M. The posterior fibulotalocalcaneal ligament complex: a forgotten ligament. *Knee Surg Sports Traumatol Arthrosc.* 2021;29(5):1627-1634.
22. Lui TH. Flexor hallucis longus tendoscopy: a technical note. *Knee Surg Sports Traumatol Arthrosc.* 2009;17:107-110.
23. Alessio-Mazzola M, Russo A, Capello AG, et al. Endoscopic calcaneoplasty for the treatment of Haglund's deformity provides better clinical functional outcomes, lower complication rate, and shorter recovery time compared to open procedures: a systematic review. *Knee Surg Sports Traumatol Arthrosc.* 2021;29(8):2462-2484.
24. Batista JP, Del Vecchio JJ, van Dijk N, Pereira H. Endoscopic FHL transfer to augment Achilles disorders. *J ISAKOS.* 2020;5:109-114.
25. van Dijk CN, van Bergen CJA. Advancements in ankle arthroscopy. *J Am Acad Orthop Surg.* 2008;11:635-646.
26. Scholten PE, Sierevelt IN, van Dijk CN. Hindfoot endoscopy for posterior ankle impingement. *J Bone Joint Surg Am.* 2008;90(12):2665-2672.
27. Nickisch F, Barg A, Saltzman CL, et al. Postoperative complications of posterior ankle and hindfoot arthroscopy. *J Bone Joint Surg Am.* 2012;94(5):439-446.
28. Zengerink M, van Dijk CN. Complications in ankle arthroscopy. *Knee Surg Sports Traumatol Arthrosc.* 2012;20(8):1420-1431.
29. Spennacchio P, Cucchi D, Randelli PS, van Dijk CN. Evidence-based indications for hindfoot endoscopy. *Knee Surg Sports Traumatol Arthrosc.* 2016;24:1386-1395.
30. Vega J, Vilá J, Batista JP, et al. Endoscopic flexor hallucis longus transfer for chronic non-insertional Achilles tendon rupture. *Foot Ankle Int.* 2018;39:1464-1472.
31. Golanó P, Vega J, Pérez-Carro L, Götzens V. Ankle anatomy for the arthroscopist. Part I: the portals. *Foot Ankle Clin.* 2006;11:253-273.
32. Kolodziej P, Glisson RR, Nunley JA. Risk of avulsion of the Achilles tendon after partial excision for treatment of insertional tendonitis and Haglund's deformity. *Foot Ankle Int.* 1999;20:433-437.
33. Pfeffer G, Gonzalez T, Zapf M, Nelson TJ, Metzger MF. Achilles pullout strength after open calcaneoplasty for Haglund syndrome. *Foot Ankle Int.* 2018;20:433-437.

26 Minimally Invasive (MIS) Repair of Achilles Tendon Ruptures

Ian Savage-Elliott and Jonathon Backus

INTRODUCTION

In this chapter, we discuss the management of Achilles ruptures using minimally invasive (MIS) repair techniques. Debate remains in the current literature regarding as to when operative repair is indicated for Achilles injuries. MIS repairs allow for the benefits of surgical repair while mitigating surgical risk. History and physical examination can be diagnostic of these injuries. However, in equivocal cases, advanced imaging may be helpful. We summarize our preferred operative management technique and then discuss outcomes, complications, alternatives, and areas of future study for these injuries.

INDICATIONS AND CONTRAINDICATIONS

Minimally invasive Achilles tendon repairs are indicated for active patients with acute ruptures choosing to undergo primary repair.[1] Nonoperative management using early functional rehabilitation is an alternative treatment that can be employed in the case of older adults, lower demand individuals, and those with medical comorbidities that may impair wound healing such as smoking or diabetes. Casting has become largely a historical treatment, limited to those who are unable to complete a functional rehabilitation program. Open surgery remains an alternative surgical option; however, it has a traditionally higher rate of complications.

BACKGROUND/ETIOLOGY

The Achilles is the largest and strongest tendon in the body, able to withstand forces of up to 12 times a person's body weight.[2] It is one of the most commonly ruptured tendons as well, with estimates suggesting 5 to 10 injuries per 100,000 people. These injuries most commonly occur in the third to fourth decade of life and have a 5 to 1 male to female predominance.[3] Three mechanisms of injury have been described: sharp, unexpected dorsiflexion moment with a strong contraction of the gastrocsoleus complex, pushing off weight bearing with knee extension, or significant dorsiflexion moment on a plantarflexed ankle.[4]

The Achilles blood supply comes from the posterior tibial artery, with a hypovascular zone or "watershed zone" described from 2 to 6 cm proximal to the calcaneal insertion. Nearly 75% of ruptures occur in this location.[5] This knowledge is imperative to the diagnosis and workup of these injuries, and any jumping or landing activities should raise suspicion for Achilles pathology.

The incidence of Achilles injuries appears to be increasing, leading to continued research into optimal nonoperative and operative management.[6] Nonoperatively treated Achilles tendon ruptures were traditionally managed with serial casting, which resulted in approximately 36% normal plantarflexion strength compared to the uninjured side.[7] This treatment has now largely been abandoned or is generally reserved for low demand patients, those with medical comorbidities or other factors that make them a poor candidate for surgery, and those who cannot complete a functional rehabilitation program. Recently, the use of aggressive functional rehabilitation acutely following injury has been developed. Similar functional outcomes to surgery have been reported with the use of this accelerated rehab protocol versus that of operative management, and it represents a viable management alternative to surgery for these injuries.[8-10]

A systematic review and meta-analysis by Wu et al found that nonoperatively managed injuries at centers using early functional rehabilitation had similar outcomes to operatively managed Achilles injuries; however, the results were inconsistent.[11] A randomized control trial by Willits et al demonstrated no difference in rerupture rates, strength, range of motion, calf circumference, or clinical outcomes (Leppilahti score) between 72 tears treated operatively and 72 tears managed using accelerated functional rehabilitation alone. In contrast to the studies mentioned above, multiple other authors have shown an increased rerupture rate and statistically significant strength differences when comparing Achilles ruptures managed nonoperatively to those managed surgically.[12-15] Therefore, there are persistent concerns that nonoperative management may lead to inferior clinical outcomes in terms of push-off strength and explosiveness, a prolonged recovery, and a reduced level of postinjury performance.

Operative management of acute Achilles ruptures includes open, "mini-open," or percutaneous MIS repairs. Open Achilles treatment was the surgical standard of care historically; however, it has been associated with wound complications in 5% to 10% of cases.[16] Percutaneous or MIS Achilles repair involves the use of smaller incisions and/or instrumentation to pass sutures through the ruptured tendon ends and provides secure fixation with minimal soft tissue disruption. Ma and Griffith were the first to describe a technique of percutaneous repair of acute Achilles rupture in 1977.[17] MIS approaches to the Achilles have grown in popularity in recent years, with numerous techniques that vary in the type of incision, number and type of sutures, and postoperative mobility and immobilization. The MIS or percutaneous repair techniques could provide the value of decreased rerupture rate with significantly fewer complications.[18-20] In this chapter, we aim to describe preoperative planning and surgical technique for MIS repairs of Achilles tendon ruptures.

PREOPERATIVE PLANNING

Obtaining a thorough history and physical examination is of paramount importance. Often, a patient will describe an audible pop in their posterior ankle or report being struck from behind. Recent reports state that roughly 82% of these injuries occur during athletic or recreational activity.[4] Pain and immediate swelling are expected. If examining in the acute setting, often a gap can be palpated, and examiners should pay particular attention to the watershed area 2 to 6 cm above the tendon's insertion. Thompson described a test by which squeezing the calf elicits a plantarflexion response of the foot when the musculotendinous unit is intact. When ruptured, the authors noted the lack of plantarflexion with squeezing the calf, which is considered a positive test.[21] Matles described placing a patient prone, flexing both knees to 90°, and observing for a change in the resting position of the foot, typically to a more neutral or dorsiflexion positioning (Fig. 26.1).[22] Numerous other tests

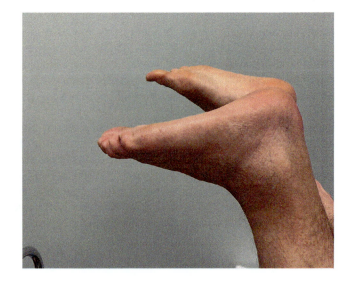

FIGURE 26.1 Matles test is performed with the patient prone and the knee flexed to 90°. Increased dorsiflexion can be seen on the right side.

have been described[23] and can be used to aid in the diagnosis in situations of high suspicion and equivocal examination findings.[24]

Although the Achilles is eponymously named for the Homeric warrior who sustained a penetrating trauma to the region resulting in his demise, injuries to the Achilles were also described in medical texts 100s of years ago.[25] Despite these descriptions, diagnosing Achilles ruptures can be difficult, and a high index of suspicion should be maintained. Differential diagnosis includes ruptures of the plantaris, gastrocnemius tears, and ankle sprains. Historically, up to 25% of Achilles injuries were missed, most commonly misdiagnosed as an ankle sprain.[26] In the face of equivocal history and examination findings, advanced imaging can be utilized; however, imaging is often unnecessary with a thorough history and clinical examination. Radiographs can be used to rule out an Achilles sleeve avulsion or tongue-type calcaneal fractures, as well as identifying any other coexisting osseous pathology. Ultrasound is a quick and inexpensive screening tool; however, results are highly user dependent.[27] MRI is the gold standard in soft tissue analysis and can be used to aid in surgical planning via estimation of the size of the defect, quality of the repair tissue, as well as characterize any other concomitant soft tissue pathology.[28] In cases where there is a history of a traumatic injury consistent with an Achilles rupture, a defect can be palpated on clinical examination, and a Thompson test fails to elicit an appropriate plantarflexion response, we consider clinical examination to be diagnostic and do not routinely obtain advanced imaging. We do not base our decision on imaging on the location of the tear. In situations where there is clinical suspicion of a large gap in the tendon, a high proximal tear at the musculotendinous junction, or severe fatty atrophy or fibrosis, MIS repair may not be possible. In these cases, surgeons may opt for an open repair or mini-open repair with or without a flexor hallucis longus tendon transfer.

OPERATIVE TECHNIQUE

Numerous techniques have been described for MIS Achilles tendon repair, including the Ma & Griffiths percutaneous repair, the Webb and Bannister repair, the Achillon device (Integra LifeSciences Corp, Princeton, New Jersey), the Tenolig device (FH Orthopedics, Heimsbrunn, France), the Wagner technique, the use of the PARS jig (Arthrex Inc, Naples, Florida), and the use of a Midsubstance Speedbridge construct (Arthrex Inc, Naples, Florida).[29] Below, we describe the authors' preferred technique employing the Percutaneous Achilles Repair System (PARS) technique (Arthrex Inc, Naples, Florida).

The patient is placed in the prone position on a standard operating room table. General anesthesia is employed. The senior author prefers the use of a nonsterile tourniquet around the operative thigh. Both extremities are prepped and draped so that the tension of the repair and carrying angle can be assessed against the contralateral side intraoperatively. Both legs are placed on a bump of blankets or pillows. The operative surgeon typically stands at the end of the table.

Approach

The limb is exsanguinated and the tourniquet inflated. A small horizontal incision of approximately 3 cm is made at the level of the tear identified by the palpable gap. We prefer that the incision is 1 cm proximal to the distal end of the tear. A horizontal incision is also preferred as this helps minimize disruption to the paratenon.[30] In cases of a previous exploration, a laceration, doubt of the level of tear, or where there is concern for converting to the open technique, a longitudinal incision or Z- versus J-shaped incision can be utilized (Fig. 26.2).[30] The sural nerve is identified alongside the short saphenous vein, at the lateral aspect of the incision and protected. The paratenon is then opened transversely and in line with the incision and is preserved for repair at the conclusion of the procedure. The Achilles tendon is grasped using two Alice or Kocher Clamps placed in vertical fashion (Fig. 26.2). Blunt dissection or a malleable retractor can be used to remove any adhesions from the tendon proximally.

Instrumentation

The PARS jig (Arthrex Inc, Naples, Florida) is adjusted on the back table to manipulate the arms to their most narrow position. It is then placed in the incision and advanced within the paratenon proximally between the tendon and paratenon (Fig. 26.3). This is essential in minimizing risk of entrapment of the sural nerve. The jig is inserted as far proximally as possible, while holding tension

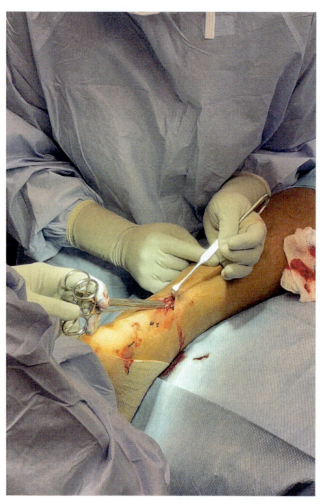

FIGURE 26.2 The proximal stump is gripped with two Alice clamps.

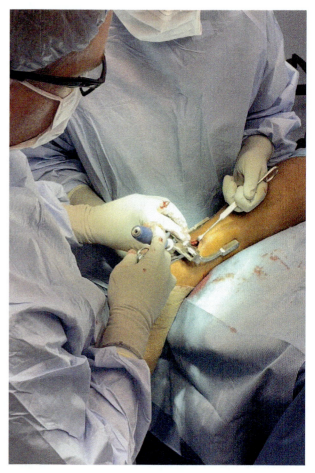

FIGURE 26.3 The PARS jig (Arthrex, Naples, Florida) is placed into the proximal aspect of the incision with care to avoid damaging the sural nerve.

on the tendon with the clamps. Typically, the jig will slide with minimal resistance if inserted within the correct layer. The device is opened enough to ensure that the tendon is between the two arms of the jig and is confirmed by palpation.

Suture Passing

A 1.6-mm guide pin ("needle") with a nitinol loop is placed in the proximal aspect of the tendon through the No. 1 hole of the jig. This provisionally fixes the jig in place and holds tension on the proximal stump. The needle is left in place without passing a suture initially. The tension on the tendon can be temporarily released to ensure that the needle is through the tendon. The second 1.6-mm guide pin is placed in the No. 2 hole of the jig (Fig. 26.4). A striped suture, typically blue and white, is placed in the loop of this needle and the needle is passed through the opposite side of the jig (Fig. 26.5). Two needles are placed in the No. 3 and No. 4 holes of the jig, which face obliquely. Two striped sutures with loops on the ends are passed in opposite directions through holes 3 and 4 of the jig, leaving the looped end on opposite sides of the leg after the needles have been passed. A striped No. 2 suture, typically white and black, is passed through the No. 5 jig hole. Lastly, a suture is placed through the No. 1 hole. There are optional No. 6 and No. 7 holes in the jig if supplemental fixation is desired. After all the sutures have been passed via the guide pins, the center wheel is turned to shorten the distance between the arms of the jig, and the jig is slowly removed from the leg, which pulls the sutures out of the incision through the Achilles tendon while staying inside the paratenon.

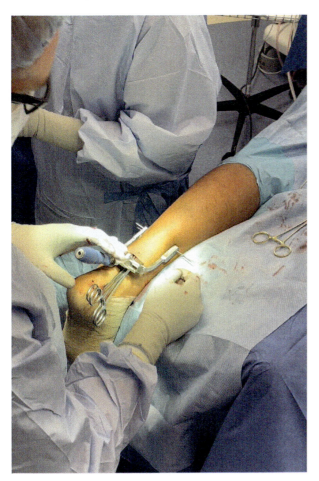

FIGURE 26.4 The setting needle is placed in the No. 1 jig, and the tension on the proximal Achilles tendon is set.

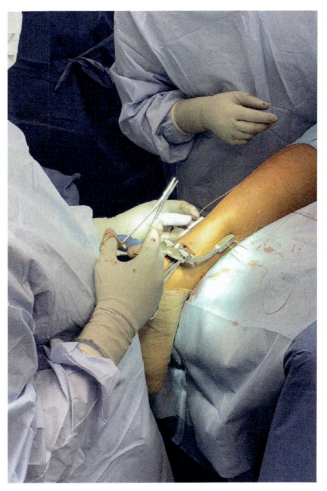

FIGURE 26.5 The sutures are passed through the jig proximally and retrieved on the opposite side of the tendon.

A hemostat can aid in the delivery of the sutures through the tendon and with removal of the jig. The surgeon is careful to avoid injury to the sural nerve while withdrawing the jig (Fig. 26.6). The sutures are then tested individually to ensure that they have adequately captured the tendon. This is done by pulling each side of the matching suture in tandem and checking to see if the tendon moves with pulling of the two sides of the same suture. If the tendons move with pulling on both sides of the suture with force, it is determined to be securely captured (Fig. 26.7). If upon testing the tendon is not secure (ie, the suture rips through the tendon or the tendon lacerates), the sutures can be removed and the procedure can be repeated, beginning again with the No. 1 hole. If a third attempt is required, it is not recommended to continue using the jig, as the proximal tissue is then felt to be inadequate to accept this form of fixation. In these cases, an additional horizontal incision is made 4 to 5 cm proximal to the first incision through the skin and paratenon (Fig. 26.8). The proximal tendon stump is delivered through the more proximal incision, where it is sutured under direct visualization (Fig. 26.9). Both a Modified Mason Allen or Krackow 2 or 4 core strand repair can be utilized with any nonabsorbable suture the treating surgeon prefers. The stump is then delivered through the distal incision (Fig. 26.9). The distal end of the tear is then either sutured through the distal incision or knotless calcaneal fixation can be undertaken, both of which are described below.

Suture Locking

After the sutures have been passed and tested, they are arranged on either side of the wound bed. The blue and white suture that was passed through the No. 2 jig hole is now locked using the two

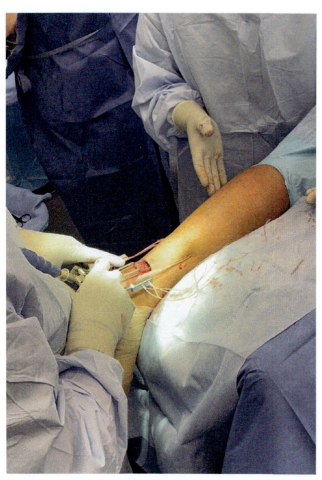

FIGURE 26.6 The jig is removed with care to bring the sutures out through the incision.

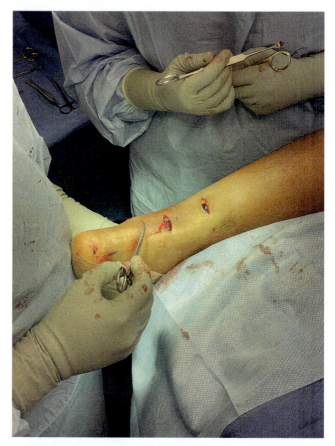

FIGURE 26.7 The use of an additional horizontal proximal incision or "bail-out" incision is used to access the proximal stump.

looped sutures in the proceeding holes. Suture management is paramount during the suture locking portion of the procedure. Once the looped sutures are passed and pulled through the tendon, the two sutures with loops can be removed from the field. The construct now has two nonlocked and one locked suture through the tendon. Again, the sutures should be tested to ensure adequate fixation. We recommend cycling of the proximal sutures can help prevent suture creep postoperatively. Two separate biomechanics study have shown that the greatest elongation of the construct occurs in the first 10 cycles of an Achilles repair regardless of the technique utilized.[31,32]

Knotless Calcaneal Fixation

One option for fixation is to employ a knotless technique in order to fix the Achilles to the calcaneus.[1,33] This works well when the tendon is torn at its distal-most aspect, or the distal stump is of poor quality for repair. Biomechanically, this knotless repair is theoretically stronger as most repairs fail at the knots.[31,32] Two small percutaneous incisions are made at the superior aspect of the tuberosity, just medial and lateral to the Achilles tendon (Fig. 26.10). A 3.5-mm drill with drill guide (Arthrex Inc, Naples, Florida) is used to drill pilot holes into the calcaneus, and then, the No. 3 and 4 loop sutures are passed on each side of the leg and back through the loop of the striped looped sutures. The No. 2 suture is then pulled through the Achilles tendon to the other side by pulling the nonlooped side of the looped sutures (No. 3 and No. 4). The No. 2 suture is then pulled and locked in place leaving two transverse sutures (No. 1 and No. 5) and the one locked No. 2 suture with the proximal Achilles tendon.[1] A Banana SutureLasso (Arthrex Inc, Naples, Florida) is passed through the distal Achilles tendon stump to retrieve the suture strands, which are then passed through the distal

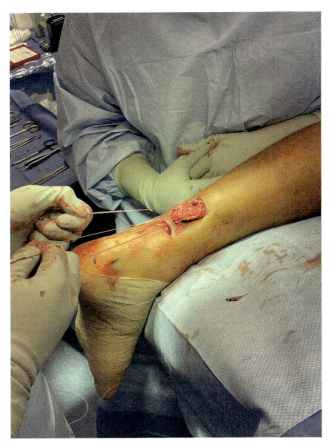

FIGURE 26.8 The proximal stump is stitched after been taken through the bail-out incision, and the sutures are pulled to ensure adequate tendon capture.

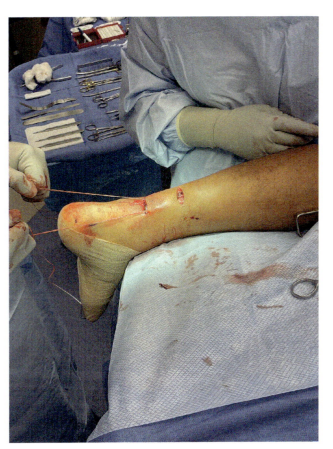

FIGURE 26.9 Once the tendon has been stitched, it is then pulled through the more distal stump back into the more distal incision.

Achilles stump, while tension is held on the distal stump using a clamp (Fig. 26.11). The strands are then secured using anchors on each side with the foot held in maximal plantarflexion (Fig. 26.12).

Knotted Technique/Midsubstance Repairs

Alternatively, the process of the proximal instrumentation process can be repeatedly distally, leaving sutures through the transverse incision and looped through both the proximal and distal stumps of the tendon. These can then be tied (No. 1 distal to No. 1 proximal, No. 2 distal to No. 2 proximal, etc.), while an assistant holds tension on the untied sutures. One suture on each side of the tendon should be tied sequentially with flat knots to maintain the tension. As with the knotless calcaneal fixation, the surgeon carefully tensions the foot to match the resting tension of the contralateral side. In the senior author's experience, a resting tension of 5° to 10° excess plantarflexion versus the contralateral side is most appropriate.[1]

Closure

A 3-0 Monocryl (Ethicon) absorbable running epitenon stitch is placed. Multiple studies have shown that an epitenon stitch increases the construct strength and cycle number to failure.[34] The wound is irrigated thoroughly and then closed in layers with 3-0 Monocryl sutures in the paratenon and subcutaneous layer and 4-0 nylon stitches in horizontal mattress fashion. A sterile dressing is applied. The patient is placed in a well-padded short leg plaster splint in plantarflexion.

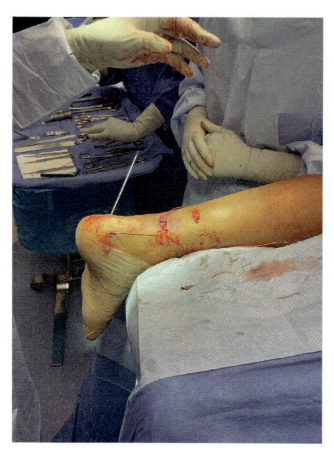

FIGURE 26.10 Two 3.5-mm drill holes have been placed in the calcaneus for distal fixation. Note the 45° angulation of the tunnels thought to be necessary to mitigate heal pain is this technique.

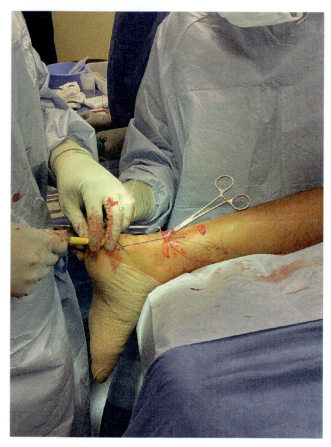

FIGURE 26.11 The Banana SutureLasso (Arthrex, Naples, Florida) is placed through the distal stump and through the distal stump of the Achilles tendon before being captured out the distal aspect of the wound.

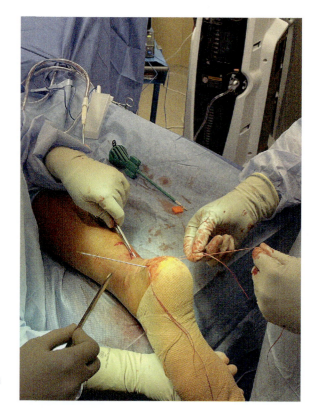

FIGURE 26.12 The sutures have now been passed through the distal stump and are secured to the calcaneus with the foot held in maximal plantarflexion.

PEARLS AND PITFALLS

We believe that tensioning of the repair is paramount. Numerous authors have found that it is better to overtension the repair, which can help accommodate for suture creep and plastic deformation at the time of rupture.[1,30,35] A typical repair may stretch 5° to 10° in the rehabilitation period, and this may be more common in the MIS technique.[1] The author's preference is for fixing the repair in maximal plantarflexion no matter the technique used; however, we believe that this is of particular importance in MIS Achilles repair.

Failure to bury the calcaneal anchor into the tunnels can present as heel pain at the anchor sites, which we have found especially prominent in younger and thinner patients. Edema may be noted around the anchor sites in this situation on MRI.[30] This condition can be treated either with a revision procedure or anchor removal once the tendon has healed. Additionally, the angle of suture placement greater than 45° can lead to disequilibrium and reduced pull-out strength of the construct versus placing the suture at a true deadman's angle or an angle that is acute relative to the load and increasing the suture's pullout strength by using a smaller angle of insertion.[36] Yet, this roughly 45° angle can result in increased and persistent heel pain in this location of the body, and therefore, we recommend inserting the anchors at 45°.

REHABILITATION

The patient is non–weight bearing until the first postoperative visit. Although patients could theoretically begin weight bearing immediately, we have found that the patient pain is often the limiting factor that abates with immobilization and time.[32] Sutures are removed at 10 to 14 days postoperatively. Patients are then transferred to a walking boot and allowed to weight bear with three 7/16 in heel wedges (Hapad, Bethel Park, Pennsylvania), and instructed to wean approximately one wedge per week in the boot. At the 7-week mark, they can begin a transition from a boot to a shoe with or without a wedge based on comfort. Physical therapy begins at the 2-week mark, with an emphasis on active plantarflexion and gradual dorsiflexion up to 5° short of the contralateral side. Strengthening can begin at the 6-week mark. No active or active-assisted dorsiflexion above neutral is permitted in the first 6 weeks of physical therapy, as this can lead to an increased risk of rerupture. There is a goal of achieving 10° of dorsiflexion by 12 weeks of rehabilitation. Full symmetric dorsiflexion is not always required for postoperative performance. We recommend that running does not commence until 16 weeks. Porter and Shadbolt found that rerupture rates are equal to the contralateral side following this time frame.[37] Sports-specific training can resume once the athlete is able to run with normal gait mechanics and functional testing shows strength within 10% of the contralateral limb.[1] Generally, athletes can return to play once symptoms and progression with physical therapy allows. Patients should be counseled that this can take a year or more to achieve.

RESULTS AND COMPLICATIONS

Randomized control trials comparing nonoperative management, open repair, and MIS repair are limited in number, sample size, and follow-up time period. A randomized control trial comparing nonoperative to MIS and open surgical treatment of acute Achilles tendon ruptures at 1 year found that there was no significant improvement in the surgical therapies when using validated patient-reported outcome measures compared with early functional rehabilitation. There was a lower risk of rerupture (0.6% versus 6.2%) in the surgical groups.[38] The MIS group also had the highest rate of nerve injuries (5.2%) versus 2.8% in the open and 1 (0.6%) in the nonoperative group. The authors concluded that Achilles surgery was not associated with a better outcome than nonoperative treatment at 12 months. Although nonoperative management may be successful, concerns remain regarding increased tendon elongation, muscle weakness, prolonged rehabilitation, and delayed return to activity.[8,13,37]

Numerous retrospective series have demonstrated excellent outcomes using MIS repair techniques. Keller et al looked at a series of 100 consecutive cases that underwent a MIS repair using a small proximal incision with sutures, noting a 98% patient satisfaction rate, no sural nerve injuries or wounds, and only two patients with reruptures.[39] Other studies have shown higher subjective clinical scores and fewer complications with MIS versus open repair.[19]

Achilles tendon repairs of all types have an excellent rate of return to activity. In a large systematic review encompassing 6,506 patients and 108 studies, Zellers et al found that 80% of athletes returned to sport following Achilles repair. The authors noted that the average time to return to play was 6 months (SD: 1.8) in the 37 studies reporting this variable.[40] The advantage of the MIS technique may be quicker return to activity, increased strength, and fewer wound complications. When comparing the MIS versus open surgical repair, Del Buono et al noted a significantly greater range of motion and fewer complications following percutaneous repair versus open surgery in a large systematic review of 375 open repairs versus 406 percutaneous repairs.[19,41] While initial results appear to demonstrate reduced morbidity as compared with open repair, further research as to the ideal technique and speed of return to play is warranted.[42]

In regard to timing of repair, a prospective study employing a modified eight-strand Bunnell and Kessler core configuration with absorbable sutures showed that MIS delayed treatment (14-30 days) may be equivalent to acute Achilles tendon repair in terms of complications or patient outcome scores at 1 year.[42] Further studies on the ideal timing of repair as well as the ideal technique for MIS repair are warranted. The authors recommend addressing these injuries as soon as possible and preferably before 14 days. Adhesions are usually minimal before this period making the surgery technically easier to perform. We have performed MIS Achilles repair in patients up to 4 weeks from injury, and it is our preferred choice for subacute Achilles ruptures. Generally, after 6 weeks, these injuries will generally be managed nonoperatively. Subacute open repairs are not typically performed in our practice.

Wu et al performed a meta-analysis of 2,060 patients in 29 randomized control trials including nonoperative treatment, MIS repairs, and open repairs. This study noted an overall major complication rate of 9.13% and found a rerupture rate of 5%, DVT rate of 2.67%, and deep infection rate of 1.5%.[43] Using a Bayesian methodology to calculate a surface under the cumulative ranking curve (SUCRA), the authors found that management consisting of MIS surgery and accelerated rehab was the safest way to treat Achilles tendon ruptures in terms of lowest risk of DVT, deep infection, and rerupture. Nonsurgical management and early immobilization ranked last.

Complications following surgery can be categorized into preoperative complications, intraoperative complications, and postoperative complications. Preoperatively, a lack of advanced imaging in the wake of an equivocal history and/or physical examination may lead to a misdiagnosis of an Achilles tear. Common differentials that can be confused for a tear include a gastrocnemius or plantaris rupture. Additionally, an Achilles sleeve avulsion can easily be mistaken for a Midsubstance Achilles rupture. In our experience, sleeve injuries may require a larger or longitudinal incision to allow for exostosis and Haglund resection in addition to bony fixation of the avulsion. Therefore, when physical examination findings are nondiagnostic, advanced imaging should be obtained to prevent misdiagnosis and/or inappropriate treatment. Similarly, a lack of knowledge of the level of the repair may lead to making a transverse incision at the wrong level. Obesity or overlying increased soft tissue can increase the difficulty of palpating the tear and make this complication more likely. Should this error occur, a second incision can be made proximally and the tendon extracted through the more proximal incision, sutures passed, and then the tendon can be repositioned subcutaneously with the sutures in place (Fig. 26.7). This can also be avoided either by pursuing advanced imaging or by using a longitudinal, Z-, or J-shaped incision in cases where a tendon defect is not palpable.

Tendon elongation is probably the most common technical error intraoperatively. Clanton et al noted that it is "virtually impossible to overtension the repair,"[31] and securing a repair in maximal tension can significantly decrease this risk. Failure to precondition the sutures may also lead to creep, with 80% of the total elongation occurring by the first 10 cycles of loading.[31] Other technical failures related to the PARS include failure of the sutures to adequately obtain purchase in the proximal tendon secondary to misplacement of the guide, failure to appropriately/maximally tension during repair, or failure to adequately fixate the anchors or knots. In a separate biomechanical comparison study, Clanton et al found that an open repair technique demonstrated significantly less elongation versus three different MIS percutaneous repair technique methods after 250 cycles ($p < .05$).[31] However, other research has shown that properly performed MIS repairs are stronger (178 N versus 128 N) than open repairs, and fail by the sutures pulling through in the MIS group versus breakage in the open group.[44]

Wound complications and/or infection have historically been one of the largest issues surrounding Achilles repair. Both of these risks are presumably decreased with the use of smaller incisions. Multiple studies have suggested that these complications are reduced with MIS techniques.[19,45-47]

Care with soft tissue handling, a shorter OR time, and appropriate patient selection all play a role in reducing wound complications and infection.

Reruptures have historically occurred during the first 4 to 12 weeks postoperatively. Maempel et al looked at the epidemiology of rerupture, noting it was more common in males and that the median time to rerupture was 98.5 days; however, 8 of 48 reruptures also occurred after 1 year.[48] Other studies have reported more acute rerupture after surgery, with a mean time to rerupture of 38.0 days.[49] Additionally, accelerated rehab programs may result in less tendon lengthening and more rapid return to running, and similar Achilles tendon total rupture scores to standard rehabilitation.[37] Biomechanical studies have found that ultimate strength of multiple different MIS repair using the author's preferred method is equivalent to open techniques. However, tendon elongation, which as mentioned above, may be more common in the MIS group versus open repairs and has been associated with an increased risk of rerupture.[50]

Traditionally, iatrogenic neurological complications have been noted to be more frequent among patients undergoing percutaneous or MIS repairs, as the sural nerve is less well visualized. Sural neuritis is quoted as high as 10% to 13% in the literature.[51,52] Cadaveric studies have also shown that even when the nerve is not damaged, a majority of cadavers had passage of a needle within 5 mm of the nerve.[53] With newer technique modifications, the sural nerve can be visualized and protected, theoretically decreasing the risk of this complication. Sural nerve damage has been noted to lead to damage and inflexibility postoperatively.[54] There is also a possibility of increased rerupture risk of the skin due to dermatosis from the transverse incision. Transverse skin ruptures have been documented postoperatively after longitudinal incisions, implying that this area may be prone to this type of skin tear.[55]

ALTERNATIVE TECHNIQUES AND AREAS OF FURTHER STUDY

There have numerous MIS techniques and variations since percutaneous repair was initially described. Technical variations include horizontal versus vertical incision, placement of incision, suture technique, type of suture, and closure. As previously mentioned, Clanton et al, performed biomechanical comparisons of 3 MIS Achilles surgeries (Achillon, PARS, and SpeedBridge) and found equivalent elongation at 250 cycles and cycles to failure.[31] Numerous authors have described technical modifications in order to avoid nerve injury, including using arthroscopic probes, endoscopic-assisted repairs, and channel-assisted repairs. Channel-assisted MIS repair techniques have also been employed, with excellent *in vitro* and preliminary results; however, further study is needed.

Most MIS repair techniques use nonabsorbable sutures including braided polyethylene terephthalate and UHMWPE sutures; however, there are reports of suture bulk, material irritation, and infection from the suture.[56] Suture has been reported to cause granulomatosis in rare cases; however, this complication has not been well quantified.[57] Kocaoglu et al performed a prospective study of the use of nonabsorbable versus absorbable sutures for a 2- to 4-cm MIS repair using a suture guide. The authors found that use of an absorbable suture was associated with a lower incidence of suture reaction versus a nonabsorbable suture and found no difference in AOFAS outcomes or rerupture rates (0 in both groups) at 1-year follow-up.[58] In cases of a traumatic laceration, the authors have used absorbable sutures passed through the PARS jig to reduce the risk of infection, using the loop sutures from the PARS jig and creating an all absorbable repair (Figs. 26.13 and 26.14).

Multiple authors have described the use of different tendon augmentation techniques for Achilles repairs. Magnussen et al looked at extracellular xenograft matrix in a cadaveric study, with 1,000 cycles of loading to 86 N and noted a higher ultimate failure load in the augmentation group and significantly less gapping after the 10th load cycle ($p < .05$).[59] Similarly, nitric oxide (NO) has been investigated for tendon healing and is frequently used in tendinopathies throughout the body.[60] A fivefold greater concentration of NO has been found in healing animal Achilles tendons, and while Glyceryl TriNitrate (GTN) patches have primarily been employed in Achilles tendinopathy, there could be a future application of these patches to augment Achilles tendon repairs in humans.[61,62] Finally, there are multiple case reports of the use of absorbable implants in conjunction with Achilles repair, which may offer accelerated healing and/or reduced elongation and higher load to failure.[63,64] Many of these technologies have had efficacy in tendon repair and tendinopathy outside of the

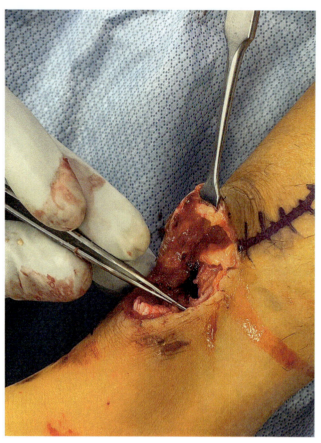

FIGURE 26.13 An example case of a traumatic laceration of the Achilles (Arthrex, Naples, Florida).

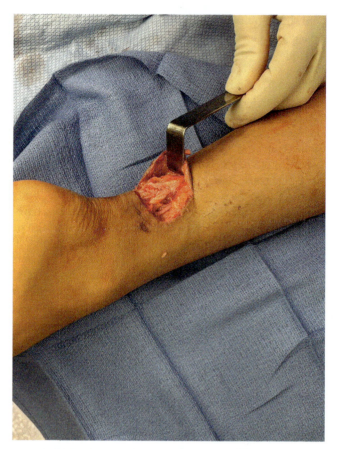

FIGURE 26.14 The final product of the traumatic laceration of the Achilles after being repaired with an absorbable suture and use of a PARS jig (Arthrex, Naples, Florida).

Achilles and offers an interesting area of future research.[65] A current randomized control trial of the use of a bioinductive implant to supplement Achilles repair is ongoing, and these techniques may be employable to MIS surgery in the future.[66]

CONCLUSION

Achilles tendon injuries are a common occurrence among both athletes and weekend warriors.

Both nonoperative and operative management with early functional rehabilitation are viable treatment options. Operative management can take the form of open versus MIS repair. MIS surgical repair offers a viable alternative to traditional open repair with a lower infection rate, wound complication rate, and lower rerupture rate when compared to nonoperative treatment. Sural neuritis remains a possible complication that should be discussed with the patient, and careful technique can mitigate this risk. Repair of delayed tendon injuries, improvements in instrumentation, and biological augmentations are currently all being studied. As techniques continue to improve and MIS surgery continues to grow, we believe that this technique will become the standard practice for care of acute Achilles tendon injuries when operative management is desired.

REFERENCES

1. Liechti DJ, Moatshe G, Backus JD, Marchetti DC, Clanton TO. A percutaneous knotless technique for acute Achilles tendon ruptures. *Arthrosc Tech.* 2018;7(2):e171-e178.
2. Doral MN, Alam M, Bozkurt M, et al. Functional anatomy of the Achilles tendon. *Knee Surg Sports Traumatol Arthrosc.* 2010;18(5):638-643.
3. Vosseller JT, Ellis SJ, Levine DS, et al. Achilles tendon rupture in women. *Foot Ankle Int.* 2013;34(1):49-53.
4. Arner O, Lindholm A. Subcutaneous rupture of the Achilles tendon; a study of 92 cases. *Acta Chir Scand Suppl.* 1959;116(Supp 239):1-51.

5. Lagergen C, Lindholm A. Vascular distribution in the Achilles tendon; an angiographic and microangiographic study. *Acta Chir Scand.* 1959;116(5-6):491-495.
6. Huttunen TT, Kannus P, Rolf C, Felländer-Tsai L, Mattila VM. Acute Achilles tendon ruptures: incidence of injury and surgery in Sweden between 2001 and 2012. *Am J Sports Med.* 2014;42(10):2419-2423.
7. Barnes MJ, Hardy AE. Delayed reconstruction of the calcaneal tendon. *J Bone Joint Surg Br.* 1986;68(1):121-124.
8. Willits K, Amendola A, Bryant D, et al. Operative versus nonoperative treatment of acute Achilles tendon ruptures: a multicenter randomized trial using accelerated functional rehabilitation. *J Bone Joint Surg Am.* 2010;92(17):2767-2775.
9. Barfod KW, Bencke J, Lauridsen HB, Ban I, Ebskov L, Troelsen A. Nonoperative dynamic treatment of acute Achilles tendon rupture: the influence of early weight-bearing on clinical outcome: a blinded, randomized controlled trial. *J Bone Joint Surg Am.* 2014;96(18):1497-1503.
10. Deng S, Sun Z, Zhang C, Chen G, Li J. Surgical treatment versus conservative management for acute achilles tendon rupture: a systematic review and meta-analysis of randomized controlled trials. *J Foot Ankle Surg.* 2017;56(6):1236-1243.
11. Wu Y, Lin L, Li H, et al. Is surgical intervention more effective than non-surgical treatment for acute Achilles tendon rupture? A systematic review of overlapping meta-analyses. *Int J Surg.* 2016;36(Pt A):305-311.
12. Wilkins R, Bisson LJ. Operative versus nonoperative management of acute Achilles tendon ruptures: a quantitative systematic review of randomized controlled trials. *Am J Sports Med.* 2012;40(9):2154-2160.
13. Lantto I, Heikkinen J, Flinkkila T, et al. A prospective randomized trial comparing surgical and nonsurgical treatments of acute Achilles tendon ruptures. *Am J Sports Med.* 2016;44(9):2406-2414.
14. Maffulli N, Longo UG, Maffulli GD, Khanna A, Denaro V. Achilles tendon ruptures in elite athletes. *Foot Ankle Int.* 2011;32(1):9-15.
15. Soroceanu A, Sidhwa F, Aarabi S, Kaufman A, Glazebrook M. Surgical versus nonsurgical treatment of acute Achilles tendon rupture: a meta-analysis of randomized trials. *J Bone Joint Surg Am.* 2012;94(23):2136-2143.
16. Bruggeman NB, Turner NS, Dahm DL, et al. Wound complications after open Achilles tendon repair: an analysis of risk factors. *Clin Orthop Relat Res.* 2004;427:63-66.
17. Ma GWC, Griffith TG. Percutaneous repair of acute closed ruptured Achilles tendon: a new technique. *Clin Orthop Relat Res.* 1977;128:247-255.
18. Alcelik I, Diana G, Craig A, Loster N, Budgen A. Minimally invasive versus open surgery for acute achilles tendon ruptures a systematic review and meta-analysis. *Acta Orthop Belg.* 2017;83(3):387-395.
19. Grassi A, Amendola A, Samuelsson K, et al. Minimally invasive versus open repair for acute achilles tendon rupture: meta-analysis showing reduced complications, with similar outcomes, after minimally invasive surgery. *J Bone Joint Surg Am.* 2018;100(22):1969-1981.
20. Kadakia AR, Dekker RG II, Ho BS. Acute Achilles tendon ruptures: an update on treatment. *J Am Acad Orthop Surg.* 2017;25(1):23-31.
21. Thompson TC, Doherty JH. Spontaneous rupture of tendon of Achilles: a new clinical diagnostic test. *J Trauma.* 1962;2:126-129.
22. Matles AL. Rupture of the tendo Achilles: another diagnostic sign. *Bull Hosp Joint Dis.* 1975;36(1):48-51.
23. Maffulli N. The clinical diagnosis of subcutaneous tear of the Achilles tendon. A prospective study in 174 patients. *Am J Sports Med.* 1998;26(2):266-270.
24. O'Brien T. The needle test for complete rupture of the Achilles tendon. *J Bone Joint Surg Am.* 1984;66(7):1099-1101.
25. Paré A. *Les Ouevres.* 9th ed. Claude rigaud et Claude Obert; 1633.
26. Ballas MT, Tytko J, Mannarino F. Commonly missed orthopedic problems. *Am Fam Physician.* 1998;57(2):267-274.
27. Weinfeld SB. Achilles tendon disorders. *Med Clin North Am.* 2014;98(2):331-338.
28. Coughlin MJ, Saltzman CL, Anderson RB. *Mann's Surgery of the Foot and Ankle.* 2014. http://site.ebrary.com/id/10785772
29. Caolo KC, Eble SK, Rider C, et al. Clinical outcomes and complications with open vs minimally invasive Achilles tendon repair. *Foot Ankle Orthop.* 2021;6(4):24730114211060063.
30. Clanton T, Stake IK, Bartush K, Jamieson MD. Minimally invasive Achilles Repair Techniques. *Orthop Clin North Am.* 2020;51(3):391-402.
31. Clanton TO, Haytmanek CT, Williams BT, et al. A biomechanical comparison of an open repair and 3 minimally invasive percutaneous Achilles tendon repair techniques during a simulated, progressive rehabilitation protocol. *Am J Sports Med.* 2015;43(8):1957-1964.
32. Backus JD, Marchetti DC, Slette EL, Dahl KD, Turnbull TL, Clanton TO. Effect of suture caliber and number of core strands on repair of acute Achilles ruptures: a biomechanical study. *Foot Ankle Int.* 2017;38(5):564-570.
33. McWilliam JR, Mackay G. The internal brace for midsubstance Achilles ruptures. *Foot Ankle Int.* 2016;37(7):794-800.
34. Shepard ME, Lindsey DP, Chou LB. Biomechanical testing of epitenon suture strength in Achilles tendon repairs. *Foot Ankle Int.* 2007;28(10):1074 1077.
35. Takahashi M, Ward SR, Marchuk LL, Frank CB, Lieber RL. Asynchronous muscle and tendon adaptation after surgical tensioning procedures. *J Bone Joint Surg Am.* 2010;92(3):664-674.
36. Burkhart SS. The deadman theory of suture anchors; observations along a south Texas fence line. *Arthroscopy.* 1995;11(1):119-123.
37. Porter MD, Shadbolt B. Randomized controlled trial of accelerated rehabilitation versus standard protocol following surgical repair of ruptured Achilles tendon. *ANZ J Surg.* 2015;85(5):373-377.
38. Myhrvold SB, Brouwer EF, Andresen TKM, et al. Nonoperative or surgical treatment of acute Achilles' tendon rupture. *N Engl J Med.* 2022;386(15):1409-1420.
39. Keller A, Ortiz C, Wagner E, Wagner P, Mococain P. Mini-open tenorrhaphy of acute Achilles tendon ruptures: medium-term follow-up of 100 cases. *Am J Sports Med.* 2014;42(3):731-736.
40. Zellers JA, Carmont MR, Grävare SK. Return to play post-Achilles tendon rupture: a systematic review and meta-analysis of rate and measures of return to play. *Br J Sports Med.* 2016;50(21):1325-1332.
41. Del Buono A, Volpin A, Maffulli N. Minimally invasive versus open surgery for acute Achilles tendon rupture: a systematic review. *Br Med Bull.* 2014;109:45-54.
42. Maffulli N, D'Addona A, Maffulli GD, Gougoulias N, Oliva F. Delayed (14-30 days) percutaneous repair of Achilles tendon ruptures offers equally good results as compared with acute repair. *Am J Sports Med.* 2020;48(5):1181-1188.
43. Wu Y, Mu Y, Yin L, Wang Z, Liu W, Wan H. Complications in the management of acute Achilles tendon rupture: a systematic review and network meta-analysis of 2060 patients. *Am J Sports Med.* 2019;47(9):2251-2260.

44. Heitman DE, Ng K, Crivello KM, Gallina J. Biomechanical comparison of the Achillon tendon repair system and the Krackow locking loop technique. *Foot Ankle Int.* 2011;32(9):879-887.
45. Cretnik A, Kosanovic M, Smrkolj V. Percutaneous versus open repair of the ruptured Achilles tendon: a comparative study. *Am J Sports Med.* 2005;33(9):1369-1379.
46. Lim J, Dalal R, Waseem M. Percutaneous vs. open repair of the ruptured Achilles tendon—a prospective randomized controlled study. *Foot Ankle Int.* 2001;22(7):559-568.
47. McMahon SE, Smith TO, Hing CB. A meta-analysis of randomised controlled trials comparing conventional to minimally invasive approaches for repair of an Achilles tendon rupture. *Foot Ankle Surg.* 2011;17(4):211-217.
48. Maempel JF, White TO, Mackenzie SP, McCann C, Clement ND. The epidemiology of Achilles tendon re-rupture and associated risk factors: male gender, younger age and traditional immobilising rehabilitation are risk factors. *Knee Surg Sports Traumatol Arthrosc.* 2022;30(7):2457-2469. doi: 10.1007/s00167-021-06824-0.
49. Jildeh TR, Okoroha KR, Marshall NE, Abdul-Hak A, Zeni F, Moutzouros V. Infection and rerupture after surgical repair of achilles tendons. *Orthop J Sports Med.* 2018;6(5):2325967118774302.
50. Costa ML, Logan K, Heylings D, Donell ST, Tucker K. The effect of Achilles tendon lengthening on ankle dorsiflexion: a cadaver study. *Foot Ankle Int.* 2006;27(6):414-417.
51. Hsu AR, Jones CP, Cohen BE, Davis WH, Ellington JK, Anderson RB. Clinical outcomes and complications of percutaneous Achilles repair system versus open technique for acute Achilles tendon ruptures. *Foot Ankle Int.* 2015;36(11):1279-1286.
52. Klein W, Lang DM, Saleh M. The use of the Ma-Griffith technique for percutaneous repair of fresh ruptured tendo Achillis. *Chir Organi Mov.* 1991;76(3):223-228.
53. McGee R, Watson T, Eudy A, et al. Anatomic relationship of the sural nerve when performing Achilles tendon repair using the percutaneous Achilles repair system, a cadaveric study. *Foot Ankle Surg.* 2021;27(4):427-431.
54. Lee SJ, Sileo MJ, Kremenic IJ, et al. Cyclic loading of 3 Achilles tendon repairs simulating early postoperative forces. *Am J Sports Med.* 2009;37(4):786-790.
55. Hanada M, Takahashi M, Matsuyama Y. Open re-rupture of the Achilles tendon after surgical treatment. *Clin Pract.* 2011;1(4):e134.
56. Ergin ÖN, Demirel M, Özmen E. An exceptional case of suture granuloma 30 years following an open repair of Achilles tendon rupture: a case report. *J Orthop Case Rep.* 2017;7(3):50-53.
57. Ollivere BJ, Bosman HA, Bearcroft PW, Robinson AH. Foreign body granulomatous reaction associated with polyethelene 'Fiberwire(®)' suture material used in Achilles tendon repair. *Foot Ankle Surg.* 2014;20(2):e27-e29.
58. Kocaoglu B, Ulku TK, Gereli A, Karahan M, Turkmen M. Evaluation of absorbable and nonabsorbable sutures for repair of Achilles tendon rupture with a suture-guiding device. *Foot Ankle Int.* 2015;36(6):691-695.
59. Magnussen RA, Glisson RR, Moorman CT 3rd. Augmentation of Achilles tendon repair with extracellular matrix xenograft: a biomechanical analysis. *Am J Sports Med.* 2011;39(7):1522-1527. doi: 10.1177/0363546510397815.
60. Bokhari AR, Murrell GA. The role of nitric oxide in tendon healing. *J Shoulder Elbow Surg.* 2012;21(2):238-244.
61. Murrell GA, Szabo C, Hannafin JA, et al. Modulation of tendon healing by nitric oxide. *Inflamm Res.* 1997;46(1):19-27.
62. Murrell GA. Using nitric oxide to treat tendinopathy. *Br J Sports Med.* 2007;41(4):227-231.
63. Kato YP, Dunn MG, Zawadsky JP, Tria AJ, Silver FH. Regeneration of Achilles tendon with a collagen tendon prosthesis. Results of a one-year implantation study. *J Bone Joint Surg Am.* 1991;73(4):561-574.
64. Gabler C, Saß JO, Gierschner S, Lindner T, Bader R, Tischer T. In vivo evaluation of different collagen scaffolds in an Achilles tendon defect model. *Biomed Res Int.* 2018;2018:6432742.
65. Thon S, Savoie FH III. Rotator cuff repair: patch the shoulder. *Arthroscopy.* 2019;35(4):1014-1015.
66. Guyton GP. *Achilles tendon repair with bioinductive implant.* 2016-2019. https://clinicaltrials.gov/ct2/show/NCT02811003

PART SIX
FLATFOOT

27 Lateral Column Lengthening and Medial Displacement Calcaneal Osteotomies for Progressive Collapsing Foot Deformity

Michael Aronow

INTRODUCTION

Progressive collapsing foot deformity (PCFD), also known as posterior tibial tendon dysfunction (PTTD) and adult acquired flat foot deformity, may be classified in different ways. In the Johnson and Strom classification system,[1] stage 1 has no planovalgus deformity; stage 2 has a flexible planovalgus deformity that is correctable to a normal arch; and stage 3 has a fixed noncorrectable deformity. Myerson[2] subsequently added a stage 4 in which ankle valgus deformity due to arthritis or deltoid ligament insufficiency is also present. In the PCFD Expert Consensus Classification System,[3,4] stage 1 is a flexible planovalgus deformity and stage 2 is a rigid deformity. There are additional classes consistent with the deformity components that can be observed: class A is a hindfoot valgus deformity; class B is a midfoot/forefoot abduction deformity; class C is a forefoot varus deformity +/− medial column instability; class D is peritalar subluxation/dislocation; and class E is ankle valgus instability.

The treatment of symptomatic PCFD depends on where in the foot any component of deformity occurs, whether the deformity is flexible or fixed, the etiology of the symptoms, and surgeon and patient preference. Nonoperative treatment includes external support with orthoses or temporary immobilization in a cast or cam walker, a home exercise or formal physical therapy program, oral and/or topical anti-inflammatory and/or analgesic medication, corticosteroid and/or biologics injections into the posterior tibial tendon sheath or lateral subtalar joint, and activity modification.

Surgical soft tissue procedures for PCFD typically address spring and/or deltoid ligament insufficiency and muscle/tendon contracture, deficiency, or imbalance. The more commonly performed procedures include spring and deltoid ligament repair, imbrication, or reconstruction; triceps surae contracture lengthening via tendo-Achilles lengthening (TAL) or gastrocnemius recession; posterior tibial tendon débridement, repair, advancement that may be performed in conjunction with accessory navicular excision, or reconstruction, most commonly with a flexor digitorum longus (FDL) transfer; and peroneus brevis to peroneus longus transfer.

Bone and joint implant procedures used to surgically treat PCFD include osteotomy, fusion, subtalar arthroereisis, and total ankle replacement. They may be performed with or without the addition of soft tissue procedures. By addressing any bone deformity present, these procedures provide biomechanical support to the soft tissue procedures and may increase the likelihood of a positive clinical outcome.

Osteotomies are typically preferred when there is a flexible deformity, particularly in younger and more-active individuals. They may also be used to augment fusions in severe deformities. Osteotomies used in PCFD include medial displacement calcaneal osteotomy (MDCO); lateral column lengthening (LCL) osteotomy within the calcaneus; medial cuneiform osteotomy with either a dorsal opening wedge (Cotton osteotomy) or a plantar closing wedge; and first metatarsal plantar closing wedge osteotomy. The latter is the author's preferred technique for plantarflexing the medial column as it may be combined with a lateral closing wedge to address concurrent hallux valgus deformity; avoids the anterior tibial tendon unlike the medial cuneiform plantar closing wedge osteotomy; and shortens the medial column, does not disrupt the intercuneiform joint, and does not require allograft or autograft unlike the Cotton osteotomy.

Fusions may be more appropriate with rigid (PCFD stage 2/Johnson and Strom stage 3) or severe deformities, particularly in more elderly and low-demand individuals, and in the presence of significant arthritis. The joints more commonly fused in the treatment of PCFD are the subtalar, talonavicular, and calcaneocuboid, either isolated or combined in a double or triple arthrodesis, naviculocuneiform, and first tarsometatarsal. In the presence of hindfoot valgus deformity secondary to advanced ankle arthritis, the ankle may be fused, although total ankle arthroplasty may be an alternative. In the presence of planovalgus deformity secondary to midfoot arthritis and collapse, the second and third tarsometatarsal joints may also be incorporated into the fusion.

INDICATIONS AND CONTRAINDICATIONS

Medial displacement calcaneal osteotomy and LCL calcaneal osteotomy are typically performed in the presence of flexible deformities (PCFD stage 1/Johnson and Strom stage 2). MDCO is typically performed to address increased hindfoot valgus (PCFD class A). By translating the calcaneal tuberosity medially, the osteotomy can realign the hindfoot to a neutral or slight physiologic valgus position. Stress is decreased on the deltoid and spring ligaments by decreasing the valgus force on the heel with weight bearing. The posterior tibialis or its replacement tendon transfer is offloaded by shifting the Achilles tendon insertion on the calcaneus medially relative to the subtalar joint axis. This medial shift makes the more powerful gastrocnemius and soleus muscles more effective supinators of the hindfoot, or in the case of severe hindfoot valgus deformity in which the Achilles tendon insertion has moved lateral to the subtalar joint axis, converts these muscles from hindfoot pronators to supinators.[9]

Lateral column lengthening is used to address midfoot/forefoot abduction and lateral peritalar subluxation at the talonavicular joint (PCFD classes B and D). The exact mechanism of how LCL works is uncertain, but proposed mechanisms include plantar ligament tensioning, peroneus longus tensioning, and medial translation of the anterior facet of the calcaneus.[10] Combining the MDCO and LCL provides increased deformity correction.[11]

Indications for MDCO and LCL include symptomatic PCFD that has failed to respond to appropriate conservative treatment. The patient's discomfort and functional limitations should be sufficient to justify the risks, recovery time, and associated discomfort of surgery to both the patient and surgeon. The threshold for surgery varies extensively between patients and surgeons and may depend upon the severity of disease, age, ability to take time off from work or family responsibilities, occupation, family and friend support, recreational interests, and individual pain/deformity tolerance. While rigid hindfoot deformities or flexible deformities associated with significant arthritis in the subtalar, talonavicular, and/or calcaneocuboid are likely more suitable for arthrodesis, adding an MDCO or LCL to a hindfoot fusion may be appropriate with severe deformity. An alternative to LCL in this situation or in PCFD with hindfoot arthritis limited to the calcaneocuboid joint is calcaneocuboid distraction arthrodesis in which the bone graft is placed in the calcaneocuboid joint instead of a calcaneal osteotomy site.[12]

Contraindications to MDCO and LCL include a patient who is not an appropriate surgical candidate due to poor vascular or skin status, active infection, medical comorbidities that would make anesthesia excessively risky, or inability or unwillingness to follow postoperative instructions. If there is no deformity or a preexisting cavovarus foot (Johnson and Strom stage 1), procedures to address the soft tissue pathology such as a posterior tibial tendon tenosynovectomy, tendon transfer, spring ligament repair, and/or gastrocnemius recession will likely be sufficient without the need for a hindfoot osteotomy or fusion. If the principal etiology of the patient's deformity is forefoot-driven hindfoot valgus, a midfoot or first metatarsal osteotomy or a midfoot fusion to correct forefoot varus is more appropriate. Relative contraindications to MDCO and LCL include poor nutritional status, significant calcaneal osteoporosis, nonambulatory status, and active smoking.

PREOPERATIVE PLANNING

The diagnosis of PCFD should be confirmed by a detailed patient history, physical examination, and appropriate radiologic studies. It is important to know what the patient's symptoms, social situation, responsibilities, constraints, expectations, and treatment goals are. Important physical examination findings include the areas of tenderness; the extent and location of the deformity; the amount of hindfoot valgus and pronation; the amount of forefoot varus with the hindfoot in neutral supination; whether the deformity is fixed or flexible; the presence of gastrocnemius and/or soleus contracture; the ability to perform a double or single limb heel raise and whether or not the heel goes into varus as it rises; and posterior tibial tendon strength. Other concurrent symptomatic foot pathology that might influence the procedures chosen to address the PCFD should be assessed. For example, if there is symptomatic hallux valgus, the surgeon might choose to address fixed forefoot supination with a Lapidus procedure over a Cotton medial cuneiform osteotomy. If there are symptomatic lesser hammertoes, a surgeon may have a lower threshold for adding an FDL transfer to decrease the deforming plantarflexing force on the lesser interphalangeal joints.

Weight-bearing bilateral Cobey or Saltzman hindfoot alignment,[13] ipsilateral ankle mortise, and ipsilateral anteroposterior (AP), lateral, and oblique foot conventional radiographs should be obtained with the ankle ideally in at least neutral dorsiflexion to avoid masking the effects of an associated equinus contracture. The Cobey hindfoot alignment view demonstrates the amount and asymmetry of hindfoot valgus present. The ankle mortise view may show whether any of the hindfoot valgus deformity is due to lateral ankle joint arthritis or deltoid ligament insufficiency. The foot radiographs may demonstrate arthritis, an accessory navicular, the extent and location of the deformity, and other associated foot pathology. The lateral foot and ankle radiographs may show anterior ankle osteophytes that may need to be removed to obtain adequate ankle dorsiflexion, closing of the sinus tarsi due to subtalar pronation, disruption of the cyma line[14] in which the calcaneocuboid joint is proximal to the talonavicular joint as opposed to at the same level, and whether there is sag in the talo-first metatarsal line and if so, is it at the talonavicular, naviculocuneiform, or plantar first tarsometatarsal joint. The AP and oblique views may also show disruption of the cyma line, an increased talo-first metatarsal angle, and uncovering of the medial talar head due to lateral peritalar subluxation.

Magnetic resonance imaging (MRI) is not mandatory if the surgeon can determine an appropriate operative plan based upon physical examination, conventional weight-bearing radiographs, and intraoperative findings. However, an MRI should be obtained when the findings may influence the operative plan. For example, an MRI may be helpful if the surgeon is trying to rule out concurrent ankle pathology that might benefit from arthroscopy or deciding between an osteotomy and a fusion based upon the extent of arthritis. A surgeon may also choose just to do an MDCO and/or LCL and not make a medial incision in a young patient with symptomatic PCFD, no medial hindfoot tenderness, normal posterior tibialis strength, and no abnormal findings in the posterior tibial tendon or spring ligament on MRI. In the author's anecdotal experience, the posterior tibial tendon appears normal when explored and the clinical results are comparable when the posterior tibial tendon is not surgically evaluated in this clinical situation.

Computed tomography (CT) scan is also not mandatory if the surgeon can determine an appropriate operative plan without it. However, it may be beneficial, in particular if the CT scan can be obtained weight bearing, for assessing the extent of peritalar subluxation, deformity, arthritis, and other foot pathology.

Once the above information has been obtained, the specific procedures to be performed are decided, some of which may be dependent upon intraoperative findings, and informed consent obtained from the patient. The surgeon should ensure that the appropriate instrumentation, implants, and, if potentially being used, allograft are available in the operating room.

Efforts should be made to minimize surgical complications including the risk of nonunion. The patient's nutritional status and endocrine function should be assessed and addressed if inadequate. A vitamin D level should be obtained, or alternatively, assumed to be low and the patient given prophylactic vitamin D supplementation. Smoking cessation is desirable, although not mandatory if the patient and surgeon are willing to take the increased risk of complications.

SURGICAL TECHNIQUE

Medial displacement calcaneal osteotomy can be performed using minimally invasive surgery techniques[15] or as discussed in this chapter, a standard open technique.[5] LCL can be performed through a variety of techniques. For the latter, a coronal plane osteotomy can be made in the calcaneus and the calcaneus lengthened by distraction osteogenesis[16] or insertion of bicortical or tricortical allograft bone, autograft bone, or metallic wedges.[17] The most commonly used osteotomy sites are in the anterior process of the calcaneus 1 to 1.5 cm from the calcaneocuboid joint for the Evans procedure[6] or between the middle and posterior facets of the subtalar joint as described by Hintermann.[18] The author prefers the osteotomy described by Hintermann over the Evans procedure as it does not violate the anterior or middle facets of the subtalar joint[19] and finds it to be more stable with a decreased need for fixation and less dorsal translation of the anterior process of the calcaneus. Z-lengthening osteotomies have also been described with the plantar and dorsal gaps anterior and posterior to the area of bone contact left open or filled with bone graft or metallic implants.[20-22]

The author's preference is to perform any associated soft tissue procedures, but not secure them, before performing the MDCO or LCL. If needed, a Hoke percutaneous TAL (Fig. 27.1) or gastrocnemius recession (Fig. 27.2) is performed first.[23] The author typically performs a gastrocnemius recession if there is a triceps surae contracture with the contracture principally in the gastrocnemius and not soleus (positive Silfverskiold test in which ankle dorsiflexion is limited with knee extension but not flexion), and in younger, more active patients in which the greater postoperative weakness after TAL is of greater concern. In the latter situation, the author will often partially release the soleus aponeurosis leaving the deep muscle fibers intact to obtain additional correction as needed. Percutaneous TAL is typically performed in patients with significant combined gastrocnemius and soleus contractures and in lower demand patients with higher surgical morbidity. If being addressed, the posterior tibial tendon and spring ligament are assessed next. If an FDL transfer is being performed, the tendon is harvested and placed through the distal posterior tibial tendon or a navicular or medial cuneiform tunnel (Fig. 27.3). Fixation of the FDL tendon as well as tying of any sutures or grafts used to repair, imbricate, or reconstruct[24] the spring ligament are deferred until after the MDCO and/or LCL have been stabilized.

For an isolated MDCO, an oblique incision is made over the posterolateral calcaneus anterior to the Achilles tendon insertion dorsally, anterior to the plantar fascia origin on the calcaneus plantarly, and posterior to the peroneal tendons (Fig. 27.4A). Taking care to protect the sural nerve, the lateral calcaneal wall is exposed (Fig. 27.4B) and the osteotomy made with a sagittal saw. The osteotomy should exit dorsally between the Achilles tendon insertion and the posterior facet and

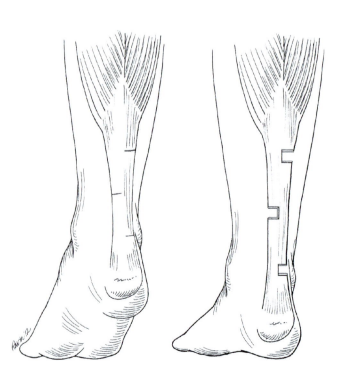

FIGURE 27.1 Hoke percutaneous tendo-Achilles lengthening. Two lateral and one intervening medial percutaneous 50% step-cuts are made in the Achilles tendon approximately 2 cm apart with the distal cut approximately 1 cm above the calcaneal insertion. The ankle is then passively dorsiflexed causing the Achilles tendon to lengthen.

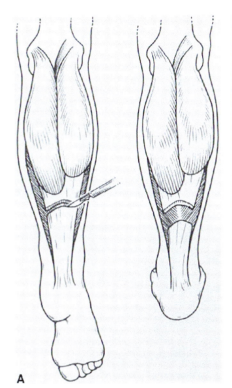
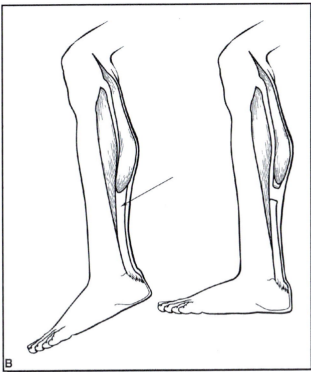
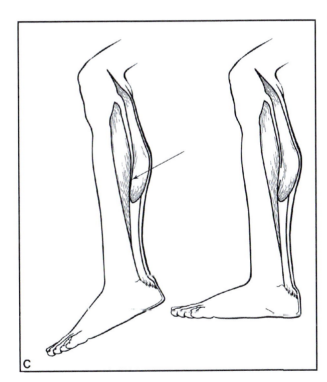

FIGURE 27.2 Gastrocnemius recession. The procedure can be performed through open or endoscopic techniques. For an open approach, a 2- to 3-cm medial incision over the gastrocnemius and soleus interval is made, which allows the patient to be in the supine position. Dissection is made through the skin, subcutaneous tissue, and deep fascia, taking care to avoid the saphenous nerve and vein. If present, the plantaris tendon is transected and a few centimeters of tendon removed. **A, B.** For a Vulpius or Strayer procedure, the skin incision is made at the level of the gastrocnemius myotendinous junction and the gastrocnemius aponeurosis transected, taking care to protect the sural nerve, which at times rests on the superficial aspect of the aponeurosis. In the Strayer procedure, the gastrocnemius aponeurosis is reattached to the soleus aponeurosis in a lengthened position, while in a Vulpius procedure, the aponeurosis is not reattached. **C.** For the Baumann procedure, the skin incision is made approximately 5 cm proximal to the gastrocnemius myotendinous junction and the gastrocnemius aponeurosis released, allowing the more superficial gastrocnemius muscle to stretch but remain intact. With all three of the above procedures, if there is still residual decreased ankle dorsiflexion with the knee in flexion, the soleus aponeurosis can also be transversely released as needed, leaving the deeper soleus muscle intact but able to stretch. The deep fascia is then either closed or released both proximally and distally to avoid subsequent muscle herniation, and the subcutaneous tissue and skin are closed per surgeon's preference (*arrows* in **B** and **C** point to gastrocnemius aponeurosis transection site).

plantarly anterior to the plantar fascia origin. Care is taken not to over penetrate medially and damage the neurovascular bundle. The osteotomy is made to, but not though, the harder medial cortex from plantar to dorsal. The medial cortex is then cut without plunging and with the initial cut avoiding the area where the neurovascular bundle runs. The osteotomy is then distracted with an osteotome and then a smooth laminar spreader to release plantar and medial soft tissue adhesions, and the posterior tuberosity shifted medially by 8 to 15 mm (average 10 mm) depending upon the amount of correction needed. It is easier to translate the tuberosity with the ankle plantarflexed and the Achilles tendon relaxed. An attempt is made to avoid superior or inferior translation of the

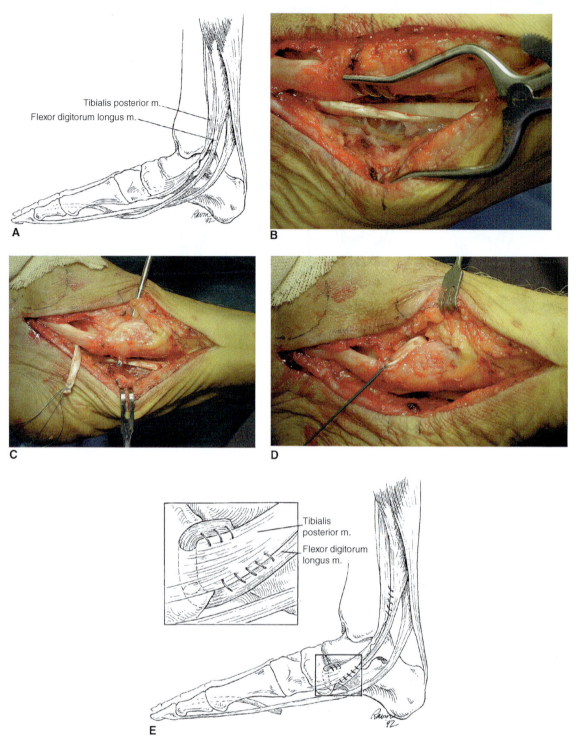

FIGURE 27.3 Flexor digitorum longus (FDL) transfer to the navicular. **A.** The posterior tibial, FDL, flexor hallucis longus, and Achilles tendons can be seen at the level of the ankle from anterior to posterior, respectively. **B.** A skin incision is typically made over the course of the posterior tibial tendon from the tip of the medial malleolus to the naviculocuneiform joint, dissecting down to the posterior tibial tendon sheath and abductor hallucis muscle. The posterior tibial tendon is then exposed and its pathology addressed with tenosynovectomy, débridement, repair, or excision. The FDL tendon is identified posterior and lateral to the posterior tibial tendon, and retracting the abductor hallucis plantarly, followed distally to just proximal to where it crosses superficial to the flexor hallucis longus tendon at the master knot of Henry. Care is taken to avoid the medial plantar nerve and medial plantar artery, which run superficial to the FDL tendon in the distal part of the incision. **C.** The FDL tendon is transected proximal to the master knot of Henry, leaving the normal connections between the FDL tendon and the flexor hallucis longus tendon at the master knot and the quadratus plantae insertion into the FDL tendon intact, and an absorbable passing suture is placed in the proximal stump. A drill hole is made in the navicular from dorsal to plantar. **D.** The FDL is passed from plantar to dorsal through the navicular tunnel and with tension applied with the ankle and hindfoot in approximately 30° of plantarflexion and supination, secured with an interference screw and/or suturing the FDL tendon back to itself as well as the distal posterior tibial tendon insertion. **E.** If the posterior tibial tendon is excised and its muscle healthy, an additional incision can be made proximal to the posteromedial ankle and the muscle tenodesed to the FDL muscle. In this situation, the FDL tendon stump is typically brought into the proximal incision and then placed through the posterior tibial tendon sheath back into the distal incision before the proximal tenodesis and subsequent navicular fixation occurs. The incisions are then closed in layers per surgeon's preference.

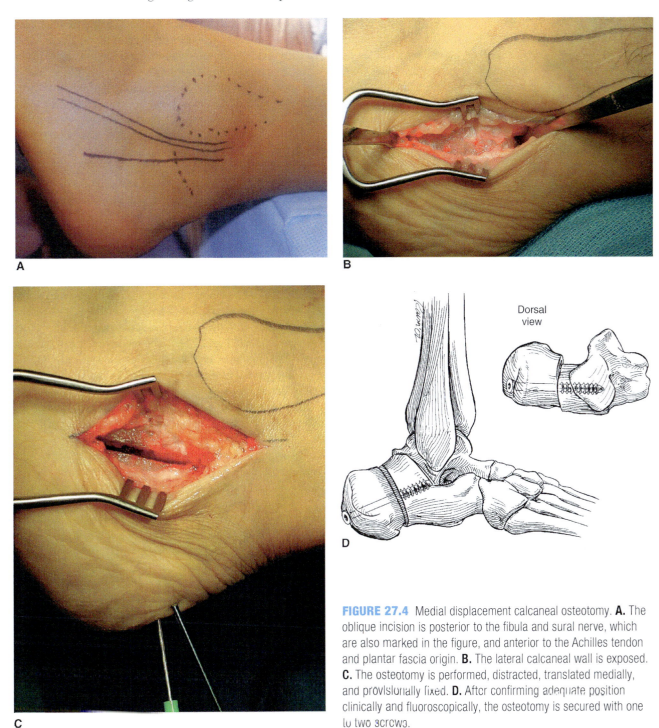

FIGURE 27.4 Medial displacement calcaneal osteotomy. **A.** The oblique incision is posterior to the fibula and sural nerve, which are also marked in the figure, and anterior to the Achilles tendon and plantar fascia origin. **B.** The lateral calcaneal wall is exposed. **C.** The osteotomy is performed, distracted, translated medially, and provisionally fixed. **D.** After confirming adequate position clinically and fluoroscopically, the osteotomy is secured with one to two screws.

tuberosity, but slight inferior translation may improve the arch at the expense of increased Achilles tendon tension. The osteotomy is then compressed, aided by ankle dorsiflexion, and stabilized with provisional K-wires or a cannulated screw guidewire(s) placed from the posterior calcaneal tuberosity (Fig. 27.4C). Axial and lateral fluoroscopic radiographs are checked for appropriate position. The osteotomy is then definitively stabilized with one or two headless, partially threaded, cannulated screws, or less commonly plate or staple fixation (Fig. 27.4D). Depending upon the amount of overlying soft tissue, the prominent overhanging lateral bone edge of the anterior fragment may be left in place, rasped or shaved smoother with a saw or bone chisel, or tamped medially after removing underlying cancellous bone with a rongeur. The incision is then closed per surgeon's preference.

For an isolated LCL using a Hintermann osteotomy, the incision is typically made from anterior to the tip of the fibula to the anterior process of calcaneus in line with the fourth metatarsal base. For an Evans osteotomy, the incision typically extends distal to the calcaneocuboid joint, which may need to be provisionally pinned with a K-wire during the procedure to decrease the risk of dorsal subluxation of the anterior process after the osteotomy. When combined with an MDCO, the LCL incision usually is translated anteriorly and the MDCO incision posteriorly to increase the skin bridge, with more extensive anterior subperiosteal dissection obtained prior to performing the MDCO (Fig. 27.5A). The LCL incision is made dorsal to the peroneal tendons, watching for a communicating branch between the sural and dorsal intermediate cutaneous branch of the superficial peroneal nerve that is sometime present. The floor of the sinus tarsi is exposed, which may involve opening the extensor digitorum brevis fascia and retracting the muscle origin dorsally. Any impinging synovitis between the posterior facet and the interosseous and lateral calcaneal ligaments is removed, and some of the fat in the sinus tarsi may be removed if needed for visualization. The lateral calcaneus is exposed inferior to the sinus tarsi by subperiosteally elevating deep to peroneal tendons and a Hohmann retractor placed deep to the peroneal tendons under the plantar calcaneus (Fig. 27.5B). A vertical osteotomy is then made with a sagittal saw anterior to the articular surface of the calcaneal posterior facet and posterior to the interosseous ligament and calcaneal middle facet (Fig. 27.5C). The medial cortex may be left intact as a hinge or completed with an osteotome or saw, with care taken not to over penetrate medially, and the osteotome is used to spread the osteotomy (Fig. 27.5D). A Hintermann distractor is then applied with the two threaded pins anterior and posterior to the osteotomy and dorsal to the peroneal tendons (Fig. 27.5E). The medial arch will recreate as the distractor is opened, and the appropriate amount of distraction, which is typically but not always 6 to 10 mm, is noted. The goal is not to prevent hindfoot eversion in an individual used to the shock absorption of a flexible planovalgus deformity but to limit it to a more normal physiological range. If the graft is too large, it may cause overcorrection or unnecessary increased load on the calcaneocuboid joint. There are also commercially available trials than simulate grafts of different width that can be used.

If an MDCO is being performed, the osteotomy is now performed as described above but not stabilized (Fig. 27.5F).

An appropriately sized graft for the LCL is then contoured using a sagittal saw. The author prefers bicortical or tricortical allograft over autograft or metallic wedges as they usually incorporate with the bone on both sides of the calcaneal osteotomy site, avoid autograft donor site morbidity, are reasonably cost-effective, and are capable of remodeling and being replaced with live bone. The graft is tapered such that it is wider dorsally than plantarly and wider laterally than medially with the cortical bone facing dorsally and laterally. The osteotomy site is distracted and the graft tamped medially into place (Fig. 27.5G). Care is taken to avoid dorsal subluxation and impingement into the sinus tarsi, which may cause pain and excessively decrease subtalar pronation, and plantar pressure is typically applied to the dorsal aspect of the graft with another instrument as it is tamped into place. Any gap plantar to the graft can be filled with autograft taken from the MDCO site or allograft removed during graft contouring. If an isolated LCL is being performed, the graft is usually stable after the distractor is removed and does not typically require internal fixation. If an MDCO is also being performed, a headless partially threaded cannulated screw is placed from a posterior calcaneal tuberosity incision across both osteotomy sites with the threads distal to the MDCO site to allow compression and spanning the LCL site to avoid graft compression (Fig. 27.5H and I). The graft and screw positions are checked by palpation, direct visualization, and lateral, AP, and axial fluoroscopy. Any plantar or lateral prominence graft impinging on the peroneal tendons is removed. A finger should comfortably fit in the sinus tarsi with slight hindfoot eversion, and any impingement against the lateral process of the talus from the graft or the dorsal aspect of the calcaneus anterior to the osteotomy site should be removed with a sagittal saw (Fig. 27.5J). The incision is then closed in layers including the EDB fascia per surgeon's preference.

A sterile, well-padded compressive dressing and a below-knee posterior and medial and lateral stirrup plaster splint is applied with the position depending on the concurrent soft tissue procedures performed. For example, the foot should be placed with the ankle in dorsiflexion if a Baumann gastrocnemius recession was performed, hindfoot inversion and ankle plantarflexion if an FDL transfer and spring ligament imbrication was performed, and neutral dorsiflexion and slight inversion if all three procedures were performed.

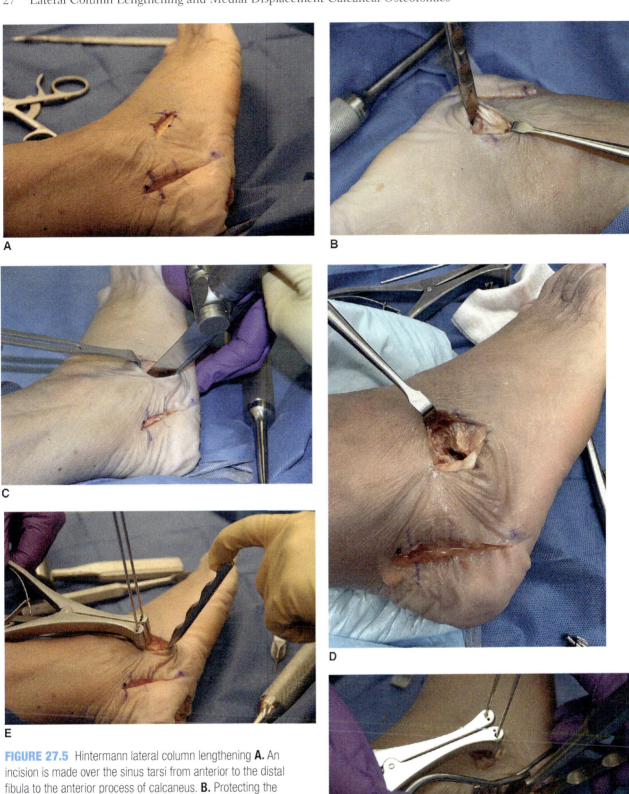

FIGURE 27.5 Hintermann lateral column lengthening **A.** An incision is made over the sinus tarsi from anterior to the distal fibula to the anterior process of calcaneus. **B.** Protecting the peroneal tendons, the lateral calcaneal wall is exposed. **C.** A vertical osteotomy is made between the posterior facet of the calcaneus and the interosseous ligament with a saw and **(D)** initially distracted with an osteotome. **E.** A Hintermann distractor is applied with dorsal pins on both sides of the osteotomy. The appropriate graft size can be assessed by measuring the amount of distraction required to recreate the desired arch while observing the medial foot. **F.** If concurrently performing an medial displacement calcaneal osteotomy (MDCO), the posterior osteotomy is now made and distracted prior to anterior graft insertion.

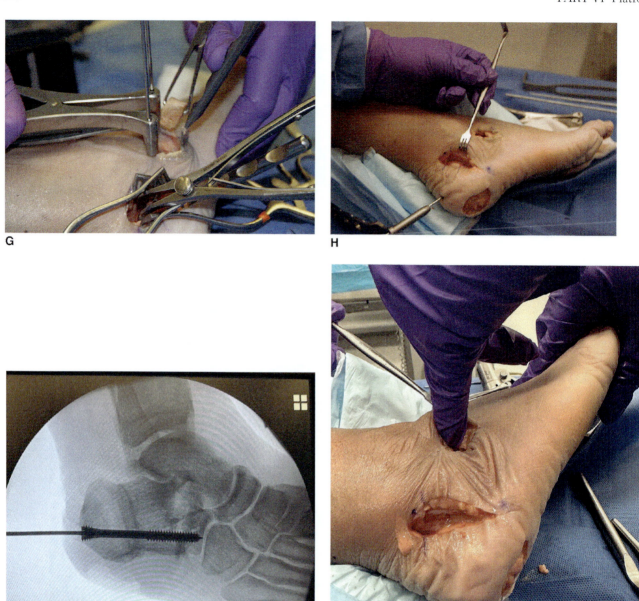

FIGURE 27.5 (Continued) **G.** The graft is then contoured such that it is wider dorsally and laterally and inserted with cortical bone facing dorsal and lateral. Care is taken to avoid graft impingement dorsally into the sinus tarsi and laterally against the peroneal tendons. **H.** If performing a concurrent MDCO, the tuberosity is shifted medially and a guidewire placed through a posterior calcaneal incision across both osteotomy sites and position of the guidewire and osteotomies confirmed clinically and fluoroscopically. **I.** A cannulated screw is placed with compression across the MDCO but not the lateral column lengthening osteotomy. In an isolated Hintermann LCL, fixation is typically not required. **J.** The surgeon's index finger should comfortably fit in the sinus tarsi with at least 5° of hindfoot pronation. If not, additional bone should be removed from the floor of the sinus tarsi to avoid impingement against the lateral process of the talus.

PEARLS AND PITFALLS

- Make sure that the procedures chosen are appropriate for the patient's pathology, capabilities, and goals.
- Confirm that the patient's expectations with respect to recovery time and final result are realistic preoperatively.
- Be happy with range of motion and foot position with simulated weight bearing while the patient is still anesthetized, prepped, and draped.
- While one can remove additional allograft bone easier than put it back, the amount of tapering required medially and plantarly in LCL is typically more than initially expected.

- Avoid sinus tarsi impingement after LCL.
- Avoid over correction, particularly in patients with mild deformity or preexisting cavovarus feet that have partially collapsed due to equinus contracture, posterior tibial tendon pathology, and/or deltoid/spring ligament pathology. Patients who have had a flexible flatfoot all their life may find a stiffer normal or cavus arch uncomfortable, in particular if asymmetric to the contralateral side.
- Avoid over penetration of the medial cortex with the saw blade.

POSTOPERATIVE MANAGEMENT

The patient is typically kept non–weight bearing with ambulation and touch down weight bearing while sitting for 6 weeks, followed by progressive weight bearing as tolerated. The initial dressing is changed at 3 to 6 days postoperatively to assess the incisions and remove any excess compression that may occur from swelling, gauze hardened by dried blood, or pressure points from the plaster splint. AP, lateral, oblique, and axial foot conventional radiographs are obtained and a short leg fiberglass cast applied. At 2 to 3 weeks postsurgery, the cast is changed, and if the incisions are sufficiently healed, the sutures are removed and Steri-Strips applied. At 6 weeks, conventional radiographs are repeated, and if the conventional radiographs and physical examination are suggestive of sufficient healing of the osteotomies and any other concurrent bone procedures performed, the patient is placed into a cam walker with the possible addition of an off the shelf orthotic insert, and physical therapy begun with any restrictions dependent about the concurrent procedures performed. If there is concern about insufficient healing or patient compliance, a walking cast is applied for another 3 to 4 weeks. The patient can advance to accommodative shoe wear with appropriate arch support when discomfort and swelling allow. Maximum recovery may take 12 to 18 months, but patients typically note significant improvement in their function and discomfort before then.

RESULTS AND COMPLICATIONS

Potential complications after MDCO and/or LCL include infection; wound dehiscence; nerve injury; malunion; nonunion; symptomatic hardware; persistent/recurrent pain, deformity, and functional loss; overcorrection of deformity; calcaneocuboid or subtalar arthritis; thromboembolic disease; complex regional pain syndrome; and anesthetic complications.[25]

Interpreting the results of MDCO and LCL in the literature is limited due to the variability of PCFD pathology between patients, the variability of the different techniques for performing the osteotomies, and the variability of the concurrent procedures performed.

Myerson et al[26] retrospectively evaluated 129 patients who underwent MDCO and FDL transfer to the navicular for flexible PCFD at mean 5.2-year follow-up. The mean American Orthopaedic Foot and Ankle Society (AOFAS) ankle-hindfoot score at follow-up was 79 points out of a 100, there was statistically significant radiographic improvement, and 118 patients were entirely satisfied, 7 patients partially satisfied, and 4 patients dissatisfied. Chadwick et al[27] evaluated 31 patients who underwent MDCO and FDL transfer for flexible PCFD at mean 15.2-year follow-up. At final follow-up, 87% of the patients were pain-free and functioning well and the mean AOFAS ankle-hindfoot score had improved to 90.3 from 48.4 preoperatively.

Hintermann et al[18] evaluated 19 patients who underwent Hintermann LCL for stage 2 to 3 PTTD at mean 23.4-month follow up. Concurrent procedures included tendon reconstruction in 18, FDL transfer in 11, deltoid ligament repair in 13, and spring ligament repair in 3. The functional score improved from 48.6 preoperatively to 91.1 postoperatively. All patients had arch correction, and there was one nonunion using iliac crest autograft. At 23.4-month follow-up, there were 17 patients with complete pain relief, 3 with minor pain, and 1 with moderate pain, but at a mean 30.1-month telephone follow-up, 19 had complete pain relief and 2 had minor pain.

Moseir-LaClair et al[11] evaluated 26 patients and 26 feet with flexible PCFD who underwent MDCO, Evans LCL, FDL transfer to the medial cuneiform, and TAL at average 5-year follow-up. There was radiographic improvement, and the mean AOFAS ankle-hindfoot score was 90 at final follow-up. There were no nonunions, and 4 feet had calcaneocuboid arthritis, one of which was symptomatic.

Saunders et al[21] retrospectively reviewed 111 patients/143 feet with flexible PCFD who underwent 65 Evans LCLO and 78 step-cut lengthening calcaneal osteotomies with at least 2-year follow-up. They found that the step-cut LCL feet had faster healing times, fewer nonunions, similar outcomes scores, and equivalent correction of deformity as compared to the Evans.

Nagy et al[22] performed a prospective randomized control trial with 17 feet undergoing combined Evans LCLO and MDCO and 17 feet undergoing a modified Malerba step-cut osteotomy in which the calcaneal tuberosity was translated medially. At 3-year follow-up, there were no statistically significant differences between the two groups with respect to AOFAS ankle-hindfoot and foot and ankle disability index outcome scores and radiographic correction, and both groups had significant improvement from preoperatively. The authors noted that calcaneocuboid subluxation, calcaneal anterior process fracture, and lateral column pain were exclusively reported in the Evans/MDCO group, but they felt that the Evans/MDCO was preferred in severe deformity due to relatively higher corrective power.

Ettinger et al[28] retrospectively reviewed 17 patients who underwent Evans LCL and 36 patients who underwent Hintermann LCL with mean follow-up of 67.7 and 40 months, respectively. Both surgical techniques resulted in a significant improvement of clinical outcome scores and led to good radiological correction of PCFD, but there was a higher rate calcaneocuboid degenerative changes following the Evans procedure.

REFERENCES

1. Johnson KA, Strom DE. Tibialis posterior tendon dysfunction. *Clin Orthop Relat Res.* 1989;239:196-206.
2. Myerson MS. Adult acquired flatfoot deformity: treatment of dysfunction of the posterior tibial tendon. *Instr Course Lect.* 1997;46:393-405.
3. Myerson MS, Thordarson DB, Johnson JE, et al. Classification and nomenclature: progressive collapsing foot deformity. *Foot Ankle Int.* 2020;41:1271-1276.
4. de Cesar NC, Deland JT, Ellis SJ. Guest editorial: expert consensus on adult-acquired flatfoot deformity. *Foot Ankle Int.* 2020;41:1269-1271.
5. Koutsogiannis E. Treatment of mobile flat foot by displacement osteotomy of the calcaneus. *J Bone Joint Surg Br.* 1971;53:96-100.
6. Evans D. Calcaneo-valgus deformity. *J Bone Joint Surg Br.* 1975;57(3):270-278.
7. Cotton FJ. Foot statics and surgery. *N Engl J Med.* 1936;214(8):353-362.
8. Ling JS, Ross KA, Hannon CP, et al. A plantar closing wedge osteotomy of the medial cuneiform for residual forefoot supination in flatfoot reconstruction. *Foot Ankle Int.* 2013;34(9):1221-1226.
9. Guha AR, Perera AM. Calcaneal osteotomy in the treatment of adult acquired flatfoot deformity. *Foot Ankle Clin.* 2012;17(2):247-258.
10. Roche AJ, Calder JD. Lateral column lengthening osteotomies. *Foot Ankle Clin.* 2012;17(2):259-270.
11. Moseir-LaClair S, Pomeroy G, Manoli A II. Intermediate follow-up on the double osteotomy and tendon transfer procedure for stage II posterior tibial tendon insufficiency. *Foot Ankle Int.* 2001;22(4):283-291.
12. Toolan BC, Sangeorzan BJ, Hansen ST Jr. Complex reconstruction for the treatment of dorsolateral peritalar subluxation of the foot: early results after distraction arthrodesis of the calcaneocuboid joint in conjunction with stabilization of, and transfer of the flexor digitorum longus tendon to, the midfoot to treat acquired pes planovalgus in adults. *J Bone Joint Surg Am.* 1999;81:1545-1560.
13. Saltzman CL, el-Khoury GY. The hindfoot alignment view. *Foot Ankle Int.* 1995;16(9):572-576.
14. Erard MUE, Sheean MAJ, Sangeorzan BJ. Triple arthrodesis for adult-acquired flatfoot deformity. *Foot Ankle Orthop.* 2019;4(3):1-12.
15. Guyton G. MIS heel slide. Chapter 31 in this book
16. Penney NT, Viselli SJ, Holmes TR, et al. Double-calcaneal osteotomy with a unilateral rail external fixator for correction of pes planus: a case report. *Foot Ankle Spec.* 2009;2(4):194-199.
17. Tsai J, McDonald E, Sutton R, et al. Severe flexible pes planovalgus deformity correction using trabecular metallic wedges. *Foot Ankle Int.* 2019;40(4):402-407.
18. Hintermann B, Valderrabano V, Kundert HP. Lengthening of the lateral column and reconstruction of the medial soft tissue for treatment of acquired flatfoot deformity associated with insufficiency of the posterior tibial tendon. *Foot Ankle Int.* 1999;20(10):622-629.
19. Ettinger S, Mattinger T, Stukenborg-Colsman C, et al. Outcomes of Evans versus Hintermann calcaneal lengthening osteotomy for flexible flatfoot. *Foot Ankle Int.* 2019;40(6):661-671.
20. Vander GR. Lateral column lengthening using a "Z" osteotomy of the calcaneus. *Tech Foot Ankle Surg.* 2008;7(4):257-263.
21. Saunders SM, Ellis SJ, Demetracopoulos CA, et al. Comparative outcomes between step-cut lengthening calcaneal osteotomy vs traditional Evans osteotomy for Stage IIB adult-acquired flatfoot deformity. *Foot Ankle Int.* 2018;39(1):18-27.
22. Nagy M, Kholeif A, Reda Mansour AM, et al. Comparison between Malerba osteotomy and combined Evans/medial displacement calcaneal osteotomies for the management of flexible pes planus in young adults: a prospective randomised control trial, three years follow-up. *Int Orthop.* 2021;45(10):2579-2588.
23. Aronow MS. Triceps surae contractures associated with posterior tibial tendon dysfunction. *Techniques In Orthopaedics.* 2000;15(3):164-173.
24. Deland J. Spring ligament reconstruction. Chapter 32 in this book
25. Obey MR, Johnson JE, Backus JD. Managing Complications of Foot and Ankle Surgery: Reconstruction of the Progressive Collapsing Foot Deformity. *Foot Ankle Clin.* 2022;27(2):303-325.
26. Myerson MS, Badekas A, Schon LC. Treatment of stage II posterior tibial tendon deficiency with flexor digitorum longus tendon transfer and calcaneal osteotomy. *Foot Ankle Int.* 2004;25(7):445-450.
27. Chadwick C, Whitehouse SL, Saxby TS. Long-term follow-up of flexor digitorum longus transfer and calcaneal osteotomy for stage II posterior tibial tendon dysfunction. *Bone Joint J.* 2015;97-B(3):346-352.
28. Ettinger S, Sibai K, Stukenborg-Colsman C, et al. Comparison of anatomic structures at risk with 2 lateral lengthening calcaneal osteotomies. *Foot Ankle Int.* 2018;39(12):1481-1486.

28 First Ray Procedures in Progressive Collapsing Foot Deformity: Cotton, Lapidus, and Lapicotton

Nacime Salomao Barbachan Mansur, Kepler Alencar Mendes de Carvalho, and Cesar de Cesar Netto

INTRODUCTION

When considering the foot tripod reestablishment in the progressive collapsing foot deformity (PCFD) scenario, first ray procedures have a crucial role.[1,2] Plantarflexion of the first ray through a medial cuneiform dorsal opening wedge osteotomy, as described by Cotton, is indicated for forefoot varus (supination after hindfoot correction) and medial column breakdown at the naviculocuneiform (NC) joint or medial cuneiform.[1,3] The Lapidus fusion aims to restructure the arch by stabilizing the first tarsometatarsal (TMT) joint, and it is traditionally indicated when the first ray is deemed unstable.[4-6] In an attempt to counterbalance the potential shortening and improve the metatarsal lever arm, the "Lapicotton" technique uses the concept of bone block fusion to reposition the collapsed column.[2,7]

Inclusion of a Cotton, Lapidus, or Lapicotton in PCFD surgical planning is expected even in mild deformities due to the high incidence of forefoot varus and medial column instability (class C—PCFD Consensus Classification) in this population.[8-10] Although traditionally performed lastly in the bone procedures list (after medial displacement calcaneal osteotomy, lateral column lengthening, or subtalar fusion), first ray procedures need to be fixed prior to soft tissue reconstruction/repair and final tensioning.[11,12] Controversy in the literature exists when deciding if a first ray procedure should be carried only when the indications (forefoot varus and medial column instability) are maintained after hindfoot correction.[9] It is the author's opinion that, when indications are present preoperatively, a first ray procedure is necessary. Further, the threshold for this decision should be low.

Correct titration can be performed intraoperatively by using trials and clinically observing the first metatarsal positioning (Fig. 28.1) in relation to the lesser metatarsals coronally.[13,14] A 1- to 2-mm lower (or at least at the same level) first metatarsal head is desirable.[7] Flexible deformities (1C) can be managed with a Cotton, Lapidus, or Lapicotton, while rigid classes (2C) should be treated with a Lapidus or Lapicotton.[9,15]

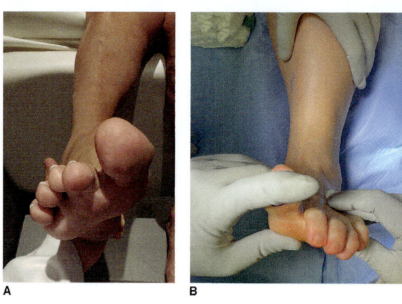

FIGURE 28.1 Forefoot varus is deemed present when forefoot supination **(A)** or first metatarsal elevation **(B)** are observed after the hindfoot is passively corrected.

COTTON

Medial Cuneiform Dorsal Opening Wedge Osteotomy

Indications

- Flexible forefoot varus (class 1C): forefoot supination or first ray elevation (Fig. 28.2A) is noted when the valgus hindfoot is corrected to neutral.[9]
- Mild first ray instability (class C): increased mobility between first ray and lateral rays (Fig. 28.3). Dorsal-plantar increase in translation.[16-18]
- Medial column sagging at the NC joint or at the cuneiform bone.[9,14]

Contraindications

- Rigid forefoot varus (class 2C).
- Severe first ray instability (subjectively and empirically determined).
- First TMT arthritis.
- Medial column sagging at the TMT joint.
- Hallux valgus in the context of PCFD (TMT instability).
- Cuneiform bone loss.

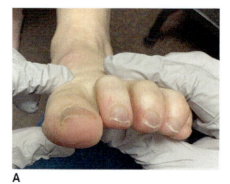 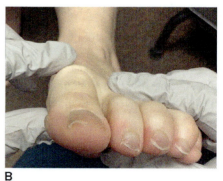

FIGURE 28.2 First ray stability evaluation performed by holding the intermediate and lateral rays with one hand and the medial ray with the other. The first ray is translated plantarly **(A)** and dorsally **(B)**. Displacements higher than 8-10 mm are considered positive for instability.

- Cotton revisions.
- Severe comorbidities impending surgery, active or latent infection at the surgical topography, poor local soft tissue coverage, or bone quality that would impair osteotomy healing.

Preoperative Planning

- Full clinical assessment focused on the PCFD scenario is necessary not only for a Cotton indication but also to determine potential additional procedures.[19]
- Forefoot varus should be evaluated with the patient seated or in supine. The hindfoot is passively corrected to neutral, and the presence of forefoot supination is observed (Fig. 28.1A). Dorsal first metatarsal displacement after the hindfoot is corrected (Fig. 28.1B) is also considered a forefoot varus sign.[9]
- First ray instability is assessed by grasping the medial column and moving it while the other columns are stabilized. A dorsal-plantar displacement higher than 8 to 10 mm is considered positive (Fig. 28.2B; Video 28.1). Other clinical findings, such as dorsal first metatarsal migration, plantar keratosis absence under the first metatarsal (or increased keratosis under the second metatarsal), and hallux pronation are also described as indirect clinical signs of first ray hypermobility. The use of external devices to measure hypermobility (Klaue, Glasoe) is described, and values above 8 mm are considered positive.[18]
- A useful test to determine first ray instability is dorsal metatarsal migration. One must check intraoperatively the amount of required plantarflexion to be performed by looking at the forefoot. With the patient seated or in supine, the provider observes the forefoot from an anterior standpoint. One of the physician's thumbs is placed under the first metatarsal head and the other under the lesser metatarsal heads (see Fig. 28.3). The ankle is positioned in neutral. A first metatarsal dorsal positioning in relation to the second and third indicates first ray incompetence in maintaining the tripod. During surgery, when testing trials, the proper size should be placed so that the first metatarsal is at the same level or slightly plantar to the lesser metatarsals.
- Gait analysis can portray first metatarsal dorsal migration, lateral forefoot overload, and pressure diminished under the first ray (Fig. 28.4).

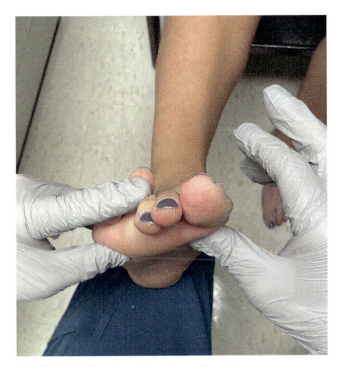

FIGURE 28.3 Dorsal metatarsal migration. The assessor observes the forefoot from an anterior perspective. The physician's thumb is positioned under the first metatarsal head and the other thumb under the lesser metatarsal heads while the ankle is placed in neutral. A dorsal first metatarsal position regarding the second and third is indicative of first ray incompetence.

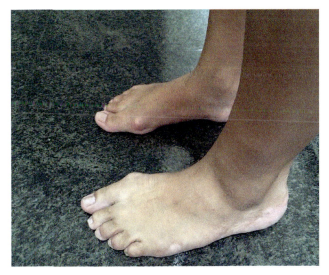

FIGURE 28.4 An indirect sign of first metatarsal instability that can be noted during stance and gait is the dorsal migration of the first ray.

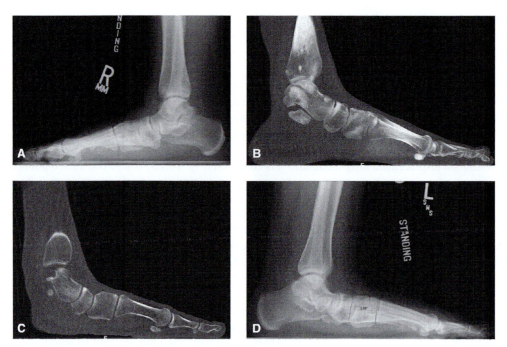

FIGURE 28.5 Plantar tarsometatarsal gapping **(A and B)** and dorsal metatarsal migration **(C)** can be identified in weight-bearing radiographs and weight-bearing computed tomography. The cuneiform articular angle can be calculated **(D)** when correcting the deformity.

- Conventional weight-bearing radiographs and weight-bearing computed tomography (WBCT) are crucial in the setting of PCFD. First ray instability can be demonstrated by the presence of NC or TMT plantar gapping (Fig. 28.5A and B), dorsal TMT subluxation (Fig. 28.5C) or increased talus-first metatarsal angle. Arthritis of the NC or TMT joints are also considered signs of instability, although their presence leads surgical indication toward fusion and not a Cotton.[20] Correction can be titrated by using the cuneiform articular angle (CAA) (Fig. 28.5D), and values greater than or equal to −2° should be targeted when performing the osteotomy.[21]

Surgical Technique

- After proper anesthesia, the patient is positioned supine with an ipsilateral small bump that rotates the limb internally, placing the dorsal foot in line with the operative table. A thigh tourniquet is applied. The limb is prepped and draped in the usual sterile fashion (Fig. 28.6). Perioperative antibiotics should be administered prior to inflation of the tourniquet. A conventional C-arm is preferred for intraoperative fluoroscopy since a good lateral imaging is needed.

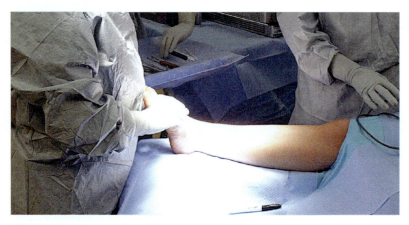

FIGURE 28.6 Example of patient positioning and preparation.

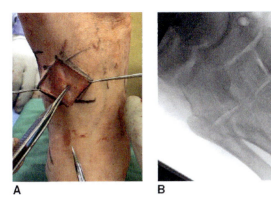
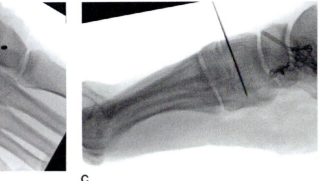

FIGURE 28.7 After a dorsal incision centered at the medial cuneiform, the extensor hallucis longus is protected **(A)**. After the cuneiform periosteum is opened and the distal and proximal joints identified, a 1.2- to 2.0-mm K-wire is introduced at the bone midpoint **(B and C)**.

- The incision is marked over the medial cuneiform, medial to the extensor hallucis longus (EHL) tendon. After the skin is carefully opened, care should be taken to protect the EHL (Fig. 28.7A) and medial branches of dorsal medial cutaneous nerve (derivate from the superficial peroneal nerve [SPN]). Proximal or distal incision extensions must contemplate the anterior tibial tendon (ATT).
- The medial cuneiform periosteum is opened. The medial NC and first TMT joints are identified. The midpoint of the cuneiform is marked and a K-wire (1.2 to 2 mm) is inserted from dorsal (Fig. 28.7B) to plantar (Fig. 28.7C), respecting the cuneiform sagittal format, as much parallel from the NC and TMT joints as possible.
- A delicate low-profile sagittal saw blade is then used to produce a straight cut using the K-wire as a guide and support. This could be done proximal or distal to the wire, depending on its position in relation to the center of the cuneiform. Saline irrigation to decrease heating injury is advisable. The cut must reach the plantar cortex without disrupting it. While a complete osteotomy might jeopardize stability and proper plantarflexion, a cut too short will not produce the desired effect and may create an intra-articular fracture during wedge placement.
- The osteotomy is checked using fluoroscopy. The trials are placed sequentially at the osteotomy site. A laminar spreader can be placed bridging the cut to facilitate trial insertion. First ray length, plantarflexion, and stability are assessed using clinical evaluation and fluoroscopy. The first metatarsal coronal positioning in relation to the second and third metatarsals should be at the same level or moderately plantar as described in the clinical evaluation section (Fig. 28.8). First metatarsophalangeal joint range of motion is also checked to prevent an overlarge wedge placement that could produce stiffness.

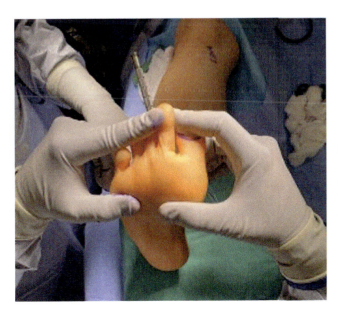

FIGURE 28.8 Intraoperative analysis of the first correction performed by placing the one thumb under the first metatarsal head and the other thumb under the lesser metatarsal heads while the toes are dorsiflexed, and the ankle is placed in neutral. A first metatarsal head at the same level or just below the lateral rays indicates an adequate correction.

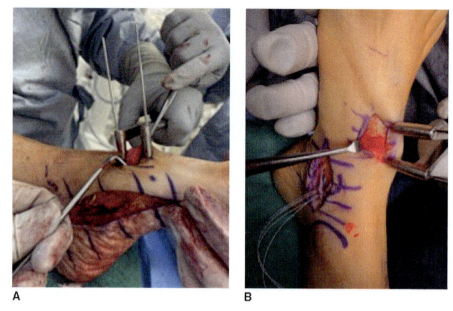

FIGURE 28.9 After the proper graft size is determined, a spreader can be utilized proximal and distal **(A)** to the osteotomy to aid in its proper placement **(B)**.

- A desirable wedge size places the first metatarsal in a *plus minus* lengthening. Correction of the Meary's angle and sinus tarsi impingement are also expected when observing a lateral fluoroscopy.
- After the proper size is selected, the allograft is thawed/activated on the side table. An alternative is to sink it into bone marrow aspirate before insertion. A Hintermann spreader can be carefully placed to facilitate graft insertion (Fig. 28.9). The graft is placed, and positioning is checked with a fluoroscopy.
- Since this is a mechanically stable procedure, we usually do not include a screw or plate fixation to the Cotton osteotomy unless the plantar cortex is disrupted inadvertently (Fig. 28.10A). Other authors report the use of a single screw, a step-off plate (with cancellous bone), staples, or a straight plate. When using metallic wedges (Fig. 28.10B), guided locking screws are commonly available inside the implant. We prefer prefabricated allograft wedges due to the facility in placing it, the nonrequirement for fixation, and potential revisions. Hardware removal can be detrimental to an already limited bone stock.
- The suture is closed in planes, and the foot is covered with dressings. A postoperative cast is placed, and patients are usually discharged the same day with conventional analgesics and deep vein thrombosis (DVT) prophylaxis.

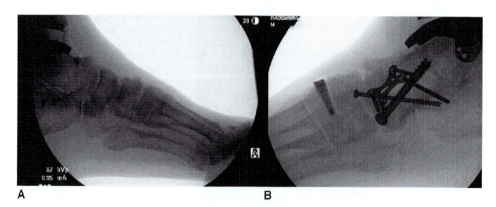

FIGURE 28.10 Examples of different Cotton osteotomies utilizing an allograft wedge **(A)** and a metallic wedge **(B)**, respectively.

Postoperative Management

- This very stable osteotomy allows early weight bearing in a boot (around 3 weeks). However, the fact that most Cotton osteotomies are usually performed in conjunction with other PCFD soft tissue reconstruction procedures could delay weight bearing and motion until the 6th postoperative week.
- A careful follow-up every 2 weeks (until the 6th week) is necessary to observe wound healing and detect potential complications. Sutures are removed around the 3rd or 4th week after surgery.
- After 6 weeks, patients are transitioned to a walking boot, and physical therapy may be initiated at this point. Around the 10th week post operation, the boot is progressively discontinued, and patients are encouraged to use stiff rocker-bottom shoes.

Pearls and Pitfalls

- A central cut in the cuneiform allows the Cotton osteotomy to have a good amount of surrounding osseous tissue, diminishing the possibility of a fracture, and improving the procedure lever arm (Fig. 28.11).
- Cuts that reach the far plantar cortex without violating it are preferable. Insufficient cuts may put the cuneiform at risk of fracture when correcting the first ray. Complete cuts destabilize the osteotomy, hindering the plantarflexion capacity and potentially translating the distal segment.
- Care should be taken when performing dissection or using the blade too laterally since there is potential for injury of the neurovascular bundle (dorsalis pedis artery and deep peroneal nerve). The intercuneiform ligaments must also be protected to avoid destabilizing this joint.
- While the osteotomy is performed, saline irrigation decreases heating injury and prevents potential late bone reabsorption. During the procedure, a meticulous protection of the surrounding skin is recommended to reduce skin complications.

Results and Complications

Cotton osteotomy was described almost a century ago with the objective of plantarflexing the first ray and reconstructing the foot's "triangle of support."[1] Several authors demonstrated the Cotton's capability in improving alignment and outcomes for PCFD patients.[9,22] Abousayed et al followed 19 patients treated with a Cotton for PCFD for at least 4 years (mean 8.6).[23] Although a mean of 30° in Meary's correction was found in the early postoperative radiographs, a 50% loss in correction was present at the final follow-up.[23] When assessing 32 feet treated with metallic Cotton wedges for PCFD, Fraser et al described improvement in radiographical parameters, one implant loosening, and no residual implant pain.[24] Romeo et al compared 18 metallic wedges with 18 allograft wedges, finding improvement in angular and clinical assessments for both groups.[25]

A retrospective evaluation of 79 feet operated with a concomitant for PCFD reconstruction by Kunas et al was able to predict that for every millimeter of a Cotton wedge, there was a 2.1° decrease of the CAA.[21] Conti et al evaluated the Cotton's postoperative CAA with patient-reported outcomes.[22] Patients with mild plantarflexion were found to have better outcomes when compared to moderate correction.[22]

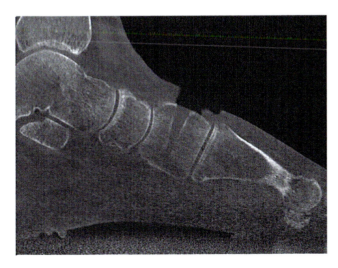

FIGURE 28.11 Example of a central cut performed at the cuneiform.

LAPIDUS

First Tarsometatarsal Arthrodesis

Indications

- Severe flexible forefoot varus (class 1C): forefoot supination or first ray elevation (see Fig. 28.1) is noted when the valgus hindfoot is corrected to neutral.[9] Although there is no available grading system to determine "severe varus," advanced deformities are an indication for first TMT fusion.
- Rigid forefoot varus (class 2C): forefoot supination or first ray elevation (see Fig. 28.1) is noted when the valgus hindfoot is corrected to neutral.[9] The deformity is deemed rigid based on the absence of clinical and radiological signs.
- First ray instability (class C): increased mobility between first ray and lateral rays (see Fig. 28.2). Dorsal-plantar increase in translation.[16-18]
- First TMT arthritis.
- Concomitant hallux valgus deformity.
- Severe plantar gapping at the TMT joint seen on weight-bearing radiographs or WBCT.

Contraindications

- Absence of first ray instability.
- Cuneiform or metatarsal bone loss.
- Lapidus revision (relative). The loss of bone stock required for a Lapidus revision (due to a malunion, nonunion, or recurrence) might place a bone block revision fusion as a better option.
- Severe comorbidities impeding surgery, active or latent infection at the surgical site, poor local soft tissues coverage, or bone quality that would impair fusion healing.

Preoperative Planning

- Full clinical assessment focused on the PCFD scenario is necessary not only for the Lapidus but also to determine the potential need for additional procedures.[19]
- Forefoot varus should be evaluated with the patient seated or in a supine position. The hindfoot is passively corrected to neutral, and the presence of forefoot supination is observed. Although there is literature proposing 15° of supination as a threshold for determining forefoot varus, many authors (including us) believe that any degree of supination is indicative of forefoot varus.[26]
- Dorsal first metatarsal displacement after the hindfoot is corrected is also considered a forefoot varus sign.[9]
- Severe rigid forefoot varus is empirically determined by a substantial supination, while the heel is passively corrected.[15,26] A rigid forefoot varus is established by an incapacity to passively reduce the forefoot deformity.
- First ray instability is assessed by grasping the medial column and moving it, while the other columns are stabilized. A dorsal-plantar displacement higher than 8 to 10 mm is considered positive. Other clinical findings, such as dorsal first metatarsal migration, the absence of plantar keratosis under the first metatarsal, and hallux pronation, are all described as indirect clinical signs of first ray instability. The use of external devices to measure hypermobility (Klaue, Glasoe) is described, and values above 8 mm are considered positive.[18]
- A useful test to determine first ray instability, to determine dorsal metatarsal migration, and to intraoperatively check the amount of plantarflexion required is performed by looking at the forefoot positioning (see Fig. 28.3). When the patient is seated or supine, the provider observes the forefoot from an anterior standpoint. One of the physician's thumbs is placed under the first metatarsal head and the other thumb under the lesser metatarsal heads. The ankle is put in a neutral position. If the first metatarsal has dorsal positioning relative to the second and third metatarsals, it indicates first ray incompetence in maintaining the tripod.
- Gait analysis can portray first metatarsal dorsal migration, medial sagging, and lateral forefoot overload. Baropodometric evaluation can show pressure diminished under the first ray.
- Conventional weight-bearing radiographs and WBCT are key to a successful evaluation in the setting of PCFD. First ray instability can be demonstrated by the presence of TMT plantar gapping, dorsal TMT subluxation, or increased talus-first metatarsal angle. Arthritis of the TMT joint is also considered instability signs, and its presence leads surgical indication toward a Lapidus fusion (Fig. 28.12).[20]

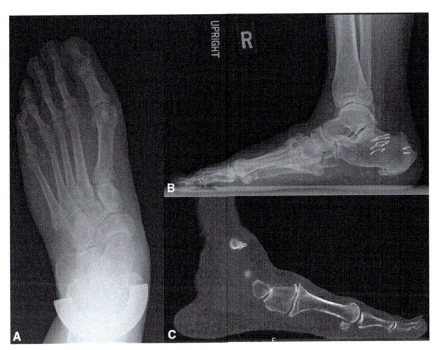

FIGURE 28.12 Indirect signs of rigid first ray instability **(C)** can be corroborated by radiographic signs of first tarsometatarsal osteoarthritis **(A and B)**. Weight-bearing computed tomography imaging is also a viable option when determining early and late degenerative changes at this joint.

- Presence of hallux valgus deformity, depicted by an increase in the intermetatarsal and hallux valgus angles, as well as the presence of sesamoid subluxation and metatarsal hyperpronation may be noted during imaging evaluation (Fig. 28.13).[27] Although the deformity may be asymptomatic, it demonstrates a high degree of first TMT instability supporting the indication for a concomitant Lapidus.

Surgical Technique

- After proper anesthesia, the patient is positioned supine with an ipsilateral small bump that rotates the limb internally, thus placing the dorsal foot in line with the operative table. A thigh tourniquet is applied. The limb is prepped and draped in the usual sterile fashion. Perioperative antibiotics should be administered prior to inflation of the tourniquet. A conventional C-arm is preferred for intraoperative fluoroscopy since a good lateral image is needed.
- The incision is marked over the first TMT joint, medial to the EHL tendon. After the skin is carefully opened, care should be taken to protect the EHL and medial branches of dorsal medial cutaneous nerve (derivate from the SPN). The ATT route and insertion must be identified and protected.

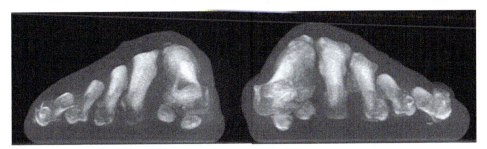

FIGURE 28.13 Hallux valgus deformity in the setting of a progressive collapsing foot deformity. Instability of the first ray might be represented also by an increase in the metatarsal pronation, as observed by the coronal weight-bearing computed tomography view.

- In case of concomitant fusions through the intermediate column (TMT 2 and 3), the incision might be placed medially.
- The first TMT joints is identified, and capsular attachments are released with care not to injury the ATT or significantly destabilize the joint. The medial NC is also identified for a proper hardware placement. Several cutting guides and implants are available on the market, and most use specific landmarks at the first metatarsal and medial cuneiform for their use.
- A delicate low-profile sagittal saw blade is then used to resect cartilages surfaces from the cuneiform and metatarsal. This can be performed free-hand or using industry cutting jigs that may account for intermetatarsal and plantarflexion correction (Fig. 28.14). A chisel can be used as an alternative to the saw.
- Considering this is a modified Lapidus without the use of a wedge, extra care should be taken to resect as little bone as possible. This will minimize first ray shortening and allow for more plantarflexion moment. The region is irrigated and cleaned.
- Subchondral preparation is achieved by doing multiple perforations at the metatarsal and cuneiform using a K-wire or small drill. Fish-scaling the surfaces is also an option if the bone quality is not poor. Preparation of the medial second metatarsal surface and the lateral aspect of the first metatarsal can be attained if a traditional Lapidus for an intercolumn instability is desired. Grafting (either autograft or allograft) is advisable to potentiate healing.
- The metatarsal is properly placed in relation to the medial cuneiform. Hallux dorsiflexion and manual pressure to close the intermetatarsal space are obtained to improve plantarflexion and axial alignment, respectively (Fig. 28.15).
- Adequate plantarflexion, checked by the talus-first metatarsal angle on the lateral fluoroscopy, and suitable axial positioning, correcting the intermetatarsal angle when appropriate and improving the talonavicular coverage, are advisable. Clinically, the first metatarsal coronal positioning

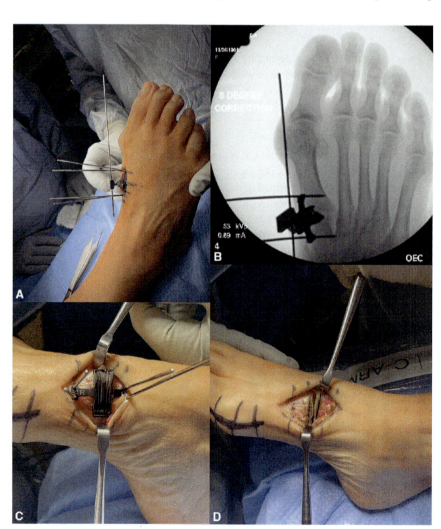

FIGURE 28.14 Example of an external cutting guide used for a Lapidus fusion aiming angular correction, more on the axial plane. The desired first metatarsal position is determined clinically **(A)** with a guide and confirmed fluoroscopically **(B)**. The longitudinal wire should be parallel to the second ray. After the amount of correction is decided, the proper cutting jig is placed **(C)** and the surfaces are resected with a saw **(D)**.

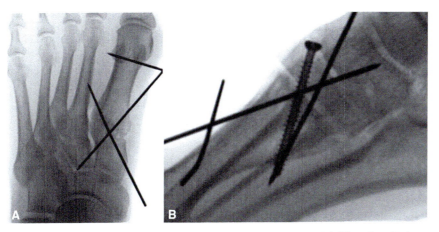

FIGURE 28.15 First metatarsal intraoperative correction in the axial **(A)** and sagittal planes **(B)**.

in relation to the second and third metatarsals should be at the same level or moderately plantar as described above (Fig. 28.16).
- The position is secured using provisional K-wires and checked. Dorsomedial, medial, or plantar plates are options for final fusion fixation. Crossing screws, staples, intramedullary nails, and post devices can also be utilized. Once performing any specific implant, proper metatarsal position should be constantly checked.
- An intercolumn screw, from the first to the second metatarsal or from the first metatarsal to the intermediate cuneiform, can be placed if an original Lapidus is desired.
- The suture is closed in planes, and the foot is covered with dressings. A postoperative cast is placed, and patients are usually discharged on the same day with conventional analgesics and DVT prophylaxis.

Postoperative Management
- Patients keep the splint until the 2nd week. It is then replaced by a postoperative boot in a non–weight-bearing regimen until the 6th postoperative week.
- A careful follow-up every 2 weeks (until the 6th week) is necessary to obverse wound healing and detect potential complications. Sutures are removed around the 3rd or 4th week after surgery.
- After 6 weeks, patients are transitioned to a walking boot, and progressive weight bearing is started. Physical therapy may be initiated at this point. Around the 10th postoperative week, the boot is progressively discontinued, and patients are encouraged to use stiff rocker-bottom shoes.

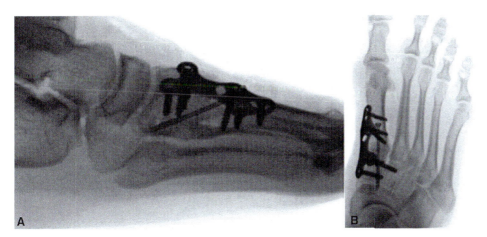

FIGURE 28.16 Lapidus fusion final construction with a proper first metatarsal position in relation to the lesser metatarsal in the sagittal **(A)** and axial planes **(B)**. Meary's and intermetatarsal angles are also corrected.

Pearls and Pitfalls
- When doing an original or a modified Lapidus fusion without the use of a structured graft, care must be taken to not over-resect bone from the cuneiform and metatarsal when preparing the joint. Although a minor loss can be overcome by an increase in plantarflexion, ray shortening is associated with worse outcomes.[28]
- The use of grafting and biological products, although not completely supported by the literature, is advised by the senior author even in the primary scenario.[29]

Results and Complications
Fusion of the first TMT joint, or Lapidus procedure,[6] is a well-accepted technique that allows correction of the first metatarsal malposition in the axial, coronal, and sagittal planes, reestablishing the medial column structural stability.[4,5,30-33] Saffo et al reported the results in 54 Lapidus procedures as having good angular correction, few complications, no transfer metatarsalgia, and several asymptomatic nonunions.[32] When reviewing 201 feet treated with a modified Lapidus, Thompson et al found a 4% nonunion a 2% revision rate.[33] The authors associated previous bunion surgery and recurrent deformity with a higher chance for nonconsolidation.[33]

On the other hand, a nonunion rate of up to 8%[34] with relative shortening and dorsiflexion of the first metatarsal are inherently possible limitations and complications associated with the procedure.[35-38] An average of 4.1 mm decrease in absolute length of the first ray is also reported in the literature.[39,40] Complications of the modified Lapidus first TMT joint arthrodesis are not rare and might reach up to 16% of cases.[36,41] Barg et al, in a systematic review for hallux valgus, described a 6.6% (95% CI, 3.9% to 9.9%) reoperation and 11.4% (95% CI, 0.3% to 35%) infection rate with the use of the modified Lapidus and an overall nonunion percentage of 3.8% (95% CI, 1.1% to 7.8%) for 261 patients from five different studies.[34]

LAPICOTTON

First Tarsometatarsal Arthrodesis Using an Interposition Bone Block
Indications
- Severe flexible forefoot varus (class 1C): forefoot supination or first ray elevation (see Fig. 28.1) is noted when the valgus hindfoot is corrected to neutral.[9] Although there is no available grading system to determine "severe," advanced deformities are an indication for a Lapicotton.
- Rigid forefoot varus (class 2C): forefoot supination or first ray elevation (see Fig. 28.1) is noted when the valgus hindfoot is corrected to neutral.[9] The deformity is deemed rigid based on the absence of clinical and radiological signs.
- First ray instability (class C): increased mobility between first ray and lateral rays (see Fig. 28.2). Dorsal-plantar increase in translation.[16-18]
- First TMT arthritis (see Fig. 28.12).
- Concomitant hallux valgus deformity (see Fig. 28.13).
- Revision (Fig. 28.17).
- Shorten first ray as a consequence of congenital, posttraumatic, iatrogenic (see Fig. 28.17), or infectious diseases.

Contraindications
- Absence of first ray instability
- Mild first ray instability
- Absence of forefoot varus
- Severe comorbidities, impending surgery, active or latent infection at the surgical topography, poor local soft tissues coverage, or bone quality that would impair fusion healing

Preoperative Planning
- Full clinical assessment focused on the PCFD scenario is necessary not only for the Lapidus but also to determine potential additional procedures.[19]
- Forefoot varus should be evaluated with the patient seated or supine as previously described (see Fig. 28.1).[26]

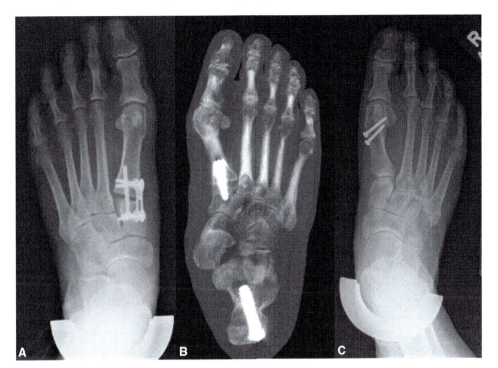

FIGURE 28.17 Tarsometatarsal arthrodesis revisions for nonunion **(A)** and malunion **(B)** are good indications for a Lapicotton procedure since surgery will produce more shortening. A shortened first metatarsal requiring fusion **(C)** will also benefit from a Lapicotton.

- Dorsal first metatarsal displacement after the hindfoot is corrected is also considered a forefoot varus sign.[9]
- Severe forefoot varus is empirically determined by a substantial supination, while the heel is passively corrected.[15,26] A rigid forefoot varus is established by an incapacity to passively reduce the deformity.
- First ray instability is assessed by grasping the medial column and moving it, while the other columns are stabilized with the contralateral hand as described in the previous sections.
- A useful test to determine first ray instability, dorsal metatarsal migration, and check intraoperatively the amount of required plantarflexion is performed by looking at the forefoot positioning as described above.
- Gait analysis can portray first metatarsal dorsal migration, lateral forefoot overload, and pressure diminished under the first ray.
- Conventional weight-bearing radiographs and WBCT can portray first ray instability and arthritis of TMT joint with the above-mentioned signs (see Figs. 28.5 and 28.12).
- Presence of hallux valgus deformity demonstrates a high degree of first TMT instability, supporting the indication (see Fig. 28.13).

Surgical Technique

- After proper anesthesia, the patient is positioned supine with an ipsilateral small bump that rotates the limb internally, placing the dorsal foot in line with the operative table. A thigh tourniquet is applied. The limb is prepped and draped in the usual sterile fashion. Perioperative antibiotics should be administered prior to inflation of the tourniquet. A conventional C-arm is preferred for intraoperative fluoroscopy since a good lateral imaging is needed.
- The incision is marked over the first TMT joint, medial to the EHL tendon (Fig. 28.18). After the skin is carefully opened, care should be taken to protect the EHL and medial branches of dorsal medial cutaneous nerve (derivate from the SPN). The ATT route and insertion must be identified and protected.
- In case of concomitant fusions through the intermediate column (TMT 2 and 3), the first TMT incision might be placed medially.

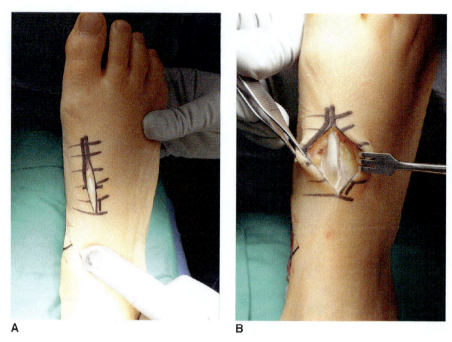

FIGURE 28.18 A. A dorsal incision is placed over the first tarsometatarsal joint. **B.** Care with the extensor hallucis longus tendon and the medial branches of the dorsal medial cutaneous nerve must be taken.

- The first TMT joint is identified, and capsular attachments are released with care taken to not injure the ATT or significantly destabilize the joint. The medial NC is also identified for a proper hardware placement (Fig. 28.19).
- Several cutting guides and implants are available on the market, and most utilize specific landmarks at the first metatarsal and medial cuneiform. Dorsomedial, medial, or plantar plates are options for final fusion fixation. Crossing screws, intramedullary nails, and post devices can also be utilized. Regardless of the specific implant, proper metatarsal position should be constantly checked.

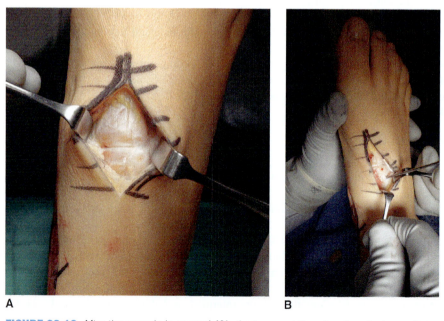

FIGURE 28.19 After the capsule is opened **(A)**, the tarsometatarsal and naviculocuneiform joints are identified **(B)**.

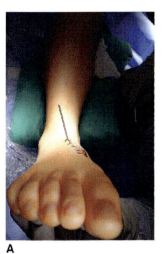 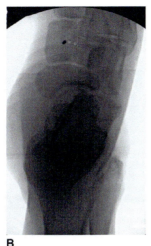 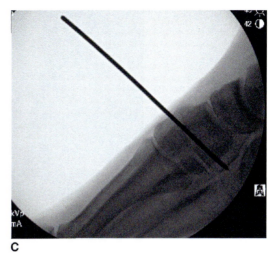

FIGURE 28.20 The guidewire for the post is inserted respecting the three different planes to avoid cuneiform fractures and optimize correction. **A.** The coronal direction is slightly lateral to medial, respecting the bone anatomy. **B.** Axially, the wire is inserted more laterally, to obtain a better structural coverage. **C.** Sagittal inclination must consider the cuneiform distal articular inclination and the desired metatarsal plantarflexion.

- It is the senior surgeon's preference to use a post configuration. The guidewire for post placement at the cuneiform is inserted. A guide for wire placement can be used by introducing the metal keel at the TMT joint and using its proximal cannulated tunnel to insert the wire. This wire should be placed centrally in the sagittal plane, respecting the cuneiform distal articular inclination (Fig. 28.20A). Axially, the wire is gently placed lateral to the bone axis (Fig. 28.20B), to have better bone coverage. Coronally, the wire is directed from dorsolateral to plantar medial, respecting the cuneiform anatomy (Fig. 28.20C).
- The position is checked, and the appropriate reamer for the post is used (Fig. 28.21A and B). Although it is preferable to not infringe on the plantar cortex with the implant, there is no real loss of stability by doing so. It is also advised to not leave a prominent dorsal post. The post is inserted and attached to an external jig containing guides for additional wires to be placed in the metatarsal, tunnels for the screws, and a distraction/compression rail (Fig. 28.21C).
- The medial segment of the jig needs to touch the medial aspect of the distal metatarsal (Fig. 28.22A). The dorsal incision is extended to allow for adequate positioning of the jig. With the medial aspect of the jig (containing the two tunnels for K-wires) in contact with the dorsomedial metatarsal cortex, two K-wires are placed to secure the jig's position (Fig. 28.22B and C).
- The external jig is then used to distract the TMT joint by using a screwdriver in a counterclockwise direction at the rail (Fig. 28.23A, ▶Video 28.2). A proximal wire, adjacent to the post, is inserted to prevent dorsal post migration when distraction is performed. About 8 to 10 mm of distraction is initially required for joint preparation (Fig. 28.23B, ▶Video 28.2).
- A delicate low-profile sagittal saw blade is then used to resect cartilaginous surfaces from the cuneiform and metatarsal. This can be performed free-hand or using an industry cutting jig that may account for intermetatarsal and plantarflexion correction (see Fig. 28.14). A chisel can be used as an alternative to the saw. The region is irrigated and cleaned.
- Subchondral preparation is completed by doing multiple perforations at the metatarsal and cuneiform using a K-wire or small drill. Fish-scaling the surfaces is also an option if the bone quality is good. The proximal medial aspect of the second metatarsal can be prepared (perforations and grafting) if intercolumn fusion is desired.
- Trials are inserted to decide the proper allograft size to be used (Fig. 28.24). The distraction is adjusted in accordance with the trial size. Available trials for this demonstrated technique are 5 mm × 5° inclination, 8 mm × 8°, 10 mm × 10°, and 12 mm × 12°. An additional parallel (no graft inclination) 14-mm graft can be used, but there is no trial offered for this configuration.
- Proper graft size is determined by using trials along with clinical and radiographical assessments. Clinically, the medial arch must be restored. Dorsal and plantar metatarsal translation should be

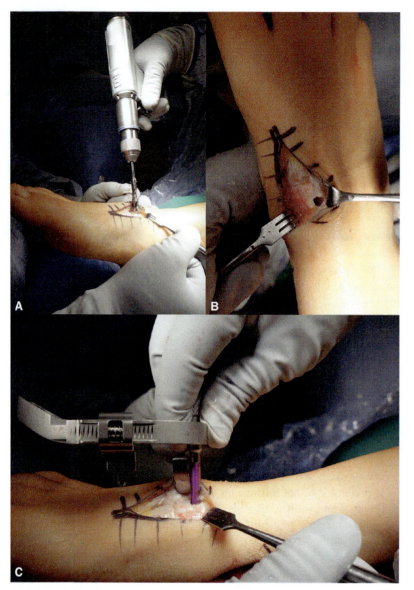

FIGURE 28.21 A, B. After wire insertion and checking, the reamer for the post is used. **C.** The post is introduced along with the external jig.

avoided. First metatarsal coronal positioning in relation to the second and third metatarsals should be at the same level or moderately plantar as described above (Fig. 28.25A). First MTP range of motion needs to be checked, and severe motion loss requires a decrease in the trial/graft length. Radiographically, Meary's angle must be reestablished, and proper length (*plus minus*) obtained (Fig. 28.25B and C). A first metatarsal medial translation or second metatarsal malposition (dislocated dorsally or laterally) could occur consequent to a graft with an excessive axial width and should be avoided. In this case, the allograft will need to be trimmed laterally before insertion.

- Suboptimal plantarflexion or ray overlength can be managed by using the saw to resect a planned slice or wedge from the metatarsal.
- After the proper graft size is chosen, the allograft is opened and placed on the preparing table. Alternatively, it can be soaked in bone marrow aspirate concentrate (Fig. 28.26). Other biological preparations and grafting (either autograft or allograft) are options to potentiate healing.
- The distraction jig is used to make room for the allograft, which might need to be trimmed laterally and plantarly to not displace the second metatarsal or cause protuberance. The allograft is inserted, and its position in relation to the surrounding structures is checked. The jig is then used

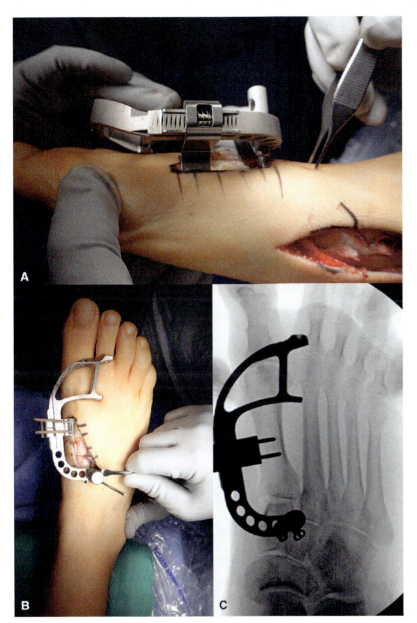

FIGURE 28.22 The medial segment of the jig is placed in contact **(A)** with the first metatarsal medial cortex. The position is secured with two bicortical K-wires **(B and C)**.

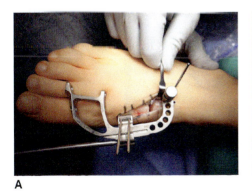
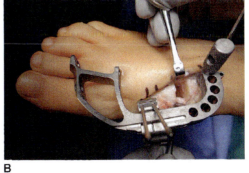

FIGURE 28.23 The jig screwdriver **(A)** is used at the rail to distract the joint about 8 to 10 mm **(B)**. The distraction will allow easier joint preparation, trials insertions, and graft placement.

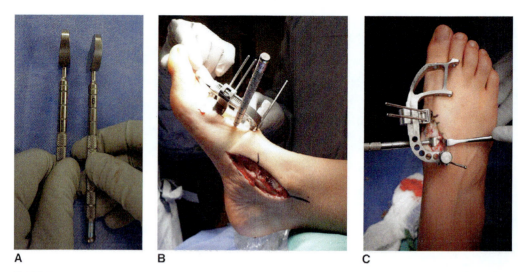

FIGURE 28.24 Wedges trials **(A)** are progressively inserted at the joint space as the distraction though the jig is adjusted accordingly **(B and C)**.

to compress the metatarsal against the graft and cuneiform (Fig. 28.27A and B). Overall reduction is maintained by dorsiflexing the hallux, manual pressure to close the intermetatarsal space, and pressure at the plantar interface between the graft and the metatarsal.
- Adequate plantarflexion, checked by the talus-first metatarsal angle on the lateral fluoroscopy, and a suitable axial positioning, correcting the intermetatarsal angle when appropriate and improving the talonavicular coverage, are advisable (Fig. 28.28). Clinically, the first metatarsal coronal positioning in relation to the second and third metatarsals should be at the same level or moderately plantar as described above.
- This position can be secured with provisional K-wires and checked. Grafting (either autograft or allograft) is advisable. By using the screws guides in the jig, percutaneous incisions are made distally, and the proper drills are used for the two post screws (Fig. 28.29). Caution should be taken for adjacent structures such as the EHL and branches of the SPN. A soft tissue protector must be used. After measurement, the post screws are inserted. There is a hard stop since the screws lock inside the intracuneiform post. The final construct is checked, and the post tamp is inserted (Fig. 28.30).
- Again, dorsomedial, medial, or plantar plates are options for final fusion fixation even when using different guides or distraction devices. Crossing screws and intramedullary nails can also be utilized (Fig. 28.31A through D).

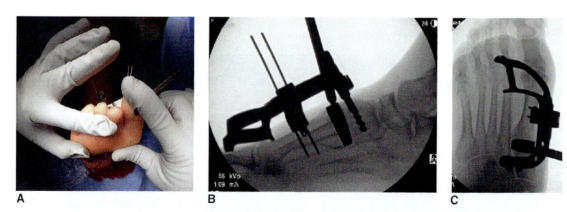

FIGURE 28.25 Intraoperative determination of the proper graft size using the different trials take into consideration the clinical coronal first metatarsal head positioning **(A)**. First metatarsophalangeal range of motion is also checked. Using the fluoroscopy, the sagittal positioning **(B)** is verified assessing the talus-first metatarsal alignment (Meary's angle) and the first ray plantarflexion in relation to the lesser rays. In the anteroposterior view, a *plus minus* configuration is desired **(C)** as well as correction of the intermetatarsal angle.

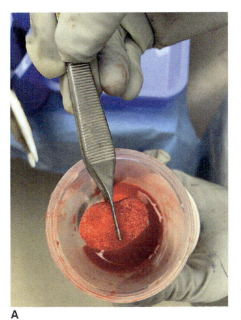
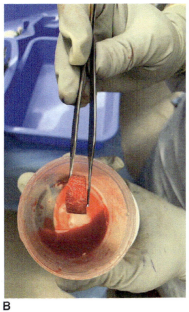

FIGURE 28.26 After the determined graft size is opened, it can be soaked into bone marrow aspirate **(A and B)** or added to any allograft or autograft to potentiate bone healing.

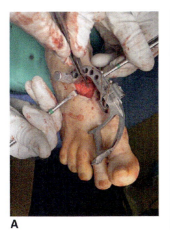
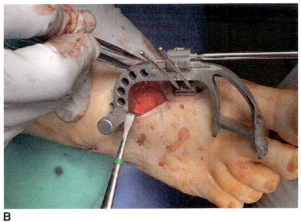

FIGURE 28.27 The graft is inserted **(A)**, and the construction is compressed using the screwdriver in a clockwise movement at the rail **(B)**. Allograft position and overall alignment are constantly checked.

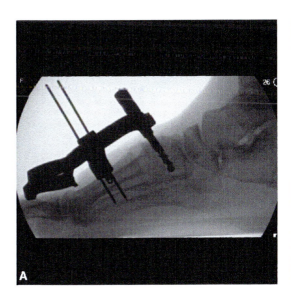
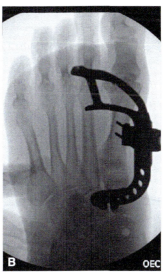

FIGURE 28.28 **A, B.** Fluoroscopic intraoperative imaging can help in determining graft positioning and overall foot alignment.

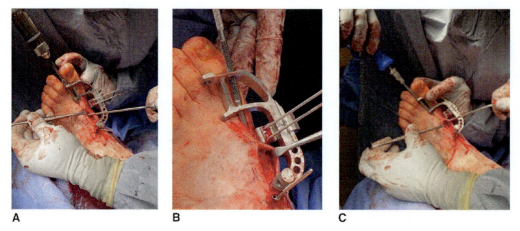

FIGURE 28.29 The skin is marked with the guides, and two small incisions are performed distally. **A.** Drilling is performed with the soft tissue protector in full contact with the metatarsal shaft. The lengths are measured **(B)**, and the post screws are inserted **(C)**.

- An intercolumn screw, from the first to the second metatarsal or from the first metatarsal to the intermediate cuneiform, can be placed if an intercolumn fixation (original Lapidus) is desired.
- The suture is closed in planes, and the foot is covered with dressings. A postoperative cast is placed, and patients are usually discharged the same day with conventional analgesics and DVT prophylaxis.

Postoperative Management

- Patients are placed in the same postoperative protocol as described for the Lapidus procedure.

Pearls and Pitfalls

- Post position is a crucial surgical step because it will dictate the direction of distraction, compression, plantarflexion, and the cuneiform integrity.
- The jig must be in contact with the medial metatarsal cortex so it can be used to distract and correct the adductus appropriately with no risk for metatarsal or cuneiform fracture.
- While using a structured graft that can be increased, care must still be taken to not over-resect bone from the cuneiform and metatarsal when preparing the joint.[28]
- Allograft trimming is important to avoid bulging and improper displacement of the second metatarsal (Fig. 28.32). When reducing and compressing the fusion, the position should always be secured and checked, avoiding metatarsal translation, dorsiflexion, or adduction.

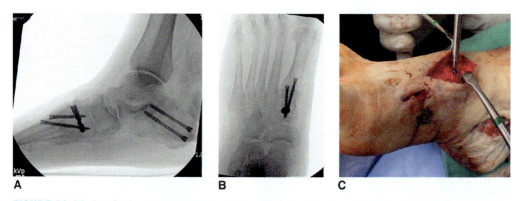

FIGURE 28.30 The final construct is checked **(A and B)**, and the tamp is inserted in the post **(C)**.

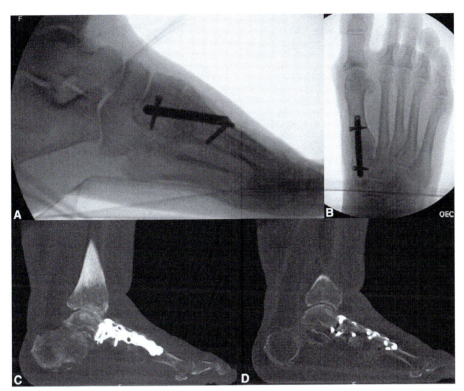

FIGURE 28.31 Examples of Lapicotton procedures carried with a post **(A and B)** and a plate configuration **(C and D)**. Weight-bearing computed tomography assessment in a progressive collapsing foot deformity patient with midfoot arthritis at 3 months postoperatively **(C and D)** demonstrates good graft healing and overall alignment.

- The use of grafting and biological products, although not completely supported by the literature, is advised by the senior author even in the primary scenario.[29]

Results and Complications

Literature is still scarce when considering Lapicotton results and complications (Fig. 28.33). De Cesar Netto et al first described the technique in a 36-year-old female with PCFD that demonstrated good clinical and radiographical outcomes, having no complications during follow-up.[2] Later, the same authors published a case series with 22 feet for several indications and a mean follow-up of 6 months.[7] The median allograft size was 8 mm (5 to 19 mm), bone healing at 3 months was found in 91% of patients, and Meary's angle improved 9.4° (95% CI, 6.7% to 12.1%). Minor complications were seen in two patients (9%) and major complications in one (4.5%).[7]

The use of a bone block for first metatarsal arthrodesis was previously described as an option after Lisfranc trauma or TMT fusion failure with a shortened first ray.[42-44] Sangeorzan et al showed the use of a structural iliac autograft in 16 patients undergoing salvage revision first TMT arthrodesis with a 18% nonunion rate, absence of major complications, and 69% of good functional results.[44] Komenda et al reported its use in a total of 11 patients of a cohort of 32 subjects with posttraumatic foot deformities with a 3% rate of nonunions and 21% of complication rate.[42] The Meary's angle improved on average from 16° to 6°.[42]

ACKNOWLEDGMENTS

We gratefully acknowledge the contribution of Ryan Jasper for his work on this chapter.

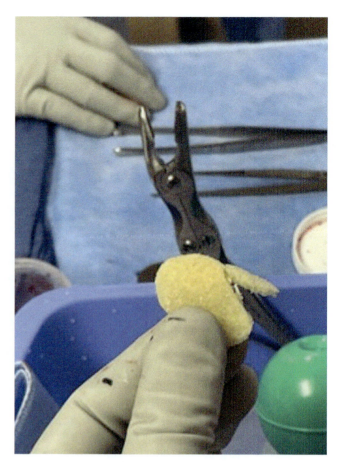

FIGURE 28.32 Trimming of the lateral aspect of the graft might be necessary to prevent first metatarsal medial translation or second metatarsal dorsal displacement.

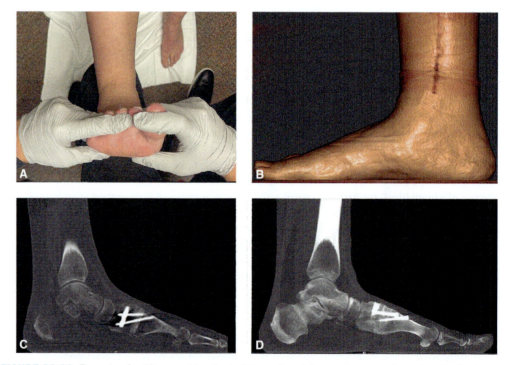

FIGURE 28.33 Example of a 43-year-old patient at 6 months status post progressive collapsing foot deformity reconstruction through a medial displacement calcaneus osteotomy, a Lapicotton and spring ligament reconstruction. **A.** Clinical assessment displays a good first ray plantarflexion. Weight-bearing computed tomography confirms the arch is restored **(B)**, the graft is completely integrated proximally and distally **(C)**, and the Meary's angle is normalized **(D)**.

REFERENCES

1. Cotton FJ. Foot statics and surgery. *N Engl J Med*. 1936;214:353-362.
2. De Cesar Netto C, Ahrenholz S, Iehl C, et al. Lapicotton technique in the treatment of progressive collapsing foot deformity. *J Foot Ankle*. 2020;14(3):301-308.
3. Hirose CB, Johnson JE. Plantarflexion opening wedge medial cuneiform osteotomy for correction of fixed forefoot varus associated with flatfoot deformity. *Foot Ankle Int*. 2004;25(8):568-574.
4. Greisberg J, Assal M, Hansen ST Jr, Sangeorzan BJ. Isolated medial column stabilization improves alignment in adult-acquired flatfoot. *Clin Orthop Relat Res*. 2005;435:197-202.
5. Lapidus PW. Spastic flat-foot. *J Bone Joint Surg Am*. 1946;28:126-136.
6. Sangeorzan BJ, Hansen ST. Modified lapidus procedure for Hallux Valgus. *Foot Ankle*. 1989;9(6):262-266.
7. De Cesar Netto C, Ehret A, Walt J, et al. Early results and complication rate of the LapiCotton procedure in the treatment of medial longitudinal arch collapse: a prospective cohort study. *Arch Orthop Trauma Surg*. 2022.
8. Gross CE, Jackson JB III. The importance of the medial column in progressive collapsing foot deformity: osteotomies and stabilization. *Foot Ankle Clin*. 2021;26(3):507-521.
9. Johnson JE, Sangeorzan BJ, de Cesar Netto C, et al. Consensus on indications for medial cuneiform opening wedge (cotton) osteotomy in the treatment of progressive collapsing foot deformity. *Foot Ankle Int*. 2020;41(10):1289-1291.
10. Myerson MS, Thordarson D, Johnson JE, et al. Classification and nomenclature: progressive collapsing foot deformity. *Foot Ankle Int*. 2020;41(10):1271-1276.
11. Deland JT, Ellis SJ, Day J, et al. Indications for deltoid and spring ligament reconstruction in progressive collapsing foot deformity. *Foot Ankle Int*. 2020;41(10):1302-1306.
12. Nery C, Lemos AVKC, Raduan F, Mansur NSB, Baumfeld D. Combined spring and deltoid ligament repair in adult-acquired flatfoot. *Foot Ankle Int*. 2018;39(8):903-907.
13. Conti MS, Chan JY, Do HT, Ellis SJ, Deland JT. Correlation of postoperative midfoot position with outcome following reconstruction of the stage II adult acquired flatfoot deformity. *Foot Ankle Int*. 2015;36(3):239-247.
14. Ellis SJ, Johnson JE, Day J, et al. Titrating the amount of bony correction in progressive collapsing foot deformity. *Foot Ankle Int*. 2020;41(10):1292-1295.
15. Sangeorzan BJ, Hintermann B, de Cesar NC, et al. Progressive collapsing foot deformity: consensus on goals for operative correction. *Foot Ankle Int*. 2020;41(10):1299-1302.
16. Cowie S, Parsons S, Scammell B, McKenzie J. Hypermobility of the first ray in patients with planovalgus feet and tarsometatarsal osteoarthritis. *Foot Ankle Surg*. 2012;18(4):237-240.
17. Hintermann B, Deland JT, de Cesar Netto C, et al. Consensus on indications for isolated subtalar joint fusion and naviculocuneiform fusions for progressive collapsing foot deformity. *Foot Ankle Int*. 2020;41(10):1295-1298.
18. Mansur NSB, de Souza Nery CA. Hypermobility in Hallux Valgus. *Foot Ankle Clin*. 2020;25(1):1-17.
19. Henry JK, Shakked R, Ellis SJ. Adult-acquired flatfoot deformity. *Foot Ankle Orthop*. 2019;4(1):2473011418820847.
20. Lee HY, Lalevee M, Mansur NSB, et al. Multiplanar instability of the first tarsometatarsal joint in hallux valgus and hallux rigidus patients: a case–control study. *Int Orthop*. 2021;46(2):255-263.
21. Kunas GC, Do HT, Aiyer A, Deland JT, Ellis SJ. Contribution of medial cuneiform osteotomy to correction of longitudinal arch collapse in stage IIb adult-acquired flatfoot deformity. *Foot Ankle Int*. 2018;39(8):885-893.
22. Conti MS, Garfinkel JH, Kunas GC, Deland JT, Ellis SJ. Postoperative medial cuneiform position correlation with patient-reported outcomes following cotton osteotomy for reconstruction of the stage II adult-acquired flatfoot deformity. *Foot Ankle Int*. 2019;40(5):491-498.
23. Abousayed MM, Coleman MM, Wei L, De Cesar Netto C, Schon LC, Guyton GP. Radiographic outcomes of cotton osteotomy in treatment of adult-acquired flatfoot deformity. *Foot Ankle Int*. 2021;42(11):1384-1390.
24. Fraser TW, Kadakia AR, Doty JF. Complications and early radiographic outcomes of flatfoot deformity correction with metallic midfoot opening wedge implants. *Foot Ankle Orthop*. 2019;4(3):247301141986897.
25. Romeo G, Bianchi A, Cerbone V, Parrini MM, Malerba F, Martinelli N. Medial cuneiform opening wedge osteotomy for correction of flexible flatfoot deformity: trabecular titanium vs. bone allograft wedges. *Biomed Res Int*. 2019;2019:1472471.
26. Bluman EM, Title CI, Myerson MS. Posterior tibial tendon rupture: a refined classification system. *Foot Ankle Clin*. 2007;12(2):233-249.
27. Lalevée M, Dibbern K, Barbachan Mansur NS, et al. Impact of first metatarsal hyperpronation on first ray alignment: a study in cadavers. *Clin Orthop Relat Res*. 2022;480(10):2029-2040.
28. Nishikawa DRC, Duarte FA, Saito GH, de Miranda BR, Fenelon EJA, Prado MP. Is first metatarsal shortening correlated with clinical and functional outcomes following the Lapidus procedure? *Int Orthop*. 2021;45(11):2927-2931.
29. Buda M, Hagemeijer NC, Kink S, Johnson AH, Guss D, DiGiovanni CW. Effect of fixation type and bone graft on tarsometatarsal fusion. *Foot Ankle Int*. 2018;39(12):1394-1402.
30. Conti MS, Willett JF, Garfinkel JH, et al. Effect of the modified lapidus procedure on pronation of the first ray in Hallux Valgus. *Foot Ankle Int*. 2020;41(2):125-132.
31. Petje G, Steinböck G, Landsiedl F. Arthrodesis for traumatic flat foot. Tarsometatarsal and medial longitudinal arch fusion by inlay grafting, 11 feet followed for 1.5 years. *Acta Orthop Scand*. 1996;67(4):359-363.
32. Saffo G, Wooster MF, Stevens M, Desnoyers R, Catanzariti AR. First metatarsocuneiform joint arthrodesis: a five-year retrospective analysis. *J Foot Surg*. 1989;28(5):459-465.
33. Thompson IM, Bohay DR, Anderson JG. Fusion rate of first tarsometatarsal arthrodesis in the modified Lapidus procedure and flatfoot reconstruction. *Foot Ankle Int*. 2005;26(9):698-703.
34. Barg A, Harmer JR, Presson AP, Zhang C, Lackey M, Saltzman CL. Unfavorable outcomes following surgical treatment of hallux valgus deformity: a systematic literature review. *J Bone Joint Surg Am*. 2018;100(18):1563-1573.
35. Busch A, Wegner A, Haversath M, Brandenburger D, Jäger M, Beck S. First ray alignment in Lapidus arthrodesis—effect on plantar pressure distribution and the occurrence of metatarsalgia. *Foot (Edinb)*. 2020;45:101686.
36. Li S, Myerson MS. Evolution of thinking of the lapidus procedure and fixation. *Foot Ankle Clin*. 2020;25(1):109-126.
37. Nishikawa DRC, Duarte FA, Saito GH, De Cesar Netto C, Miranda BRD, Prado MP. Correlation of first metatarsal sagittal alignment with clinical and functional outcomes following the Lapidus procedure. *Foot Ankle Surg*. 2022;28(4):438-444.
38. Toth K, Huszanyik I, Kellermann P, Boda K, Rode L. The effect of first ray shortening in the development of metatarsalgia in the second through fourth rays after metatarsal osteotomy. *Foot Ankle Int*. 2007;28(1):61-63.

39. Foran IM, Mehraban N, Jacobsen SK, et al. Radiographic impact of lapidus, proximal lateral closing wedge osteotomy, and suture button procedures on first ray length and dorsiflexion for Hallux Valgus. *Foot Ankle Int*. 2020;41(8):964-971.
40. Greeff W, Strydom A, Saragas NP, Ferrao PNF. Radiographic assessment of relative first metatarsal length following modified lapidus procedure. *Foot Ankle Int*. 2020;41(8):972-977.
41. Thomas T, Faroug R, Khan S, Morgan S, Ballester JS. Comparison of Scarf-Akin osteotomy with Lapidus-Akin fusion in cases of Hallux Valgus with a disrupted Meary's line: a case series study. *Foot (Edinb)*. 2020;49:101747.
42. Komenda GA, Myerson MS, Biddinger KR. Results of arthrodesis of the tarsometatarsal joints after traumatic injury. *J Bone Joint Surg Am*. 1996;78(11):1665-1676.
43. Mittlmeier T, Haar P, Beck M. Reconstruction after malunited Lisfranc injuries. *Eur J Trauma Emerg Surg*. 2010;36(3):217-226.
44. Sangeorzan BJ, Verth RG, Hansen ST. Salvage of Lisfranc's tarsometatarsal joint by arthrodesis. *Foot Ankle*. 1990;10(4):193-200.

29 Subtalar Fusion for Progressive Collapsing Foot Deformity

Tonya An, Scott Ellis, and Matthew M. Roberts

INTRODUCTION

Subtalar fusion is a surgical option for the pathological flexible planovalgus foot with severe deformity and/or subtalar instability/impingement, as well as for the arthritic and rigid flatfoot deformity.[1] A concomitant medializing calcaneal osteotomy (MCO) can be performed to further correct the hindfoot axis. The goal of surgery is to provide pain relief and restore hindfoot alignment to a biomechanically neutral position.[2]

Novel understanding of pes planus pathology, especially through study of weight-bearing computed tomography (CT), has led to new terminology "progressive collapsing foot deformity (PCFD)," to replace adult acquired flatfoot deformity (AAFD).[3] PCFD is recognized as a complex, 3-dimensional deformity composed of distinct constituent parts involving the different segments of the foot. The new classification system of PCFD includes class A: hindfoot valgus, class B: midfoot abduction, class C: forefoot varus, class D: peritalar subluxation, and class E: ankle instability.[4] The classes do not necessarily progress in a stepwise fashion, and each deformity may occur in isolation or combined with others. The stages I and II reflect flexibility or rigidity, respectively, of each deformity.

For flexible disease or milder deformity, joint-sparing reconstructive techniques involving lateral column lengthening, calcaneal osteotomy with flexor digitorum longus (FDL) tendon transfer have achieved predictable outcomes.[5] Preservation of motion in the hindfoot joints is preferred. However, select flexible deformities that also feature advanced arthritis at the subtalar joint, symptomatic subtalar impingement at the angle of Gissane, or severe joint instability due to incompetent soft tissue have more predictable outcomes when treated with isolated subtalar arthrodesis.[1,6] The subtalar fusion addresses both joint pathology and hindfoot deformity associated with peritalar subluxation.

Despite some reduction achieved through the subtalar arthrodesis, deformity magnitude or lack of soft tissue mobility may limit one's ability to achieve the desired hindfoot alignment. Therefore, a MCO can be performed concurrently to realign the hindfoot. The MCO has been shown to achieve greater correction of hindfoot alignment than lateral column lengthening, with each millimeter of medialization correlating to 1.52 mm of hindfoot correction.[7] The calcaneal osteotomy also offers the advantage of correcting hindfoot valgus without supinating the forefoot, which can occur with excessive inversion to reduce the subtalar joint.[8] Of note, derotation of the talus through the subtalar joint may not be sufficient to correct forefoot abduction and varus, if present; those deformities often require a Cotton osteotomy or other fusions of the medial column.[1]

INDICATIONS

- The primary indication for an isolated subtalar arthrodesis in the setting of PCFD with a flexible hindfoot is excess joint instability along with a moderate to severe deformity (stage I, classes A, B, and D). Pain at the lateral hindfoot in the sinus tarsi (subtalar) or subfibular regions suggests instability and impingement.[2] A weight-bearing CT identifies peritalar subluxation through incongruency of the middle facet and impingement at the sinus tarsi.[9] An MRI typically demonstrates edema around the angle of Gissane.[10]

- Alternatively, a rigid deformity with arthrosis at the subtalar joint (stage II, classes A and D) can be treated with isolated subtalar fusion to eliminate arthritis pain and attempt to spare the talonavicular joint.[11] A CT scan is best to reveal the extent of arthritis at the subtalar joint and adjacent joints. Weight-bearing CT, when available, is also useful for determining standing alignment preoperatively.
- In both instances described above, instability or arthritis pain from the subtalar joint would likely persist after a joint-sparing reconstructive procedure. This chapter's technique describes combined subtalar arthrodesis with MCO. The need for a MCO is assessed after preparing and provisionally fixing the subtalar joint fusion site or planned in advance based on the deformity severity.

CONTRAINDICATIONS

- A subtalar arthrodesis is contraindicated in cases of flexible PCFD if the deformity can be reduced with joint-sparing procedures.
- If arthrodesis is indicated for the reasons listed above, a relative contraindication to isolated subtalar arthrodesis includes severe PCFD deformities with symptomatic arthritis at the talonavicular joint or tibiotalar joint. In these cases, avoiding a talonavicular fusion may not provide adequate deformity correction or pain relief. An arthritic tibiotalar joint must be assessed for the need for ankle replacement or fusion.
- An absolute contraindication to MCO is a hindfoot that is already in neutral or varus alignment. If appropriate alignment can be achieved through the subtalar fusion alone, as in cases of mild PCFD, additional calcaneal osteotomy is not necessary.
- Poor or over-tensioned soft tissue envelope at the lateral hindfoot may restrict the use of a second incision for the calcaneal osteotomy.
- Other relative contraindications include poorly systemic disease, active or latent infection at the surgical site, poor local soft tissues or bone quality that would impair arthrodesis, or osteotomy healing.

PREOPERATIVE PLANNING

- Preoperative evaluation of patients presenting with PCFD requires a thorough history and physical examination. The primary site of symptoms should be localized, especially eliciting for posterior tibial tendon pain versus subfibular and sinus tarsi impingement pain. Patients should also be assessed for prior treatments, such as orthotics, braces, physical therapy, and injections and their response to these modalities.
- The physical examination involves inspection of the foot and ankle while weight bearing, both standing and ambulating. Clinical hindfoot valgus and ability to perform a single and double limbed heel rise are indicative of the magnitude and flexibility of the deformity as well as function of the flexor tendons. Gastrocnemius contracture is frequently present and can be examined by the Silfverskiold test.
- Active and passive range of motion testing at the subtalar joint is critical. The clinician should attempt passive correction of the hindfoot to neutral to determine if the deformity is flexible or rigid. Pain elicited with this passive motion examination may reflect advanced arthritis that poses a contraindication to joint-sparing reconstruction. Furthermore, it is important to examine for forefoot varus, first ray hypermobility, or hallux valgus deformity. These findings may indicate the need for a Cotton osteotomy or modified Lapidus procedure.
- Our preferred radiographic evaluation of the PCFD involves anteroposterior (AP), oblique and lateral foot radiographs, an AP ankle radiograph, and a bilateral hindfoot alignment view. All radiographs should be performed while weight bearing to best evaluate the deformity under physiologic loading. Talonavicular uncoverage on the AP foot radiograph is indicative of forefoot abduction. Meary's angle on the lateral view offers an estimate of the severity of arch collapse. The AP ankle radiograph is critical to rule out talar tilt from chronic deltoid insufficiency, which would require intervention at the time of surgery (Fig. 29.1A through E). The radiographic findings identify the isolated or combined deformity classes present according to recent consensus nomenclature.[4]
- Advanced imaging of the foot provides useful diagnostic information for surgical planning. If accessible, a weight-bearing CT scan offers unique information about joint alignment and morphology under loading conditions.[9] Subluxation of the middle facet has been shown to be highly associated with symptomatic PCFD and may be considered as an indication for subtalar fusion.[10,12] Extra-articular impingement as well as degenerative changes at the subtalar joint and

29 Subtalar Fusion for Progressive Collapsing Foot Deformity

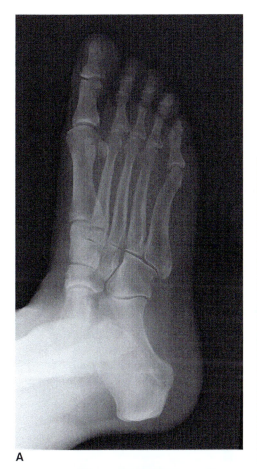

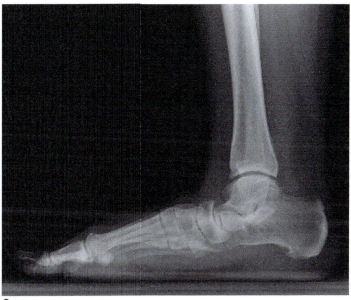

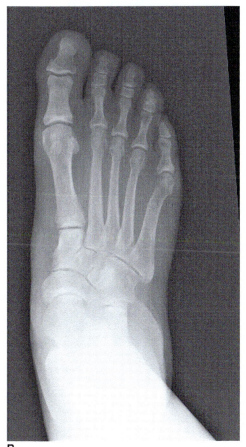

FIGURE 29.1 Illustrative case example of a patient with right-sided symptomatic flatfoot, status post left-sided correction. Preoperative radiographs of including **(A)** oblique, **(B)** anteroposterior (AP), and **(C)** lateral foot—weight bearing, AP ankle-weight bearing, bilateral hindfoot alignment views. Forefoot abduction with talar uncoverage is best seen on the AP view. The lateral view shows an abnormal Meary's angle associated with sagging at the talonavicular joint due to peritalar subluxation.

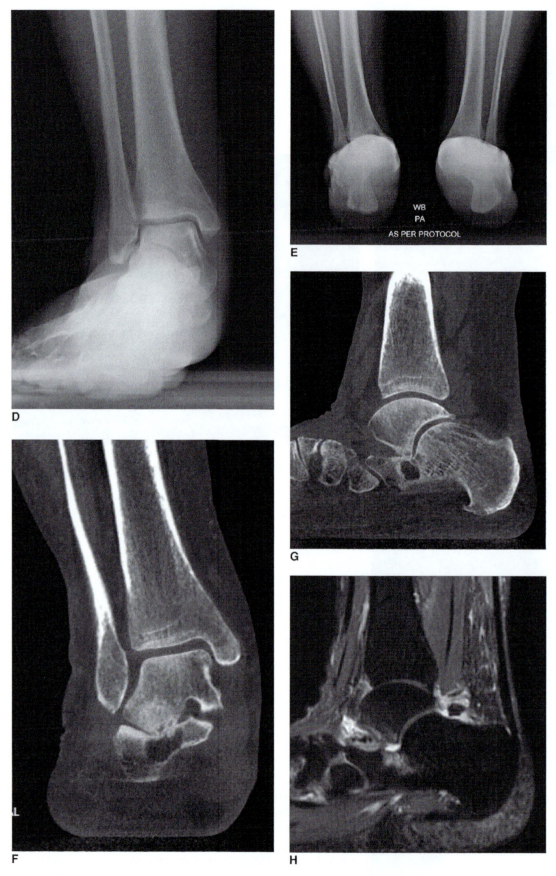

FIGURE 29.1 *(Continued)* **D.** The hindfoot alignment is in severe valgus with weight bearing. **E.** No talar tilt is observed on the AP ankle radiograph. **F,G.** Weight-bearing CT scan reveals significant middle facet subluxation and subtalar arthrosis with cysts, as well as impingement at the angle of Gissane. **H.** MRI also demonstrates impingement and reactive bone marrow edema at the angle of Gissane.

other adjacent joints are best seen on CT (Fig. 29.1F and G).[13-16] An MRI allows for visualization of the posterior tibial tendon, spring ligament, interosseous ligament of the subtalar joint, and may reveal bony edema associated with sinus tarsi impingement (Fig. 29.1H).

SURGICAL TECHNIQUE

With an appropriate perioperative analgesia protocol, PCFD correction by subtalar arthrodesis with MCO can be safely performed as an outpatient procedure. Select patient cases may require inpatient stays for postoperative pain control or physical therapy. The typical anesthesia is either parenteral or spinal anesthesia combined with peripheral nerve block. Our preferred institutional protocol consists of outpatient surgery with spinal anesthesia and a long-acting popliteal nerve block, administered under ultrasound guidance.

The patient is positioned in a semidecubitus position on a surgical table using a bump under the ipsilateral hip so that the operative leg is internally rotated at least 20° to 30°. The operative heel rests at the end of the table and a nonsterile thigh tourniquet is applied as proximally as possible. The limb is prepped and draped in the usual sterile fashion with the leg exposed up to the knee. Perioperative antibiotics should be administered within 60 minutes of incision and prior to inflation of the tourniquet. An Esmarch wrap is used to exsanguinate the limb before the pneumatic thigh tourniquet is inflated to 250 to 300 mm Hg. A mini C-arm is positioned on the ipsilateral side of the patient for intraoperative fluoroscopy.

- Since the surgical procedure requires two lateral hindfoot incisions, these should be carefully marked out in advance (Fig. 29.2).
  - The incision to expose the subtalar joint extends from the tip of the lateral malleolus toward the fourth metatarsal base. The sinus tarsi is palpable in the center of this incision.
  - The calcaneal osteotomy incision runs obliquely from a palpable "soft spot" posterior to the calcaneal tuberosity and deep to the Achilles tendon insertion to a second "soft spot" plantar to the tuberosity.[17]
  - Even though the bridge between incisions may only be 2 to 3 cm, it is the authors' experience that skin necrosis and wound complications are rare as long as tissues are handled carefully.

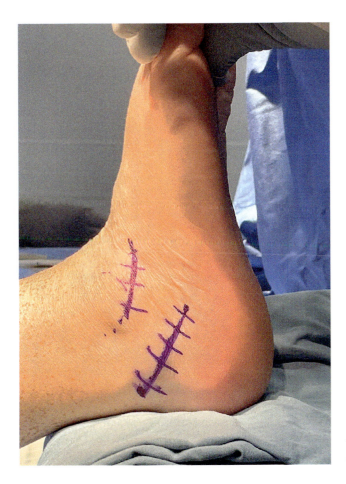

FIGURE 29.2 Planned incisions for subtalar exposure and calcaneal osteotomy.

Subtalar Joint Preparation

- The skin is incised over the sinus tarsi, and exposure of the posterior facet of the subtalar joint is performed by dissecting through the subcutaneous tissues and splitting the fascia of the extensor digitorum brevis muscle distally. The peroneal tendons that travel along the lateral wall of the calcaneus should be visualized and retracted plantarly.
- Débridement of the sinus tarsi fat pad and resection of the cervical and interosseous ligaments facilitates better access to the subtalar joint. A smooth lamina spreader may be inserted at the sinus tarsi to distract and visualize the joint space (Fig. 29.3A and B).
- The subtalar joint is prepared by denuding any residual cartilage with osteotomes and curettes. Bleeding subchondral bone should be encountered on both calcaneal and talar surfaces with minimal areas of sclerosis remaining (Fig. 29.4). Complete exposure and preparation of the posterior facet can be confirmed if the FHL tendon is visualized medially. It is important to maintain the anatomic contour of the joint surface.
- The middle and anterior facets are not always directly visualized or prepped.
- A 1.6-mm K-wire or 2.0-mm drill bit (or both) is used to penetrate into the subchondral bone to prepare the joint for fusion. Additional roughened surfaces can be created using the tip of a ¼ in curved osteotome in a fish-scale pattern.
- At this point, the surgeon may decide to proceed with a calcaneal osteotomy based off of preoperative templating or reduce and provisionally fixate the subtalar joint to make an intraoperative assessment of the hindfoot alignment.[7,8]

Calcaneal Osteotomy

- An incision is made over the previously planned calcaneal osteotomy site (Fig. 29.5A). When dissecting through proximal subcutaneous tissues, branches of the sural nerve are identified and protected.

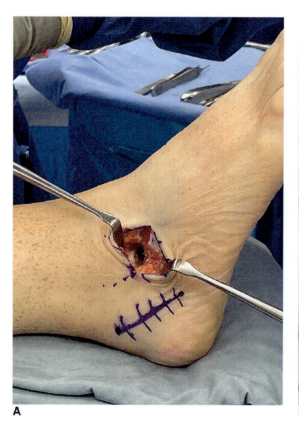 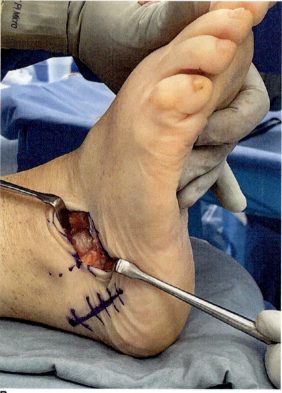

FIGURE 29.3 Manipulation reveals impingement at the subtalar joint when the foot is brought from **(A)** plantarflexion/inversion to **(B)** dorsiflexion/eversion.

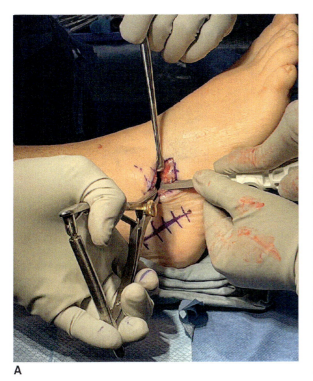
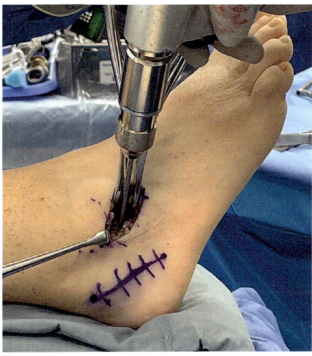

FIGURE 29.4 A. The posterior facet is prepared by removing residual cartilage with osteotome and **(B)** drilling the subchondral plate with a 2.0-mm drill bit. A smooth lamina spreader is repositioned as needed to gain joint distraction and exposure.

- The lateral wall of the posterior tuberosity can be exposed sharply or with electrocautery. A portion of the periosteum in line with the incision is cleared using a small periosteal elevator. Bennet retractors are inserted superior and inferior to the posterior tuberosity to protect soft tissues.
- Planning for the oblique calcaneal osteotomy can be guided by inserting two 1.6-mm K-wires unicortically in the orientation of the osteotomy and obtaining a lateral fluoroscopic radiograph (Fig. 29.5B and C). The pins are cut short and protected with yellow pin caps.
- If satisfied with the planned osteotomy orientation, the pins are removed, leaving the pin holes visible. The calcaneal osteotomy is performed using a no. 40 saw blade on pneumatic power (Fig. 29.6A). The saw blade connects the pin hole tracts on the lateral cortex and aims slightly distal medially by dropping one's hand.
- The osteotomy can be completed with the saw blade or a wide Hoke osteotome (Fig. 29.6B). Care should be taken to not advance too far beyond the medial wall of the calcaneus and damaging medial neurovascular structures.[17]
- Soft tissue release at the superior calcaneus and plantar fascia or temporary distraction with a smooth lamina spreader may aid in mobilization of the posterior tuberosity fragment.

Reduction and Fixation

- The posterior tuberosity is translated medially by the desired amount (usually ranging from 7 to 15 mm) while holding the foot in plantarflexion and inversion. Then, the foot is brought back into neutral and slight eversion to prevent superior translation of the posterior tuberosity. The clinical position of the hindfoot can be checked after this provisional reduction. The optimal position of the heel has been suggested to be 0 to 5 mm varus, due to an association with improvement in foot ankle outcome score (FAOS) pain score.[18] Anecdotally, a slight residual valgus may also prevent patient complaints of lateral column overload. The MCO has a strong, significant correlation with ultimate hindfoot alignment. Every millimeter of medialization at the calcaneal osteotomy leads to 1.52 mm of change in the hindfoot moment arm, making it the most predictive variable of hindfoot position.[7]
- While manually holding the osteotomy reduction, two parallel 1.6-mm K-wires are partially inserted into the posterior tuberosity fragment. These typically start just lateral to midline at the posterior heel and aim perpendicular to the osteotomy site and toward the body and neck of the talus. These wires provisionally fix the osteotomy site but do not cross the subtalar joint yet.

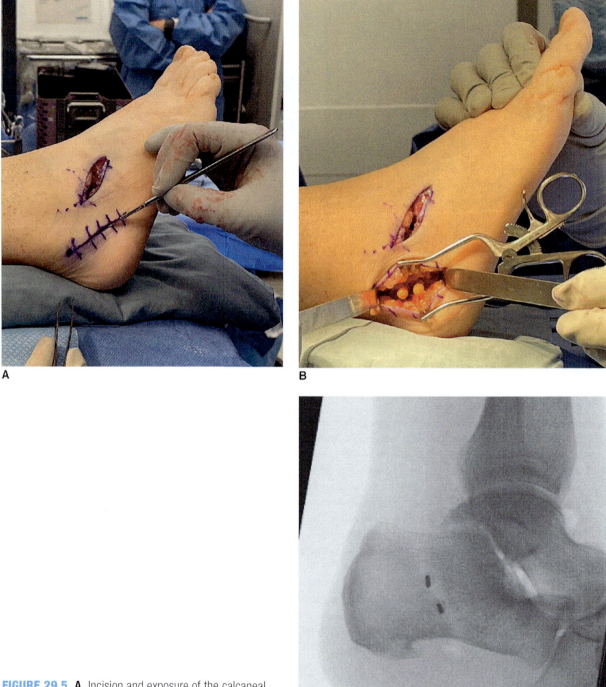

FIGURE 29.5 A. Incision and exposure of the calcaneal osteotomy site. **B.** Pins (with yellow pin caps) are inserted to plan the osteotomy. **C.** This orientation is verified on lateral fluoroscopy.

- At this point, bone autograft or biologic material is inserted to the subtalar joint fusion site while maintaining distraction with a lamina spreader (Fig. 29.7).
- The subtalar joint is reduced by manipulating the calcaneus anteriorly on the talus to oppose and compress the posterior facet. The position of the subtalar joint should be in neutral with approximately a finger-breadth's space at the sinus tarsi. Alternatively, a lamina spreader at the sinus tarsi, which pushes the talus posteriorly and proximally relative to the calcaneus, can aid in reduction. This maneuver effectively internally rotates the calcaneus under the talus, which reduces the peritalar subluxation deformity. The two K-wires, previously crossing the osteotomy, are advanced across the subtalar joint into the talus.

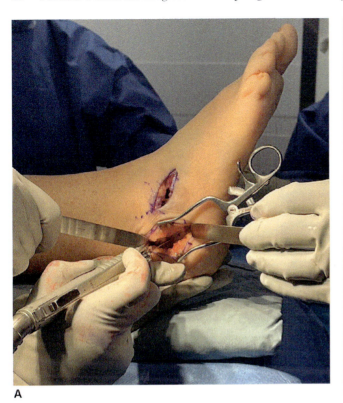
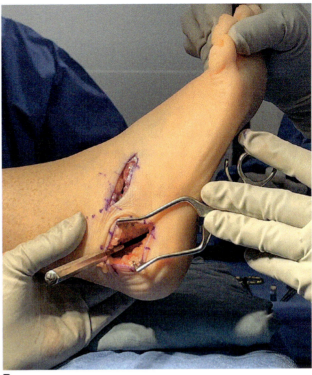

FIGURE 29.6 A. Osteotomy cut performed with micro-oscillating saw blade and **(B)** completed with a Hoke osteotome. Soft tissues proximally and distally are protected with Hohmann retractors.

- Alternatively, the subtalar joint can first be reduced as described above and fixed with provisional K-wires inserted from the talar neck and across the subtalar joint. This allows for intraoperative assessment of the hindfoot alignment to determine whether an MCO is required. If so, the calcaneal osteotomy is performed, translated, and secured with pins spanning both osteotomy and subtalar joint.
- Hindfoot alignment and the magnitude of correction is clinically checked and verified with fluoroscopic AP and lateral views of the ankle, as well as a hindfoot alignment view (Fig. 29.8A through C).

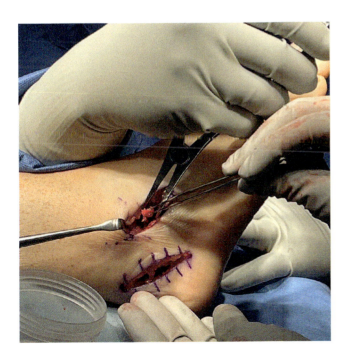

FIGURE 29.7 Insertion of autograft into the subtalar fusion site.

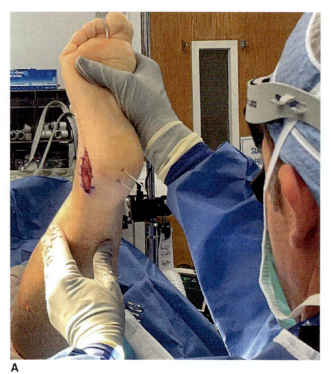
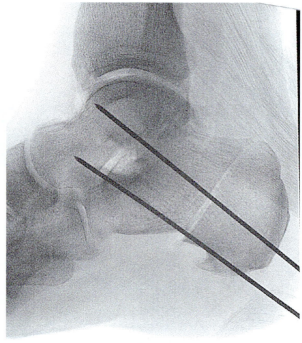

FIGURE 29.8 A. Clinical assessment of hindfoot is performed after provisional fixation. **B.** Lateral fluoroscopy confirms opposition of subtalar joint and osteotomy site without translation of the posterior tuberosity. **C.** The anteroposterior ankle radiograph confirms appropriate pin placement in the lateral one-third body of the talus.

- If using cannulated screws for fixation, new appropriate guidewires are inserted in addition to the provisional K-wires. These should be parallel and be centered in the calcaneal body on an axial heel radiograph. The tips are inserted to the subchondral bone of the talar neck and body, taking care not to penetrate into the ankle joint by confirming on AP and lateral ankle fluoroscopic views (Fig. 29.9A through C).
- After making poke-hole incisions in the heel, the guidewires are drilled with a cannulated drill bit across the entire length of the wire. Our practice involves using fully threaded, variable pitch,

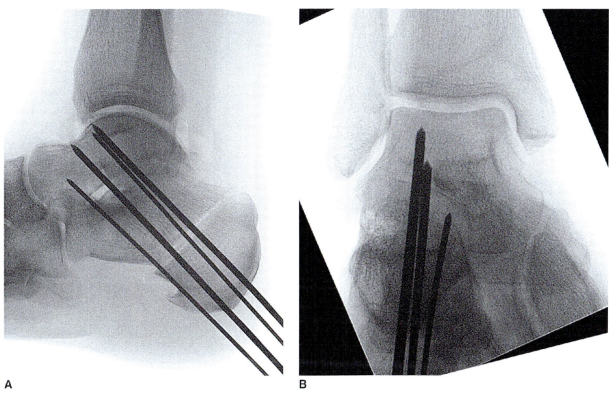
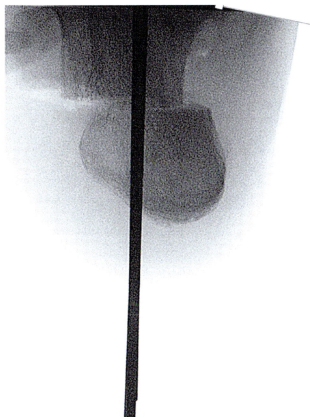

FIGURE 29.9 A through C. Lateral ankle, anteroposterior ankle, and Harris heel intraoperative radiograph confirming position of guidewires for cannulated screws.

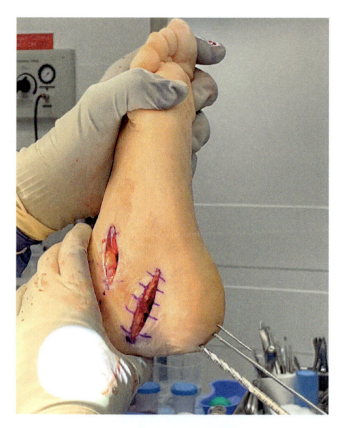

FIGURE 29.10 After confirming placement of guidewires, each is sequentially drilled and fixed with a cannulated screw.

headless cannulated 7.0-mm compression screws for fixation (Arthrex, Naples, Florida). The more superior screw is drilled and inserted first because there is more robust bone along its trajectory for compression (Fig. 29.10).
- Multiplanar fluoroscopic views verify appropriate length of screws and excellent compression across the osteotomy and subtalar joint (Fig. 29.11A through C). The screws are countersunk into bone to avoid hardware irritation.
- Prominent lateral bone, just anterior to the osteotomy site, is scored or partially cut through the cortex with an oscillating blade and removed with an osteotome and rongeur (Fig. 29.12).
- After irrigation and hemostasis. Incisions are closed with 4-0 Monocryl for deep dermal sutures and 4-0 running nylon suture. The poke-hole heel incisions are closed with horizontal mattress or simple nylon suture.
- Sterile dressings and a well-padded non–weight-bearing short leg splint is applied to maintain the ankle in neutral.

POSTOPERATIVE MANAGEMENT

- Patients return to the office 10 to 14 days after surgery for their first postoperative visit. Sutures are removed if the incisions are healing well, and the patient is converted into a tall controlled ankle motion (CAM) walker boot. The typical duration of non–weight bearing is 6 weeks from the time of surgery. However, the patient may perform daily ankle dorsiflexion and plantarflexion exercises out of the boot after 2 weeks. Showering is also allowed after the splint and sutures are removed.
- At the 6-week postoperative visit, simulated weight-bearing (the patient putting on a small amount of weight to emulate stance) radiographs are obtained to look for evidence of bony bridging. Patients are instructed to start progressive weight bearing in the CAM boot over a 4-week period. Formal physical therapy starts at this point.

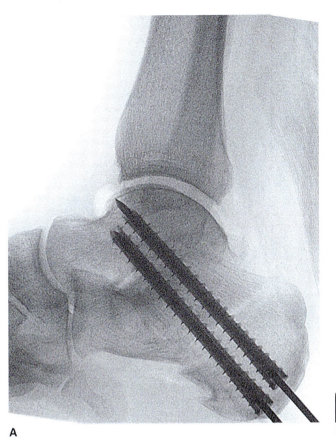
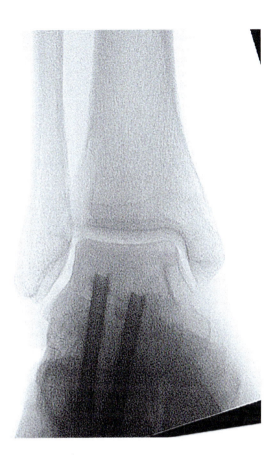
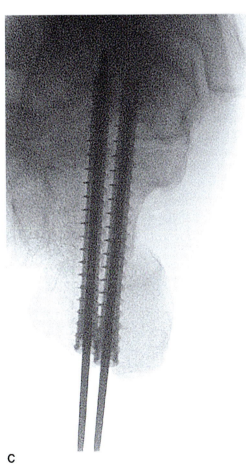

FIGURE 29.11 **A.** Lateral ankle. **B.** Anteroposterior ankle. **C.** Harris heel intraoperative radiograph confirming position of final length and position of cannulated screws.

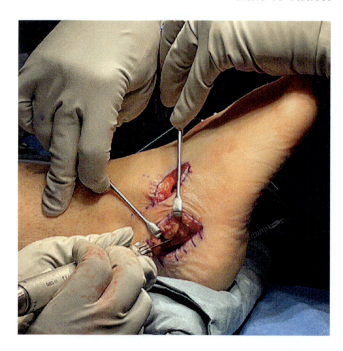

FIGURE 29.12 Removal of prominent ridge of lateral bone at the calcaneal osteotomy site.

- By 12 weeks, patients are full weight bearing, wearing sneakers, and continue in formal physical therapy for additional range of motion, strengthening, and gait training. Formal weight-bearing radiograph are repeated (Fig. 29.13).
- All patients are prescribed deep vein thrombosis prophylaxis during the time they remain non–weight bearing, typically aspirin 81 mg twice daily.

PEARLS AND PITFALLS

- The initial surgical step in PCFD correction is typically a gastrocnemius recession (which can be performed off tourniquet) to relieve equinus contracture and facilitate mobilization of the hindfoot.
- Meticulous joint preparation and maintenance of the subtalar joint contour will allow for compression at the arthrodesis site and successful bone healing.
- Autograft from the proximal tibia, distal tibia, or calcaneus (through the osteotomy cut) can help promote arthrodesis union and fill in small bony defects. Bone marrow aspirate concentrate from the iliac crest may be added to the graft material. Additional biologic products such as platelet-derived growth factor (PDGF) or bone morphogenic protein-2 may be used selectively for patients at higher risk for nonunion, such as those with diabetes or smoking history.
- Avoid overcorrection of the PCFD, as evidenced by talonavicular overcoverage on AP foot radiograph or clinically restricted motion in eversion. Patients with overcorrection may experience symptomatic stiffness or lateral column overload.[19,20]
- Following hindfoot correction, the forefoot position should be carefully assessed for residual varus. A Cotton osteotomy or first tarsometatarsal joint fusion may be necessary if the first ray is elevated.

RESULTS AND COMPLICATIONS

The goal of treatment in PCFD is to improve hindfoot biomechanics and eliminate pain, often arising from subtalar arthrosis or subfibular impingement.[21] The technique of realignment subtalar fusion has been evaluated for management of stage IIB AAFD, in which there is flexible talonavicular uncoverage and hindfoot motion at the subtalar joint.[22,23] In contemporary reclassification based on distinct deformity components, this is analogous to class D involving peritalar subluxation, with flexible (D1) and rigid (D2) subclasses.[4,24] Davies et al compared subtalar fusion to lateral column lengthening for cases of flexible hindfoot valgus.[6] They found that patients who underwent isolated

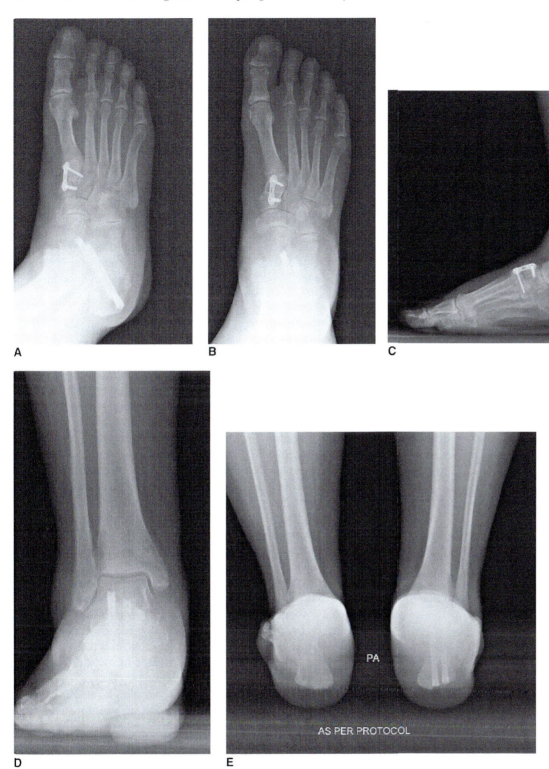

FIGURE 29.13 A through C. Postoperative oblique, anteroposterior (AP), and lateral foot radiograph showing radiographic fusion across the subtalar joint and healing of the calcaneal osteotomy. In addition to subtalar fusion with calcaneal osteotomy, this patient also underwent Cotton osteotomy to correct forefoot varus. **D.** The ankle joint is congruent on an AP ankle film. **E.** Hindfoot alignment view demonstrates a neutral position similar to the contralateral side.

subtalar fusion had worse preoperative talonavicular uncoverage but achieved excellent correction of both hindfoot valgus and forefoot abduction. Despite being older and heavier, improvement in both radiographic parameters and patient-reported outcomes was greater in patients who underwent subtalar fusion than lateral column lengthening.

Recent imaging evaluation using weight-bearing CT in PCFD has identified subluxation at the middle and posterior facets of the subtalar joint to be highly associated with pathology.[9,12,25] These findings suggest peritalar instability and chronically altered biomechanics at the subtalar joint, which may not be adequately addressed with a joint-sparing procedure such as lateral column lengthening. Compared to triple arthrodesis, which eliminates all motion of the hindfoot, subtalar arthrodesis reduces the motion at the transverse tarsal joint by 40%.[26] Therefore, patients with flexible deformities, especially those of older age or higher body mass indexes, may benefit from a repositional subtalar arthrodesis to address malalignment while still preserving partial motion at the transverse tarsal joint.[6] A recent expert consensus statement advocates that subtalar joint fusion can correct the position of the talus on the calcaneus, but forefoot abduction and varus deformity must still be addressed, if present.[1] The authors note that a completely ruptured posterior tibial tendon would necessitate FDL transfer in addition to subtalar fusion to stabilize the talonavicular joint.

The MCO can be performed concomitantly with subtalar arthrodesis to improve the hindfoot alignment.[8] The ideal magnitude of hindfoot correction is still under investigation. Conti et al retrospectively evaluated hindfoot position and associated FAOS scores in PCFD.[18] They found that correction to 0° to 5° of varus was associated with the greatest degree of patient-reported improvement. Especially in severe valgus deformities, achieving a neutral to mild varus correction may not be possible through the subtalar joint alone, and therefore, a calcaneal osteotomy is indicated. Biomechanically, the MCO also normalizes forces at the talonavicular joint and the converts the Achilles tendon from an eversion deforming force to an advantageous hindfoot inverter.[27] Overcorrection by excessive medialization, however, may lead to lateral column overload, stiffness, and pain.[28]

Multiple types of calcaneal osteotomy procedures including simple oblique, wedge resection, and the opening wedge osteotomy have been described.[29,30] All help achieve the goal of restoring the hindfoot axis by biomechanically shifting the hindfoot moment arm by 1.5 mm for every 1 mm of medial translation. The average translation in a clinical cohort of 30 flatfoot patients was 10.4 mm.[7] By realigning the hindfoot, there is decreased stress on the spring ligament and medial arch in reconstructive cases, and decreased stress on the deltoid ligament complex in subtalar fusion cases. As described in the surgical technique, our preferred method is a simple oblique osteotomy, which limits the extent of soft tissue dissection while facilitating adequate translation of the posterior tuberosity.

As with any arthrodesis procedure, nonunion is a concerning complication. One series of 21 feet undergoing subtalar arthrodesis for pes planus without bone graft had 100% union and significant improvement in hindfoot position.[31] However, 11 of 21 patients still had some persistent pain. A larger series of 184 feet demonstrated a 86% successful fusion rate after primary arthrodesis.[32] This series included patients with primary or posttraumatic subtalar arthritis and avascular necrosis. Smoking, avascular necrosis, and use of structural bone graft were risk factors for subtalar nonunion. Meticulous joint preparation is critical, along with compression across the fusion site. Modifiable risk factors such as smoking must be addressed to minimize this complication. There are limited data on the union rates of subtalar arthrodesis with calcaneal osteotomy. Davies et al reported 11% (3/27) subtalar nonunion, but concomitant calcaneal osteotomy did not seem to increase this risk. Their study found no nonunions among the 17 patients who had subtalar fusion with calcaneal osteotomy.[6]

While calcaneal osteotomy union rates are very high, wound healing complications are more prevalent.[33] Recently, minimally invasive calcaneal osteotomy has gained recognition with lower wound complications, with reported rates of 6% versus 28% in an open osteotomy cohort.[34,35] Medializing calcaneal osteotomies have been reported to have lower complication rates compared to lateralizing procedures, possibly due to a reduced degree of tension on the lateral soft tissues and the sural nerve.[36] Regardless, meticulous dissection and wound closure should be performed to mitigate risk of wound dehiscence and infection.

In summary, the subtalar fusion is a reliable alternative procedure for rigid as well as severe PCFD that feature subtalar arthrosis or considerable peritalar instability/subluxation, especially in older or heavier patients. An MCO can be performed concomitantly to achieve the desired neutral hindfoot alignment. Preoperative planning and intraoperative assessment, along with careful joint preparation and tissue handling, are key components of a successful outcome.

REFERENCES

1. Hintermann B, Deland JT, de Cesar Netto C, et al. Consensus on indications for isolated subtalar joint fusion and naviculocuneiform fusions for progressive collapsing foot deformity. *Foot ankle Int.* 2020;41(10):1295-1298.
2. Henry JK, Shakked R, Ellis SJ. Adult-acquired flatfoot deformity. *Foot Ankle Orthop.* 2019;4:1.
3. de Cesar NC, Deland JT, Ellis SJ. Guest editorial: expert consensus on adult-acquired flatfoot deformity. *Foot Ankle Int.* 2020;41(10):1269-1271.
4. Myerson MS, Thordarson DB, Johnson JE, et al. Classification and nomenclature: progressive collapsing foot deformity. *Foot ankle Int.* 2020;41(10):1271-1276.
5. Sangeorzan BJ, Hintermann B, de Cesar Netto C, et al. Progressive collapsing foot deformity: consensus on goals for operative correction. *Foot Ankle Int.* 2020;41(10):1299-1302.
6. Davies JP, Ma X, Garfinkel J, et al. Subtalar fusion for correction of forefoot abduction in stage II adult-acquired flatfoot deformity. *Foot Ankle Spec.* 2022;15(3):221-235.
7. Chan JY, Williams BR, Nair P, et al. The contribution of medializing calcaneal osteotomy on hindfoot alignment in the reconstruction of the stage II adult acquired flatfoot deformity. *Foot Ankle Int.* 2013;34(2):159-166.
8. Schon CL, de Cesar Netto C, Day J, et al. Consensus for the indication of a medializing displacement calcaneal osteotomy in the treatment of progressive collapsing foot deformity. *Foot Ankle Int.* 2020;41(10):1282-1285.
9. de Cesar Netto C, Myerson MS, Day J, et al. Consensus for the use of weightbearing CT in the assessment of progressive collapsing foot deformity. *Foot Ankle Int.* 2020;41(10):1277-1282.
10. de Cesar Netto C, Silva T, Li S, et al. Assessment of posterior and middle facet subluxation of the subtalar joint in progressive flatfoot deformity. *Foot Ankle Int.* 2020;41(10):1190-1197.
11. Conti MS, Ellis SJ. Spare the talonavicular joint! The role of isolated subtalar joint fusion in the treatment of progressive collapsing foot deformity. *Foot Ankle Clin.* 2021;26(3):591-607.
12. De Cesar NC, Godoy-Santos AL, Saito GH, et al. Subluxation of the middle facet of the subtalar joint as a marker of peritalar subluxation in adult acquired flatfoot deformity: a case-control study. *J Bone Jt Surg Am.* 2019;101(20):1838-1844.
13. Ellis SJ, Deyer T, Williams BR, et al. Assessment of lateral hindfoot pain in acquired flatfoot deformity using weight-bearing multiplanar imaging. *Foot Ankle Int.* 2010;31(5):361-371.
14. Malicky ES, Crary JL, Houghton MJ, Agel J, Hansen ST, Sangeorzan BJ. Talocalcaneal and subfibular impingement in symptomatic flatfoot in adults. *J Bone Joint Surg Am.* 2002;84(11):2005-2009.
15. Lalevée M, Barbachan Mansur NS, Rojas EO, et al. Prevalence and pattern of lateral impingements in the progressive collapsing foot deformity. *Arch Orthop Trauma Surg.* 2023;143(1):161-168.
16. Jeng CL, Rutherford T, Hull MG, Cerrato RA, Campbell JT. Assessment of bony subfibular impingement in flatfoot patients using weight-bearing CT scans. *Foot Ankle Int.* 2019;40(2):152-158.
17. Talusan PG, Cata E, Tan EW, Parks BG, Guyton GP. Safe zone for neural structures in medial displacement calcaneal osteotomy. *Foot Ankle Int.* 2015;36(12):1493-1498.
18. Conti MS, Ellis SJ, Chan JY, Do HT, Deland JT. Optimal position of the heel following reconstruction of the stage II adult acquired flatfoot deformity. *Foot ankle Int.* 2015;36(8):919.
19. Ellis SJ, Johnson JE, Day J, et al. Titrating the amount of bony correction in progressive collapsing foot deformity. *Foot Ankle Int.* 2020;41(10):1292-1295.
20. Hadfield MH, Snyder JW, Liacouras PC, et al. Effects of medializing calcaneal osteotomy on achilles tendon lengthening and plantar foot pressures. *Foot Ankle Int.* 2003;24(7):523-529.
21. Deland JT. Adult-acquired flatfoot deformity. *J Am Acad Orthop Surg.* 2008;16(7):399-406.
22. Stephens HM, Walling AK, Solmen JD, Tankson CJ. Subtalar repositional arthrodesis for adult acquired flatfoot. *Clin Orthop Relat Res.* 1999;365(365):69-73.
23. Bluman EM, Title CI, Myerson MS. Posterior tibial tendon rupture: a refined classification system. *Foot Ankle Clin.* 2007;12(2):233-249.
24. Lalevée M, Barbachan Mansur NS, Lee HY, et al. A comparison between the Bluman et al. and the progressive collapsing foot deformity classifications for flatfeet assessment. *Arch Orthop Trauma Surg.* 2023;143(3):1331-1339.
25. Lôbo CFT, Pires EA, Bordalo-Rodrigues M, de Cesar Netto C, Godoy-Santos AL. Imaging of progressive collapsing foot deformity with emphasis on the role of weightbearing cone beam CT. *Skeletal Radiol.* 2022;51(6):1127-1141.
26. Mann RA, Beaman DN, Horton GA. Isolated subtalar arthrodesis. *Foot ankle Int.* 1998;19(8):511-519.
27. Nyska M, Parks BG, Chu IT, Myerson MS. The contribution of the medial calcaneal osteotomy to the correction of flatfoot deformities. *Foot Ankle Int.* 2001;22(4):278-282.
28. Chan JY, Greenfield ST, Soukup DS, Do HT, Deland JT, Ellis SJ. Contribution of lateral column lengthening to correction of forefoot abduction in stage IIb adult acquired flatfoot deformity reconstruction. *Foot Ankle Int.* 2015;36(12):1400-1411.
29. Guha AR, Perera AM. Calcaneal osteotomy in the treatment of adult acquired flatfoot deformity. *Foot Ankle Clin.* 2012;17(2):247-258.
30. Greenfield S, Cohen B. Calcaneal osteotomies: pearls and pitfalls. *Foot Ankle Clin.* 2017;22(3):563-571.
31. Kitaoka HB, Patzer GL. Subtalar arthrodesis for posterior tibial tendon dysfunction and pes planus. *Clin Orthop Relat Res.* 1997;345:187-194. http://www.ncbi.nlm.nih.gov/pubmed/9418639
32. Easley ME, Trnka HJ, Schon LC, Myerson MS. Isolated subtalar arthrodesis. *J Bone Joint Surg Am.* 2000;82(5):613-624.
33. Abbasian A, Zaidi R, Guha A, Goldberg A, Cullen N, Singh D. Comparison of three different fixation methods of calcaneal osteotomies. *Foot Ankle Int.* 2013;34(3):420-425.
34. Kendal AR, Khalid A, Ball T, Rogers M, Cooke P, Sharp R. Complications of minimally invasive calcaneal osteotomy versus open osteotomy. *Foot ankle Int.* 2015;36(6):685-690.
35. Gutteck N, Zeh A, Wohlrab D, Delank KS. Comparative results of percutaneous calcaneal osteotomy in correction of hindfoot deformities. *Foot Ankle Int.* 2019;40(3):276-281.
36. Madeley NJ, Kumar CS, Alenezi A. Complications of calcaneal osteotomy: are they equal between different osteotomy types? *Foot Ankle Orthop.* 2022;7(1):2473011421S0033.

30 Minimally Invasive Osteotomies of the Calcaneus

Gregory P. Guyton

INDICATIONS AND CONTRAINDICATIONS

Medial Displacement Calcaneal Osteotomy

Osteotomies of the calcaneus were first described for the surgical treatment of the planovalgus foot in 1893 by Gleich[1] but have only more recently become more popular. The contribution of posterior tibial tendon dysfunction to progressive collapsing foot deformity (PCFD) was appreciated in the 1980s by Mann and Thompson[2] and Johnson and Strom,[3] who independently proposed the flexor digitorum longus (FDL) tendon transfer to the navicular as a surgical solution. Although the FDL transfer alone often resulted in symptomatic relief, it offered no correction of the foot deformity. Promising results had more recently been demonstrated with the medial displacement calcaneal osteotomy (MDCO) in the pediatric flatfoot by Koutsogiannis et al in 1971,[4] and several authors subsequently proposed that the osteotomy be added to the FDL transfer to provide an element of bony deformity correction to the procedure.[5-7] The indications for the procedure today in the planovalgus remain the same: to provide correction of the longitudinal arch and coronal plane deformity, either in conjunction with an FDL tendon transfer in the case of an adult case of PCFD or in a flexible pediatric deformity.

The MDCO functions through both static and dynamic mechanisms. Essentially, the foot can be viewed as a tripod with limbs striking the ground at the first metatarsal head, fifth metatarsal head, and the center of the heel (calcaneal tuberosity). In a planovalgus deformity, that tripod sags to the medial side. An MDCO shifts the posterior limb of that tripod medially, correcting the sag. A distal displacement of the tuberosity fragment can also be performed to allow for an increase in the calcaneal inclination and overall longitudinal arch.

A dynamic component for the role of the MDCO has also been proposed.[7] When the hindfoot sags into valgus, the line of pull of the Achilles tendon moves laterally, which tends to pull the calcaneus into further valgus and accentuate the deformity. The osteotomy brings the Achilles insertion back toward the midline, decreasing the valgus deforming force of the Achilles tendon and potentially reducing the forces on the reconstructed posterior tibialis tendon medially.

The contraindications to the procedure are identical to those for the FDL tendon transfer itself and include a rigid PCFD and/or hindfoot arthritis. In those cases, a hindfoot fusion is preferred because it provides a more powerful correction and addresses the arthritis if needed. Even then, an MDCO can be added with hindfoot fusion for more severe deformities.

The Lateral Displacement Calcaneal Osteotomy

In much the same way that the medial displacement calcaneal osteotomy corrects the static tripod of the planovalgus foot, the lateral displacement calcaneal osteotomy (LDCO) can be used to shift the center of the heel laterally and provide a static correction for the cavovarus foot. Lateral calcaneal shifts were first described in 1959 by Dwyer,[8] who proposed removing a laterally based wedge of bone and hinging the osteotomy on the intact medial cortex. Variations on the Dwyer osteotomy have been proposed, and larger corrections are possible by completing the osteotomy medially and allowing it to both close and shift.[9] Although somewhat less powerful, a simple sliding lateral displacement osteotomy can also be used and is easily adapted to minimally invasive techniques.

The primary contraindication to all lateralizing calcaneal osteotomies is a rigid hindfoot. Sufficient subtalar motion should be present for the calcaneus to achieve at least a slight valgus position following the osteotomy and completion of any ancillary procedures. If this is not expected to be possible, strong consideration should be given to hindfoot fusion as a more powerful alternative.

The Malerba osteotomy is an alternative to a wedge or sliding osteotomy. Although correction with this osteotomy can be powerful, it requires substantially more dissection in the region of the peroneal tendons and the sural nerve.

Minimally Invasive Techniques

Minimally invasive approaches for calcaneal osteotomies have been proposed to diminish the potential for nerve injury, avoid wound complications, and potentially speed healing of the osteotomy itself. In the case of the LDCO, the minimal incision also facilitates the use of parallel adjacent incisions for other ancillary procedures, particularly peroneal tendon reconstruction or lateral ankle ligament reconstruction.

The indications for the use of a minimal incision are identical to those for the osteotomy itself, and there are no contraindications specific to the minimal approach. There is no additional functional limitation on the degree of shift for either the MDCO or the LDCO when using minimally invasive techniques compared to an open approach. Experientially, shifts up to 13 mm are readily accomplished through the minimally invasive surgical (MIS) approach. Admittedly, the minimally invasive approach is best suited to a simple shift. If an additional wedge resection is desired, such as in a traditional Dwyer osteotomy, it will be more technically challenging than with open techniques.

PREOPERATIVE PLANNING

All calcaneal osteotomies play the same role in the correction of deformity whether they are performed open or through a minimally invasive approach. The specific planning for an MIS approach revolves around avoiding neurovascular structures. The sural nerve is traditionally considered the most at risk, but as a practical matter, the small lateral calcaneal branches projecting posteriorly from the sural nerve are sometimes unavoidable.

Talusan et al[10] defined a desired "safe zone" for localizing MIS calcaneal osteotomies based upon the lateral fluoroscopic projection. Those investigators initially dissected the sural nerve laterally and the medial and lateral plantar nerves medially and then applied fine radio-opaque wires to their surface. Accounting for radiographic magnification, that study noted a safe zone to avoid these nerves extends anteriorly for 11 mm from the line connecting the plantar fascia origin and the posterior apex of the calcaneus on a perfect lateral projection (Fig. 30.1). Following this guideline

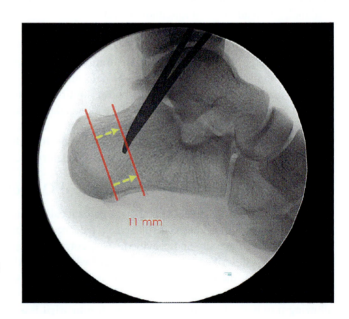

FIGURE 30.1 The safe zone to avoid the sural nerve and medial neurovascular structures can be visualized on a perfect lateral fluoroscopy image. A line between the plantar fascia origin and posterosuperior apex of the calcaneus can be projected anteriorly 11 mm to define the area.

30 Minimally Invasive Osteotomies of the Calcaneus

does not avoid potential injury to the lateral calcaneal branches, but the smaller incision of the MIS approach along with limited distraction of the skin margin minimizes this risk.

SURGICAL TECHNIQUE (▶ VIDEO 30.1)

- A bump is placed under the ipsilateral hip to internally rotate the operative leg.
- A perfect lateral projection of the hindfoot is obtained. Typically, this involves ensuring that the medial and lateral projections of the talus perfectly overlap on the image.
- The starting point of the osteotomy is localized on the lateral heel with a small snap or elevator. This is placed in the center of the calcaneus tuberosity at the anterior margin of the radiographic safe zone. This location is 11 mm anterior to a line projecting from the plantar fascia origin to the posterosuperior angle of the calcaneus (Fig. 30.2). An oblique incision 5 to 7 mm in length is made along the desired path of the osteotomy. As a guide, the surgeon may place their index finger just anterior to the Achilles tendon and their thumb underneath the inferior border of the calcaneal tuberosity.
- A hemostat is used to spread down to the lateral periosteum of the calcaneus. This should be done in a vertical path parallel to the course of the sural nerve.
- A small elevator is used to lift the periosteum along the anticipated course of the osteotomy in both the plantar and dorsal directions. This course should pass over the superior margin of the calcaneus and below the inferior margin of the tuberosity (Fig. 30.3).
- A 0.062 K-wire is now placed at the anticipated center of the osteotomy in a path normal to the lateral wall of the calcaneus. The wire should be placed along the anterior margin of the incision. The goal is to both template the location of the osteotomy and provide an additional measure of protection for the nerve while the initial cut is made. Lateral and axial calcaneal views are obtained to check the starting point and orientation (Fig. 30.4). A long, thin, narrow microsagittal saw is used to create an initial path for the osteotomy. The blade is placed immediately posterior to the templating K-wire along the desired angle of the cut. A blade measuring 5.5 × 25 mm with a 0.5-mm kerf is appropriate. The kerf of a saw cut is the thickness of the utilized saw blade. Initially, this should be placed only to a depth of 2 to 3 mm and then removed from the trinkle (attachment between a power motor and its working device). A lateral flouoroscopic image is now taken to confirm the angle of the osteotomy. If this is acceptable, the K-wire is removed, and the saw blade driven to its full depth. This creates an appropriately oriented channel for the micro-reciprocating saw to complete the cut (Fig. 30.5).
- As the microsagittal saw is removed, a micro-reciprocating saw is immediately placed into the channel. The blade should be long enough to cross the calcaneal tuberosity, typically 30 to 35 mm. The technique depends on the ability of a reciprocating blade to follow its own path as

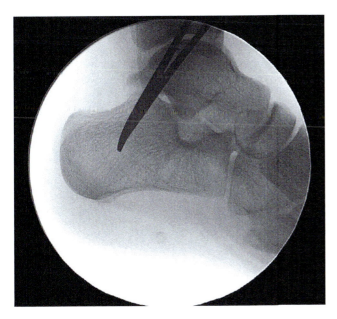

FIGURE 30.2 The starting point at the midportion of the calcaneal tuberosity and at the anterior margin of the safe zone is marked using a small hemostat while obtaining a perfect lateral image.

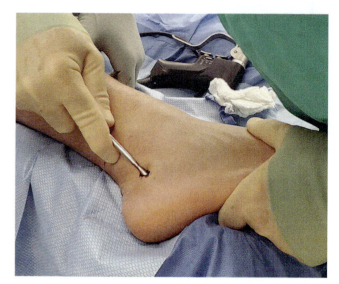

FIGURE 30.3 An incision 5 to 8 mm in length is made parallel to the expected path of the osteotomy oblique to the long axis of the calcaneus. A small elevator is then used to lift the periosteum dorsally and plantarly along this path.

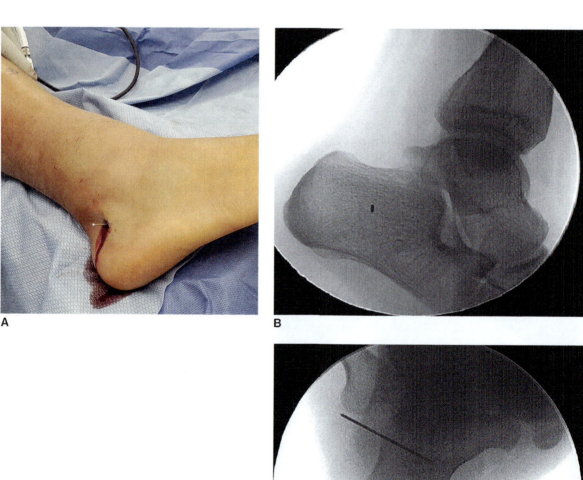

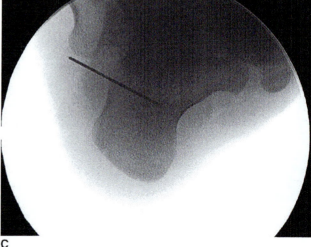

FIGURE 30.4 A 0.062-inch K-wire is placed at the anterior margin of the incision, perpendicular to the long axis of the calcaneus. This helps template the center of the cut and, because the saw will enter posterior to it, provides further protection for the sural nerve. Clinical photograph **(A)** and lateral **(B)** and axial **(C)** fluoroscopy image.

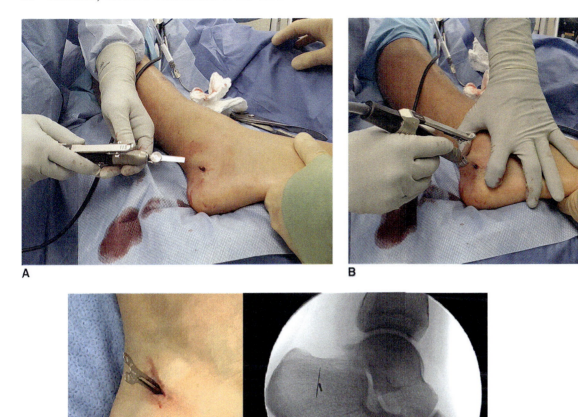

FIGURE 30.5 A microsagittal saw **(A)** is placed into the bone along the anticipated line of the osteotomy to a depth of 2 to 3 mm **(B)**. It is removed from the trinkle and the orientation checked **(C)**. If acceptable, the K-wire is removed, and the saw driven across the calcaneus to create a central channel.

it progresses, and a stiffer saw blade with a kerf of 0.5 to 0.7 mm is appropriate. Thinner blades will more easily fit into the channel created by the microsagittal saw but may tend to wander as the cut is made (Fig. 30.6).
- Typically, the kerf of the micro-reciprocating blade is very slightly greater than the microsagittal saw used to create the channel. If the blade does not readily advance down the channel, usually a gentle application of power will allow it to move forward.
- It is not critical to complete the channel across the medial cortex with the initial microsagittal cut. While the second micro-reciprocating blade is technically not an end-cutting device, when the blade is powered it will still be possible to advance it through the medial cortex.
- The inferior portion of the osteotomy is initially completed in a plantar direction. The surgeon should use an angular motion with the saw to complete the cut. In addition to the tactile sensation of a completed cut, the fifth toe may twitch as the blade comes through the cortex and touches the surface of the abductor digiti quinti (Fig. 30.7).
- The micro-reciprocating blade is now removed, flipped to face superiorly, and placed back in the cut. The superior portion of the osteotomy is now completed. Although the blade will tend to follow the previous cut, care should be taken to avoid deviating posteriorly. When the osteotomy completes and becomes mechanically loose, a small release of blood and marrow fat may be seen at the wound.
- The ankle is plantarflexed to relax the Achilles tendon and the posterior fragment moved medially or laterally (medial or lateral displacement osteotomies, respectively). The blade typically cuts the periosteum on the far (medial) side of the cut sufficiently to mobilize the posterior fragment. If the osteotomy is complete but an adequate shift cannot be achieved, a narrow Cobb elevator may be inserted to gently distract the tuberosity fragment and achieve displacement (Fig. 30.8).

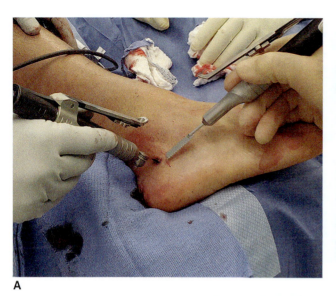
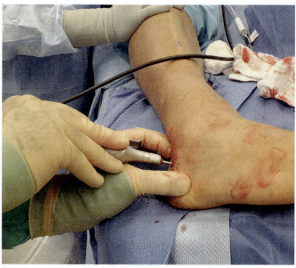

FIGURE 30.6 The microsagittal saw is exchanged for a micro-reciprocating saw oriented inferiorly **(A)**. This is used to create the inferior limb of the osteotomy **(B)**. The saw is then flipped, reinserted, and used to create the superior portion.

- In the rare case that the tuberosity fragment cannot be displaced sufficiently by hand, a narrow Cobb elevator may be placed underneath the anterior cortical margin of the cut to lever it medially or underneath the cortical margin of the tuberosity of itself to lever it laterally. The tuberosity displaces more easily in the medial direction. Up to 13 mm of displacement can be achieved with medial displacement, and up to 8 mm can be achieved laterally. The degree of displacement can be determined fluoroscopically on an axial calcaneal view.
- Two guide pins for headless 5.5-mm screws are now placed into the tuberosity spaced 1 cm apart. These should be oriented toward the hard subchondral bone underneath the posterior facet rather than down the anterior process. This location is better for bone stock and helps avoid any concurrent lateral column lengthening procedure. Although one screw is often sufficient, using two pins helps ensure that the fragment does not spin or angulate as the screw is placed. The starting point should be made by reference to the center of the body of the calcaneus. For instance, to place a screw directly up the calcaneus when the tuberosity is displaced 10 mm medially, the starting point should be relatively lateral in the tuberosity fragment (Fig. 30.9).
- Lateral and axial images are used to confirm pin placement. A headless 5.5-mm screw is then placed into whichever of the two pin locations is preferred. If adequate purchase is achieved, one screw is sufficient. There is no concern if a few threads of a headless compression screw remain across the osteotomy site as long as it closes radiographically. The bone in the center of the osteotomy site has minimal holding power and will not prevent compression in most cases (Fig. 30.10).
- A second screw can be placed, or larger screws used if the bone quality is poor.

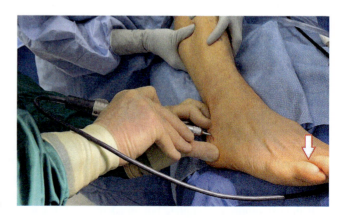

FIGURE 30.7 Photograph from different case. In addition to the tactile sensation of a completed cut, the fifth toe (*arrow*) may twitch as the blade comes through the cortex and touches the surface of the abductor digiti quinti.

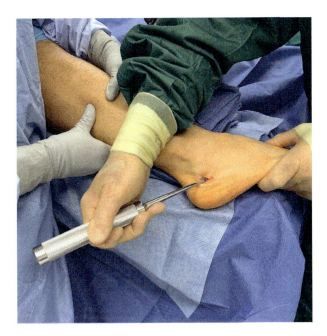

FIGURE 30.8 Photograph from same patient shown in Figure 30.7. If the osteotomy is complete but an adequate shift cannot be achieved, a narrow Cobb elevator may be inserted to gently distract the tuberosity fragment and achieve displacement.

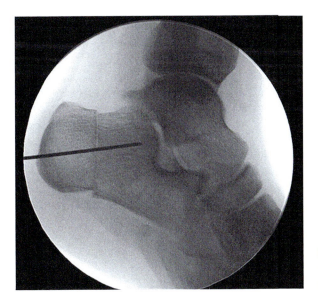

FIGURE 30.9 The osteotomy is displaced medially or laterally as required. One or two guide pins for 5.5-mm screws are placed normal to the osteotomy. If two are used, they should be spaced at least 1 cm apart.

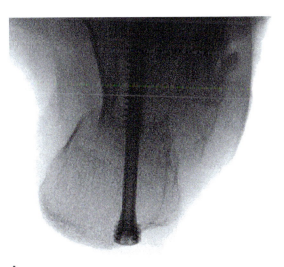
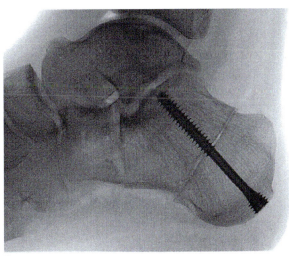

A B

FIGURE 30.10 One or two headless axial 5.5-mm screws are used for fixation. Axial **(A)** and lateral **(B)** fluoroscopy image.

PEARLS AND PITFALLS

- If additional correction is desired in the sagittal plane, the tuberosity may be displaced dorsally or plantarly. This is most commonly used in correction of a cavus foot with a high calcaneal pitch and accomplishes the same effect as the historic Samilson crescentic osteotomy[11] once used for the correction of polio deformity.
- The saw technique for an MIS calcaneal osteotomy provides a reliable and regular cut with minimal bone resection while still allowing for displacement. If the surgeon wishes to use a Shannon burr instead, only slight modifications are required. Instead of using a K-wire to localize the center of the osteotomy, the burr itself may be used and temporarily disconnected to check position. A sweeping motion is used to create the osteotomy along the desired path. Because the burr removes a kerf of bone between 2.5 to 3 mm along its path, considerable heat may be generated. Constant irrigation is recommended. Commercial jigs to create an even cut using a spinning burr were previously available but are no longer marketed. The saw is preferred because the cut tends to template itself, cuts more quickly and more efficiently, and removes far less bone than the burr and thus generates less heat.
- As a general rule, greater displacement for both medial and lateral osteotomies can be achieved as the cut is moved more anteriorly in the bone. The plantar fascia restrains motion of the tuberosity fragment if the cut is made too far posterior. However, the risk to the neurovascular structures increases with anterior positioning.
- Regardless of the technique used to make the cut, care should be taken to avoid lengthening the calcaneus as it will make it harder to shift. For instance, a cut that exits farther posteriorly on the medial side of the bone will inhibit a medial shift.
- If greater displacement of the tuberosity is needed, an angular correction can be added. For the lateralizing osteotomy, the Shannon burr may be used to remove bone from the lateral side of the osteotomy to create a closing wedge similar to an open Dwyer osteotomy. For a medializing osteotomy, the burr may be used to shave bone away from the deep (medial) side of the tuberosity fragment.
- A theoretical risk of iatrogenic tarsal tunnel syndrome exists with lateralizing calcaneal osteotomies, particularly if they are made in a more anterior location in the middle third of the calcaneus. This concern was originally described in a cadaveric model by Bruce et al,[12] who demonstrated decreased tarsal tunnel volume with lateralizing osteotomies. Despite this concern, a subsequent clinical paper by VanValkenburg et al[13] did not find a protective effect from prophylactically performing a tarsal tunnel release in conjunction with the LDCO. While the surgeon should be aware of the possibility of an iatrogenic tarsal tunnel syndrome in the postoperative patient, a prophylactic open release is not required.
- If an osteotomy is made that inadvertently exits dorsally into the retrocalcaneal bursa, a prominence may be present when the tuberosity is shifted medially. This should be carefully examined clinically after fixation of the osteotomy. If prominent, a small open exostectomy should be performed and will have no impact on the correction.
- Carefully avoid an osteotomy cut that passes through a plantar enthesophyte. The osteotomy will heal uneventfully, but the enthesophyte may not and symptoms of plantar fasciitis may persist for many months after surgery.
- If using a Shannon burr to create the osteotomy, both simple flat cut and chevron (V-shaped) osteotomies have been described. A recent biomechanical study by Gutteck et al[14] found no difference in stiffness between the two techniques, and no clinical difference has been described. The simpler flat cut technique is recommended (Fig. 30.11).

POSTOPERATIVE MANAGEMENT

The calcaneal osteotomy has a large surface area and heals rapidly. If other concurrent procedures do not dictate otherwise, full weight bearing in a boot is allowed at 1 month postoperatively. Regular footwear may be initiated at 2 months. Physical therapy is not required for an isolated calcaneal osteotomy but is commonly required as part of a combined correction of the cavus or planovalgus foot. Tendon transfers alone do not require any additional period of limited weight bearing. Other osteotomies such as an Evans procedure are typically protected for 6 weeks.

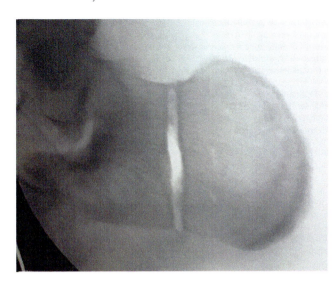

FIGURE 30.11 If a Shannon burr is used to create the osteotomy, a substantial kerf of bone will be resected and much more heat will be generated. A simple flat cut is sufficient.

RESULTS AND COMPLICATIONS

Calcaneal osteotomies overall heal reliably whether performed by MIS or open techniques. Kheir et al[15] reported no nonunions in a case series of 30 patients using a Shannon burr. Kendal et al[16] performed a case-control study in which nonunion occurred in 1/31 MIS procedures and 0/50 open procedures. Gutteck et al[17] performed a similar study in with no nonunions in either 64 MIS procedures or 64 open procedures. In the largest series in the literature, Coleman et al[18] reviewed 189 MIS calcaneal osteotomies, which included a combination of procedures with the Shannon burr and the reciprocating saw technique described in detail in this chapter. A short case cluster of nonunions was identified likely relating to a mechanical issue with the burr driver. Outside of that cluster, a 0.7% overall rate of nonunion was found. No cases of nonunion occurred with the micro-reciprocating saw technique.

Wound complications are rare but may be related to heat necrosis if a burr is used. They have nevertheless been noted to be reduced with the MIS technique in those studies that have compared it with open techniques.[16,17] In the largest series, Coleman et al[18] found a 3% incidence of wound complications that occurred solely in the Shannon burr group compared with a 0% incidence when a micro-reciprocating saw was used.

In practice, the kerf of a burr cut is 2.5 to 3 mm and generates a significant amount of heat. Continuous irrigation is recommended. The use of a saw removes a typical kerf of only 0.5 mm, and irrigation is not critical.

Nerve injury has been variably reported after calcaneal osteotomy. Kendal et al[16] reported 0/30 sural nerve injuries in their MIS procedures compared with 3/51 in their open procedures. Coleman et al[18] noted an overall nerve injury incidence of 2%, including some that were confined only to lateral calcaneal branches. Nerve injury in that series was associated with concomitant Strayer procedures or Evans procedures. This raises the possibility of a double crush syndrome in some cases in which a partial sural nerve injury at two levels has a cumulative effect. Alternatively, some cases of sural nerve injury may have simply been due to the other procedure alone.

REFERENCES

1. Gleich A. Beitrag zur operativen plattfussbehandlung. *Arch Klin Chir*. 1893;46:358-362.
2. Mann RA, Thompson FM. Rupture of the posterior tibial tendon causing flat foot. Surgical treatment. *J Bone Joint Surg Am*. 1985;67:556-561.
3. Johnson KA, Strom DE. Tibialis posterior tendon dysfunction. *Clin Orthop*. 1989;239:196-206.
4. Koutsogiannis E. Treatment of mobile flat foot by displacement osteotomy of the calcaneus. *J Bone Joint Surg Br*. 1971;53(1):96-100.
5. Guyton GP, Jeng C, Krieger LE, Mann RA. Flexor digitorum longus transfer and medial displacement calcaneal osteotomy for posterior tibial tendon dysfunction: a middle-term clinical follow-up. *Foot Ankle Int*. 2001;22(8):627-632.
6. Myerson MS, Corrigan J. Treatment of posterior tibial tendon dysfunction with flexor digitorum longus tendon transfer and calcaneal osteotomy. *Orthopedics*. 1996;19:383-388.
7. Myerson MS, Corrigan J, Thompson F, Schon LC. Tendon transfer combined with calcaneal osteotomy for the treatment of posterior tibial tendon insufficiency: a radiological investigation. *Foot Ankle Int*. 1995;16:712-718.
8. Dwyer FC. Osteotomy of the calcaneum for pes cavus. *J Bone Joint Surg Br*. 1959;41:80-86.

9. An TW, Michalski M, Jansson K, Pfeffer G. Comparison of lateralizing calcaneal osteotomies for varus hindfoot correction. *Foot Ankle Int*. 2018;39(10):1229-1236.
10. Talusan PG, Cata CE, Tan EW, Parks BG, Guyton GP. Safe zone for neural structures in medial displacement calcaneal osteotomy: a cadaveric and radiographic investigation. *Foot Ankle Int*. 2015;36(12):1493-1498.
11. Samilson RL. Crescentic osteotomy os calcis for calcaneovarus feet. In: Bateman JE, ed. *Foot Science*. WB Saunders Co; 1976:18.
12. Bruce BG, Bariteau JT, Evangelista PE, Arcuri D, Sandusky M, DiGiovanni CW. The effect of medial and lateral calcaneal osteotomies on the tarsal tunnel. *Foot Ankle Int*. 2014;35(4):383-388.
13. VanValkenburg S, Hsu RY, Palmer DS, Blankenhorn B, Den Hartog BD, DiGiovanni CW. Neurologic deficit associated with lateralizing calcaneal osteotomy for cavovarus foot correction. *Foot Ankle Int*. 2016;37(10):1106-1112.
14. Gutteck N, Haase K, Kielstein H, Delank KS, Arnold C. Biomechanical results of percutaneous calcaneal osteotomy using two different osteotomy designs. *Foot Ankle Surg*. 2020;26(5):551-555.
15. Kheir E, Borse V, Sharpe J, Lavalette D, Farndon M. Medial displacement calcaneal osteotomy using minimally invasive technique. *Foot Ankle Int*. 2015;36(3):248-252.
16. Kendal AR, Khalid A, Ball T, Rogers M, Cooke P, Sharp R. Complications of minimally invasive calcaneal osteotomy versus open osteotomy. *Foot Ankle Int*. 2015;36(6):685-690.
17. Gutteck N, Zeh A, Wohlrab D, Delank KS. Comparative results of percutaneous calcaneal osteotomy in correction of hindfoot deformities. *Foot Ankle Int*. 2018;40(3):276-281.
18. Coleman MM, Abousayed MM, Thompson JM, Bean BA, Guyton GP. Risk factors for complications associated with minimally invasive medial displacement calcaneal osteotomy. *Foot Ankle Int*. 2021;42(2):121-131.

31 Spring Ligament Reconstruction

Jaeyoung Kim and Jonathan Deland

The spring ligament complex is the principal stabilizer of the talonavicular (TN) joint,[1] and its degeneration can result in plantarflexion and adduction of the talar head,[2] causing the medial longitudinal arch to collapse.[3] Magnetic resonance imaging (MRI) investigation has indicated that the spring ligament complex is the most commonly involved ligament in progressive collapsing foot deformity (PCFD).[4] Due to unfavorable clinical and radiographic outcomes associated with direct repair of the spring ligament,[5-7] tendon graft reconstruction of the spring ligament complex has been reported.[7-13] One of the reasons for performing spring ligament reconstruction (SLR) is to potentially avoid a fusion of the TN joint, a vital joint in triple joint motion with also important connections with the ankle joint.[5,14] Another reason may be to decrease the amount of lateral column lengthening (LCL) performed in cases where the SLR procedure is implemented. Several surgical techniques of SLR utilizing a variety of graft options, including autograft, allograft, synthetic materials, and tendon transfer, have been explored[7-13,15-18]; clinical and radiological data indicate that this gives further correction when combined with PCFD reconstruction.[10,12,16] However, outcome studies of the procedure are limited by short-term follow-up or expert opinion and by the complex nature of PCFD reconstruction with the many components of deformity and accessory procedures generally carried out in the same setting. Accordingly, patient selection is of equal importance to optimize SLR surgical outcomes.

INDICATION AND CONTRAINDICATION

Since the spring ligament complex limits abduction and dorsiflexion at the TN joint, prominent instability/subluxation at the TN joint in PCFD has been described as an indication for SLR.[14] In addition, it should be remembered that it has recently been demonstrated that the talus is also moving out of place in PCFD, adducting in the ankle mortise;[3,19] therefore, correction of abnormal talar rotation is likely also an indication for SLR. Since the tendon graft goes from the medial malleolus of the tibia to the plantar aspect of the navicular, we refer to our technique described in this chapter as reconstruction of the spring and superficial deltoid ligaments.[20] These two ligaments are in continuity with one another, together encompassing part of the ligament support of the medial, plantar, and dorsal parts of the TN joint. In a biomechanical study, this technique, which incorporates proximal fixation of the graft to the tibia, demonstrated superior TN joint correction ability compared to a more anatomic SLR or isolated TN joint reconstruction,[13] where the graft would have its proximal fixation in the sustentaculum tali and insert distally at the plantar navicular tuberosity. Although preoperative foot anteroposterior (AP) radiographs may indicate the need for concurrent SLR at the time of PCFD reconstruction, the final decision to add a SLR is recommended to be made in the operating room after the bony procedures (usually LCL and medial displacement calcaneal osteotomy. However, other procedures could be used in conjunction such as the medial column stabilization with flexor hallucis longus tendon transfer[21] or Lapicotton procedure[22,23]) have been completed.[24] Once all planned bony procedures have been performed and the amount of improvement in TN joint coverage is insufficient, but there is more than 50% of talar head coverage on simulated foot AP weight-bearing fluoroscopy intraoperatively with the foot stressed into eversion, SLR is an excellent surgical option for achieving a more optimal correction.[14] However, if following all the bony procedures but there is more than 50% of talar head left uncovered on intraoperative simulated weight-bearing fluoroscopy findings, it is the author's opinion that there is a high probability of failure or undercorrection of the TN joint abduction deformity. Then, TN fusion should

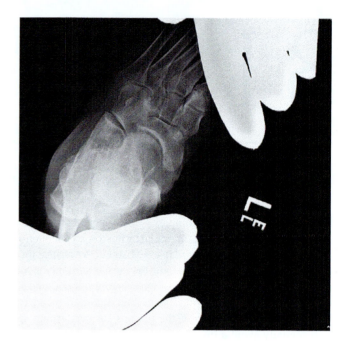

FIGURE 31.1 A preoperative adduction stress radiograph demonstrates that the talonavicular joint is flexible enough to allow full correction of the abduction deformity.

be considered. The patient's foot must be sufficiently flexible to allow the navicular to return to an adducted position in order to cover the talar head; this possibility can be evaluated preoperatively with a stress radiograph (Fig. 31.1).[14]

Severe arthritic changes that result in a stiff TN joint are not a good indicator for SLR. Such cases would warrant fusion. Also, if the triple joints of the foot are rigid, necessitating TN fusion to reconstruct a good tripod of the foot, it would be preferable to choose fusion to correct deformity at the TN joint rather than performing a SLR, as good alignment, stability, and control of arthritic pain would be preponderant. Additionally, it is believed that the talocalcaneal interosseous ligament (TCIL) should be intact for a successful SLR and LCL.[14] Once the TCIL is insufficient to maintain the subtalar joint relationship, multidirectional subtalar joint instability of peritalar subluxation occurs,[25] and hindfoot fusion options should be explored. The TCIL ligament can be palpated with a freer elevator at surgery to confirm it is tight and intact. Subfibular impingement in the ankle standing AP radiographs or weight-bearing computed tomography suggests multidirectional subtalar joint instability and severe peritalar subluxation[25]; hence, the possibility of subtalar fusion should be strongly considered.

PREOPERATIVE PLANNING

Foot standing/weight-bearing AP radiographs are most commonly used to evaluate the severity of abduction deformity. If the patient is not fully weight bearing during a foot AP radiograph (holding the arch up), it may result in an underestimation of the deformity's severity, compared to when the patient is standing directly over their foot and allowing it to relax. The surgeon should examine the patient's foot to confirm considerable TN subluxation by observing the patient standing. In the standing position, patients may have severe medial protrusion of the talar head or callus formation underneath the TN joint, which may be painful enough to necessitate correction. There are several parameters for assessing the severity of forefoot abduction deformity in foot AP radiographs;[26-29] talonavicular coverage (TNC) angle is likely the most frequently used metric.[29] In the majority of the senior author's practice, SLR is not performed in isolation, rather it is performed with LCL. Preoperative stress radiographs should confirm that the TN joint can go into adduction with a supine radiograph taken while the foot is pushed into inversion. Whether the TN joint is sufficiently flexible and allows for appropriate inversion/adduction correction; if it does not go into at least neutral or some adduction, a TN fusion should be considered. MRI may reveal a tear or attenuation of the spring ligament complex, but it does not necessarily determine preoperatively whether reconstruction of the spring ligament is going to be required. There are instances in which there is no tear but attenuation in the spring ligament in the setting of severe abduction deformity.

Conversely, there are instances in which the abduction deformity is mild, but there is a spring ligament tear. Prior to surgery, it must be determined which graft or materials will be used if a SLR is necessary. It is possible to utilize a hamstring tendon autograft, an Achilles or semitendinosus tendon allograft, or synthetic materials. Performing a peroneus longus tendon transfer is a further feasible alternative.[9] Regardless of the graft used, the bony deformity must be properly corrected, and a restored foot tripod must be achieved for the success of the SLR surgery and the maintenance of the desired correction.

SURGICAL TECHNIQUE

- Position the patient supine with a bump on the operating side to allow for both a medial and lateral approach.
- A medial longitudinal incision is made, beginning over the navicular and extending proximally to the medial malleolus, including the distal/medial aspect of the tibia (Fig. 31.2).
- Dissect the subcutaneous layer to expose the navicular and identify the naviculocuneiform joint at the distal end and the TN joint at the proximal end to locate the navicular tunnel (Fig. 31.3A).
- Insert a guidewire into the navicular from superior-distal to inferior-proximal (Fig. 31.3B) and use a fluoroscopy to determine if the wire is appropriately centered (Fig. 31.3C).
- Drill with a smaller-sized reamer and switch to a larger-sized reamer based on the size of the graft. Protect the muscles and neurovascular structures on the plantar side with a retractor while reaming the tunnel (Fig. 31.3D). Depending on the size of the navicular, with proper positioning of the hole, the hole is usually in the range of 7 to 8 mm. When using 7- to 8-mm graft, the graft should go through the 8-mm hole. This can be confirmed with an interference screw sizer. Fluoroscopic images are needed to judge the upper limit of the size of the hole (Fig. 31.3E).
- Insert a 3.5-mm screw into the navicular dorsolateral to the hole (Figs. 31.3F and 31.3G). This screw serves as a post to secure the permanent sutures that have been woven into the end of the tendon graft.
- Locate the tip of the medial malleolus by dissecting its inferior aspect. Next, identify the space between the anterior and posterior colliculi of the medial malleolus. Place a guidewire in the intercollicular area and insert it up into the apex of the intercollicular notch. After doing so, confirm that there is adequate bone on either side to avoid break out into the medial gutter or medial cortex and judge the size of the reamer that can be used by sizing the graft with the interference screw sizer (Figs. 31.4A and 31.4B). An 8- to 8.5-mm hole can usually be achieved, but AP ankle fluoroscopic view with a K-wire driven into the medial malleolus along the proposed path can be used to confirm proper position and avoid breakout into the medial gutter of the ankle.

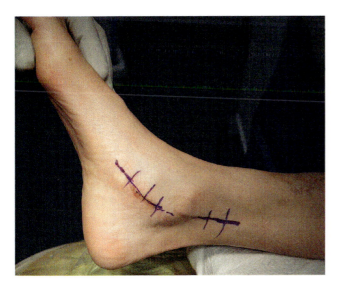

FIGURE 31.2 The incision is made over the navicular to the medial malleolus and proximally to the distal tibia. The distal incision can be extended for harvesting a flexor digitorum longus or flexor hallucis longus tendon when tendon transfers are indicated.

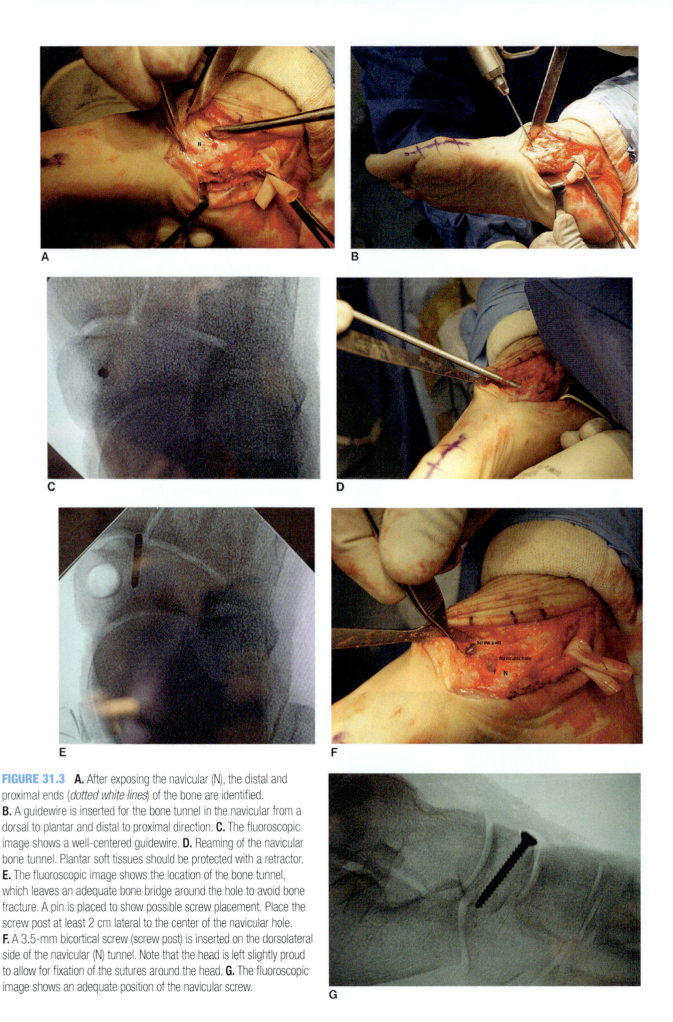

FIGURE 31.3 **A.** After exposing the navicular (N), the distal and proximal ends (*dotted white lines*) of the bone are identified. **B.** A guidewire is inserted for the bone tunnel in the navicular from a dorsal to plantar and distal to proximal direction. **C.** The fluoroscopic image shows a well-centered guidewire. **D.** Reaming of the navicular bone tunnel. Plantar soft tissues should be protected with a retractor. **E.** The fluoroscopic image shows the location of the bone tunnel, which leaves an adequate bone bridge around the hole to avoid bone fracture. A pin is placed to show possible screw placement. Place the screw post at least 2 cm lateral to the center of the navicular hole. **F.** A 3.5-mm bicortical screw (screw post) is inserted on the dorsolateral side of the navicular (N) tunnel. Note that the head is left slightly proud to allow for fixation of the sutures around the head. **G.** The fluoroscopic image shows an adequate position of the navicular screw.

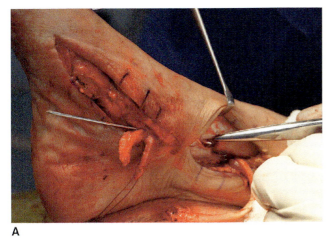
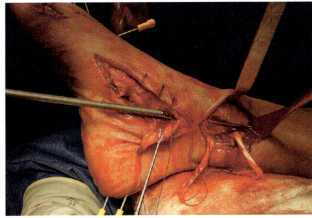
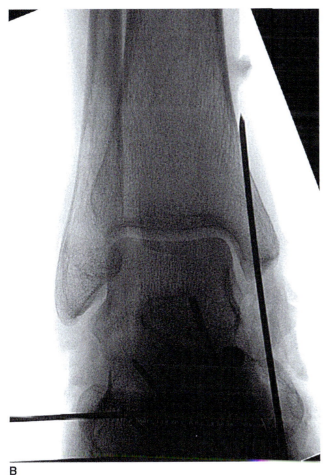

FIGURE 31.4 **A.** A guidewire is inserted into the medial malleolus, exactly at the medial tibial metaphysis. **B.** Fluoroscopic image shows that the guidewire is well centered in the medial malleolus. **C.** Tibial bone tunnel reaming.

- Drill the medial malleolar hole of an appropriate size relative to the width of the medial malleolus (often 7- to 8-mm drill bit). Confirm the location of the hole with the C-arm prior to drilling (Fig. 31.4C).
- After the navicular and medial malleolar tunnels are completed, the length of the graft is measured using a clamped suture from the navicular hole to the outlet of the medial malleolus. The graft length chosen is usually 1 cm longer than the string measurement from the dorsal navicular hole to the exit of the malleolar hole at the medial and dorsal metaphysis, with the foot in neutral. Before the tendon fixation, all bony procedures, including LCL, medial displacement calcaneal osteotomy, and medial column procedures, must be completed and fixed.
- Achilles tendon allograft is prepared on a side table (Fig. 31.5A). The width of the tendon is equivalent to that of the tunnel created in the navicular or medial malleolus; however, both ends

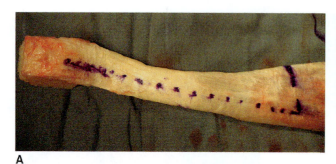
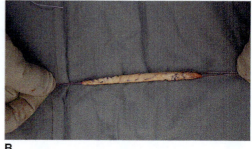

FIGURE 31.5 A. On a side table, an Achilles tendon allograft is thawed and prepared. The graft's width when sutured as a tube if necessary is slightly smaller than the width of the bone tunnels. **B.** Allograft Achilles tendon after preparation. Two sutures are placed on each end for ease of tensioning and screw post fixation. If there is difficulty passing the graft through the tunnel, it may be necessary to wrap the graft with an absorbable suture to make it a round shape. In this case, absorbable wrapping was unnecessary.

may be tapered to a narrower width to allow for easy passage into the tunnels. On each end, we place two sutures, one for initial fixation to the screw post and the other for tensioning the tendon during tendon fixation (Fig. 31.5B). The author has used the Achilles tendon because a larger graft was once preferred, this potentially could be achieved with a doubled over hamstring graft.

- Before the fixation of the tendon on the navicular tuberosity tunnel, the proximal end of the tendon graft is passed through the medial malleolar tunnel, with the tendon end visible at the top of the tunnel, in order to adjust the amount of graft placed in both bone tunnels (Fig. 31.6A). The sutures of the graft are pulled through first which guide the attached tendon into the tunnel. Both sutures are tied down to the screw post making sure that the tip of the tendon graft remains on the top of the tunnel (Fig. 31.6B).
- After tendon fixation on the navicular side, the tendon's proximal end is passed deep to the posterior tibial tendon if it is being retained and then up through the medial malleolar tunnel using a loop wire. After determining good tension of the graft, the position of the proximal screw post on the tibia is determined and a 3.5-mm cortical screw is inserted (Fig. 31.6C and D).
- The proximal free end of the tendon is then secured to the tibial side screw post. Before tying down the two sutures, make sure that no screw threads are cutting into the sutures. Tension the graft with the ends of one of the sutures while the foot is in a slightly inverted and plantarflexed position. Then, tie the ends of the other suture to the screw post to achieve good tensioning (slightly adducted) as there will be a small amount of creep during healing. Check AP foot fluoroscopy with eversion stress to confirm the good position of the TN joint. Slight overcorrection can be present on the fluoroscopic view, but considerable undercorrection after the first tie of the first set of sutures should not be present. Tie down the other set of sutures. More tension can be applied if needed for good position of the TN joint (Fig. 31.6E through I.)
- The wound is then irrigated and closed layer by layer.
- If the surgeon is using the navicular to medial malleolus technique with no plantar limb from the navicular to the sustentaculum, it is particularly important to check the lateral foot everted fluoroscopic view to make sure there is minimal plantar sag at the TN joint remaining. If the plantar TN joint sag remains considerable, a plantar limb is added to the SLR from navicular to the sustentaculum or a subtalar fusion is performed. For the plantar limb, a 5- to 6-mm drill hole in the sustentaculum can be used, but careful positioning of the guidewire for the drill is necessary. Both exposing a portion of the dorsal and inferior aspect of the sustentaculum for targeting when placing the guidewire and checking guidewire position under fluoroscopy is helpful. With the graft placed in the navicular tunnel from dorsal to plantar, the 2-0 permanent sutures in the navicular end of the graft are tied to a dorsal navicular screw. The graft is then placed through the bicortical tunnel from the sustentaculum exiting at the lateral calcaneus. The TN joint is pinned dorsally with slight overcorrection to allow for a creep of the graft. The graft is then tensioned by pulling on the sutures at the end of the graft at the lateral calcaneus and a biotenodesis screw is placed into the sustentaculum. Tie down to a lateral screw in the calcaneus is also possible but rarely necessary.

31 Spring Ligament Reconstruction

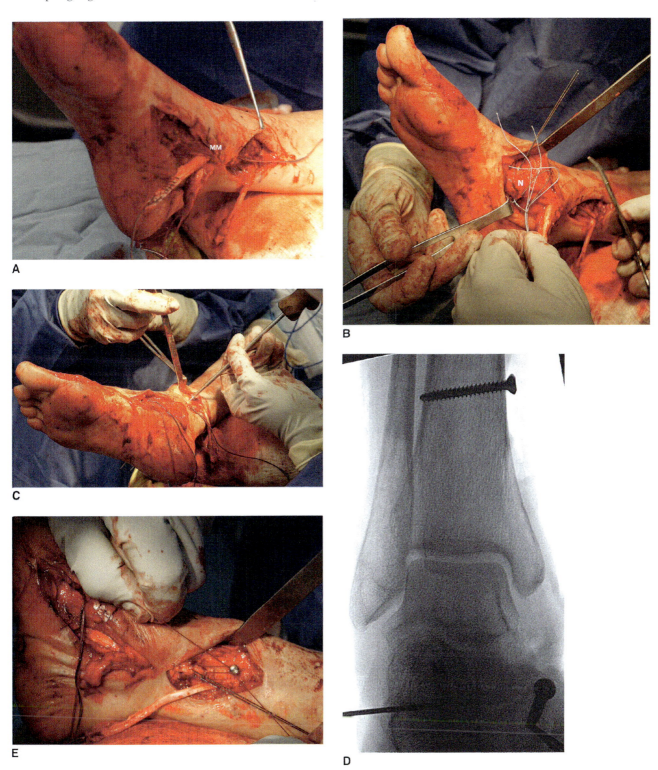

FIGURE 31.6 **A.** The proximal end of the graft is passed through the medial malleolar (MM) tunnel before the distal fixation of the tendon to the navicular tunnel to adjust the amount of graft placed in both bone tunnels. **B.** The distal end of the graft is pulled through the navicular (N) tunnel from plantar to dorsal and tied to the navicular screw post. **C.** For proximal tendon graft fixation, a 3.5-mm bicortical screw is inserted into the tibial shaft, after performing an initial tensioning with the foot in slight inversion and the ankle in neutral to make sure screw placement is proximal enough to allow suture tie down to the screw when the graft is taut. **D.** The position of the proximal screw is shown in a fluoroscopic image. The screw position is chosen once the tendon has been secured to the navicular post and the graft under tension. In this manner, the surgeon can make sure the screw is not too low and there is adequate room to tie the graft to the screw under tension. **E.** The proximal end of the tendon graft is tied to the screw post, with the end of one suture held tight while graft is tied by the other suture.

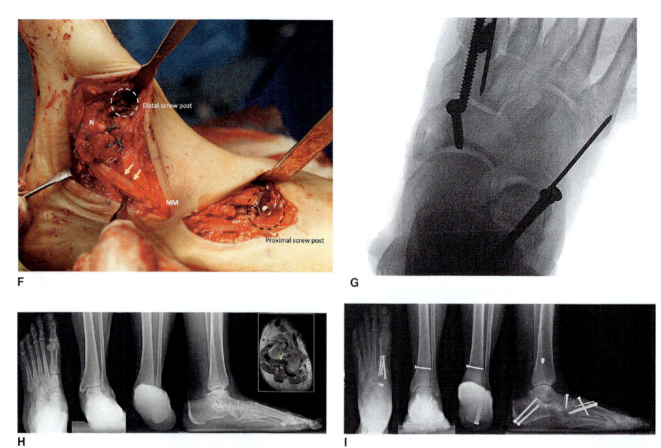

FIGURE 31.6 (*Continued*) **F.** The final appearance of the spring/superficial deltoid ligament reconstruction. The tendon graft (*yellow arrows*) extends from the navicular (N) tunnel to the medial malleolar (MM) tunnel and is tied to both distal and proximal screw posts. **G.** Fluoroscopic image after tendon graft tensioning. The abduction deformity at the talonavicular (TN) joint is corrected, and slight adduction is acceptable as the graft will creep during healing. **H.** Preoperative radiographs of a patient with progressive collapsing foot deformity who had spring ligament reconstruction. Oblique coronal magnetic resonance imaging (*white box*) shows severe degeneration and attenuation of the superomedial fibers of the spring ligament (*arrow*). **I.** Postoperative radiographs of the patient depicted in **(H)**. Note that abduction deformity and sag at the TN joint have been successfully corrected, and that the heel has been neutralized in relation to the tibial axis.

PEARLS AND PITFALLS

- The decision to add SLR is typically made intraoperatively, and the TN joint left uncovered after bony procedures should be less than 50%.
- Fluoroscopic monitoring to ensure a central positioning of the navicular and medial malleolar tunnels is required to prevent breakage of the cortex. However, the senior author has not yet had a failure of the navicular or medial malleolus tunnels.
- The tendon is secured in a slightly inverted and plantarflexed foot position. However, normal hindfoot eversion motion should be maintained. Eversion motion should be checked prior to the ligament reconstruction when choosing of the size of the wedge for LCL. It should also be confirmed when tying down the SLR. Subsequently, tie down the first suture end at the tibial screw.

POSTOPERATIVE MANAGEMENT

Postoperatively, patients are immobilized in a short-leg splint for at least 2 weeks after surgery, until the sutures are removed. Following this, a transition to a short leg cast for an additional 4 weeks is advised. At 6 to 8 weeks postoperatively, patients may begin physiotherapy with progressive weight bearing in a removable walking boot. At 12 weeks, patients should wean out of the boot to a sneaker transition to regular footwear and gradually resume previous activities.

RESULTS AND COMPLICATIONS

Unfortunately, it is difficult to determine the efficacy of SLR alone because it is almost typically performed in conjunction with other bony and soft tissue reconstructive procedures.[10,12] The senior author has used it in two situations.[30] First, it is most commonly used when a LCL or subtalar fusion has given inadequate correction at the TN joint on the AP foot everted fluoroscopic view, but 50% of the abduction deformity was corrected by the bony procedure. For example, if it is corrected in the operating room from 44° of TNC angle to 30° of TNC angle by the LCL or subtalar fusion, the deformity was approximately 50% corrected or more and the surgeon can proceed the SLR. If not, TN fusion is suggested. The SLR caused the TN joint to have good correction, which has held up overtime.[12,14] The senior author has not used SLR without a LCL or subtalar fusion in cases of severe deformity. Second, it has been used to restore good tissue to the spring ligament in instances where deformity has been well corrected by the bony procedure, but there is a greater than 2-cm full-thickness hole in the ligament (talar head is visible). Techniques and grafts vary among surgeons and reports.[7,9-12,15,16] However, the majority of published research do indicate that SLR can give extra TN correction, which is also good for patient-reported outcomes.[10,12] Nevertheless, those results are limited by a small sample size and a lack of long-term follow-up. In our recent study, we reported the outcomes of nonanatomic SLR using allograft tendon in 27 feet of 26 patients, with a mean follow-up period of 8 years. The surgical technique employed was consistent with the description provided in this chapter. The study demonstrated successful correction of abduction deformity, as well as the sustained maintenance of correction observed during the early postoperative period (mean 11.6 months). Furthermore, none of the patients required conversion to TN fusion or subtalar fusion throughout the follow-up period. This finding suggests that SLR with PCFD correction possesses the potential to correct and maintain the correction of severe abduction deformities in the long term. Moreover, this approach may contribute to the preservation of the TN joint in patients presenting with significant abduction deformities.[20]

Regarding complications, there is a chance of fracturing the cortex of the navicular or the medial malleolus when creating a hole for the tendon tunnel; however, this has not occurred in the author's practice. Fluoroscopic imaging checks help prevent this problem. Overtightening the tendon graft may limit eversion motion of the foot. This should be carefully examined with manual assessment. If the LCL is used, be sure that it leaves good eversion prior to proceeding with the SLR. It should be explained to the patients preoperatively that SLR can fail possibly necessitating TN fusion, which senior author rarely has to do.

REFERENCES

1. Vadell AM, Peratta M. Calcaneonavicular ligament: anatomy, diagnosis, and treatment. *Foot Ankle Clin*. 2012;17(3):437-448.
2. Jennings MM, Christensen JC. The effects of sectioning the spring ligament on rearfoot stability and posterior tibial tendon efficiency. *J Foot Ankle Surg*. 2008;47(3):219-224.
3. Henry JK, Hoffman J, Kim J, et al. The foot and ankle kinematics of a simulated progressive collapsing foot deformity during stance phase: a cadaveric study. *Foot Ankle Int*. 2022;10711007221126736.
4. Deland JT, de Asla RJ, Sung I-H, Ernberg LA, Potter HG. Posterior tibial tendon insufficiency: which ligaments are involved? *Foot Ankle Int*. 2005;26(6):427-435.
5. Astion DJ, Deland JT, Otis JC, Kenneally S. Motion of the hindfoot after simulated arthrodesis. *JBJS*. 1997;79(2):241-246.
6. Gazdag AR, Cracchiolo III A. Rupture of the posterior tibial tendon. Evaluation of injury of the spring ligament and clinical assessment of tendon transfer and ligament repair. *JBJS*. 1997;79(5):675-681.
7. Palmanovich E, Shabat S, Brin YS, Feldman V, Kish B, Nyska M. Anatomic reconstruction technique for a plantar calcaneonavicular (spring) ligament tear. *J Foot Ankle Surg*. 2015;54(6):1124-1126.
8. Deland JT, Arnoczky SP, Thompson FM. Adult acquired flatfoot deformity at the talonavicular joint: reconstruction of the spring ligament in an in vitro model. *Foot Ankle*. 1992;13(6):327-332.
9. Lee W-C, Yi Y. Spring ligament reconstruction using the autogenous flexor hallucis longus tendon. *Orthopedics*. 2014;37(7):467-471.
10. Brodell JD Jr, MacDonald A, Perkins JA, Deland JT, Oh I. Deltoid-spring ligament reconstruction in adult acquired flatfoot deformity with medial peritalar instability. *Foot Ankle Int*. 2019;40(7):753-761.
11. Choi K, Lee S, Otis JC, Deland JT. Anatomical reconstruction of the spring ligament using peroneus longus tendon graft. *Foot Ankle Int*. 2003;24(5):430-436.
12. Williams BR, Ellis SJ, Deyer TW, Pavlov H, Deland JT. Reconstruction of the spring ligament using a peroneus longus autograft tendon transfer. *Foot Ankle Int*. 2010;31(7):567-577.
13. Baxter JR, LaMothe JM, Walls RJ, Prado MP, Gilbert SL, Deland JT. Reconstruction of the medial talonavicular joint in simulated flatfoot deformity. *Foot Ankle Int*. 2015;36(4):424-429.
14. Deland JT, Ellis SJ, Day J, et al. Indications for deltoid and spring ligament reconstruction in progressive collapsing foot deformity. *Foot Ankle Int*. 2020;41(10):1302-1306.

15. Acevedo J, Vora A. Anatomical reconstruction of the spring ligament complex: "internal brace" augmentation. *Foot Ankle Spec*. 2013;6(6):441-445.
16. Heyes G, Swanton E, Vosoughi AR, Mason LW, Molloy AP. Comparative study of spring ligament reconstructions using either hamstring allograft or synthetic ligament augmentation. *Foot Ankle Int*. 2020;41(7):803-810.
17. Grunfeld R, Oh I, Flemister S, Ketz J. Reconstruction of the deltoid-spring ligament: tibiocalcaneonavicular ligament complex. *Techniques in Foot & Ankle Surgery*. 2016;15(1):39-46.
18. Ellis SJ, Williams BR, Joseph CY, Deland JT. Spring ligament reconstruction for advanced flatfoot deformity with the use of an Achilles allograft. *Oper Tech Orthop*. 2010;20(3):175-182.
19. Kim J, Rajan L, Henry J, et al. Axial plane rotation of the talus in progressive collapsing foot deformity: a weightbearing computed tomography analysis. *Foot Ankle Int*. 2023;44(4):281-290.
20. Kim J, Mizher R, Sofka CM, Ellis SJ, Deland JT. Medium-to long-term results of nonanatomic spring ligament reconstruction using an allograft tendon in progressive collapsing foot deformity with severe abduction deformity. *Foot Ankle Int*. 2023;44(4):363-374.
21. Kim J, Kim J-B, Lee W-C. Dynamic medial column stabilization using flexor hallucis longus tendon transfer in the surgical reconstruction of flatfoot deformity in adults. *Foot Ankle Surg*. 2021;27(8):920-927.
22. de Cesar NC, Ehret A, Walt J, et al. Early results and complication rate of the LapiCotton procedure in the treatment of medial longitudinal arch collapse: a prospective cohort study. *Arch Orthop Trauma Surg*. 2023;143(5):2283-2295.
23. de Cesar NC, Ahrenholz S, Iehl C, et al. Lapicotton technique in the treatment of progressive collapsing foot deformity. *J Foot Ankle Surg*. 2020;14(3):301-308.
24. Nery C, Baumfeld D. Current trends in treatment of injuries to spring ligament. *Foot Ankle Clin*. 2021;26(2):345-359.
25. de Cesar NC, Saito GH, Roney A, et al. Combined weightbearing CT and MRI assessment of flexible progressive collapsing foot deformity. *Foot Ankle Surg*. 2021;27(8):884-891.
26. Ellis SJ, Yu JC, Williams BR, Lee C, Chiu Y-l, Deland JT. New radiographic parameters assessing forefoot abduction in the adult acquired flatfoot deformity. *Foot Ankle Int*. 2009;30(12):1168-1176.
27. Chadha H, Pomeroy G, Manoli A. Radiologic signs of unilateral pes planus. *Foot Ankle Int*. 1997;18(9):603-604.
28. Deland JT. Adult-acquired flatfoot deformity. *JAAOS-Journal of the American Academy of Orthopaedic Surgeons*. 2008;16(7):399-406.
29. Sangeorzan BJ, Mosca V, Hansen ST Jr. Effect of calcaneal lengthening on relationships among the hindfoot, midfoot, and forefoot. *Foot Ankle*. 1993;14(3):136-141.
30. Kim J, Deland JT. Progressive collapsing foot deformity–flatfoot. *Foot and Ankle Disorders*. Springer; 2022:537-554.

32 Double/Triple Arthrodesis

James W. Brodsky and Andrew P. Thome Jr

INDICATIONS

Introduction

The triple arthrodesis is a fundamental (and historic) procedure in foot and ankle surgery. It was one of the most commonly performed operations in all of orthopaedics during and after the polio epidemic 70 years ago. It is still indicated today for neurologic deformity, hindfoot arthritis of every cause, congenital and developmental abnormalities, posttraumatic deformity, and more. Combined arthrodesis of the subtalar (ST), talonavicular (TN), and calcaneocuboid (CC) joints is the single most powerful, durable, and versatile operation to correct severe deformity and advanced arthritis of the hindfoot. Properly performed, it can correct deformities in all three planes and is equally useful for opposing deformities, that is, valgus or varus, inversion or eversion, abduction or adduction, and combinations thereof.

INDICATIONS

The indications are a symptomatic patient with deformity, arthritis, or instability of the hindfoot, of varying degrees of severity.[1]

- **Deformity.** Increasingly indicated in proportion to the severity of the deformity and to the severity of its associated pain and loss of function.
- **Arthritis.** The most definitive and predictable relief of advanced hindfoot arthritis, regardless of underlying pathogenesis.
- **Instability.** Usually a result of loss of tibialis posterior or peroneal tendon function, and sequelae thereof, or neuromuscular disease (eg, Charcot-Marie-Tooth [CMT] disease, spinal pathology, stroke). Chronic cases often present primarily as deformity, due to progressive rigidity of the imbalanced limb.

The causes of hindfoot deformity are innumerable, from very common to esoterically rare. Regardless of cause, deformity correction is indicated according to criteria, which include a nonplantigrade hindfoot, severe pain, impaired standing, walking, or transfers, difficulty with shoewear or bracing, and failure of nonsurgical therapies. This is equally true in varus as valgus, cavus as planus, adduction as abduction, and inversion as eversion.

Deformity and arthritis of the hindfoot are often seen in combination, and the triple arthrodesis procedure is capable of addressing both these issues simultaneously. Whether the arthritis is a result of trauma, rheumatic diseases, congenital (eg, clubfoot) or developmental (eg, tarsal coalition) abnormality, rigid progressive collapsing foot deformity (PCFD), infection, or as a result of injury or deformity in an adjacent area (eg, tibial or ankle malunion), triple arthrodesis is the definitive procedure for pain relief.

Dynamic instability of the hindfoot due to tendon weakness or loss of inversion (tibialis posterior) or eversion (peroneal) may be particularly indicated when very severe deformity results, in morbidly obese patients, or the patient is unlikely to be able to rehabilitate a soft tissue and bone reconstruction.

In many patients requiring triple arthrodesis, the indications are two or three of the above categories. Prior to proceeding with arthrodesis, attempts should be made to determine if the patient is a candidate for a joint preserving procedure such as osteotomies, tendon transfers, and ligament reconstructions.

CONTRAINDICATIONS[2]

- A dysvascular limb
- An active osteomyelitis, local soft tissue infection, extensive soft tissue loss, or other factor that would substantially interfere with healing
- Medical comorbidities that portend an unacceptably high surgical risk
- Inability to comply with postoperative care, especially restrictions of weight bearing

Relative contraindications may include the following:

- Poorly controlled diabetes mellitus (attempts should be made to optimize HbA1c less than 7.5% or lower)[3]
- Smoking[4]
- Peripheral neuropathy, because of the increased risk of nonunion and malunion

PREOPERATIVE PLANNING

History

At every visit, ask your patient, "What's new with you?" Then pause to encourage an answer. You could hear about resolution of their orthopaedic symptoms, new medical problems that may preclude or delay surgery, or a family crisis, which would fundamentally change the plans for any treatment. Of course, the history comes first, followed by physical exam. Make it your habit not to look at the radiographs or imaging until after you have completed both. With rigorous adherence to this routine, one's diagnostic skills cannot help but sharpen, as you compare your own findings and working diagnoses to the imaging. Pay attention to the location and distribution of arthritic symptoms in lower extremities. Are the symptoms proximal and distal, or bilateral? Assess alleviating and aggravating factors.

The patient's history is the single most important determinant of the indication for surgery. Certainly the severity of physical or radiographic/imaging findings must meet a threshold for consideration of surgery, but one must determine in what ways are the patient's function and/or quality of life is affected. What losses in physical activity, exercise, work, companionship, social interactions, or activities of daily living are the result of this orthopaedic problem?

Surgeons (and their patients) want good surgical outcomes. Despite proper indications, well-executed surgical technique, and outstanding patient compliance, other factors can and often do lead to surgical complications or failures. Not all but many can be avoided or diminished by routine attention to the patient's surgical and medical history, medical comorbidities, quality of social support for postoperative recovery, obstacles to non–weight bearing in the home, lack of transportation, or psychiatric impediments to recovery. Ask your patient at the preoperative evaluation, "Who is going to help you after surgery?" because lack of understanding of the (universal) need for assistance postoperatively and lack of the support itself are shortcuts to poor results. Medications and past history bear directly on surgical outcomes. Examples include cardiac disease, diabetic control, tobacco and vaping, history of pulmonary embolism or deep vein thrombosis, and current anticoagulation.

History specific to disorders treated with triple arthrodesis include a rigid deformity in combination with the below complaints:

- Imbalance or perceived weakness due valgus hindfoot or abduction through TN and CC joints ("my foot is not under my leg").
- Lateral border of foot overload and pain, most often under base of the fifth metatarsal, usually due to varus deformity of hindfoot.
- Inability to walk on inclined and irregular surfaces.
- Painful shoewear at points of deformity in the hindfoot and midfoot. In severe PCFD, the foot can be so deformed that the patient is ambulating on their talus medially.

Physical Examination

Create and use a routine for the physical exam. Self-discipline in adhering to a routine produces provides fundamental information quickly and reduces impactful oversights and omissions. Making not just the right diagnosis but all the relevant diagnoses improves decision-making and the surgical plan and outcomes. Examine the area of known interest last.

Principles

- Bilateral, always.
- Socks off, not just shoes.
- Roll pants to knee, or wear exam shorts.
- Examine the entire musculotendinous unit: up to the knee, always.
- Examine the patient at every visit because the patient's clinical manifestations and/or what one observes often change.

Stance

Observe from all four directions. Look for deformities in the standing position, and this is easier with the patient standing on a platform or step stool. Examine from proximal to distal. Is there scoliosis? Is the pelvis level and what is the alignment of the knees? Follow with alignment of ankles, then segments of the foot. It can be difficult or impossible at this point to distinguish the ankle versus hindfoot as a source of coronal plane deformity. All deformity is easier to see if asymmetric. If the deformity is bilateral, but subtle, look for a change in markers of normal alignment such as loss of varus of the first metatarsal, or curvature of the lateral border of the foot especially as seen from plantar.

In a collapsed foot with hindfoot valgus, differentiate valgus at the hindfoot from abduction occurring through the midfoot, namely the TN joint. These appear different clinically and radiographically. Look for elevation or plantarflexion of first ray. In a cavus foot, note the height of the arch, the position of heel as seen from posterior with the patient standing and compare this to nonstanding.

Gait Evaluation

One should have the patient walk fast because it reduces the unconscious compensatory mechanisms that may obscure or reduce gait abnormalities. Their gait may be abnormal due to mechanical problems or due to pain. One should carefully evaluate their proximal deformity as well, including spine, pelvis, knees, and legs.

Have the patient sit down, and examine the pulses, skin, affect, breathing, and expression of pain. Then, have the patient point to the location(s) of greatest and most consistent symptoms, and pain.

Range of Motion

Test range of motion (ROM) every time, the same way, in the same order, bilaterally, and write it down: dorsiflexion/plantarflexion of the ankle; inversion/eversion of the hindfoot; adduction-abduction of the transverse tarsal joints (TN + CC); and hallux metatarsophalangeal joint.

Inversion/eversion with the ankle relaxed is a composite of motions at the triple joint complex with a contribution from the ankle joint. In order to get an accurate exam of isolated ST motion, bend the knee to relax the gastrocnemius and leg and then passively hold the ankle in maximum dorsiflexion while testing inversion-eversion. Otherwise undiagnosed talocalcaneal tarsal coalitions are discovered in this way because the life-long ST stiffness often produces compensatory ankle laxity in inversion. Decreased ROM at the ankle, crepitus, or ankle pain on exam should be carefully explored as fusing the triple joint complex may have detrimental effects on the ankle.

Deformity

Determine if the deformity is flexible or fixed. If a cavus deformity is present and you observe heel varus standing, determine if the heel still in varus while sitting and prone. If there is a difference, then there is a significant element of forefoot-driven hindfoot varus. The fixed plantarflexion of the first ray pushes a flexible or somewhat flexible hindfoot into varus once the pronated forefoot is placed on the floor. In this case, a first metatarsal osteotomy will be appropriate and necessary to prevent tendency of recurrent varus, even after triple arthrodesis. Tenderness, callus, bursa under fifth metatarsal base, and/or head are caused by proximal varus until proven otherwise. Examination by an experienced surgeon can differentiate the subtleties of varus deformities. Is varus present in all three hindfoot joints, or just the ST? Is there also a fixed supination at the Chopart joint—this is particularly subtle, so use radiographic correlation. In cavus feet, as knee position is changed, look only at the plantar surface of the heel for change in ankle dorsiflexion, because severe cavus feet have equinus at the midfoot.

In valgus deformities of the hindfoot, look for rigidity. A fixed valgus deformity, that is, loss of hindfoot motion, is a strong indication to correct using a triple arthrodesis (and concomitant procedures for gastrocnemius and first ray position), even in the absence of radiographic joint damage or osteoarthritis. Theoretically, medial column or first ray instability can lead to hindfoot valgus, but that is rare. The opposite is the overwhelmingly more common process, that is, hindfoot valgus leads to elevation of the first ray. There are two reasons. First, hindfoot valgus deformities are very common, and second, it is rare to have sufficiently severe first ray instability to change hindfoot position in the absence of hindfoot pathology, for example, loss of the static (ligamentous) constraints of hindfoot alignment. Perhaps it is easier to imagine in the context of posttraumatic dorsiflexion deformity of the first metatarsal. Severe hindfoot valgus is almost always associated with a gastrocnemius or Achilles tendon contracture. Examine the gastrocnemius with the patient standing and then compare to sitting or supine examination for valgus deformities that are not rigid. Examine both limbs for comparison. Hold the hindfoot with one hand, and with the other, the knee. If ankle dorsiflexion is reduced as the knee moves from flexion to extension, there is a gastrocnemius contracture (Silfverskiöld test). This test is best performed by holding the hindfoot locked in inversion while testing ankle dorsiflexion. Because hindfoot eversion is a complex multiplanar motion, which includes dorsiflexion, if one allows the hindfoot to evert during the test, at full knee extension it will incorrectly appear to be ankle dorsiflexion, resulting in a false-negative Silfverskiöld test. If the fixed flexion deformity at ankle is unchanged by knee position, then the contracture is distal to the gastrocnemius, that is, the Achilles tendon or ankle joint itself (Figs. 32.1A and B and 32.2).

Strength

Weakness and asymmetry of strength and tendon excursion are particularly relevant to deformities and dysfunction of the hindfoot. Look for calf asymmetry and do not hesitate to measure and document calf circumference preoperatively. It indicates chronicity and severity and dispels doubts postoperatively regarding the presence of muscle atrophy at the time of presentation. Exam of the calf is valuable in CMT disease, showing selective wasting of anterior and lateral compartments of leg.

Test for sensation manually, and if necessary with monofilaments, if there is suspicion of peripheral neuropathy. Peripheral neuropathy dramatically increases the risk of surgical complications in the foot and ankle, especially nonunion.

Compare retrofibular and hindfoot swelling to the unaffected ankle and foot. Swelling along the peroneal tendons is almost always associated with chronic partial or split tears of the peroneals, especially the peroneus brevis. While frequently associated with hindfoot varus, this can occur in valgus with chronic fibular-calcaneal impingement.

In PCFD, examine for tibialis posterior function. While the single-limb standing test is applicable, it is nonspecific in our experience. Anything made painful with elevation on the toes, for example, midfoot arthritis, or any other relevant weakness, for example, of the triceps surae will confound the examination. The physical test that is specific to the tibialis posterior weakness is, with the ankle in plantarflexion, manual strength testing of inversion of the hindfoot from an everted position, such that the foot moves across the midline of the limb. In plantarflexion, and starting from maximal eversion, the tibialis anterior contribution to inversion is eliminated.

Ankle Instability

Anterior drawer and inversion stress are complementary tests of the anterior talofibular (ATFL) and calcaneofibular ligaments, respectively. Performance of the test under radiographic control provides an objective basis to indicate surgical reconstruction of instability. It is advisable to test ankle stability on preoperative physical exam. If positive, then stress radiographs should be performed, including the contralateral ankle, for comparison. Iatrogenic ankle instability can be a complication of triple arthrodesis because the attachment of the ATFL to the talus is close to the lateral approach to the ST joint. Surprisingly, a fair number of patients with valgus hindfoot deformity may have lateral ligamentous instability at the ankle, which may be worsened or exposed by correction of the hindfoot deformity. It is also important to scrutinize for deltoid insufficiency at the ankle both on exam and clinically as this can influence treatment options and predispose a patient to potential worsening of their valgus deformity at the ankle after triple arthrodesis. Clinically, this presents as increased laxity with valgus stress at the ankle and can be further evaluated with dynamic stress imaging or magnetic resonance imaging (MRI) to evaluate the competency of the deltoid ligament.

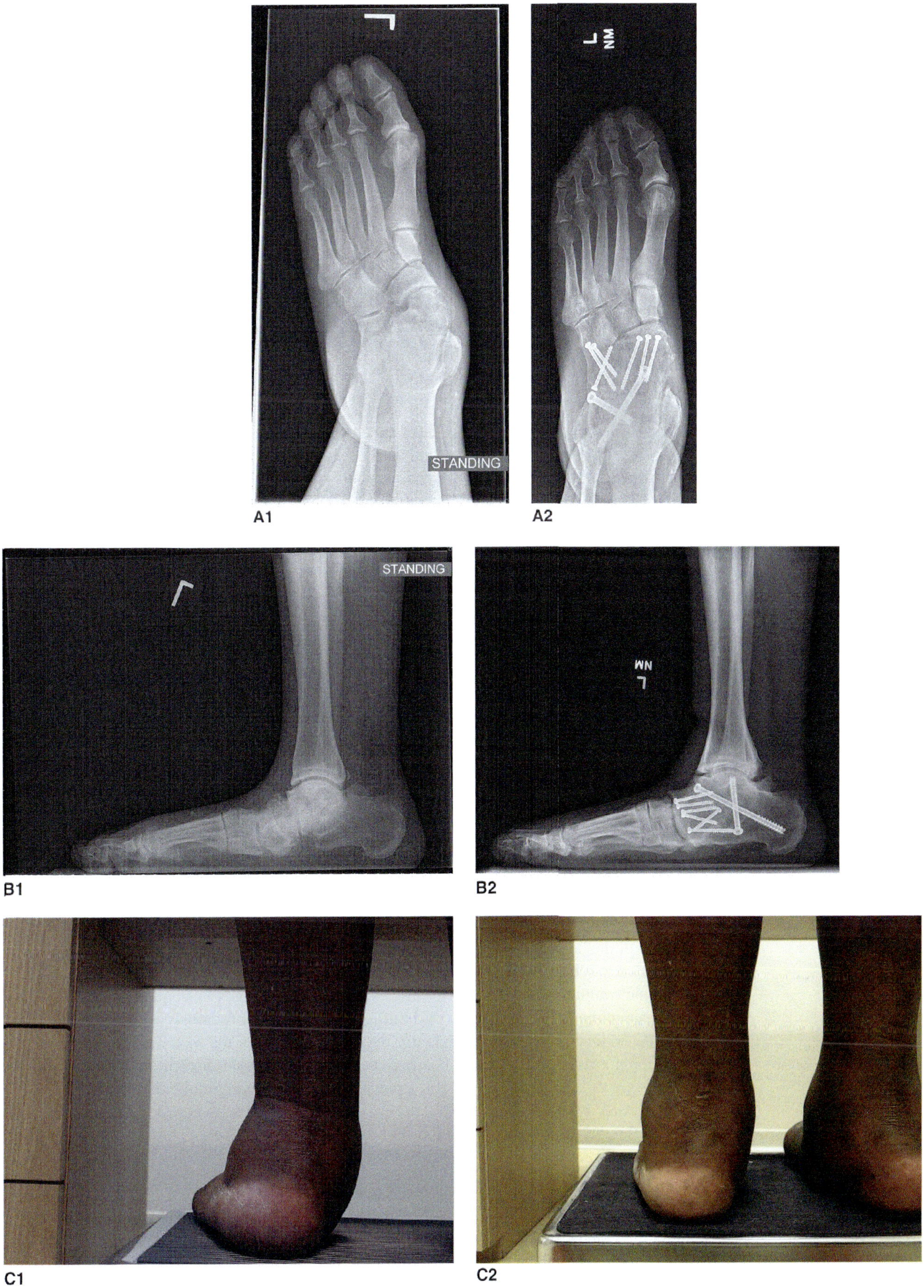

FIGURE 32.1 **A, B.** Progressive collapsing foot deformity. **A.** Photo A1, preoperative AP radiograph; photo A2, postoperative AP radiograph. **B.** Photo B1, preoperative lateral radiograph; photo B2, postoperative lateral radiograph. **C.** Photo C1, preoperative hindfoot view; photo C2, postoperative hindfoot view.

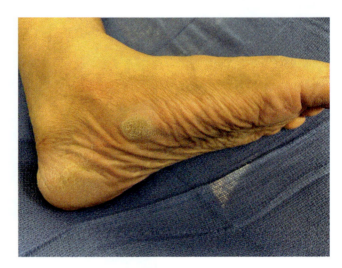

FIGURE 32.2 Clinical photograph demonstrating plantar-medial callus over the talar head due to severe hindfoot valgus, medial column collapse, and midfoot abduction deformity.

Radiographs

After the history and physical exam, evaluate conventional weight-bearing radiographs and the need for advanced imaging. It is commonly valuable to do a quick and very selective re-examination of a specific physical exam finding, to compare to the radiographs or imaging.

Radiographs in evaluation for hindfoot surgery should include the following:

- Five weight-bearing views of the ankle and foot (anterior/posterior [AP], mortise of the ankle and AP, oblique, lateral of the foot).
- The lateral view must include the ankle and whole foot.
- If both feet and ankles are assessed, each should be imaged separately, with the radiograph beam centered as if it were a unilateral exam, so that the radiographic technique is always the same, for accuracy.
- Contralateral comparison views can be very helpful, especially in evaluating subtle findings (eg, missed tarsal coalition).
- In some cases (proximal deformity on exam, prior trauma or arthroplasty), long limb length films are helpful to evaluate alignment.
- Lateral radiographs tend to underrepresent the severity of ST arthritis because the posterior facet is highly curved, and because it is not possible to obtain a second, orthogonal view as is the case for the TN and CC joints. The reason for this is that radiographs show the part of the curved surface, which is perpendicular to the beam of the radiograph. Much of the joint can, therefore, be missed.
- Assessment and measurement of hindfoot varus and valgus is important, and complex. This can be assessed on a hindfoot alignment view radiograph. It also includes AP and lateral talocalcaneal angles, lateral talus-first metatarsal angle, and calcaneal pitch; on lateral films, the overlap or lack thereof of the talus and calcaneus, TN and CC joints, and the morphologic appearance of the individual bones, which is highly affected by rotational deformity.
- Radiographic evaluation of the severity of flexible hindfoot valgus is frequently inaccurate because the patient has medial hindfoot and midfoot pain and unconsciously externally rotates the tibia in order to invert the hindfoot and raise the medial border of the foot. The problem is eliminated by doing a single-limb weight-bearing lateral on the affected side, often with contralateral comparison views. Standing on one foot, a patient cannot externally rotate the tibia.
- Severe or chronic hindfoot varus and valgus are often associated with concomitant or compensatory plantarflexion or dorsiflexion of the first metatarsal, respectively. This should be routinely observed (Fig. 32.3A through D).

Cross-Sectional Imaging

Computed tomography (CT) is exceptionally useful for evaluating the extent of arthritis and the three-dimensional details of osseous deformity. CT frequently shows deformity and arthritis in the adjacent ankle and midfoot, which are unclear or underrepresented on conventional radiographs. The most common examples include talocalcaneal coalition, or arthritis of one portion of the

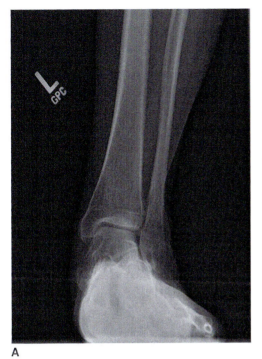
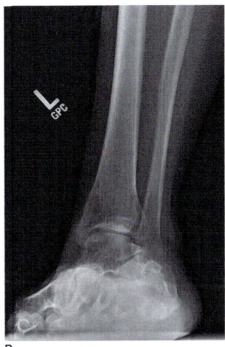
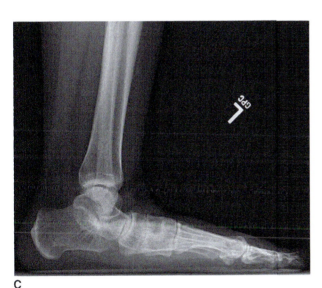
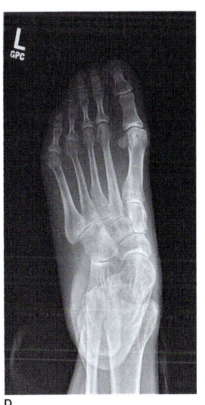

FIGURES 32.3 A, B. AP and mortise left ankle radiographs demonstrating severe left hindfoot valgus deformity. Of note, there is no evidence of valgus deformity at the ankle. **C.** Lateral left foot radiograph demonstrating plantarflexion of the talus and planus deformity. There is mild dorsal translation of the first metatarsal at the first tarsometatarsal joint. **D.** AP left foot radiograph demonstrating forefoot abduction with talar head uncoverage.

tibiotalar joint. It is difficult to overestimate the utility of CT as a guide and map for surgical planning of osseous reconstruction of the hindfoot. Weight-bearing CT can further enhance knowledge of the underlying deformity and severity of arthritis at specific joints with weight bearing.

Magnetic resonance imaging is usually not needed to diagnosis the presence of an acquired hindfoot valgus due to ruptured tibialis posterior tendon. But MRI is very valuable, even in cases of obvious deformity, to identify other lesions, which are commonly concomitant with PCFD such as calcaneonavicular ligament tear; a subradiographic occult osteochondral lesion of the talar dome, or within the triple joints; peroneal tendon tears; or focal or subtle arthritic changes in the ankle and hindfoot.

SURGICAL PREPARATION

In some patients, all three of the hindfoot joints are not equally affected. How many joints should be fused? If the patient has isolated ST arthritis, and the TN and CC joints are unaffected, isolated ST fusion is appropriate. If the primary arthritis is in the TN or CC joint, isolated fusion of only one joint has a theoretically increased risk of nonunion, because the débridement for the arthrodesis creates shortening of either the medial or lateral column. If only the medial (TN) or lateral (CC) column is shortened, the other column tends to distract the arthrodesis. The difference must be made up with generous grafting of the isolated fusion. Alternatively, in our experience, it is more predictable and has a lower nonunion rate to fuse both the TN and CC if only one is affected because of the decreased stress on the fusion construct. This gives more power to correct deformity in all planes, especially pronation-supination and adduction-abduction. Some surgeons will fuse the TN or CC plus the ST joint for similar considerations.

If the patient has ipsilateral knee deformity, especially in the coronal plane, the knee should be corrected first. This is to prevent the need to revise the ankle and hindfoot following the magnified effects of angular change at the knee.

The TN and CC joints that are flexible and unaffected can be flexible after ST arthrodesis, but once the TN is fused, neither the CC nor the ST will have clinically meaningful motion (75% reduction in motion), reinforcing the principle of augmenting isolated TN arthrodesis at an adjacent joint.[5]

Further Considerations

Do the history and symptoms correspond in severity and location to the physical findings and to the radiographic and imaging findings? If these are not concordant, review everything again, including selective parts of the exam, to resolve the discrepancy, or establish a plan for additional information for such resolution.

Social assessment is an underreported but incredibly impactful aspect of obtaining a good surgical result. Is the patient's desire for surgery appropriate and proportional to the objective findings? The surgeon who routinely assesses the patient's ability to endure the rigors of postoperative recovery will have fewer complications and problems given the prolonged non–weight-bearing period afterward. Ask the patient who will help them after surgery, and who is their main source of support in general. Are those people nearby and available? What resources does the patient have or lack, as this can be the deciding factor in surgical outcomes? (Fig. 32.4A through C)

SURGICAL TECHNIQUE

General Principles

Skin complications, especially over the lateral hindfoot, are common. A longer incision creates less skin tension when retracting. Sharp (scalpel) dissection is the least traumatic and the method primarily used by the authors. Where possible, full-thickness flaps reduce the potential for wound healing issues. Place retractors deep and minimize retracting on the skin alone. Remove retractors from the wound when not actively working in that area.

Setup and Positioning

- Preoperative popliteal and adductor blocks are typically performed by the anesthesia department in the absence of contraindications. The effect of the former may be extended by an indwelling block catheter for postoperative pain control.

32 Double/Triple Arthrodesis

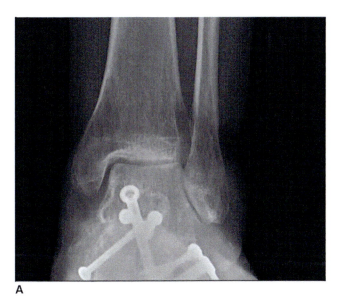
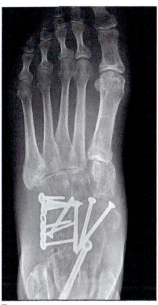
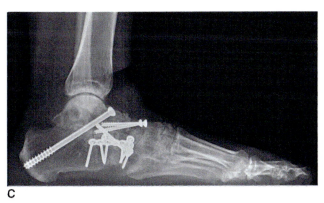

FIGURES 32.4 A-C. AP and lateral conventional radiographic images demonstrating excellent restoration of talar position and talar head coverage after a triple arthrodesis.

- The patient is positioned supine with padding for the contralateral malleoli and the common peroneal nerve at the proximal fibula. A pneumatic tourniquet is applied to the proximal thigh and protected from the prep solution with adhesive plastic drapes. General anesthesia is used for tourniquet pain, but patients may need less intraoperative narcotics as result of the regional blocks. Spinal anesthesia could be considered; however, predicted length of case is important to consider. A "bump" of folded blankets or sheets is placed under the ipsilateral hip and sacrum to internally rotate the limb for access to the lateral hindfoot. This may result in an effective external rotation of the shoulder, so a bump may be placed under the torso, and the ipsilateral arm positioned across the chest to protect the brachial plexus.
- The authors prefer mini C-arm fluoroscopy positioned on the operative side, for its superior maneuverability in imaging multiple planes quickly. The large C-arm, positioned on the opposite side of the table, requires elevation of the operative leg for clearance above the contralateral limb.
- Antibiotic prophylaxis is routinely used per institutional protocol.

Gastrocnemius Recession

- If the patient has a gastrocnemius contracture, this is addressed first. The choice between a recession at the anterior fascia of the muscle (modified Baumann) and at the musculotendinous junction (modified Strayer) is based on the severity of the contracture and expectations of the patient's future activity level. The former is preferred for more mild deformity and higher activity level, and vice versa. This is performed prior to osseous reconstruction in order to reduce the tension on the heel that impedes positioning of the triple arthrodesis.

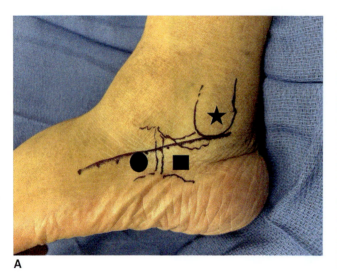
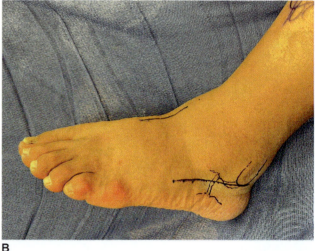

FIGURE 32.5 A. Clinical picture with the skin demarcated for a lateral incision for subtalar (ST) exposure and calcaneocuboid (CC) joint exposure from the tip of the fibula extending distally to the base of the fourth metatarsal. The distal fibula (*star*) is outlined as are the anterior process of the calcaneus (*square*) and cuboid (*circle*). **B.** Relationship between lateral ST/CC incision and medial talonavicular incision.

Subtalar Joint

- The lateral incision begins at or just posterior to the tip of the fibula along a line toward the fourth metatarsal base. The incision may be extended proximal to the fibula along a gentle curve for exposure of the peroneal tendons, and distally according to the required exposure of the cuboid. It is rather extensile as it also allows lateral exposure of the TN joint (Fig. 32.5A and B).
- The incision should be superior to the peroneal tendons and the sural nerve, which is inferior to the tendons proximally. Gently identify the major branches of the sural nerve, which cross the incision from inferior-proximal to superior-distal. There will always be some very small branches interrupted, and most patients have at least a transient area of diminished sensation dorsolateral over the midfoot-forefoot after surgery.
- The muscle belly of the extensor digitorum brevis (EDB) is incised from medial to lateral with a #15 scalpel along the superior margin of the anterior process of the calcaneus, just proximal to the CC joint. Its fascia is incised laterally along the margin of the peroneals, and medially in parallel fashion, taking care to protect the EDL tendon and superficial peroneal nerve. The EDB muscle belly is sharply elevated subperiosteally off the calcaneus from proximal to distal in a single flap and reflected distally. Care is taken to maintain its integrity for closure over the CC arthrodesis (Fig. 32.6A and B).
- The soft tissue in the sinus tarsi is excised with a scalpel and rongeur, and the interosseous ligaments are divided in the horizontal plane, perpendicular to its fibers. Division of the cervical ligament improves joint distraction. The capsule of the posterior facet is incised along its lateral margin by retracting the peroneal tendons. The calcaneofibular ligament is included. The peroneal tendons are protected with the short end of the army-navy retractor.
- The joint is distracted with a sharp-toothed lamina spreader, while separating the surfaces by levering with an osteotome or elevator. It is placed in the anterior joint or sinus tarsi. Two lamina spreaders are required in order to exchange their position between the anterior and posterior parts of the joint, while maintaining distraction (Fig. 32.7).
- Débridement of the posterior facet is done with a combination of osteotomes, curettes, and rongeurs until clear bony surfaces are achieved on the opposing sides of talus and calcaneus. Visualization of the undersurface of the talus is facilitated by temporary Trendelenburg position of the table. All cartilage and soft tissue are removed, exposing the underlying subchondral bone. The areas most often missed or inadequately prepared are those closest to surgeon and shielded by the marginal curvature of the bone.

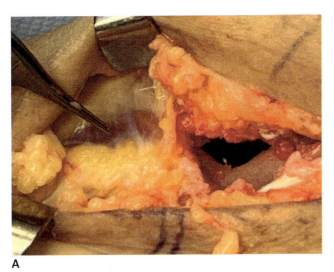
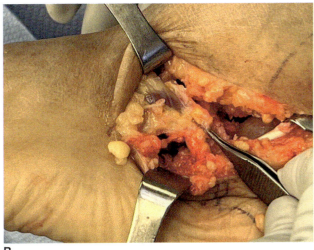

FIGURE 32.6 A. Intraoperative photo of the intact extensor digitorum brevis (EDB) prior to detachment from anterior calcaneus. **B.** Intraoperative photo of mobilized EDB.

- The flexor hallucis longus tendon is identified posteromedially. The bundle is just anterior to it at the level of the medial joint. A curette is the safest instrument here, pulling and twisting from the medial margin in a lateral direction (Fig. 32.8).
- The second lamina spreader is inserted into the posterior facet and the lamina spreader in the sinus removed.
- Preparation of the middle and anterior facets, which are usually confluent, is done with the same instruments, though predominantly with large, long curettes.
- Fragments of cartilage, bone, and soft tissue are removed during débridement.

Calcaneocuboid Joint

- The CC joint is prepared next trough the distal part of the same later incision. Sharply release the ligaments at the plantar lateral corner of the joint. Release the medial capsule as needed for exposure, keeping in mind that the joint curves in two planes: proximally from lateral to medial and dorsally from plantar to dorsal. An osteotome is inserted into the joint and turned 90° to provide space to insert a lamina spreader. The lamina spreader is inserted first plantar for dorsal joint preparation, then vice versa. Be mindful of achieving complete joint preparation, especially medially, using the same instruments as for the ST joint. Surface preparation is detailed below (Fig. 32.9A through C).

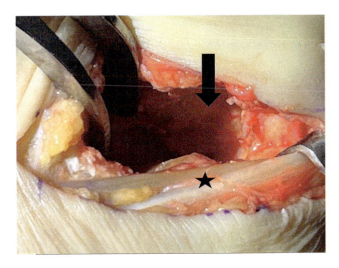

FIGURE 32.7 Intraoperative view of the lamina spreader placement for preparation of the posterior facet. The peroneals are demonstrated inferior in the field and retracted. *Solid arrow*—posterior facet of the talus. *Solid star*—peroneal tendons.

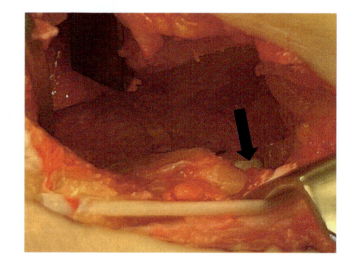

FIGURE 32.8 Intraoperative view after preparation of the subtalar joint. The flexor hallucis longus tendon is visualized in the inferior and right aspect of the image (*black arrow*).

Talonavicular Joint

- The lateral (and sometimes all of the) TN joint can be prepared from the lateral approach, depending on the deformity and flexibility of the soft tissues. Be aware of the skin when doing so.
- It is usually best to approach the TN joint from a dorsal incision, centered over the neck of the talus and TN joint. A dorsal approach is chosen because of the wider exposure and visualization of the entire TN joint, especially the lateral side, than a medial incision, although it can be used as

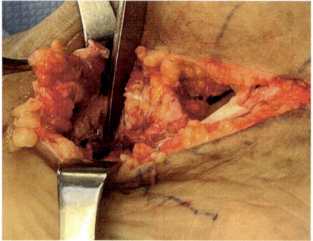
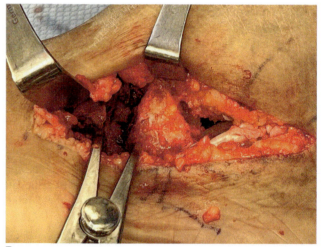
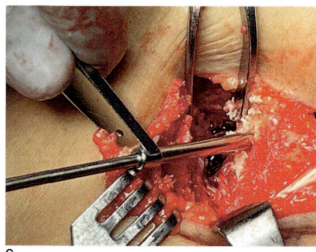

FIGURE 32.9 **A.** Osteotome is used to first pry open the calcaneocuboid (CC) joint. **B.** CC joint is distracted with lamina spreader. **C.** Drilling of the CC joint during joint preparation.

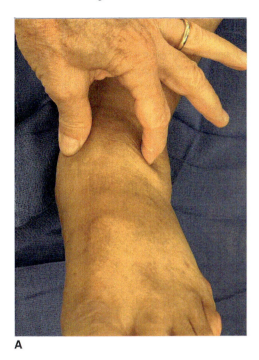 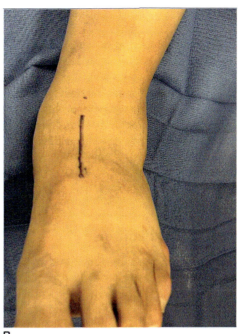

FIGURE 32.10 **A.** Palpating the talar neck for talonavicular (TN) incision placement. **B.** Distal view of TN incision placement.

well. Correction of severe deformity is primary, and it is often necessary to accept that the opposing surfaces of the talus and navicular may not match perfectly or be offset. Reduction medially may require grafting laterally, hence a centered dorsal incision. Dissection is performed between the EHL and tibialis anterior tendons extending distally to the margin of the navicular-cuneiform joints. Dissection is carried to the bone, reflecting the joint capsule in line with the medial and lateral flaps created. Stay on the bone. The neurovascular bundle is retracted laterally keeping in mind that the bundle traverses the navicular between its central point, and the junction of its medial 2/3 and lateral 1/3, quite close to the TN joint preparation (Fig. 32.10A and B).

- Initial access is gained to the joint with an osteotome than a lamina spreader. Preparation of the TN joint is the most difficult of the three because of the curved surfaces and it is in our experience the most likely to develop nonunion, a fact that is likely not unrelated. It is difficult to see the entire navicular articular surface. The subchondral bone of the talus is dense.
- Usually curettes are most effective to prepare the navicular. Special effort is required to see "around the corner" medially and dorsally. The rule is once you have finished scraping, scrape some more. Leverage is better with straight curettes, so the joint can be pushed apart while curetting. If an assistant is unavailable to hold the lamina spreader, a pin distractor can be useful.
- Routinely prepare the navicular before the talus, because once the thin subchondral bone of the talar head is removed and the soft cancellous bone beneath is exposed, distraction is difficult.
- Convex surfaces are easier to prepare than concave ones. Application of the convex side of a curved rongeur to the convex talar head exerts both the greatest force (two circles meet at one point) and accuracy for preparation of the talus. The most common error is plunging and removing too much bone.

Surface Preparation

- Surface prep correlates to union. Perseverance and fastidious attention to detail yields higher union rates. The goal is to expose the cancellous bone to enhance healing, while maintaining the surface morphologies for alignment and apposition.
- After thorough preparation of all three joints and four bones is completed, each joint is irrigated and suctioned to remove all particles of tissue, cartilage, and bone. Begin with the TN, then CC, then ST so that gravity works in your favor.

- Irrigation of each joint must be done while distracting with a lamina spreader in order to remove all residual debris.
- For each joint, the subchondral bone is prepared by extensive perforation of the surface with a 3.2-mm drill bit, which is commonly longer than a 3.5-mm one. A drill sleeve is essential to protect the soft tissue and to hold the drill point accurately against the bone while covering the surface with more holes than residual smooth bone.
- Include the calcaneal surface of the sinus tarsi, and the opposing talar surface of the sinus canal as an extra-articular augmentation, if desired. The authors do this routinely. The tips of a medium rongeur are used to remove additional hard subchondral bone by inserting the jaws in adjacent drill holes. Alternatively, a long ¼-inch osteotome can be used to connect the holes or fish scale the surface (Fig. 32.11A).
- Be particularly thorough on the navicular, and either drill the dorsal edge of the subchondral bone or trim it with a rongeur to expose cancellous bone.

Reduction and Fixation

- The order of reduction and fixation is always:
  - Subtalar → talonavicular → calcaneocuboid
- The ST is performed first in order to establish heel position, upon which the alignment of the other joints depends. The TN must be second because it determines adduction-abduction of the transverse tarsal joints (TN + CC) and pronation-supination of the midfoot and forefoot. Additional sagittal plane correction at the TN can increase or decrease plantarflexion of the midfoot-forefoot on the hindfoot. Each joint is reduced and fixed, sequentially.
- Whenever a TN joint is reduced and fixed first, neither of other hindfoot joints will have sufficient motion to allow correction of deformities therein. It is easier to obtain satisfactory heel alignment first, and easier to adjust the CC position to the TN after than vice versa.
- Grafting of the arthrodesis sites is done to augment healing, to fill in irregularities and defects of the opposing bone surfaces, and to include the sinus tarsi in the ST arthrodesis. Currently, the authors usually use allograft with a biologic component, for ease and reduced morbidity compared to autograft (Fig. 32.11B).

Subtalar Joint

- Hindfoot valgus is reduced by holding the heel in one hand (right hand if a left foot, left hand if a right foot). Check for inadvertent translation medially or laterally. Correction of varus-valgus is done primarily by rotation through the joint of the calcaneus relative to the talus (which is fixed in the mortise). The shape of the posterior facet matches this screw-like mechanism.
- Internal rotation of the calcaneus opens the sinus tarsi and produces varus (Fig. 32.12A).

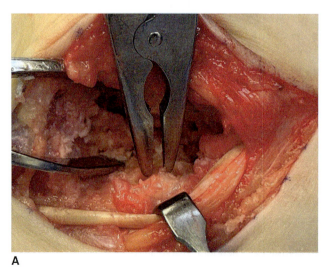
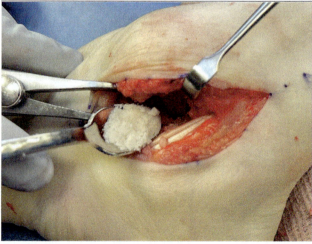

FIGURE 32.11 **A.** Utilization of a rongeur between drill holes for further subtalar (ST) joint preparation. **B.** Placement of allograft into ST joint after joint preparation.

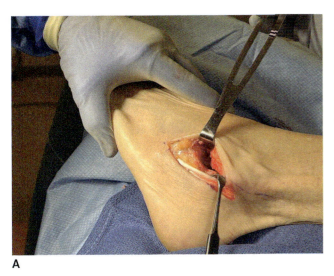 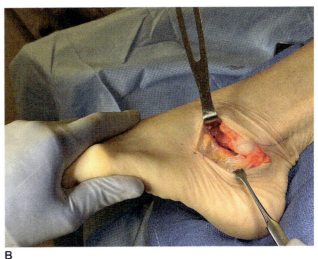

FIGURE 32.12 **A.** Internal rotation of the calcaneus relative to the talus opens the sinus tarsi and produces hindfoot varus. **B.** External rotation of the calcaneus relative to the talus closes the sinus tarsi and produces hindfoot valgus.

- External rotation of the calcaneus closes the sinus and produces valgus (Fig. 32.12B).
- Additional correction is sometimes required or possible by using a lateral closing wedge and/or translation of the calcaneus. There are no jigs to assist the surgeon. Three-dimensional alignment of the triple arthrodesis is challenging and has a definite learning curve.
- Judgment of heel position depends on the following:
  - Surgeon feels the alignment of the heel.
  - Looking at the heel position relatively to the leg by raising the limb in the air.
  - The opening or closing of the sinus tarsi width (space between anterior surface of the talar body and the posterior surface of the anterior process of the calcaneus).
  - Intraoperative fluoroscopy, especially the Harris axial heel view and on lateral view with the foot on a sterile flat surface to simulate weight bearing.
- Once the ST joint is reduced manually, a guidewire for a large, cannulated screw is placed to hold the reduction and determine the position of the first screw. The pin position is assessed on lateral and axial heel fluoroscopic images, and adjusted as necessary. Sometimes provisional K-wire fixation may be necessary based on the deformity, but usually the guidewire is adequate to hold the ST reduction prior to screw placement. The pin is directed from the dorsum of the talar neck through the TN incision, directed posteriorly, inferiorly, and plantarly, aiming at the posterolateral corner of the calcaneal tubercle. The pin should start sufficiently distal to avoid impinging on the anterior ankle. Drilling is occasionally needed, but the exception. A large, partially threaded cannulated screw with a long thread, at least 6.5 mm diameter in all but the smallest patients, is advanced along the pin. A screw is selected that is approximately 10 mm shorter than measured with the depth gauge to accommodate compression (Fig. 32.13).
- A second screw is usually placed from the inferolateral margin of the anterior calcaneus, directed medially and proximally into the body of the talus. This is a short thread version of the same screw. Extreme care is taken to avoid penetration of the ankle joint two ways: inserting under fluoroscopic control in AP and lateral projections of the ankle and using a threaded pin to prevent pin penetration upon screw insertion (Fig. 32.14).

Talonavicular Joint

- The TN joint is the most difficult both to reduce and to fix. It is difficult to reduce because correction must be achieved in three planes at once. It is difficult to fix because the shallow depth of the navicular from proximal to distal along with the curved joint shape make it difficult to achieve fixation in this tight space.
- Reduction of the TN and CC joints are related because the lengths of the medial and lateral columns must be gauged and adjusted to one another in addition to the alignment in three

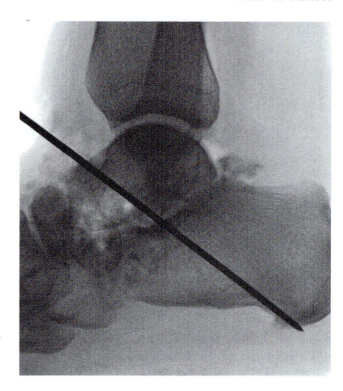

FIGURE 32.13 Intraoperative lateral fluoroscopic image demonstrating appropriate wire placement for subtalar screw fixation from dorsal talar neck to plantar calcaneal body.

planes. Thus, bone grafting ranges from very helpful to utterly essential. If the medial column is longer or shorter than the lateral, the foot can be abducted or adducted, respectively, once compression is applied. Also, compression at the TN and CC joints must be done judiciously.

- The TN joint requires a two-handed reduction, which once achieved is best held by the surgeon while provisionally fixed by an assistant using wires or pins.
- In the reduction maneuver, one hand is held firmly to stabilize the heel with the thumb on the medial side of the talar neck. The other hand reduces the foot to the talus with a combination of first adduction, then pronation, and then dorsiflexion-plantarflexion (Fig. 32.15A and B).
- The authors' preference is to use the threaded guidewires for 4.0- or 4.5-mm partially threaded cannulated screws, directed from distal (navicular) to proximal (talus). The pins for the partially threaded cannulated screws are used to temporarily hold reduction. Care must be taken to ensure adequate spread of the screws but also to remain away from previously placed dorsal ST screw. The pins are inserted at or near the naviculocuneiform (NC) joint, and the screws

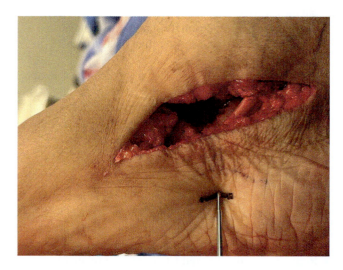

FIGURE 32.14 Placement of the second subtalar screw from the inferolateral aspect of the calcaneus to the superomedial talar dome.

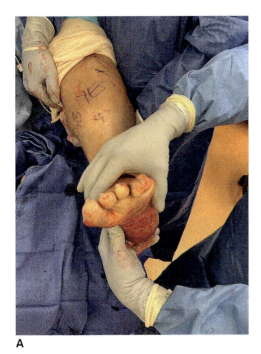 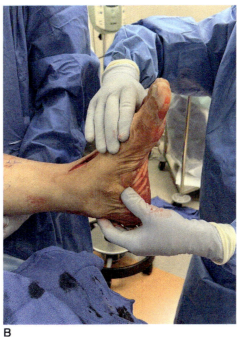

FIGURE 32.15 **A.** Distal view showing pronation and adduction maneuver during reduction. **B.** Medial view showing plantarflexion, pronation, and adduction during reduction.

- countersunk into the navicular for compression and reduced prominence or impingement of the screw heads. Reduction and screw position are evaluated on AP and lateral fluoroscopic images of the foot (Fig. 32.16A through C).
- The goal is clinical correction of the deformity and restoration of plantigrade alignment, not perfect fluoroscopic reduction, because this is done in the context of deformity and bone abnormality. There is wide variety in surgeons' preferences for type of fixation, and many different methods are effective given adherence to the principles above. Experience is very helpful.

Calcaneocuboid Joint

- Final resolution of a discrepancy in length between the medial (TN) and lateral (CC) columns is now done at the CC arthrodesis. This is usually by bone grafting but could also be performed by bone trimming. Grafting is also used to correct deficiency in apposition of the surfaces.
- Proper alignment of the CC joint is necessary to achieve a straight midfoot to forefoot relationship and to avoid overload of the lateral border of the foot.
- Lateral overload can occur even if the heel is in an ample degree of valgus because supination through the CC joint has a very similar effect. Thus, care must be taken to align the CC joint in all three planes.
- First determine the abduction adduction. From the plantar side of the elevated limb confirm that the lateral border of the foot is straight. Then align flexion and pronation. If the CC arthrodesis is positioned in flexion, the patient will have pain on the plantar-lateral border of the foot. This is most easily prevented by pushing on the plantar surface under the cuboid so that it is elevated some amount relative to the anterior calcaneus. On lateral fluoroscopy, one should see both the dorsal translation of the cuboid and plantarflexion at the joint (Fig. 32.17).
- Fixation of the CC joint can be done in numerous ways. Compression is difficult, and the focus should be on rigidity of the properly aligned construct. The authors currently favor a T-shaped plate with a combination of cortical and locking screws but also have extensive experience with screws alone.

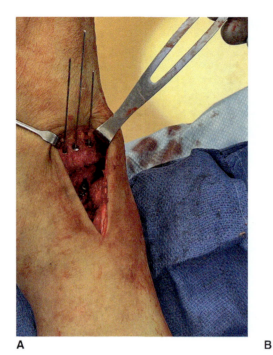
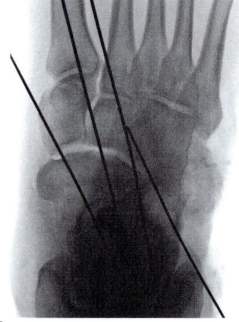
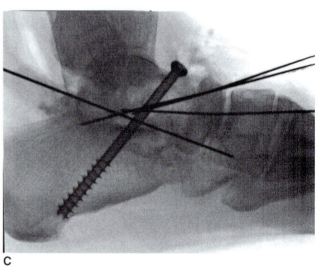

FIGURE 32.16 A. Clinical photograph (superior view) demonstrating cannulated screw fixation placement for talonavicular (TN) arthrodesis. **B, C.** AP and lateral fluoroscopic images of wire placement for cannulated screws for TN arthrodesis. In this particular case, only one subtalar screw was utilized.

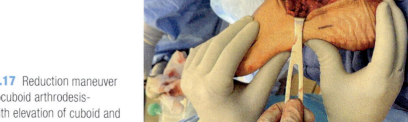

FIGURE 32.17 Reduction maneuver for calcaneocuboid arthrodesis-pronation with elevation of cuboid and plantar angulation.

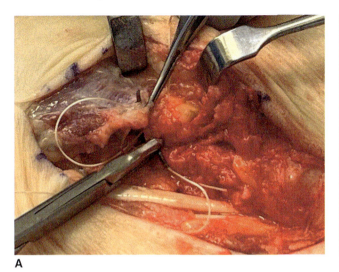
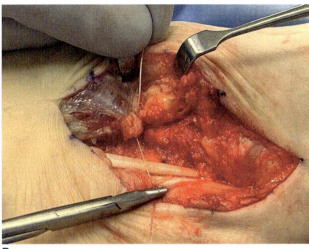

FIGURE 32.18 **A.** Suture repair of the extensor digitorum brevis (EDB) origin with 2-0 Vicryl, ensuring adequate bites of the fascia. **B.** Tying of EDB repair.

Final Steps

- Closure: Remaining bone graft is applied to arthrodesis sites. Each area of graft is covered with surgical gelatin foam to prevent dislodgement of graft during closure.
- The EDB is sutured back to its origin, sewing the proximal tendon and fascial edges to the adjacent tissue with 2-0 Vicryl. Next, the dermis is closed with 3-0 Monocryl in a buried, interrupted fashion. The skin is closed with 3-0 nylon in an interrupted vertical mattress fashion (Fig. 32.18A and B).
- Once all fixation is placed and confirmed on fluoroscopy, position of the first ray is reassessed. With finger pressure under the fourth metatarsal head pushing dorsally to a neutral ankle position, the position of the first ray is evaluated for malalignment in the sagittal plane. Feet with preoperative cavovarus deformity begin with forefoot pronation, that is, plantarflexion of the first ray. Conversely, valgus feet characteristically have compensatory forefoot supination, that is, dorsiflexion of the first ray. Either can be corrected with first tarsometatarsal arthrodesis, or first metatarsal basilar wedge osteotomy, using the surgeon's favored method of fixation, usually screws or plate and screw fixation.
- Ankle stability may need to be reassessed and possibly even surgically corrected. Careful fluoroscopic stress tests of the ankle can be done as needed.

PEARLS

- Placing the ST screw from the dorsal talus to the plantar calcaneus gives access to more bone for longer screw threads and better fixation. It also avoids hardware prominence at the heel and has a lower risk of ankle joint penetration.
- Threaded guidewires for cannulated screws decrease the risk of the wire dislodging or inadvertent advancement into adjacent joints.
- Surgical foam on arthrodesis sites protects bone graft and prevents loss and dislodgement.
- If there is difficulty placing lamina spreaders into the sinus, then more release and débridement of the sinus should be performed.
- Preparation of the sinus tarsi on the calcaneus and the tarsal canal on the talus augments the triple arthrodesis by incorporation of these extra-articular areas.
- In some deformities, there is lateral translation of the calcaneus in addition to rotational deformities. This may require medial translation of the calcaneus to correct the deformity. This may be the key when there is difficulty reducing the CC and TN joints.
- Speed of and confidence in radiographic signs of bone healing postoperatively are proportional to the removal of subchondral bone.
- Although varus hindfoot deformity is associated with peroneal pathology, there can be peroneal tendon tears in valgus deformity because of impingement.[6]

- The order of fixation should always be respected, ST then TN then CC.
- In a large deformity correction, it is unlikely that the medial and lateral column will be balanced. It is often necessary to bone graft to compensate and bridge the defect (usually at the CC joint).
- The position of the heel is achieved primarily by rotation of the calcaneus relative to the talus.
- The best way to judge abduction and adduction alignment is by inspecting the lateral border of foot from the plantar surface.
- Experience is essential and there are no templates such as in total joint arthroplasty.
- Correction of alignment is crucial, followed by appropriate bone grafting of defects.
- While some have advocated double arthrodesis of the ST and TN joints, that technique is contingent on the absence of CC joint pain and arthritis, and the ability to achieve equivalent deformity correction despite omitting the CC arthrodesis. While surgical decisions must be tailored to each patient, triple arthrodesis is the most proven and reported technique for achieving correction of severe and, especially of rigid, hindfoot deformity.[7] Decision-making benefits by adhering to anatomic and biomechanical principles. The "triple joints" function as a complex unit.

PITFALLS AND COMPLICATIONS

- Insufficiently prepped joints, especially with sclerotic bone, will not fuse.
- Wound healing is the most common complication. Be mindful of soft tissue handling, particularly on the lateral side.
- Overcorrection of preoperative hindfoot valgus is poorly tolerated because of lateral overload.
- Hindfoot deformities can produce secondary deformity at the ankle.
- Compliance with non–weight bearing after arthrodesis really matters. Early weight bearing can cause fixation failure and nonunion.
- Identify secondary changes at the midfoot, which may alter forefoot position secondary to hindfoot deformity correction.
- Identify lateral ligamentous instability, which can lead to varus deformity at the ankle after triple arthrodesis (Fig. 32.19).

POSTOPERATIVE CARE

- The patient is placed into a well-padded splint. Initial follow-up is typically performed at 2 weeks for conventional radiographs and removal of sutures. At that time, patients are transitioned into a cast for another 4 weeks with continued non–weight bearing. They are next evaluated at the 6-week postoperative mark with radiographs. At that time, based on radiographic progression and

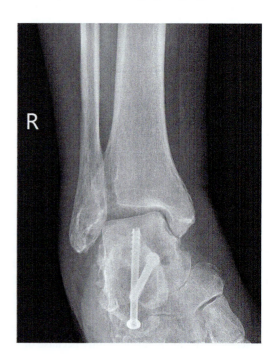

FIGURE 32.19 AP ankle demonstrating the development of varus instability due to lateral ligamentous instability status post revision triple arthrodesis.

intraoperative findings, the patient is typically allowed to begin weight bearing in a controlled ankle motion type boot. This is a gradual process with approximately 25% weight bearing the first week followed by 50% the following week, etc. Physical therapy is typically only ordered for patients who are having difficulty progressing on their own.

OUTCOMES

Triple arthrodesis is a powerful tool for correction of hindfoot deformity, and for a predictable relief of the pain of hindfoot arthritis. It is a durable, long-lasting construct, has versatility for alignment in all three planes, and is applicable to a wide range of pathologies.[7]

In a 2000 study by Pell et al, 111 patients undergoing a total of 132 triple arthodeses for a variety of pathologies including cavovarus and PCFD were followed for a minimum of 2 years postoperatively with an average follow-up of 5.7 years. Ankle arthritis was more severe postoperatively than preoperatively, with 69 patients (60%) demonstrating signs of progressive arthritis of the ankle joint ($P < .01$). Overall satisfaction was 8.3 out of a 10 point scale, with 101 of the 111 patients (91%) stating that they would have the procedure performed again under similar circumstances. One of the most important conclusions of this study was that there was an association between patient satisfaction and improved postoperative alignment, which highlights the need for careful attention to deformity correction intraoperatively. With regard to complications, there were only three nonunions (2%) and four superficial wound problems (3%).[8] The TN joint is the most common site of nonunion with nonunion rates reported between 10% and 20%.[9]

Triple arthrodesis performed for PCFD has been shown to lead to improvements in clinical outcomes scores, alignment, and pain. Coetzee and Hansen demonstrated a 31° improvement in lateral talus-first metatarsal angle, 25° improvement in AP talus-first metatarsal angle, and 11° improvement in calcaneal pitch with triple arthrodesis ($P < .01$). Average time to bony fusion was 14 weeks (9 to 21 weeks). There were two delayed unions and four wound problems with delayed healing and one superficial infection. AOFAS scores improved from 30 points preoperatively to 74 points postoperatively, and pain score improved from 11/40 to 33/40.[10]

A dual incision (medial and lateral) approach in a cadaveric study demonstrated improved access to the CC joint without disruption of the vascular supply to the talus. The single medial incision approach did not afford adequate access to the CC joint for cartilage removal and also consistently disrupted the blood supply to the talar body. We recommend the dual incision technique discussed in detail, as above.[11]

In summary, triple arthrodesis affords unparalleled deformity correction in all three planes and allows for a durable correction in the appropriate patient. Careful preoperative examination and planning are keys to a positive surgical outcome.

REFERENCES

1. Wapner KL. Triple arthrodesis in adults. *J Am Acad Orthop Surg.* 1998;6(3):188-196.
2. Louwerens JWK. Triple arthrodesis. *Techniques Foot Ankle Surg.* 2012;11(4):181-188.
3. Thevendran G, Wang C, Pinney SJ, Penner MJ, Wing KJ, Younger ASE. Nonunion risk assessment in foot and ankle surgery. *Foot Ankle Int.* 2015;36(8):901-907.
4. Ishikawa SN, Murphy GA, Richardson EG. The effect of cigarette smoking on hindfoot fusions. *Foot Ankle Int.* 2002;23(11):996-998.
5. Savory KM, Wulker N, Stukenborg C, Alfke D. Biomechanics of the hindfoot joints in response to degenerative hindfoot arthrodeses. *Clin Biomech.* 1998;13(1):62-70.
6. Danna NR, Brodsky JW. Diagnosis and operative treatment of peroneal tendon tears. *Foot Ankle Orthop.* 2020;5(2):2473011420910407.
7. Saltzman CL, Fehrle MJ, Cooper RR, Spencer EC, Ponseti I. Triple arthrodesis. *J Bone Joint Surg Am.* 1999;81(10):1391-1402.
8. Pell RF, Myerson MS, Schon LC. Clinical outcome after primary triple arthrodesis. *J Bone Joint Surg Am.* 2000;82(1):47-57.
9. Klassen LJ, Shi E, Weinraub GM, Liu J. Comparative nonunion rates in triple arthrodesis. *J Foot Ankle Surg.* 2018;57(6):1154-1156.
10. Coetzee JC, Hansen ST. Surgical management of severe deformity resulting from posterior tibial tendon dysfunction. *Foot Ankle Int.* 2001;22(12):944-949.
11. Phisitkul P, Haugsdal J, Vaseenon T, Pizzimenti MA. Vascular disruption of the talus. *Foot Ankle Int.* 2013;34(4):568-574.

PART SEVEN
ANKLE OSTEOARTHRITIS

33 Ankle Distraction Arthroplasty

Austin T. Fragomen and Brian Joseph Page

INTRODUCTION

Ankle distraction arthroplasty (ADA) and subtalar (ST) joint distraction are limb salvage options introduced to preserve arthritic joints in the lower extremity. These procedures mechanically unload arthritic joints to unlock the biological healing potential of subchondral bone and articular cartilage. Mechanically unloading an arthritic joint allows the patient's physiological healing potential to be optimized while preserving joint motion. ADA and ST joint distraction are utilized as an alternative to joint-sacrificing procedures (ie, ankle and/or ST arthrodesis, total ankle arthroplasty) to improve pain and function in patients with posttraumatic ankle arthritis.

Mechanically unloading an arthritic joint is a biomechanical treatment modality that initiates a healing response in subchondral bone and articular cartilage. This is accomplished through joint distraction, but it was initially performed in the hip[1] and was later trialed in the foot and ankle.[2,3] ADA was first introduced in 1995 by van Valburg and van Roermund in order to reverse clinical and radiographic findings commonly seen in posttraumatic ankle arthritis.[4] The procedure was performed by application of a circular external fixator spanning the ankle joint followed by gradual distraction across the joint until 5 mm of distraction was measured on radiographs. The external fixator was worn for 3 (or more) months to achieve the desired results. This group went on to popularize the technique and publish numerous reports on the benefits of joint distraction including radiographic improvement, reduction in subchondral bone sclerosis, and increase in joint space.[5] This was further supported by research that identified positive changes in proteoglycan metabolism and a decrease in joint inflammation.[6] A randomized trial found that joint débridement combined with distraction produced superior results when compared with débridement alone.[7] This patient population yielded consistent results with success in the 70% range.[8,9]

The mechanism of action for joint distraction has been studied clinically and in animal research. The procedure has been observed to reduce the density of the sclerotic subchondral bone and improve subchondral cysts as seen on radiographs[5] and computed tomography (CT) scan.[10] The radiographic joint space has been noted to increase and be sustained for years after completion of the procedure.[5,11] Subchondral cysts have been seen to decrease in size and ossify on pre- and postoperative CT scans, which has been correlated with clinical improvement.[10] Magnetic resonance imaging (MRI) changes have also been observed to increase joint space.[11,12] Joint distraction seems to enable the arthritic ankle's natural ability to regenerate, which may be due to a combination of the absence of mechanical stress with intermittent fluid pressure created within the joint. Distraction has also been shown to alter cartilage proteoglycan metabolism including an increase in proteoglycan synthetic activity.[13,14] A cadaver model analyzed the amount of distraction required for treatment and determined that a distraction gap of 5.8 mm measured on weight-bearing radiographs would ensure an absence of articular contact in an average weight person.[15] However, it is not currently known if the absence of joint contact is required to obtain good results. Most studies cite that 5 mm of joint space is adequate to achieve lasting pain relief.

INDICATIONS AND CONTRAINDICATIONS

Posttraumatic osteoarthritis is the primary indication for ADA. There have been reports of using joint distraction to treat hemophilic arthritis.[16] To predict the suitable candidate for joint distraction, various risk factors have been analyzed including female sex, osteonecrosis, ankle joint deformity, obesity, and age. Female sex has been found to slightly reduce success relative to males,[17,18] and osteonecrosis of the talus was associated with poorer outcome.[17] Patients with ankle joint deformity greater than 5° and obesity were seen to negatively affect outcome.[19] However, when the deformity is corrected with supramalleolar osteotomy (SMO) at time of distraction, the results improved dramatically.[20] Increasing age has not been seen to correlate with failure.[9,21] In general, patients with severe ankle stiffness are treated with an arthrodesis procedure. Preoperative ankle range of motion (ROM) has not been associated with a poor outcome.

There are not any absolute contraindications, but there are relative contraindications. It is not recommended to perform distraction arthroplasty in patients with inflammatory arthritis unless the ankle has clear signs of an osteoarthritic component. Distraction arthroplasty surgery is contraindicated in an actively infected joint. Once appropriate treatment for the infection is addressed, a staged approach for postinfectious arthritis may be appropriate. Distraction surgery does not appear to facilitate revascularization of osteonecrosis of the talus or tibial plafond, but distraction can improve surface cartilage and can be considered on a case-by-case basis. Other relative contraindications include bone collapse, gross deformity of the talus, and ankle arthrofibrosis. If the talus and plafond have maintained their general shape, then necrotic areas may be amenable to autografting or even local vascularized pedicle grafting to reperfuse the damaged bone. However, in severely stiff joints, arthrodesis may be the optimal treatment modality.

PREOPERATIVE PLANNING

Preoperative planning for distraction involves a thorough clinical and radiological examination. The addition of advanced imaging including CT and/or MRI can aid in surgical planning in select patients. Preoperative planning begins with a history of the patient's injury, surgeries, limitations, and pain. It is also important to note the locations of previous incisions and any remaining hardware. Physical examination helps to determine where the pain is located and helps correlate imaging findings with clinical findings. It is helpful to have a mental plan of pain locations (ie, ankle joint, ST joint, midfoot, etc.) prior to a thorough review of the available imaging. If there is a question of which joint is the pain generator, selective targeted intra-articular injection may be used.

Radiographs should be evaluated for osteophyte location and correlated with the clinical examination to determine the optimal surgical approach. Large posterior osteophytes may be asymptomatic, or they may be painful and limit plantarflexion. In patients with concern for areas of avascular necrosis or osteochondral defects, advanced imaging may aid in planning. Lastly, joint alignment should be evaluated and considered for surgical planning. This may be addressed with an SMO.

SURGICAL TECHNIQUE

Ankle Distraction Arthroplasty

An anterior approach to the ankle joint provides the best exposure for osteophyte resection and reshaping of the anterior ankle joint. However, each patient must be considered on a case-by-case basis considering their symptomatology and location of osteophytes. In patients with posterior osteophytes, a posterolateral or posteromedial approach may be best. However, an anterior approach provides excellent access to the subchondral bone for drilling and bone marrow injection, microfracture, and open grafting of large subchondral cysts. Additionally, osteophyte excision may be performed arthroscopically if preferred. However, large anterior osteophytes are common and are difficult to safely address arthroscopically. In patients with minimal osteophytes, distraction may be performed in isolation without an open arthrotomy.

The joint can be minimally débrided,[7] or aggressive removal of osteophytes and fibrous tissue[22] with routine microfracture or subchondral drilling[17] can be performed (Fig. 33.1). Ankle contracture

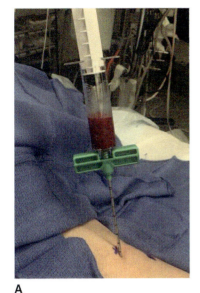
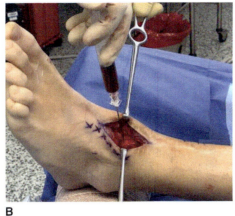
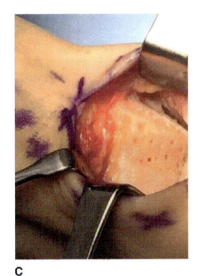

FIGURE 33.1 Ankle distraction arthroplasty (ADA) biologics: **(A)** bone marrow is aspirated form the iliac crest and later centrifuged to produce concentrated stem cells; **(B)** open arthrotomy with osteophyte resection and subchondral drilling is performed, and the stem cells are then injected into the subchondral bone under pressure; **(C)** microfracture of the talar surface is a popular treatment for ankle osteoarthritis and is often paired with ADA.

with a tight gastrosoleus tendon should be addressed to achieve the appropriate distraction and allow for ankle ROM.[17,22,23] This can be done with a percutaneous lengthening of the Achilles or using a gastrosoleus recession depending on the etiology of the contracture. Bone marrow aspirate concentrate has been shown to improve clinical results, and microfracture may negatively impact results, but that is debated.[24] Recombinant human growth hormone,[25] stem cell injection,[23] and hyaluronic acid have all been trialed to improve the outcomes of ankle distraction without any direct comparisons. Platelet-rich plasma may improve results over distraction alone.[26]

There are several technical considerations in ADA to ensure safety and maintain diastasis throughout treatment, specifically patient size and stiffness of the ankle should be considered. These two factors increase the force needed to be generated by the external fixator to distract the joint. More fixation should be used in larger patients to counter the increased force on the external fixator. The external fixator can be constructed to be a fixed/static fixator or to be an articulated fixator with hinges to allow for ankle ROM. For the latter, the accuracy of the placement of the axial joints in accordance with the axis of flexion/extension of the ankle joint is paramount (Fig. 33.2). However, literature reports on the optimal construct are contradictory; both constructs seem to achieve similar results.[21,27] There has been no evidence that 3 months of ankle distraction, fixed or hinged, is associated with long-term stiffness of the ankle or ST joint. In fact, it has been shown that preoperative ROM is equal to postoperative ROM on average.[9]

The author's preferred mounting details for the ankle hinged frame have been previously described in the literature.[23] In patients with a concomitant coronal or sagittal plane malalignment, an SMO

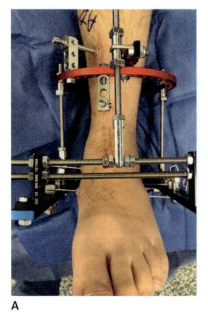
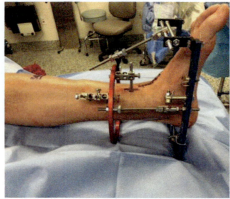
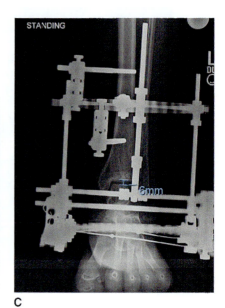
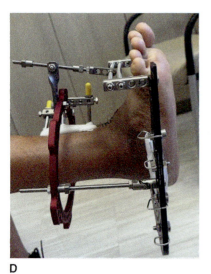
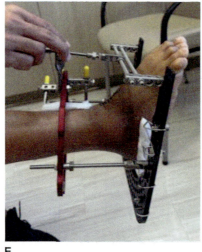
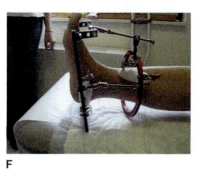

FIGURE 33.2 Ankle distraction arthroplasty (ADA) technique. **A.** A completed frame is shown on the front view. **B.** Lateral view of complete frame. The universal hinge allows for ankle motion immediately post-surgery. **C.** Distraction is applied gradually until 5 to 6 mm of space is seen in the tibiotalar joint on standing radiographs. **D.** Unlocked ADA frame in dorsiflexion. **E.** Unlocked ADA frame in plantarflexion. **F.** A video still showing a hinged ADA frame in motion.

is added to the procedure.[28] This procedure requires placement of an additional circular ring at the proximal tibia, with the distraction tibial ring closer to the ankle joint (Fig. 33.3). The SMO begins with the patient in a supine position on a radiolucent table. A bump is placed under the ipsilateral buttock to ensure that the limb is in neutral rotation (ie, patella facing upward). The external fixator is typically divided into two divisions: (1) the proximal hexapod frame for the SMO and deformity correction and (2) the distal ankle distraction external fixator. These two divisions share the middle ring centered at the distal ankle joint. Upon completion of the distraction frame, the inferior foot ring may be removed to allow further healing at the SMO site. Further information is found below in the subsection titled, "Supramalleolar Osteotomy."

The application of the ankle distraction external fixator begins by choosing a tibial ring (proximal ring) that allows for two fingerbreadths of space circumferentially between the skin and the ring (see Fig. 33.2). The medial malleolus and the anterior and posteromedial border of the distal tibia are palpated and marked. The proximal ring is then secured with a minimum of two 6-mm hydroxyapatite-coated pins.[29,30] The first pin is placed approximately 6 cm proximal to the medial malleolus directly anterior in the tibial crest using a 4.8-mm drill bit. Intraoperative fluoroscopy is typically used to

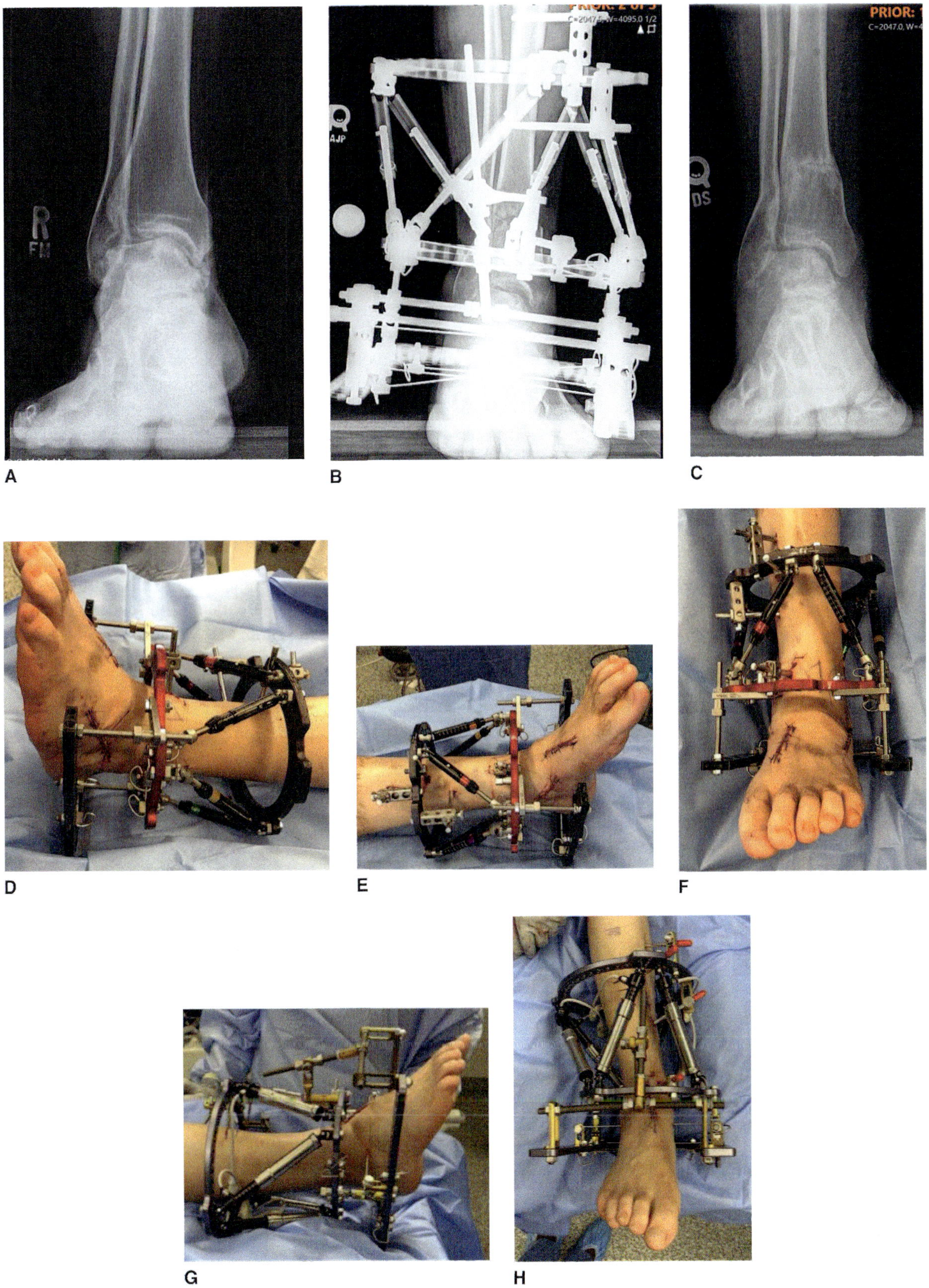

FIGURE 33.3 Supramalleolar osteotomy (SMO) with ankle distraction arthroplasty (ADA). **A.** Preoperative radiograph of varus ankle deformity and posttraumatic osteoarthritis. The majority of the varus originates from the joint line obliquity. **B.** Combined articulated ankle distraction frame and a hexapod frame for SMO was used to correct the foot alignment through the tibia. **C.** Postoperative radiographs with improved joint alignment and joint space. The tibia has been partially deformed to improve talar alignment, but a future total ankle replacement can still be carried out if needed. The SMO is performed first and then the ADA frame is attached to the distal ring. **D.** Lateral view of a completed SMO frame with static ADA frame. **E.** Medial view of completed SMO frame with static ADA frame. **F.** Anterior view of complete SMO frame with static ADA. **G.** Lateral view of a complete SMO frame with a hinged ADA frame. **H.** Anterior view of a complete SMO frame with a hinged ADA frame.

confirm the pin is placed orthogonally to the shaft of the tibia. The pin is then secured in place with a three-hole cube attached to the distal end of the proximal ring. Prior to final tightening of the pin to the ring, intraoperative fluoroscopy is used to make adjustments to the ring to ensure that it is positioned perpendicular to the axis of the tibial shaft. Typically, an additional one to two pins are placed on the proximal end of the proximal ring off axis from the first pin to improve stability of the ring (see Fig. 33.2A). A temporary K-wire is then inserted into the talus in line with the ankle joint axis of motion as a guide for the hinge location. This is done by placing it from the tip of the lateral malleolus exiting at the tip of the medial malleolus, in a posterolateral-to-anteromedial trajectory (Fig. 33.4). Universal hinges are then applied in line with the wire and then the wire is subsequently removed.

A footplate (distal ring) is then selected and secured 2 to 3 cm proximal to the plantar aspect of the foot. It is important to place the footplate parallel to the plantar aspect of the foot to not impede ambulation. Two opposing olive wires are then placed into the calcaneus and secured to the foot ring and tensioned. A talus wire is then placed from medial-to-lateral and attached to the foot ring and tensioned. A midtarsal wire maybe be inserted to control forefoot position and protect the talus wire from excess stress secondary to midfoot motion if desired. Two rods are used to close the foot ring, minimizing ring deflection with wire tensioning, prior to the tensioning of wires. A locking rod then connects the footplate to the proximal adjustable ring, which allows for gradual dorsiflexion to correct equinus contractures when needed and allows for ankle ROM. The ring is typically unlocked four times daily for ROM exercises (15 repetitions/session).

The ankle can be acutely distracted 3 mm in the operating room by turning the square nuts on the proximal ring. The safest method is to avoid all acute distraction. If equinus has been acutely corrected, then no distraction is applied in the operating room, due to the potential for nerve injury. Fluoroscopy is used to confirm that the distraction gap is congruent on the AP and lateral views. Further acute distraction is discouraged due to risk for neurologic traction injury. Acute correction of an equinus contracture is avoided for the same reason. In a patient with scarring over the tibial nerve, all distraction is performed gradually. Typically, the patient is evaluated on postoperative day 1 to assess for normal plantar sensation. Once confirmed, additional distraction is usually performed at 1-mm intervals on sequential postoperative days for a total of 7 mm of nut distraction. (Applying 7 mm of distraction to the nuts will usually yield 5 mm of new joint space on radiographs.) At the 2-week clinic visit, using calibrated radiographs, the distraction gap is assessed. If needed, additional distraction is prescribed to the patient at home at 1 mm/day to minimize nerve traction injury.

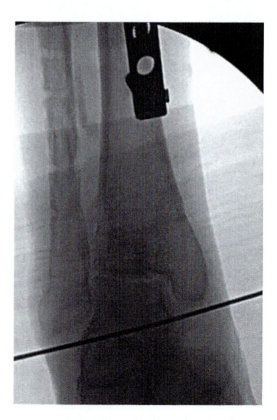

FIGURE 33.4 Wire placement for hinge.

33 Ankle Distraction Arthroplasty

A biomechanical study found that a relative increase of 5.8 mm of joint space should be obtained relative to the preoperative standing radiograph to ensure that the articular surfaces of the tibial plafond and talar body do not come in contact during weight bearing.[15]

The patient is typically allowed full weight bearing as tolerated with crutches immediately postoperatively. The neutral position (ie, ankle dorsiflexion) is marked on the hinge so that the patient can lock the frame in the appropriate position when not performing ROM exercises. The physical therapist teaches the patient how to unlock the hinge to perform active-assisted ROM exercises of the ankle joint with a foot strap. However, once patients are comfortable, they are encouraged to ambulate with the frame's hinge unlocked. Unfortunately, there is not a reliable means of allowing ST ROM during treatment. Animal models support the use of the frame in distraction for at least 8 weeks, and no added benefit has been seen beyond 12 weeks.[6,31] It is our practice to leave the frame on for approximately 12 weeks.

Subtalar Distraction

Subtalar distraction (SD) arthroplasty is a nice option for patients with ST arthritis wanting to avoid arthrodesis. It has gained popularity for treating ST joint osteoarthritis in younger patients who do not want to give up hindfoot mobility. This is common in rock climbers who have sustained calcaneus fractures and have developed posttraumatic arthritis of the posterior facet but want to continue climbing, which requires lateral motion at the ST joint. Fusion is unacceptable in this and other populations (Fig. 33.5).

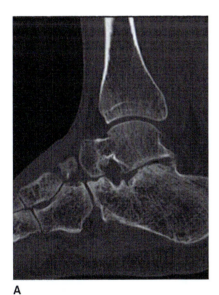
A

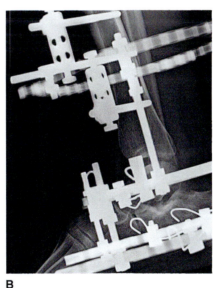
B

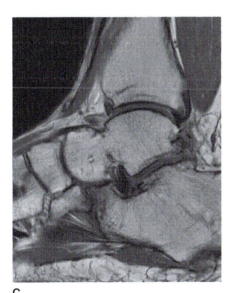
C

FIGURE 33.5 Subtalar distraction frame. This 40-year-old male sustained a calcaneus fracture while rock climbing and developed debilitating subtalar (ST) joint arthritis. **A.** The preoperative CT scan shows moderate posterior facet degeneration. **B.** ST joint distraction was performed by distracting both the ankle and posterior facet joints. **C.** An MRI performed 1 year after surgery shows restoration of much of the ST cartilage, which correlated with great improvement in pain.

Contrary to ADA in SD, typically the posterior facet is approached via a sinus tarsi approach. A Hintermann retractor can be utilized to distract the ST joint to aid in visualization and provide space for microfracture and/or subchondral drilling. There is also the option to inject bone marrow aspirate in the subchondral bone and the ST joint as in ADA. Interestingly, the ST joint often distracts unintentionally in the normal course of ADA. This is one of the reasons to add a talus wire to prevent ST widening when performing ankle distraction. In select cases, a talar wire is not placed in ankle distraction to allow for distraction of the ankle and ST joints (Fig. 33.6).

Subtalar joint distraction arthroplasty is not performed with a hinge. Frame construction with a hinge for the ST joint would be extremely technically challenging considering it would require the external fixator to include the ankle joint. To mount a ST frame, two wires are placed into the talus and two wires into the calcaneus. The first talus wire is placed transversely through the talar neck anterior to the medial and lateral malleoli. The second talus wire is placed from the posterolateral (just posterior to the peroneal tendons) and exits anteromedially avoiding the talonavicular joint. The midfoot can be added for increased stability if desired.

To finely control distraction of the ankle and ST joints separately, a special frame using two-foot rings can be utilized. This construct has a dedicated talus ring and a dedicated calcaneal ring. This allows control over the ankle and ST joints individually. The frame does not typically include hinges for the purpose of simplicity and to improve the efficiency of the distraction. This static frame is highly effective in achieving its goals.

Including the ankle provides the needed stability to achieve adequate distraction and will greatly increase patient comfort. Articulated ankle distraction is possible, but the talus ring used in SD occupies the typical location of the ankle hinges. This is achieved by building the frame outward with plates, but this weakens the construct's ability to achieve distraction. The author's preference

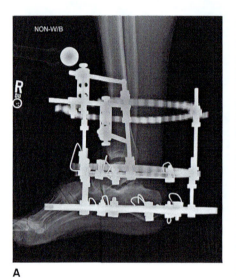
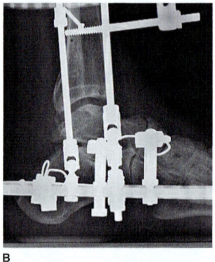
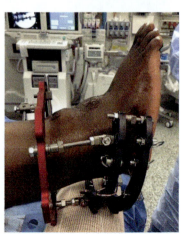

FIGURE 33.6 Subtalar distraction (SD) technique. **A.** Distraction of both the subtalar joint and the ankle joint can be achieved with great control using a double foot-ring setup allowing for individualized control over each joint. **B.** The talus neck wire helps control unwanted SD when using only one foot ring for ankle distraction. Casual SD occurs with this weak talar neck wire. **C.** Lateral view of SD frame.

is the double foot ring set up connected to a tibial ring without the use of hinges. This is a strong, nonarticulated frame, which is quite effective at obtaining and maintaining distraction of the ankle and ST joints.

The ST joint is distracted for 12 weeks, as in ankle distraction. Acute distraction is limited to avoid nerve injury as well. SD is applied gradually typically at a rate of 1 mm/day for up to 7 days. The ankle joint needs to be distracted as well to avoid compression of the ankle joint secondary to distraction of the ST joint. Serial radiographs are obtained at 2-week intervals to ensure that the desired distraction has been achieved and maintained in both joints.

Subtalar joint distraction outcomes are similar to ankle distraction outcomes. Most patients have good results with significant improvement in ankle arthritis scores (AOS) in pain and disability. Positive outcomes are seen at a minimum of 1 year postoperatively.[3]

Supramalleolar Osteotomy

As mentioned earlier, an SMO may be combined with distraction arthroplasty when significant deformity is present.[17,28] This technique is used to correct varus, valgus, and sagittal plane distal tibia and intra-articular deformity with reliable functional improvement.[20,32] An acute, opening wedge osteotomy is an option but requires a large incision with extensive soft tissue stripping. The choice of bone graft is important with acute correction. Allograft wedges are readily available but are slow to incorporate with native bone. Autograft unites much more quickly and reliably; it is the preferred bone graft for this method. However, distraction across the ankle creates tension at the osteotomy site in cases where a plate is used, which has the potential to negatively affect bone healing. The author's preferred method is to perform a percutaneous SMO and gradual correction technique using an all-frame stabilization technique.

SMO shows reliable healing when performed using a corticotomy technique and gradual correction. A latency of 10 days is standard, and the correction is performed at 0.5 mm/day. Patients perform the adjustments at home and follow up every 2 weeks. At the completion of the correction program, the foot and ankle are evaluated for radiographic and clinical alignment. Clinical confirmation that the foot is flat on the ground is important. Upon completion of the hexapod schedule, if any further deformity remains, a residual schedule is prescribed to the patient to fine-tune the correction.

A fibular osteotomy is recommended in addition to an SMO to ensure that the tibia can realign without obstruction into its ideal position. An intact fibula may block the correction and/or compress the mortise during SMO correction. This is commonly performed at the start of the case with skin closure for ease once the frame application proceeds.

Careful planning on how much to correct the alignment of the distal tibia must be considered during the preoperative planning. If the deformity is entirely in the distal tibia, then a full correction is optimal and will not negatively impact the ankle joint or future procedures; however, if the deformity is secondary to joint obliquity, an undercorrection may be optimal. This is because if the deformity is being corrected through the tibia, then the SMO will have to deform the tibia in order to reorient the joint. This osteotomy is challenging because it requires translation at the tibia osteotomy site and malaligns the malleoli. This will make future total ankle replacement more complicated. SMO for an intra-articular deformity may make a total ankle replacement impossible. Commonly, ankle deformity will be partially due to distal tibia malalignment and partially due to joint obliquity. SMO can be used to overcorrect the tibia deformity to improve the articular alignment. The surgeon must consider how much overcorrection of the tibia is acceptable to prevent jeopardizing future prosthetic arthroplasty (see Fig. 33.3).

Hinges are a challenge to position when combined with an SMO hexapod frame (see Fig. 33.3). A good principle is to create two frames with a shared central ring—a proximal SMO frame and a distal distraction frame. After setting up the proximal hexapod, it is ideal to connect the distal tibial ring with two points of fixation prior to set the hinges. After this is complete, additional fixation can be added to provide the necessary stability. This technique will help from blocking holes in the ring that need to be used for hinge placement. Another option is to not use hinges and create a fixed/static frame when performing an SMO with distraction.

Careful consideration to the order of distraction adjustments is important when combining SMO with distraction. Attempts at simultaneous ankle distraction and osteotomy adjustments may place too much tension on the nerves and/or may be too painful for the patient. The author's preference is to perform ankle distraction at 1 mm/day for approximately 7 days starting the day after surgery and once complete start the osteotomy frame adjustments on days 7 to 10.

PEARLS AND PITFALLS

Pearls

- The distraction can be placed across the joint acutely or gradually. While it is tempting to simply "crank" the frame out 5 to 6 mm in the operating room, there is no patient feedback to notify the surgeon if the tibial nerve is being overstretched.
- Ankle ROM is typically started the day after surgery by unlocking the hinged external fixator.
- Weight bearing as tolerated ambulation can be started immediately after surgery. Some patients prefer to keep the external frame unlocked during ambulation, which is safe.
- Patients should be given a modified postoperative shoe to walk. Alternatively, a walking plate maybe be bolted underneath the foot to allow weight bearing without the foot touching the ground or experiencing any load.[33]
- The talus should be captured with a wire to prevent unwanted SD. This is especially important when correcting concomitant equinus with ankle distraction. This wire is typically inserted transversely through the talar neck. A very powerful option is inserting a talus wire posterior to the fibula and exiting the anteromedial talus.
- Patients who need to stand at work will be well served working no more than 3 days a week throughout the 3-month distraction period. The days-off will be best spent with the leg elevated.
- Nonsteroidal anti-inflammatory drugs (NSAIDs) and acetaminophen are typically adequate to provide pain control and help reduce the need for narcotics. It is preferred to have patients stop NSAIDs after 1 month if possible due to unknown effects on tissue regeneration.
- The external fixator is kept on the leg for a total of 3 months at which point it is removed in the operating room under sedation. After removal of the external fixation, the patient is provided a walking boot for support for 2 to 6 weeks.
- Patients are followed every 3 months for the first year and then once yearly afterward. Most patients reach peak improvement 1 to 2 years post-frame removal. It is helpful to council the patient prior to the procedure on this expectation. Radiographs are obtained at these visits where joint space is measured and subchondral bone sclerosis is noted (see Fig. 33.8).

Pitfalls

- When correcting concomitant equinus with ankle distraction, no acute distraction should be performed to mitigate the risk for tibial nerve neuropraxia.
- Improper hinge placement may make ankle ROM painful and/or impossible. Careful attention to this step is paramount.
- The hinges may rotate when applying distraction to the ankle joint. A wrench should hold the hinge rotation during distraction.
- Patients must be able to apply distraction to their frame and make any necessary adjustments in the postoperative period. It is prudent to only recruit compliant patients to maximize the success of the procedure.
- Deep vein thrombosis (DVT) prophylaxis for the first month, while the patient is increasing mobility, is important to decrease the risk for DVT.
- A standard talus pin through the talar neck may be inadequate to resist SD. Placing a stronger posterolateral to anteromedial wire will better stabilize the talus (Fig. 33.7).
- A tibial nerve stretch injury is possible during distraction. A thorough neurovascular examination at each encounter is necessary. A numb plantar foot suggests tibial neuropraxia and can be treated with immediate reversal of distraction. If sensation returns relatively quickly, a short break from distraction is recommended followed by careful distraction as needed. If sensation does not return, then the tarsal tunnel should be released surgically (Fig. 33.7C). A tibial nerve injury can also result from acute equinus correction and acute ankle distraction simultaneously.
- Broken wires and loosening of the half pins can occur but are not common. Broken wires can be managed in the office by reattachment to the ring (or removal if not critical). Adding an extra wire at the index surgery will allow for later removal of a broken wire in the case of wire fracture without affecting frame stability.
- Loss of distraction can occur later in treatment, which will be recognized by a reduction in joint space on radiographs. Monitoring the joint space with calibrated radiographs serially throughout the treatment is paramount for addressing this issue.

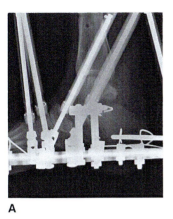 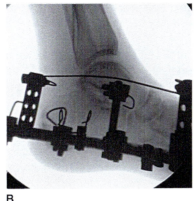 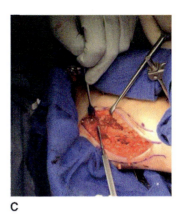

FIGURE 33.7 Complications. **A.** The talus neck wire may be inadequate to protect the subtalar (ST) joint for equinus correction and ankle distraction. Here, the posterior facet is seen with significant widening. **B.** For high stress cases, a stronger posterolateral to anteromedial wire will better stabilize the talus. The wire was added in the same patient to regain control of the ST joint. **C.** Injury to the tibial nerve is possible with rapid distraction. Open tarsal tunnel release may be required if acute ankle distraction results in recalcitrant tibial neuralgia. The instrument is pointing to the tibial nerve in the image above.

POSTOPERATIVE MANAGEMENT

All patients should be evaluated on postoperative day 1 and subsequent days to assess for normal plantar sensation. Once confirmed, additional distraction is usually performed at 1-mm intervals on sequential postoperative days for a total of 7 mm of nut distraction (applying 7 mm of distraction to the nuts will usually yield 5 mm of new joint space on radiographs). Typically, patients are made weight bearing as tolerated with crutches immediately postoperatively. This can be performed on a hinged frame, either in the locked or unlocked position, or on a static frame. On a hinged frame, the neutral position (ie, ankle dorsiflexion) is marked on the hinge so that the patient can lock the frame in the appropriate position when not performing ROM exercises. While in the hospital, the physical therapist teaches the patient how to unlock the hinge to perform active-assisted ROM exercises of the ankle joint with a foot strap.

Serial radiographs are obtained at 2-week intervals to ensure that the desired distraction has been achieved and maintained in both joints. At the 2-week clinic visit, using calibrated radiographs, the distraction gap is assessed. If needed, additional distraction is prescribed to the patient at home at 1 mm/day to minimize nerve traction injury. The ankle or ST joint is distracted for approximately 12 weeks at which point the frame is removed in the operating room and the pin sites are debrided.

RESULTS AND COMPLICATIONS

Ankle and ST joint distraction arthroplasty requires the use of an external fixator for 3 months. The risk of a pin site infection is high and should be expected. This should be discussed with the patient prior to the procedure. Fortunately, these irritations are easily treated with local pin care and with short courses of oral antibiotics. Prophylactic antibiotics are not recommended.[34] In addition to pin care, the patients must be able to apply distraction to their hexapod frame and make the necessary adjustments if an SMO is necessary. It is prudent to only recruit compliant patients to maximize the success of the procedure.

Postoperative swelling is common if patients are on their feet all day; elevation is required every day. Venous thrombosis is a potentially lethal complication, but it can usually be prevented with the routine use of aspirin for 1 month following surgery. The talar pin may not be strong enough to protect against SD. This can be alleviated by adding a stronger posterolateral to anteromedial wire, which will better stabilize the talus (see Fig. 33.7).

A tibial nerve stretch injury is possible but not well documented in the literature. Postoperatively, a thorough neurovascular examination should be performed on each encounter. A numb plantar foot suggests tibial neuropraxia and can be treated with immediate reversal of distraction. If sensation returns relatively quickly, a short break from distraction is recommended followed by careful distraction as needed. If sensation does not return, then the tarsal tunnel should be released surgically (Fig. 33.7C). A tibial nerve injury can also result from acute equinus correction and acute ankle distraction simultaneously.

Broken wires and loosening of the half pins can occur but are not common. Broken wires can be managed in the office by reattachment to the ring (or removal if not critical). Adding an extra wire at the index surgery will allow for later removal of a broken wire in the case of wire fracture without affecting frame stability. Loose pins can be seen at the time of frame removal and are benign. The distal tibia pin in cancellous bone tends to be most at risk for loosening. Adding a third pin at the index surgery will ensure no problems from loosening.

Loss of distraction can occur later in treatment, which will be recognized by a reduction in joint space on radiographs. Monitoring the joint space with calibrated radiographs serially throughout the

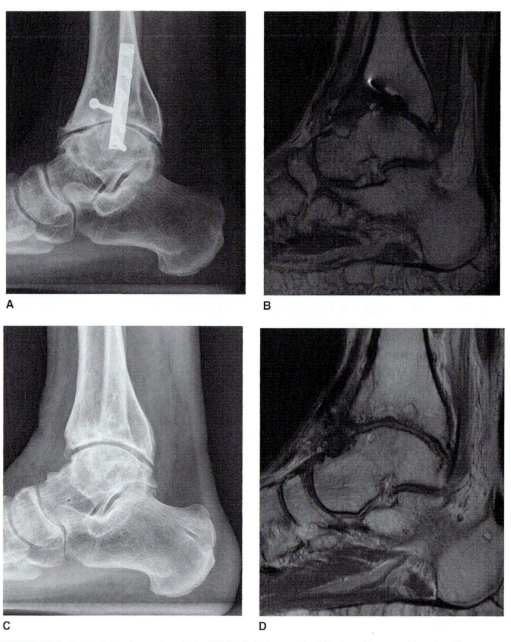

FIGURE 33.8 Ankle distraction arthroplasty (ADA) clinical example. This is a 40-year-old male with posttraumatic ankle osteoarthritis as seen on a lateral ankle radiograph **(A)** and on preoperative T2 sagittal MRI scan **(B)**. The patient underwent ADA. The radiographs taken 2 years post-surgery show an increase in tibiotalar joint space **(C)**. The T1 sagittal MRI taken 1-year post-frame removal shows an increase in joint space due to reparative cartilage growth **(D)**.

treatment is paramount for addressing this issue. Further distraction can be provided in the clinic, and the patient can be taught to apply further distraction at home. It is important to closely monitor the distraction as it not uncommon for this to occur late in the treatment (ie, 8 to 10 weeks).

Ankle distraction is a joint-preserving procedure that does not "burn any bridges" for future procedures. There is no permanent fusion of the articular surfaces or resection of the joint. If the benefits of the surgery wear off over time and the patient wishes to proceed with other treatment options, they are still able to receive a total ankle replacement or arthrodesis. Additionally, they may undergo repeat distraction.

Most patients will experience an increase in joint space following surgery. Radiographs usually show improved joint space and resolution of subchondral cysts (Fig. 33.8).

REFERENCES

1. Judet R, Judet T. The use of a hinge distraction apparatus after arthrolysis and arthroplasty (author's transl). *Rev Chir Orthop Reparatrice Appar Mot.* 1978;64(5):353-365.
2. Dabash S, Buksbaum JR, Fragomen A, Rozbruch SR. Distraction arthroplasty in osteoarthritis of the foot and ankle. *World J Orthop.* 2020;11(3):145-157.
3. Ghasemi SA, Zhang D, Fragomen A, Rozbruch SR. Subtalar distraction arthroplasty with bone marrow aspirate concentrate (BMAC), preliminary results of a new joint preservation technique. *Foot Ankle Surg.* 2021;27(1):87-92.
4. van Valburg AA, van Roermund PM, Lammens J, et al. Can Ilizarov joint distraction delay the need for an arthrodesis of the ankle? A preliminary report. *J Bone Joint Surg Br.* 1995;77(5):720-725.
5. Marijnissen AC, Vincken KL, Viergever MA, et al. Ankle images digital analysis (AIDA): digital measurement of joint space width and subchondral sclerosis on standard radiographs. *Osteoarthritis Cartilage.* 2001;9(3):264-272.
6. van Valburg AA, van Roermund PM, Marijnissen AC, et al. Joint distraction in treatment of osteoarthritis (II): effects on cartilage in a canine model. *Osteoarthritis Cartilage.* 2000;8(1):1-8.
7. Marijnissen AC, Van Roermund PM, Van Melkebeek J, et al. Clinical benefit of joint distraction in the treatment of severe osteoarthritis of the ankle: proof of concept in an open prospective study and in a randomized controlled study. *Arthritis Rheum.* 2002;46(11):2893-2902.
8. Ploegmakers JJ, van Roermund PM, van Melkebeek J, et al. Prolonged clinical benefit from joint distraction in the treatment of ankle osteoarthritis. *Osteoarthritis Cartilage.* 2005;13(7):582-588.
9. Tellisi N, Fragomen AT, Kleinman D, O'Malley MJ, Rozbruch SR. Joint preservation of the osteoarthritic ankle using distraction arthroplasty. *Foot Ankle Int.* 2009;30(4):318-325.
10. Intema F, Thomas TP, Anderson DD, et al. Subchondral bone remodeling is related to clinical improvement after joint distraction in the treatment of ankle osteoarthritis. *Osteoarthritis Cartilage.* 2011;19(6):668-675.
11. Haleem AM, Galal S, Nwawka OK, et al. Short-term Results of magnetic resonance imaging after ankle distraction arthroplasty. *Strategies Trauma Limb Reconstr.* 2020;15(3):157-162.
12. Lamm BM, Gourdine-Shaw M. MRI evaluation of ankle distraction: a preliminary report. *Clin Podiatr Med Surg.* 2009;26(2):185-191.
13. Lafeber FPJG, Veldhuijzen JP, Van Roy JL, HuberBruning O, Bijlsma JWJ. Intermittent hydrostatic compressive force stimulates exclusively the proteoglycan synthesis of osteoarthritic human cartilage. *Br J Rheumatol.* 1992;31:437-442.
14. Van Valburg AA, Van Roy JLAM, Lafeber FPJG, Bijlsma JWJ. Beneficial effect of intermittent fluid pressure, of a low but physiological magnitude, on cartilage and inflammation in osteoarthritis. *J Rheumatol.* 1998;25:515-520.
15. Fragomen AT, McCoy TH, Meyers KN, Rozbruch SR. Minimum distraction gap: how much ankle joint space is enough in ankle distraction arthroplasty? *HSS J.* 2014;10(1):6-12.
16. Van Meegeren ME, Van Veghel K, De Kleijn P, et al. Joint distraction results in clinical and structural improvement of haemophilic ankle arthropathy: a series of three cases. *Haemophilia.* 2012;18(5):810-817.
17. Greenfield S, Matta KM, McCoy TH, Rozbruch SR, Fragomen A. Ankle distraction arthroplasty for ankle osteoarthritis: a survival analysis. *Strategies Trauma Limb Reconstr.* 2019;14(2):65-71.
18. Marijnissen AC, Hoekstra MC, Pré BC, et al. Patient characteristics as predictors of clinical outcome of distraction in treatment of severe ankle osteoarthritis. *J Orthop Res.* 2014;32(1):96-101.
19. Zhao H, Qu W, Li Y, et al. Functional analysis of distraction arthroplasty in the treatment of ankle osteoarthritis. *J Orthop Surg Res.* 2017;12(1):18.
20. Zhao HM, Wen XD, Zhang Y, et al. Supramalleolar osteotomy with medial distraction arthroplasty for ankle osteoarthritis with talar tilt. *J Orthop Surg Res.* 2019;14(1):120.
21. Nguyen MP, Pedersen DR, Gao Y, Saltzman CL, Amendola A. Intermediate-term follow-up after ankle distraction for treatment of end-stage osteoarthritis. *J Bone Joint Surg Am.* 2015;97(7):590-596.
22. Paley D, Lamm BM. Correction of the cavus foot using external fixation. *Foot Ankle Clin.* 2004;9(3):611-624. x
23. Bernstein M, Reidler J, Fragomen A, Rozbruch SR. Ankle distraction arthroplasty: indications, technique, and outcomes. *J Am Acad Orthop Surg.* 2017;25(2):89-99.
24. Gianakos AL, Haring RS, Shimozono Y, Fragomen A, Kennedy JG. Effect of microfracture on functional outcomes and subchondral sclerosis following distraction arthroplasty of the ankle joint. *Foot Ankle Int.* 2020;41(6):631-638.
25. Paley D, Lamm BM, Purohit RM, Specht SC. Distraction arthroplasty of the ankle—how far can you stretch the indications? *Foot Ankle Clin.* 2008;13(3):471-484. ix
26. Li K, Wang P, Nie C, Luo H, Yu D. The effect of joint distraction osteogenesis combined with platelet-rich plasma injections on traumatic ankle arthritis. *Am J Transl Res.* 2021;13(7):8344-8350.
27. Saltzman CL, Hillis SL, Stolley MP, Anderson DD, Amendola A. Motion versus fixed distraction of the joint in the treatment of ankle osteoarthritis: a prospective randomized controlled trial. *J Bone Joint Surg Am.* 2012;94(11):961-970.
28. Horn DM, Fragomen AT, Rozbruch SR. Supramalleolar osteotomy using external fixation with six-axis deformity correction of the distal tibia. *Foot Ankle Int.* 2011;32:986-993.
29. Moroni A, Cadossi M, Romagnoli M, Faldini C, Giannini S. A biomechanical and histological analysis of standard versus hydroxyapatite-coated pins for external fixation. *J Biomed Mater Res B Appl Biomater.* 2008;86(2):417-421.

30. Pizà G, Caja VL, González-Viejo MA, Navarro A. Hydroxyapatite-coated external-fixation pins. The effect on pin loosening and pin-track infection in leg lengthening for short stature. *J Bone Joint Surg Br.* 2004;86(6):892-897.
31. Yanai T, Ishii T, Chang F, Ochiai N. Repair of large full-thickness articular cartilage defects in the rabbit: the effects of joint distraction and autologous bone-marrow-derived mesenchymal cell transplantation. *J Bone Joint Surg Br.* 2005;87(5):721-729.
32. Nozaka K, Miyakoshi N, Kashiwagura T, et al. Effectiveness of distal tibial osteotomy with distraction arthroplasty in varus ankle osteoarthritis. *BMC Musculoskelet Disord.* 2020;21(1):31.
33. Barg A, Amendola A, Beaman DN, Saltzman CL. Ankle joint distraction arthroplasty: why and how? *Foot Ankle Clin.* 2013;18(3):459-470.
34. Fragomen AT, Miller AO, Brause BD, Goldman V, Rozbruch SR. Prophylactic postoperative antibiotics may not reduce pin site infections after external fixation. *HSS J.* 2017;13(2):165-170.

34 Open Ankle Arthrodesis Utilizing Anterior Plating

David M. Walton and James R. Holmes

INTRODUCTION

The ankle joint experiences the highest contact pressure and is the most commonly injured joint in the body; however, primary ankle osteoarthritis is relatively uncommon in comparison to other major lower extremity joints.[1] Tibiotalar arthritis occurs predominantly in the setting of previous trauma, chronic instability, sequelae of mechanical alignment abnormalities, and underlying inflammatory arthropathy.[1] Recent advances in total ankle arthroplasty (TAR) have resulted in increased utilization; however, ankle arthrodesis (AA) remains an excellent treatment option for patients with ankle arthritis, especially in the young and high-demand patients.

Historically, unacceptable rates of recurrent deformity and pseudoarthrosis with cast immobilization alone led to the development of external fixation, namely the Charnley external fixator. Subsequent evolution to internal fixation with transarticular screws resulted in improved patient tolerance, fewer complications, and improved union rates.[2] These techniques allow for compression of the arthrodesis site as well as an increase in construct stiffness with regard to bending and torsional forces. Transfibular and arthroscopically assisted approaches to arthrodesis have become popular in the past decades, typically stabilized with screws placed in a crossing fashion. However, the addition of anterior plating to transarticular screws, typically through an anterior incision, has been shown to increase construct rigidity.[3] Additionally, preservation of the fibula aids in construct stability, rotational reproducibility, and better allows for the possibility of later conversion to arthroplasty if indicated in the future. Utilization of this approach in TAR has increased surgeons experience and confidence for its use in arthrodesis.

INDICATIONS AND CONTRAINDICATIONS

Ankle arthrodesis is predominantly indicated for arthritis of the tibiotalar joint. Other common indications are profound and recalcitrant ankle instability, foot drop refractory to other measures, and talar avascular necrosis. TAR has been performed increasingly over the past several decades. However, AA continues to be preferred in a number of clinical situations. These include a relatively younger and more active patient, severe deformity, bone loss, history of previous infection, neuromuscular compromise, neuropathy, or other evidence of end-organ damage secondary to diabetes.[4]

Contraindications to AA include open wounds, active infections, inability to remain non–weight bearing and vascular insufficiency. In addition, relative contraindications include poorly controlled diabetes, active use of nicotine products, and patients with significant renal disease. Arthroplasty may be considered a better alternative in patients with contralateral AA, ipsilateral hindfoot arthrosis, or inflammatory arthropathies.

With regard to anterior plating of AA in particular, the biomechanical advantages of this construct may be mitigated if not nullified by patients with a poor anterior soft tissue envelope, posterior talar station, or insufficient talar neck area. In these situations, an alternative arthrodesis construct is likely more appropriate.

PREOPERATIVE PLANNING

Preoperative planning starts with a careful history and physical examination. Care should be taken to understand the etiology of the arthrosis as primary ankle osteoarthritis is relatively uncommon. When causal, underlying inflammatory disease should be optimized and immune-suppressing medications altered, when possible, in concert with other partners on the health care team. Previous ankle procedures, including incisions, soft tissue quality, and underlying hardware, must be evaluated as these may alter the preferred approach. In the setting of previous surgery or a history of open wounds or fractures, a workup to rule out potential persistent infection should be performed. This includes laboratory evaluation of C-reactive protein, erythrocyte sedimentation rate, white blood cell count with differential, and ankle aspiration for cell count and culture if indicated. Finally, and importantly, patient expectations should be addressed with a clear and mutual understanding of postoperative motion, acceptable activities, expected limitations, and functional status. The authors choose to demonstrate to the patients the contributions of motion from the hindfoot articulations compared to the tibiotalar joint in both the sagittal and coronal plane. Additionally, it is recommended that they restrict activity to low-impact exercise such as walking on level surfaces, cycling, and water aerobics. Careful explanation of progression of adjacent joint disease is also included.

Careful radiographic examination should include evaluation of the presence of deformity (Fig. 34.1). Coronal plane deformity can be mostly isolated to the soft tissues where there is minimal bone loss in

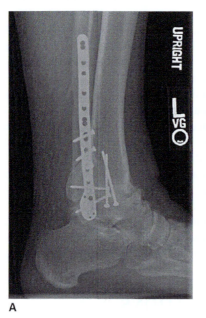
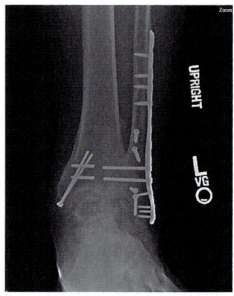
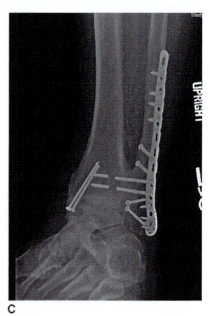

FIGURE 34.1 Lateral **(A)**, anteroposterior **(B)**, and mortise **(C)** standing radiographs of a patient with posttraumatic arthrosis with minimal coronal plane deformity, however, mild anterior talar station.

the setting of ligamentous unbalance. However, in long-standing instability or in the setting of trauma, the talus or tibial plafond may have significant bone loss, which often requires a combination of bone grafting and osteoplasty of the opposite plafond to achieve appropriate alignment. A direct lateral approach is often considered in cases of severe coronal plane deformity or bone loss as well as in settings with poor anterior soft tissues. In the sagittal plane, the talar station should be noted. Anterior talar station is relatively accommodated from an anterior approach; however, posterior talar station leads to difficulty with exposure joint preparation, reduction, and implant fixation anteriorly. The foot should also be assessed for deformity or instability as a proximal correction at the tibiotalar joint may lead to exacerbation or compensatory deformities, some of which may require concurrent intervention.

SURGICAL TECHNIQUE

Patient Positioning

The patient is positioned supine with the feet to the end of a radiolucent table. Fluoroscopy is planned to enter on the opposite side of the surgical extremity. The operative extremity is elevated above the contralateral extremity on blankets to allow clear lateral fluoroscopic evaluation. The contralateral extremity is examined to assess their normal ankle and hindfoot alignment. Typically, the authors prefer general anesthesia as they employ a thigh tourniquet, although other options such as spinal or regional anesthesia may be considered by surgeon preference and patient variables. After anesthesia is induced, a hip bump should be placed to align the tibial crest perpendicular to the floor. A nonsterile thigh tourniquet is placed, and the patient is prepped and draped in the usual sterile manner. The authors prefer to isolate the toes with a nonadhesive bandage.

Approach

The incision is planned 10 to 15 cm proximal to the tibiotalar joint lined 1 cm lateral to the tibial crest extending distally to the talonavicular joint (Fig. 34.2). Next, full-thickness skin flaps are created with care to identify the superficial peroneal nerve (SPN) as it courses from lateral to central near the tibiotalar joint line. This is often found in subcutaneous fat and should be carefully freed distally and retracted laterally (Fig. 34.3). Patients are counseled for the potential numbness in this distribution as on occasion a medial branch of the SPN is sacrificed for adequate exposure. At

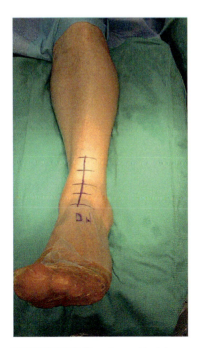

FIGURE 34.2 The planned incision has been marked lateral to the tibial crest from a point 10 cm proximal to the joint line extending distally to the talonavicular joint.

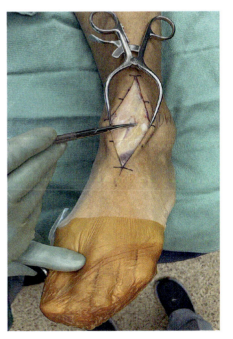

FIGURE 34.3 The superficial peroneal nerve is identified as it travels proximal-lateral to inferomedial, crossing the incision near the joint line.

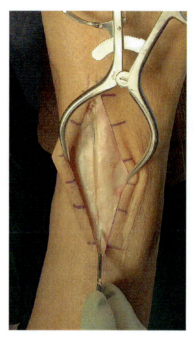

FIGURE 34.4 The extensor retinaculum is sharply divided though its thickest portions just lateral to the tibialis anterior sheath.

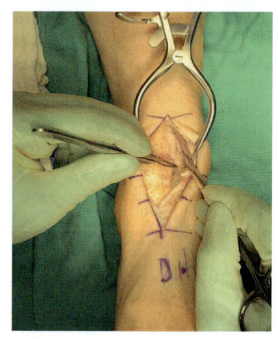

FIGURE 34.5 The deep neurovascular bundle is identified and gently retracted laterally. There are frequently veins, crossing transversely, as seen here, which may be cauterized and released to aid in mobilization of the bundle.

this point, the extensor retinaculum is exposed and should be sharply incised lateral to the tibialis anterior (TA) sheath over the extensor hallucis longus (EHL) tendon (Fig. 34.4). It can be noted that there is variable thickness to the retinaculum, and if possible, the incision should go through the thickest part to aid in closure. Care should be taken to avoid damaging the TA sheath. The interval between the TA and the EHL can be bluntly developed. The neurovascular bundle can then be identified under the EHL and gently retracted laterally (Fig. 34.5). There are typically crossing veins that can be cauterized medial to the bundle, which aids in its mobility.

A capsulotomy is then performed sharply along the distal tibia to the neck of the talus elevating the periosteum and the joint capsule as one layer. This is done medially and laterally to expose the entire tibiotalar joint including the medial and lateral gutters. A deep retractor is placed; the authors prefer a Gelpi to avoid pressure on the wound edges. An osteotome is then used to resect the anterior osteophytes from the distal tibia (Fig. 34.6). A more aggressive resection may be performed for better exposure or to allow improved contouring of an anterior plate.

At this time, coronal plane deformity can be addressed. In the setting of varus deformity, often a deltoid "peel" can be performed with care to avoid injury to the posterior tibial tendon. This is performed by extending the medial capsular layer subperiosteally, elevating to expose the medial malleolus. This is done proximally and distally to release contracted tissues.

Joint Preparation

The joint is distracted either by small laminar spreaders or a pin distractor to expose the surfaces of the distal tibia and talar body (Fig. 34.7). The residual cartilage is then removed. This can be done utilizing a chisel, curettes, curved osteotomes, or power burr. If a burr is chosen, reduced speed and continuous irrigation is recommended to avoid thermal damage. The subchondral bone is preserved to provide structural support. The medial and lateral gutters are similarly prepared, often without the need for distraction or with the distractor placed perpendicular to the gutter. The subchondral plate is then perforated to promote fusion; the authors prefer a 2.5-mm drill bit as it generates less heat than K-wires.[5] Reamings from the drill remain in the joint for bone graft. Next, a small osteotome is used to "fish scale" the surface connecting the drill holes (Fig. 34.8). In cases where bone graft is indicated or there is deformity, bone graft is then placed.

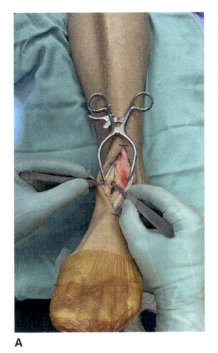
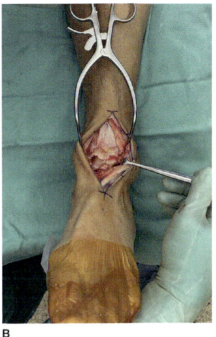
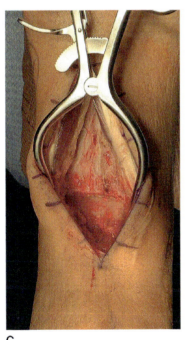

FIGURE 34.6 Sharply exposing the joint. **A.** Using an "inside-out" technique, the joint capsule is sharply elevated medially and laterally to the extend that both gutters are easily visualized and accessible. **B.** Exposure is satisfactorily complete when both the medial and lateral gutters are visualized. **C.** The anterior osteophytes are removed with an osteotome to improve access to the joint and aid in roduction and position of the plate.

Joint Reduction

Ideal position for tibiotalar arthrodesis is in neutral dorsiflexion, 5° to 7° of hindfoot valgus, and 5° to 10° of external rotation or to match the contralateral extremity.[6] This position should be intraoperatively confirmed both clinically and radiographically. Assessing the sagittal alignment can be misleading on lateral radiographs as there is combined motion from the hindfoot joints; the authors find it helpful to assess the talus position on preoperative standing lateral radiographs compared to fluoroscopic imaging combined with clinically positioning. The talar station should be neutral as determined by the central portion of the talar dome in line with the central axis of the tibia. The wear patterns of standard arthrosis may lead to anterior station, and commonly more posterior tibial plafond débridement is required for positioning of the talus to avoid increasing the lever arm by leaving the talus anteriorly. After appropriate alignment is achieved, the ankle should be temporarily

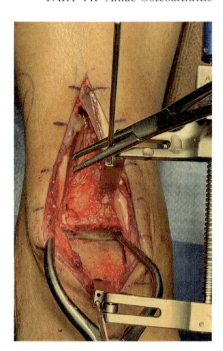

FIGURE 34.7 A pin distractor is placed to improve access to the joint. At this point, soft tissue retraction should be adjusted as the combination of two plane tension can damage tissues. Continued awareness of retraction, especially self-retaining, and the soft tissue envelope is important.

stabilized with crossed 2.5-mm K-wires from the central anterior tibia into the posterior talus and medal tibia to lateral talus. If the appropriate dorsiflexion is difficult to achieve, a gastrocnemius recession or achilles lengthening is performed as indicated.

Internal Fixation

There are several techniques for application of internal fixation while utilizing anterior plating for ankle fusion (Video 34.1). The authors prefer utilization of a posterolateral compression screw followed by compression and stabilization with an anterior plate. This technique secures the talus posteriorly to avoid anterior translation while providing initial compression. Subsequent compression anteriorly increases both compression and stability with less concern for gapping posteriorly with anterior plate compression. Some plating systems have specific guide arms to facilitate placement of compression screws that can be placed independent from the plate.

Approximate trajectory is drawn utilizing a surface K-wire in conjunction with fluoroscopy after confirming position (Fig. 34.9). Next, a 2-cm incision is made posteriorly between the peroneals and achilles tendon. This can be done with an assistant elevating the leg or a large towel bump under the heel. The subcutaneous tissue is bluntly divided with care to protect the sural nerve. Next, the deep fascia is penetrated bluntly, and deep blunt dissection is carried down to the posterior tibia. This location is confirmed fluoroscopically. Once the location is identified with manual compression on the ankle and maintaining appropriate position, a K-wire is placed. Fluoroscopy is used to confirm that it resides in appropriate position at the metaphyseal flare of the posterior tibia into the talar neck. After countersinking and measuring for the appropriate length, a compression or lag screw is placed

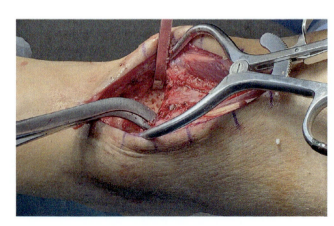

FIGURE 34.8 Joint preparation has been performed initially by fenestration with a 2.5-mm drill, and presently a small osteotome is being used to additionally "fish scale" the surface. The distractor has been swapped for lamina spreader.

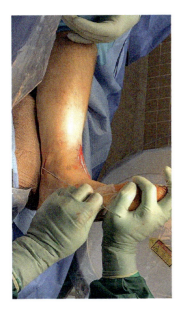 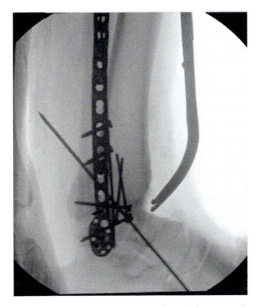

FIGURE 34.9 The trajectory of the posterolateral (PL) screw is planned and confirmed fluoroscopically.

(typically 6.5 or 7 mm in diameter), with care to remove the previous temporary K-wires prior to final compression. Position is again confirmed clinically and fluoroscopically (Fig. 34.10).

The anterior plate is then applied and pinned in place with an olive wire. The anterior tibia and talar necks can be contoured with a rongeur or osteotome to ensure optimal placement. Care should be taken to ensure that the holes intended for the talar neck are centered to allow best purchase as in many systems there are limited talar screw options. The next steps vary depending on the type of implant, either a transarticular lag screw is placed to aide in compression or the plate is fixated into the talus and a standard compression slot is utilized in the tibia (Fig. 34.11). Some systems allow a transarticular screw to be placed through the plate; this is often utilized to facilitate compression after initial plate fixation. Regardless of the order after initial fixation, radiographs should be obtained to ensure proper joint apposition, hardware position, and ankle position before the remaining holes are filled. Final radiographs are then obtained to ensure appropriate placement of all hardware, and care is taken to ensure none of the talar screws penetrate the subtalar joint (Fig. 34.12).

Screw configuration can vary widely depending on implant. If the posterolateral screw was not utilized, the authors opt for a medial transarticular leg screw centered on the long axis of the tibia into the talar body.

Closure

Closure is then performed in a standard layered manner with an attempt to cover the hardware with the capsule to avoid adhesions. The extensor retinaculum is closed to avoid tendon bowstringing, utilizing a careful approach closing through the most substantial tissue. Subcutaneous and skin closure is performed in a standard manner. Sterile dressings are then applied, and a well-padded three-sided splint is applied in neutral dorsiflexion.

PEARLS AND PITFALLS

- Examine the contralateral leg for alignment comparison.
- Bump the ipsilateral hip to minimize need for assistance.
- Generous proximal and distal exposure will allow distraction and plate placement.
- During exposure, open the extensor retinaculum strategically through the thickest portion for ease of closure.
- Fully expose the joint for ease in distraction and preparation.
- Use a pin distractor that will allow visualization of the entire joint during distraction.
- Use of a curved osteotome allows efficient débridement of posterior tibia plafond and talus.
- Maintain the subchondral architecture during preparation of the joint surfaces to avoid deformity or shortening during fixation and compression.

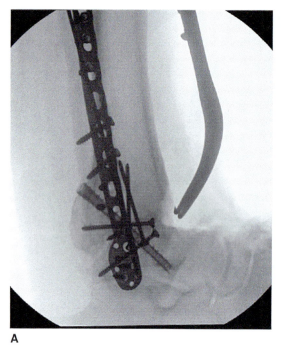
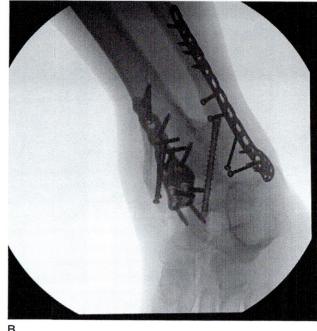
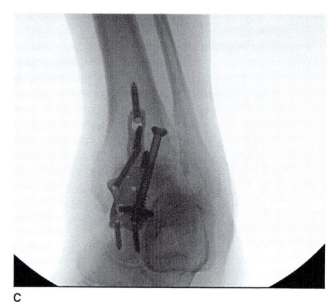

FIGURE 34.10 **A.** Position of the ankle is confirmed radiographically and clinically after placement of the PL compression screw. **B.** An oblique view of the ankle allows visualization of the posterior flare of the tibia noting the placement of the screw. **C.** Another case representation of a more anteroposterior view of the foot to confirm trajectory of the posterolateral screw into the talar neck.

- Use preoperative weight-bearing lateral ankle radiographs for assistance talar position when determining neutral dorsiflexion is challenging.
- Careful positioning of temporary K-wires allows for ease of lag screw insertion.
- Aligning the lateral malleolus and lateral heel pad allows for generally appropriate valgus.
- Avoid anterior subluxation or talar station by posterior joint preparation and posterolateral lag screw.
- If the talus continues to position anteriorly, place bumps under tibia and not the heel to provide posterior pressure to the foot and to translate talus posteriorly.
- Careful plate alignment prior to compression will avoid coronal deformity when compressing through the plate.
- When compressing through a compression slot, it can be helpful to utilize a screw longer than necessary for improved metaphyseal purchase and subsequently swap out after other holes are filled.

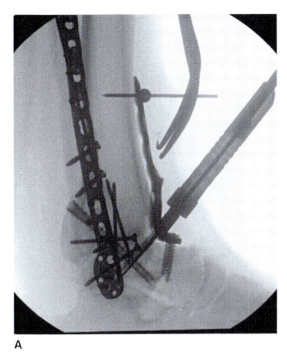 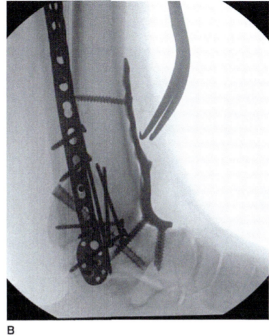

FIGURE 34.11 Plate fixation. **A.** The talar screws in this case are placed first, and position (plate and anatomic) is confirmed fluoroscopically. Portions of the distal tibia may be removed to aid in conforming to the plate contours providing more anatomic fit. **B.** Next, the compression slot is utilized to add further compression across the prepared joint.

POSTOPERATIVE MANAGEMENT

The patient remains in the intraoperative splint for 2 weeks with strict elevation. At 2 weeks, the splint is removed, and dressings are changed, and the wound is assessed. Non–weight-bearing ankle radiographs are obtained. Sutures are removed, and the patient is then placed into a short leg cast and

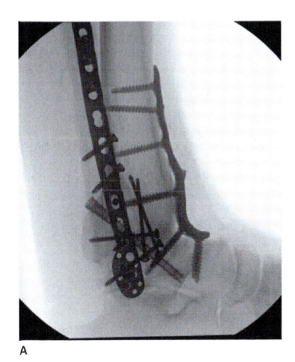 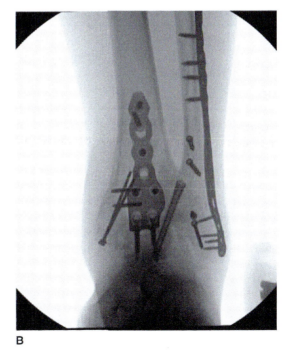

FIGURE 34.12 Final anteroposterior **(A)** and lateral **(B)** radiographs demonstrate appropriate position of the ankle arthrodesis and hardware, especially ensuring that the subtalar joint has not been violated by any screws.

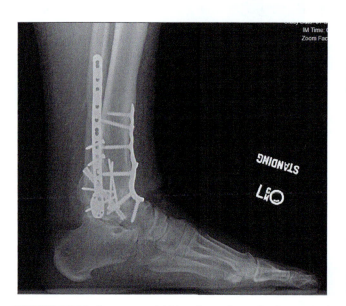 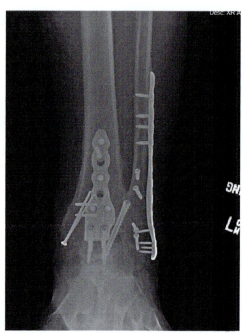

FIGURE 34.13 One-year weight-bearing radiographs demonstrating appropriate alignment and positioning of the ankle as well as healing of the arthrodesis.

instructed to be non–weight bearing. At 6 weeks, the patient returns for cast removal and standing radiographs. If appropriate signs of healing are present and the patient is without significant comorbidities or nonunion risks, they are then allowed to progress to full weight bearing as tolerated in a controlled ankle motion (CAM) boot over the nest 2 to 4 weeks. At 12 weeks, the patient returns for weight-bearing radiographs, and if appropriate radiographic and clinically healing is identified, the patient may transition from the CAM boot into ankle support brace (Fig. 34.13). It is suggested that patients initially use a rocker style athletic shoe. However, they may wean from both as tolerated. Compliance with venous thromboembolism prophylaxis should be assessed at each visit.

RESULTS AND OUTCOMES

Overall, the literature reports favorable outcomes after AA. Good to excellent results are achieved in up to 90% of patients, and the majority of dissatisfaction are related to nonunion and ipsilateral hindfoot arthritis.[7] Nonunion rates have historically been as high as 40%. However, with contemporary techniques and implants, several series have shown fusion rates greater than 90%.[1] Of these patients, many of them have associated risk factors such as history or current infection, tobacco use, impaired vascularity, neuropathy, avascular necrosis, and postoperative noncompliance.[8] Two recent systematic reviews report greater than 96% union rates for AA, which utilize anterior plating techniques.[9,10]

Patients who undergo successful AA tend to be satisfied with their gait. However, gait analysis does detect significant abnormalities including decreased knee flexion before heel strike, less time in single-limb stance, reduced sagittal ground-reaction force, and increased external rotation if the ankle is fused in equinus.[11,12] This exemplifies the importance of appropriate positioning of the arthrodesis as well as preoperative patient education as it relates to expectations. Lastly, progression of hindfoot degeneration is likely to be accelerated after AA.[13]

REFERENCES

1. Thomas RH, Daniels TR. Ankle arthritis. *J Bone Joint Surg Am*. 2003;85-A:923-936.
2. Moeckel BH, Patterson BM, Inglis AE, Sculco TP. Ankle arthrodesis. A comparison of internal and external fixation. *Clin Orthop Relat Res*. 1991;268:78-83.
3. Tarkin IS, Mormino MA, Clare MP, Haider H, Walling AK, Sanders RW. Anterior plate supplementation increases ankle arthrodesis construct rigidity. *Foot Ankle Int*. 2007;28:219-223.
4. Morash J, Walton DM, Glazebrook M. Ankle arthrodesis versus total ankle arthroplasty. *Foot Ankle Clin*. 2017;22: 251-266.

5. Yao L, Belmont B, Wang Y, Tai B, Holmes J, Shih A. Notched K-wire for low thermal damage bone drilling. *Med Eng Phys*. 2017;45:25-33.
6. Buck P, Morrey BF, Chao EY. The optimum position of arthrodesis of the ankle. A gait study of the knee and ankle. *J Bone Joint Surg Am*. 1987;69:1052-1062.
7. Mann RA, Rongstad KM. Arthrodesis of the ankle: a critical analysis. *Foot Ankle Int*. 1998;19:3-9.
8. Perlman MH, Thordarson DB. Ankle fusion in a high risk population: an assessment of nonunion risk factors. *Foot Ankle Int*. 1999;20:491-496.
9. van den Heuvel SBM, Doorgakant A, Birnie MFN, Blundell CM, Schepers T. Open ankle arthrodesis: a systematic review of approaches and fixation methods. *Foot Ankle Surg*. 2021;27:339-347.
10. Kusnezov N, Dunn JC, Koehler LR, Orr JD. Anatomically contoured anterior plating for isolated tibiotalar arthrodesis: a systematic review. *Foot Ankle Spec*. 2017;10:352-358.
11. Wu W-LFCS, Cheng YM, Huang PJ, Chou YL, Chou CK. Gait analysis after ankle arthrodesis. *Gait Posture*. 2000;11:54-61.
12. King HA, Watkins TB, Samuelson KM. Analysis of foot position in ankle arthrodesis and its influence on gait. *Foot Ankle Int*. 1980;1:44-49.
13. Coester LM, Saltzman CL, Leupold J, Pontarelli W. Long-term results following ankle arthrodesis for post-traumatic arthritis. *J Bone Joint Surg Am*. 2001;83-A:219-228.

35 Ankle Fusion With External Fixation

Justin Orr

INTRODUCTION

Current recommendations for primary and revision tibiotalar (ankle) joint arthrodesis favor internal compression techniques using internal fixation, with satisfactory outcomes being reported for most patients. Similarly, when there is concomitant subtalar joint arthritis, current recommendations for primary and revision tibiotalocalcaneal (TTC) arthrodesis favor internal fixation or retrograde TTC intramedullary nail internal fixation. Numerous authors report comparable union rates and results of primary and revision tibiotalar arthrodeses using circular external fixation techniques.[1-6] In select patients, ankle and TTC arthrodesis with internal fixation may be limited or even contraindicated given insufficient bone stock to adequately support implants, an abundance of avascular bone, a history of deep infection or osteomyelitis, in cases of prior failed total ankle replacement with significant osseous defects, or in cases when previous ankle or TTC arthrodesis has failed. Circular external fixation may facilitate clinically acceptable limb salvage in these complex cases. This chapter will discuss the indications/contraindications, surgical technique, and postoperative management for ankle arthrodesis using circular external fixation; however, these principles apply equally to TTC arthrodesis. A description of the modifications in surgical technique necessary for TTC arthrodesis using circular external fixation in cases where subtalar joint arthritis is present is described as well.

Advances have been made in recent years for management of advanced ankle arthritis recalcitrant to nonoperative treatment in cases where other options are not available. Results of ankle arthrodesis using internal fixation for stability and compression are consistently favorable, and internal fixation for ankle arthrodesis is the technique of choice in most cases. However, surgeons occasionally encounter cases of ankle arthritis with or without concomitant subtalar joint arthritis that should be managed with arthrodesis but does not lend itself well to internal fixation. External circular fixation represents an attractive alternative in such situations. A recent cadaveric biomechanical study demonstrated equal bending stiffness and a twofold increase in torsional stiffness using a circular external fixator for TTC arthrodesis compared to retrograde intramedullary nailing, providing biomechanical support for circular external fixation.[7] Other authors have found similar results.[8]

INDICATIONS/CONTRAINDICATIONS

The most common indication for ankle arthrodesis is severe, destructive arthritis that fails nonoperative management, most commonly posttraumatic in origin. Less frequently, ankle arthritis is caused by primary or inflammatory arthropathies. Currently, severe ankle arthritis can be managed with total ankle replacement or allograft reconstruction as well as distraction arthroplasty in select cases, but ankle arthrodesis remains an option in appropriate patients. Regardless of the method of fixation, ankle arthrodesis is contraindicated in patients with peripheral vascular disease until adequate circulation for healing can be re-established.

Typically, ankle arthrodesis can be effectively performed with internal fixation. External fixation may confer advantages over internal fixation in several situations. Specifically, external fixation for ankle arthrodesis may be considered with (1) a history of septic arthrosis or osteomyelitis; (2) a compromised soft tissue envelope about the ankle; (3) inadequate bone stock at the arthrodesis site to support internal fixation limited to the tibia and talus; (4) a leg length discrepancy that is inadequately treated with a shoe modification, requiring potential distraction osteogenesis for limb lengthening[9]; (5) failed prior ankle arthrodesis using internal fixation; (6) neuropathic joint arthropathy; and (7) anticipated patient noncompliance with postoperative weight-bearing restrictions. A series by Easley et al reported an 85% fusion rate with use of circular external fixation for revision and re-revision ankle arthrodesis and noted that circular external fixation is a valuable alternative to internal fixation in complex cases where internal fixation is limited or contraindicated. The authors of that study selected history of infection at the nonunion site or patient noncompliance with weight-bearing restrictions as absolute indications for circular external fixation in cases of revision ankle fusion. While contraindications to ankle arthrodesis are few, relative contraindications to external fixation for ankle arthrodesis are patients with indwelling total joint arthroplasties, as potential pin tract infections may lead to periprosthetic infection, and sensory neuropathy of the contralateral leg, as the external fixator may cause wounds to the contralateral lower extremity unbeknownst to the patient.

PREOPERATIVE PLANNING

Patient history, clinical evaluation, and routine ankle radiographs establish the diagnosis of symptomatic ankle arthritis. Particular attention is paid on examination to associated malalignment deformities and/or presence of ankle equinus contracture, as adjunctive deformity corrective procedures or Achilles tendon lengthening may be necessary. Weight-bearing radiographs of the ankle usually confirm the diagnosis. The soft tissue envelope about the ankle and the vascular status must be evaluated. Poor soft tissues about the ankle, often secondary to trauma and/or prior surgery, typically necessitate a less invasive exposure for joint preparation. Compromised perfusion of the extremity should prompt vascular consultation to optimize the chance for union and proper soft tissue healing.

Routine weight-bearing AP, mortise, and lateral ankle radiographs suffice, but if there is any suspicion on clinical evaluation for limb malalignment or foot pathology, then mechanical axis, hip and knee, and foot radiographs should also be evaluated. Computed tomography (CT) and magnetic resonance imaging (MRI) are not routinely required. In select cases, CT may help identify hindfoot arthritis/deformity if plain radiographs of the foot and ankle fail to reveal these clinical findings. MRI should be considered if osteonecrosis of either the tibial plafond or talus is suggested by the radiographs; this may dictate how much bone resection is required at the arthrodesis site to access vascular surfaces for fusion, although CT scan can often suffice for this purpose.

Simply placing a tibiotalar arthrodesis in neutral plantarflexion/dorsiflexion (0°), subtle hindfoot valgus (0° to 5°), and avoidance of internal rotation will generally result in a functional, plantigrade foot. However, disregard for whole limb and foot alignment may lead to a poor functional outcome, despite successful ankle fusion.[10] Limb malalignment may need to be addressed before or simultaneous to ankle arthrodesis. A powerful advantage of arthrodesis with circular external fixation in the setting of proximal or distal malalignment or limb length discrepancy is that simultaneous combined procedures can be performed, such as proximal tibial corticotomy with lengthening/realignment and ankle arthrodesis or concomitant ankle and foot procedures.

Preoperative expectations are critical to a successful result, and certain realities should be addressed in preoperative counseling, to include the risks of wound healing complications, pin tract infections, failure of fusion and requirement for additional procedures, neurovascular risks, and infection. Regarding pin tract infection, it is critical that the patient understands that pin tract infections are an inherent risk of circular external fixation and do not represent an unexpected complication nor necessitate automatic hardware removal; however, use of one or more cycles of oral antibiotics during the period of circular fixator frame wear is often typical.

Daily living with an applied circular external fixator frame can be an intimidating and frustrating experience for some patients. Therefore, it is paramount that every potential patient understands thoroughly what the external fixator frame will look like and has a full appreciation for and understanding of the potential burdens and benefits of the frame prior to application. It is helpful to maintain one or two previously removed, sanitized frames in the office or clinic to provide as exhibits for the patient who is considering ankle or TTC arthrodesis with circular external fixation. It is also helpful to provide direct lines of communication with other consenting patients who also have an attached external circular fixator or previously did.

SURGERY: ANKLE ARTHRODESIS

A proximal regional anesthetic and general anesthesia typically suffice for both ankle and TTC arthrodeses using circular external fixation. Tourniquet (thigh) use is limited to the approaches for joint preparation. External fixation alone cannot produce fusion; proper joint preparation is essential. Tourniquet use is not recommended during application of the external fixator, particularly while drilling wires and half pins, as it can contribute to thermal necrosis during predrilling.

Positioning

The patient is positioned supine with a support under the hip of the operative leg. The goal is to orient the lower leg perpendicular to the operating table and floor to facilitate proper placement of the external fixator. A sterile proximal calf support (bump) should be created to suspend the lower leg during external fixator placement. The lower leg is prepared and draped in usual sterile fashion, and the leg is exsanguinated according to the surgeon's preference.

Surgical Approach and Joint Preparation

The ankle joint is approached using the surgeon's preferred exposure, considering prior incisions and the status of the existing soft tissue envelope. The author prefers to perform ankle arthrodesis through a direct anterior approach when possible, utilizing the interval between the tibialis anterior (TA) and extensor hallucis longus (EHL) tendons, with preservation of the medial and lateral malleoli. The author prefers to preserve the malleoli in most cases, as it improves the available surface area for fusion and provides a more "anatomic" fusion without bone loss. In select cases—such as severe deformity, osteomyelitis, Charcot arthropathy, or in cases where ankle arthroplasty later will not be possible—the author is amenable to resecting one or both malleoli if necessary for appropriate alignment and bony apposition. In cases of extreme deformity, resection of one or both malleoli allows for easier correction of sagittal plane deformity correction. When malleolar resection is performed, surgical approaches can be performed directly lateral or medial.

Make a longitudinal midline incision over the anterior ankle, starting approximately 10 cm proximal to the ankle joint and 1 cm lateral to the tibial crest, just along the lateral border of the palpable TA tendon (Fig. 35.1). Extend the incision distally to just proximal to the talonavicular joint. Utilize deep, full-thickness retraction as soon as possible to limit the risk of skin compromise. The author prefers early use of self-retaining retractors, and at no point should direct tension be placed on the skin margins. Protect the traversing branch of the superficial peroneal nerve, which is often identifiable as it crosses directly over or immediately proximal to the ankle joint. The extensor retinaculum

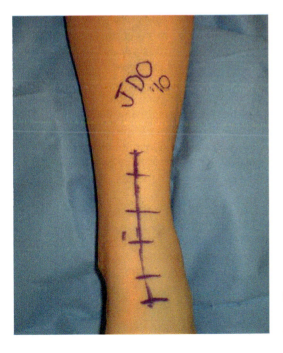

FIGURE 35.1 Incision for anterior approach to the ankle, utilizing the interval between the tibialis anterior and extensor hallucis longus tendons.

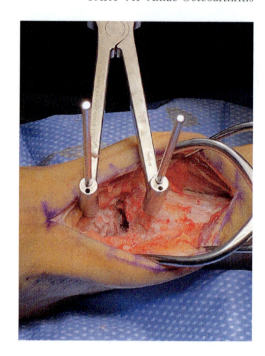

FIGURE 35.2 Anterior ankle joint fully exposed with self-retaining retractors and invasive joint distractor.

is identified and divided directly over the EHL tendon. It is best to maintain integrity of the TA tendon sheath. The EHL and TA tendons are retracted laterally and medially, respectively, with deep self-retaining retractors. The dissection is continued deep, and the deep anterior neurovascular bundle is identified and safely retracted laterally or medially with the EHL or TA tendons. Incise the joint capsule and periosteum over the distal tibia and dorsal talar neck longitudinally, sharply dissect the periosteum off the bone, and retract the capsule and periosteum medially and laterally, exposing the ankle joint fully. Visually inspect the ankle joint, removing any loose bodies and anterior tibial or talar osteophytes, as necessary.

Once the ankle joint is fully exposed, attention is now turned to meticulous joint preparation. Again, just as with ankle arthrodesis using internal fixation, external fixation does not obviate the need for thorough joint preparation. The author routinely uses joint distraction with either lamina spreaders or an invasive joint distractor placed over anterior smooth pins in the distal tibia and talar head-neck junction (Fig. 35.2). Remaining articular cartilage is removed with a sharp elevator, osteotome, or chisel. The author prefers to maintain the architecture of the subchondral bone of the tibial plafond and talar dome, which facilitates easy adjustment of coronal and sagittal plane alignment without compromising limb length or bony apposition. On the contrary, flat cuts sacrifice limb length and make alignment adjustments more challenging. In the setting of malalignment, some deformity correction may need to be made through the joint with limited sacrifice of the subchondral osseous anatomy. This can be accomplished by resection of appropriate wedges of bone from the tibiotalar joint to ensure normal alignment. The subchondral bone is penetrated with a drill bit and/or narrow chisel (Fig. 35.3A and B). This promotes fusion by increasing surface area, delivering autogenous bone graft to the arthrodesis site, and encouraging bridging trabeculae for fusion. The malleoli are preserved when possible, and the medial and lateral gutters are prepared as described above to further increase the arthrodesis surface area. Autogenous or allograft bone grafting is performed at the discretion of the individual surgeon, but excessive use of bone graft might prevent bony apposition and should be avoided when possible. In addition, the author selectively supplements limited bone graft with appropriate antibiotic powder.

Once the joint is prepared, attention is then turned to ankle joint reduction and provisional alignment prior to the application of the external fixator. The author finds that provisional fixation with a single large-diameter Steinmann pin maintains ideal position prior to application of the circular external fixator (Fig. 35.4A through C). While this does violate the subtalar joint, the author does not find this exposes increased the risk of subtalar arthritis postoperatively. Alternatively, a pin can be placed across only the tibiotalar joint to spare the subtalar joint. Provisional fixation should maintain adequate reduction of the prepared talus within the prepared ankle mortise. Optimal function and potential for fusion is established with maximum contact between the arthrodesis surfaces, avoiding

35 Ankle Fusion With External Fixation

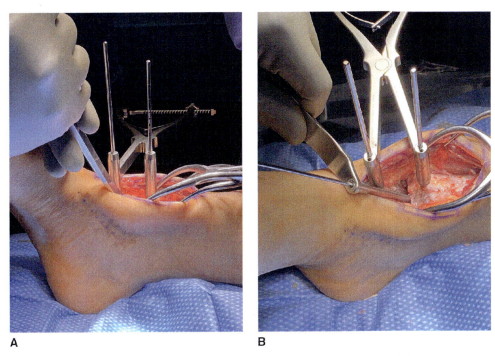

FIGURE 35.3 Use of an osteotome **(A)** and drill bit **(B)** for appropriate arthrodesis joint preparation.

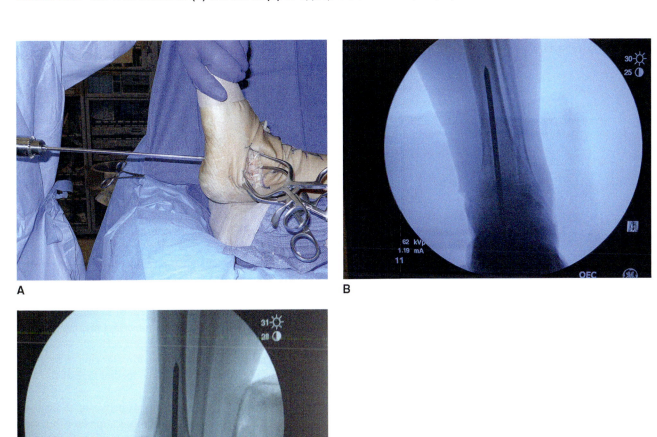

FIGURE 35.4 Drilling of provisional pin fixation to control arthrodesis alignment prior to circular fixator placement **(A)**, with confirmation on AP **(B)** and lateral **(C)** radiographs.

anterior translation of the talus within the ankle mortise. Valgus is established in the hindfoot; varus malalignment at the ankle joint must be avoided. Furthermore, calcaneus or equinus positioning must be corrected to a neutral alignment. Finally, the second metatarsal should be in line with the tibial crest to ensure proper rotational positioning, avoiding internal rotation.

The wound is then gently irrigated and meticulously closed in a layered fashion, making sure to reapproximate the extensor retinaculum and subcutaneous skin. The skin is closed in a tension-free manner, using nonbraided suture. The author recommends closing the wound before applying the external fixator because access to the wound becomes challenging with the circular external fixator applied. If the individual surgeon chooses to close the wound after application of the circular external fixator, one or two anterior fixator struts or threaded rods can be retracted or removed to allow adequate access to the wound(s). The author does not routinely use a deep suction drain. Judicious use of incisional negative pressure wound therapy dressings is at the discretion of the individual surgeon and may have a role in cases of prior infection or tenuous soft tissue envelope.

Safe Insertion of Transosseous Wires and Half Pins

With any use of external fixation, adherence to safe, proper transosseous wire and half pin placement is quintessential to avoid untoward injury to soft tissues and neurovascular structures at risk. For ankle and TTC arthrodesis, a thorough understanding of cross-sectional anatomy of distal lower extremity is paramount to safe use of transosseous fixation. In general, the author recommends use of 1.8- to 2.0-mm thin wires and 5- or 6-mm hydroxyapatite (HA)-coated half pins for ankle and TTC external fixator arthrodesis. Threaded half pins should be meticulously placed to ensure that threads engage the tibia in a bicortical manner, avoiding transcortical drilling. Drilling and placement of half pins should always include the use of blunt dissection to bone and the use of tissue-protecting guides or sleeves placed against the bone. Saline solution should always be utilized during drilling to prevent thermal bone necrosis. Admittedly, a comprehensive discussion of transosseous fixation is beyond the scope of this chapter; however, useful anatomical atlases have been published demonstrating safe zones for transosseous fixation techniques.[11]

For the purposes of ankle and TTC arthrodesis, the author recommends a two-circular ring proximal tibial block, which will be described below. Alternatively, it is appropriate to use a single circular ring. The top, or proximal-most, circular ring in the tibial block is placed just distal to the midshaft of the tibia (Fig. 35.5A and B). The bottom, or distal-most, circular ring in the tibial block is placed in the distal third of the tibia, well proximal to the metaphyseal flare. The tensioned reference wire for the proximal-most circular ring is placed orthogonally to the long axis of the tibia, and two half pins are placed directly perpendicular to the medial face of the tibia. Alternatively, to enhance external fixator rigidity through multiplanar pin placement, one of the half pins can be placed more anteroposterior, starting just medial to the tibial crest (Fig. 35.5C). The author recommends at least one anterior, one anteromedial, and one medial half pin and avoid laterally based half pins through the anterior muscle compartment. This wire-pin configuration confers excellent stability to the construct and avoids risk of soft tissue or neurovascular injury. The tensioned reference wire for the distal-most circular ring is placed parallel to the frontal plane of the tibia, perpendicular to the long axis of the tibia. It is helpful to place this wire just posterior to the tibial crest to avoid thermal bone necrosis associated with drilling directly through the cortical tibial crest. The concept of a "reference wire" is to ensure that the proximal ring is orthogonal in reference to the anatomic and mechanical axis of the tibia. This wire is placed under direct fluoroscopic guidance is placed perfectly orthogonal to the tibia on the AP radiograph. As with the top circular ring, the bottom circular ring in the tibial block is further stabilized with one or two half pins placed directly into the medial face of the tibia or anteroposterior just medial to the tibial crest (Fig 35.5D).

As discussed below, the author recommends attaching the foot plate with two or three forefoot wires and two calcaneal wires. Figure 35.6 demonstrates standard configurations for thin wire placement in the foot. The author recommends one transosseous thin wire traversing the first and second metatarsals and one thin wire traversing the fifth through third (or second) metatarsals. It is not advisable to attempt to capture all five metatarsals with a single thin wire, as this can lead to unwanted flattening of the normal cascade of the forefoot. If additional stability is desired, a midfoot thin wire can be placed most easily through the cuboid and lateral two cuneiforms. Thin wire placement in this manner is typically safe and avoids unnecessary risk of important anatomic structures.

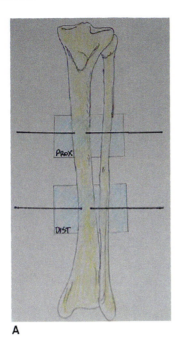
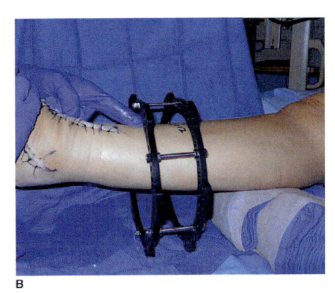
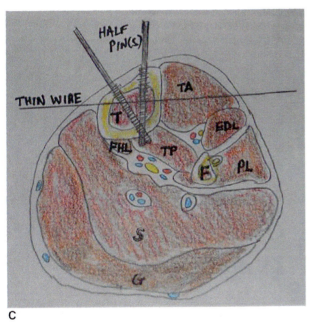
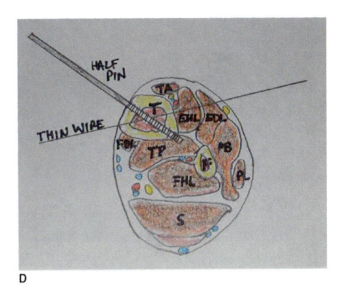

FIGURE 35.5 Diagram by the author **(A)** and actual intraoperative representation **(B)** of appropriate placement and spacing for tibia circular ring block. Diagram by the author of appropriate cross sectional anatomy pin placement for **(C)** proximal and **(D)** distal most tibia circular external fixator rings.

Application of External Fixator

Most ankle circular external fixators have consistent components: (1) a proximal (tibial) circular block (Fig. 35.7A and B), (2) an intermediate (talar) circular ring and connectors (Fig. 35.7C), and (3) a foot plate (Fig. 35.8). The proximal circular block usually consists of one or two circular rings attached to the distal tibia. The intermediate (talar) circular ring serves to support thin wires secured to the talus. The foot plate connects directly to the hindfoot, and in most constructs, to the midfoot and forefoot as well. The individual components are secured to their respective bones using either thin wires or a combination of half pins and thin wires. The components of the external fixator are attached to one another by threaded rods, adjustable struts, or sockets. The connectors between the components that span the ankle joint must be able to compress, using either adjustable struts or threaded compression rods.

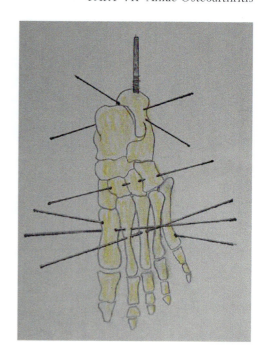

FIGURE 35.6 Diagram by the author of standard configurations for circular fixator foot wire placement.

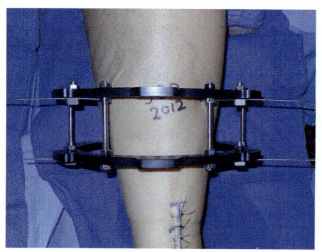

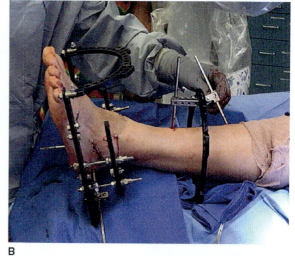

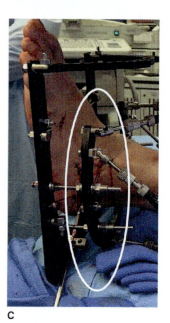

FIGURE 35.7 Proximal tibia ring block **(A)** and single tibia ring **(B)** with associated connectors **(C)** that connect rings and plates.

35 Ankle Fusion With External Fixation

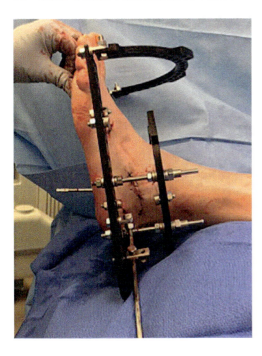

FIGURE 35.8 Standard foot and ankle circular fixator "foot plate."

The external fixator can be constructed and applied in two basic ways: (1) preassembled and applied en bloc or (2) step-by-step assembly as it is applied on the patient. Theoretically, prebuilding the external fixator may save time and guarantees a symmetrical frame construct, with limited modifications to connect the various circular rings (Fig. 35.9). Moreover, if the prebuilt external fixator has been symmetrically assembled, it serves as a template for proper lower leg and foot alignment. One challenge with a prebuilt frame is that it may be difficult to position both the proximal circular rings orthogonally with the tibia and the foot plate parallel with the foot. Alternatively, if the external fixator is assembled in a stepwise manner, the proximal (tibial) circular block is attached first. The foot plate is then applied, with or without an intermediate (talar) circular ring or connection for the talar wires. As an alternative method, some surgeons prefer to slide the tibia ring block up the leg and assemble the foot plate first, followed by the tibia block. Either method is acceptable. Lastly, the proximal circular block is connected to the distal construct. In assembling the frame in this graduated fashion, it may be useful to place threaded rods longitudinally between the proximal and distal blocks to facilitate proper positioning of the 3 to 4 threaded rods that will ultimately be used for

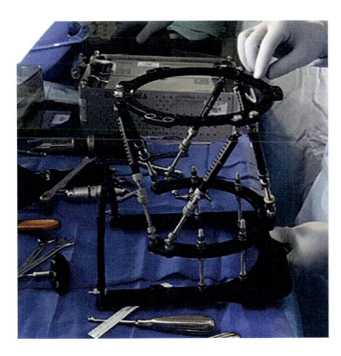

FIGURE 35.9 Preassembled ankle circular fixator hexapod frame.

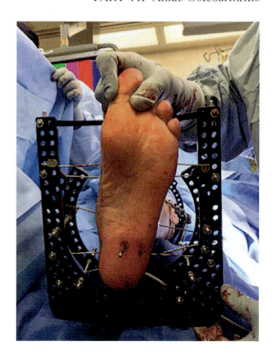

FIGURE 35.10 Applied circular fixator foot plate with appropriate spacing between posterior heel and posterior foot plate.

compression across the arthrodesis site. Telescopic hexapod struts are not required for ankle fusion but does facilitate running a computerized compression and deformity correction program.

There are numerous technique tips that facilitate appropriate circular ring application and typically avoid intraoperative fixator revisions:
1. Ensure adequate spacing between tibial circular rings and posterior soft tissue. This can be facilitated by placing the tibial circular block with only two finger breadths above the tibial crest.
2. Allow adequate room between the posterior heel and the foot plate. This space does not need to be more than 2 cm, as almost no swelling occurs directly posteriorly at the calcaneus, irrespective of how extensive the surgery is (Fig. 35.10).
3. Be sure that the actual foot is plantar to the foot plate. The plantar foot pad is thicker than it appears, and if the foot plate is positioned too low, it will not be possible to pass the thin wires through the bones of the foot, only the plantar soft tissues (Fig. 35.11).

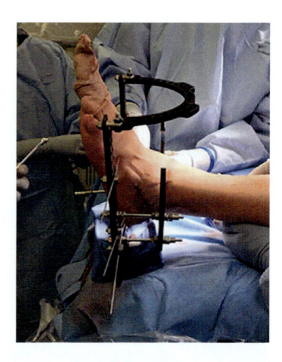

FIGURE 35.11 Applied circular fixator foot plate, demonstrating plantar-based position of actual foot with regard to fixator foot plate.

APPLYING A PREBUILT EXTERNAL FIXATOR

The author does not suggest that a prebuilt external fixator is the favored method for ankle arthrodesis using external fixation, but particularly for the surgeon inexperienced with traditional techniques of external fixation, this method may best facilitate the procedure. After satisfactory joint preparation, this sequence of steps could be considered:

1. Provisional pin fixation of the arthrodesis site.
2. Intraoperative fluoroscopy to confirm satisfactory position of the ankle arthrodesis site (Fig. 35.4B and C).
3. Support under the calf using towels or any mechanical bump to elevate the leg off the table and positioning of the prebuilt external fixator.
4. Position the foot plate portion symmetrically about the foot, avoiding contact between the posterior heel and the foot plate.
5. Next, thin wires and half pins are added to the construct. For ankle arthrodesis, smooth or olive wires are used. Both wires and half pins should be inserted without tensioning the skin. Cool saline irrigation or a moist sponge to gently hold the thin wire should be used to cool the wire during insertion. Once the thin wire has exited the opposite cortex, a mallet should be used to complete the insertion. Half pin insertion requires a small stab incision; thin wires can be placed directly through the skin without an incision.
6. Attach the foot plate (Fig. 35.10). Suspend the foot plate from a single wire or two forefoot wires. Traditional positioning of forefoot wires is one wire through the first and second metatarsals and the second wire through the fifth through the third metatarsals. This orientation is safe and stable but necessitates that the wires extend above and below the foot plate, which may make weight bearing more difficult. Alternatively, a single forefoot wire can be placed from the fifth metatarsal to the first. This wire is usually placed obliquely to the foot plate and often needs to be connected off the medial side using an extended connector ("post") to avoid excessive plantar flexion of the first ray. Two oblique calcaneal wires are placed. A fourth thin wire is placed in the midfoot/forefoot.
7. The foot wires are tensioned (Fig. 35.12A). I recommend closing the foot plate prior to tensioning the foot wires by adding an additional two-thirds (2/3)-circular ring to the anterior foot plate. The 2/3-circular ring can be placed perpendicularly or in line with the foot plate. Closing the foot

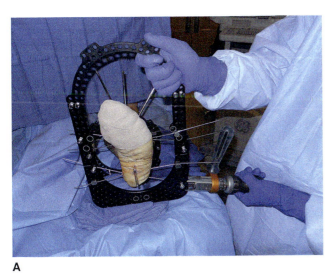
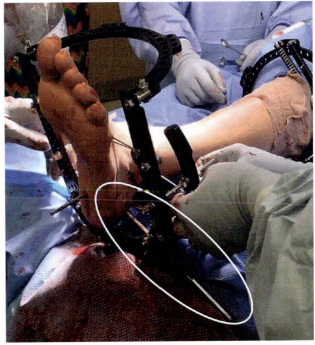

FIGURE 35.12 Tensioning of foot plate wires **(A)** and demonstration of laterally based calcaneal half pin for additional foot plate fixation **(B)**.

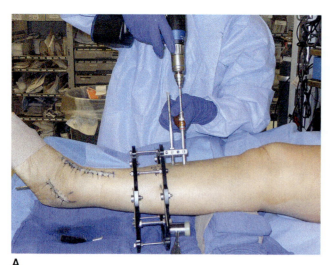 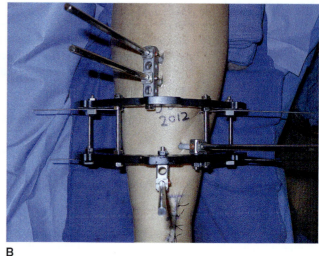

FIGURE 35.13 Use **(A)** and spacing **(B)** of hydroxyapatite (HA)-coated half pins for circular ring tibia fixation.

plate prior to wire tensioning prevents bending the plate during tensioning and ensures that tension is maintained through the wires. Because the foot plate is open anteriorly, it is "closed" with an additional quarter ring or threaded rod built off the foot plate. If the foot plate is not "closed" prior to tensioning, the plate will undergo permanent deformation and risk biomechanical stability of the construct. If there is an open foot plate construct distally, then the forefoot wires need to be tensioned before the calcaneal wires to ensure that tension is maintained in all foot wires. If the calcaneal wires are tensioned before the forefoot wires are tensioned, the calcaneal wires may lose tension, depending on the inherent stiffness of the foot plate. Consideration may be given to a supplemental half pin placed posterior to anterior in the calcaneus and attached to the foot plate (Fig. 35.12B). The author does not routinely place a calcaneal half pin.

8. With the foot plate securely applied to the foot, the proximal circular block is secured to the tibia. Although provisional fixation remains across the ankle joint, subtle adjustments are still possible (ie, slightly greater dorsiflexion or a shift in rotation can be accomplished). The proper proximal circular ring position can be maintained with a transverse thin wire that is tensioned. Proximal circular fixation can be performed solely with the use of thin wires, as originally described, but half pins or some combination of half pins and wires are also a preferable option (Fig. 35.13A and B). Different combinations of pins are possible. Generally, if a single circular ring is used, three half pins are possible and provides ample fixation rigidity. If additional rigidity is required, a two-ring block allows for two half pins on each circular ring. Regardless, half pins are best placed in multiple orientations.

9. With the thin wires properly tensioned and the half pins secured, compression can now be applied across the ankle arthrodesis site. In a patient with a prior subtalar fusion, compression between the calcaneus and distal tibia is sufficient. However, in patients with a normal subtalar joint, compression should only be applied across the ankle arthrodesis site. To accomplish this, a fixed "distal circular block" is applied to isolate the talus from the calcaneus and protect the subtalar joint. Through either extended connectors from the foot plate or an additional intermediate 2/3-circular ring about the talus, one or preferably two thin wires are placed in the talus and appropriately tensioned. Care must be taken to ensure that the pins are indeed in the talus and do not incorporate the malleoli. If an intermediate 2/3-circular ring is used, it is connected to the foot plate with threaded rods or other fixed connectors. No compression is applied across the subtalar joint. The author prefers the use of the talus intermediate ring (Fig. 35.14A and B). While it may seem counterintuitive to include a foot plate in a patient that is only undergoing ankle arthrodesis, the addition of the foot plate provides enhanced stability to the construct by introducing additional distal points of fixation.

10. Compression may be applied across the ankle joint after all components of the external fixator have been tightened, and all thin wires have been tensioned. Compression can be applied equally effectively with telescopic struts or threaded rods. Calibrated adjustable struts that facilitate individualized online computer software-directed dynamic multiplanar correction are available

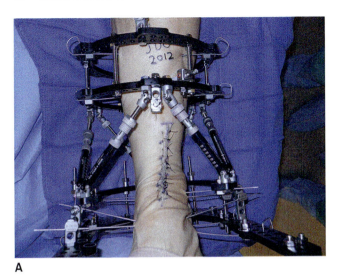 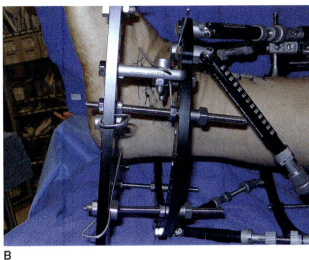

FIGURE 35.14 Demonstration of talus intermediate 2/3-circular ring to isolate subtalar and ankle joints **(A)** and use of connector components for intermediate ring **(B)**.

from various manufacturers. Whereas traditional external fixator frame constructs allow only immediate and subsequent compression at the arthrodesis site, a hexapod frame readily affords angular, rotational, and translational correction to fine-tune the relative positions of the tibia and talus for fusion. The details of this technique are beyond the scope of this chapter. The author finds that use of adjustable struts affords greater ease making intraoperative gross alignment and compression adjustments as well as fine adjustments postoperatively; however, the use of adjustable struts carries a greater financial cost. As with threaded rods, compression across the joint with adjustable struts requires initial manual axial compression of the foot plate followed by incremental tightening of individual struts to obtain smaller increases in compression.

11. Intraoperative fluoroscopy is used to confirm adequate bony apposition and alignment at the arthrodesis site and proper pin position (Fig. 35.15).
12. If there is concern for inadequate compression or a tendency toward varus malalignment at the ankle joint, consideration should be given to a fibular osteotomy if it was not already cut or resected during the approach. The author prefers an oblique osteotomy at the junction of the middle and distal thirds of the fibula, proximal lateral to distal medial through a 2 to 3 cm incision.
13. The wires are appropriately cut flush with the rings and plates or bent over the rings or plates. Bending the wires over the frame allows for later retensioning in clinic if necessary. The author finds this scenario to be exceedingly rare, and therefore typically cuts or breaks off wires flush with the ring/plate wire fixation points.

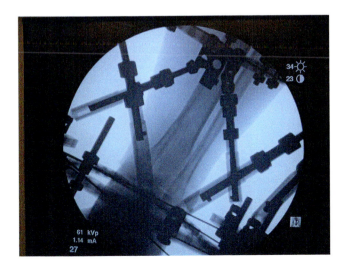

FIGURE 35.15 Intraoperative fluoroscopy confirming adequate bony apposition and alignment at ankle arthrodesis site.

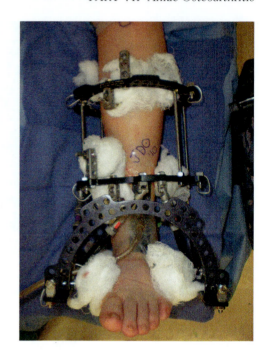

FIGURE 35.16 Sterile dressings applied with sterile gauze wrapped tightly around pins and wires at interface of skin at the conclusion of external fixator application. Alternatively, commercial silver-coated absorbent sponges can be applied at pin/wire-skin interface.

14. Sterile dressings are applied and wrapped tightly over the pins to provide stability at the skin/wire interface to decrease the likelihood of pin tract infections (Fig. 35.16); alternatively, several manufacturers provide silver-coated absorbent sponges that can be secured at the skin-pin interface. The author recommends overwrapping the entire construct with elastic ACE bandages or a bias wrap (Fig. 35.17).

TRADITIONAL STEP-BY-STEP EXTERNAL FIXATION METHOD

1. The same general principles described above for placing thin wires and half pins, aligning the circular rings, and securely attaching the external fixator to the thin wires and half pins applies for the traditional method.

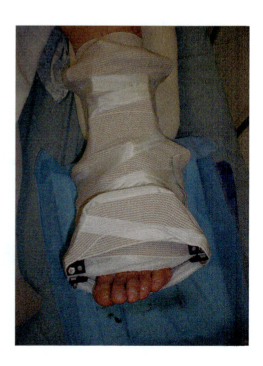

FIGURE 35.17 Entire external fixator construct overwrapped with elastic dressings.

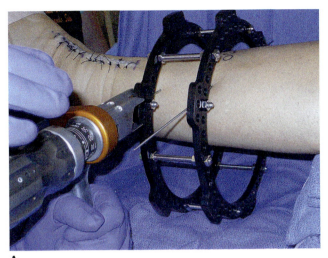 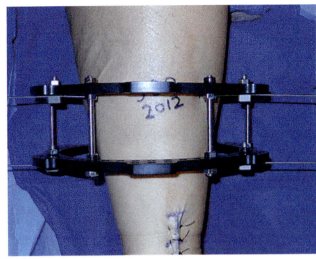

FIGURE 35.18 Tensioning of tibia block reference wire **(A)** and completely attached two ring tibia block **(B)**.

2. The proximal (tibial) circular block is usually attached first. A reference (thin) wire can be placed perpendicular to the anatomical axis of the tibia. The proximal circular ring is attached to this reference wire and tensioned accordingly (Fig. 35.18A). If placing two thin wires on the same circular ring, one should be above and the other below the circular ring. If the pins are placed on the same side of the circular ring, they will collide and displace. These thin wires are tensioned. A second circular ring can be placed and secured in a similar manner. The two circular rings are connected by sockets or short threaded rods (Fig. 35.18B). The spacing between these two circular rings is variable and should allow for adequate stability (ie, adequate space should be left to permit half pin placement between the circular rings). To ensure that the two circular rings are symmetrically oriented, it may be easier to first connect the two circular rings, slide them onto the lower leg, have the assistant hold the circular rings in an orthogonal position, and place thin wires in both circular rings to maintain proper position. Half pins may then be added to both proximal circular rings if desired. Half pins stiffen the construct but are not essential. In fact, traditional Ilizarov teaching does not include half pins. The author typically adds two half pins from the most proximal circular ring attached to a clamp and at least one additional half pin from the lower circular ring. Spacing between the proximal circular block and the distal construct should allow for compression.
3. The foot plate is attached to the foot in the manner described for the prebuilt external fixator frame above.
4. An intermediate partial, or 2/3, circular ring or connectors from the foot plate are incorporated to attach to one or preferably two talar wires as described above (Fig. 35.14A and B). The talar wires are tensioned after the intermediate partial circular ring or connectors have been secured to the foot plate. Next, the proximal (tibial) circular block and distal blocks are connected, and compression is applied across the ankle joint. As noted above, either threaded rods or adjustable struts can be used to connect the proximal and distal blocks and apply compression across the ankle joint. If the threaded rods do not line up congruently/symmetrically with both portions of the external fixator, then various connectors and plates can easily be added to the proximal and distal blocks to allow for longitudinal threaded rods or adjustable struts that can be used for compression across the ankle joint (Fig. 35.19). This is not problematic when using adjustable struts.

SURGERY: TIBIOTALOCALCANEAL ARTHRODESIS

Positioning

The patient is positioned, prepped, and draped just as described for the ankle arthrodesis technique. Access to the subtalar joint approach and preparation may require use of a larger temporary support under the operative hip as well as temporary rotation ("airplaning") of the operative table.

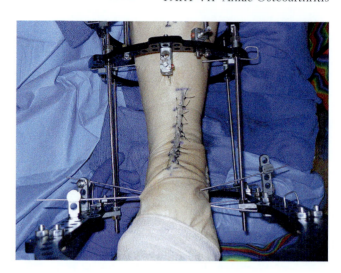

FIGURE 35.19 Use of threaded rods to span ankle and subtalar joints as opposed to telescoping hexapod struts.

Surgical Approach and Joint Preparation

Just as with ankle arthrodesis, the author recommends joint preparation before application of the external fixator. The ankle joint is prepared in the same manner as described above for ankle arthrodesis (Figs. 35.1 through 35.3). The subtalar joint is then approached through a standard oblique incision centered over the sinus tarsi, extending from the tip of the lateral malleolus, distally to the base of the fourth metatarsal (Fig. 35.20A). The subcutaneous tissue is incised in line with the skin incision, exposing the underlying extensor digitorum brevis (EDB) muscle belly, peroneal tendon sheath, and fat pad overlying the sinus tarsi. The fat pad overlying the sinus tarsi is sharply incised and preserved if possible. The EDB muscle belly is retracted dorsally, and the peroneal tendon sheath and its contents are retracted plantarly with self-retaining retractors (Fig. 35.20B). If necessary, the insertion of the EDB muscle belly overlying the calcaneus is carefully dissected proximal to distal to better expose the sinus tarsi and anterior process of the calcaneus. In cases where there is no need to preserve the malleoli (eg, prior infection and not a candidate for later total ankle replacement conversion), it is reasonable to approach both joints through a single lateral approach with a fibular ostectomy.

Once the subtalar joint is fully exposed, attention is now turned to meticulous joint preparation. Just as with subtalar joint arthrodesis using internal fixation, external fixation does not obviate the need for thorough joint preparation. The author routinely uses joint distraction with either lamina spreaders or an invasive joint distractor placed over anterior smooth pins in the lateral calcaneus and lateral talar body. Remaining articular cartilage is removed with a sharp elevator, osteotome, or chisel (Fig. 35.20C and D). As with ankle joint preparation, maintain the contour and architecture of the subchondral bone of the talus and posterior facet of the calcaneus. The subchondral bone is penetrated with a drill bit and/or narrow chisel (Fig. 35.20E). As with the ankle, bone grafting of the prepared subtalar joint is at the discretion of the individual surgeon, avoiding excessive use.

Once both joints are prepared, attention is then turned to ankle and subtalar joint reduction and provisional alignment prior to application of the external fixator. As described above, provisional fixation with a single large-diameter (4 to 6 mm) smooth Steinmann pin facilitates maintenance of ideal position prior to application of the circular external fixator. Ankle joint alignment is the same as described above. Specifically for the subtalar joint, appropriate alignment places the subtalar joint in a neutral to slight valgus position, with care to ensure that the subtalar joint is never aligned in varus. Both wounds are then gently irrigated and meticulously closed in a layered fashion. The ankle wound is closed as described previously. When closing the deep layers of the subtalar joint wound, it is important to attempt to reapproximate the EDB muscle and its aponeurosis with absorbable sutures. Skin is closed in a tension free manner, using nonbraided suture. As noted previously, the author recommends closing the wounds before applying the external fixator.

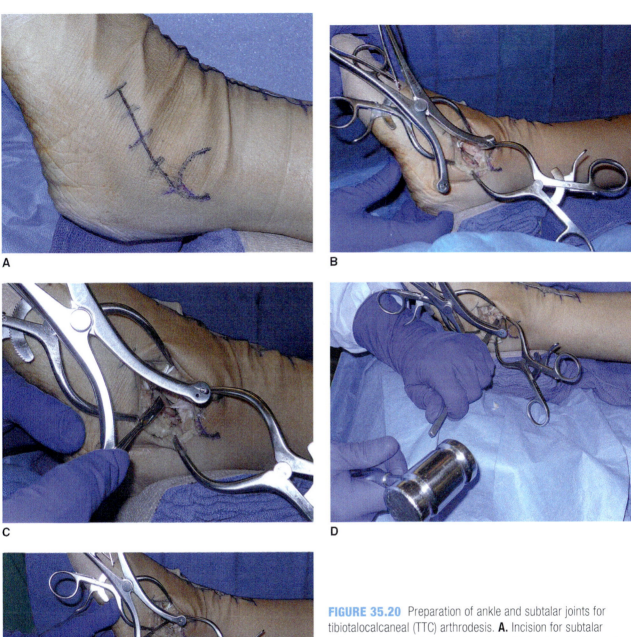

FIGURE 35.20 Preparation of ankle and subtalar joints for tibiotalocalcaneal (TTC) arthrodesis. **A.** Incision for subtalar arthrodesis approach, beginning at tip of lateral malleolus and extending distally to the base of the fourth metatarsal. **B.** Self-retaining retractor, fully exposing subtalar joint laterally, with EDB retracted dorsally and peroneal tendon sheath retracted plantarly. **C.** Sharp osteotome used to remove remaining articular cartilage from subtalar joint surfaces. **D.** Sharp osteotome used to perforate and "fish scale" the remaining subchondral bone at the subtalar joint surfaces. Every effort is made to maintain the articular contour and architecture of the subtalar joint surfaces. **E.** Perforation of the subchondral surfaces at the subtalar arthrodesis site with a drill bit to promote fusion.

Application of External Fixator

Application of a circular external fixator for TTC arthrodesis is much the same as with ankle arthrodesis with minor adjustments. The standard components of the external fixator are the proximal (tibial) circular block and a foot plate. In select cases, which will be discussed, an intermediate (talar) circular ring may be used but is not always necessary. The author contends that the traditional

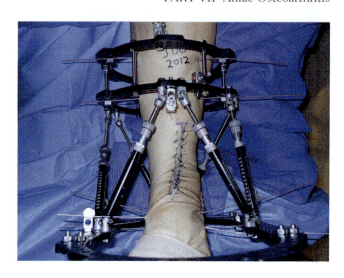

FIGURE 35.21 Use of telescoping adjustable struts to span the ankle and subtalar joints as opposed to threaded rods.

step-by-step assembly of the external fixator is the most dependable. The following description demonstrates placement of a circular external fixator in a traditional step-by-step manner for TTC arthrodesis, highlighting subtle differences unique to TTC arthrodesis.

1. The same general principles described above for placing thin wires and half pins, aligning the circular rings, and securely attaching the external fixator to the thin wires and half pins applies for TTC arthrodesis.
2. In the exact same manner as described above for ankle arthrodesis, the proximal (tibial) circular block is attached first.
3. The foot plate is attached to the foot in the manner described above for ankle arthrodesis external fixators.
4. For TTC arthrodesis with circular external fixation, there are two options, with or without an intermediate talar circular ring. While placement of an intermediate (talar) 2/3-circular ring can be more cumbersome, the author recommends its use in most cases, as it allows for independent compression across the subtalar joint and independent compression across the ankle joint. In appropriate cases where there is minimal bone loss at the ankle and subtalar joints, threaded compression rods or adjustable struts may be placed directly between the proximal tibial block and foot plate without an intermediate talar circular ring, spanning the ankle and subtalar joints completely (Fig. 35.21). This technique will permit equal, simultaneous compression across both joints as the rods or struts are compressed. This technique is not recommended when there is a disparity in bone stock between the ankle and subtalar joints.

In most cases, it is advisable to place an intermediate (talar) partial circular ring, connected to the foot plate by threaded compression rods and connected to the proximal tibial block by threaded compression rods or adjustable struts. The purpose of the intermediate circular ring for TTC arthrodesis is different than for ankle arthrodesis. In ankle arthrodesis circular external fixation, the intermediate talar 2/3-circular ring is placed between the tibial block and foot plate to isolate the ankle joint and prevent subtalar joint compression, utilizing static connectors between the foot plate and the intermediate circular ring. However, in TTC arthrodesis circular external fixation, dynamic compression connectors are placed between the foot plate and intermediate circular ring to allow for independent compression across the subtalar joint (Fig. 35.22).

As described above, the intermediate talar circular ring is placed in line with the mid-axis of the talus on AP and lateral radiographs, and one or preferably two thin wires are placed through the talus, making sure to avoid incorporation of the malleoli. Intraoperative fluoroscopy is critical to ensure proper wire placement in the talus. The thin wire(s) are then attached to the intermediate partial circular ring and tensioned after the circular ring has been secured to the foot plate with threaded compression rods. Next, the proximal (tibial) circular ring block and intermediate talar circular ring are connected, and compression is applied independently across the ankle and subtalar joints. As with ankle arthrodesis, either threaded compression rods or adjustable struts can be used to connect the proximal and distal blocks and apply compression across the ankle joint. Compression of the subtalar and ankle joints is the same as previously described for ankle arthrodesis. If the threaded rods do not line up congruently/symmetrically between any portions of the proximal and distal

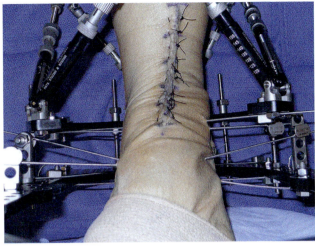

FIGURE 35.22 Use of talus intermediate 2/3-circular ring to isolate subtalar and ankle joints for TTC arthrodesis.

blocks, then various connectors and plates can easily be built off the external fixator to allow for longitudinal passage of the rods (Fig. 35.23). This is typically not problematic when using adjustable struts.

Intraoperative fluoroscopy is used to confirm adequate bony apposition and alignment at the arthrodeses sites and proper pin position.

POSTOPERATIVE MANAGEMENT

Surgical sites must be protected adequately until sealed. Pin care will be discussed below. Skin compromise can be kept to a minimum by maintaining mild pressure on the skin at the pin site. Problems arise if the pin-skin interface is unstable. The author delays weight bearing until the surgical wound(s) is healed. Select manufacturers provide a prefabricated walking platforms that can similarly be attached to the foot plate to facilitate weight bearing (Fig. 35.24). Frequently, by 4 to 6 weeks after ankle arthrodesis, full weight bearing is tolerated by the patient in the external fixator. The author routinely compresses an additional 1 to 2 mm at two to three subsequent follow-up visits, particularly if there is a suggestion of incomplete bony apposition at the ankle arthrodesis site. Removal of the external fixator is determined based on follow-up radiographs and the suggestion of bridging trabeculation in at least two planes at the arthrodesis site. If the arthrodesis site is obscured by the external fixator on follow-up radiographs, a limited CT scan in the coronal and sagittal planes aids in assessing fusion. If healing is suggested radiographically, then the individual surgeon should plan for external fixator removal between 12 and 16 weeks. If healing is delayed radiographically, more axial compression is added, and follow-up is set for 3 to 4 more weeks. External fixator removal is always delayed until healing is evident radiographically.

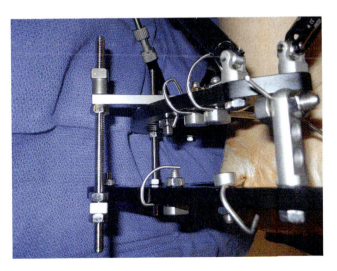

FIGURE 35.23 When threaded rods cannot be longitudinally passed between rings and plates, strategic use of various connectors can be implemented to ensure longitudinal alignment of the rods. In this example, two prefabricated extension plates extend from the intermediate (talar) ring and foot plate to ensure longitudinal alignment of a threaded compression rod across the subtalar joint.

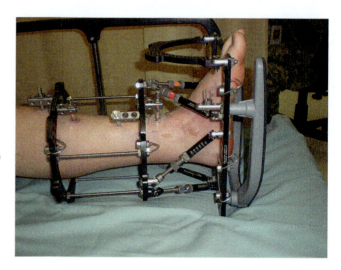

FIGURE 35.24 Patients are allowed to weight bear in external fixator, typically after 4 to 6 weeks, using specially applied walking platforms or plates. Shown is a prefabricated walking platform connected to the foot plate to allow for weight bearing.

While circular fixators can be removed in clinic, the author recommends that fixators relying on HA-coated half pins be removed in the operating room. Removal of HA-coated pins can be extremely uncomfortable for the unanesthetized patient. Following removal, the author recommends that patients wear a walking cast for 3 to 4 weeks progress to an ankle foot orthosis for an additional 3 to 4 weeks. A permanent rocker bottom shoe is often required postfusion for comfortable gait.

COMPLICATIONS

Intraoperative

Pin placement, particularly thin wire application, cannot be haphazard. Safe zones have been established to avoid neurovascular injury. Pins should be placed with the skin in a relaxed, tensionless position. If excessive skin tension occurs, the pin should be replaced. Alternatively, a small relaxing incision can be made. The author recommends cool saline irrigation or holding pins with moistened sponges during pin placement to decrease the risk of bone and/or skin necrosis that may lead to pin tract infections, pin loosening, and osteomyelitis.

Short-Term Postoperative

Poor pin care will invariably lead to pin tract infections and, potentially, osteomyelitis. Pin sites should be cleaned regularly, and the skin needs to be stabilized around the pin sites. There is no consensus on best method for pin care. Some authors, the current included, have gravitated toward just encouraging patients to allow soapy water to run over the frame during normal showering. Others, and specifically for higher risk patients, advocate use of gently applying chlorhexidine soap with cotton tip applicators once daily around all the pins and wires. If a pin tract should become infected and fails to respond to proper pin care and oral antibiotic management, the involved pin will need to be removed and replaced with a different pin in a minor operative procedure. Proper pin and wire placement, particularly avoiding transcortical placement and thermal necrosis during drilling, is paramount to avoidance of pin tract infections. Wound dehiscence is rare because the external fixator maintains excellent stability of the ankle arthrodesis site, but just like for any surgical procedure, infections occasionally occur. The advantage is that no implant is located at the arthrodesis site; instead, all wires are far removed from the arthrodesis site. Another advantage is that the infection can often be managed without removing the external fixator, thereby maintaining compression at the arthrodesis site.

Ankle arthrodesis, regardless of technique, may go on to delayed union, nonunion, and malunion. Delayed union is effectively managed with further compression applied to the arthrodesis site in the office setting. The risk of malunion (equinus, varus, and excessive valgus), as for arthrodesis using internal fixation, is typically avoided by proper intraoperative positioning of the ankle joint. The advantage of external fixation is that subtle adjustments are typically still possible postoperatively. After external fixator removal, the patient should be protected in a walking cast, boot, or brace until the tibial pin sites have healed. With the stiffness at the ankle arthrodesis site, immediate full weight bearing after external fixator removal may lead to stress fracture through a tibial pin site. Patients are encouraged to maintain low-impact activities for at least 3 months after removal.

Intermediate/Long-Term Postoperative

Adjacent joint arthritis invariably develops over time but is not consistently symptomatic. Simultaneous subtalar compression of the talus into the calcaneus may accelerate the development of subtalar arthritis and should be avoided with the proper frame construct.

RESULTS

Numerous authors have reported good results using circular fixation for salvage ankle and TTC arthrodesis. A study by Easley et al[12] showed that in revision and re-revision ankle and TTC arthrodesis with prior failures, healing rates were highest with circular fixation compared to other techniques. Another study by Morasiewicz et al[13] demonstrated possibly increased fusion rates with circular fixation in similar cases (100% with circular fixation versus 88% with standard internal fixation techniques) and overall improvement in sagittal plane alignment. Finally, a comprehensive study by Fragomen et al[14] in 101 patients with "complex" ankle fusion—which included smokers and diabetics, Charcot patients, and patients with prior osteomyelitis—who underwent circular fixation ankle arthrodesis, produced an 85% fusion rate. The authors noted an 80% healing rate in Charcot patients and found that smoking was a major predictor of failure. Coincidentally, the authors did not find that proximal lengthening, in cases of bone transport, impacted healing rates. Various authors have also demonstrated that circular fixation is superior biomechanically to more traditional fixation techniques.[7,8] Based on these results, and others, it is safe to assume that use of circular fixation for complex ankle and TTC fusion salvage is a reliable procedure that can lead to acceptable healing rates in the appropriate patient and with a surgeon skilled in this technique.

ILLUSTRATIVE CASES

Case 1: Septic Nonunion of Primary Ankle Arthrodesis

A 65-year-old man with osteoarthritis of the right ankle underwent primary ankle arthrodesis with internal fixation at another institution. Eight weeks after surgery, he presented with lateral incision wound dehiscence and purulent drainage with proximally spreading erythema. Complete work-up revealed positive blood cultures; elevated erythrocyte sedimentation rate, C-reactive protein, and white blood cell count; and clinical signs of early sepsis. Initial radiographs are shown, demonstrating incomplete ankle fusion (Fig. 35.25A and B). The patient was taken to the

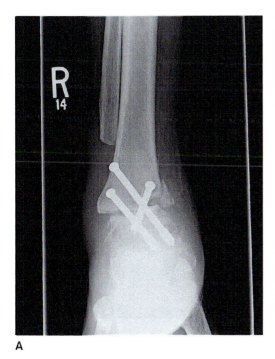
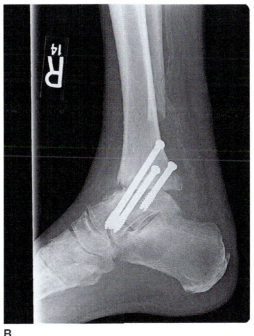

FIGURE 35.25 AP **(A)** and lateral **(B)** radiographs at initial presentation in a patient who has developed an infected, nonhealing ankle arthrodesis.

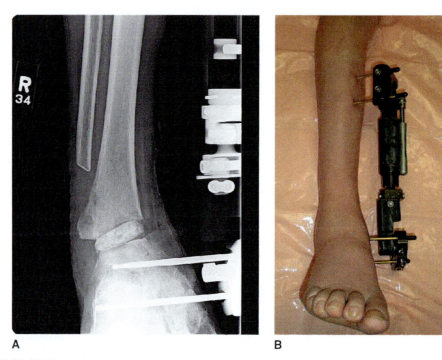

FIGURE 35.26 The patient underwent placement of ankle-spanning monolateral external fixation and antibiotic spacer placement to treat an infected ankle joint. Postoperative radiograph **(A)** and photograph **(B)** shown here.

operating room that evening by the on-call orthopaedic surgeon for irrigation and débridement, removal of hardware, placement of broad-spectrum antibiotic spacer, and monolateral ankle spanning external fixator (Fig. 35.26A and B). After completing a 12-week course of species-directed intravenous antibiotics, he was taken to the operating room by the author for definitive treatment. Given his history of infection and failed ankle fusion, the patient was indicated for revision ankle arthrodesis using a circular external fixator (Fig. 35.27A through C). At the 6-week follow-up appointment, the patient was walking on his external fixator frame (Fig. 35.28), and CT scan at the 5-month follow-up revealed completely healed ankle fusion (Fig. 35.29A and B). It is not

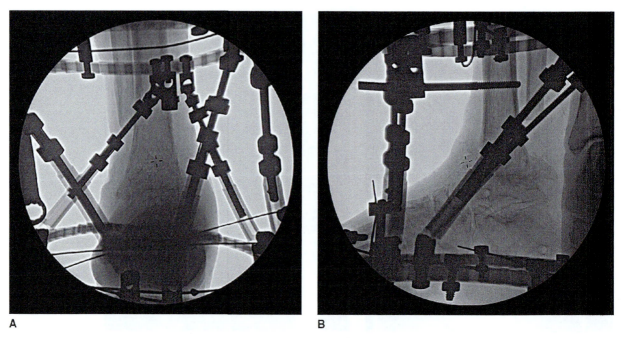

FIGURE 35.27 Intraoperative radiographs **(A, B)** during placement of ring external fixation, spanning the ankle and subtalar joints. Given the patient's radiographic evidence of subtalar arthrosis, the subtalar joint was spanned without placement of an intermediate talar ring **(C)**.

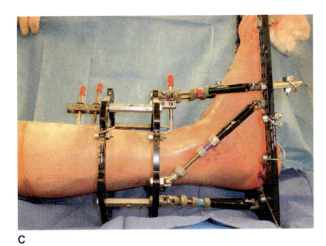

C

FIGURE 35.27 (*Continued*)

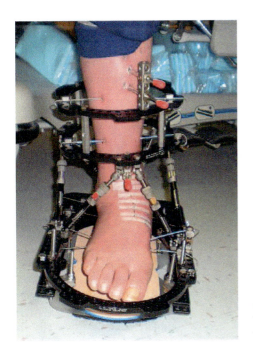

FIGURE 35.28 Patient walking weight bearing in external fixator at 6 weeks postoperatively with use of an applied foot plate with tread.

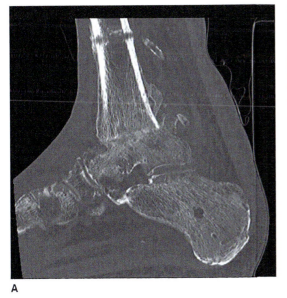

A

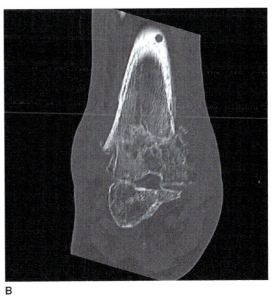

B

FIGURE 35.29 Five months after placement of the external fixator, the ankle joint is solidly fused without complications on coronal (**A**) and sagittal (**B**) plane CT scan, allowing for removal of the frame.

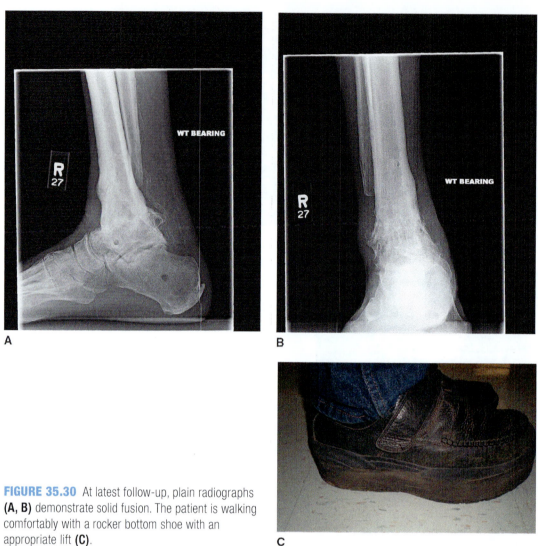

FIGURE 35.30 At latest follow-up, plain radiographs **(A, B)** demonstrate solid fusion. The patient is walking comfortably with a rocker bottom shoe with an appropriate lift **(C)**.

uncommon for frame fusion to require up to 6 months before complete healing, especially in patients with prior infection or comorbidities and risk factors that preclude robust osseous healing. At 2-year follow-up, the clinical result is excellent, and the patient is back working on his farm with a rocker bottom shoe (Fig. 35.30A through C).

Case 2: Symptomatic Ankle Arthritis With Malalignment and History of Osteomyelitis

A 37-year-old female presented to the author's clinic with debilitating left ankle pain secondary to posttraumatic osteoarthritis and 30° valgus tibiotalar deformity. Ten years prior, she underwent open reduction and internal fixation of a closed bimalleolar ankle fracture and developed osteomyelitis per report, requiring hardware removal after 6 months (Fig. 35.31A and B). Given her history of infection and debilitating osteoarthritis with severe deformity, the patient was indicated for primary ankle arthrodesis using a circular external fixator (Fig. 35.32A through C). The patient was comfortably walking in her external fixator frame at 4 weeks postoperatively, using a prefabricated walking "horseshoe" attached to the foot plate (Fig. 35.33). CT scan at 2-month follow-up revealed completely healed ankle fusion (Fig. 35.34A and B). At 2 years, the clinical result is excellent, and the patient is wearing a normal shoe with minimal daily discomfort (Fig. 35.35A through E).

35 Ankle Fusion With External Fixation

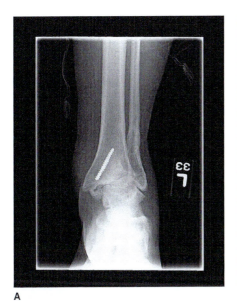
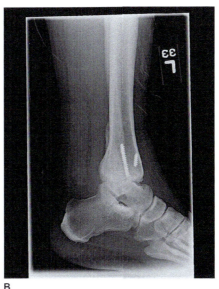

FIGURE 35.31 AP **(A)** and lateral **(B)** radiographs at initial presentation in a patient who has developed valgus ankle arthritis with a history of osteomyelitis following distant ankle fracture ORIF.

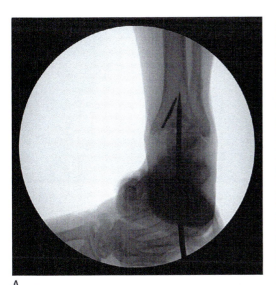
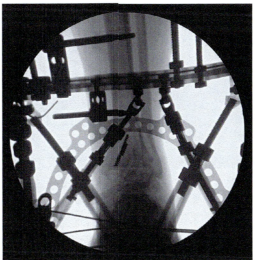
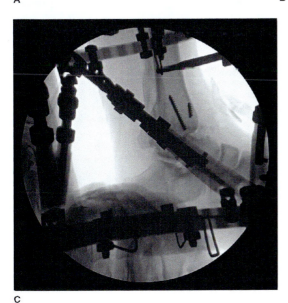

FIGURE 35.32 Intraoperative radiographs during placement of ring external fixation, spanning the ankle and subtalar joints. **A.** Placement of smooth Steinmann pin to provisionally align the ankle joint. **B, C.** Completed ring external fixator for ankle arthrodesis.

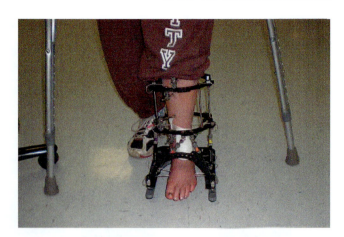

FIGURE 35.33 Patient walking with weight bearing in external fixator at 6 weeks postoperatively with use of a prefabricated walking platform connected to the foot plate.

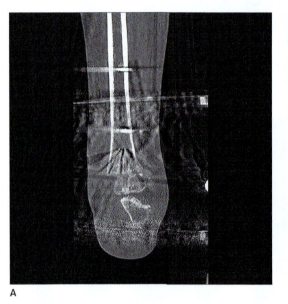
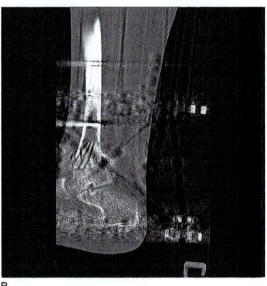

FIGURE 35.34 Two months after placement of the external fixator, the ankle joint is solidly fused without complications on coronal **(A)** and sagittal **(B)** plane CT scan, allowing for removal of the frame.

FIGURE 35.35 At 2 years postoperative, plain radiographs **(A, B)** demonstrate solid fusion. Ankle alignment is normal clinically **(C, D)**. The patient is walking comfortably with a normal shoe (no rocker bottom) with minimal built-in lift **(E)**.

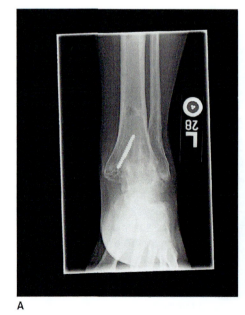
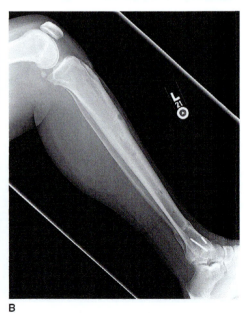

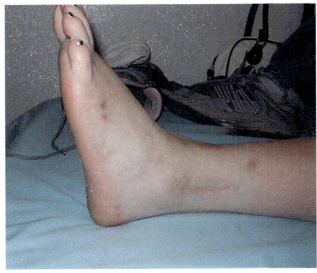
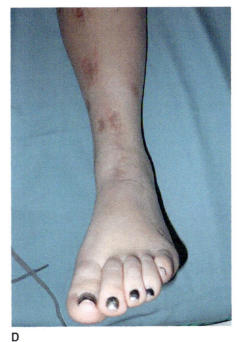
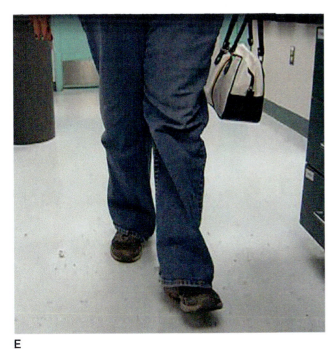

FIGURE 35.35 (Continued)

REFERENCES

1. Calif E, Stein H, Lerner A. The Ilizarov external fixation frame in compression arthrodesis of large, weight bearing joints. *Acta Orthop Belg.* 2004;70:51-56.
2. Easley M, Looney C, Wellman S, Wilson J. Ankle arthrodesis using ring external fixation. *Techniques Foot Ankle Surg.* 2006;5(3):150-163.
3. Hawkins BJ, Langermann RJ, Anger DM, et al. The Ilizarov technique in ankle fusion. *Clin Orthop Relat Res.* 1994;217-225.
4. Katsenis D, Bhave A, Paley D, et al. Treatment of malunion and nonunion at the site of an ankle fusion with Ilizarov apparatus. *J Bone Joint Surg Am.* 2005;87:186-191.
5. Monroe MT, Beals TC, Manol A II. Clinical outcome of arthrodesis of the ankle using rigid internal fixation with cancellous screws. *Foot Ankle Int.* 1999;20:227-231.
6. Paley D, Lamm BM, Katsenis D, et al. Treatment of malunion and nonunion at the site of an ankle fusion with the Ilizarov apparatus. Surgical technique. *J Bone Joint Surg Am.* 2006;88:119-134.
7. Santangelo JR, Glisson RR, Garras DN, Easley ME. Tibiotalocalcaneal arthrodesis: a biomechanical comparison of multiplanar external fixation with intramedullary fixation. *Foot Ank Int.* 2008;29(9):936-941.

8. Ogut T, Glisson RR, Chuckpaiwong B, Le IL, Easley ME. External ring fixation versus screw fixation for ankle arthrodesis: a biomechanical comparison. *Foot Ankle Int.* 2009;30(4):353-360.
9. Sakurakichi K, Tsuchiya H, Uehara K, et al. Ankle arthrodesis combined with tibial lengthening using the Ilizarov apparatus. *J Orthop Sci.* 2003;8:20-25.
10. Thomas R, Daniels TR, Parker K. Gait analysis and functional outcomes following ankle arthrodesis for isolated ankle arthritis. *J Bone Joint Surg Am.* 2006;88:526-535.
11. Catagni MA. *Atlas for the Insertion of Transosseous Wires and Half-Pins (Ilizarov Method).* 6th ed. Medicalplastic srl (in conjunction with Smith and Nephew, Inc.); 2007.
12. Easley ME, Montijo HE, Wilson JB, Fitch RD, Nunley JA. Revision tibiotalar arthrodesis. *J Bone Joint Surg Am.* 2008;90:1212-1223.
13. Morasiewicz P, Dejnek M, Urbański W, Dragan SŁ, Kulej M, Dragan SF. Radiological evaluation of ankle arthrodesis with Ilizarov fixation compared to internal fixation. *Injury.* 2017;48(7):1678-1683.
14. Fragomen AT, Borst E, Schachter L, Lyman S, Rozbruch SR. Complex ankle arthrodesis using the Ilizarov method yields high rate of fusion. *Clin Orthop Relat Res.* 2012;470(10):2864-2873.

36 Arthroscopic Ankle Arthrodesis

Oliver J. Gagne and Alastair S. E. Younger

INDICATIONS AND CONTRAINDICATIONS

The advances made with arthroscopy between 1960 and 1980 allowed for progressive expansion of the possibilities of surgeries that could be performed arthroscopically. Ankle arthrodesis has been a long-standing gold standard when it comes to the treatment of end-stage ankle arthritis (ESAA). Ankle arthroplasty has been popularized and become a reliable treatment for ESAA only in the last 15 years and still faces some limitation with longevity of the implants and risk of reoperation and revisions. The truth remains that while the role and the value of ankle arthroplasty has grown over the past 20 years, ankle arthrodesis will always remain a reliable option for specific indications, which are wider than the patient selection required for ankle arthroplasty.[1]

The advent of arthroscopic technique for ankle arthrodesis have been described in the literature from 1991 when Myerson et al reported on a first cohort of 33 patients and compared outcomes of an open group with an arthroscopic group.[2] Following this study, a variety of smaller case series reported on the early favorable outcomes of arthroscopic ankle arthrodesis including time to fusion and a lower risk of complications.[3-7] More recently, clearer consensus has been reached with this procedure. While it is recognized that open ankle fusion was the standard for many years and is well understood, the authors support a learning curve volume of 20 to 30 cases prior to reaching a superior level of comfort with larger deformities and efficiency around the posterior joint preparation.

The etiology of ankle arthritis can range from posttraumatic, postinfectious, talar avascular necrosis (AVN), neuropathy, inflammatory arthropathy, hemophilia, and rarely acutely in the setting of an unsalvageable traumatic injury.[8] In our practice, out of the patients presenting for foot and ankle opinion with ESAA, those who are 50 or 55 years old and younger are likely to be offered an arthroscopic ankle fusion as they will require a reliable ankle that can withstand the higher demands of an active life.

Patients seen with Canadian Orthopaedic Foot and Ankle Society (COFAS) 1-3 tibiotalar arthritis are eligible for arthroscopic ankle fusion (Figs. 36.1 through 36.3)[9] (Table 36.1). Patients with COFAS 4 (ankle arthritis and ipsilateral hindfoot arthritis requiring surgical intervention) are usually indicated for staged hindfoot reconstruction and ankle arthroplasty or pantalar fusion if not eligible for a total ankle arthroplasty (nerve injury, infection). If these patients (COFAS 1-3) develop ipsilateral adjacent hindfoot arthritis in the subtalar or talonavicular joint after an arthrodesis, they might be a candidate for a conversion of ankle fusion to ankle replacement, which would be performed open with concomitant or staged hindfoot arthrodesis.[10]

One of the other major advantages and consideration to pursue arthroscopic ankle arthrodesis is the minimal disruption of the soft tissue, which is a strong indication in patients with concomitant diabetes, previous flap and soft tissue coverage, or previous incisions in the area. This is also an advantage in patients with a decreased vascularity in smokers, patients with a vascular disease, or patients who have previous had a diagnosis of AVN. While some of those considerations cannot be changed, there should be a real effort to change the modifiable risk factors such as smoking and diabetes in order to decrease the risk of wound complications as will be shown in a subsequent case in this chapter (case 3, Figs. 36.4 and 36.5).

The contraindications for this procedure include an active infection or previous history of infection that could represent a dormant infection. Surgeons must exercise a thoughtful patient selection with the risk factors listed above. Surgeons can be apprehensive to perform an arthroplasty in patients with

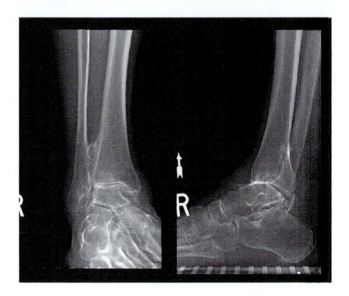

FIGURE 36.1 Preoperative radiographs of a COFAS 1 patient with concentric isolated tibiotalar arthritis. (Courtesy of Alastair S. E. Younger.)

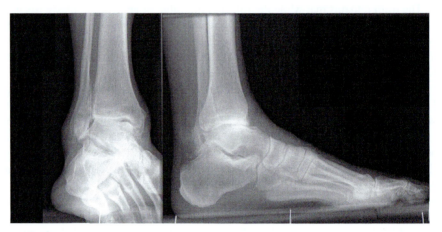

FIGURE 36.2 Preoperative radiographs of a COFAS 2 patient with nonconcentric isolated tibiotalar arthritis. (Courtesy of Alastair S. E. Younger.)

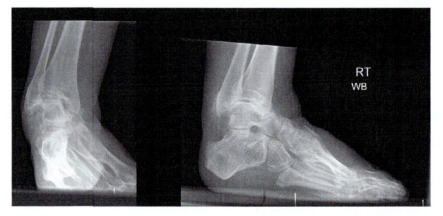

FIGURE 36.3 Preoperative radiographs of a COFAS 3 patient with nonconcentric tibiotalar arthritis with an associated hindfoot deformity in varus and cavus foot. (Courtesy of Alastair S. E. Younger.)

TABLE 36.1 The Canadian Orthopaedic Foot and Ankle Society COFAS Preoperative and Postoperative Classification System for End-Stage Ankle Arthritis

	Type 1	Type 2	Type 3	Type 4
Preoperative classification	Isolated ankle arthritis	Ankle arthritis with intra-articular varus or valgus deformity, ankle instability, and/or a tight heel cord	Ankle arthritis with hindfoot deformity, tibial malunion, midfoot abductus or adductus, supinated midfoot, plantarflexed first ray, etc.	Types 1-3 plus subtalar, calcaneocuboid, or talonavicular arthritis
Postoperative classification	Arthroscopic ankle arthrodesis (AAA) or total ankle replacement (TAR) with no procedure requiring a second incision except syndesmosis fusion	AAA or TAR with a soft tissue procedure requiring a separate incision	AAA or TAR with an additional osteotomy including midfoot arthrodesis	AAA or TAR with an additional hindfoot arthrodesis
Concurrent procedures	None, hardware removal	Deltoid ligament release, ligament reconstruction, tendo achilles lengthening, gastrocnemius recession, tendon transfer, capsule release, forefoot reconstruction, metatarsal osteotomy, dissection of neurovascular structures	Fibular osteotomy, calcaneal osteotomy, midtarsal arthrodesis	Arthrodesis: triple, subtalar, talonavicular, calcaneocuboid

From Krause FG, Di Silvestro M, Penner MJ, et al. Inter- and intraobserver reliability of the COFAS end-stage ankle arthritis classification system. *Foot Ankle Int.* 2010;31(2):103-108. Copyright © 2010 by the American Orthopaedic Foot & Ankle Society. Reprinted by permission of SAGE Publications, Inc.

a previous history of infection; however, tibiotalar arthrodesis can be considered if the infection is remote and serological markers are normal as will be seen in a subsequent case (case 2, Figs. 36.6 and 36.7). While this procedure can bring positive clinical benefits to patients with isolated tibiotalar arthritis, patients who suffer from ipsilateral talonavicular or subtalar arthritis would be better treated with an ankle arthroplasty and selective hindfoot fusions in order to prevent a pantalar fusion down the road. One other relative contraindication is if the preoperative coronal deformity is larger than 15° as it makes the reduction technique harder to obtain a neutral tibiotalar joint arthroscopically.[11] However, this has recently been debated in the literature and demonstrated that the tibial plafond angle is more likely to dictate if a case needs to be performed open as opposed to the overall coronal deformity as this allows the use of structural bone graft if needed.[12] Bone graft can be inserted arthroscopically assisted through a larger portal if significant bone loss or in the context of AVN.

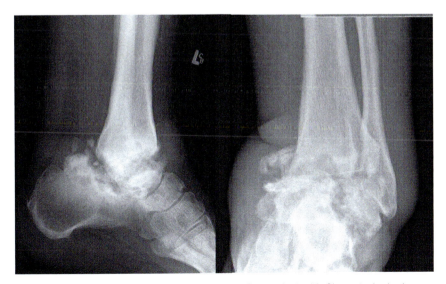

FIGURE 36.4 Preoperative radiographs of case 3, a patient with Charcot who had enough bone stock on the calcaneus to qualify for a tibiotalocalcaneal fusion with the joint preparation performed through the scope. The decision to do this arthroscopically was also in keeping with minimizing the soft tissue disruption in this area. (Courtesy of Alastair S. E. Younger.)

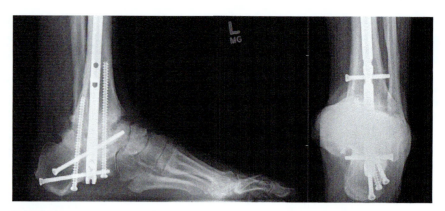

FIGURE 36.5 Postoperative radiographs of case 3 with adequate reduction and alignment. (Courtesy of Alastair S. E. Younger.)

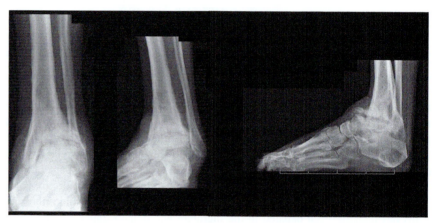

FIGURE 36.6 Preoperative radiographs of case 2 with posttraumatic end-stage ankle arthritis and remote history of infection. Significant hindfoot varus deformity. (Courtesy of Alastair S. E. Younger.)

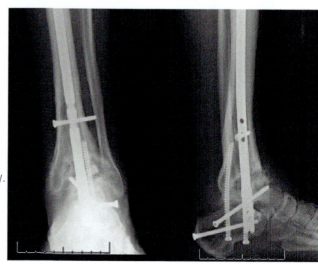

FIGURE 36.7 Postoperative radiographs of case 2 with a tibiotalocalcaneal fusion with the joint preparation completed arthroscopically. In this case, the subtalar joint was not prepared however was included to increase the construct stability since the talar bone stock was marginal. (Courtesy of Alastair S. E. Younger.)

PREOPERATIVE PLANNING

Patients should be counselled and explore nonsurgical treatment solutions as well as joint preserving treatment options including distal tibia osteotomies, which can give them a better outcome in a younger age.

Careful physical examination for scars from prior surgeries should be completed as well as a dedicated neurovascular examination. The examiner should record the hindfoot, midfoot, and forefoot position as well as the range of motion in the adjacent joints.

Investigations needed for preoperative templating include weight-bearing radiographs of bilateral anteroposterior ankle, ipsilateral mortise, a full lateral including the forefoot and the distal half of the tibia, as well as a hindfoot alignment film to assess for segmental deformity through the calcaneus, subtalar joint, or the tibiotalar joint. In selected cases, a long leg view hip to ankle weight-bearing radiograph can be helpful to assess the overall leg coronal and sagittal deformity. A computed tomography (CT) is part of the standard of care for preoperative preparation in order to recognize the cystic component of the arthritis as well as adjacent arthritis in the ipsilateral hindfoot joints. A SPECT CT can be helpful in discriminating the pain generator in a patient with multiple areas with pathology. Magnetic resonance imaging (MRI) can be helpful to look at surrounding structures that can be associated with the coronal deformity such as the peroneal tendon pathology in varus hindfoot and posterior tibialis tendon in the progressive collapsing flatfoot deformity patients. MRI can also be helpful in determining the viability of bone segments in the setting of AVN of the talus or the distal tibia.

Patients with ipsilateral knee arthritis might elect to undergo knee arthroplasty or corrective osteotomy first as the limb alignment needs to be corrected from a proximal to distal fashion.

SURGICAL TECHNIQUE

Patient positioning can be accomplished in a few different ways. The most common described method includes a leg bolster under the thigh in order to bring the knee to 90° and apply an ankle noninvasive distractor to stabilize the ankle and gain an additional level of distraction in the joint. Different authors will prefer only using a bean bag in order to internally rotate the leg so that the foot is pointing up and use a strapped traction around the surgeon's waist, which allows for control of ankle dorsiflexion and plantar flexion while making it more difficult to alternate operators once the body traction is set up (Fig. 36.8). A thigh tourniquet is preferred as it allows for access to the proximal tibia if there is a need for bone grafting. Alternatively, if the surgery is performed under regional anesthesia, a high calf tourniquet can be used recognizing that it would tighten the gastrocnemius-soleus complex, limit the ankle range of motion, and restrict joint distraction. The table needs to be set up to allow for fluoroscopy to be performed while inserting the hardware. The leg can be prepped

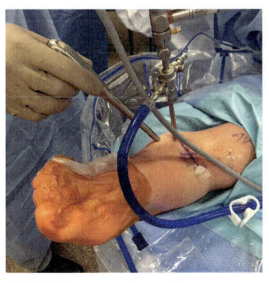 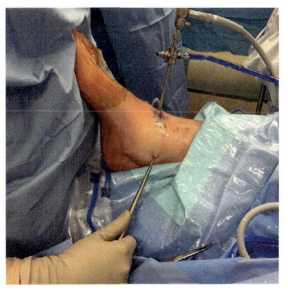

FIGURE 36.8 Intraoperative use of the arthroscopy and a curette to prepare the joint and the gutter.

up to the midportion of the calf or below the thigh tourniquet if a need for proximal tibial bone graft has been determined.

Traditional ankle arthroscopy portals can be used: anteromedial and anterolateral. Additional portals along the lateral and medial gutters can be added to gain better access. The addition of a posteromedial or posterolateral portal can allow for a thorough preparation of the posterior talus and improve the posterior fusion mass. As this joint will have anterior osteophyte and a decreased joint space, access might be difficult. Careful percutaneous fluoroscopically assisted anterior joint débridement can be performed with a curette, a chisel (Fig. 36.9), or a Shannon or Wedge burr prior to inserting the camera. This is performed mostly using palpation and intraoperative fluoroscopy. Care must be taken to lift the soft tissue from the anterior tibia and talus in order to prevent neurovascular injuries. Once this is completed, a shaver can be inserted to débride the anterior ankle from the thickened synovium and obtain proper visualization of the ankle (Fig. 36.10). The joint can then be prepared and the cartilage needs to be removed in its entirety up to the subchondral bone is seen (Fig. 36.11). A combination of burr and curved curette can be used in conjunction with a shaver to remove the debris. While obtaining a fusion in the gutter is not essential for the treatment of the condition and to obtain a reliable fusion, it might be necessary in the setting of severe valgus or varus in order to create the room to allow the reduction of the tibiotalar joint back into a neutral coronal alignment. Preservation of the gutters if not needed to accomplish a fusion can be seen as an advantage for later conversion to ankle replacement with the standard referencing technique and does not make a difference when a patient-specific instrumentation is used. Once the whole cartilage has been removed, the articular surface for fusion is prepared using a bur to roughen the surface in a golf ball–like texture and provoke some bleeding from the subchondral plate (Fig. 36.12).

As the joint is prepared, careful position of the foot needs to be achieved. Placement of bone graft or bone substitute can be performed prior to achieving compression through the future arthrodesis site (Fig. 36.13). If the preoperative deformity requires additional procedures, these need to be performed at this stage. For instance, the authors will use a percutaneous tendoachilles lengthening to increase the dorsiflexion of the talus.

The optimal position of fusion for the ankle is physiologic hindfoot valgus of 5° to 10°. This position allows for the natural biomechanics of the foot to unlock the transverse tarsal joint.[13] Dorsiflexion needs to be neutral with specific attention given to prevent the talus from being in an

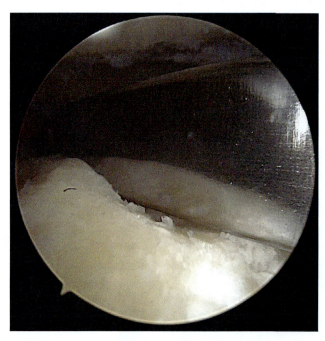

FIGURE 36.9 Arthroscopic use of the chisel to prepare the joint surfaces as well as removing the anterior osteophytes that can block dorsiflexion of the joint and its access. (Courtesy of Andrea Veljkovic.)

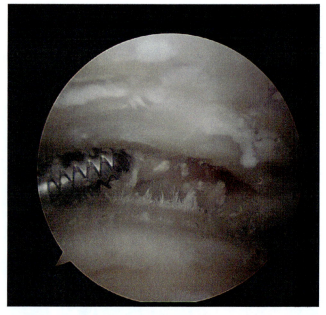

FIGURE 36.10 Arthroscopic visualization upon insertion of the tibiotalar arthritic joint surfaces and the need for débridement using a combination of shaver, bone dissector, and burrs. (Courtesy of Alastair S. E. Younger.)

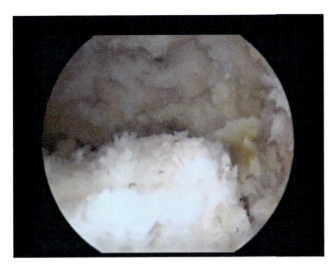

FIGURE 36.11 Arthroscopic visualization of the tibiotalar joint after thorough débridement of the cartilage and perforation of the subchondral plate has been completed. (Courtesy of Alastair S. E. Younger.)

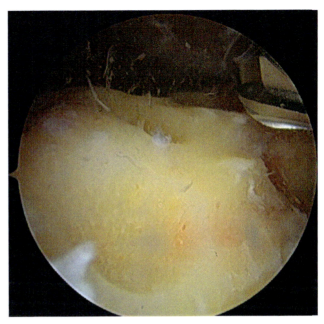

FIGURE 36.12 Arthroscopic visualization of the tibiotalar joint after using the burr and creating a golf ball–like pattern and perforating of the subchondral plate. (Courtesy of Andrea Veljkovic.)

equinus position as this can lead to an inability to stand with the knee straight, midfoot break, metatarsalgia, and recurvatum of the knee. In a dorsiflexed ankle arthrodesis, the midfoot can add up to 10° of plantarflexion hence normalizing the gait cycle and making this malunion more forgiving.[14] External rotation can be within 5° to 10° compared to the tibial tubercle and can be compared to the other side preoperatively. The talar position can be brought posteriorly in order to decrease the lever arm effect of the foot.

While the position of fusion is achieved as noted above, a variety of fixation sequences have been popularized. In general, in trying to minimize the soft tissue dissection, partially and fully threaded cannulated screws of 6.7 or 6.5 mm can be used in different configuration. While the K-wires will be

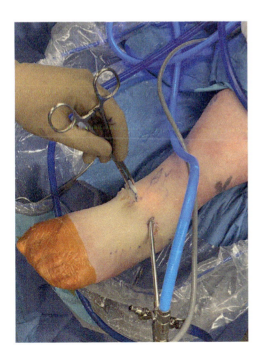

FIGURE 36.13 Intraoperative positioning of the foot with the use of a central portal to insert a piece of bone graft if required in the setting of bone loss and deformity. (Courtesy of Andrea Veljkovic.)

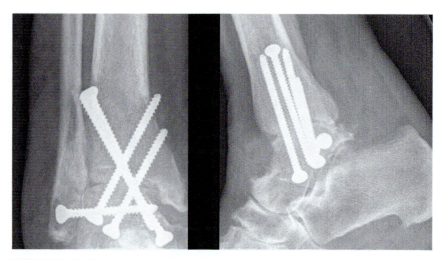

FIGURE 36.14 Postoperative radiographs of a typical screw configuration by the senior author with bony opposition of the surfaces and compression. (Courtesy of Alastair S. E. Younger.)

first inserted to maintain the position of fusion, the order in which they are inserted can be based on the deformity, with the first screw being inserted at the site where the most compression is required to prevent recurrence of the deformity. Lateral compression is used for varus deformities and medial compression for valgus deformities. Additional screws can be placed to neutralize the joint with full threads hence using the strength of the subchondral bone to immobilize the ankle joint on both sides. A typically described "home run screw" will be placed posterolaterally and aim in the anterior and distal direction to capture the talar neck and head.[15] Intraoperative fluoroscopy needs to be used extensively for the wire positioning as well as the screw selection between short and long threads (Fig. 36.14 and case 2: Figs. 36.15 and 36.16).

Finally, the incisions are closed and the tourniquet is deflated. Final fluoroscopy is completed, and the patient is splinted with a sterile dressing and a well-padded plaster of Paris splint.

PEARLS AND PITFALLS

- Positioning is key: Ensure that the leg is internally rotated to assist in portal placement and fusion positioning.
- Use a thigh tourniquet as a calf tourniquet will compress the calf muscles and prevent opening of the joint and may plantarflex the fusion position.

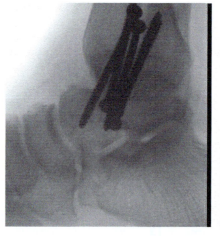
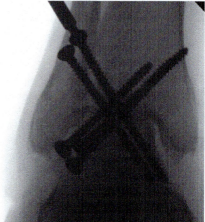

FIGURE 36.15 Intraoperative fluoroscopy of case 1 with adequate bony opposition of the fusion mass and compression of the joint surfaces. (Courtesy of Alastair S. E. Younger.)

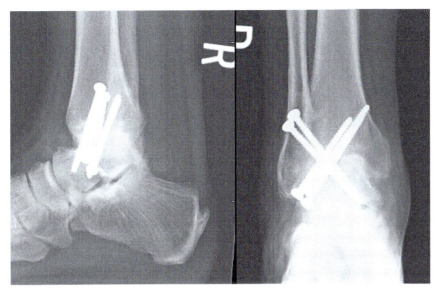

FIGURE 36.16 Postoperative radiographs of case 1, 6 months after index procedure. Interval bridging of the fusion mass. (Courtesy of Alastair S. E. Younger.)

- Correctly place the portals over the joint line.
- Use blunt dissection and a nick and spread technique to avoid nerve damage.
- Perform a complete cartilage removal to ensure high fusion rates, and remove all cartilage debris.
- More portals are better to ensure visualization.
- Anterior osteophytes should be removed to improve access and allow reduction.
- Avoid plantarflexion, anterior translation, and varus during fixation of the fusion.
- Use at least two screws to ensure control of the fusion site.
- Fully threaded screws will result in fixation of the subchondral bone and better fusion site stability.
- Use one screw to compress and two other fully threaded, nonvariable pitch screws using the smaller drill (ie, 3.2 drill for a 4.5 cortical screw) on both sides of the joint to fixate the subchondral bone on both sides of the joint.
- Use bone graft, bone marrow aspirate concentrate, or bone graft substitute for at-risk patients (elderly, patients with diabetes, previous smokers).

POSTOPERATIVE MANAGEMENT

This procedure is performed as an outpatient procedure when the regional pain service locally administers a perineural nerve block and an adequate pain regimen is set in place. Patients are advised to maintain elevation in order to prevent swelling and pain. An outpatient appointment is set up at least 14 days after the procedure to assess the status of the skin, remove the stitches, and convert the patient out of the splint into a removable orthopaedic boot. Some surgeons use a short leg cast at this point if there are concerns of patient reliability. Patients remain non–weight bearing for at least 6 to 8 weeks. When the patient is allowed to weight bear, a progressive return to full weight bearing is set up with increments of 25% of body weight over 4 weeks. A CT scan is not the standard of care, but rather radiographs at the 6 weeks, 3 months, 6 months, and 1-year postoperative follow-up. Physical therapy referral is made at the 6-weeks postoperative mark in order to assist with gait training and proprioception and balance training. The orthopaedic boot is worn up to the 10-week postoperative time point.

RESULTS AND COMPLICATIONS

While patients are aware of the loss of sagittal range of motion that is to come with the tibiotalar arthrodesis, compensatory range of motion will come from the midfoot, subtalar, and the talonavicular joint. Specifically, when looking at the outcomes of this procedure, patients had significant improvements in the ankle osteoarthritis scale (AOS) score, SF-36 mental component summary between the preoperative and the first and second year postoperative values. Arthroscopic cases performed better than the open cases in the AOS score and SF-36 physical component summary scores.[16] Many studies have noted a shorter time to fusion, reduced blood loss, and decrease cost of the procedure.[17] The reported rate of union ranges from 87% to 91% up to 100%.[18] The rate of major reoperation after arthroscopic ankle arthrodesis has been reported 4%, whereas it is 7% in the open group and 24% in the ankle arthroplasty group used a comparator.[19]

CASES

Case 1: A 56-year-old male. Working in a construction site with a remote chronic history of ankle sprains. We discussed performing an ankle arthroplasty however the patient was going to stay employed for an additional 10 years (see Figs. 36.15 and 36.16).

Case 2: A 65-year-old male with a previous history of posttraumatic ankle osteoarthritis and a remote history of infection. He was deemed a high risk ankle arthroplasty. A tibiotalocalcaneal (TTC) construct was used in order to maximize the amount of distal fixation since the talar bone stock was minimal. The subtalar joint cartilage was not denuded.

Case 3: A 72-year-old female with a previous history of Charcot and rapidly degenerating foot pain who was high risk from wound complication as such an arthroscopic TTC fusion was completed (see Figs. 36.4 and 36.5).

CONCLUSION

In summary, arthroscopic ankle arthrodesis allows for arthrodesis to be performed in a larger number of patients with similar outcomes, less wound complications, and decreased cost. We encourage surgeons to consider transitioning to this and include it in their armamentarium.

REFERENCES

1. O'Brien TS, Hart TS, Shereff MJ, Stone J, Johnson J. Open versus arthroscopic ankle arthrodesis: a comparative study. *Foot Ankle Int*. 1999;20(6):368-374.
2. Myerson MS, Quill G. Ankle arthrodesis. A comparison of an arthroscopic and an open method of treatment. *Clin Orthop Relat Res*. 1991;268:84-95.
3. Corso SJ, Zimmer TJ. Technique and clinical evaluation of arthroscopic ankle arthrodesis. *Arthroscopy*. 1995;11(5):585-590.
4. De Vriese L, Dereymaeker G, Fabry G. Arthroscopic ankle arthrodesis. Preliminary report. *Acta Orthop Belg*. 1994;60(4):389-392.
5. Dent CM, Patil M, Fairclough JA. Arthroscopic ankle arthrodesis. *J Bone Joint Surg Br*. 1993;75(5):830-832.
6. Ogilvie-Harris DJ, Lieberman I, Fitsialos D. Arthroscopically assisted arthrodesis for osteoarthrotic ankles. *J Bone Joint Surg Am*. 1993;75(8):1167-1174.
7. Turan I, Wredmark T, Fellander-Tsai L. Arthroscopic ankle arthrodesis in rheumatoid arthritis. *Clin Orthop Relat Res*. 1995;320:110-114.
8. Le V, Veljkovic A, Salat P, Wing K, Penner M, Younger A. Ankle arthritis. *Foot Ankle Orthop*. 2019;4(3):2473011419852931.
9. Krause FG, Di Silvestro M, Penner MJ, et al. Inter- and intraobserver reliability of the COFAS end-stage ankle arthritis classification system. *Foot Ankle Int*. 2010;31(2):103-108.
10. Chu AK, Wilson MD, Houng B, Thompson J, So E. Outcomes of ankle arthrodesis conversion to total ankle arthroplasty: a systematic review. *J Foot Ankle Surg*. 2021;60(2):362-367.
11. Fitzgibbons TC. Arthroscopic ankle debridement and fusion: indications, techniques, and results. *Instr Course Lect*. 1999;48:243-248.
12. Schmid T, Krause F, Penner MJ, Veljkovic A, Younger ASE, Wing K. Effect of preoperative deformity on arthroscopic and open ankle fusion outcomes. *Foot Ankle Int*. 2017;38(12):1301-1310.
13. Mann RA. Surgical implications of biomechanics of the foot and ankle. *Clin Orthop Relat Res*. 1980;146:111-118.
14. King HA, Watkins TB Jr, Samuelson KM. Analysis of foot position in ankle arthrodesis and its influence on gait. *Foot Ankle*. 1980;1(1):44-49.
15. Holt ES, Hansen ST, Mayo KA, Sangeorzan BJ. Ankle arthrodesis using internal screw fixation. *Clin Orthop Relat Res*. 1991;268:21-28.
16. Townshend D, Di Silvestro M, Krause F, et al. Arthroscopic versus open ankle arthrodesis: a multicenter comparative case series. *J Bone Joint Surg Am*. 2013;95(2):98-102.
17. Peterson KS, Lee MS, Buddecke DE. Arthroscopic versus open ankle arthrodesis: a retrospective cost analysis. *J Foot Ankle Surg*. 2010;49(3):242-247.
18. Manke E, Yeo Eng Meng N, Rammelt S. Ankle arthrodesis—a review of current techniques and results. *Acta Chir Orthop Traumatol Cech*. 2020;87(4):225-236.
19. Veljkovic AN, Daniels TR, Glazebrook MA, et al. Outcomes of total ankle replacement, arthroscopic ankle arthrodesis, and open ankle arthrodesis for isolated non-deformed end-stage ankle arthritis. *J Bone Joint Surg Am*. 2019;101(17):1523-1529.

37 Supramalleolar Osteotomy

Jaeyoung Kim and Woo-Chun Lee

INDICATIONS AND CONTRAINDICATIONS

In general, a supramalleolar osteotomy (SMO) is indicated when the distal tibia or talus is malaligned relative to the tibial axis. This malalignment is not limited to a single plane deformity; it can be coronal,[1] sagittal,[2-4] or axial.[5,6] Malalignment in the coronal plane includes varus/valgus and/or medial/lateral translation of the talus relative to the axis of the tibia. The fundamental principle of joint preservation surgery is to transfer weight-bearing load to the uninvolved side of the joint.[7-9] Therefore, joint preservation surgery can generally be attempted if more than 50% of cartilage remains in the ankle joint.[10,11]

In varus ankle arthritis with bone-on-bone contact and a greater degree of talar tilt, joint preservation surgery has been suggested to be unsuccessful.[12,13] Since the advent of weight-bearing computed tomography (WBCT), the axial plane orientation of the talus has been studied in relation to varus ankle arthritis. Specifically, a WBCT study of varus ankle arthritis revealed that the talus is internally rotated in the axial plane.[5] In response to this finding, some authors have attempted to derotate or oppose the rotational force by transferring the tibialis posterior tendon or fusing the subtalar joint following repositioning of the talocalcaneal relationship, with positive short-term results.[14,15] Although these studies demonstrated that a joint with a greater degree of talar tilt can be preserved, the decision to pursue joint preservation surgery for ankles with greater deformities should be made after carefully weighing the risks and benefits compared to alternative treatments.

In valgus ankle arthritis, SMOs have been performed mostly for posttraumatic valgus deformities of the distal tibia. Conversely, supramalleolar correction in valgus arthritic ankles not associated with fracture deformities has rarely been documented. However, a recent study suggests that valgus ankle arthritis may occur in combination with malalignment of the distal tibia or lower limb[2,16] and that SMO may be a useful option for joint preservation.

PREOPERATIVE PLANNING

When planning an SMO with preoperative radiographs, it is crucial to assess the center of rotation and angulation (CORA) as well as the orientation and degree of deformity. In ankle arthritis unrelated to a fracture deformity, the CORA is typically located near the level of the ankle joint. Therefore, the angle between the tibial axis and distal tibial plafond, the medial distal tibial angle (MDTA), is the essential angle to be assessed in the coronal plane. Talar tilt angle is another indicator that can be used to quantify the degree of deformity and predict the success of joint preservation. It has been reported that a greater talar tilt angle is associated with a higher failure rate of joint preservation surgery. However, radiologic stage should be considered along with talar tilt because the talar tilt often decreases as the arthritis progresses. Ankle stress (either varus or valgus) radiographs are useful for determining the reducibility of the ankle joint, although an irreducible joint is not a contraindication for joint preservation surgery. Coronal plane malalignment includes translational deformity of the talus relative to the tibial axis, where talar center migration is used to express the location of the talus.[17] On the sagittal plane, the anterior distal tibial angle is measured, which is the angle between the tibial axis and the tibial plafond. Talus location relative to the tibial axis in the sagittal plane can be measured using the tibia axis to talar ratio (T-T ratio)[18] or lateral talus center migration.[19] Axial plane rotation is difficult to determine preoperatively with plain radiographs; therefore, the rotation of the ankle mortise should be examined clinically by palpating the bimalleolar axis with the patellar facing forward. If available, a WBCT is useful for evaluating axial plane deformities of the talus in ankle mortise.

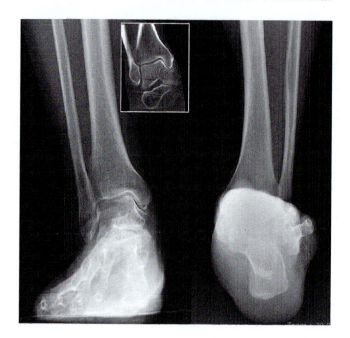

FIGURE 37.1 Varus ankle arthritis with valgus hindfoot alignment. Lateral impingement symptoms may develop from valgus angulation and lateral translation of the ankle joint following medial opening wedge supramalleolar osteotomy. Therefore, medial displacement calcaneal osteotomy should be considered.

Since the abnormal hindfoot alignment may be compensatory to the proximal deformity, evaluation of entire lower limb alignment should be included in the assessment of the hindfoot. Hindfoot alignment can be assessed with the hindfoot alignment angle to assess angulation and the hindfoot moment arm or hindfoot alignment ratio to assess the translation of the heel relative to the tibial axis. Hindfoot alignment after SMO is often difficult to predict preoperatively; however, severe valgus deformity in varus ankle arthritis may need to be corrected with a medial displacement calcaneal osteotomy, since the lateral translation of the hindfoot will cause lateral impingement at the sinus tarsi[13] (Fig. 37.1).

Weight-bearing computed tomography is useful for understanding the tibiotalar deformity and rotational alignment of the foot and ankle in three dimensions in a standing position. Typically, WBCT reveals greater deformity of talar tilt or angulation of the distal tibial plafond, suggesting that plain radiographs frequently underestimate the true degree of ankle joint deformity.[20] WBCT scanners that allow imaging of the hip, knee, ankle, and lower extremities may help in gaining a comprehensive understanding of ankle deformities, especially in the weight-bearing axis and axial plane rotation. Whole lower limb radiographs should be incorporated into preoperative planning, not just the local geometry presented in ankle radiographs. Recent studies have described joint preservation techniques for the ankle joint while considering the alignment of the entire lower limb.[7,8,21]

Selecting the specific type of distal tibial osteotomy is typically determined by the alignment of the whole limb and the orientation of the tibial plafond. Globally (in the whole lower limb view), the ankle must be translated closer to the hip-knee line. Locally (in the ankle radiograph), the tibial plafond is angulated to a slightly overcorrected position relative to the tibial axis opposite to the original deformity. In general, wedge-type osteotomies (whether opening or closed) are accompanied by translation of the distal fragment, whereas dome-type osteotomies feature sole angulation without translation when the center of the dome is located within the ankle joint. When a loose circled dome osteotomy line is created with the center of the circle located distal to the ankle joint, rotation of the dome osteotomy is accompanied by translation and axial plane rotation in addition to the angular correction. This chapter describes a procedure for performing a loose circled dome osteotomy,[7] which differs from the classic focal dome osteotomy.[22,23] The various combinations of tibial plafond and lower limb deformities listed below explain how to select the type of osteotomy based on the orientation of the distal tibia and the lower limb.

- *Varus* distal tibial plafond with *varus* lower limb mechanical axis (Fig. 37.2A): In this combination of deformities, valgus angulating the distal tibia and laterally translating the ankle to meet the hip-knee line should be the goal. To accomplish this goal, medial opening wedge SMO of both the tibia and fibula is preferred, as it laterally translates the ankle and valgus angulates the distal tibial plafond.
- *Varus* distal tibial plafond with *valgus* lower limb mechanical axis (Fig. 37.2B): In this combination, a medial opening wedge SMO to correct varus distal tibia may worsen preexisting lower limb alignment because it will translate the ankle joint laterally. Therefore, in the authors' practice,

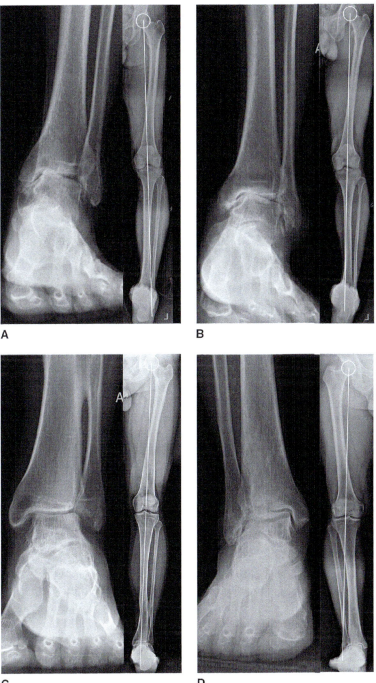

FIGURE 37.2 A. Varus distal tibial plafond with varus lower limb mechanical axis. **B.** Varus distal tibial plafond with valgus lower limb mechanical axis. **C.** Valgus distal tibial plafond with valgus lower limb mechanical axis. **D.** Valgus distal tibial plafond with varus lower limb mechanical axis.

dome osteotomy (distally concave) is preferred for medial translation of the ankle while valgus angulation of the distal tibial plafond.
- *Valgus* distal tibial plafond with *valgus* lower limb mechanical axis (Fig. 37.2C): Varus angulation of the distal tibia and medial translation of the ankle joint are required to align the hip-knee-ankle line. Therefore, a medial closing wedge SMO is preferred for medially translating the ankle and varus angulating the distal tibial plafond.
- *Valgus* distal tibial plafond with *varus* lower limb mechanical axis (Fig. 37.2D): In this combination, a medial closing wedge osteotomy to varus angulate the distal tibia may exacerbate the preexisting lower limb varus deformity because it will medially translate the ankle joint. To translate the ankle laterally and achieve varus angulation, a reverse dome osteotomy (U-shaped) can be performed in conjunction with sawing out the medial aspect of the osteotomy site.

Lateral closing wedge osteotomy is indicated when the ankle needs to be laterally translated and valgus angulated. Since the lateral closing wedge osteotomy involves deeper dissection across the lower leg from the fibula, and leg length is shortened, its use is limited to circumstances in which an anterior or medial approach cannot be performed due to poor soft tissue in the anterior or medial aspects of the lower leg and ankle.

In general, it is advised to slightly overcorrect the distal tibial angle to the opposite orientation of the underlying deformity; however, caution must be given to avoid too much overcorrection. Potentially, patient-specific osteotomy guides can help in attaining a more precise correction than the free-hand osteotomy technique; nevertheless, their clinical significance must be investigated further.[24]

SURGICAL TECHNIQUE

Medial Opening Wedge Supramalleolar Osteotomy

There is still uncertainty regarding whether tibia-only osteotomy or tibia-and-fibula osteotomy should be performed. Some surgeons opt for tibia-only osteotomy, whereas fibular osteotomy is done to obtain additional correction or to prevent lateral impingement. When the fibula is concurrently osteotomized, medial opening of the tibia can be achieved without a complete osteotomy to the lateral cortex; however, tibia-only osteotomy requires a complete osteotomy to achieve medial opening and correction. In a tibia-only osteotomy, the osteotomy site may be more unstable than in an incomplete osteotomy, which may result in a delayed union in some patients.[25] In most cases, the authors perform tibia-and-fibula osteotomy to achieve the desired distal tibial angle as well as the successful medial and lateral shift of the weight-bearing axis. In the authors' practice, tibia-only osteotomy is performed in select patients to narrow the widened ankle mortise when the talus is significantly displaced medially relative to the tibial axis.[26] For osteotomy fixation, one medial side plate is typically used; however, if the osteotomy appears unstable due to a lateral hinge fracture or a large medial opening gap, a second plate might be placed to provide further stability.

Technique

1. Position: Patient supine on the operating table with a bump on the ipsilateral hip.
2. Lateral incision: When concurrent tibial and fibular osteotomy is planned, the fibular osteotomy with a lateral incision is performed first. A 5-cm longitudinal incision is made, centered on the imaginary osteotomy site (Fig. 37.3A). The typical osteotomy site for the fibula is approximately 3 cm proximal to the ankle joint line just above the syndesmosis. In order to efficiently accomplish medial opening wedge osteotomy of the tibia, the fibular osteotomy must be at the same level as the tibial osteotomy or proximal to it. If the fibular osteotomy is located far distal to the tibial osteotomy, the fibula will inhibit the tibia from opening as if it were an unosteotomized fibula. Two 1.6-mm K-wires distanced by 2 to 4 mm are introduced into the probable fibular osteotomy site from the lateral proximal side to the medial distal side to assess the fibular osteotomy level (Fig. 37.3B). These two wires help determine the level of the osteotomy.
3. Medial incision: An incision is made along the medial border of the tibia, from approximately 7 cm proximal to the lower end of the medial malleolus and slightly anteriorly curved along the posterior aspect of the medial malleolus (Fig. 37.3C). After subcutaneous tissue is incised and retracted along the same line, the periosteum is exposed. Approximately 3 cm proximal to the ankle joint, a perpendicular incision is made in the periosteum, allowing for exposure of the bone with a curette or small periosteal elevator. A K-wire is inserted slightly obliquely from the proximal medial to the distal lateral toward the upper tibiofibular syndesmosis margin (Fig. 37.3D). Like the fibula, two K-wires are inserted 2 to 4 mm apart to assess the level of the osteotomy with the fluoroscopy. On the fibular side, an osteotomy is performed in an oblique direction, whereas on the tibia side, wires are inserted slightly less obliquely in a direction that is nearly parallel to the articular surface.
4. Determining the osteotomy level using fluoroscopy: An osteotomy line is made just proximal to the tibiofibular syndesmosis (Fig. 37.4). If the osteotomy is performed too proximally, hard cortical bone may result in a complete osteotomy, resulting in an unstable construct and union problems. If the osteotomy is performed too distally, the osteotomy may violate the tibiofibular syndesmosis. Moreover, there would be insufficient space for screw placement distal to the osteotomy, resulting in less secure stabilization.

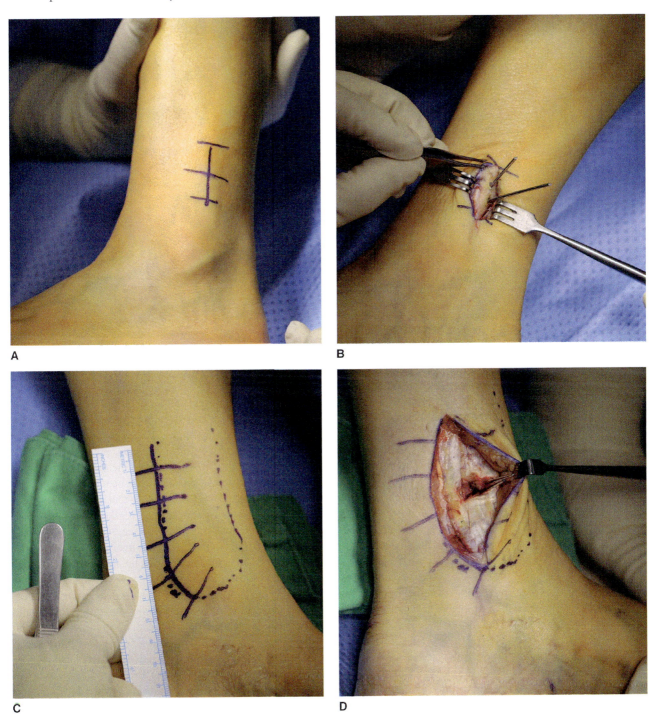

FIGURE 37.3 A. Lateral incision over the fibula in the case when tibia-and-fibula osteotomy is performed for medial opening wedge osteotomy for varus arthritic ankles. **B.** Kirschner wires are inserted to determine the level of the fibular osteotomy. **C.** Medial incision over the tibia. **D.** K-wires are inserted to determine the level of the tibial osteotomy.

5. Fibular osteotomy and temporary fixation with a plate: Place a small Hohmann retractor on the osteotomy site and cut the fibula with a saw while protecting the soft tissue (Fig. 37.5A). Cut only two-thirds of the fibula's circumference by inserting the saw from lateral to medial. If the fibula is completely fractured at this time, it may float and be unstable, making plate fixation slightly more challenging. The four-hole metal plate must be slightly curved in order to accommodate the slightly valgus corrected fibula after the osteotomy (Fig. 37.5B). First, insert a screw just proximal to the osteotomy, then insert and fully tighten the second screw proximal to the osteotomy line (Fig. 37.5C). The two previously inserted screws are then unscrewed approximately 5 mm in reverse, as the metal plate can later impede the lateral translation of the SMO. The

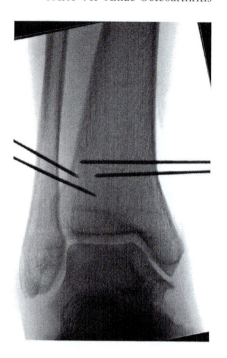

FIGURE 37.4 Using fluoroscopy to determine the osteotomy level. Ensure that the osteotomy line is positioned just proximal to the tibiofibular syndesmosis.

Hohmann retractor is then repositioned at the osteotomy site, and the osteotomy is completed with a small osteotome through an interval between the plate and the fibula (Fig. 37.5D). Then, the fibula is completely osteotomized and can be freely angulated or displaced laterally.

6. Tibia osteotomy and plate fixation: Expose the predetermined osteotomy site on the medial side while protecting the anterior and posterior sides of the tibia with a Hohmann retractor. The anterior, medial, and posterior cortices of the tibia are osteotomized using the previously inserted K-wire as a guide, while leaving the lateral cortex (Fig. 37.6A). After this incomplete osteotomy, attach a 7-hole metal plate. The distal portion of the metal plate should be bent slightly, between the third and fourth holes, and the distal end should also be bent slightly so that it fits well with the medial surface of the tibia and the medial malleolus to prevent irritation over the medial malleolus (Fig. 37.6B). The metal plate is positioned over the exposed tibial surface, while the proximal-distal location is adjusted to allow for the insertion of four screws proximally and three screws distal to the osteotomy. The metal plate is less bent than the curvature of the medial tibial surface, and there is some gap between the plate and the bone, so that when the screws are tightened to the proximal segment of the osteotomy, the distal portion of the plate pushes the distal fragment laterally to spread the osteotomy (Fig. 37.6C). First, drill a hole just above the osteotomy (fourth hole from the distal end) and insert a screw of the appropriate length (typically 36 mm) to secure the plate (Fig. 37.6D and E). Insert and tighten the proximal screws afterward (Fig. 37.6F). If the gap is not created or insufficient to achieve correction, place a thin osteotome on the front and back of the metal plate and gently tap to widen the gap (Fig. 37.6G). Usually, the 3- to 4-mm gap at the medial opening site results in a 6°-to-8° valgus correction; however, this can vary depending on the size of the tibia (Fig. 37.6H).[27] The distal fragment is fixed with screws. First, insert the second screw (approximately 40 mm from the distal end) into the corresponding hole. The distal most screw is then inserted (Fig. 37.6I). At this time, the screw must be inserted obliquely to prevent it from entering the ankle joint. After stabilization of the tibial osteotomy, the proximal screws on the fibula side are fully tightened, then the distal screws are inserted (Fig. 37.6J). This is to stabilize the fibula in a position angulated and translated by the tibial osteotomy. Using fluoroscopy, confirm that the degree of correction and screw length are appropriate. The degree of correction is determined by the MDTA and the talus position relative to the tibial axis. The ideal MDTA angle is neutral to slight overcorrection of normal control, which is about 88° to 92°.[28,29] Not only must the angle of the distal tibia be approximately neutral, but the talus must also be slightly lateral to the tibial axis, with the tibial axis passing slightly medial to the center of the talus (Fig. 37.6K and L). The wound is closed once the medial opening gap has been filled with demineralized bone matrix. Bone graft is typically unnecessary if the lateral tibial hinge is intact and the opening gap is between 3 and 4 mm; however, if a larger correction with a larger gap is created, filling the gap with bone graft can promote healing and improve stability.

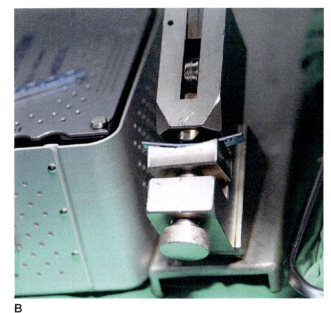
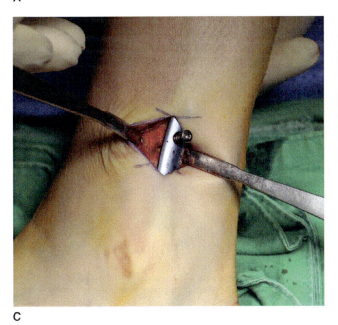
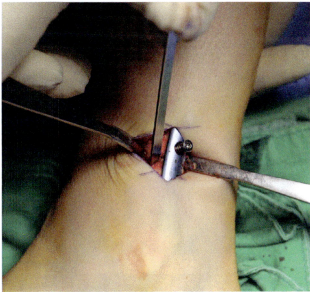

FIGURE 37.5 A. A superolateral to inferomedial fibular osteotomy is performed while a small Hohmann retractor is used to protect the soft tissue at the osteotomy site. **B.** The fibular plate is slightly bent to accommodate valgus angulation of the fibula after the osteotomy. **C.** Insertion of screws proximal to the osteotomy. **D.** The osteotomy is completed with a small osteotome through an interval between the plate and the fibula.

Medial Closing Wedge Supramalleolar Osteotomy

Compared to a medial opening wedge osteotomy, precise correction is a little more difficult in a medial closing wedge osteotomy. Additionally, it is technically difficult to bend the metal plate to fit along the sharply angled medial contour of the tibia after osteotomy. Patient positioning and skin incisions are identical to the medial opening wedge osteotomy. The procedure's sequence is as follows: lateral incision and insertion of two K-wires to determine the level of fibular osteotomy; medial incision and insertion of two K-wires to determine the level of osteotomy; fluoroscopic evaluation of the osteotomy level; fibular osteotomy and plate and screw fixation; tibial osteotomy (wedge resection) and plate fixation.

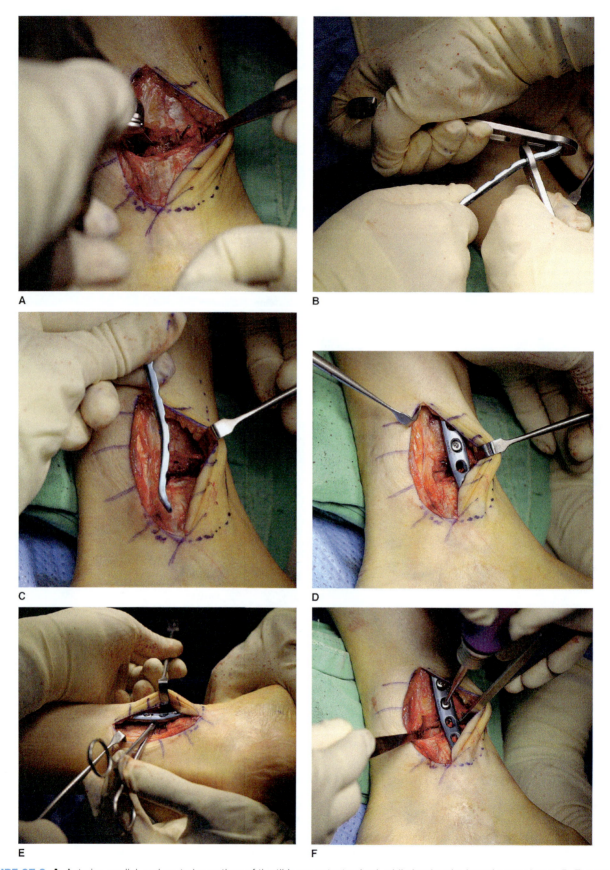

FIGURE 37.6 **A.** Anterior, medial, and posterior cortices of the tibia are osteotomized, while leaving the lateral cortex intact. **B.** To prevent irritation over the medial malleolus, the tibial plate is curved to fit well with the medial surface of the tibia and the medial malleolus. **C.** Shape of the plate after bending. **D.** The first screw is inserted just above the osteotomy. **E.** Note the space between the tibial plate and the tibia. When screws are placed into the plate's holes, it will widen the osteotomy and push the distal fragment laterally. **F.** Insertion of another proximal screw.

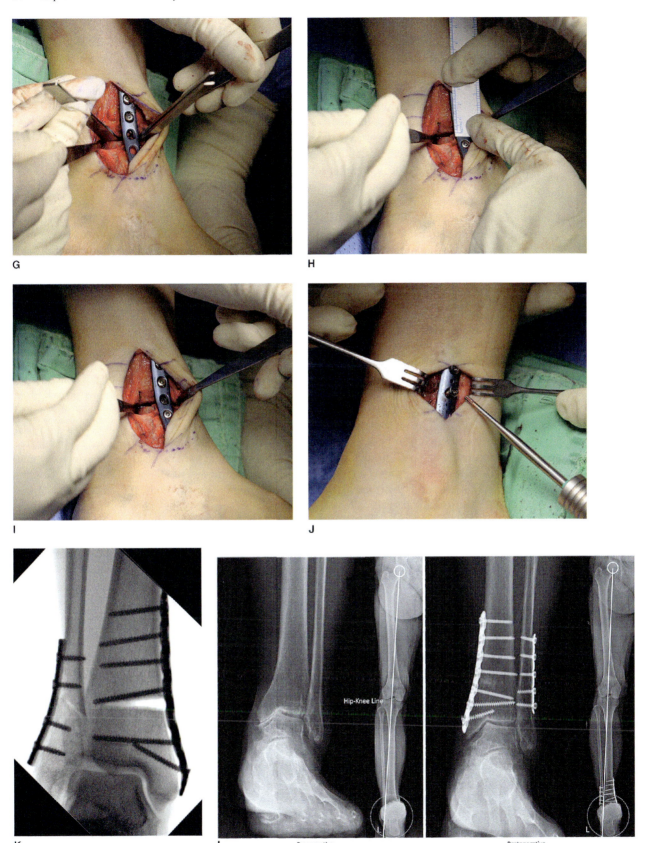

FIGURE 37.6 (*Continued*) **G.** Thin osteotomes can be used to open the medial gap. **H.** Usually, 3 to 4 mm of opening would suffice to achieve the desired correction of the distal tibia. **I.** Insertion of distal screws. **J.** Fixation of the fibula plate after tibial fixation has been completed. **K.** Fluoroscopic image demonstrates the correction of the distal tibial angle and the lateralization of the talus with respect to the tibial axis. **L.** Preoperative and postoperative whole lower limb radiographs of a patient with varus arthritic ankle who underwent a medial opening wedge osteotomy. The medial opening wedge osteotomy can translate the ankle joint laterally, bringing it closer to the hip-knee line (*dotted circle*). However, compared to proximal osteotomies such as high tibial osteotomy, the efficacy of supramalleolar osteotomy in realigning whole limb alignment is relatively minimal.

Technique

1. Determining level of osteotomy: On the fibular side, a K-wire is introduced from the distal lateral to the proximal medial direction aiming at the upper border of syndesmosis. On the tibial side, a K-wire is inserted along the line parallel to the tibial plafond at the anticipated osteotomy level. Then, a second wire is inserted approximately 4 mm proximal to the first wire aiming at the lateral end of the distal wire. The K-wires can be inserted under fluoroscopy as a guide (Fig. 37.7A).
2. Osteotomy and fixation of the fibula and tibia: If the osteotomy site is determined using fluoroscopy, cut the fibula and insert a metal plate and two screws proximal to the osteotomy site. Since the medial closing wedge osteotomy entails an opening wedge osteotomy to the fibula, the metal plate on the fibular side is slightly bent in the opposite direction of the medial opening wedge osteotomy. Complete the fibular osteotomy after placing the metal plate. Since the tibia osteotomy has not yet been performed, the screw proximal to the osteotomy remains slightly loosened. In the tibial osteotomy, a metal plate must be bent to match its final shape. A sharp contour is formed on the medial side, and the distal end of the medial plate tends to protrude excessively medially after fixation. The distal contour of the plate must be adjusted once the plate has been bent to meet the osteotomy location. A Hohmann retractor is inserted between the anterior and posterior cortical bones of the tibia to protect the soft tissue during osteotomy. Cut four-fifths of the entire tibial circumference, leaving only a small portion on the lateral side while utilizing the previously inserted K-wires as a guide. Between the two osteotomy lines, an appropriate-sized wedge-shaped bone fragment is then removed. The wedge-shaped bone fragment between the two osteotomy lines is then removed. Throughout medial closure, the osteotomy plane may become unstable, allowing the distal bone fragment to rotate in the axial plane. Creating one or two saw marks across the osteotomy line is useful for identifying the rotation and realigning it. To close the osteotomy site, place a bolster beneath the lateral malleolus with the lower limb in an externally rotated and abducted position while applying compressive pressure over the medial surface of the proximal segment. If, at this point, the osteotomy gap does not close properly, the remaining cortical bone must be trimmed with a saw. Using fluoroscopy, assess the degree of correction and perform fine adjustments by introducing the saw blade in the osteotomy gap. Once the correction seems appropriate, which is usually 88° to 90° of MDTA while the talus translates medial to the tibial axis, insert two 2.0-mm Steinmann pins for temporary stabilization, one from the lateral malleolus to the proximal medial tibial cortex and another from the medial malleolus to the proximal lateral tibial cortex. Finally, the tibial plate is applied over the medial surface (Fig. 37.7B).

Returning to the lateral side, completely tighten the proximal screws before inserting two distal screws into the distal fragment of the fibula. Confirm by fluoroscopy that the intended degree of correction has been achieved, and add the remaining screws to the plate. Postoperative care is similar to the medial opening wedge SMO (Fig. 37.7C and D).

Dome Supramalleolar Osteotomy (Distally Concave Dome)

The shape of a dome osteotomy can be either focal or loose circled. Focal dome osteotomy, which centers the CORA at the level of the ankle joint, is conventionally described and commonly used to minimize translation after the osteotomy while obtaining enough angular correction.[22,23] In the authors' practice, a loose circled dome osteotomy is preferred when the alignment of the lower leg and the distal tibial plafond are in opposition.[7] This permits substantial angular correction, rotation in the axial plane, and medial or lateral translation of the ankle joint.

Technique

1. Position: Supine with a bump under the operating side.
2. Skin incision: An anterior midline incision is made approximately 7 cm proximal to 3 cm distal to the ankle joint line (Fig. 37.8A). The distal tibia is exposed through the interval between the tibialis anterior and extensor hallucis longus tendons. Then, the anterior neurovascular structures are retracted laterally. Using a Mosquito clamp, the level of the ankle joint is determined, and if necessary, the spur in the anterior distal tibia or the talus is excised.
3. Determining the level of osteotomy: A T-shaped, seven-hole plate is placed on the anterior surface of the distal tibia, with the plate's distal margin approximately 5 mm above the joint line. The plate serves as a template for determining the site of the tibial and fibular osteotomies (Fig. 37.8B).

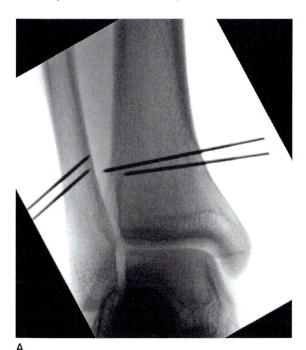
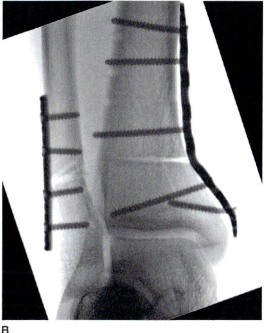
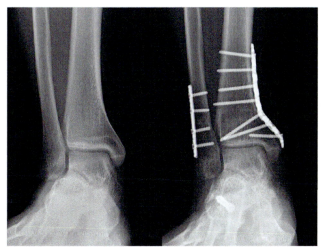
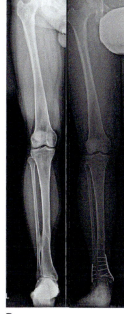

FIGURE 37.7 A. Kirschner wires are inserted to determine the osteotomy level. **B.** Following the fixation of the osteotomy. As seen, the tibial plate must be bent to accommodate the medial contour of the tibia following osteotomy. **C.** Preoperative and postoperative radiographs demonstrate correction of the distal tibial angle and medialization of the talus with respect to the tibial axis. **D.** Preoperative and postoperative whole lower limb radiographs of a patient who underwent a medial closing wedge osteotomy. Due to fracture malunion, the distal tibia was displaced laterally preoperatively (image on the *left*); therefore, a medial closing wedge osteotomy was performed to medially translate the ankle joint.

Typically, the tibial osteotomy apex is set at the level between the second and third hole from the distal end of the plate. The apex of the osteotomy is located around 3 cm proximal to the ankle joint, which is about 5 mm proximal to the upper margin of the syndesmosis while the medial and lateral margin of the tibial osteotomy is at the level of the syndesmosis (Fig. 37.8C). On the distal tibia and skin over the anterior and lateral aspects of the supramalleolar region, a curved line is drawn using a marking pen. Typically, the thickness of the tibia at the apex of the osteotomy is 30 to 35 mm; therefore, the osteotomy is accomplished with a 35-mm-long saw blade.

4. Osteotomy of the fibula: A 5-cm longitudinal incision is made laterally over the fibula, based on the curved line that crosses the fibula (Fig. 37.9A). K-wires can be put into the fibula to determine the level and direction of the osteotomy, which aim at the proximal margin of the syndesmosis. Complete fibular osteotomy is performed, allowing the fibula to freely move, resulting in subsequent free movement of the distal tibial segment (Fig. 37.9B).

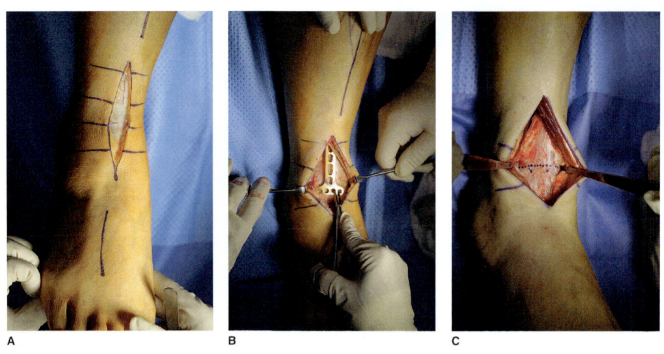

FIGURE 37.8 **A.** Anterior midline incision for the dome osteotomy. **B.** A T-shaped plate with seven holes acts as a template for establishing the location of the tibial and fibular osteotomies. **C.** Drawing an osteotomy line on the anterior tibia.

5. Osteotomy of the tibia: Using a thin saw blade, two or three short marks are made across the planned osteotomy line drawn over the anterior tibia (Fig. 37.10A). These marks are used to determine the amount of displacement after angular correction. The tibial osteotomy is then accomplished with a micro sagittal saw blade (Fig. 37.10B). After measuring the anteroposterior distance of the distal tibia with a drill at the osteotomy's apex, the length of the saw blade is adjusted. Clockwise rotation of the distal segment is accompanied by valgus angulation, medial translation, and internal rotation in the axial plane. Approximately 1 cm displacement of the saw marks and a grossly slightly valgus angulated heel indicates adequate correction. Radiological confirmation is done after provisional fixation with K-wires (Fig. 37.10C and D). A T-shaped plate is reapplied and screwed into place (Fig. 37.10E and F). A one-third tubular plate secures the fibular osteotomy (Fig. 37.10G). When necessary, a bone graft is used to fill the osteotomy site. Postoperative care is similar to wedge-type SMOs.

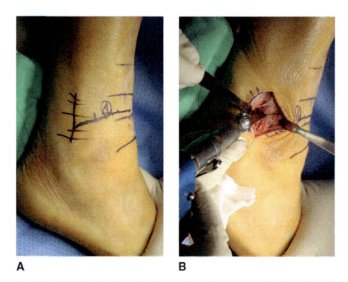

FIGURE 37.9 **A.** Lateral incision for fibular osteotomy when the dome osteotomy is performed. **B.** The fibula is osteotomized. The osteotomy is performed from inferolateral to superomedial to align with the tibial osteotomy.

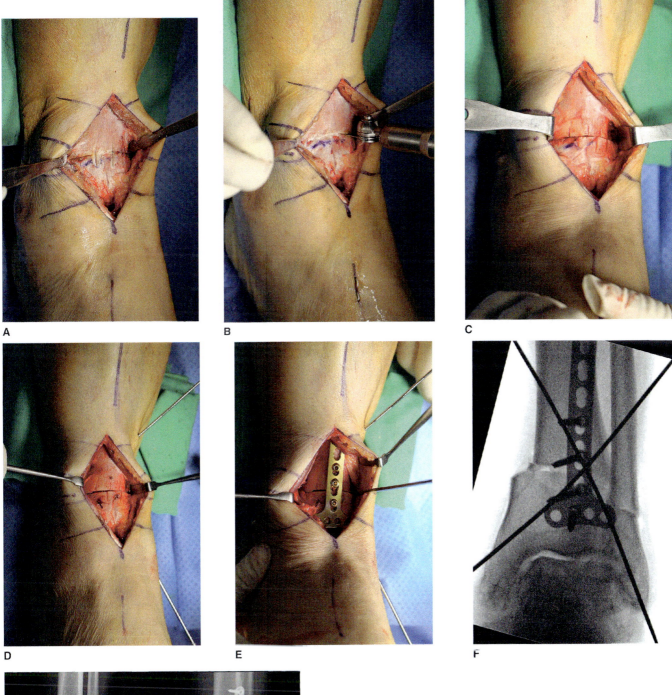
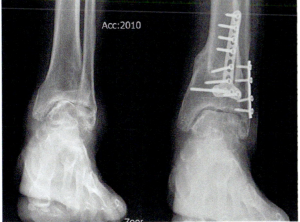

FIGURE 37.10 A. To determine the degree of displacement, two to three short marks are made across the osteotomy line. **B.** A micro sagittal saw blade is used to perform a tibial osteotomy along the planned osteotomy line, while avoiding injury to the neurovascular structures at the posteromedial corner. **C.** Simultaneous valgus angulation of the distal fragment and the medial displacement. **D.** After performing the provisional fixation, the correction is evaluated using fluoroscopic images. **E.** On the anterior aspect of the tibia, the T-shaped plate is placed, and screws are inserted. **F.** The fluoroscopic image shows both valgus angulation and the medial translation. **G.** Radiographs taken before and after a dome osteotomy for varus ankle deformity.

Reverse Dome Supramalleolar Osteotomy (U-Shaped Dome)

This is the reverse shape of the dome osteotomy (which is distally convex) that the authors employ on occasion. In contrast to the limited ability of a distally concave dome osteotomy to translate the distal fragment laterally, this reverse dome would easily translate the distal fragment laterally (Fig. 37.11A). This also permits simultaneous rotation in the axial plane.

Technique

The surgical approach and method of the reverse dome osteotomy are identical to those of the distally concave dome osteotomy (Fig. 37.11B and C). The lowest point of the dome is located where the highest point of the dome is in the distally concave dome osteotomy (Fig. 37.11D). As the tibial plafond becomes valgus as it is laterally rotated (in varus ankles), a saw can be introduced at the location of the medial osteotomy (Fig. 37.11E and F). Depending on the targeted correction, the degree of valgus angulation can be adjusted. The fixation process is identical to the distally concave dome osteotomy. After the osteotomy fixation, the distal medial aspect of the proximal tibia and the proximal lateral aspect of the distal fibular segment are trimmed with a saw (Fig. 37.11G and H).

Lateral Closing Wedge Supramalleolar Osteotomy

Theoretically, this osteotomy can be used to correct varus angulation of the distal tibia while also laterally translating the ankle joint (Fig. 37.12A through C); however, this results in greater soft tissue dissection as well as leg length shortening; hence, it is only performed when other types of osteotomies cannot be performed due to extensive scarring over the anterior and medial aspects of the distal tibia.

Technique

A 10-cm longitudinal incision is made laterally over the fibula. Using small Hohmann retractors, the lateral portions of the tibia and fibula are exposed. The level of the osteotomy is determined using K-wires. The lateral aspects of the fibula and tibia are resected with a predetermined amount of bone, but the medial cortex of the tibia should be retained. Next, a valgus angulating force is applied to close the lateral gap. For temporary fixation, two Steinmann pins are utilized, one from distal medial to proximal lateral and the other from distal lateral to proximal medial. To stabilize the tibia and fibula, a narrow dynamic compression plate is placed over the fibular osteotomy site, and screws are introduced all the way into the tibia.

PEARLS AND PITFALLS

- The type of osteotomy should be carefully chosen based on the most appropriate method to align the whole limb and the ankle joint.
- The angle of the tibial plafond should not be the only goal of correction. The position of the talus in reference to the tibial axis should also be examined to validate the shift of the weight-bearing load intraoperatively.
- The lateral cortex of the tibia should be kept unbroken in tibia-and-fibula SMO. If the bone is cut all the way through, it may compromise the correction and result in healing problems such as delayed union or nonunion. If the lateral hinge is fractured and the osteotomy appears unstable, another plate might be added anteriorly or posteriorly to the original plate.
- Overcorrecting the distal tibial angle does not necessarily result in a greater correction of the talar tilt. Overcorrecting the deformity could alter the shape of the ankle and make it more difficult to do a total ankle arthroplasty if the joint preservation surgery fails.

37 Supramalleolar Osteotomy

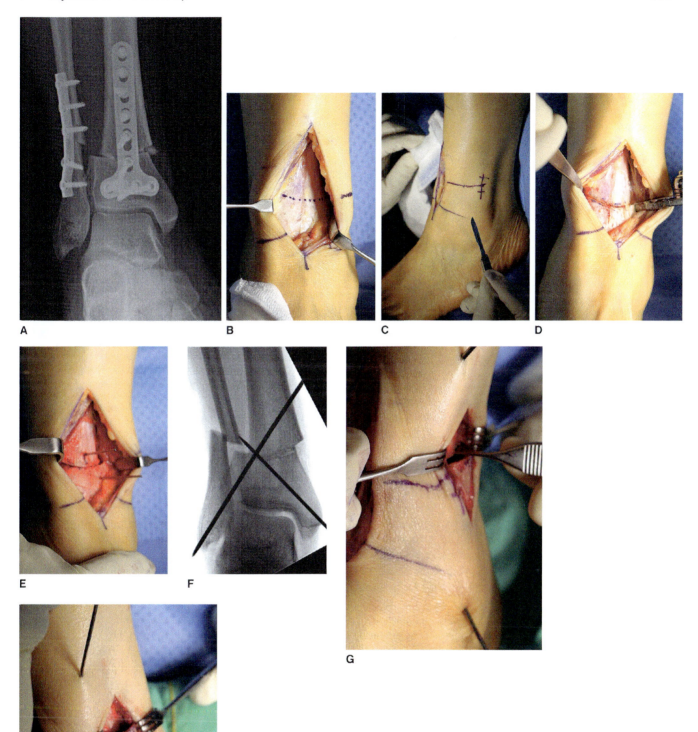

FIGURE 37.11 **A.** Reverse dome osteotomy is utilized for both angular correction of the distal tibia and lateral ankle translation. **B.** For the reverse dome osteotomy, an anterior approach is utilized, and a U-shaped osteotomy line is created just above the distal tibiofibular syndesmosis. **C.** Lateral side incision for the fibular osteotomy when a U-shaped osteotomy is performed. A 5-cm longitudinal incision is made laterally over the fibula, based on the curved tibial osteotomy line that crosses the fibula. **D.** U-shaped osteotomy. **E.** Simultaneous angular correction with lateral translation of the distal fragment. **F.** The fluoroscopic image reveals lateral translation of the ankle in relation to the axis of the tibia. **G.** After the tibial correction, the distal fibula is translated laterally. **H.** For the placement of the metal plate and to prevent irritation, the fibular prominence is trimmed.

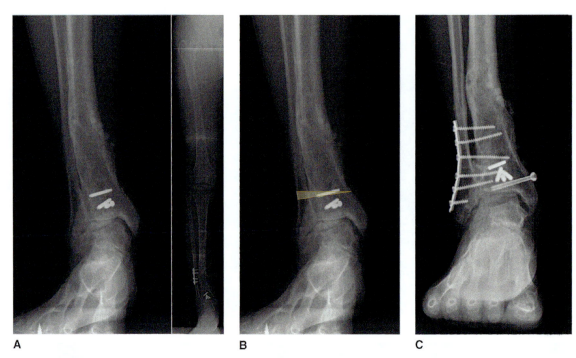

FIGURE 37.12 A. Preoperative ankle standing anteroposterior view (*left*) and whole lower limb alignment view (*right*) of a patient with distal tibial varus and a medially positioned ankle relative to the lower limb axis. **B.** To correct the distal tibial plafond varus and translate the ankle laterally, a lateral closing wedge osteotomy was planned. The *yellow triangle* indicates the bone wedge that will be resected during the osteotomy. **C.** After the lateral closing wedge supramalleolar osteotomy, the postoperative radiograph demonstrates valgus angulation of the distal tibia and lateral translation of the ankle joint.

POSTOPERATIVE MANAGEMENT

The postoperative regimen is the same regardless of the osteotomy type whether tibia-only osteotomy or tibia-and-fibula osteotomy. The initial clinical and radiographic assessments after surgery are often performed at 6 weeks, and radiographs are taken until clinical and radiographic union has been demonstrated. At 1 year, the authors obtain radiographs to assess overall alignment correction. The postoperative protocol can vary depending on the amount of correction, patient characteristics, and the stability of osteotomy fixation. Usually, patient remains in a splint until the 3rd postoperative day (POD), when they are switched to a detachable orthosis or walker brace and allowed active ankle range of motion. At this point, partial weight bearing is allowed (one-third of body weight). At POD 7 weeks, tolerable weight bearing with crutches is allowed, followed by full weight bearing 11 weeks after surgery. When stable radiographic union is confirmed 3 months after surgery, more strenuous activities can be started.

RESULTS

The severity of preoperative deformity appears to impact the clinical and radiological outcomes of SMO for the treatment of ankle arthritis, according to prior research findings.[12-14] Since the SMO is performed in conjunction with other bony or ligamentous procedures in realignment surgery, it is impossible to determine the influence of SMO alone on clinical outcomes. In general, clinical studies have established the radiographic and clinical success of joint preservation surgery with SMOs[2,7,12-14,19,26]; nevertheless, a well-designed study with longer-term survival is required to clarify the efficacy of joint preservation surgery with SMOs.

COMPLICATIONS

Intraoperative Complications

Nerve injuries, such as to the superficial peroneal nerve over the distal fibula and the saphenous nerve over the medial distal tibia surface, are possible. If an opening wedge osteotomy is used to perform a large amount of angular correction, tarsal tunnel syndrome may develop. When a larger angular correction is necessary, a lateral closing wedge osteotomy or dome osteotomy may be considered.

Tendon injuries are rare. However, the posterior tibial tendon should be protected with a Hohmann retractor when cutting the posteromedial corner of the distal tibia. Vascular injuries during SMOs are extremely rare.

Overcorrection of the distal tibia may result in lateral impingement at the subfibular region, either at the talofibular or talocalcaneal area. Overcorrection of the tibial plafond into valgus may have a negative effect on a future total ankle arthroplasty. In a valgus-angulated tibial plafond, more bone cutting is required during the arthroplasty procedures, and if the ankle mortise is translated too laterally, lateral overloading may result after total ankle arthroplasty. In the tibia-only osteotomy, medial opening of the tibia might lead to medial translation of the talus relative to the tibial axis, resulting in an ineffective weight-bearing load transfer.

Postoperative Complications

Infection and wound healing issues are uncommon. However, the incision over the medial tibial surface should be placed posterior to the tibial plate in order to decrease the stress applied over the incision and to prevent exposure of the plate in the event of a wound healing problem. Patients may still experience medial, anteromedial, or lateral pain despite satisfactory radiographic correction. In such cases, insufficient or unmanaged ankle spurs could be the source of the pain. Therefore, it is recommended to remove spurs at the time of the osteotomy when present. To avoid impeding blood flow to the talus, however, it is preferable to minimize dissection. When the tibia is completely osteotomized without a concurrent fibular osteotomy, delayed union or nonunion can sometimes occur. When the fibula is not osteotomized, angulation at the tibial osteotomy site tends to break the lateral cortex of the tibia. In the tibia-only osteotomy, a bone graft may be necessary, as well as a longer period of non–weight bearing and protective partial weight bearing.

REFERENCES

1. Pagenstert GI, Hintermann B, Barg A, Leumann A, Valderrabano V. Realignment surgery as alternative treatment of varus and valgus ankle osteoarthritis. *Clin Orthop Relat Res.* 2007;462:156-168.
2. Kim J, Kim J-B, Lee W-C. Outcomes of joint preservation surgery in valgus ankle arthritis without deltoid ligament insufficiency. *Foot Ankle Int.* 2021;42(11):1419-1430.
3. Kim J, Lee W-C. Joint preservation surgery for varus and posterior ankle arthritis associated with flatfoot deformity. *Foot Ankle Clin.* 2022;27(1):115-127.
4. Kim J, Kim J-B, Lee W-C. Eccentric ankle arthritis in the sagittal plane: a novel description of anterior and posterior ankle arthritis. *Foot Ankle Surg.* 2021;27(8):934-941.
5. Kim J-B, Yi Y, Kim J-Y, Cho J-H, et al. Weight-bearing computed tomography findings in varus ankle osteoarthritis: abnormal internal rotation of the talus in the axial plane. *Skelet Radiol.* 2017;46(8):1071-1080.
6. Song JH, Kang C, Kim TG, et al. Perioperative axial loading computed tomography findings in varus ankle osteoarthritis: effect of supramalleolar osteotomy on abnormal internal rotation of the talus. *Foot Ankle Surg.* 2021;27(2):217-223.
7. Kim J, Henry JK, Kim J-B, Lee W-C. Dome supramalleolar osteotomies for the treatment of ankle pain with opposing coronal plane deformities between ankle and the lower limb. *Foot Ankle Int.* 2022;43(4):474-485.
8. Haraguchi N, Ota K, Tsunoda N, Seike K, Kanetake Y, Tsutaya A. Weight-bearing-line analysis in supramalleolar osteotomy for varus-type osteoarthritis of the ankle. *J Bone Joint Surg Am.* 2015;97(4):333-339.
9. Hintermann B, Knupp M, Barg A. Supramalleolar osteotomies for the treatment of ankle arthritis. *J Am Acad Orthop Surg.* 2016;24(7):424-432.
10. Easley ME. Surgical treatment of the arthritic varus ankle. *Foot Ankle Clin.* 2012;17(4):665-686.
11. Barg A, Pagenstert GI, Leumann AG, Müller AM, Henninger HB, Valderrabano V. Treatment of the arthritic valgus ankle. *Foot Ankle Clin.* 2012;17(4):647-663.
12. Tanaka Y, Takakura Y, Hayashi K, Taniguchi A, Kumai T, Sugimoto K. Low tibial osteotomy for varus-type osteoarthritis of the ankle. *J Bone Joint Surg Br.* 2006;88(7):909-913.
13. Lee W-C, Moon J-S, Lee K, Byun WJ, Lee SH. Indications for supramalleolar osteotomy in patients with ankle osteoarthritis and varus deformity. *J Bone Joint Surg Am.* 2011;93(13):1243-1248.
14. Park CH, Kim JB, Kim J, Yi Y, Lee W-C. Joint preservation surgery for varus ankle arthritis with large talar tilt. *Foot Ankle Int.* 2021;42(12):1554-1564.
15. Park CH, Kim J, Kim JB, Lee W-C. Repositional subtalar arthrodesis combined with supramalleolar osteotomy for late-stage varus ankle arthritis with hindfoot valgus. *Foot Ankle Int.* 2022;43(2):203-210.
16. Kim J, Rajan L, Kumar P, Kim J-B, Lee W-C. Lower limb alignment in patients with primary valgus ankle arthritis: a comparative analysis with patients with varus ankle arthritis and healthy controls. *Foot Ankle Surg.* 2023;29(1):72-78.
17. Yi Y, Cho J-H, Kim J-B, Kim J-Y, Park S-Y, Lee WC. Change in talar translation in the coronal plane after mobile-bearing total ankle replacement and its association with lower-limb and hindfoot alignment. *J Bone Joint Surg Am.* 2017;99(4):e13.
18. Tochigi Y, Suh J-S, Amendola A, Pedersen DR, Saltzman CL. Ankle alignment on lateral radiographs. Part 1: sensitivity of measures to perturbations of ankle positioning. *Foot Ankle Int.* 2006;27(2):82-87.
19. Kim J, Kim J-B, Lee W-C. Clinical and radiographic results of ankle joint preservation surgery in posterior ankle arthritis. *Foot Ankle Int.* 2021;42(10):1260-1269.
20. Ahn J-Y, Park C-H, Jung JW, Lee W-C. Plain radiographs underestimate varus deformity of the tibial plafond. *J Foot Ankle Surg.* 2022;61(4):836-840.

21. Burssens AB, Buedts K, Barg A, et al. Is lower-limb alignment associated with hindfoot deformity in the coronal plane? A weightbearing CT analysis. *Clin Orthop Relat Res.* 2020;478(1):154.
22. Easley ME, Park YU, Park JY, Kim HN. Use of a locking plate and drill sleeves to guide dome-shaped supramalleolar osteotomy: technique tip. *Foot Ankle Int.* 2021;42(9):1185-1190.
23. Wagner P, Colin F, Hintermann B. Distal tibia dome osteotomy. *Tech Foot Ankle Surg.* 2014;13(2):103-107.
24. Faict S, Burssens A, Van Oevelen A, Maeckelbergh L, Mertens P, Buedts K. Correction of ankle varus deformity using patient-specific dome-shaped osteotomy guides designed on weight-bearing CT: a pilot study. *Arch Orthop Trauma Surg.* 2021;143(2):791-799.
25. Suh JW, Park KH, Lee JW, Han SH. Outcomes of oblique supramalleolar osteotomy without fibular osteotomy for congruent-and incongruent-type medial ankle arthritis. *Foot Ankle Surg.* 2022;28(5):603-609.
26. Ahn T-K, Yi Y, Cho J-H, Lee W-C. A cohort study of patients undergoing distal tibial osteotomy without fibular osteotomy for medial ankle arthritis with mortise widening. *J Bone Joint Surg Am.* 2015;97(5):381-388.
27. Warnock KM, Johnson BD, Wright JB, Ambrose CG, Clanton TO, McGarvey WC. Calculation of the opening wedge for a low tibial osteotomy. *Foot Ankle Int.* 2004;25(11):778-782.
28. Lee W-C, Moon J-S, Lee HS, Lee K. Alignment of ankle and hindfoot in early stage ankle osteoarthritis. *Foot Ankle Int.* 2011;32(7):693-699.
29. Hayashi K, Tanaka Y, Kumai T, Sugimoto K, Takakura Y. Correlation of compensatory alignment of the subtalar joint to the progression of primary osteoarthritis of the ankle. *Foot Ankle Int.* 2008;29(4):400-406.

38 Tibiotalocalcaneal Fusion

Braden Boyer, John Wunn Cancian, and Clayton C. Bettin

INTRODUCTION

Patients with end-stage arthritis of the tibiotalar and subtalar joints are best treated with tibiotalocalcaneal (TTC) arthrodesis. Achieving adequate fixation in the correction of severe deformity or trauma in the ankle and hindfoot can be challenging. In cases with complex deformity of the tibiotalar joint, the subtalar joint (although not arthritic) is sacrificed to obtain a more robust fixation construct. These patients often have poor bone quality secondary to osteoporosis, diabetes, and renal osteodystrophy. Such challenges can be compounded by a poor soft tissue envelope about the ankle, including previous traumatic wounds or surgical incisions. Due to age and comorbidities, many patients will struggle to maintain non–weight-bearing precautions. For such patients, TTC arthrodesis may be the most predictable treatment to return function.

Numerous treatment strategies have been attempted for these complicated patients. Fixation options include screws-only, locking plates, and blade plates. These are reasonable options in some scenarios; however, their load-sharing nature may limit their success. External fixation can be added to any construct; however, the challenges of external fixation are well known to include infection and poor patient tolerance.

Tibiotalocalcaneal arthrodesis with the use of a hindfoot intramedullary nail (IMN) can be useful in these salvage situations to achieve a plantigrade foot and pain-free ambulation. This procedure can be performed less invasively and can respect a poor soft tissue envelope. The use of a load-sharing device reduces the risk of failure in patients who may bear weight early as well as provide sufficiently rigid fixation in severe deformity. Supplemental fixation, including additional screws or a locked lateral plate, can be added to provide additional strength to the construct in those with particularly poor bone quality.

Numerous approaches are feasible to use with this procedure. Posterior approaches have the advantage of allowing for a simultaneous approach to the tibiotalar and subtalar joints and allow for a robust soft tissue envelope; however, the prone positioning of the patient may be problematic. Anterior and medial approaches are useful in conjunction with other approaches for subtalar joint preparation. A lateral approach allows for easy access to both the ankle and subtalar joints and may be performed in a fibula-sparing or sacrificing manner. Although the fibula may be completely spared by anterior tissue retraction and preparing the tibiotalar joint around the intact fibula, we generally perform a fibula osteotomy to enhance joint visualization and/or deformity correction. Portions of the fibula may be utilized as graft to aid in restoration of structural defects or as an onlay strut for additional bridging fixation. If an onlay strut is planned, maintaining the posterior soft tissue attachments to the fibula will enhance vascularization of the strut. The lateral approach is our preferred surgical approach. We often use combined approaches, particularly the combination of medial and lateral, to facilitate deformity correction. Minimally invasive and arthroscopic approaches are also described,[1] and in certain patients (ie, geriatric ankle fractures), preparation of the joints for arthrodesis may not be required.[2]

Hybrid fixation, composed of IMN and locking plates, is a concept that is gaining traction in the trauma community, particularly in the treatment of complex periarticular fractures in the elderly, which are at high risk of nonunion, including distal femur fractures, proximal tibia, and proximal humerus. Biomechanical studies show that this construct combines the strengths of the load-sharing nature of the IMN with the torsional strength of a plate making it superior to either as shown in both biomechanical[3] and canine models.[4] In distal femur fractures, patients with a plate/nail combination are allowed immediately full-weight bearing, which is a significant benefit to elderly patients.[5] Hybrid fixation may prove especially useful in patients with neuropathic arthropathy where poor bone quality, combined with inability to maintain protected weight-bearing precautions, significantly increases the risk of complications postoperatively.

INDICATIONS AND CONTRAINDICATIONS

The primary indication for TTC arthrodesis is as salvage procedure in the treatment of severe tibiotalar and hindfoot arthritis, deformities, and/or trauma. Specific indications include combined ankle and subtalar osteoarthritis, severe posttraumatic osteoarthritis and deformity including nonunion or malunion, severe flatfoot deformity (Bluman stage IV or progressive collapsing flatfoot deformity stage 2E), avascular necrosis of the talus, Charcot neuroarthropathy, rheumatoid arthritis, or failed ankle arthroplasty. Deformities that cause ulceration are a good indication for TTC arthrodesis.[6] A TTC nail may also be indicated for severe ankle and pilon fractures, especially fracture/dislocations in minimally ambulatory elderly patients[7,8] or diabetics.

Contraindications primarily include active infection, poor vascularity, or significant tibial deformity. This procedure is relatively contraindicated in the younger, more active patient as TTC arthrodesis may be poorly tolerated in the high-demand patient; however, it may be appropriate as an attempt at limb salvage. The use of a fibular-sparing technique should be considered to permit conversion to an ankle arthroplasty in an appropriate patient. For patients with severe bone loss, the inclusion of bulk allograft (frequently femoral head allograft[9,10]) or a 3D-printed arthrodesis cage[11] may be needed to prevent excessive shortening. While peripheral neuropathy is a risk factor for nonunion, the salvage nature of this procedure does not make this a contraindication.[12] In the setting of severe osteoporosis, neuropathy, or likely patient noncompliance, we typically add a lateral locking plate to the construct to improve rigidity. In our practice, we routinely use supplemental fixation with either additional screws or locked plating in addition to IMN.

PREOPERATIVE PLANNING

We begin preoperative evaluation with a standard history and physical examination. In the patient's history, we risk stratify the patient noting any history and severity of diabetes, osteoporosis, thyroid dysfunction, nicotine use, or other systemic conditions, which will inhibit bone healing. Risk factors that are modifiable, such as nicotine use, are optimized prior to surgical intervention. If there is a history of previous surgery with retained hardware, we routinely obtain infection labs to evaluate for septic nonunion. If needed, preoperative medical clearance is obtained from the patient's primary care physician.

On physical examination, particular attention is paid to the soft tissue envelope as well as the vascular status of the extremity. Previous surgical incisions and other wounds are noted, and incisions kept away if possible. If good pulses are not palpated, we send patients for vascular evaluation. Sensation testing with 5.07-gauge monofilament is performed as is a motor examination. Deformity is noted along with its ability to be passively corrected, and the neurologic status of the extremity is documented. It is important to evaluate the entirety of the extremity for more proximal concomitant deformities or surgeries (eg, stemmed total joint arthroplasty).

Standard weight-bearing radiographs are obtained of the foot, ankle, and tibia. Computed tomography (CT) scan is essential for preoperative planning, and if available, we prefer weight-bearing CT. Magnetic resonance imaging may be considered in cases of avascular necrosis. We evaluate the imaging for several key factors; most importantly, we evaluate the overall deformity and preoperatively plan for deformity correction. The source of deformity is crucial, whether tibiotalar, hindfoot, or a combination of the two. In planning for our construct, we evaluate the amount of bone stock available and consider whether structural autograft or allograft will be required (or, in rare cases, a 3D-printed cage). A discussion is held with the patient regarding the planned shortening required to obtain primary bone contact; if the patient is not amenable to shoe wear modifications to make up for the length inequality, a structural graft or cage is templated accordingly. Arthritis and joint deformity are evaluated. Previous hardware is noted, and consideration is given to hardware removal or retention.

Preoperatively, the surgeon must consider the required deformity correction. If the deformity is primarily through the ankle joint, osteotomy of the distal tibia and/or talus may be sufficient. Deformity in the hindfoot requires correction through the subtalar joint.

An array of IMNs is available from various manufacturers. Some are straight, while others include a valgus bend; either are reasonable depending on surgeon preference.[13-15] Valgus nails may allow

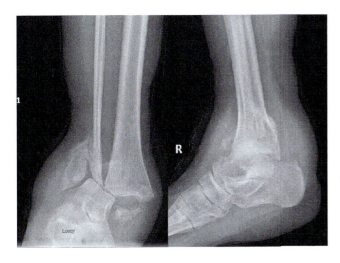

FIGURE 38.1 Preoperative anteroposterior and lateral radiographs demonstrate chronic ankle fracture dislocation with significant valgus deformity and callus formation.

for more fixation within the calcaneus but require manipulating the hindfoot into a neutral position for reaming and allowing the nail to return the hindfoot to slight valgus; straight nails can be placed with the ankle and hindfoot held reduced in the desired position. Nails are available with and without internal compression mechanisms; no difference has been shown to date with either technique.[16]

The following case example is a 48-year-old homeless neuropathic patient with renal disease who presented 5 months after a fall with persistent deformity to her extremity. She was found to have a fracture dislocation of the ankle with significant callus formation (Fig. 38.1). After discussion of options and medical optimization, we elected to proceed with TTC arthrodesis using a hybrid IMN and lateral locked plate technique due to her difficulty following non–weight-bearing precautions in the postoperative period.

SURGICAL TECHNIQUE

- Positioning
  - Based on surgeon preference and patient's pathology, the operation may be performed in a supine, lateral, or prone position. Bring the patient to the end of the bed so the foot hangs over the edge for ease of access to the heel.
  - Minimize tension on the Achilles tendon by keeping the knee in slight flexion. This can be accomplished by using a ramp bone foam. A bump is placed under the ipsilateral hip to point the tibial tubercle directly upward. A tourniquet is placed on the upper thigh. The body and bone foam are secured to the table with appropriate belts and tape (Fig. 38.2).

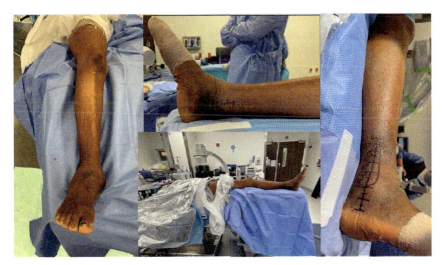

FIGURE 38.2 Patient is positioned supine with leg on a foam ramp and bump under the hip. Longitudinal lateral and curvilinear surgical incisions are shown.

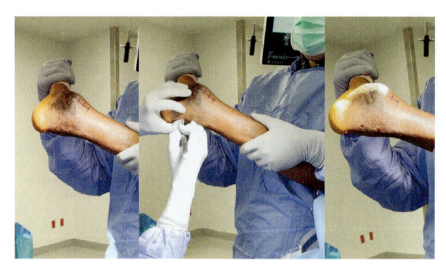

FIGURE 38.3 Triple hemisection of the Achilles tendon is performed to correct any equinus contracture.

- Place the fluoroscopy unit on the side of the contralateral leg and the view screens on the operative side positioned near the head of the OR table.
- The leg is prepped and draped in a standard sterile fashion, and the leg is exsanguinated with an elastic bandage and the tourniquet insufflated to desired pressure.
- Approaches and dissection
  - We routinely begin with a triple Hoke hemisection of the Achilles tendon to prevent equinus contracture from adequate joint positioning for fusion (Fig. 38.3).
  - A variety of approaches can be used and are dictated by physician preference, implants used, soft tissue compromise, and secondary procedures to be performed during the operation. A lateral approach provides easy access to both ankle and subtalar joints and is most used. A medial approach can be added to improve joint preparation particularly the medial gutter in varus ankle arthritis. A posterior approach may be appropriate when compromised lateral skin and soft tissue is present.
  - Numerous designs and constructs can be utilized including compression screws, IMNs, blade plates, locking plates, external fixation, and combination or hybrid fixation. The approach, joint preparation, and deformity correction are the same regardless of the method of fixation. The choice of the fixation construct is made based on patient factors, surgeon experience, and preference to bring about a successful outcome.
  - Laterally, the transfibular approach can be completed with or without fibular strut graft. A fibular onlay strut graft brings an added measure of stability and vascular supply to the fusion site while also serving as a guide to proper rotation and positioning.
  - A longitudinal incision is made centered over the fibula and carried distally 2 cm past the tip of the fibula and then curved to the base of the fourth metatarsal. If a lateral locked plate is to be used alone or in conjunction with an IMN, the incision should be extended longitudinally in line with the fibula to the plantar surface of the calcaneal tuberosity and not curved anteriorly (Fig. 38.4). This will allow better access to the posterior tuberosity for locking screw placement through the plate. Care is taken to protect the superficial peroneal nerve proximally and the sural nerve distally. The peroneal tendons are identified and retracted (Fig. 38.5).
  - Release the ATFL and CFL to allow mobility of the talus.
  - Dissection is carried over the anterior surface of the tibia and a deep retractor is placed. Large visible osteophytes are removed.
  - A medial incision is made, and the medial malleolus is skeletonized to allow medial gutter débridement and to protect the posterior neurovascular bundle if the medial malleolus is planned to be excised (Fig. 38.6).
  - Transect the fibula with a microsagittal saw approximately 5 to 7 cm proximal to the tibial plafond. Make a second parallel cut that allows removal of 1 cm of fibula.

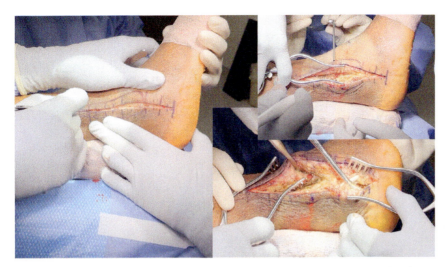

FIGURE 38.4 Lateral incision is performed, and peroneal tendons are exposed and protected as needed.

- The anterior syndesmotic ligaments are released using Bovie. A lamina spreader between the tibia and fibula can put these ligaments on tension for ease of release. Release can also be facilitated by advancing an osteotome down the incisura anteriorly (Fig. 38.7). Care is taken to maintain the posterior syndesmotic ligaments and fibular blood supply if a fibular onlay is planned later in the procedure. If the fibula is to be excised for placement of a lateral plate, that is performed at this time (Fig. 38.8).
- Stabilize the fibula with towel clips and make a longitudinal cut in the sagittal plane in order to remove the medial half of the fibula. Maintain the lateral half with the intact posterior syndesmotic ligaments and periosteum and allow it to fall out of the way posteriorly. This lateral portion may later be fixed to the tibia and talus as an onlay graft after nail construct is complete using two 3.5-mm lag screws, or excised if planning to apply a lateral TTC plate (see Fig. 38.33).

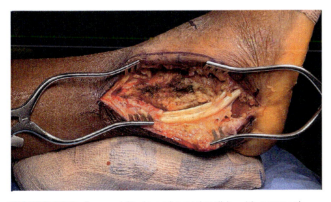

FIGURE 38.5 Exposed fibula and anterior tibia with peroneal tendons visible and Weitlaner retractors positioned.

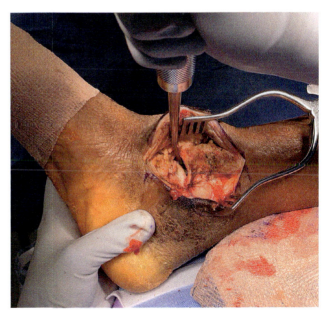

FIGURE 38.6 Medial exposure performed, and a Cobb elevator is used to mobilize and expose the ankle.

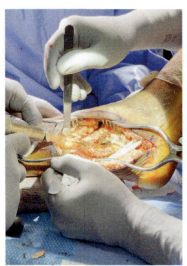
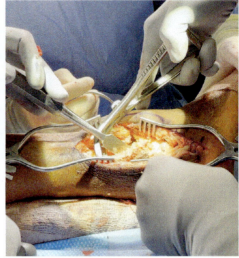

FIGURE 38.7 A fibular osteotomy is performed with a saw and syndesmotic ligaments are released with osteotomes and electrocautery.

- Place a pin distractor with large K-wires laterally centered about the tibiotalar joint with handles posterior to aid in retraction of the fibula. The ankle joint is then opened and prepared (Fig. 38.9).
- The pin distractor is adjusted to be centered over the subtalar joint for distraction and joint preparation (Fig. 38.10). Ensure that the interosseous talocalcaneal ligament is released in order to visualize and prepare the medial facet of the subtalar joint.
- Joint preparation
  - There are a variety of techniques for joint preparation, but union outcome is heavily dependent on the primary principles of removing all cartilage, devitalized bone, and soft tissue within the joint in order to provide an environment of bony apposition.
  - OR light positioning and use of a headlight can aid in visualizing all remaining cartilage. Gentle motion of the joint during preparation can also reveal areas of remaining cartilage.
  - If minimal deformity correction is required, joint preparation is best completed by removing cartilage with a knife, sharp osteotomes, curettes (both cupped and ringed), and rongeurs. Curved instruments can help clear the gutters and follow the curvature of the bone.

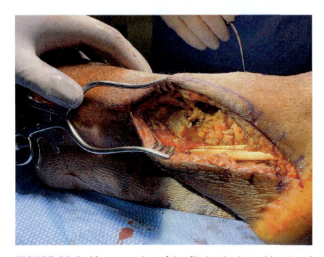

FIGURE 38.8 After resection of the fibula, the lateral border of the tibia is visualized.

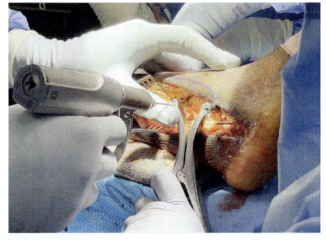

FIGURE 38.9 Hintermann distractor is placed at tibiotalar joint with large K-wires.

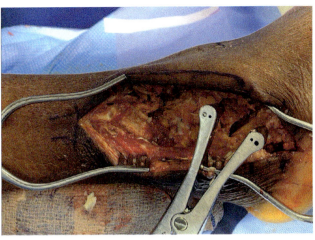

FIGURE 38.10 Subtalar joint is distracted for joint preparation using an additional Hintermann distractor.

- If major deformity correction is required, flat cuts that preserve bone can be performed but should achieve neutral extension, slight external rotation, and neutral to slight valgus. If flat cuts are made be sure to dissect posteriorly around the medial and lateral tibia and protect the medial neurovascular bundle with large Hohmann retractors. The medial malleolus can be excised in line with the tibial plafond to aid in medial translation of the hindfoot under the mechanical axis of the tibia.
- Perform thorough irrigation of joints prior to preparation in order to avoid postpreparation flush of cancellous graft.
- Subchondral bone should be prepared in order to optimize healing via increased bone surface area, vascular channels, and inflammatory response setting the stage for union. This is completed through any combination of subchondral drilling with a 2.0-mm drill bit, fenestration with a 4-mm powered burr at low speed (20,000 rev/min) and "fish-scaling" with a small osteotome.
- Rongeurs and a bone mill may be utilized to morselize large pieces of removed noninfected bone into graft to be placed into joints for fusion (Fig. 38.11).
- Place any acquired autograft, morselized graft from the fibula, or allograft adjuncts within the joints (Fig. 38.12).
- If there are major tibial or talar bone deficiencies, structural bone graft such as portions of the fibula, femoral head allograft, iliac crest autograft, or 3D-printed wedges may be

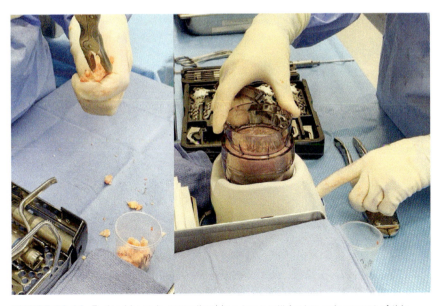

FIGURE 38.11 Excised bone is morselized in a bone mill for later placement of this autograft into any bone voids.

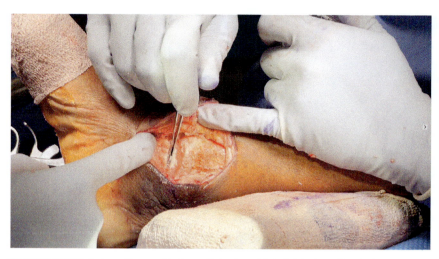

FIGURE 38.12 Autograft or synthetic graft is placed into joints for arthrodesis.

used. The talar head and neck should be preserved in order to maintain talonavicular joint function.
- Reduction and alignment
  ○ The goal in positioning of the joints is to create a plantigrade alignment. The ankle and subtalar joint are adjusted to neutral dorsiflexion-plantarflexion, approximately 5° external rotation to the tibial tubercle, about 5° of valgus, neutral medial-lateral translation of the talus, and neutral to slight posterior translation of the talus. The slight posterior translation of the talus can help avoid a gait pattern described as "vaulting" over the foot. Avoid extension, varus, or internal rotation at the ankle as these are poorly tolerated (Figs. 38.13 to 38.15).
  ○ The tibiotalar and subtalar joints are held in the desired reduced position and held with provisional K-wire fixation. The position of the sinus tarsi space is adjusted by using a lamina spreader between the lateral process of the talus and anterior process of the calcaneus. Opening the laminar spreader will lengthen the lateral column. This technique of lengthening the

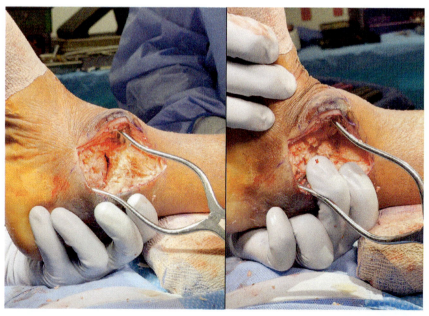

FIGURE 38.13 The ankle and subtalar joints are manually reduced and positioned for arthrodesis.

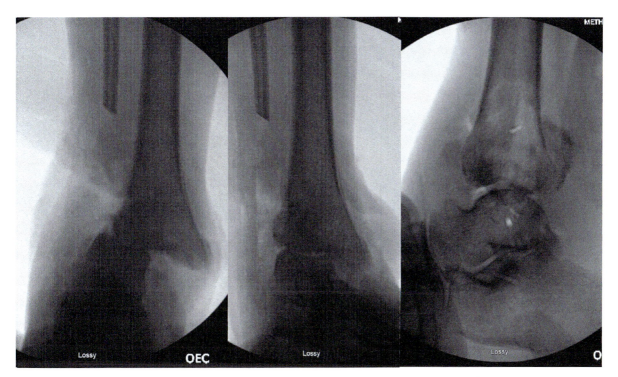

FIGURE 38.14 Intraoperative fluoroscopy shots show joint reduction and positioning for arthrodesis.

lateral column may also be performed by manually manipulating the K-wires placed through the Hintermann distractor. This pushes the calcaneus back under the tibia without gapping the subtalar joint as it would when a varus moment is applied instead. Ensure that wires are placed with the hindfoot nail and associated outrigger in mind to avoid traffic and blockage of final fixation. We prefer one wire from the posterior calcaneal tuberosity into the posterior tibia, one from the anterior process of the calcaneus into the lateral anterior tibia, and one wire from the medial tibia into the anterior process of the calcaneus. These wires are clipped

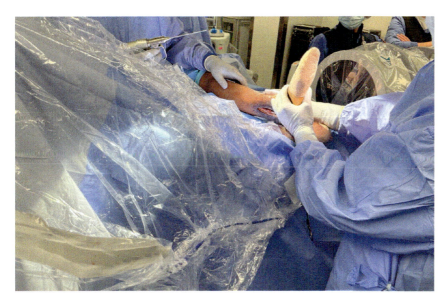

FIGURE 38.15 Joints are held in desired position for arthrodesis under arthroscopy while an assistant prepares to place provisional fixation.

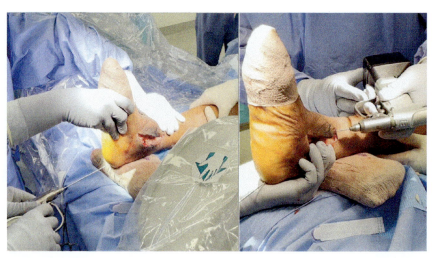

FIGURE 38.16 Provisional fixation is placed from posterior calcaneus into the tibia and medial anterior tibia into anterior process of the calcaneus.

several centimeters away from the skin to allow removal but to avoid the outrigger of the IMN (Figs. 38.16 to 38.20).
- The contralateral foot and ankle can also be evaluated preoperatively in order to establish appropriate specific alignment for any given patient.
• Intramedullary nail steps
  - There are many hindfoot nail manufacturers, and appropriate care should be taken to understand the given technique and follow the manufacturer guidelines. However, there are basic steps consistent with each hindfoot nail implant.
  - Similar with other nailing procedures of long bones, the positioning and alignment in the final result is largely dependent on the start point of the guide pin with little room left for adjustments once the canal is reamed. The start point should first be identified on the lateral fluoroscopic view to ensure that the pin is at least 2.5 cm posterior to the calcaneal cuboid joint. The start point varies per implant, but the trajectory should ensure a center-center position at the tibiotalar

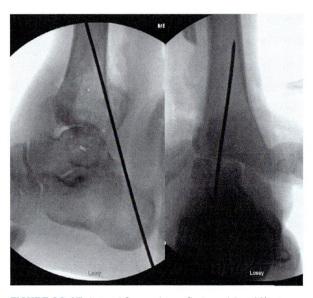

FIGURE 38.17 Lateral fluoro shows first provisional K-wire placed from posterior calcaneus to the tibia.

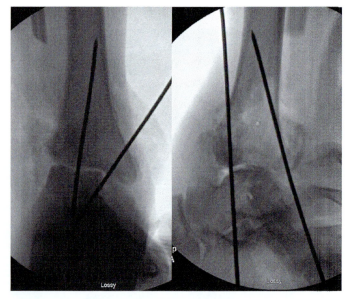

FIGURE 38.18 Anteroposterior fluoro shows placement of second provisional K-wire from medial tibia to anterior process of the calcaneus, out of path of planned nail placement.

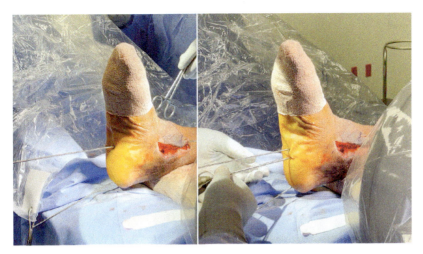

FIGURE 38.19 Additional provisional fixation placed from anterior process calcaneus into anterior tibia prior to obtaining starting point for intramedullary nail.

joint seen in both the anteroposterior and lateral fluoroscopic images and allow the nail to pass into the center of the tibial diaphysis (Fig. 38.21). An axial view of the calcaneus can also be used to evaluate guide pin position. In the sagittal plane, a line is drawn from the second toe to the center of the heel. In the coronal plane, line is drawn at the junction of the anterior and middle thirds of the heel pad. Where they intersect indicates the entry portal for the nail, but this should be verified under fluoroscopy.

- We prefer a nail length that permits the proximal end of the nail to be engaged with diaphyseal bone for increased construct stability, which is generally a 20-cm implant length. A nail that ends in the distal metaphysis has the potential to "windshield washer" in patients with poor bone quality. We try to end the nail below where a standard transtibial amputation would be performed so as to not interfere with that additional surgery should significant complications occur in the future.
- Correction of alignment should be made at each joint before crossing with the guide pin. With the ankle and hindfoot alignment held, the pin is advanced into the tibial metaphysis and position using fluoroscopy.

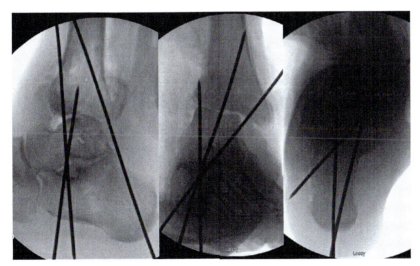

FIGURE 38.20 Fluoro of three provisional K-wires for stabilization outside of intended path of intramedullary nail.

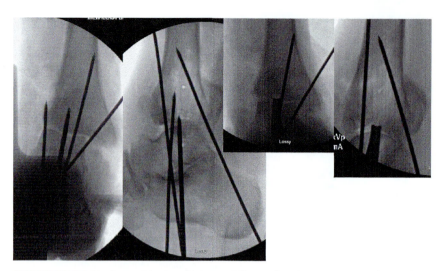

FIGURE 38.21 Starting guidewire of intramedullary nail and entry reamer advanced into center-center position of the tibia.

- A 2-cm horizontal or longitudinal plantar heel incision is made at the level of the pin. We prefer a transverse incision as it is in line with the Langer lines of the foot and allows easier medial-lateral correction of the starting point. Bluntly dissect down to the calcaneus. Care must be taken to protect the plantar neurovascular structures.
- An entry reamer is then used through a soft tissue sleeve to dilate the proximal end. The guide pin is then replaced by a ball-tip guidewire and advanced past the isthmus of the tibia. Sequential reaming is then performed ensuring to ream at least 2 to 3 cm beyond the proposed tip of the nail with each passing of the reamer. Reaming is typically completed at 1 to 1.5 cm larger than the selected diameter of the nail. Larger diameter nails will have more resistance to breakage but have increased risk of periprosthetic fracture (Figs. 38.22 to 38.24).
- After reaming is completed, the nail is assembled per manufacturer guidelines to the corresponding jig and impacted by hand into the foot until it is not easily advanced. At which point, a mallet is used to impact until the nail is flush with or slightly inside the plantar aspect of the calcaneus as compression will bring the nail just outside the cortex (Figs. 38.25 and 38.26).
- Interlocking screws are placed using outriggers or perfect circle techniques with a variety of internal and external compression methods (Figs. 38.27 to 38.30).
• Compression
- The interlocking screws for IM are typically designed to be placed distally through outriggers followed by the application of axial compression externally, internally, or both.

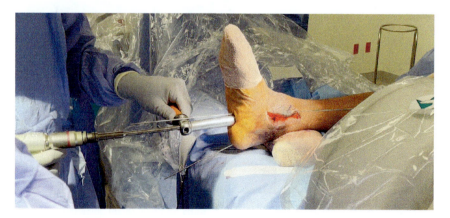

FIGURE 38.22 Entry reamer through calcaneus, talus, and into the distal tibia.

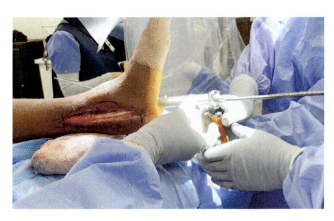

FIGURE 38.23 Flexible reamer placed to ream diaphysis of the tibia.

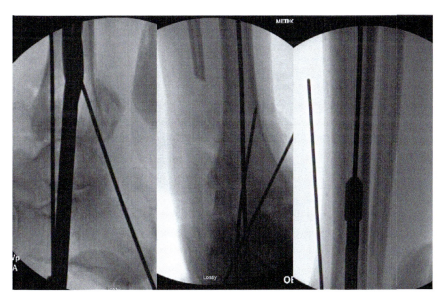

FIGURE 38.24 Lateral and anteroposterior of intramedullary reaming.

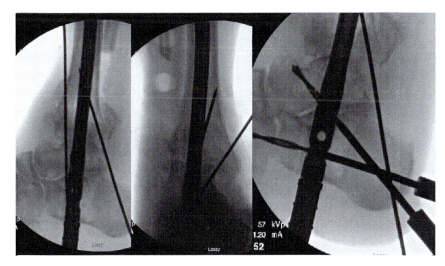

FIGURE 38.25 Fluoro of nail insertion depth and interlocking drills.

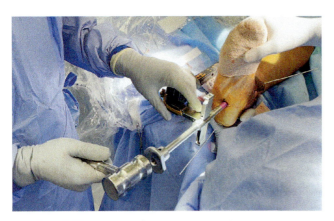

FIGURE 38.26 Insertion of intramedullary nail.

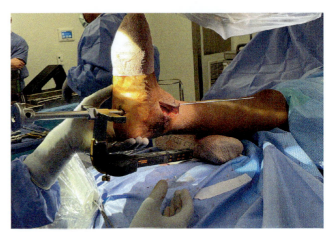

FIGURE 38.27 Positioning for interlocking screws.

- External compression is applied via impaction after distal interlocking and prior to proximal interlocking by hitting the nail or outrigger with a heavy mallet (see Fig. 38.29). Internal compression may be applied in appropriate nails through implant designs such as tightening compression rods or nitinol sustained compression.
- Ensure that the distal end of the IMN is not plantar or below the weight-bearing surface of the calcaneus.
- Once the depth of the nail is confirmed on the lateral fluoroscopic view, rotation and alignment should be checked.
- Proximal and distal interlocking screws are placed as per the manufacturer's technique guide and following directions for any internal and external compression desired. Once distal fixation is complete, additional compression is applied at the tibiotalar joint through impaction. Proximal screws from medial to lateral are then placed either in static or dynamic slots. Static slots will lock the rotation and maintain the current compression, while the dynamic slots allow the nail to settle more proximally with a goal to sustain bone-to-bone apposition at the fusion site.

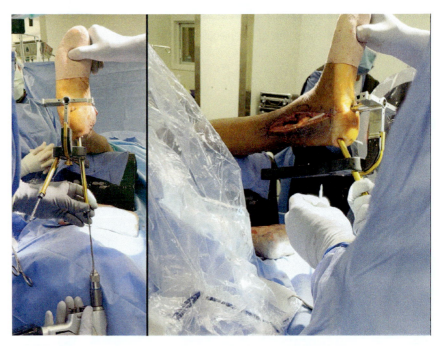

FIGURE 38.28 A radiolucent triangle is useful to support the leg so that the outrigger is not manipulated during interlocking screw placement.

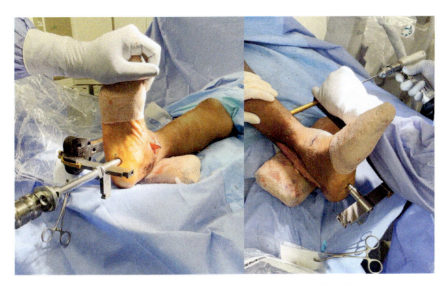

FIGURE 38.29 Impaction of intramedullary nail prior to proximal interlocking screw placement.

- Prior to placing these screws, ensure appropriate rotation of the foot. While holding the rotation and maintaining tibiotalar compression, place the proximal interlocking screws.
- Supplemental fixation
  - Additional cannulated screws outside the nail crossing the fusion sites or lateral locking plates may be used to increase strength and stability of the construct.
  - For supplemental fixation, cannulated 7.0-mm screws may be placed from the posterior calcaneus into the tibia and from the medial tibia into the anterior process of the calcaneus. Some implants have outrigger guides to place these screws out of the path of the nail, but a freehand technique may also be performed.
  - A TTC locking plate can be used in a nail-plate construct fashion with linking screws above and below the IMN interlocks as is often seen in the trauma world with distal femur fracture. This is particularly helpful in patients with poor bone quality such as those with osteoporosis, diabetes, or in patients poorly compliant with postoperative protocols. If a locking plate is to be used in conjunction with the IMN, we recommend a 10-mm-wide IMN and a locking plate with variable angle capability in all holes so that screws may be inserted around the IMN

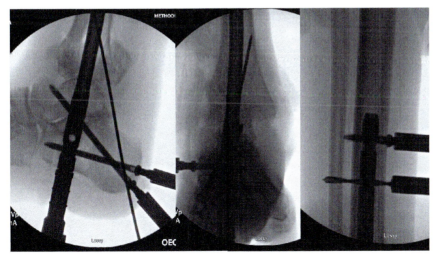

FIGURE 38.30 Fluoro of interlocking screw placement.

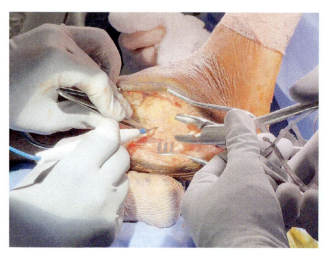

FIGURE 38.31 Clearing lateral tissue from tibia for lateral locked plate placement.

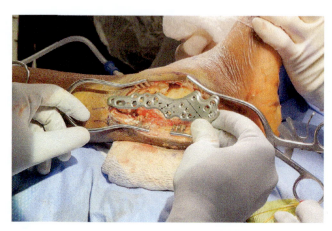

FIGURE 38.32 Plate selection for lateral variable angle locked plate for supplemental fixation.

(Figs. 38.31 through 38.36). Placement of a plate will preclude an onlay fibular strut, so one must balance enhanced construct rigidity at the expense of removing available bone stock. In cases of severe deformity, anticipated patient noncompliance with restricted weight-bearing precautions, and an amenable soft tissue envelope, we prefer to excise the fibula and place a supplemental plate for enhanced fixation.
- If the fibula is maintained, it can then be fixated to the talus and tibia as a lateral strut with 3.5-mm cortical screws and washers.
- Supplemental graft is placed as desired, vancomycin powder is placed into the deep wounds, and the wounds are closed in a layered fashion.
- Lateral locking plate
  - If a lateral locked plate is chosen instead of an IMN, the initial procedure is the same as identified above until the foot is pinned into a reduced position.
  - Prior to placing the lateral plate, we prefer to place 7.0-mm partially threaded screws from the medial tibia into the calcaneus to provide initial compression.
  - A lateral locked plate may then be applied to the tibia, talus, and calcaneus with bicortical locking screws.
  - Lateral locked plates in isolation may be most useful in large deformity cases where medial incisions are not desired as it may be difficult to line up the calcaneus under the tibia to permit IMN fixation.
  - Caution, though, is necessary as the locked plate is a load-bearing implant that is subject to failure in patients noncompliant with weight-bearing precautions.
- External fixation
  - In cases of significant infection where amputation is refused and a single-stage procedure is desired, the procedure is the same until provisional reduction and pinning is performed.

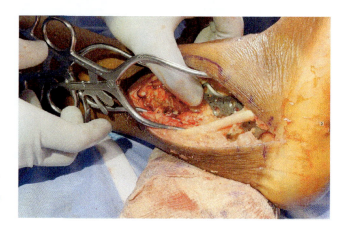

FIGURE 38.33 Positioning plate deep to peroneal tendons.

38 Tibiotalocalcaneal Fusion

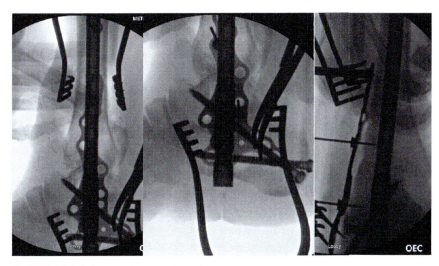

FIGURE 38.34 Fluoro of lateral plate placement.

- At this point, we place vancomycin powder into the wounds and close the surgical wounds.
- A three ringed static Ilizarov fixator is applied with fine wires only in neuropathic patients due to the increased risk of fracture with half-pins. We prefer one ring around the midtibia level, one ring around the distal tibia, and a foot plate. We use three olive or smooth wires per level in the tibia, three in the calcaneus, and two in the forefoot. Compression across the fusion site is applied through threaded rods after removing the provisional K-wire fixation. Please refer to the chapter on ankle arthrodesis with external fixation for further details.

PEARLS AND PITFALLS

- Accurate guidewire placement is essential. Avoid aiming the wire posterior into the tibia for an IMN as this will cause the nail to hit the posterior tibia leading to fracture or causing the foot to go into an equinus position.
- Provisional K-wire fixation should be placed out of the planned path of the IMN.
- Use visual inspection and fluoroscopy to confirm optimum alignment. Avoid a plantarflexion or varus alignment.
- Be aware of tibial nerve location just medial to flexor hallucis longus to avoid injury.
- Avoid overreaming or aggressive reaming particularly in osteopenic bone.

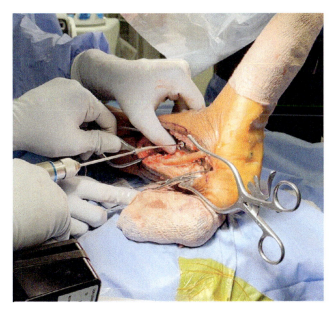

FIGURE 38.35 Screw placement in lateral locked plate.

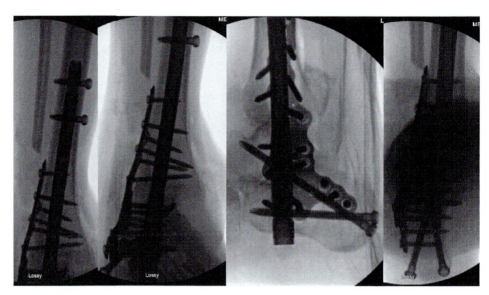

FIGURE 38.36 Final fluoroscopic images including mortise, lateral, and axial views.

- Properly prepare both ankle and subtalar joints for fusion.
- Avoid plantar heel irritation from a prominent nail or calcaneal interlocking screw.
- Compression is helpful but avoid overcompression.

POSTOPERATIVE MANAGEMENT

Immediately postoperatively, patients are placed in a well-padded splint and made non–weight bearing. We provide the patient with deep vein thrombosis prophylaxis, usually oral aspirin depending on their risk factors, as well as routine pain control and vitamin D3 supplementation. Sutures are removed at 3 to 4 weeks, and the patient is kept in a splint, which is worn an additional 4 to 8 weeks until the ankle and subtalar joint is healed clinically and radiographically (Fig. 38.37). Casts are avoided as a loosening cast can act as a weight on the arthrodesis site and possibly increase the risk of a nonunion. We aim for a total of 10 weeks of non–weight bearing; however, we recognize that

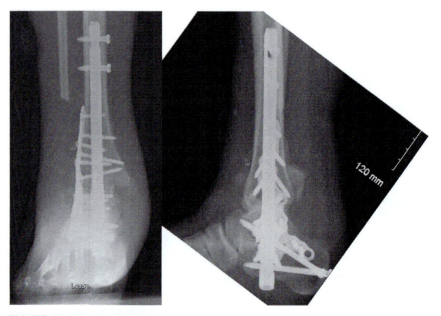

FIGURE 38.37 Final mortise and lateral radiographs.

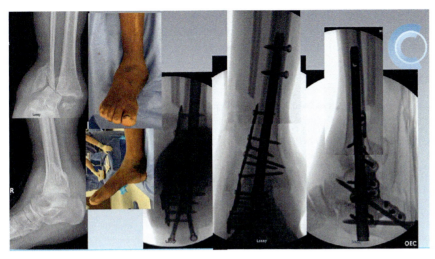

FIGURE 38.38 Before and after tibiotalocalcaneal intramedullary nail with lateral locked plate.

these patients often struggle to maintain a non–weight-bearing status and may begin ambulating on the operative extremity immediately. This high rate of patient inability to comply with postoperative non–weight bearing has driven our inclination to add a lateral locking plate to a TTC nail (Fig. 38.38).

When the splint is removed, the patient is fitted with a walking boot for an additional 4 weeks. At this point, the patient can be fitted for a rocker bottom shoe as needed. Physical therapy for gait training is added as needed.

RESULTS AND COMPLICATIONS

In these challenging operative cases, complications are common, and results can be mixed. One systemic review of outcomes following TTC found an overall 86.7% union rate, with union on average at 4.5 months. A high 55.7% complication rate was noted as well as a 22% reoperation rate, including 1.5% amputation rate.[17] A series of 41 patients reported common complications to include ankle nonunion (20%), tibial stress fracture (17%), wound infection and healing problems (9.7%), and subtalar nonunion (5%).[18]

The most significant, and common, complication with TTC IMN is nonunion. There are several risk factors for nonunion. Neuropathy is a significant risk factor for nonunion, causing bone resorption and loss of compression.[12] Other risks can include poor joint preparation or deep infection. If nonunion occurs, most nails offer the option for dynamization. A screw through the oblong dynamic proximal hole in a nail allows for compression of the nail with ambulation but will prevent rotation. If this is going to be utilized, however, it is crucial that the surgeon ream deeper than the planned nail to allow for the compression.

Implant failure is indicated by backing out of the fixation screws distally or breaking of the locking screws proximally. In most instances, this is due to delayed union or malunion, which will allow micromotion of the components or proximal migration of the nail. Prominent screws should be removed and replaced with the proximal screw in the dynamic position to prevent foot rotation but allow axial migration of the nail. Bone graft may be added to the nonunion site. Sometimes, patients who have screw breakage will progress to solid union.

Stress fractures have been reported after ankle arthrodesis with or without subtalar arthrodesis, although they may be more common in TTC arthrodesis. The origin of these stress fractures is related to the abnormal forces caused by the changes in ambulation secondary to the loss of ankle motion, likely similar to the cause of adjacent joint disease. They are common at the proximal end of hardware[19] and in patients with plantarflexed foot position; longer nails (spanning to the proximal metaphysis) may be protective.[20] Most can be treated successfully nonoperatively; unstable fractures may need to be treated with a longer nail and/or repositioning of the arthrodesis.

One large series of patients in whom TTC arthrodesis was used for limb salvage found an 88% rate of successful limb salvage. Diabetes was the greatest risk factor for amputation, and others included age, preoperative ulceration, and revision setting.[21]

REFERENCES

1. Carranza-Bencano A, Tejero S, Del Castillo-Blanco G, Fernández-Torres JJ, Alegrete-Parra A. Minimal incision surgery for tibiotalocalcaneal arthrodesis. *Foot Ankle Int.* 2014;35(3):272-284.
2. Kulakli-Inceleme E, Tas DB, Smeeing DPJ, et al. Tibiotalocalcaneal intramedullary nailing for unstable geriatric ankle fractures. *Geriatr Orthop Surg Rehabil.* 2021;12:21514593211020705.
3. Başcı O, Karakaşlı A, Kumtepe E, Güran O, Havıtçıoğlu H. Combination of anatomical locking plate and retrograde intramedullary nail in distal femoral fractures: comparison of mechanical stability. *Eklem Hastalik Cerrahisi.* 2015;26(1):21-26.
4. von Pfeil DJ, Déjardin LM, DeCamp CE, et al. In vitro biomechanical comparison of a plate-rod combination-construct and an interlocking nail-construct for experimentally induced gap fractures in canine tibiae. *Am J Vet Res.* 2005;66(9):1536-1543.
5. Liporace FA, Yoon RS. Nail plate combination technique for native and periprosthetic distal femur fractures. *J Orthop Trauma.* 2019;33(2):e64-e68.
6. Newton WN, Hoch C, Gross CE, Scott D. No effect of preoperative ulceration on outcomes of tibiotalocalcaneal arthrodesis. *Foot Ankle Surg.* 2022;28(8):1235-1238.
7. Georgiannos D, Lampridis V, Bisbinas I. Fragility fractures of the ankle in the elderly: open reduction and internal fixation versus tibio-talo-calcaneal nailing: short-term results of a prospective randomized-controlled study. *Injury.* 2017;48(2):519-524.
8. Srinath A, Matuszewski PE, Kalbac T. Geriatric ankle fracture: robust fixation versus hindfoot nail. *J Orthop Trauma.* 2021;35(Suppl 5):S41-S44.
9. Bussewitz B, DeVries JG, Dujela M, McAlister JE, Hyer CF, Berlet GC. Retrograde intramedullary nail with femoral head allograft for large deficit tibiotalocalcaneal arthrodesis. *Foot Ankle Int.* 2014;35(7):706-711.
10. Jeng CL, Campbell JT, Tang EY, Cerrato RA, Myerson MS. Tibiotalocalcaneal arthrodesis with bulk femoral head allograft for salvage of large defects in the ankle. *Foot Ankle Int.* 2013;34(9):1256-1266.
11. Abar B, Kwon N, Allen NB, et al. Outcomes of surgical reconstruction using custom 3D-printed porous titanium implants for critical-sized bone defects of the foot and ankle. *Foot Ankle Int.* 2022;43(6):750-761.
12. Patel S, Baker L, Perez J, Vulcano E, Kaplan J, Aiyer A. Risk factors for nonunion following tibiotalocalcaneal arthrodesis: a systematic review and meta-analysis. *Foot Ankle Surg.* 2022;28(1):7-13.
13. Budnar VM, Hepple S, Harries WG, Livingstone JA, Winson I. Tibiotalocalcaneal arthrodesis with a curved, interlocking, intramedullary nail. *Foot Ankle Int.* 2010;31(12):1085-1092.
14. Lucas YHJ, Abad J, Remy S, Darcel V, Chauveaux D, Laffenetre O. Tibiotalocalcaneal arthrodesis using a straight intramedullary nail. *Foot Ankle Int.* 2015;36(5):539-546.
15. Mückley T, Klos K, Drechsel T, Beimel C, Gras F, Hofmann GO. Short-term outcome of retrograde tibiotalocalcaneal arthrodesis with a curved intramedullary nail. *Foot Ankle Int.* 2011;32(1):47-56.
16. Taylor J, Lucas DE, Riley A, Simpson GA, Philbin TM. Tibiotalocalcaneal arthrodesis nails: a comparison of nails with and without internal compression. *Foot Ankle Int.* 2016;37(3):294-299.
17. Jehan S, Shakeel M, Bing AJ, Hill SO. The success of tibiotalocalcaneal arthrodesis with intramedullary nailing—a systematic review of the literature. *Acta Orthop Belg.* 2011;77(5):644-651.
18. Pellegrini MJ, Schiff AP, Adams SB Jr, DeOrio JK, Easley ME, Nunley JA II. Outcomes of tibiotalocalcaneal arthrodesis through a posterior achilles tendon-splitting approach. *Foot Ankle Int.* 2016;37(3):312-319.
19. Thordarson DB, Chang D. Stress fractures and tibial cortical hypertrophy after tibiotalocalcaneal arthrodesis with an intramedullary nail. *Foot Ankle Int.* 1999;20(8):497-500.
20. Noonan T, Pinzur M, Paxinos O, Havey R, Patwardhin A. Tibiotalocalcaneal arthrodesis with a retrograde intramedullary nail: a biomechanical analysis of the effect of nail length. *Foot Ankle Int.* 2005;26(4):304-308.
21. DeVries JG, Berlet GC, Hyer CF. Predictive risk assessment for major amputation after tibiotalocalcaneal arthrodesis. *Foot Ankle Int.* 2013;34(6):846-850.

39 Total Talus Replacement

Albert T. Anastasio, Amanda N. Fletcher, and Selene G. Parekh

INTRODUCTION

Management of avascular necrosis (AVN) or traumatic loss of significant portions of the talus remains a challenging problem for foot and ankle surgeons, and numerous techniques have been described for the treatment of these pathologies. In brief, treatment modalities are dependent on the extent or stage of AVN (partial versus complete talar body involvement, presence of subchondral collapse), involvement of the surrounding articular surfaces (ie, tibiotalar, talonavicular, or subtalar arthritis), and patient-specific factors (ie, age and functional goals). In the setting of AVN, procedures to induce revascularization such as core decompression, drilling procedures, and vascularized bone grafting techniques have been developed, with reasonable success for partial talar body involvement.[1] However, in patients with complete talar body involvement and subchondral collapse, revascularization techniques prove unsuccessful, and existing interventions focus largely on arthrodesis procedures of the tibiotalar and subtalar joints. This includes tibiotalocalcaneal (TTC) arthrodesis with or without bone block augmentation to restore length and fill bony voids. While TTC arthrodesis may relieve pain and corrects the deformity associated with talar collapse, it is associated with a high complication rate including nonunion,[2] infection, and limb shortening. Additionally, as a joint-scarifying procedure, the loss of motion may result in functional limitation and adjacent joint arthritis.[3]

The first synthetic talar body prosthesis was reported in 1997.[4] After concern for late collapse of the talar head, total talar prostheses were subsequently developed in 2005.[5,6] Total talus replacement (TTR) has emerged as a novel solution for the treatment of patients with end-stage talar AVN with significant collapse and without tibiotalar, talonavicular, or subtalar arthritis. This procedure aims to alleviate pain, restore plantigrade alignment, maintain motion, and limit the functional morbidity of a concomitant hindfoot arthrodesis procedure. With advancement in manufacturing capabilities, modern technology has allowed for 3D-printing of anatomic talar replacement componentry. Initial results prove promising as implant technology continues to develop and surgical techniques are refined, but reports including long-term follow-up are limited.[5-12] In this chapter, we aim to discuss the indications, examination, and imaging workup of the patient who is being considered for a TTR. We then aim to provide a step-by-step surgical technique for TTR including the postoperative care and a brief review of the literature evaluating outcomes following this procedure.

INDICATIONS

The indications for TTR in the patient with isolated AVN remain broad at this time: patients of any age with AVN of the talus can theoretically be considered for TTR. However, younger, active patients may have a high rate of progression of adjacent joint degenerative arthritis and therefore may be poor candidates for TTR. The aforementioned joint-sparing procedures such as core decompression and vascularized bone grafting should be considered for patients with partial talar body involvement and integrity of the articular dome and for the younger patient. A total talus is indicated for lower functional demand patients with end-stage talar AVN and subchondral collapse with minimal coronal malalignment and who desire to preserved motion in the ankle and hindfoot.

Consideration of the adjacent joints (tibiotalar, subtalar, and talonavicular joints) is imperative when evaluating a patient for candidacy for TTR. In cases where there is concomitant talonavicular or subtalar joint arthritis, talonavicular or subtalar joint arthrodesis can be performed at the time of TTR through the use of undersurface porous coating and custom-printed drill holes for placement of arthrodesis screws. Given the high rates of concomitant tibiotalar arthritis following traumatic talus injuries or AVN-induced collapse of the articular margin, a combined total ankle-TTR may be considered. This encompasses adding the tibial component of a total ankle arthroplasty above the total talus component. An articulating polyethylene component is then placed between the total talus and the tibial component of the total ankle arthroplasty to preserve motion at the tibiotalar joint. In this chapter, we will focus on isolated TTR, but the reader should be aware of the potential for combined total ankle-TTR in the patient with talar collapse and concomitant tibiotalar arthritis who is interested in preserving motion through the ankle. Additional contraindications for isolated TTR include active infection or greater than 5° of coronal malalignment, which is not correctable with soft tissue procedures or by varus or valgus-producing osteotomies. Finally, osteonecrosis with either impending or active collapse of the distal tibia, calcaneus, and navicular precludes isolated TTR.

HISTORY AND PHYSICAL EXAMINATION

The history and physical examination remain important components of the diagnosis of talar AVN and subsequent treatment considerations. Relevant question with regard to patient history include duration of symptoms, specific location of pain(s), history of trauma or ankle infection, functional limitations, and current versus desired activity level. Patient comorbidities, history of tobacco use, or use of immunosuppressive agents should also be identified as these may contribute to postoperative complications if not optimized preoperatively. Additional questions should also be asked to identify common risk factors for AVN-corticosteroid use, alcohol abuse, or foot and ankle trauma. Careful consideration of the patient's current occupation and hobbies is imperative, as arthrodesis may remain the appropriate management for a young and active individual with a physically demanding occupation who is likely to overuse their TTR.

A complete orthopedic examination of the lower extremity should then be performed. The affected foot and ankle should be examined while the patient is standing and should be compared to the contralateral extremity. Any clinically apparent coronal deformity should be noted. Observation of gait should be performed, and the patient's normal gait should be evaluated as well as during both tiptoe and heel walking. During gait evaluation, the physician should pay careful attention to lack of ankle and subtalar mobility, coronal imbalance, and excessive inversion or eversion of the foot. A careful vascular examination should be performed, as peripheral vascular disease and advanced diabetes mellitus may lead to poor wound healing following TTR. Range of motion (ROM) examination should be performed, with special emphasis on dorsiflexion, plantarflexion, inversion, and eversion through the tibiotalar and subtalar joints. In the setting of limited tibiotalar dorsiflexion, Silfverskiold testing should be performed to evaluate the need for tendo-Achilles lengthening versus gastrocnemius recession at the time of surgery. In the event of limited dorsiflexion, gastrocnemius recession may be favored, given potential for decreased plantarflexion strength after tendo-Achilles lengthening in total ankle arthroplasty.[13] The effect of tendo-Achilles lengthening versus gastrocnemius recession in the case of the total talus has not been evaluated in a direct comparison, but surgeons should consider the trade-off between the stability of the final implant and the degree of dorsiflexion when choosing whether or not to proceed with one of these adjunctive procedures. Finally, a thorough examination of the forefoot and midfoot as well as overall foot and ankle alignment should be obtained, as deformities may require additional procedures such as Cotton osteotomy or calcaneal slide osteotomy to fully restore a plantigrade foot and the native joint kinematics.

If considering a TTR for a patient, a patient-centered discussion should focus on patient education and expectation management. Patients must understand postoperative limitations including avoidance of strenuous endurance activities, especially open chain activities such as running and jumping, heavy lifting through the lower extremity, and other high-impact activities. Acute surgical risks as well as long-term risks should be addressed including the risk of degenerative arthritis throughout the tibiotalar, subtalar, and talonavicular joint, which may necessitate subsequent procedures in the future. In the patient who desires the intervention with the greatest likelihood of reducing need for secondary surgical procedures, a TTC or pantalar arthrodesis may remain the optimal technique. Attention to expectation management and patient activity modification can greatly improve the lifespan of the total talus component and limit patient dissatisfaction after this procedure.

39 Total Talus Replacement

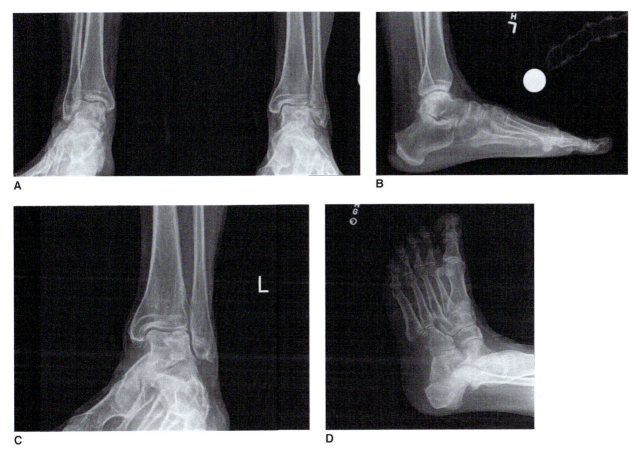

FIGURE 39.1 Initial workup for total talus replacement should include standard radiographic imaging, such as the **(A)** anteroposterior weight-bearing radiograph, **(B)** lateral radiograph, **(C)** mortise view, and **(D)** oblique view of the foot.

Imaging

The imaging workup should begin with initial weight-bearing radiographs to include the anteroposterior (Fig. 39.1), lateral, Saltzman hindfoot alignment, ankle mortise, and dorsiflexion/plantarflexion ankle views. Bilateral computed tomography (CT) scans of the ankle and hindfoot are obtained for all patients as the contralateral CT scan is used to develop the 3D-printed total talus component. Furthermore, the CT scan provides additional evaluation for degenerative change of the tibiotalar, subtalar, and talonavicular joints. 3D reconstructions also allow for quantitative analysis of bone loss and can further elucidate the presence of talar collapse. Magnetic resonance imaging (MRI) of the ankle and hindfoot is also obtained for the planned operative extremity. MRI is particularly useful in the setting of AVN, as it allows for accurate representation of the current vascularization status of the talus in addition to evaluation for degenerative cartilaginous change of the tibiotalar, subtalar, and talonavicular joints. Our authors favor a multifactorial approach involving patient history and demographic factors such as age and activity level, physical examination, CT, MRI, and intraoperative assessment when making the decision to proceed with isolated TTR.

Implants

With regard to engineering and subsequent manufacturing of the final 3D-printed total talus component, a few medical device companies currently provide 3D printing services for this componentry: Paragon 28, Inc. (Dr. Englewood, CO), restor3d (Durham, North Carolina), and 4WEB Medical (Frisco, Texas). After careful screening of a patient for appropriateness for TTR, the device representative obtains the bilateral CT scans from the treating physician (Fig. 39.2). The scans are then sent to the manufacturing site where the 3D-printed implants are produced. In total, three to four implants are created including nominal, small, and large sizes. The nominal implants are identical

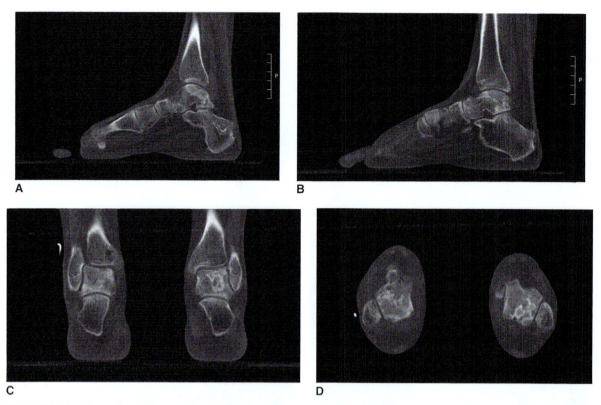

FIGURE 39.2 CT scan confirms the extent of talar avascular necrosis (AVN) and allows for evaluation for the presence of degenerative change in the adjacent joints. CT is utilized in creating size-matched total talus implants, which are sized based on the contralateral talus, in the event of talar collapse. Several cuts from the CT confirm extensive talar AVN and maintenance of joint space: **(A)** medially based sagittal cut, **(B)** sagittal cut at the level of the talonavicular joint, **(C)** coronal cut, and **(D)** axial cut.

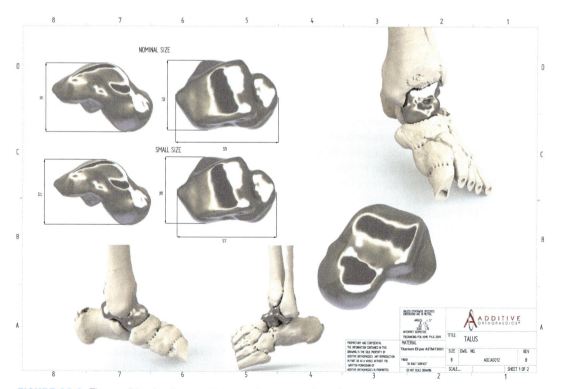

FIGURE 39.3 The small implant is created to be volumetrically 2 mm² smaller than nominal implant. The small implant allows for size reduction in the event of overstuffing. (Courtesy of Additive Orthopaedics. Reproduced with permission from Paragon 28, Inc.)

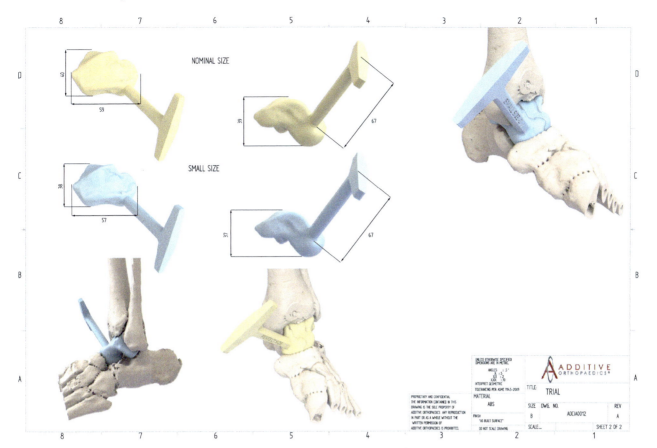

FIGURE 39.4 Plastic trial total talus components with handles attached for easy insertion and removal are also included in the manufacturer kit. (Courtesy of Additive Orthopaedics. Reproduced with permission from Paragon 28, Inc.)

in size to the contralateral, unaffected talus. The small and large implants are created to be volumetrically smaller and larger than the nominal implants, respectively. The small implant allows for implant size reduction in the event of overstuffing (Fig. 39.3). Larger implants can limit ROM but may enhance stability and restore ankle height in the setting of a talar collapse. Plastic trial total talus components are also created with handles attached for easy insertion and removal (Fig. 39.4). Care is taken to ensure an appropriately sized implant is chosen. Most commonly, the implants are made of either a cobalt-chromium alloy or a titanium alloy with a titanium nitride coating. Titanium alloys are corrosion resistant and have a modulus of elasticity similar to bone.[14] However, titanium exhibits poor wear properties when coupled with polyethylene[14] and should therefore not be used in the setting of a combined total ankle-TTR.

SURGICAL TECHNIQUE

Once the surgeon and staff have ensured that all 3D-printed componentry is available and appropriately sterilized without obvious manufacturing defect, the patient is brought to the operating room and anesthesia is induced. A regional block in combination with monitored anesthesia care *in lieu* of general anesthesia and intubation is typically preferred. Typically, general anesthesia and paralysis is not required for insertion of the implant after talar removal. Regional block with liposomal bupivacaine provides the added benefit of improved postoperative pain control.[15] The patient is positioned supine on a standard operating room table, and a tourniquet is applied at the thigh. A bump can be utilized under the hip of the operative extremity if there is significant external rotation of the limb. The extremity is then prepped and draped following standard sterile protocol. A timeout is performed.

A direct anterior approach to the ankle is utilized (Fig. 39.5). A midline skin incision is marked from 4 cm proximal to the tibiotalar joint and 2 cm distal past the level of the talonavicular joint. Incision is made with a No. 15 blade, and dissection is carried sharply down to the level of the

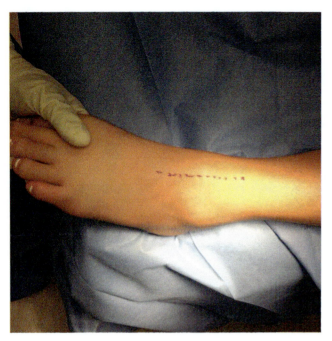

FIGURE 39.5 A direct anterior approach to the ankle is utilized as the approach for total talus replacement. A midline skin incision is marked from 4 cm proximal to the tibiotalar joint and 2 cm distal past the level of the navicular tuberosity.

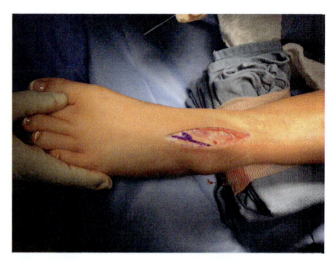

FIGURE 39.6 The superficial peroneal nerve is identified and a marking pen is utilized to mark the nerve to draw attention to maintaining protection of the nerve proper as well as crossing branches if possible.

extensor hallucis longus tendon sheath. The superficial peroneal nerve is identified, and attention is given to maintaining protection of the superficial peroneal nerve proper and as many crossing branches as possible (Fig. 39.6). The nerve may be highlighted with a marking pen to allow for easy identification throughout the case and closure. In some circumstances, a crossing branch of the superficial peroneal nerve will need to be sacrificed to obtain adequate access to the talus.

After retracting the superficial peroneal nerve, the extensor hallucis longus tendon is identified in its sheath underneath the extensor retinaculum, and the tendon sheath is opened longitudinally. The extensor hallucis longus tendon is retracted laterally. The tibialis anterior tendon is maintained within its sheath and retracted medially. The deep anterior neurovascular bundle containing the deep peroneal nerve and anterior tibial artery is then identified, carefully mobilized via dissection medial to the bundle, and ultimately protected with lateral retraction. Mobilization of the neurovascular bundle often requires cauterization of leash vessels, which travel medially from the neurovascular bundle. Next, sharp dissection can then safely be used to gain access to the tibiotalar joint with either a No. 15 blade or the electrocautery device. Full-thickness capsular flaps should then be developed both medially and laterally. The capsular flaps will ultimately be utilized after the procedure for a robust capsular closure, which is imperative in maintaining stability of the ankle and preventing infection. The dissection is then carried just distal to the level of the talonavicular joint, and all capsuloligamentous attachments of the talus are freed off the dorsal aspect of the navicular. Care should be taken to make a clean, longitudinal incision in the talonavicular capsuloligamentous complex, which allows for closure over the talonavicular joint after placement of the total talus. A large Gelpi retractor is then placed into the wound and used to maintain exposure. The Gelpi should be placed as deep as possible at the level of the talar neck to avoid excessive skin traction (Fig. 39.7).

First, attention is turned toward removing the talar head and neck. An osteotomy perpendicular to the long axis of the talus is then made at the distal talar neck initially with an oscillating saw (Fig. 39.8) and completed using a 1-inch straight osteotome (Fig. 39.9). After the initial talar neck osteotomy, another osteotomy is made with the oscillating saw at approximately 1.5 to 2 cm proximal on the talar neck in a converging direction. This second osteotomy is then completed with the osteotome to create a dorsal "closing wedge" osteotomy in the talar neck to facilitate removal. A Cobb is then placed in the talonavicular joint, with the sharp side pointed away from the

39 Total Talus Replacement

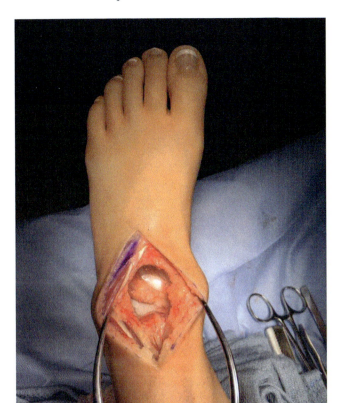

FIGURE 39.7 A large Gelpi retractor is placed as deep as possible at the level of the talar neck to avoid excessive skin traction.

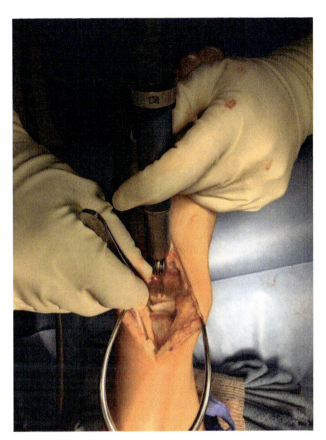

FIGURE 39.8 A horizontal osteotomy is made at the distal talar neck initially with an oscillating saw.

talonavicular joint cartilage, and the talonavicular ligaments and joint capsule are then released from medial to lateral. The osteotomized talar head and neck is removed with a rongeur.

Next, the exposed talar body and dome are then carefully excised in piecemeal fashion. To complete the talar excision, three parallel vertical osteotomies are then performed to segment the remaining talar dome and body for ease of removal (Fig. 39.10). With a rongeur, the "alligator roll" technique can then be utilized to remove the remaining portions of the talus after these bony fragments have been released from their deltoid ligament attachments medially and their anterior talofibular ligament insertions laterally. After performing the above steps, the most inferior fragments of the talus often remain attached to the interosseous ligament between the calcaneus and the

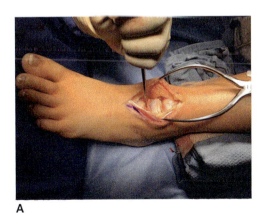

A

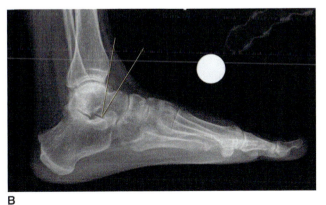

B

FIGURE 39.9 **(A)** The horizontal osteotomy is then finished using a 1-inch straight osteotome, and **(B)** a dorsal "closing wedge" osteotomy at the talar neck is completed to facilitate removal of the talus. Cuts are made approximately as shown on the lateral radiograph of the ankle.

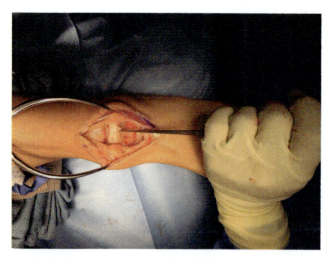

FIGURE 39.10 To complete the talar excision, three parallel vertical osteotomies are then performed to segment the remaining talar dome and body for ease of removal.

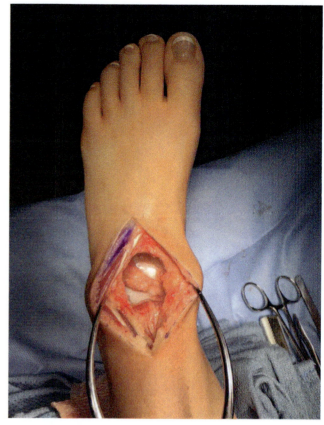

FIGURE 39.11 Once the talus has been removed, thorough inspection is warranted to ensure that all remaining bony fragments have been excised and that the talar resection is complete. The posterior facet of the calcaneus can also be visualized and is found to be free of degenerative change.

talus. This ligament typically needs to be sharply released in order to free up the remaining pieces, which can then be removed sequentially with use of a rongeur.

The excision of the native talus is the most technically challenging step of the procedure. During the entire process of talus removal, careful attention is required to avoid violation of the articular cartilage of the tibia, calcaneus, and navicular to minimize risk for postoperative development of adjacent joint arthritis. As a further point of emphasis, the portions of the deltoid ligament not inserting on the talus should be preserved as much as possible during removal of the talus. Namely, the tibionavicular and tibiocalcaneal portions of the deltoid ligament should be preserved, but the anterior tibiotalar portion of the deltoid ligament must be sacrificed to allow for complete talar removal. Another consideration is the distorted anatomy and talar collapse, which indicates this procedure. It is imperative to identify the talonavicular joint and ensure that the navicular is protected when resecting the talar head. A final point of caution when resecting the talar head is to consider the proximity of the medial resected bone to the plantar calcaneonavicular (Spring) ligament. Both the Spring ligament and calcaneofibular ligament should be maintained.

After performing the above steps, thorough inspection is warranted to ensure that all remaining bony fragments have been excised and that the talar resection is complete (Fig. 39.11). Small fragments of bone cannot only prevent proper reduction of the trial and malpositioning of the final component but can also act as loose bodies, potentially accelerating postoperative degenerative arthritis of the surrounding joints.

Once adequate resection of the talus has been achieved, the next step is to select one of the trial implants. As previously mentioned, there is often nominal, small, and large implants constructed (see Fig. 39.3). The 3D-printed total talus trial implants are made with a handle to aid in insertion and removal of the component (Fig. 39.12). A combination of plantarflexion of the foot and

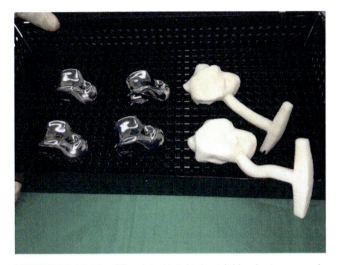

FIGURE 39.12 The 3D-printed total talus trial implants are made with a handle to aid in insertion and removal of the component. Typically, a nominal, small, and large implant is constructed.

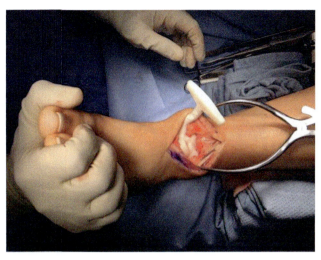

FIGURE 39.13 A combination of plantarflexion of the foot and longitudinal traction through the ankle facilitates reduction of the talar trial.

longitudinal traction through the ankle allows reduction of the talar trial (Fig. 39.13). ROM and stability is then clinically accessed with the different size talar trials, starting first with the nominal trial. After appropriate reduction of the trial talar component into the bony void, the ankle is taken through a full ROM to evaluate fit, stability, and estimated degree of plantarflexion, dorsiflexion, eversion, and inversion. As some ligamentous loosening is expected postoperatively, we prefer to err on the side of tighter fit as opposed to looser fit to minimize risk of postoperative dislocation or instability events. Preoperative assessment of the contralateral ankle and hindfoot ROM is imperative to match the motion of the operative side to that of the unaffected, contralateral side, such that the operative hindfoot and ankle does not exhibit excessive or inhibited ROM. Generally speaking, the implant size that allows for best replication of contralateral ROM is the ideally sized implant. An implant that is too large may result in overstuffing, decreased ROM, and acceleration of degenerative arthritis of the adjacent joints. Conversely, a component that is too small may induce instability or subsequent formation or arthrofibrosis leading to increased pain and stiffness through the midfoot and hindfoot.

After final selection of the appropriately sized trial, the wound is copiously irrigated, and the matching final 3D-printed implant is inserted into the bony defect (Fig. 39.14). ROM is again assessed to ensure appropriate matching to the contralateral hindfoot and ankle. Once satisfied with the TTR, the surgeon should proceed with any additional corrective soft tissue or bony procedures to ensure stable, plantigrade foot positioning. Any residual malalignment will result in failure of the TTR. Tendo-Achilles lengthening or gastrocnemius recession may be helpful to improve dorsiflexion and should be considered as well.

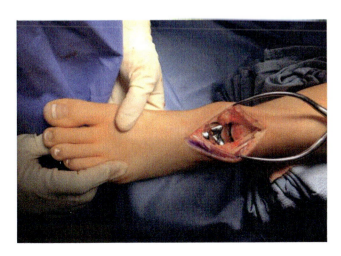

FIGURE 39.14 The final 3D-printed implant is inserted into the bony defect created from talus removal.

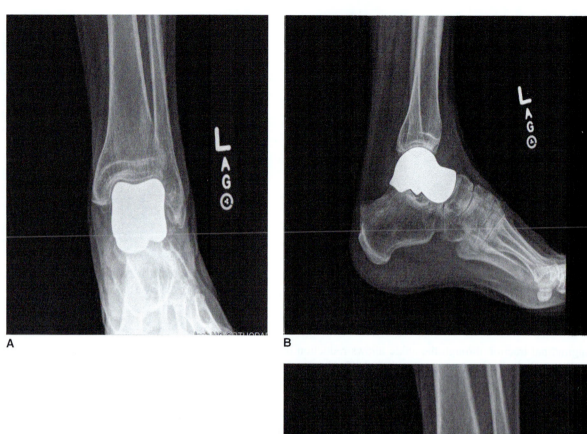
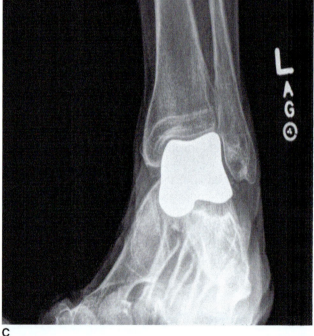

FIGURE 39.15 Sample radiographs of a total talus replacement obtained at 6 months postoperatively confirm stability of the implant and maintenance of the joint space: **(A)** anteroposterior weight-bearing radiograph, **(B)** lateral radiograph, and **(C)** mortise view.

Following irrigation, a layered closure is undertaken, starting with the full-thickness capsular flaps of both the tibiotalar and talonavicular joints. Capsular closure is essential to decrease risk of infection and to ensure stability of the total talus implant. The extensor retinaculum of the extensor hallucis longus is then closed, followed by the subcutaneous layer and skin layer. Following skin closure, an incisional vacuum may be placed over the wound if there is concern for postoperative wound complications or poor patient protoplasm. Alternatively, if there is less concern about wound breakdown, a routine sterile dressing can be used. The limb is then placed into a well-padded immobilizing splint such as a plaster-based posterior slab and sugar tong U-splint with significant bulky wrap to decrease skin pressure points.

POSTOPERATIVE CARE

The patient remains non–weight bearing in the plaster splint for 3 weeks postoperative. This immobilization allows for swelling control and soft tissue healing. The patient should be encouraged to elevate the operative extremity as much as possible. At 3 weeks, the splint and sutures are removed. At this time, the patient is allowed to shower with water running over the incision. The patient is cautioned, however, to avoid scrubbing or full water immersion of the operative extremity for 1 month or until wounds are fully healed. The patient is then placed into a removable controlled ankle motion (CAM) boot and is cleared to begin weight bearing as tolerated. The patient is instructed to slowly wean from the use of crutches between postoperative weeks 3 to 6 with a goal of ambulating without an assistive device at 6 weeks postoperatively. The CAM boot should remain on while weight bearing but can come off for ROM and strengthening activities (described below). At 6 weeks postoperatively, the patient can begin weaning out of the CAM boot and begins transition to phase 1 of physical therapy. It is recommended to decrease CAM boot utilization by 2 hours each subsequent day until the patient is free from the boot entirely. Patients are seen in clinic for both clinical and radiographic evaluation at the following time points: 3 weeks, 6 weeks, 3 months, 6 months, 1 year, and annually thereafter. Sample images obtained at 6 months postoperatively from TTR are shown in Figure 39.15.

As it pertains to the physical therapy regimen, TTR formal therapy activities begin at 6 weeks postoperative. Formal, instructional therapy at least 2 to 3 times weekly with active participation in a daily home exercise regimen is recommended. The therapist should graduate the therapy protocol based on patient progression and should leave room for individual modifications as needed on a patient-to-patient basis. We have outlined a generalized, three-phase protocol, which a therapist practitioner can utilize as a guideline for rehabilitation after TTR.

Phase 1

Phase 1 is initiated at 6 weeks postoperative and begins with ROM, including active ROM of the foot and ankle through dorsiflexion and plantarflexion, ankle circle exercises, and alphabet exercises. Intrinsic foot musculature stretching and strengthening is begun at this time with light toe towel scrunch exercises. Careful attention is placed on edema control with elevation, ice, and compressive stockinettes, with the therapist demonstrating appropriate utilization of these techniques and encouraging the patient to consistently practice edema control at home as well. As the patient progresses, ankle strengthening activities can then be introduced around 8 weeks postoperative. The Thera-Band (Akron, Ohio) is an effective modality to provide graduated degrees of resistance during ankle movement activities. Aerobic conditioning should then be introduced, starting with a stationary bicycle and graduating ultimately to proprioceptive exercises utilizing the seated Biomechanical Ankle Platform System board. As phase 1 comes to a close, the individual therapist and patient are encouraged to evaluate for specific weaknesses and attempt to address these weaknesses before graduation to phase 2. The patient begins weaning out of the CAM boot at 6 weeks postoperative and should be tolerating normal shoe wear by the end of phase 1.

Phase 2

Phase 2 begins 10 to 14 weeks postoperative. Patients may begin weight-bearing proprioceptive exercises on static and dynamic surfaces with a goal of ultimately progressing to single limb stance exercises, plyoball exercises, and four-way Thera-Band exercises while standing on the operative limb. Strengthening exercises should continue to increase in intensity throughout phase 2, and the patient should work up to performing standing heel raises, squats, lunges, and step-ups. As phase 2 ends, the patient should be full weight bearing as tolerated in their usual shoe wear without the use of assistive devices and able to participate in most of their day-to-day activities. At 3 months postoperative, the patient is seen by their surgeon, and the surgeon should evaluate for wound healing, progression of ROM, as well as need for potential corrective orthotic device.

Phase 3

Finally, phase 3 should be implemented around 14 to 16 weeks postoperative and should include higher-intensity duration activities such as lunges and semicircles. The therapist should continue to progress the difficulty of the proprioceptive exercises and can utilize dynamic surfaces to increase the intensity of such activities. The patient should be reminded that, while participation in lower-level plyometric activity can be necessary to ensure adequate maintenance of ROM in the postoperative state, high-level activities such as hopping and jumping should be significantly reduced or eliminated following TTR to prevent postoperative degenerative arthritis to the surrounding joints.

Goals of formal physical therapy should include working toward achieving a normal gait without an assistive device and reduced pain throughout normal activities of daily living. There should be minimal joint effusion and adequate neuromuscular control and proprioceptive awareness to allow for participation in basic stabilization exercises as well as completion of light sport or recreation-related activities.

EXPECTED OUTCOMES

While there is still a relative paucity of literature on TTR, especially when directly compared to alternative options such as arthrodesis, early results have been promising. Theoretic benefits of TTR include preservation of hindfoot motion, less adjacent joint arthritis, and eliminating the risk of nonunion. Numerous case reports and case series have outlined positive results.[5-12] To demonstrate the breadth of indications and use, Ando et al. reported use of a third-generation aluminum ceramic TTR for idiopathic talar AVN in a 72-year-old female with excellent American Orthopedic Foot and Ankle Society (AOFAS) scores at 2 years postoperatively.[11] Similarly, Angthong reported excellent outcomes after the use of a custom anatomic stainless steel total talar prosthesis in a 25-year-old male who had sustained a traumatic loss of the talus; the patient ultimately had an excellent outcome, with improvement of visual analog scale (VAS) scores and maintenance of ankle ROM.[16]

While larger patient sample analyses remain limited, several series have recently been published demonstrating good results. Taniguchi and colleagues reported on a series of 51 patients who underwent TTR with alumina ceramic total talus implant. These authors report promising results at a mean follow-up of 52.8 months, with all patients returning to full activities of daily living. No amputations or revisions were required in this cohort, and inversion stress, eversion stress, and anterior drawer examinations demonstrated excellent stability of the ankle joint. Despite excellent clinical results, radiographs at final follow-up showed sclerosis in the distal tibia (44%), navicular (9%), and calcaneus (35%).

Scott et al. published a case series of early outcomes on 15 patients who underwent a custom, 3D-printed TTR comprised of cobalt-chrome at an average of 13-month follow-up.[9] Foot and Ankle Outcome Scores, VAS scores, and ROM data showed statistically significant improvements postoperatively as compared with preoperative scores. There was a substantial decrease in VAS pain scores from 7.0 preoperatively to 3.6 postoperatively. At an average of 22 months of follow-up, these initial positive outcomes were obtained in a total of 27 patients.[17] There were only three complications requiring reoperation in this cohort (11.1%). Mid- to long-term follow-up is planned in this cohort to allow for assessment of the survivorship of the 3D-printed implants. With regard to the titanium oxide–coated additive TTR, Abramson et al. recently published a series of eight patients who underwent this procedure. AOFAS and SF-36 scores showed improvement, and no revision surgeries had been performed at final mid-term follow-up of 23 months. In the patient with the longest follow-up (49 months), there was evidence of tibiotalar joint degeneration, but the patient was symptom free.[18] It is postulated that 3D technology may be superior to alternative prosthesis options given enhanced anatomic configuration of the printed models. It is imperative that surgeons have appropriate strict indications for this procedure, practice meticulous surgical technique, and continue to assess and report mid- to long-term patient outcomes as well as comparative outcomes to alternative procedures.

REFERENCES

1. Dhillon MS, Rana B, Panda I, Patel S, Kumar P. Management options in avascular necrosis of talus. *Indian J Orthop.* 2018;52(3):284-296.
2. Dujela M, Hyer CF, Berlet GC. Rate of subtalar joint arthrodesis after retrograde tibiotalocalcaneal arthrodesis with intramedullary nail fixation: evaluation of the RAIN database. *Foot Ankle Spec.* 2018;11(5):410-415.
3. Jung HG, Parks BG, Nguyen A, Schon LC. Effect of tibiotalar joint arthrodesis on adjacent tarsal joint pressure in a cadaver model. *Foot Ankle Int.* 2007;28(1):103-108.
4. Harnroongroj T, Vanadurongwan V. The talar body prosthesis. *J Bone Joint Surg Am.* 1997;79(9):1313-1322.
5. Taniguchi A, Takakura Y, Tanaka Y, et al. An alumina ceramic total talar prosthesis for osteonecrosis of the talus. *J Bone Joint Surg Am.* 2015;97(16):1348-1353.

6. Tonogai I, Hamada D, Yamasaki Y, et al. Custom-made alumina ceramic total talar prosthesis for idiopathic aseptic necrosis of the talus: report of two cases. *Case Rep Orthop.* 2017;2017:8290804.
7. Hussain RM. Metallic 3D printed total talus replacement: a case study. *J Foot Ankle Surg.* 2021;60(3):634-641.
8. Bejarano-Pineda L, DeOrio JK, Parekh SG. Combined total talus replacement and total ankle arthroplasty. *J Surg Orthop Adv.* 2020;29(4):244-248.
9. Scott DJ, Steele J, Fletcher A, Parekh SG. Early outcomes of 3D printed total talus arthroplasty. *Foot Ankle Spec.* 2020;13(5):372-377.
10. Taniguchi A, Tanaka Y. An alumina ceramic total talar prosthesis for avascular necrosis of the talus. *Foot Ankle Clin.* 2019;24(1):163-171.
11. Ando Y, Yasui T, Isawa K, Tanaka S, Tanaka Y, Takakura Y. Total talar replacement for idiopathic necrosis of the talus: a case report. *J Foot Ankle Surg.* 2016;55(6):1292-1296.
12. Magnan B, Facci E, Bartolozzi P. Traumatic loss of the talus treated with a talar body prosthesis and total ankle arthroplasty. A case report. *J Bone Joint Surg Am.* 2004;86(8):1778-1782.
13. Jeng CL, Campbell JT, Maloney PJ, Schon LC, Cerrato RA. Effect of Achilles tendon lengthening and gastrocnemius recession on radiographic tibiotalar motion following total ankle replacement. *Foot Ankle Int.* 2021;42(4):476-481.
14. Hu CY, Yoon TR. Recent updates for biomaterials used in total hip arthroplasty. *Biomater Res.* 2018;22:33.
15. Beiranvand S, Moradkhani MR. Bupivacaine versus liposomal bupivacaine for pain control. *Drug Res (Stuttg).* 2018;68(7):365-369.
16. Angthong C. Anatomic total talar prosthesis replacement surgery and ankle arthroplasty: an early case series in Thailand. *Orthop Rev (Pavia).* 2014;6(3):5486.
17. Kadakia RJ, Akoh CC, Chen J, Sharma A, Parekh SG. 3D printed total talus replacement for avascular necrosis of the talus. *Foot Ankle Int.* 2020;41(12):1529-1536.
18. Abramson M, Hilton T, Hosking K, Campbell N, Dey R, McCollum G. Total talar replacements short-medium term case series, South Africa 2019. *J Foot Ankle Surg.* 2021;60(1):182-186.

PART EIGHT
FOREFOOT/LESSER TOES

40 Crossover Toe Correction

Phinit Phisitkul

INTRODUCTION

Crossover toe is a condition where there is an overlap between toes, most commonly the second toe crossing over the great toe, especially when a hallux valgus is present (Fig. 40.1).[1] It is more common in females over the age of 50 years. The deformity represents a spectrum of damage to the forefoot that has insidious onset but can also be traumatic. An attenuation or rupture of the plantar plate with or without collateral ligament(s) damage describes the primary pathomechanics of the crossover toe deformity.[2] Once the lesser metatarsal joint drifts into dorsiflexion at the metatarsophalangeal joint, a secondary hammertoe deformity occurs with flexion of the interphalangeal joints. The flexible deformity at the proximal interphalangeal joint becomes rigid over time. The tear in the plantar plate is usually located laterally, adjacent to the insertion to the base of the proximal phalanx. This tear can propagate across the entire plantar plate in varieties of patterns and can involve the lateral collateral ligament complex or, less commonly, the medial side.[3] As the second metatarsophalangeal is vulnerable to both sagittal and coronal plane deformities, the deformity is usually progressive, starting from painful instability without a deformity to a complete metatarsophalangeal joint dislocation. In the sagittal plane, intrinsic muscles counteract against all extrinsic flexors and extensors in keeping the lesser metatarsophalangeal joint in flexion. Unfortunately, the intrinsic muscles become ineffective as plantar flexors when the joint is in a dorsiflexed position. Deviation of the great toe into valgus alignment further prevents the second toe from proper engagement with the ground. In the coronal plane, the prominent lateral condyle of the second metatarsal head can abut against the lateral aspect of the plantar plate. Over time, the flexor digitorum longus tendon can pull the torn plantar plate and the base of the proximal phalange medially as it subluxates medial to the metatarsal head. The lumbricals on the medial side of the metatarsophalangeal joint can also add to the deforming force.

Diagnosis of a crossover toe is usually based on clinical evaluation and weight-bearing radiographs. The present of a plantar plate tear can be diagnosed with a combination of a gradual onset of forefoot pain, edema, and a positive drawer sign.[4] It is important to recognize extrinsic factors leading to the overload of the second metatarsophalangeal joint such as rheumatoid arthritis, repetitive jumping activities, gastrocnemius contracture, an unstable first ray, hallux valgus, and hallux rigidus deformity.[5] An isolated treatment to the second ray alone without addressing underlying problems can lead to failure or recurrence.

NONOPERATIVE TREATMENTS

Multiple nonsurgical treatments are available to treat a patient with a crossover lesser toe, including silicone toe sleeves, toe straighteners, taping, insoles, shoe modification, rocker shoes, calf stretching, and activity modification.[6] An early initiation of treatment when there is no or minimal deformity is paramount.[7] Once a deformity is present, nonsurgical care can still help mitigate symptoms but will not correct the deformity. Taping is highly effective in the protection of the affected toe, but it can take up to 6 months for pain to subside (Fig. 40.2).[7] A cortisone injection is not recommended as

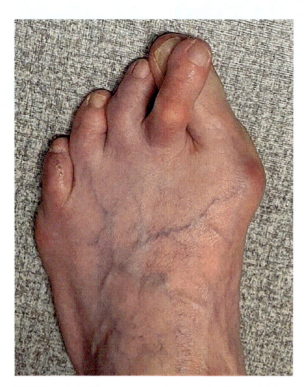

FIGURE 40.1 Clinical picture of a patient with a painful crossover second toe. A severe hallux valgus deformity and coronal plane deviation of adjacent toes are observed.

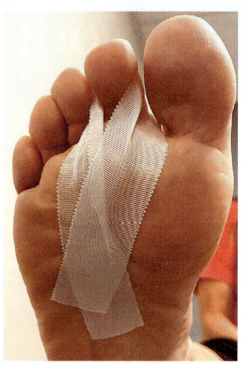

FIGURE 40.2 Plantar view of a taping technique to protect second toe in a patient with a plantar plate rupture.

it can mask pain and possibly attenuate ligamentous structures leading to accelerated development of metatarsophalangeal joint dislocation.[8]

OPERATIVE TREATMENTS

Surgical treatments of crossover toe deformity have gone through multiple paradigm shifts along with the growth of a body of knowledge led by dedicated work by leaders in the foot and ankle subspecialties.[1-4,9-17] The list of possible surgical options are shown in Table 40.1. Prior to the recognition of plantar plate injury, the treatment of crossover toe was similar to the treatment of complex hammertoe focusing on the fusion or resection arthroplasty of the proximal interphalangeal joint together with deforming soft tissue release and stabilization with K-wires.[12,13] Stiffness from the prolonged K-wire fixation must be balanced against early recurrence from early K-wire removal or inadequately balanced toes. Decades of exploration in pathomechanics and improvement in surgical techniques allowed understanding of the importance of the plantar plate and collateral ligaments in joint stability. Deformity correction, however, was indirect with numerous options of tendon transfer using various donors and recipients.[12,13,17-21] The most widely used technique is a Girdlestone-Taylor flexor digitorum longus transfer to the extensor hood. Stability of the toe in sagittal plane is effectively restored but suffered from toe stiffness and residual joint subluxation. More recent techniques using an extensor digitorum brevis tendon transferred underneath the intermetatarsal ligament aim to more anatomically restore the stability from the lateral plantar plate and lateral collateral ligament. While the plantar plate could be accessed from the plantar incision more directly, this approach has been limited due to the concern of painful scarring and the need for an additional dorsal approach for concomitant procedures. Development of specialized joint distractors and suture passers have allowed adequate access for plantar plate and collateral ligament repair from the dorsal approach.[22] A dorsal intermetatarsal approach was described for access to address the lateral collateral ligament and lateral side of the plantar plate in cases without joint dislocation.[23] The role of metatarsal osteotomy has been highlighted to improve surgical exposure to the plantar plate tear, shorten the long second metatarsal, and realign the bone to balance coronal plane deformity.[10,24,25] Orthopedic surgeons equipped with minimally invasive surgical principles may adopt a wide array of arthroscopic options and percutaneous bony realignment. Toe amputation is an option in a low-demand patient with severe deformities who want to return to function quickly.[26]

TABLE 40.1 Surgical Treatment Options for Crossover Toe Deformity

Metatarsophalangeal joint release
Partial excision of metatarsal head
Extensor tendon lengthening
Flexor digitorum longus tendon transfer
Extensor digitorum brevis transfer
K-wire fixation
Percutaneous tenodesis
Distal metatarsal osteotomy
Proximal phalangeal base excision
Partial metatarsal condylectomy
Plantar plate and collateral ligament repair
Minimally invasive correction
Dermodesis
Syndactyly
Resection arthroplasty of the proximal interphalangeal joint
Release of the flexor digitorum brevis and proximal interphalangeal joint

INDICATIONS AND CONTRAINDICATIONS (TABLE 40.2)

TABLE 40.2

Indications	Contraindications
Recalcitrant pain	Arterial insufficiency
Impending ulceration	Active infection
Difficulties in shoe wear	

PREOPERATIVE PLANNING

Clinical evaluation is the most important step in the preoperative planning. Overall lower limb alignment should be accessed especially in patients with valgus alignment with possible progressive collapsing foot deformity. Isolated gastrocnemius contracture and gastrocsoleus contracture can increase force in the forefoot during a late stance-phase of gait.[26] A Silfverskiold test should be performed. It is critical to carefully analyze alignment and stability issues of the first ray, such as hallux valgus deformity, instability, and hallux rigidus, as uncorrected first ray pathology may lead to failure of surgical correction of the lesser ray crossover toes. A discussion should be made with the patient regarding the risks and benefit of first ray correction especially when it is not painful.

A crossover toe deformity may or may not be associated with a painful instability at the metatarsophalangeal joint. A drawer test is critical to determine whether instability is present and more importantly if the instability is associated with pain.[4] It has been the author's experience that patients with painful instability benefit more from an anatomic repair of the plantar plate and collateral ligaments. Patients with plantar overloading at the second metatarsal head may only need a shortening osteotomy of the second ray with or without stabilization of the first ray. This can also decrease irritation on the interdigital nerve in the second web space. Patients with impingement symptoms from the toe deformity without pain at the second metatarsal head or metatarsophalangeal joint may be treated with just a realignment osteotomy of the second toe proximal phalanx.

Weight-bearing radiographs of the foot are essential in the determination of surgical options (Fig. 40.3). Conditions of the first ray should be critically analyzed. The length of the lesser metatarsals should be assessed to determine whether shortening osteotomies are needed to unload the affected rays and recreate a more natural forefoot parabola. The second metatarsophalangeal joint must be evaluated for alignment and subluxation. A frank dislocation of the metatarsophalangeal joint is demonstrated by the loss of parallel subchondral lines at the metatarsal head and the proximal phalanx. Coronal metatarsophalangeal alignment commonly demonstrates varus alignment, but it could also be valgus or neutral. Mild coronal plane deformities are usually not critical as long as they are in line with surrounding toes. Arthritis is not usually well seen on the anteroposterior

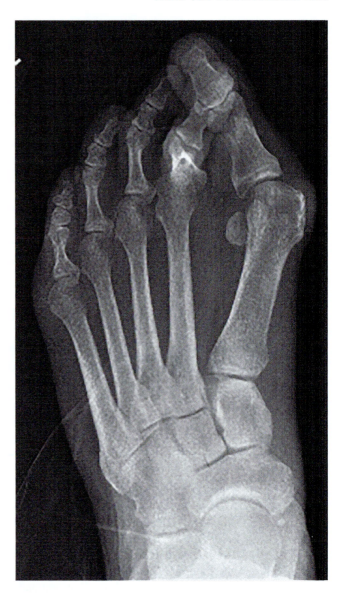

FIGURE 40.3 Weight-bearing radiograph of the left foot from the same patient as in Figure 40.1 is shown. Severe hallux valgus deformity is observed. The second metatarsal is relatively long. There is a dislocation of the second metatarsophalangeal joint. A gun-barrel sign is seen at the proximal phalanx of the second toe indicating severe dorsiflexion of the metatarsophalangeal joint.

radiographs as joint subluxation can obscure the view, but osteophytes or erosion of the metatarsal head could be observed on lateral or oblique views. When there is evidence of arthritis at the lesser metatarsophalangeal joint, emphasis should be made to decompress the joint with a metatarsal shortening osteotomy.

A diagnostic injection using local anesthetic agent could be helpful in differentiating multiple causes of forefoot pain, for example, plantar plate injury, interdigital neuritis, Freiberg infarction, and peripheral neuropathy.[14] Magnetic resonance imaging (MRI) is found to be reliable in the diagnosis of plantar plate tears with 95% sensitivity, 100% specificity, 100% positive predictive value, and 67% negative predictive value.[27] While clinical evaluation is usually sufficient, MRI still has a role for cases with uncertain diagnosis.

SURGICAL TECHNIQUES

Although it is beyond the scope of this chapter, repair of associated conditions leading to overload of the second ray is paramount. Procedures such as gastrocnemius recession, bunion reconstruction, and first ray stabilization may be considered during the same surgical setting with and prior to a crossover toe repair.

In each case, a systematic algorithm is used to determine the required procedures (Fig. 40.4). The sequence of procedures may or may not follow this chart. For instance, a metatarsal osteotomy may be performed first to assist with the exposure of the plantar plate repair, or the extensor digitorum brevis may be spared for possible use as a donor in a tendon transfer at the end.

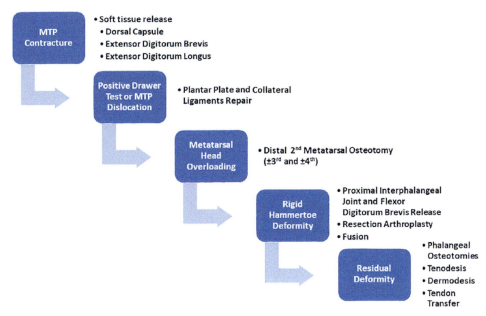

FIGURE 40.4 Diagram indicates systematic algorithm for the selection of procedures to address a crossover toe deformity.

Metatarsophalangeal Joint Soft Tissue Release

- Prior to a soft tissue release, the surgeon should be confident that a tendon transfer is not planned or those structures could be sacrificed precluding subsequent use as a donor tendon such as extensor digitorum longus tendon, extensor digitorum brevis tendon, or flexor digitorum longus tendon.
- The extension contracture at the metatarsophalangeal joint is corrected by a release of the dorsal capsule and extensor tendons.[25] A dorsal incision is made at the level of the metatarsophalangeal joint medial or lateral to the extensor tendons. Under gentle distraction, a beaver blade is inserted into the joint to release the dorsal capsule.
- The blade is turned dorsally while the joint is held in plantarflexion to complete the tenotomies.
- Manipulation is then performed once more to break any residual adhesions.
- Release of the medial collateral ligament is rarely indicated to avoid further instability of the joint except when joint stabilization procedures such as plantar plate repair, collateral ligament repair, or tendon transfer is concomitantly performed.
- Flexor digitorum longus is rarely released due to the concern about loss of toe purchase to the ground. The flexor digitorum longus tendon contracture is usually indirectly relieved by the shortening effect of the proximal phalangeal osteotomy (Fig. 40.5). It also should be kept intact as a possible donor if a tendon transfer is required.

Plantar Plate and Collateral Ligament Repair

- Plantar plate repair is performed using a dorsal approach when there is a flank dislocation of the metatarsophalangeal joint or when both medial and lateral collateral ligaments are involved.[22]
- A curvilinear incision is made over the affected lesser metatarsophalangeal joint (Fig. 40.6).
- The extensor digitorum longus is split longitudinally.
- A synovectomy is performed using a rongeur.
- The dislocated joint is reduced with a conservative release of the plantar plate. An attempt should be made to preserve as much plantar plate tissue as possible. In an irreducible joint with extensive adhesion between the plantar plate and the metatarsal head, a McGlamry elevator can be carefully used to mobilize the plantar plate proximally.
- Pin distractors are used to distract the joint, using a 1.4-mm K-wire placed in the proximal phalanx metaphysis and a second wire placed in the metatarsal head.
- The plantar plate and both collateral ligaments are sharply cut at the level of the metatarsal head so that a repair will tighten the soft tissue further. This step is carefully performed to ensure that there is no injury to the flexor digitorum longus tendon immediately plantar to the plantar plate.

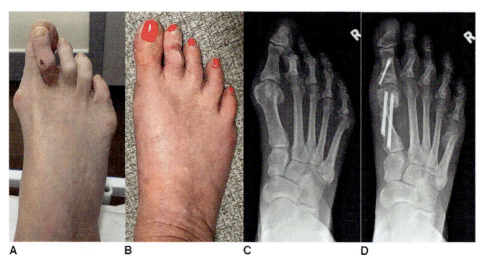

FIGURE 40.5 Preoperative and 3-month postoperative photographs of a patient with a crossover second toe, hallux valgus, bunionette, and hammer toe deformity of second, third, and fourth toes **(A, B)**. Excellent deformity correction is observed with normal postoperative swelling. The second toe is treated with a proximal phalangeal osteotomy plus flexor digitorum brevis tendon release. Preoperative and 3-month postoperative anteroposterior radiographs are demonstrated **(C, D)**.

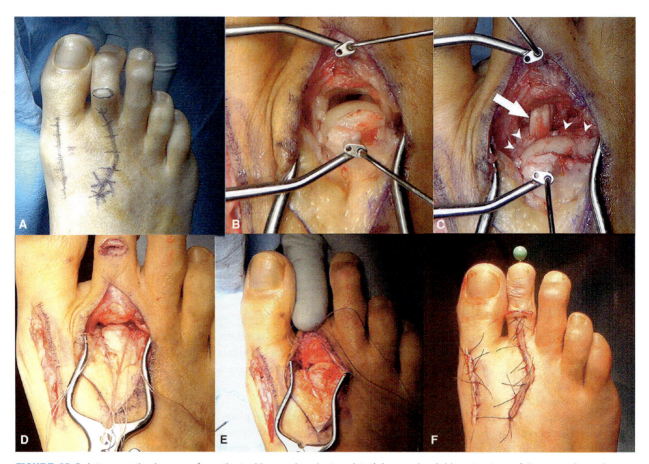

FIGURE 40.6 Intraoperative images of a patient with complex plantar plate injury and a rigid contracture of the second toe. A dorsal curvilinear incision is used for the plantar plate repair **(A)**. Surgical exposure after a metatarsal neck osteotomy is shown **(B)**. Plantar plate and collateral ligaments are demonstrated (**C**, *arrow heads*) dorsal to the flexor tendons (**C**, *solid arrow*) after a complete soft tissue release. Four sets of 2/0 nonabsorbable sutures are placed to grasp the medial and lateral parts of the plantar plate and both collateral ligaments **(D)**. The plantar plate sutures and collateral ligament sutures are shuttled through bone tunnels at the base of the proximal phalanx and tied together **(E)**. Wound closure is shown after a second ray repair plus proximal phalangeal fusion with a K-wire **(F)**.

- The joint is further distracted after the complete soft tissue release. The pattern of plantar plate tear is analyzed.
- A grasping suture is placed using a customized suture passer (HAT-TRICK Lesser Toe Repair System, Smith & Nephew, Andover, Massachusetts) at the medial and lateral portion of the plantar plate on each side of the tunnel for the flexor digitorum longus tendon.
- A grasping suture is placed on each collateral ligament.
- If there is a complex or longitudinal tear at the plantar plate, a side-to-side stitch can be placed and incorporated to the repair. This suture should not be tied until all other sutures have been placed as the working area will be diminished afterward.
- The pin distractor is removed to allow dorsal subluxation of the proximal phalangeal base. Débridement is performed along the medial, lateral, and plantar edges of the proximal phalangeal base to promote ligamentous healing onto bone.
- Using Phalangeal Drill Guides, two bone tunnels are created from dorsal to plantar-medial and plantar-lateral aspects of the proximal phalangeal base. Plantar plate and collateral ligament grasping sutures from ipsilateral sides are shuttled from plantar to dorsal. Sutures are now tensioned without a secured knot to demonstrate final alignment.
- A Weil osteotomy can be performed at this stage or even earlier to assist in surgical exposure to the plantar plate, if needed. The saw blade should be parallel to the sole of foot to prevent relative plantar prominence of the metatarsal head. The Weil osteotomy is fixed using a screw with 3 mm of shortening and 3 mm of medial translation to decompress the metatarsal head and promote more valgus alignment of the toe.
- The plantar plate sutures from the bone tunnels are tied together while the metatarsophalangeal joint is held reduced and plantarflexed. The collateral ligament grasping sutures are tied together with the toe held in neutral coronal plane alignment.
- Back-up fixation using 1.6-mm threaded PEEK interference wire is inserted into the suture-tunnel interface to further secure the construct.
- When only the lateral side of the plantar plate and lateral collateral ligament are injured, a more limited approach from the intermetatarsal interval is preferred (Figs. 40.7 through 40.9).[23] A small laminar spreader is placed between the second and third metatarsal space to improve working space.
- The joint is approached just lateral to the extensor digitorum longus tendon. A pin distractor is inserted in the same fashion but only ipsilateral collateral ligament is release together with the

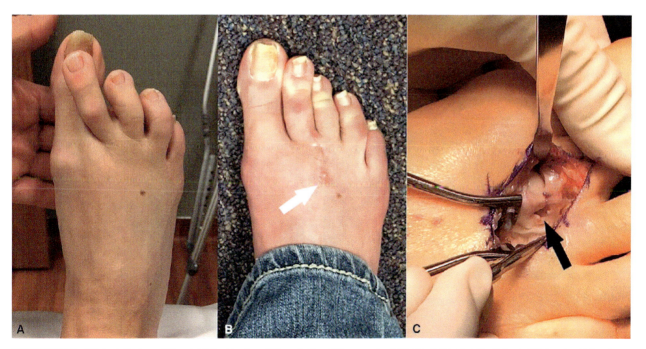

FIGURE 40.7 Clinical photos of the right foot before **(A)** and after **(B)** a surgical repair of the plantar plate and lateral collateral ligament using the intermetatarsal approach **(C)**. The *white arrow* indicates the surgical scar at 3 months postoperatively. The *black arrow* indicates a rupture of the lateral collateral ligament and the lateral aspect of plantar plate.

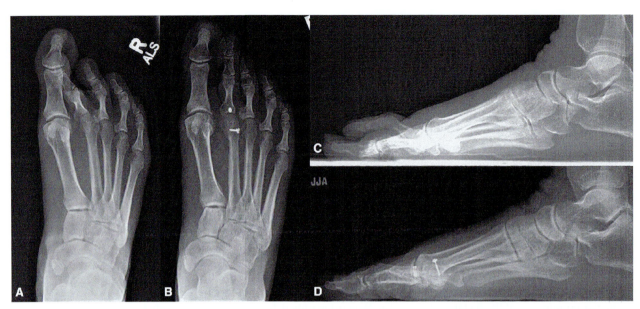

FIGURE 40.8 Preoperative **(A, C)** and postoperative **(B, D)** radiographic images of the same patient as in Figure 40.7 demonstrate improvement of coronal and sagittal plane alignments of the second toe. A cannulated screw is used for securing sutures from the plantar plate and collateral ligament repair. The second metatarsal osteotomy is fixed in slightly medial translated position using a snap-off screw.

lateral half of the plantar plate. A grasping suture is placed into the released plantar plate and collateral ligament stumps. Only a single bone tunnel is made dorsally toward the plantar-lateral edge of the proximal phalange. Fixation is performed by tying sutures over a cannulated screw (HAT-TRICK Lesser Toe Repair System, Smith & Nephew, Andover, Massachusetts).

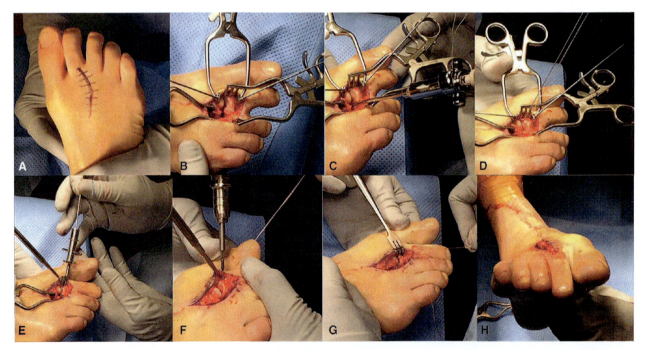

FIGURE 40.9 Intraoperative images of a patient with an injury to the lateral collateral ligament and lateral aspect of the plantar plate. A dorsal intermetatarsal approach is used **(A)**. Exposure is facilitated by the use of self-retaining retractors **(B)**. A suture passer is used to place 2/0 nonabsorbable sutures into the lateral aspect of the plantar plate and the lateral collateral ligament **(C)**. Two sets of 2/0 nonabsorbable sutures are placed to grasp the lateral plantar plate and the lateral collateral ligament **(D)**. A suture shuttle assembly is inserted through the proximal phalange drill guide to facilitate the retrieval of 2/0 sutures **(E)**. Cannulated screw is inserted along the axis of the bone tunnel with one limb from each of the plantar plate and collateral ligament sutures through the handle, driver, and screw assembly **(F)**. Knots are tied over the shoulder of the screw to complete the repair **(G)**. The satisfactory final alignment of the second toe is shown **(H)**.

Percutaneous Distal Metatarsal Osteotomy

Distal metatarsal osteotomy can be used to relieve overloading underneath the metatarsal head, restore metatarsal parabola, correct medial or lateral deviation of the toe, and facilitate exposure to the plantar plate of the metatarsophalangeal joint (see Fig. 40.6). When shortening is desired to decrease overloading of the lesser metatarsal heads without a plantar plate repair, an osteotomy can be performed using a minimally invasive technique (Figs. 40.10 through 40.12).[25] The mechanics of the osteotomy can be adjusted such as tilting the osteotomy plane medially or laterally to allow medial-lateral translation or keeping the plane of the osteotomy more parallel to the plantar border of the foot to promote more shortening (Figs. 40.13 and 40.14). A medial crossover second toe may be supported better with the osteotomy that allows medial translation of the second metatarsal head.

- To avoid thermonecrosis of the bone, tourniquet should be avoided or released and copious irrigation should be used. For all percutaneous bur use, a high-torque, low-speed system should be utilized as well.
- A dorsal lateral or dorsal medial stab incision is made at the level of the metatarsophalangeal joint just proximal to the web space.
- A 2 × 12 mm bur is then advanced toward the neck of the metatarsal. An osteotomy is then performed along the plane of 45° with the metatarsal axis. At the end of the osteotomy, the surgeon should have rotated the bur 90° so that the final part of the osteotomy is across the top of the metatarsal head and neck junction.

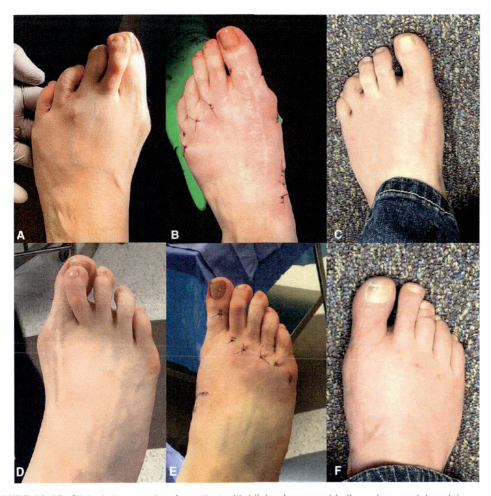

FIGURE 40.10 Clinical photographs of a patient with bilateral recurrent hallux valgus, metatarsalgia, and crossover second toe deformities at preoperative **(A, D)**, immediately postoperative **(B, E)**, and final follow-up of 5 months **(C)** and 3 months **(F)** postoperatively.

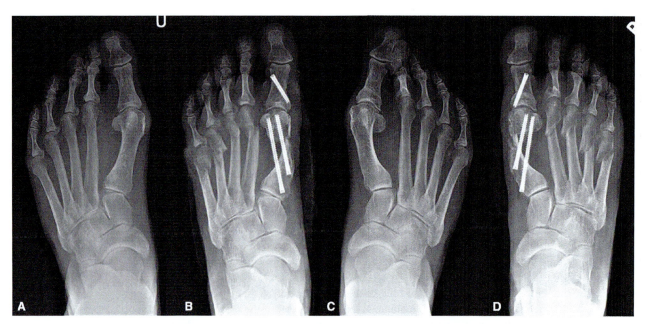

FIGURE 40.11 Preoperative weight-bearing radiographs **(A, C)** and 6-week postoperative weight-bearing radiographs **(B, D)** of the same patient as in Figure 40.10. Both sides require a minimally invasive chevron and Akin osteotomy and all distal lesser metatarsal osteotomies. The right side also requires a proximal phalangeal osteotomy of the second toe.

- A Fluoroscan is then used to assess completion of the osteotomy as well as the alignment of the adjacent metatarsals. Additional osteotomies may be required if bony prominence is appreciated on the plantar aspect of the third or fourth metatarsal heads upon direct palpation in a simulated weight-bearing position.
- Fixation of the osteotomy is not recommended.

When only one metatarsal dorsiflexion osteotomy is desired to relieve plantar pressure, a 2-mm bur can be used to create an osteotomy of the dorsal cortex while preserving the plantar cortex allowing the metatarsal head to migrate dorsally for 2 to 3 mm (Fig. 40.15).[28] This osteotomy will not effectively shorten or deviate the affected metatarsal but will only elevate the bone in sagittal plane.

- A dorsal stab incision is made at the level of the metatarsophalangeal joint line.

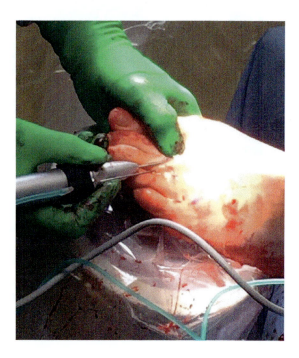

FIGURE 40.12 Intraoperative images of a minimally invasive distal metatarsal osteotomy of the second ray are demonstrated.

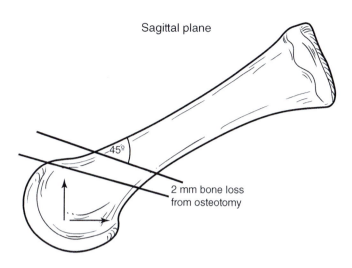

FIGURE 40.13 Diagram of a minimally invasive distal metatarsal osteotomy in sagittal plane is demonstrated. The metatarsal head is allowed to migrate proximally and dorsally.

- A 2 × 12 mm bur is inserted obliquely 30° from the axis of the metatarsal shaft until the plantar cortex is reached. A Fluoroscan is used to document the trajectory of the osteotomy using a lateral or oblique view.
- The osteotomy is then completed for dorsal, medial, and lateral cortices while leaving the plantar cortex intact.
- A dorsally directed pressure is then applied at the affected metatarsal head to complete the osteotomy.
- Fixation is not required.

Correction of Hammertoe Deformity

Flexor Digitorum Brevis Release

At the level of proximal interphalangeal joint, a flexible deformity correction can be obtained by soft tissue release of the plantar plate and the flexor digitorum brevis insertions.[29]

- A medial or lateral stab incision is made at the level of proximal phalangeal neck (Fig. 40.16).
- The Beaver blade is then advanced toward the base of the middle phalanx. The plantar plate is then released while the toe is held in extension.
- The surgeon then walks the tip of the Beaver blade along the plantar surface of the middle phalangeal base and releases the two insertions of the flexor digitorum brevis tendons directly from bone.
- The proximal interphalangeal joint is then manipulated into full extension. Although uncommon, residual sharp bony edges on the dorsal aspect can be percutaneously removed using a 2 × 8 mm bur.

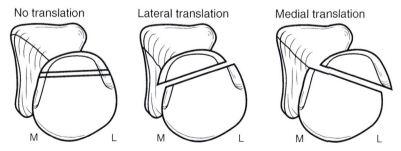

FIGURE 40.14 Diagram of a minimally invasive distal metatarsal osteotomy in coronal plane is demonstrated. The obliquity of the osteotomy promotes medial or lateral translation of the metatarsal head.

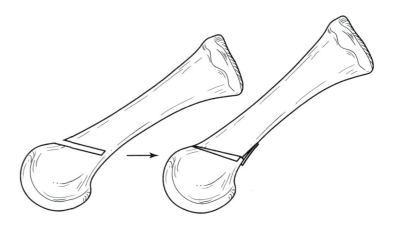

FIGURE 40.15 Diagram of a minimally invasive distal metatarsal dorsal closing wedge osteotomy in sagittal plane is demonstrated.

Resection Arthroplasty

Alternatively, the hammertoe correction can be corrected using a resection arthroplasty technique, particularly when the deformity is rigid (see Fig. 40.6).

- A dorsal transverse incision is made at the level of the proximal phalangeal head.
- The soft tissue release is performed for the dorsal capsule and collateral ligament.
- A power saw or a rongeur is used to remove the distal 4 to 5 mm of the proximal phalangeal head.
- Articular cartilage at the base of the middle phalange may be removed using a curette if a fusion is desired.
- Fixation is made using K-wires, a screw, or other implant of choice in 10° of plantarflexion.

Residual Deformity

Proximal Phalanx Osteotomy

Proximal phalangeal osteotomy is a workhorse for the correction of crossover toe deformity, with or without a plantar plate repair, due to its power of correction of severe deformity or fine-tuning

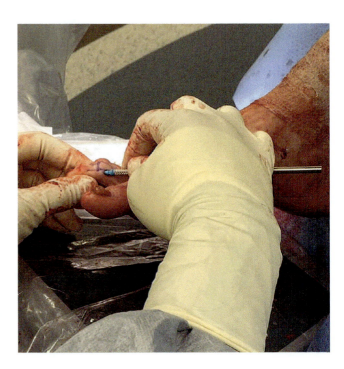

FIGURE 40.16 A percutaneous release of the plantar plate and the flexor digitorum brevis insertions at the proximal interphalangeal joint of the right second toe is demonstrated.

residual deformities. Open exposure is possible, but a minimally invasive approach is preferred (see Figs. 40.5 and 40.11).[25]

- This portion of surgery is performed without a tourniquet.
- A dorsolateral approach is used when the lesser toe is deviated medially and vice versa for a lateral deviation.
- A 3-mm incision is made just lateral to the base of the proximal phalange.
- A 2 × 8 mm bur is inserted through the base of the proximal phalange in an oblique plane extra-articularly under fluoroscopic guidance.
- For a mild deformity, the dorsolateral cortex can be preserved to allow a plantar-lateral closing wedge osteotomy.
- In severe cases, a complete osteotomy is performed followed by a manipulation of the affected toe laterally and plantarly. Surgical fixation is not required and not recommended.
- Sterile adhesive strips are used to keep the toe in proper coronal plane alignment while keeping the interphalangeal joints in relative extension. The toe must be kept in slightly more plantarflexed position compared to adjacent toes. Surgeons should avoid circumferential constriction around the toe to avoid vascular compromise.

Flexor to Extensor Transfer

If a tendon transfer is contemplated using a flexor digitorum longus, extensor digitorum longus, or extensor digitorum brevis, they should be preserved so that an appropriate harvest can be performed. The author has found that the need for a tendon transfer is extremely limited having all the less invasive techniques as described above. However, a transfer of the flexor digitorum longus tendon can be used as a salvage procedure and may assist in the stabilization of the metatarsophalangeal joint when plantar plate is not repairable.[10]

- The long flexor tendon is identified at the proximal toe crease plantarly. The distal insertion is percutaneously released at the plantar aspect of the distal interphalangeal joint.
- The tendon is then retrieved from the proximal incision and sharply separated into medial and lateral strips.
- Each strip is then separately transferred to a dorsal incision through a plane right on bone while avoiding strangulation of neurovascular structures.
- The two tendon ends are then sutured together or to the extensor apparatus.

Dermodesis

Some residual deformity of the metatarsophalangeal joint may be corrected further using dermodesis.[17]

- Remove an elliptical-shaped section of the skin to further pull the metatarsophalangeal joint into more plantarflexion and possibly slight medial or lateral deviation.
- This section of the skin is removed including the epidermis and dermis without dissection into subcutaneous tissue to minimize the risk of neurovascular injury.
- The skin is repaired in a tightened position, aiding in plantarflexion of the digit.

Toe Amputation

Trans-metatarsophalangeal amputation is an option that allows patient to fully weight bear immediately postoperatively with minimal postoperative care (Fig. 40.17).

- A "fishmouth" incision is made sharply down to bone, creating dorsoplantar or mediolateral flaps.
- Soft tissue structures at the base of the proximal phalanx are sharply released until the toe is disarticulated.
- Hemostasis is performed, and the soft tissue flaps are approximated and closed with simple nylon sutures.

POSTOPERATIVE MANAGEMENT

The patients may require a walking boot after a gastrocnemius recession or other associated procedures in the hindfoot and the ankle joint. Otherwise, a postoperative hard-sole shoe is sufficient for most patients. Patients are typically allowed to bear a minimum of 50% weight bearing for most

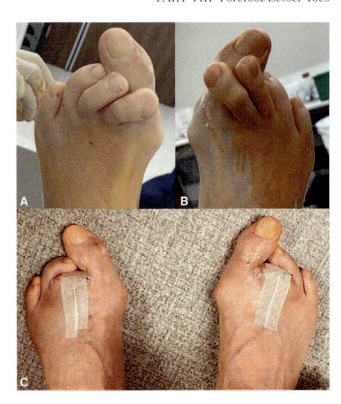

FIGURE 40.17 Bilateral crossover lesser toes are demonstrated in an elderly man with low demand **(A, B)**. The patient is allowed to bear full weight on both feet. Complete wound healing is shown at the 2-week follow-up **(C)**.

surgical reconstructions as described above. The patient can advance to full weight bearing between 2 to 4 weeks depending on the complexity of reconstruction. It is important that the patient keep the dressing clean and dry. Dressing change and taping is usually required to be meticulously performed by the operating surgeon at 2- and 4-week follow-up visits in order to maintain alignment, especially when percutaneous procedures without fixation were performed (see ▶ Video 40.1). Elevation for the first 2 weeks at least 50% of the time is encouraged to minimize postoperative swelling. Postoperative weight-bearing radiographs are performed at 6-week follow-up or sooner if needed. Dressing and taping can be discontinued after 6 weeks, and a silicone spacer can be used as needed.

RESULTS AND COMPLICATIONS

In 1987, Michael Coughlin described a surgical treatment of crossover second toe in 17 patients with an average age of 60 years.[12] All toes were treated with extensor tenotomy or lengthening, a metatarsophalangeal capsulotomy, and K-wire fixation. Toes with more advanced deformities required a combination of lateral capsule reefing, a flexor digitorum longus tendon transfer, and a metatarsophalangeal joint resection arthroplasty. A proximal interphalangeal joint deformity was corrected with a resection arthroplasty. The patients reported a good or an excellent result in 93% with only 7% fair results. The author highlighted the benefit of early recognition and operative intervention to avoid more severe subluxation and dislocation that would be more difficult to treat. In 1993, Thompson and Deland reported on surgical correction of painful instability of the second toes in 11 patients.[13] All the toes underwent a metatarsophalangeal dorsal capsulotomy, flexor digitorum longus transfer, K-wire fixation, and mostly proximal interphalangeal joint resection arthroplasty. All but one patient were satisfied with the results. Stiffness appeared to be the source of the mild residual pain. All toes, including six toes with preoperative medial crossover toe deformity, were corrected into valgus alignment with adjacent toes. A more rapid postoperative mobilization was recommended to reduce postoperative uncomfortable stiffness.

Numerous variations of tendon transfer have been proposed to realign the crossover second toes. Haddad et al reported on the surgical treatment of crossover toe deformity in 31 patients using either an extensor digitorum brevis or a flexor digitorum longus transfer.[18] Twenty-four patients were completely satisfied with the surgical correction, six were satisfied with reservations, and one was dissatisfied. The authors found that the extensor digitorum brevis transfer underneath the intermetatarsal ligament to itself was powerful in coronal plane correction, had less postoperative stiffness, but was not as effective in rigid deformities. It is also contraindicated in those with deficient intermetatarsal ligament such as after a decompression of the interdigital neuritis. Barca and Acciaro reported the use of an extensor digitorum brevis transfer underneath the intermetatarsal ligament to the proximal phalanx with 83% good or excellent results.[20] One recurrence of deformity was related to a premature removal of K-wire by the patient. Lui et al described a modification of the extensor digitorum brevis transfer with the incorporation of extensor digitorum longus transfer and a bone tunnel at the proximal phalanx to minimize supination of the toe and improve strength of tendon anastomosis.[21] Ellis et al reported a modification of the extensor digitorum brevis transfer using bone tunnels at both the proximal phalangeal base and the metatarsal neck.[17] Nine of 11 patients were either highly satisfied or moderately satisfied. The average metatarsophalangeal joint angle was 4.5° in the varus direction, which changed to 14.2° in the valgus direction postoperatively. The authors recommended against overtightening the reconstruction to avoid overcorrection of deformity.

Flint et al reported a prospective case series on plantar plate repair in 97 feet with 138 plantar plate tears.[30] A combination of dorsal approach with a Weil osteotomy was used. Hallux valgus correction and management of hallux rigidus were required in 57% of cases. Eighty percent of patients scored "good" to "excellent" satisfaction scores at 12 months. The mean visual analog scale pain score decreased from 5.4/10 to 1.5/10, postoperatively. The mean American Orthopedic Foot and Ankle Society scores increased from 49 to 81 points. There was no complication reported.

A minimally invasive arthroscopic approach for the correction of crossover toe deformity has been extensively described by Lui et al.[31-35] The techniques included a combination of plantar plate tenodesis using PDS sutures, extensor digitorum brevis transfer, and arthroscopic release of the medial capsuloligamentous complex and the lumbrical tendon. A 1.9-mm arthroscopy of the second metatarsophalangeal joint was used to assist with suture passage into the plantar plate. Eleven patients underwent combined plantar plate tenodesis and extensor digitorum brevis transfer with successful correction of crossover second toe deformity in all.[32] Two patients had residual mild residual claw toe deformity. Complexity of the procedures may require surgeons to have some experience in small joint arthroscopy and percutaneous techniques.

Minimally invasive surgery using low-speed, high-torque burs has been popularly adopted in Europe and more recently in the United States. Although there has been no dedicated clinical study focusing on the correction of crossover toes using minimally invasive osteotomy techniques, a basic principle of osteotomy and deformity correction could allow this application to be used as an adjunct. It has been the author's experience (level V) that minimally invasive osteotomies and soft tissue releases are quite helpful for a number of clinical scenarios as described in prior sections with less stiffness and faster recovery noted compared to open procedures.

PEARLS AND PITFALLS

- Meticulous foot and ankle examination is required to identify pain generators and pathomechanics of the crossover toe deformity.
- Crossover toe deformity is often a complex, long-standing overload of the lesser metatarsophalangeal joint. Associated conditions especially gastrocnemius contracture, unstable first ray, and hallux valgus should be treated to maximize success.
- A normal foot appearance and alignment may not always be restored. Surgeons should at least aim for final toe alignment that fit with adjacent toes in the coronal plane while avoiding cockup deformity at the metatarsophalangeal joint.
- Manage expectations appropriately to ensure that the patient understands the realistic surgical goals and recovery. Balance should be made between a complex reconstruction and an amputation.
- The importance of postoperative immobilization cannot be overstated. Meticulous postoperative care is required especially for dressing changes and taping.
- Familiarity with minimally invasive treatment and the use of burs is advantageous.
- A well-planned surgical strategy is required. Certain steps should be done in order such as a tendon transfer prior to a tenotomy. Soft tissue release is also more easily performed prior to an osteotomy.

- Lesser metatarsophalangeal joints have a natural tendency to contract in extension. Soft tissue balance is important both intraoperatively, during postoperative taping, and during postoperative stretching exercise.
- Open repair of the plantar plate is powerful but requires meticulous surgical techniques and customized instruments.

CONCLUSION

A crossover toe deformity is a challenging clinical problem that requires complete understanding of the pathology at the level of the metatarsophalangeal joint as well as other extrinsic factors. A systematic approach to the bone and soft tissue conditions is described. Multiple options are available to fine-tune the residual toe deformity. The advancement in the repair of the plantar plate and the use of minimally invasive techniques may allow patients to achieve superior outcomes with early recovery.

REFERENCES

1. Kaz AJ, Coughlin MJ. Crossover second toe: demographics, etiology, and radiographic assessment. *Foot ankle Int.* 2007;28(12):1223-1237.
2. Deland JT, Sung IH. The medial crossover toe: a cadaveric dissection. *Foot ankle Int.* 2000;21(5):375-378.
3. Coughlin MJ, Baumfeld DS, Nery C. Second MTP joint instability: grading of the deformity and description of surgical repair of capsular insufficiency. *Phys Sportsmed.* 2011;39(3):132-141.
4. Klein EE, Weil L, Weil LS, Coughlin MJ, Knight J. Clinical examination of plantar plate abnormality: a diagnostic perspective. *Foot Ankle Int.* 2013;34(6):800-804.
5. Akoh CC, Phisitkul P. Plantar plate injury and angular toe deformity. *Foot Ankle Clin.* 2018;23(4):703-713.
6. Federer AE, Tainter DM, Adams SB, Schweitzer KM. Conservative management of metatarsalgia and lesser toe deformities. *Foot Ankle Clin.* 2018;23(1):9-20.
7. Kinter CW, Hodgkins CW. Lesser metatarsophalangeal instability: diagnosis and conservative management of a common cause of metatarsalgia. *Sports Health.* 2020;12(4):390-394.
8. Ito E, Shima H, Togei K, et al. Dislocations of the second and third metatarsophalangeal joints after local steroid injection in patients with refractory metatarsalgia: a case report. *SAGE Open Med Case Reports.* 2021;9.
9. Doty JF, Coughlin MJ. Metatarsophalangeal joint instability of the lesser toes. *J Foot Ankle Surg.* 2014;53(4):440-445.
10. Doty JF, Coughlin MJ, Weil L, Nery C. Etiology and management of lesser toe metatarsophalangeal joint instability. *Foot Ankle Clin.* 2014;19(3):385-405.
11. Jastifer JR, Coughlin MJ. Exposure via sequential release of the metatarsophalangeal joint for plantar plate repair through a dorsal approach without an intraarticular osteotomy. *Foot Ankle Int.* 2015;36(3):335-338.
12. Coughlin MJ. Crossover second toe deformity. *Foot Ankle.* 1987;8(1):29-39.
13. Thompson FM, Deland JT. Flexor tendon transfer for metatarsophalangeal instability of the second toe. *Foot Ankle.* 1993;14(7):385-388.
14. Coughlin MJ, Schenck RC, Shurnas PJ, Bloome DM. Concurrent interdigital neuroma and MTP joint instability: long-term results of treatment. *Foot Ankle Int.* 2002;23(11):1018-1025.
15. Johnson A, Aibinder W, Deland JT. Clinical tip: partial plantar plate release for correction of crossover second toe. *Foot Ankle Int.* 2008;29(11):1145-1147.
16. Coughlin MJ, Schutt SA, Hirose CB, et al. Metatarsophalangeal joint pathology in crossover second toe deformity: a cadaveric study. *Foot Ankle Int.* 2012;33(2):133-140.
17. Ellis SJ, Young E, Endo Y, Do H, Deland JT. Correction of multiplanar deformity of the second toe with metatarsophalangeal release and extensor brevis reconstruction. *Foot ankle Int.* 2013;34(6):792-799.
18. Haddad SL, Sabbagh RC, Resch S, Myerson B, Myerson MS. Results of flexor-to-extensor and extensor brevis tendon transfer for correction of the crossover second toe deformity. *Foot Ankle Int.* 1999;20(12):781-788.
19. Myerson MS, Jung HG. The role of toe flexor-to-extensor transfer in correcting metatarsophalangeal joint instability of the second toe. *Foot Ankle Int.* 2005;26(9):675-679.
20. Barca F, Acciaro AL. Surgical correction of crossover deformity of the second toe: a technique for tenodesis. *Foot Ankle Int.* 2004;25(9):620-624.
21. Lui TH, Chan KB. Technique tip: modified extensor digitorum brevis tendon transfer for crossover second toe correction. *Foot Ankle Int.* 2007;28(4):521-523.
22. Watson TS, Reid DY, Frerichs TL. Dorsal approach for plantar plate repair with weil osteotomy: operative technique. *Foot Ankle Int.* 2014;35(7):730-739.
23. Phisitkul P, Hosuru Siddappa V, Sittapairoj T, Goetz JE, Den Hartog BD, Femino JE. Cadaveric evaluation of dorsal intermetatarsal approach for plantar plate and lateral collateral ligament repair of the lesser metatarsophalangeal joints. *Foot Ankle Int.* 2017;38(7):791-796.
24. Devos Bevernage B, Deleu PA, Leemrijse T. The translating Weil osteotomy in the treatment of an overriding second toe: a report of 25 cases. *Foot Ankle Surg.* 2010;16(4):153-158.
25. Cordier G, Nunes GA. Minimally invasive advances: lesser toes deformities. *Foot Ankle Clin.* 2020;25(3):461-478.
26. Sundaram RO, Walsh HPJ. Amputation of a crossover 2nd toe in the presence of hallux valgus. *Foot.* 2003;13(4):196-198.
27. Sung W, Weil L, Weil LS, Rolfes RJ. Diagnosis of plantar plate injury by magnetic resonance imaging with reference to intraoperative findings. *J Foot Ankle Surg.* 2012;51(5):570-574.
28. Lui TH. Percutaneous dorsal closing wedge osteotomy of the metatarsal neck in management of metatarsalgia. *Foot (Edinb).* 2014;24(4):180-185.

29. Frey S, Hélix-Giordanino M, Piclet-Legré B. Percutaneous correction of second toe proximal deformity: proximal interphalangeal release, flexor digitorum brevis tenotomy and proximal phalanx osteotomy. *Orthop Traumatol Surg Res.* 2015;101(6):753-758.
30. Flint WW, Macias DM, Jastifer JR, Doty JF, Hirose CB, Coughlin MJ. Plantar plate repair for lesser metatarsophalangeal joint instability. *Foot Ankle Int.* 2017;38(3):234-242.
31. Lui TH. Correction of crossover toe deformity by arthroscopically assisted plantar plate tenodesis. *Arthrosc Tech.* 2016;5(6):e1273-e1279.
32. Lui TH. Correction of crossover deformity of second toe by combined plantar plate tenodesis and extensor digitorum brevis transfer: a minimally invasive approach. *Arch Orthop Trauma Surg.* 2011;131(9):1247-1252.
33. Lui TH, LiYeung LL. Modified double plantar plate tenodesis. *Foot Ankle Surg.* 2017;23(1):62-67.
34. Lui TH, Chan YLC. Correction of severe crossover toe deformity by plantar plate tenodesis, arthroscopic release of lumbrical and plication of lateral capsuloligamentous complex. *Arthrosc Tech.* 2021;10(8):e1921-e1927.
35. Lui TH, Ng CK. Correction of crossover toe deformity by plantar plate tenodesis and arthroscopic release of lumbrical. *Arthrosc Tech.* 2021;10(6):e1621-e1626.

41 Lesser Toes Metatarsophalangeal Plantar Plate Tears: Dorsal Direct Repair in Combination With Weil Osteotomy

Caio Nery and Daniel Baumfeld

INTRODUCTION

Plantar plate tears have been established as the main affected anatomic structure for a range of lesser metatarsophalangeal (MTP) conditions including metatarsalgia, instability, frank dislocation, crossover toe, and toe deviation. As clinical experience with plantar plate repair grows, the indications, role, and outcomes are becoming better defined with more consistent results.[1-3]

The results obtained with plantar plate tears by direct repair through a dorsal approach combined with a Weil metatarsal osteotomy have already been proved to be the most valuable combination of techniques to manage this problem.[2,4]

INDICATIONS AND CONTRAINDICATIONS

Initially in the course of the pathology, the clinical picture could reveal only pain and light inflammatory signals sign such as swelling and thickening of the MTP joint capsule that resemble an acute arthritic condition. In a few days, the widening of the interdigital space is noticed, and pain can be intense (Fig. 41.1A).[1,5] The progression of the deformity will take place if some protective treatment is not initiated. As the condition progresses, dorsal, dorsomedial, or dorsolateral deviation of the toe occurs, followed by a loss of contact of the toe with the ground (ground touch) and a loss of power of the toe (digital purchase); a flexible or fixed hammertoe may develop with time and, in the end, different degrees of the classic "crossover toe" may be found (Fig. 41.1B and C).[6]

The inconsistent results observed in the literature with the various conventional techniques based on the combination of interphalangeal joints resection arthroplasties, release of collateral ligaments and dorsal joint capsule, in addition to lengthening the contracted tendons, with or without fixation of the toes with Kirschner wires, acted as the main impulse for the deepening of the knowledge of these deformities and for the search for new surgical techniques.

The MTP joint drawer test is one of the most important objective sign of MTP joint instability. The involved toe should be plantarflexed 20° during the MTP joint drawer test, and a comparison with the normal toes is recommended. The stability of the joint is rated as follows: G0 = stable joint; G1 = light instability (<50% subluxable); G2 = moderate instability (>50% subluxable); G3 = gross instability (displaceable joint); G4 = dislocated joint (Fig. 41.2A and B).[6-8]

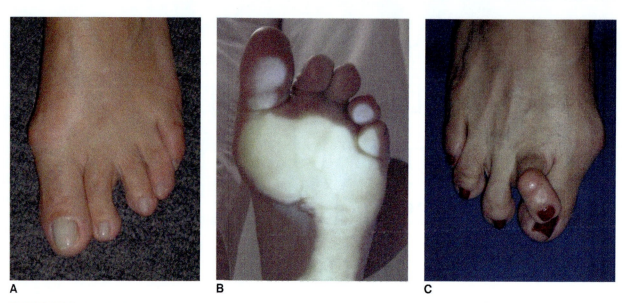

FIGURE 41.1 **A.** Widening of the second interdigital space—one of the earliest signs of plantar plate injury. **B.** Podoscopic image of the left foot of a patient with 2nd and 3rd toe plantar plate tears showing the absence of "ground touch" of both toes. **C.** Gross crossover toe deformity—late stage of the lesser metatarsophalangeal joint instability.

Table 41.1 shows the most important clinical findings, its relative frequency as well as the importance and significance of each one in typifying and grading the MTP joint instability. After the clinical evaluation, each patient is classified according to the anatomical grading for plantar plate dysfunction which grades the evolution of the deformity in five stages—0 to 4.[9]

Imaging of lesser MTP joints is needed to assess and help confirm plantar plate injuries as well as identify associated injuries. Standing anteroposterior and lateral radiographs can demonstrate the magnitude of the MTP joint angular deformity, joint incongruity, the presence of MTP joint arthritis, and determining the existence of some metatarsal protrusion—commonly the second ray—causing a break of the ideal metatarsal parabola (Fig. 41.3A and B).[10] Magnetic resonance imaging (MRI) is essential to the differential diagnoses and to confirm the initial stages of the pathology (Fig. 41.4A and B). The sensitivity of MRI is up to 87%, and the efficiency of the method can be improved through the use of intra-articular contrast or by combining MRI with ultrasound.[8,11-13]

Each type of plantar plate tear has a particular treatment. We proposed a plantar plate treatment algorithm that is essentially based on the clinical and anatomical findings. The anatomic grading system helps the surgical planning and management of plantar plate ruptures.[6,8]

The rationale of the surgical treatment indication is based on the failure of the conservative treatment in a patient who has appropriate vascular status and no comorbidities that contraindicate surgery.[14] The plantar plate repair with metatarsal osteotomy is often indicated in patients with lesions grades 1-3 according to the anatomical grading system with second and/or third metatarsal

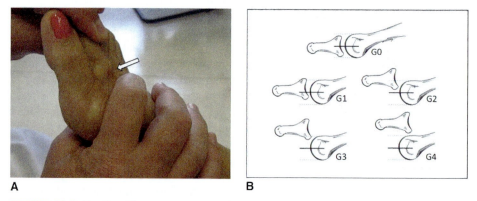

FIGURE 41.2 Hamilton-Thompson metatarsophalangeal (MTP) drawer test. **A.** The maneuver—the *arrow* points to the dorsal subluxation of the proximal phalanx. **B.** Degrees of MTP joint instability—G0 = stable joint; G1 = light instability (<50%); G2 = moderate instability (>50%); G3 = gross instability (dislocatable joint) and G4 = dislocated joint.

TABLE 41.1 Relative Frequency and Statistical Significance of the Clinical Findings in Plantar Plate Lesions

Parameter	Incidence (%)	Grade 0	Grade 1	Grade 2	Grade 3	Grade 4	Statistical Significance
Drawer test	100	1	1	2	2/3	3/4	(*) High
Pain under MT head	94	—	—	—	—	—	No significance
Toe dorsal elevation	93	√	—	—	—	—	(*) Low
Toe purchase	92	√	—	—	—	—	(*) High
Varus/valgus	84	√	√	√	√	√	(*) Low
Interdigital widening	77	—	—	√	√	√	(*) Low
Ground touch	77	√	√	√	√	√	(*) High
Crossover toe	77	—	—	—	√	√	(*) High
Acute pain onset	69	—	—	√	√	—	(*) High
High-heeled shoes	62	—	—	—	—	—	No significance
Local edema	38	—	—	—	—	—	No significance
Toe supination	29	—	—	√	√	√	(*) High
Mulder signal	26	—	—	—	—	—	No significance
Sportive trauma	16	—	—	—	—	—	No significance

*All clinical findings that were statistically significant help decisively in the grading of plantar plate injuries. MT, metatarsophalangeal.
Reprinted with permission from Nery C, Coughlin MJ, Baumfeld D, et al. Classification of metatarsophalangeal joint plantar plate injuries: history and physical examination variables. *J Surg Orthop Adv.* 2014;23(4):214-223.

protrusion that cause alteration of metatarsal parabola, who lead to a third rocker metatarsalgia and overload of the lesser MTP joint.[2,4,8]

Plantar plate grade 0 and grade 4 are not suitable for plantar plate repair, and the procedure described in this text is not indicated for these types of lesions.

PREOPERATIVE PLANNING

The surgery can be done under regional block anesthesia and lower thigh tourniquet, but different types of anesthetic procedures can also be recommended according to the surgeon's criteria. The examination under anesthesia is recommended and allows for better evaluation of the MTP joint instability as a whole.[14]

We usually start the surgical procedure by performing an MTP joint arthroscopy that has two distinct objectives:

- The first is to confirm our clinical and radiological assessment of the plantar plate tears (Fig. 41.5A).

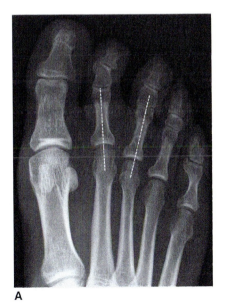
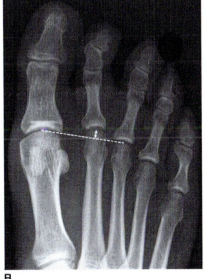

FIGURE 41.3 **A.** Anteroposterior plain radiograph showing a widening of the second interdigital space in a patient in the early stage of plantar plate tear. **B.** Second metatarsal head protrusion is positively related to metatarsophalangeal joint overload and plantar plate injury.

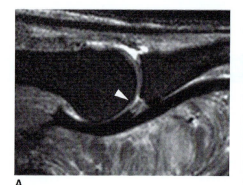
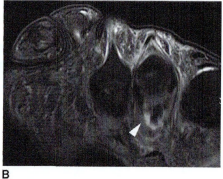

FIGURE 41.4 MR T2 images of the second metatarsophalangeal joint (**A.** sagittal plane; **B.** coronal plane) showing the hyperintense signal (*arrowheads*) that corresponds to a discontinuity of the plantar plate at the base of the proximal phalanx.

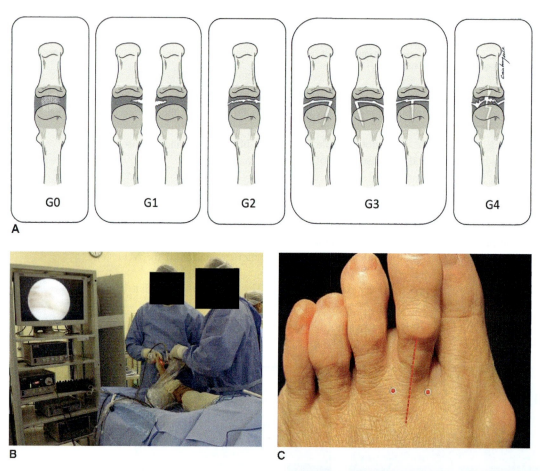

FIGURE 41.5 A. Anatomic grading system of the plantar plate tears (schematic representing the right second metatarsophalangeal [MTP] joint): grade 0—thinning and attenuation of the plantar plate; G1—partial transverse lesion involving the lateral or medial border; G2—complete transverse rupture; G3—combination of a transverse and a longitudinal lesion forming "7," inverted "7" or "T" figures; grade 4—random combination of plantar plate tears in different directions. **B.** Positioning the patient and the surgical team to perform the arthroscopic step of the evaluation of the MTP joints. **C.** Dorsal arthroscopic portals to the MTP joint—medial and lateral. **D.** Composition of arthroscopic images of a right second MTP joint in which complete transverse tear (G2) of the plantar plate is observed: the probe tip is inside the lesion that spans the entire width of the plantar plate. The rounded ivory-colored structure seen in the lower portion of the images corresponds to the metatarsal head.

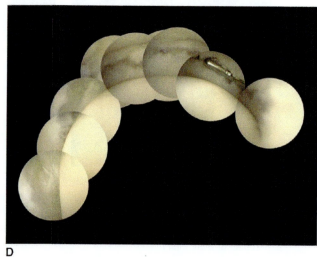

- The second is to remove the intra-articular hypertrophic and inflamed synovial tissue and the fringes of fibrous tissue from the torn plantar plate tears in addition to possible intra-articular free bodies resulting from old injuries.

In our treatment algorithm, the plantar plate repair with metatarsal osteotomy is indicated as 1 to 3 grade lesions, and this type of lesion will be the focus of this chapter.

SURGICAL TECHNIQUE

The patient is placed supine on the operating table. The surgeon starts the procedure facing the dorsal aspect of the forefoot, whereas their first assistant faces the sole of the foot (Fig. 41.5B). In some steps of the procedure, they will change their positions to make feasible the surgical maneuvers.

Two dorsal arthroscopic portals are used to perform the lesser MTP joint arthroscopy: the dorsomedial and dorsolateral portals. Both are placed at or slightly distal to the MTP articular joint line, medially, and laterally 4 to 5 mm equidistant from the extensor digitorum longus (EDL) tendon (Fig. 41.5C). Conventional arthroscopic view makes it possible to easily identify the base of the proximal phalanx with its concave articular facet, the metatarsal head with its convex articular facet, and the accessory collateral ligaments functioning as the medial and lateral walls of the joint. Composing the background of the image, we have the plantar plate that appears in the normal individual as a pearly structure with a shiny and smooth surface (Fig. 41.5D).

To perform the open repair of the lesser MTP plantar plate through the dorsal approach, one can use:

- A dorsal longitudinal incision centered over the MTP joint (especially when the arthroscopic step of the procedure is not performed) or
- An S-shaped dorsal incision that encompasses the arthroscopic portals

In our experience, the "S" shape dorsal incision is used routinely, and it could be extended over the third and the fourth toes if necessary (Fig. 41.6A). The extensor digitorum brevis and longus are retracted medially in mild deformities, but it could be necessary to lengthen the extensor tendons if there is a gross and stiff deformity of the toe. A longitudinal capsulotomy is performed to expose the affected MTP joint followed by a partial collateral ligament release to improve visualization. A distal metatarsal Weil osteotomy, using a sagittal saw, is performed. The saw cut is made parallel to the plantar aspect of the foot, starting at a point 2 to 3 mm below the top of the metatarsal articular surface (Fig. 41.6B). In the presence of a plantar keratosis beneath the metatarsal head, a small slice of bone is removed to achieve a subtle elevation of the metatarsal head. It is recommended to resect 2 or 3 mm of the distal metaphyseal flare to improve the plantar plate visualization. The capital fragment is pushed proximally as far as possible (8 to 10 mm) and held in this position temporarily with a small vertical K-wire (Fig. 41.6C). Care must be taken not to capture the plantar plate with the wire during this step of the technique in order to avoid the impairment of its free mobilization. Longitudinal traction to the toe helps to distract the joint, creating space to the next steps of the procedure.

The plantar plate is then inspected, and the type of lesion is confirmed. If some portion of the plantar plate remains connected to the inferior border of the proximal phalanx, it is cut carefully with a small scalpel avoiding lesions to the flexor digitorum longus tendon.

It is important to release the distal margin of the plantar plate from any soft tissue adhesions especially at the plantar surface, creating room for the introduction of the instruments used to grasp the free border of the plantar plate and to help with the sutures.

The MTP plantar plate is 2.0 to 2.5 mm thick in its anterior border, and care must be taken not to delaminate the plantar plate during the intent to free the margins of this structure.

Any residual tissue is excised from the plantar margin of the proximal phalanx with a small rongeur or curette, creating a roughened surface for optimal attachment of the plantar plate.

If a longitudinal tear of the plantar plate is detected (grade 3 T- or 7-shaped lesions), it can be repaired through interrupted nonabsorbable 3.0 sutures placed with the help of a small needle holder or other surgical instruments specially created for this purpose.

There are different and efficient ways to suture the distal border of plantar plate, in all of them the main objective is to attach the sutures in as viable tissue as proximal as possible at the free border of the plantar plate.

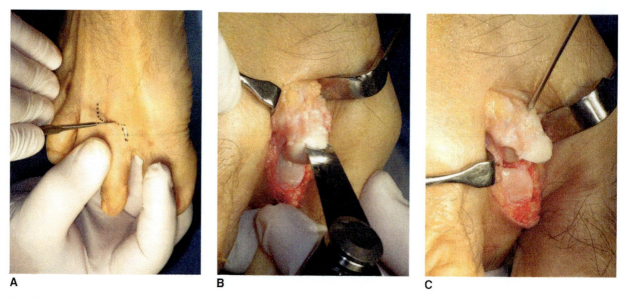

FIGURE 41.6 A. S-shape skin incision. **B.** Weil metatarsal osteotomy. **C.** The cephalic fragment is pushed as proximal as possible and held with a K-wire.

A joint distractor can be used to help the visualization of all anatomical reference sites before passing the sutures. It could be placed over the proximal phalanx and the retracted metatarsal head with the help of K-wires to support the distraction.

To perform the suture, one can use a mechanical suture passer or a micro "pig-tail" suture passer (Mini SutureLasso, Arthrex, Naples, Florida). With this, the surgeon can easily and safely place horizontal or longitudinal mattress or laced sutures in the plantar plate.

The horizontal mattress stitch may be the biomechanically superior configuration in plantar plate repairs. The mattress and luggage tag configuration demonstrated better peak load-to-failure force compared with the Mason-Allen suture (Fig. 41.7).

There are several options of mechanical or manual suture passers in the market (Mini Scorpion and VIPER, Arthrex; HAT-TRICK, Smith & Nephew; GoSTRoPP, CrossRoads), but when they are not available, there is an alternative surgical technique that has been called the "ugly technique."

In this technique, before starting to pass the main sutures through the anterior border of the plantar plate, we have to build a "snake-headed NINJA instrument" from a 1-mm K-wire as shown in Figure 41.8.

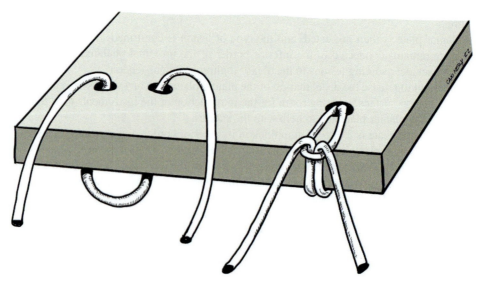

FIGURE 41.7 The "mattress suture" on the left side and the "luggage tag suture" on the right side.

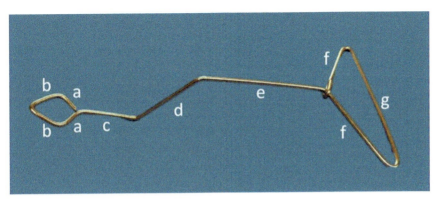

FIGURE 41.8 The snake-headed NINJA instrument obtained by bending a 1.0-mm K-wire with a strong surgical needle holder: head ($a = 3$ mm; $b = 5$ mm); neck ($c = 10$ mm); step 1 (first step angle $= 45°$); bridge ($d = 15$ mm); step 2 (second step angle $= 45°$); stem ($e = 20$ mm); handle ($f = 15$ mm/$g = 20$ mm). Our tribute to Michelle Reichter Geronimo—"Miss NINJA"—for the design of this instrument.

The head of the NINJA instrument is positioned under the anterior border of the plantar plate, in its lateral or medial half, taking care to avoid injury to the flexor tendons. It is important to reach the healthiest area of the plantar plate to be repaired in order to place sutures in strong and vitalized tissue capable of healing and attaching to the proximal phalanx (Fig. 41.9A).

A straight handheld suture passer (SutureLasso, Arthrex, Naples, Florida) or an 18-gauge needle is passed from dorsal to plantar through the plantar plate, into the snake-head of the NINJA instrument, and through the soft tissue of the sole until it is exteriorized at the plantar face of the foot (Fig. 41.9B).

A flexible wire loop is introduced into the needle or suture passer from dorsal to plantar. A folded 2.0 nonabsorbable suture is then passed through the wire loop and pulled up through the plantar plate. The loop of the suture involves the handle of the NINJA instrument, while the free suture tails are firmly kept in the plantar face of the foot by the assistant (Fig. 41.9C). With this maneuver, a lace will be created while the NINJA instrument is pulled out of the surgical field at the same time that the suture tails are released by the assistant (Fig. 41.9D). The same sequence is repeated for the other half of the plantar plate. At the end, we have two sutures firmly passed through the remaining healthy tissue from the MTP plantar plate (Fig. 41.10A through H).

With the use of a 1.5-mm K-wire or a drill bit, two vertical and parallel drill holes are made medially and laterally in the base of the proximal phalanx from the dorsal cortex to the plantar rim of the proximal phalanx, matching the sutures placed over the plantar plate (Fig. 41.11A). The same flexible wire loop used in the previous steps is passed from dorsal to plantar through

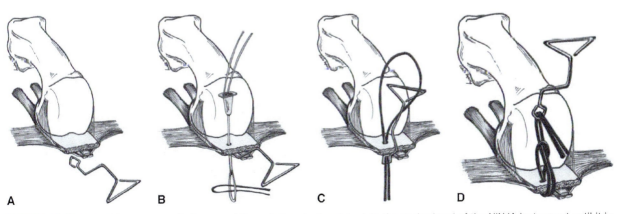

FIGURE 41.9 A. An 18-gauge needle is passed through the plantar plate, into the snake-head of the NINJA instrument until it is exteriorized at the plantar face of the foot. **B.** A flexible wire loop is introduced into the needle. **C.** The loop of the suture involves the handle of the NINJA instrument. **D.** The NINJA instrument is pulled out of the surgical field to create a luggage tag–type suture.

the holes of the phalanx base and then used to catch and pull the sutures through the dorsal side (Fig. 41.11B through E).

The Weil osteotomy is fixed in the desired position with one small snap-off self-tapping vertical screw or any other type of micro screw available (Fig. 41.11F and G). The metatarsal shortening is determined in the preoperative planning to achieve a regular metatarsal parabola. Normally, only 2 or 3 mm of metatarsal shortening is required. Care must be taken with metatarsal shortenings greater than 3 mm that can cause transference metatarsalgia and must be avoided.

Once the Weil osteotomy is fixed, the sutures are tied over the bone bridge at the proximal phalanx, attaching the plantar plate at the base of the phalanx while the toe is held in 20° of plantarflexion (Fig. 41.11H).

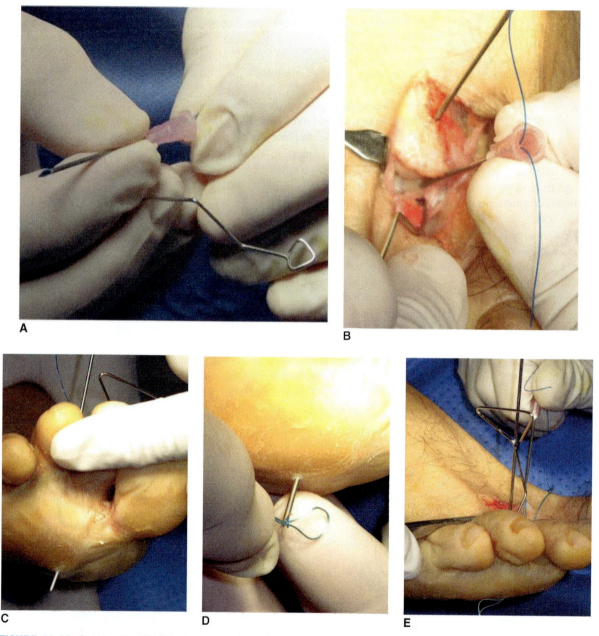

FIGURE 41.10 **A.** Using the NINJA instrument and an 18-gauge needle with a flexible wire loop inside, the plantar plate sutures could start. **B.** The 18-gauge needle is passed through the plantar plate and the snakehead of the NINJA instrument that was positioned under the plantar plate, externalizing through the plantar skin **(C)**. **D.** A folded suture is passed through the wire loop that is inside the 18-gauge needle. **E.** The needle is pulled up through the plantar plate.

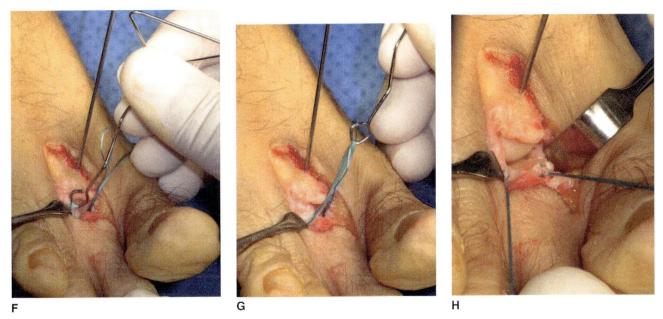

FIGURE 41.10 *(Continued)* **F.** The loop of the suture involves the handle of the NINJA instrument creating a lace. **G.** The NINJA instrument is pulled out. **H.** The suture firmly locks in the plantar plate margin. The entire process is repeated to obtain two firm sutures on the free edge of the plantar plate.

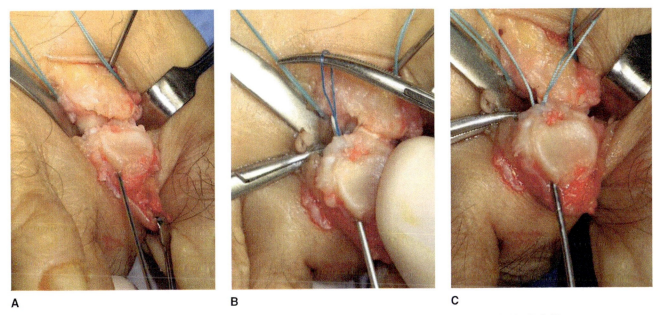

FIGURE 41.11 **A.** Two bone tunnels are made at the base of the phalanx with a 1.5-mm K-wire or a drill bit. **B-E.** The sutures are passed through the bone tunnels with the help of the 18-gauge needle used before.

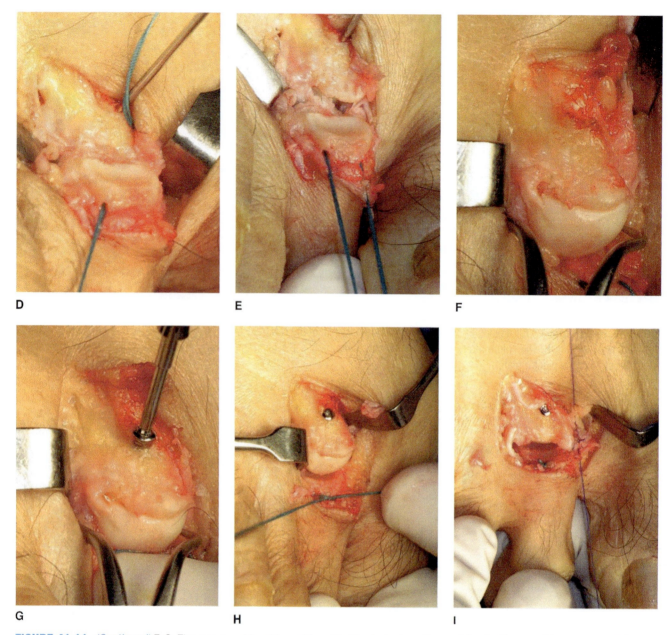

FIGURE 41.11 *(Continued)* **F, G.** The metatarsal head is positioned in the desired position and fixed with a small bone screw. **H.** The sutures are tied while the toe is kept in 20° of plantarflexion. **I.** Careful soft tissue and ligament repair.

Lateral and medial soft tissue reefing is performed to repair any collateral ligamentous insufficiency and transverse plane deformities (Fig. 41.11I). The articular capsule is closed and the EDL tendon is sutured in the appropriate length if elongation was performed.

At this moment, it is important to release the tourniquet and to proceed to a careful hemostasis of the dorsal region of the MTP joints. Substantial bleeding can result from the small dorsal vessels, and the hematoma formed can compromise the soft tissue coverage of the region with potential skin necrosis with dehiscence of the surgical incision. After routine wound closure, a postoperative compression dressing is applied with the affected toes held in 20° of plantarflexion (Fig. 41.12A and B).

Figure 41.13 shows images of a patient with hallux valgus and plantar plate injuries in the second and third MTP joints, in addition to the clinical and radiological results at 9 years postoperatively.

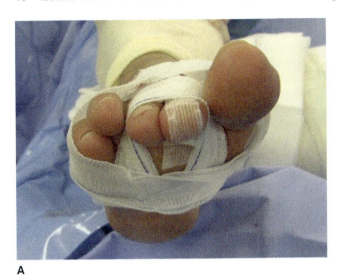
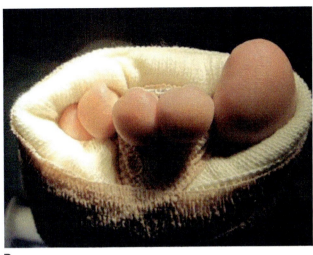

FIGURE 41.12 A. Intraoperative dressing in which the position of the operated toes is maintained at 20° of flexion with sterile adhesive tapes. **B.** The successive changes of postoperative dressings aim to keep the operated toes in a 20° of flexion position, for 6 weeks, with elastic bandages.

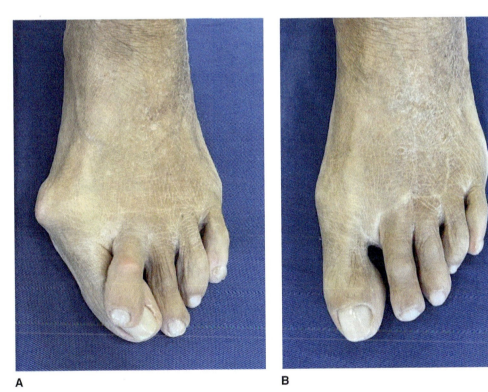

FIGURE 41.13 Clinical and radiographic aspect of a patient with hallux valgus and a grade 2 plantar plate lesion of the second metatarsophalangeal (MTP) joint (with severe crossover toe deformity) and a grade 1 plantar plate lesion of the third MTP joint of the left foot. The images shown on the *left* were obtained preoperatively and the images shown on the *right* were obtained 9 years after surgery. **A.** Preoperative dorsal clinical appearance. **B.** Dorsal clinical view of the foot in the late postoperative period.

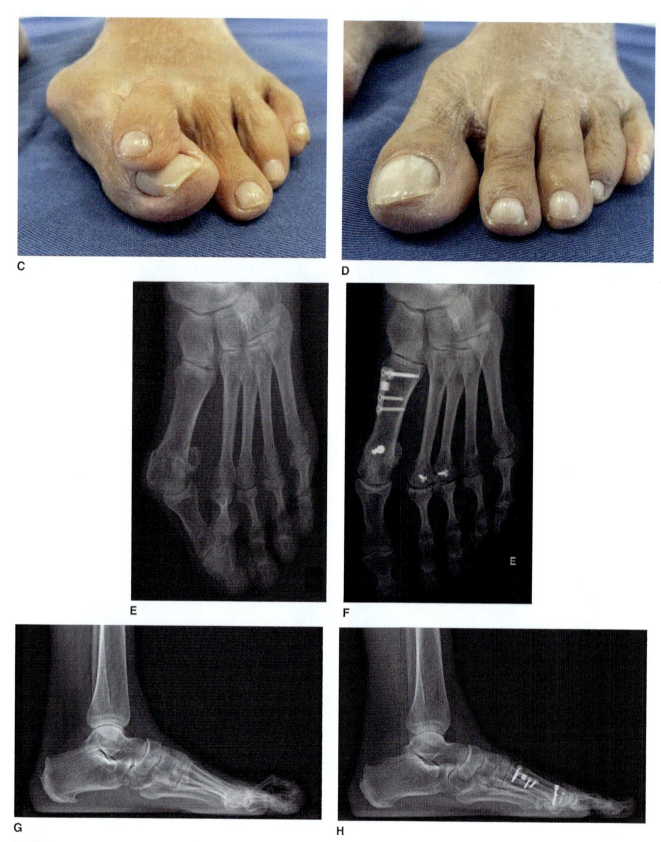

FIGURE 41.13 *(Continued)* **C, D.** Clinical anterior axial view of the left foot in both periods (C = preoperative and D = postoperative). **E, F.** Plain dorsoplantar weight-bearing radiographs of the left foot pre- and postoperatively, respectively. On the first ray, a basilar opening wedge osteotomy was performed in combination with a triplanar chevron osteotomy (to correct for exaggerated metatarsal pronation). In the second MTP joint, the plantar plate repair was performed combined with a Weil osteotomy according to the technique mentioned in this text (note the image of the bone tunnels at the base of the proximal phalanx—9 years after the procedure). The plantar plate of the third MTP joint was treated through shrinkage using radiofrequency (performed arthroscopically before the index surgery) in combination with a Weil osteotomy. **G, H.** Plain lateral weight-bearing radiographs of the left foot of the same patient in both periods. The correct alignment in the sagittal plane of the second and third toes in the postoperative image can be verified.

PEARLS AND PITFALLS

Diagnosis
- Think "plantar plate lesion" is the first step to diagnose correctly.
- Intimacy with the regional anatomy is paramount to understand and propose the right treatment regimen.
- Acute pain under the affected metatarsal head, widening of the web space, and the positive MTP drawer test are the most important and reliable findings in MTP joint instability.
- The clinical staging system and its correlation with the anatomic grading system for the MTP plantar plate lesions proved to be very important in the treatment decision-making process.
- Due to the intense interrelationship between the structures of the forefoot, especially the great and the lesser toes, it is highly recommended to treat all the deformities at the same time, redistributing the pressures and avoiding the deleterious action of an untreated deformity on the newly corrected segments. This observation is particularly important when we are faced with the most frequent combination of hallux valgus and second cross-over toe deformity.

Skin Incision
- The S-shaped dorsal incision can be elongated to expose two or three MTP joints at the same time.

EDL Tendon
- Depending on the amount of the toe deformity, consider elongating the extensor tendons.

Weil Osteotomy
- Try to keep the osteotomy cut as parallel as possible with the sole of the foot, avoiding an undesirable amount of descending of the metatarsal head.
- Take off a thin slice of bone if you attempt to elevate the metatarsal head and reduce its overload.
- Beware of metatarsal shortenings >3 mm.

Plantar Plate Repair
- Remove all fibrous tissue from the free border of the plantar plate lesion.
- Be sure to free the plantar plate from its adhesions to the plantar fat pad before passing the sutures.
- Be sure to pass the sutures in a healthy tissue.
- Be sure to identify and suture any longitudinal tear of the plantar plate.

Preparing the Phalanx
- Be extremely careful when orienting the K-wire or the drill bit to make the bone holes at the base of the proximal phalanx.
- Leave, at least, 1 mm of bone between the articular cartilage and the bone hole.
- Take care not to jeopardize the metatarsal head while doing the phalangeal bone holes.

Fixing the Weil Osteotomy
- Beware of rotational deviation of the metatarsal head while fixing the osteotomy. Use two screws if you feel it is necessary.
- Be gentle while bending the screwdriver of the powered machine at the end of the screw insertion. You can cause a bone fracture at this moment.

Tie the Sutures
- Keep the toe in a 20° plantarflexion at the MTP joint while fixing the sutures over the proximal phalanx.
- Be sure that the MTP joint is stable and aligned at the end of this step.
- If not, complete the procedure by reefing the collateral ligaments and the articular capsule.
- Suture the tendons at the appropriate length.

Before Closing

- Take caution with the hemostasis before closing the wound.

Dressing

- Keep the affected toes in 20° of plantarflexion for 6 weeks after the surgery.

POSTOPERATIVE MANAGEMENT

The operated toe is held in 20° of plantarflexion to provide adequate healing of the repaired plantar plate during the first 6 weeks (Fig. 41.14A and B). The patient is allowed to ambulate in a postoperative shoe for 6 weeks with no weight bearing on the forefoot. After 6 weeks, dressings are discontinued, and comfortable shoes are permitted.

An aggressive and early physical therapy program that mainly aims to strengthen the flexor tendons and the foot-core muscles is started after the 2nd postoperative week. The patient is not allowed to perform dorsiflexion of the fingers until 6 weeks after surgery. It is not advisable to wear high-heeled shoes for 6 months after the surgery.

RESULTS AND COMPLICATIONS

The objective of plantar plate repair is to restore the stability of the MTP joint and preserve the joint function and motion. Surgical repair of the plantar plate through a dorsal approach has a reported success rates of 68% to 93%.[2,3,15]

With the combination of plantar plate repair and a Weil metatarsal osteotomy, over 63% of the patients have the ability to perform digital purchase.[2]

Regarding the stability, some authors found that 68% of the patients were completely stable after this treatment (grade 0 of the stability classification) and 32% had an unstable MTP joint grade 1 or mild instability with no clinical implications.[2]

The most undesired complication is recurrence of symptoms; this may be due to an incorrect diagnosis, incomplete repair of the plantar plate, or true incorrect alignment of the metatarsal parabola. Painful prominent hardware can also occur after fixation of the Weil osteotomy.[3] Dorsal hematoma formation and healing skin problem, scaring and retraction of the surgical incisions, persistent edema (long lasting), and elevated and insufficient toes are also complications reported in the literature.[2,4,15,16]

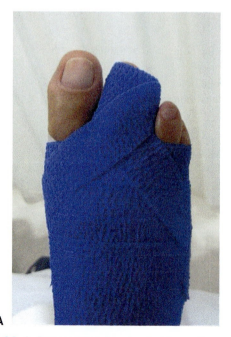
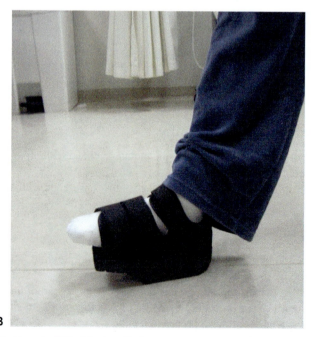

FIGURE 41.14 A. Postoperative dressing that keeps the operated toes in 20° of flexion. **B.** Postoperative shoe with a "short" sole in its anterior portion that allows the toes to be kept in a flexed position during the postoperative period.

REFERENCES

1. Mendicino RW, Statler TK, Saltrick KR, et al. Predislocation syndrome: a review and retrospective analysis of eight patients. *J Foot Ankle Surg.* 2001;40:214-224.
2. Nery C, Coughlin MJ, Baumfeld D, et al. Lesser metatarsophalangeal joint instability: prospective evaluation and repair of plantar plate and capsular insufficiency. *Foot Ankle Int.* 2012;33:301-311.
3. Suero EM, Meyers KN, Bohne WH. Stability of the metatarsophalangeal joint of the lesser toes: a cadaveric study. *J Orthop Res.* 2012;30:1995-1998.
4. Weil L Jr, Sung W, Weil LS Sr, et al. Anatomic plantar plate repair using the Weil metatarsal osteotomy approach. *Foot Ankle Spec.* 2011;4:145-150.
5. Nery C, Umans H, Baumfeld D. Etiology, clinical assessment, and surgical repair of plantar plate tears. *Semin Musculoskelet Radiol.* 2016;20(2):205-213.
6. Coughlin MJ, Baumfeld DS, Nery C. Second MTP joint instability: grading of the deformity and description of surgical repair of capsular insufficiency. *Phys Sportsmed.* 2011;39:132-141.
7. Bouche RT, Heit EJ. Combined plantar plate and hammertoe repair with flexor digitorum longus tendon transfer for chronic, severe sagittal plane instability of the lesser metatarsophalangeal joints: preliminary observations. *J Foot Ankle Surg.* 2008;47:125-137.
8. Nery C, Coughlin MJ, Baumfeld D, et al. MRI evaluation of the MTP plantar plates compared with arthroscopic findings: a prospective study. *Foot Ankle Int.* 2013;34:315-322.
9. Nery C, Coughlin MJ, Baumfeld D, et al. Classification of MTPl joint plantar plate injuries: history and physical examination variables. *J Surg Orthop Adv.* 2014;23(4):214-223.
10. Mann TS, Nery C, Baumfeld D, Fernandes EA. Is second metatarsal protrusion related to metatarsophalangeal plantar plate rupture? *AJR Am J Roentgenol.* 2021;216(1):132-140.
11. Nery C, Baumfeld D, Umans H, Yamada AF. MR imaging of the plantar plate: normal anatomy, turf toe, and other injuries. *Magn Reson Imaging Clin N Am.* 2017;25(1):127-144.
12. Gregg J, Silberstein M, Schneider T, et al. Sonographic and MRI evaluation of the plantar plate: a prospective study. *Eur Radiol.* 2006;16:2661-2669.
13. Yamada AF, Crema MD, Nery C, et al. Second and third metatarsophalangeal plantar plate tears: diagnostic performance of direct and indirect MRI features using surgical findings as the reference standard. *AJR Am J Roentgenol.* 2017;209(2):W100-W108.
14. Doty JF, Coughlin MJ. Metatarsophalangeal joint instability of the lesser toes. *J Foot Ankle Surg.* 2014;53(4):440-445.
15. Yu GV, Judge MS, Hudson JR, et al. Predislocation syndrome. Progressive subluxation/dislocation of the lesser metatarsophalangeal joint. *J Am Podiatr Med Assoc.* 2002;92:182-199.
16. Kaz AJ, Coughlin MJ. Crossover second toe: demographics, etiology, and radiographic assessment. *Foot Ankle Int.* 2007;28:1223-1237.

42 Ankle Fracture Late Syndesmosis Repair

Fernando Raduan and John Y. Kwon

INTRODUCTION

Ankle fractures are among the most commonly treated injuries by orthopedic surgeons.[1] Achieving anatomic syndesmotic reduction remains a significant challenge. Over 50% of lower extremity fractures occur at the ankle, and they make up approximately 14% of fracture-related hospital admissions.[1,2] A large percentage have concomitant syndesmotic lesions.[3,4] Poor functional outcomes usually arise from malreduction[5-11] as it leads to altered kinematics and the development of osteoarthritis.[12] While it is well established that anatomic reduction is crucial,[11] the most accurate and reproducible means to reduce the syndesmosis is still not clear.[13]

When symptomatic syndesmotic malalignment or instability results, regardless of initial treatment, revision surgery is often warranted. While late revision can be described as subacute or chronic, these terms are relative as syndesmotic malalignment may be detected near immediately after the index procedure. Similarly, instability may be detected earlier or later in the postoperative or recovery period. It is important, however, to understand key aspects of initial assessment, reduction, and stabilization to understand iatrogenic causes for malalignment and how to correct them. Many of the concepts discussed in this work apply similarly for primary or revision syndesmotic stabilization.

INDICATIONS AND CONTRAINDICATIONS

Per Lauge-Hansen mechanistic theory regarding supination-external rotation ankle fractures, initial injury occurs at the anterior inferior tibiofibular ligament and/or an avulsion fracture at either the fibular or tibial insertions. If supraphysiologic external rotational forces continue, an oblique fibular fracture occurs followed by injury to the posterior structures (either the posterior malleolus or the posterior syndesmotic ligaments). In the final stage of injury, the medial malleolus is fractured and/or a deltoid ligament rupture occurs.[4,14] Approximately 20% of supination-external rotation injuries present with syndesmotic lesions, and an even higher incidence arises from pronation external rotation-type injuries.[15]

Syndesmotic injuries lead to impairment of ankle kinematics altering tibiotalar contact areas and pressures.[16-21] Abnormal kinematics leads to pathologic loading, which results in long-term loss of function and degenerative joint disease.[7,11,12] Classic studies published by Ramsey and Hamilton, which were corroborated by other authors, demonstrated that 1 to 2 mm of loss of mortise congruency leads to pathologic loading and may be considered as a relative indication for surgical anatomic reduction and fixation.[17,18,22-24] Fibular rotation and sagittal reduction are important for ankle kinematics[17,21] and should be restored as soon as the diagnosis is made regardless of chronicity.

Syndesmotic injuries are associated with worse functional outcomes in patients with ankle fractures.[25] Weening and Bhandari demonstrated that syndesmotic malreduction was the sole important predictor of clinical outcomes in a retrospective study analyzing 51 patients.[5] Sagi et al demonstrated significantly worse outcomes in patients with poorly reduced syndesmosis[7] regardless of injury severity at a minimum follow-up of 24 months.[7,26] In another retrospective series of 120 patients published by Ray et al, the independent predictor for the development of degenerative changes was again syndesmotic malreduction.[12] A study published by Andersen et al, which evaluated 87 patients with minimum 2-year follow-up, demonstrated that a threshold of 2 mm for malreduction was indeed a predictor of poor results.[11]

Anatomic syndesmotic reduction is imperative since the biomechanics of the tibiotalar joint are only reestablished when original anatomy and stability is restored.[27] This concept applies to acute and nonanatomically reduced fractures. While multiple relative contraindications exist for revision syndesmotic fixation, active infection should be considered an absolute contraindication necessitating a staged approach in which infection eradication is necessary prior to reconstruction.

PREOPERATIVE PLANNING

For decades, objective and seemingly reproducible radiographic parameters published by Harper-Keller were used to diagnose syndesmotic injuries.[28] However, subsequent studies have challenged the sole use of tibiofibular overlap (TFO) and clear space to define anatomic tibiofibular relationships.[29]

Bilateral computed tomography (CT) scan may prove to be a better diagnostic tool since it can not only evaluate specific portions of the syndesmosis in particular in the axial plane (anterior syndesmosis, posterior syndesmosis, widening of the tibiofibular clear space [TFCS]) but also compares these parameters with the contralateral, uninjured side. Weight-bearing CT scan, according to Osgood et al, may be even more accurate in detecting subtle pathology and can show different measurement values when compared to non–weight-bearing CT scans.[30] The increased accuracy from bilateral weight-bearing CT scans is even more valuable when evaluating patients who have undergone previous surgery.

Linear (two-dimensional) syndesmotic measurements on CT scan have already been demonstrated to be more accurate when compared to plain radiographic measurements.[31] However, some authors have recently examined calculation of syndesmotic areas and volumes postulating that these measurement techniques may be even more accurate to diagnose subtle lesions.[32,33] While further research is required, this increased ability to detect malalignment may be even more crucial in revision cases.

While these newer means of analyzing syndesmotic malalignment are intriguing, they remain static modalities and some patients may only demonstrate late instability when the syndesmosis is stressed. Arthroscopic syndesmotic evaluation has been studied by multiple authors, and work in this area continues in particular to define thresholds. While technically demanding and invasive, it may prove to be an even more accurate and reliable way to diagnose syndesmotic lesions and instability.[34-36] While traditional assessments have focused on coronal plane motion, some authors have increasingly demonstrated that sagittal plane mobility (and malalignment) may be of increasing importance.[37-39]

SURGICAL TECHNIQUE

Intraoperatively, the syndesmosis should be stressed after fibular fixation to assess its integrity.[40,41] Significant disruption leads to instability and is occasionally detected on preoperative stress radiographs, especially for Maisonneuve or ligamentous-equivalent injuries. The most common intraoperative tests are the Cotton and the external rotation stress tests.[42] Even though it has been shown that abnormal medial clear space (MCS) (usually caused by deltoid lesions) may overestimate the level of syndesmotic instability, the Cotton test is still one of the most popular intraoperative tests[43] (Fig. 42.1). Force applied and ankle position can influence the radiographic evaluation,[44,45] and per Ingall et al, adequate distraction force should be applied so as not to underdiagnose instability.[46] These techniques can also be applied in chronic cases, in particularly when residual syndesmotic instability is suspected.

While TFO and TFCS have some known limitations in assessing anatomic syndesmotic reduction, the contralateral ankle should be used as a template. Whether primary or revision cases, it is

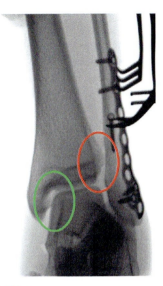

FIGURE 42.1 Cotton test demonstrating pathologic diastasis at the medial clear space (*green oval*) and tibiofibular articulation (*red oval*) consistent with a combined syndesmotic and deltoid ligament disruption.

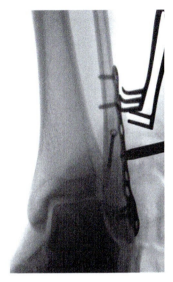

FIGURE 42.2 Counterpressure being applied when drilling for syndesmotic fixation by inverting/reducing the mortise. Note how this technique ensures appropriate medial clear space distance. Counterpressure should not be applied on the medial foot as it can cause subtle mortise displacement.

crucial to obtain contralateral fluoroscopic images (perfect mortise and lateral with ankle in neutral position) prior to prepping and draping for reference intraoperatively. It is our preference to obtain these intraoperatively as contralateral radiographs taken in the clinic setting often differ in foot position and rotation. Reference images may be the best parameters to use intraoperatively when reducing and fixing the syndesmosis in the absence of the availability of intraoperative CT and/or when concomitant arthroscopy is not being performed.[8,28,47-51]

When anatomically reducing the syndesmosis, several intraoperative details should be taken into consideration to avoid iatrogenic malreduced fixation. While a complete description is beyond the scope of this work, direct visualization, in particular anteriorly, has been shown to decrease malreduction rates.[52,53]

Ankle Positioning

Ankle position (dorsi/plantarflexion) at the time of fixation, and its possible influence on syndesmotic reduction, has been widely debated in the literature.[54,55] Although plantarflexion during syndesmotic fixation was believed to predispose to overcompression given previous understanding of talar mortise geometry,[56] multiple studies showed no effect of ankle position during fixation of the syndesmosis.[62,63] Placing the ankle in a neutral position when stabilizing the syndesmosis is advisable as is passively dorsiflexing and plantarflexing after fixation to ensure smooth, unencumbered motion. To date, there are no studies investigating the relative risk of malreduction comparing patients in supine versus prone positioning, but the majority of techniques for achieving and evaluating syndesmotic reduction have been described for use in the supine position. A support under the heel during syndesmotic reduction, according to Boszczyk and colleagues, could predispose to anterior malreduction especially in grossly unstable cases.[55] Similar to ankle lateral ligament repair, one must be careful to avoid iatrogenically applying an anterior drawer displacement.

Similarly, special consideration should be given when applying counterpressure when drilling for the planned implant of choice. It is our preference to apply counterpressure to the tibia (or with the foot inverted and the mortise in a reduced position) so as not to iatrogenically displace the talus laterally by applying pressure on the foot when countering drilling (Fig. 42.2).

Screw Trajectory

It has been long recommended that screws should be placed 2 cm proximal and parallel to the tibial plafond, inserted obliquely posterior to anterior at an angle of approximately 30° to the transaxial axis.[57] While based on a general presumption of incisural anatomy, these initial recommendations did not take into consideration anatomic variation, technical aspects nor were supported by any substantive clinical/radiographic/functional outcomes studies.[58,59] The distal tibiofibular axis, according to Mendelsohn et al, is 32° ± 6° externally rotated from the transepicondylar axis.[60] Putnam et al correlated CT imaging to plain radiographs and found that the trans-syndesmotic angle (TSA) was aimed 21.5° anterior to the plane of the lateral radiograph.[61] When evaluating 200 normal ankles by CT imaging, Kennedy et al determined that the optimal force vector for anatomic reduction and fixation passed through the fibula within 2.5 mm of the lateral cortical apex and the anterior half of the medial malleolus.[62] They suggested that the anterior half of the medial malleolus is a reliable aiming point when starting the screw on the lateral cortical fibular ridge.

Traditionally, in order to avoid theoretical iatrogenic fibular shortening or lengthening, screws (one or two) are placed parallel to the tibial joint line.[62] Furthermore, the level of syndesmotic screw fixation (in relation to the plafond) has also been studied with several authors demonstrating no differences in clinical or radiological outcomes between supra or trans-syndesmotic screw placement.[63-66] Currently, it appears that acceptable outcomes can be achieved by placing screws between 2 and 5 cm proximal to the tibial plafond. While traditional teaching has recommended that screws be placed in parallel to both the plafond and each other in both the coronal and axial planes, rigidity of the construct can be enhanced following simple biomechanical principles by placing screws divergent in multiple planes (Fig. 42.3A and B).

In the revision setting, previous screw tracts and/or osteolytic loosening may be present in the tibia if previous syndesmotic fixation was performed. As long as syndesmotic reduction is anatomic, various screw trajectories in multiple planes (to avoid previous screw tracts) can be utilized to ensure rigid osseous tibial fixation.

Clamping and Indirect Reduction

Several different techniques to indirectly reduce the syndesmosis have been described. Clamp reduction prior to fixation is a well-described technique.[67,68] While another long-standing recommendation, several authors have demonstrated the risk of iatrogenic malreduction.[54] Miller et al, using CT scan in a cadaveric study, demonstrated that clamp angles of 0°, 15°, and 30° starting at the

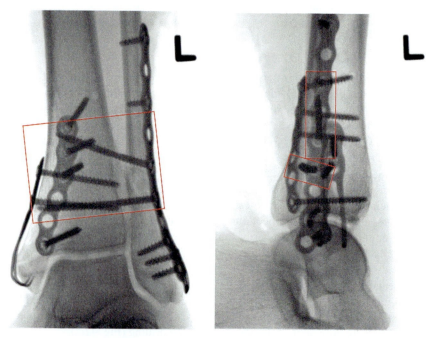

FIGURE 42.3 Syndesmotic screws (*red rectangles*) placed divergently in multiple planes to increase construct rigidity.

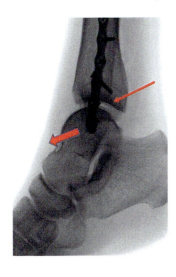

FIGURE 42.4 Example of iatrogenic syndesmotic malreduction. The radiographic syndesmosis reduction parameters are within normal limits, but axial CT imaging demonstrates anterior displacement. *Thick red arrow* demonstrates anterior talar shift. *Thin red arrow* demonstrates anterior fibular malpositioning.

posterolateral fibular corner resulted in syndesmotic malreduction[67,69] and concluded that accurate reduction cannot be reliably achieved only with a clamp.[69] Cosgrove and colleagues concluded that sagittal plane reduction is highly sensitive to clamp malpositioning with a high risk of iatrogenic malreduction.[67]

Trying to facilitate clamp positioning according to the TSA, Putnam and colleagues analyzed CT scans of 45 normal patients and concluded that the average TSA was 21.5° anterior to a lateral view of the ankle. After placing the lateral clamp tine over the fibular ridge, the medial tine should be placed 23% of the distance from anterior to posterior medial tibial cortex on the lateral view.[61] Anterior talar subluxation can be a subtle sign of syndesmotic malreduction. Hoshino et al described this pattern in three patients in their series and hypothesized that this was a result of posterior fibular tine placement leading to anterior fibular malreduction and rotation (Fig. 42.4).

It is our preference to avoid clamp placement whenever possible given the increased risk of malreduction. If considerable force is required by clamp application to restore normal TFO and/or medialization of the talus, usually additional débridement or evacuation of soft tissue imposition (at the medial gutter, incisura, or both) is needed.[70] Kaiser et al suggested that placing a laminar spreader between the tibia and the fibula to remove soft tissue interposition with a pituitary or a rongeur can be helpful for syndesmotic débridement.[71] If fibular fixation has occurred and similarly aggressive clamp application is required to restore normal parameters, fibula fracture malalignment should be considered.

Direct Open Reduction

Assessing fibula positioning in the incisura visually, by palpation, or both are methods of open direct reduction, which have been demonstrated by several authors to decrease malreduction rates.[52,70] Both techniques use the anterior syndesmosis as a parameter, and this can be facilitated curving the incision anteriorly when performing the surgical approach. Tibial plafond contact forces, areas, and pressures were studied by LaMothe and colleagues using three different reduction and fixation techniques: indirect clamp and screw reduction, indirect reduction using a suture-button (SB) implant, and thumb reduction (manual palpation) and subsequent screw placement. While none of the tested reduction techniques restored normal kinematics, thumb reduction proved to be significantly better than the indirect reduction techniques tested.[52] Miller et al utilized CT to compare the reduction quality of patients treated with open reduction via direct visualization versus 25 historical controls treated with indirect intraoperative fluoroscopic reduction. The direct visualization group had a malreduction rate of 16%, while the indirect reduction group demonstrated a 50% malreduction rate.[70]

At the level of the joint, the anterior aspect of the syndesmosis is the parameter used when open reduction under direct visualization is being performed to more accurately ensure reduction.[70] Pang and colleagues found no differences when comparing direct visualization and blind palpation of the reduction at this location in a cadaver study.[72] In another cadaver study, Tornetta et al suggested that one can more accurately access the anterior syndesmosis via direct open reduction visualization through a separate small anterior incision.[53] Reb and colleagues attempted to establish the "tibiofibular line" as a method to objectively judge the quality of direct open syndesmotic reduction.[73] Relatively poor intra- and interobserver reliability of this technique, however, illustrates the subjective nature of judging reduction despite direct visualization and palpation. Although overall conclusions are limited by variations in methods between studies, direct open reduction leads to better reduction when compared to indirect visualization reduction techniques.[59,70]

In the revision setting, careful analysis of the anterior tibial tubercle and posterior malleolus is warranted. In the presence of a malunited Chaput fragment and/or posterior malleolus, abnormal anatomy should be considered when utilizing direct visualization for reduction.

Intraoperative Evaluation of Reduction

Several fluoroscopic techniques have been published in the past to help achieve appropriate reduction intraoperatively. Furthermore, the combination of (1) fluoroscopic assessment, (2) use of contralateral templating, and (3) a thorough knowledge of techniques to avoid malreduction will likely be the preferred strategies available to most surgeons to ensure anatomic reduction. While assessment in three-dimensions to ensure proper sagittal, coronal and axial plane alignment is the goal, this remains difficult without the aid of intraoperative CT capabilities, which are still not uniformly available at most institutions. Aside from cost and institutional availability, radiation exposure as well as acquisition times are considerations (Fig. 42.5).

Fluoroscopy

The utility of traditional radiographic parameters has been investigated not only for detecting syndesmotic injury[88] but also to evaluate intraoperative reduction.[29,74] While TFO and TFCS remain important radiographic parameters to assess, limitations exist. Marmor et al showed in their cadaveric study that plain radiographs have limitations detecting rotational malreduction.[29] When assessing various degrees of intentional malalignment, they demonstrated that up to 30° of external rotation malreduction can go undetected when utilizing TFCS and TFO.[29] To evaluate fibular rotation, Chang et al suggested two new parameters on anteroposterior (AP) radiograph evaluating the details of the distal fibula contour and the appearance of the malleolar fossa.[75] Futamura found high sensitivity and specificity of three indices for detecting malreduction including TFCS, anterior tibiofibular interval, and fibular rotation, always comparing images with contralateral uninjured AP radiograph. They did not describe parameters for assessing sagittal plane reduction.[76]

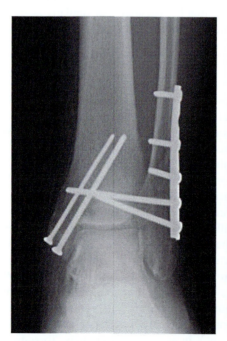
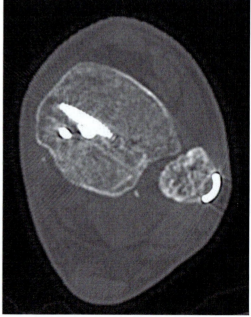

FIGURE 42.5 Example of iatrogenic syndesmotic malreduction. The radiographic syndesmosis reduction parameters are within normal limits, but the CT scan shows anterior translation of the fibula, out of the incisura.

Other parameters for assessing sagittal plane reduction on fluoroscopy have been published.[77-79] Loizou et al demonstrated that the anterior fibular line ratio (AFL ratio) and posterior fibular line distance (PFL distance) to assess sagittal reduction according to the relationship to the posterior tibial articular margin on lateral views had excellent reliability.[78] Similarly, Grenier et al described the anteroposterior tibiofibular ratio, which determines where the anterior fibular cortex crosses the tibial growth plate scar.[79] In a cadaver study, Koenig et al asked fully trained trauma surgeons to evaluate different amounts of malreduction (on lateral radiographs) in iatrogenically malreduced ankles comparing to a normal contralateral radiograph. Anterior translation and greater magnitudes of displacement in general showed to be most easily diagnosed to a threshold of 2.5 mm. Posterior displacement of 2.5 mm imposed the most difficulty to reviewers in detecting malalignment. However, as previously emphasized, the use of comparative contralateral radiographs increased surgeons' accuracy in detecting malalignment.[74] Summers et al described a technique for obtaining accurate syndesmotic reduction by comparison to mortise and lateral fluoroscopic views of the uninjured ankle. They obtained provisional fixation and then used intraoperative CT to confirm reduction. CT changed their reduction in only 1 of 18 patients, indicating their technique may obviate the need for intraoperative CT.[80] Finally, sagittal translational malreductions detected on CT scan may not be detected measuring the TFCS and TFO, according to Baek et al indicating once again the importance of intraoperative lateral radiographs.[81]

Implant Choice

While many means of stabilization have been described, metal syndesmotic screws (SS) and SB devices have proven to be the mainstay for surgical stabilization. According to multiple prior studies and systematic reviews, screw diameter, number of screws, and number of cortices engaged do not influence clinical outcomes in general and no definitive correlation with loss of syndesmotic reduction has been demonstrated.[66,82] Despite this, individual patients may benefit from specific fixation strategies. Screws may be superior to SBs when extra stability is needed depending on the injury pattern and/or in highly comorbid patients. Furthermore, screws are more effective at maintaining length especially in the setting of axially unstable (fibular shortening) fractures.[83,84] If axial length is not restored by internal plate fixation, SB devices may be inadequate to prevent fibular shortening, resulting in valgus talar tilt and lateral talar displacement.[85] Screws have also been shown to have better torsional resistance to sagittal fibular translation, and since the screws provide an overall sturdier fixation, it is frequently the best choice for revisions.[83,84] On the other hand, screws have higher rates of reoperation and implant breakage in acute primary cases.[86,87]

Several level one studies have compared reduction and clinical outcomes after SS versus SB fixation for syndesmotic injuries, and SB devices may provide improved functional outcomes with lower rates of malreduction.[86] In a recent prospective multicenter randomized control trial (RCT) Sanders et al found higher malreduction rates with SS (39%) versus SB fixation (15%). While functional outcome scores were similar in both groups, the study was of limited power.[34] In the retrospective series by Miller et al mentioned previously, the authors found an 18% malreduction rate with SS fixation under direct visualization,[70] and this is a similar number to the one reported for SB in the RCT by Sanders. Direct comparison between the studies is difficult, but experienced surgeons can probably achieve similarly low malreduction rates with screws under direct visualization. While the previously mentioned studies were performed on acute syndesmotic injuries and not revision surgery, the SB may still hold benefit in revision cases due to its ability to aid in accurate syndesmotic reduction. As such, hybrid constructs (SB placed initially followed by SS) may have played a role in revision syndesmotic stabilization.

In general, late syndesmotic reconstruction should be stabilized with metal screws given their increased rigidity. Furthermore, augmentation of chronically disrupted ligamentous structures should be considered.

Débridement

While arthroscopy should be utilized in revision cases to assess and treat intra-articular pathology, open débridement of the syndesmosis is commonly required. Our preferred technique is to place a laminar spreader between the fibula and tibia approximately 6 to 8 cm proximal to the incisura as previously discussed. Care must be taken to avoid iatrogenic injury to the lateral talar cartilage when debriding this area. As adequate exposure for débridement requires transecting any remnant anterior syndesmotic ligaments, augmentation can be performed. Our preference is to reconstruct and supplement the anterior syndesmotic ligaments using a nonabsorbable suture tape (Fig. 42.6A through D).

Syndesmotic Arthrodesis

Syndesmotic fusion may be warranted if significant arthritic changes at the incisura are demonstrated on CT imaging. While reduction and stabilization may be considered, patients may have continued pain localized to this area despite revision surgery. While beyond the scope of this work, adequate bone grafting, rigid internal fixation, and limiting early postoperative motion is advised. Similarly, overcompression of the syndesmosis during arthrodesis should be avoided as this may increase lateral gutter pressures and adversely affect ankle kinematics even more so than what is imparted by the fusion itself.

PEARLS AND PITFALLS

- *Preoperative imaging*
  Patients with suspected syndesmotic malalignment based on plain radiographs should undergo bilateral ankle CT imaging especially in revision situations. Weight-bearing CT, if available, may be helpful due to application of physiologic load. Subtle syndesmotic displacement may be only appreciated when comparing area or volume measurements between injured and healthy sides.
- *Intraoperative contralateral fluoroscopy*
  Obtain a contralateral perfect mortise and lateral fluoroscopic image in the operating room prior to prepping and draping as a template to assist with anatomic syndesmotic reduction. These images help determine normal TFO, TFCS, MCS, fibular length, fibular rotation, as well as sagittal plane tibiofibular alignment. Carefully examine these radiographic parameters both before and after syndesmotic realignment.

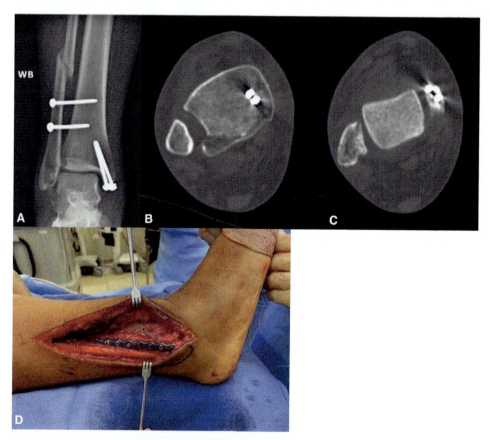

FIGURE 42.6 A-D. A 39-year-old female 9 months s/p ankle and syndesmotic stabilization with a shortened, malrotated fibular malunion with syndesmotic diastasis. After revision surgery was performed, the anterior syndesmosis was reconstructed utilizing a nonabsorbable suture tape construct.

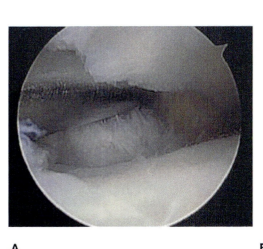 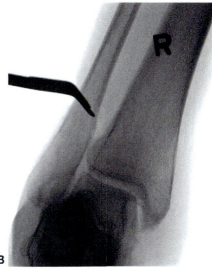

FIGURE 42.7 A, B. A 45-year-old male with chronic ankle pain. Arthroscopic image demonstrates insertion of a 5-mm probe into the incisura strongly suggestive of syndesmotic instability. Confirmation demonstrated fluoroscopically in the same patient by Cotton test showing significant instability.

- *Ankle arthroscopy*

  Ankle arthroscopy should be considered for all revision cases given the high rate of intra-articular pathology associated with ankle fractures and syndesmotic injury such as osteochondral lesions, synovitis, loose bodies, arthrofibrosis, and impingement. Furthermore, ankle arthroscopy is a valuable tool to aid in assessment and reduction of syndesmotic pathology (Fig. 42.7A and B). While the use of noninvasive traction facilitates access, it may mask possible instability. Therefore, when analyzing syndesmotic instability, ankle distraction should be removed. While arthroscopy is helpful for gutter debridement, revision cases often require formal arthrotomy for gutter débridement as well as syndesmotic débridement.

- *Approaches*

  Usually the previous fibular approach may be used during revision surgery especially when hardware needs to be removed. In cases where the arthroscopy shows medial soft tissue interposition that could not be cleaned arthroscopically, a medial incision should be made. The surgeon must be able to check the anterior ridge of tibiofibular articulation to ensure anatomic reduction. If it cannot be accessed through the original approach, a distal anterior curve or small separate longitudinal anterolateral incision can be utilized (Fig. 42.8A and B).

- *Fibula fracture reduction/fibular malunion*

  Restoring fibular length and rotation are crucial for subsequent syndesmotic reduction. Syndesmotic malalignment cannot be appropriately improved if an established fibular malunion is present. If a fibular malunion is present, osteotomy with correction of length and rotation is warranted. Length can be confirmed by examining the relative distance between the tip of the fibula and the lateral talar process keeping the ankle in neutral position as compared to the contralateral ankle.[88] Rotation can be determined by examining symmetry of the lateral clear space as well as distal fibular morphology.

- *Deltoid ligament repair*

  Residual deltoid ligament incompetence if often associated with chronic syndesmotic pathology. MRI may be helpful for preoperative planning. However, if any diastasis of MCS exists, it is our preference to repair the deltoid ligament formally at time of revision surgery (see Fig. 42.1).

- *Assessing final reduction*

  At the completion of surgery, we obtain a perfect AP, mortise, and lateral views with comparison to contralateral fluoroscopy obtained at the start of the procedure to mitigate limitations of traditional measurements as previously discussed. To examine for potential subtle syndesmotic displacement, the lateral radiograph is initially obtained holding only the leg without

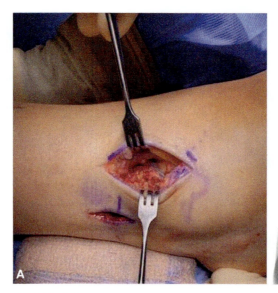
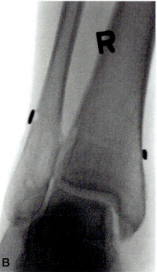

FIGURE 42.8 A, B. An anterolateral incision is made to allow for direct visualization for syndesmotic reduction and placement of a nonabsorbable suture tape construct. A separate lateral incision was made for placement of a suture-button device.

any pressure or force applied to the foot. Pressure on the foot and/or manual dorsiflexion can artificially reduce the talus posteriorly and hide subtle sagittal plane malreduction. If the talus is subluxated within the mortise and/or sagittal plane, TFO appears incorrect, malreduction is possible, and fixation is revised.

It is helpful to assess these radiographic parameters, in particularly sagittal fibular-tibial relationships prior to syndesmotic realignment. After appropriate reduction, reassessment fluoroscopically should demonstrate improved osseous relationships.

POSTOPERATIVE MANAGEMENT

Patients are kept in a splint for 2 to 3 weeks with strict non–weight bearing. Given the need for revision surgery, often in highly comorbid patients, wounds are checked at 7 to 10 days and sutures are typically removed 2 to 3 weeks after surgery. Patients are casted an additional 2 weeks if a concomitant Achilles lengthening/Strayer procedure has been performed. If not, patients are placed into a removable fracture boot with initiation of gentle passive and active ankle range of motion as guided by a physical therapist. Weight bearing is typically initiated after 6 weeks, and patients are transitioned to full weight bearing by 10 to 12 weeks with subsequent transition into a regular shoe. Low-impact activities are allowed after 3 months, and patients are cleared for higher-impact activities at 6 months.

If syndesmotic arthrodesis is performed, we prefer cast immobilization for 6 weeks at which time range of motion and initial weight bearing is initiated.

RESULTS AND COMPLICATIONS

While we discussed multiple papers examining outcomes after syndesmotic malreduction, the literature is lacking on clinical investigations examining results after syndesmotic revision. However, it is intuitive that the interval between initial surgery and revision likely impacts the damage done to the joint and may be an important prognostic factor. The longer the ankle is stressed with its biomechanics altered by syndesmotic instability or malreduction, the higher the chance for severe degenerative changes and poor results. Therefore, revision surgery is indicated as soon as malreduction is identified. While no current investigation has examined timing of revision surgery, timely revision is recommended to prevent the detrimental effects of altered ankle kinematics.

Complications, whether for primary syndesmotic stabilization or for revision surgery, are similar to other surgical interventions. These include infection, wound dehiscence, delayed/nonunion, and the effects from malalignment.

REFERENCES

1. Shibuya N, Davis ML, Jupiter DC. Epidemiology of foot and ankle fractures in the United States: an analysis of the National Trauma Data Bank (2007 to 2011). *J Foot Ankle Surg.* 2014;53(5):606-608.
2. Jennison T, Brinsden M. Fracture admission trends in England over a ten-year period. *Ann R Coll Surg Engl.* 2019;101(3):208-214.
3. Haynes J, Cherney S, Spraggs-Hughes A, McAndrew CM, Ricci WM, Gardner MJ. Increased reduction clamp force associated with syndesmotic overcompression. *Foot Ankle Int.* 2016;37(7):722-729.
4. Dattani R, Patnaik S, Kantak A, Srikanth B, Selvan TP. Injuries to the tibiofibular syndesmosis. *J Bone Joint Surg Br.* 2008;90(4):405-410.
5. Weening B, Bhandari M. Predictors of functional outcome following transsyndesmotic screw fixation of ankle fractures. *J Orthop Trauma.* 2005;19(2):102-108.
6. Kennedy JG, Soffe KE, Dalla Vedova P, et al. Evaluation of the syndesmotic screw in low Weber C ankle fractures. *J Orthop Trauma.* 2000;14(5):359-366.
7. Sagi HC, Shah AR, Sanders RW. The functional consequence of syndesmotic joint malreduction at a minimum 2-year follow-up. *J Orthop Trauma.* 2012;26(7):439-443.
8. Roberts RS. Surgical treatment of displaced ankle fractures. *Clin Orthop Relat Res.* 1983;172:164-170.
9. Reckling FW, McNamara GR, DeSmet AA. Problems in the diagnosis and treatment of ankle injuries. *J Trauma.* 1981;21(11):943-950.
10. Leeds HC, Ehrlich MG. Instability of the distal tibiofibular syndesmosis after bimalleolar and trimalleolar ankle fractures. *J Bone Joint Surg Am.* 1984;66(4):490-503.
11. Andersen MR, Diep LM, Frihagen F, Castberg Hellund J, Madsen JE, Figved W. Importance of syndesmotic reduction on clinical outcome after syndesmosis injuries. *J Orthop Trauma.* 2019;33(8):397-403.
12. Ray R, Koohnejad N, Clement ND, Keenan GF. Ankle fractures with syndesmotic stabilisation are associated with a high rate of secondary osteoarthritis. *Foot Ankle Surg.* 2019;25(2):180-185.
13. Hak DJ, Egol KA, Gardner MJ, Haskell A. The "not so simple" ankle fracture: avoiding problems and pitfalls to improve patient outcomes. *Instr Course Lect.* 2011;60:73-88.
14. Massri-Pugin J, Lubberts B, Vopat BG, Wolf JC, DiGiovanni CW, Guss D. Role of the deltoid ligament in syndesmotic instability. *Foot Ankle Int.* 2018;39(5):598-603.
15. Ebraheim NA, Elgafy H, Padanilam T. Syndesmotic disruption in low fibular fractures associated with deltoid ligament injury. *Clin Orthop Relat Res.* 2003;409:260-267.
16. Fitzpatrick DC, Otto JK, McKinley TO, Marsh JL, Brown TD. Kinematic and contact stress analysis of posterior malleolus fractures of the ankle. *J Orthop Trauma.* 2004;18(5):271-278.
17. Lloyd J, Elsayed S, Hariharan K, Tanaka H. Revisiting the concept of talar shift in ankle fractures. *Foot Ankle Int.* 2006;27(10):793-796.
18. Ramsey PL, Hamilton W. Changes in tibiotalar area of contact caused by lateral talar shift. *J Bone Joint Surg Am.* 1976;58(3):356-357.
19. Kelly M, Vasconcellos D, Osman WS, et al. Alterations in tibiotalar joint reaction force following syndesmotic injury are restored with static syndesmotic fixation. *Clin Biomech (Bristol, Avon).* 2019;69:156-163.
20. Hunt KJ, Goeb Y, Behn AW, Criswell B, Chou L. Ankle joint contact loads and displacement with progressive syndesmotic injury. *Foot Ankle Int.* 2015;36(9):1095-1103.
21. Stroh DA, DeFontes K, Paez A, Parks B, Guyton GP. Distal fibular malrotation and lateral ankle contact characteristics. *Foot Ankle Surg.* 2019;25(1):90-93.
22. Macko VW, Matthews LS, Zwirkoski P, Goldstein SA. The joint-contact area of the ankle. The contribution of the posterior malleolus. *J Bone Joint Surg Am.* 1991;73(3):347-351.
23. Vrahas M, Fu F, Veenis B. Intraarticular contact stresses with simulated ankle malunions. *J Orthop Trauma.* 1994;8(2):159-166.
24. Kimizuka M, Kurosawa H, Fukubayashi T. Load-bearing pattern of the ankle joint. Contact area and pressure distribution. *Arch Orthop Trauma Surg (1978).* 1980;96(1):45-49.
25. Egol KA, Pahk B, Walsh M, Tejwani NC, Davidovitch RI, Koval KJ. Outcome after unstable ankle fracture: effect of syndesmotic stabilization. *J Orthop Trauma.* 2010;24(1):7-11.
26. Sagi C, Shah A. In response. *J Orthop Trauma.* 2013;27(10):e247-e248.
27. Scolaro JA, Marecek G, Barei DP. Management of syndesmotic disruption in ankle fractures: a critical analysis review. *JBJS Rev.* 2014;2(12):e4.
28. Harper MC, Keller TS. A radiographic evaluation of the tibiofibular syndesmosis. *Foot Ankle.* 1989;10(3):156-160.
29. Marmor M, Hansen E, Han HK, Buckley J, Matityahu A. Limitations of standard fluoroscopy in detecting rotational malreduction of the syndesmosis in an ankle fracture model. *Foot Ankle Int.* 2011;32(6):616-622.
30. Osgood GM, Shakoor D, Orapin J, et al. Reliability of distal tibio-fibular syndesmotic instability measurements using weightbearing and non-weightbearing cone-beam CT. *Foot Ankle Surg.* 2019;25(6):771-781.
31. Ng N, Onggo JR, Nambiar M, et al. Which test is the best? An updated literature review of imaging modalities for acute ankle diastasis injuries. *J Med Radiat Sci.* 2022;69(3):382-393.
32. Hagemeijer NC, Chang SH, Abdelaziz ME, et al. Range of normal and abnormal syndesmotic measurements using weightbearing CT. *Foot Ankle Int.* 2019;40(12):1430-1437.
33. Bhimani R, Ashkani-Esfahani S, Lubberts B, et al. Utility of volumetric measurement via weight-bearing computed tomography scan to diagnose syndesmotic instability. *Foot Ankle Int.* 2020;41(7):859-865.
34. Bejarano-Pineda L, DiGiovanni CW, Waryasz GR, Guss D. Diagnosis and treatment of syndesmotic unstable injuries: where we are now and where we are headed. *J Am Acad Orthop Surg.* 2021;29(23):985-997.
35. Lubberts B, Guss D, Vopat BG, et al. The arthroscopic syndesmotic assessment tool can differentiate between stable and unstable ankle syndesmoses. *Knee Surg Sports Traumatol Arthrosc.* 2020;28(1):193-201.

36. Massri-Pugin J, Lubberts B, Vopat BG, Guss D, Hosseini A, DiGiovanni CW. Effect of sequential sectioning of ligaments on syndesmotic instability in the coronal plane evaluated arthroscopically. *Foot Ankle Int.* 2017;38(12):1387-1393.
37. Hagemeijer NC, Elghazy MA, Waryasz G, Guss D, DiGiovanni CW, Kerkhoffs GMMJ. Arthroscopic coronal plane syndesmotic instability has been over-diagnosed. *Knee Surg Sports Traumatol Arthrosc.* 2021;29(1):310-323.
38. Elghazy MA, Massri-Pugin J, Lubberts B, et al. Arthroscopic characterization of syndesmotic instability in the coronal plane: exactly what measurement matters? *Injury.* 2021;52(7):1964-1970.
39. Bhimani R, Lubberts B, Sornsakrin P, et al. Do coronal or sagittal plane measurements have the highest accuracy to arthroscopically diagnose syndesmotic instability? *Foot Ankle Int.* 2021;42(6):805-809.
40. Stark E, Tornetta P, Creevy WR. Syndesmotic instability in Weber B ankle fractures: a clinical evaluation. *J Orthop Trauma.* 2007;21(9):643-646.
41. Hunt KJ, Phisitkul P, Pirolo J, Amendola A. High ankle sprains and syndesmotic injuries in athletes. *J Am Acad Orthop Surg.* 2015;23(11):661-673.
42. Matuszewski PE, Dombroski D, Lawrence JT, Esterhai JL, Mehta S. Prospective intraoperative syndesmotic evaluation during ankle fracture fixation: stress external rotation versus lateral fibular stress. *J Orthop Trauma.* 2015;29(4):e157-e160.
43. Jiang KN, Schulz BM, Tsui YL, Gardner TR, Greisberg JK. Comparison of radiographic stress tests for syndesmotic instability of supination-external rotation ankle fractures: a cadaveric study. *J Orthop Trauma.* 2014;28(6):e123-e127.
44. Saldua NS, Harris JF, LeClere LE, Girard PJ, Carney JR. Plantar flexion influences radiographic measurements of the ankle mortise. *J Bone Joint Surg Am.* 2010;92(4):911-915.
45. Park SS, Kubiak EN, Egol KA, Kummer F, Koval KJ. Stress radiographs after ankle fracture: the effect of ankle position and deltoid ligament status on medial clear space measurements. *J Orthop Trauma.* 2006;20(1):11-18.
46. Ingall EM, Kaiser P, Ashkani-Esfahani S, Zhao J, Kwon JY. The lateral fibular stress test: high variability of force applied by orthopaedic surgeons in a biomechanical model. *Foot Ankle Orthop.* 2022;7(2):24730114221106484.
47. Harper MC. An anatomic and radiographic investigation of the tibiofibular clear space. *Foot Ankle.* 1993;14(8):455-458.
48. Ostrum RF, De Meo P, Subramanian R. A critical analysis of the anterior-posterior radiographic anatomy of the ankle syndesmosis. *Foot Ankle Int.* 1995;16(3):128-131.
49. DeAngelis JP, Anderson R, DeAngelis NA. Understanding the superior clear space in the adult ankle. *Foot Ankle Int.* 2007;28(4):490-493.
50. Switaj PJ, Mendoza M, Kadakia AR. Acute and chronic injuries to the syndesmosis. *Clin Sports Med.* 2015;34(4):643-677.
51. Shah AS, Kadakia AR, Tan GJ, Karadsheh MS, Wolter TD, Sabb B. Radiographic evaluation of the normal distal tibiofibular syndesmosis. *Foot Ankle Int.* 2012;33(10):870-876.
52. LaMothe J, Baxter JR, Gilbert S, Murphy CI, Karnovsky SC, Drakos MC. Effect of complete syndesmotic disruption and deltoid injuries and different reduction methods on ankle joint contact mechanics. *Foot Ankle Int.* 2017;38(6):694-700.
53. Tornetta P, Yakavonis M, Veltre D, Shah A. Reducing the syndesmosis under direct vision: where should I look? *J Orthop Trauma.* 2019;33(9):450-454.
54. Tornetta P. Invited commentary related to: a novel indirect reduction technique in ankle syndesmotic injuries: a cadaveric study. *J Orthop Trauma.* 2018;32(7):367-368.
55. Boszczyk A, Kordasiewicz B, Kiciński M, Fudalej M, Rammelt S. Operative setup to improve sagittal syndesmotic reduction: technical tip. *J Orthop Trauma.* 2019;33(1):e27-e30.
56. Tornetta P, Spoo JE, Reynolds FA, Lee C. Overtightening of the ankle syndesmosis: is it really possible? *J Bone Joint Surg Am.* 2001;83(4):489-492.
57. Buckely RE, Moran CG, Apivatthakakul T. *AO Principles of Fracture Management.* 3rd ed. AO Publishing; 2017.
58. Boszczyk A, Kwapisz S, Krümmel M, Grass R, Rammelt S. Correlation of incisura anatomy with syndesmotic malreduction. *Foot Ankle Int.* 2018;39(3):369-375.
59. Cosgrove CT, Spraggs-Hughes AG, Putnam SM, et al. A novel indirect reduction technique in ankle syndesmotic injuries: a cadaveric study. *J Orthop Trauma.* 2018;32(7):361-367.
60. Mendelsohn ES, Hoshino CM, Harris TG, Zinar DM. CT characterizing the anatomy of uninjured ankle syndesmosis. *Orthopedics.* 2014;37(2):e157-e160.
61. Putnam SM, Linn MS, Spraggs-Hughes A, McAndrew CM, Ricci WM, Gardner MJ. Simulating clamp placement across the trans-syndesmotic angle of the ankle to minimize malreduction: a radiological study. *Injury.* 2017;48(3):770-775.
62. Kennedy MT, Carmody O, Leong S, Kennedy C, Dolan M. A computed tomography evaluation of two hundred normal ankles, to ascertain what anatomical landmarks to use when compressing or placing an ankle syndesmosis screw. *Foot (Edinb).* 2014;24(4):157-160.
63. Stuart K, Panchbhavi VK. The fate of syndesmotic screws. *Foot Ankle Int.* 2011;32(5):S519-S525.
64. Kukreti S, Faraj A, Miles JN. Does position of syndesmotic screw affect functional and radiological outcome in ankle fractures? *Injury.* 2005;36(9):1121-1124.
65. McBryde A, Chiasson B, Wilhelm A, Donovan F, Ray T, Bacilla P. Syndesmotic screw placement: a biomechanical analysis. *Foot Ankle Int.* 1997;18(5):262-266.
66. Peek AC, Fitzgerald CE, Charalambides C. Syndesmosis screws: how many, what diameter, where and should they be removed? A literature review. *Injury.* 2014;45(8):1262-1267.
67. Cosgrove CT, Putnam SM, Cherney SM, et al. Medial clamp tine positioning affects ankle syndesmosis malreduction. *J Orthop Trauma.* 2017;31(8):440-446.
68. Cherney SM, Haynes JA, Spraggs-Hughes AG, McAndrew CM, Ricci WM, Gardner MJ. In vivo syndesmotic overcompression after fixation of ankle fractures with a syndesmotic injury. *J Orthop Trauma.* 2015;29(9):414-419.
69. Miller AN, Barei DP, Iaquinto JM, Ledoux WR, Beingessner DM. Iatrogenic syndesmosis malreduction via clamp and screw placement. *J Orthop Trauma.* 2013;27(2):100-106.
70. Miller AN, Carroll EA, Parker RJ, Boraiah S, Helfet DL, Lorich DG. Direct visualization for syndesmotic stabilization of ankle fractures. *Foot Ankle Int.* 2009;30(5):419-426.
71. Kaiser PB, Bejarano-Pineda L, Kwon JY, DiGiovanni CW, Guss D. The syndesmosis, part II: surgical treatment strategies. *Orthop Clin North Am.* 2021;52(4):417-432.
72. Pang EQ, Coughlan M, Bonaretti S, et al. Assessment of open syndesmosis reduction techniques in an unbroken fibula model: visualization versus palpation. *J Orthop Trauma.* 2019;33(1):e14-e18.
73. Reb CW, Hyer CF, Collins CL, Fidler CM, Watson BC, Berlet GC. Clinical adaptation of the "tibiofibular line" for intraoperative evaluation of open syndesmosis reduction accuracy: a cadaveric study. *Foot Ankle Int.* 2016;37(11):1243-1248.

74. Koenig SJ, Tornetta P, Merlin G, et al. Can we tell if the syndesmosis is reduced using fluoroscopy? *J Orthop Trauma*. 2015;29(9):e326-e330.
75. Chang SM, Li HF, Hu SJ, Du SC, Zhang LZ, Xiong WF. A reliable method for intraoperative detection of lateral malleolar malrotation using conventional fluoroscopy. *Injury*. 2019;50(11):2108-2112.
76. Futamura K, Baba T, Mogami A, et al. Malreduction of syndesmosis injury associated with malleolar ankle fracture can be avoided using Weber's three indexes in the mortise view. *Injury*. 2017;48(4):954-959.
77. Schreiber JJ, McLawhorn AS, Dy CJ, Goldwyn EM. Intraoperative contralateral view for assessing accurate syndesmosis reduction. *Orthopedics*. 2013;36(5):360-361.
78. Loizou CL, Sudlow A, Collins R, Loveday D, Smith G. Radiological assessment of ankle syndesmotic reduction. *Foot (Edinb)*. 2017;32:39-43.
79. Grenier S, Benoit B, Rouleau DM, Leduc S, Laflamme GY, Liew A. APTF: anteroposterior tibiofibular ratio, a new reliable measure to assess syndesmotic reduction. *J Orthop Trauma*. 2013;27(4):207-211.
80. Summers HD, Sinclair MK, Stover MD. A reliable method for intraoperative evaluation of syndesmotic reduction. *J Orthop Trauma*. 2013;27(4):196-200.
81. Baek JH, Kim TY, Kwon YB, Jeong BO. Radiographic change of the distal tibiofibular joint following removal of transfixing screw fixation. *Foot Ankle Int*. 2018;39(3):318-325.
82. Michelson JD, Wright M, Blankstein M. Syndesmotic ankle fractures. *J Orthop Trauma*. 2018;32(1):10-14.
83. Clanton TO, Whitlow SR, Williams BT, et al. Biomechanical comparison of 3 current ankle syndesmosis repair techniques. *Foot Ankle Int*. 2017;38(2):200-207.
84. Ebramzadeh E, Knutsen AR, Sangiorgio SN, Brambila M, Harris TG. Biomechanical comparison of syndesmotic injury fixation methods using a cadaveric model. *Foot Ankle Int*. 2013;34(12):1710-1717.
85. Riedel MD, Miller CP, Kwon JY. Augmenting suture-button fixation for maisonneuve injuries with fibular shortening: technique tip. *Foot Ankle Int*. 2017;38(10):1146-1151.
86. Shimozono Y, Hurley ET, Myerson CL, Murawski CD, Kennedy JG. Suture button versus syndesmotic screw for syndesmosis injuries: a meta-analysis of randomized controlled trials. *Am J Sports Med*. 2019;47(11):2764-2771.
87. Laflamme M, Belzile EL, Bédard L, van den Bekerom MP, Glazebrook M, Pelet S. A prospective randomized multi-center trial comparing clinical outcomes of patients treated surgically with a static or dynamic implant for acute ankle syndesmosis rupture. *J Orthop Trauma*. 2015;29(5):216-223.
88. Panchbhavi VK, Gurbani BN, Mason CB, Fischer W. Radiographic assessment of fibular length variance: the case for "fibula minus". *J Foot Ankle Surg*. 2018;57(1):91-94.

43 Arthroscopic-Assisted Open Reduction and Internal Fixation Ankle

Arianna L. Gianakos, Stephanie Maestre, Niall Smyth, and Amiethab Aiyer

INTRODUCTION

Ankle fractures are common injuries in the adult population traditionally managed with open reduction and internal fixation (ORIF) when displacement is present. Although clinical outcomes following ankle ORIF have been favorable, previous studies have demonstrated residual symptoms as a result of various intra-articular pathologies including chondral defects or ligamentous injury.[1,2] Studies have found a prevalence of intra-articular lesions in patients sustaining an ankle fracture between 20% and 79%.[3,4] In addition, up to 55% of ankle fractures may have a resultant loose body that cannot be addressed with standard open management.[5]

The use of arthroscopy to assist in the evaluation and management of ankle surgical fixation has gained increased attention (see ▶ Video 43.1). Arthroscopy-assisted ORIF affords the orthopedic surgeon the ability to directly visualize and potentially address intra-articular injuries without formal arthrotomy.[4] In addition, formal lavage and débridement of the ankle joint can also be performed, which may help improve postoperative range of motion (ROM) and expedite return to activity.[6] This chapter will provide an overview for the use of ORIF in the surgical management of ankle fractures. The authors' surgical technique will be described, and this article will provide technical tips and tricks for success.

INDICATIONS AND CONTRAINDICATIONS

ORIF is indicated when direct visualization of the articular surface may be warranted. Visualization of the talus is often limited when performing ORIF for most ankle fractures. ORIF is useful when there is concomitant pathology that can be addressed at the time of surgery. This includes patients with an osteochondral lesion or an osteochondral fracture of the talus that can be microfractured or fixed. In addition, ORIF is useful in patients who have a loose body affording the ability to remove the loose fragments. Lastly, ORIF can improve the evaluation of ligamentous injury, particularly that of the syndesmosis, which can then be addressed and fixed concomitantly. ORIF can afford direct visualization of chondral injury as well assess the integrity of the syndesmosis and deltoid ligament complex. ORIF can also be useful in determining whether there is an impaction injury of the medial malleolus not evident on plain radiographs, particularly with supination adduction injuries or any shear injuries through the medial malleolus from talar inversion and axial loading. Relative contraindications to arthroscopy may include open injury, vascular injury, and a poor soft tissue envelope limiting the ability to establish portal sites as well as increasing the risks related to fluid extravasation and potential compartment syndrome.

PREOPERATIVE PLANNING

Soft Tissue Status

The clinical examination of the patient is crucial for preoperative planning. The integrity of the soft tissues around the ankle, particularly around the portal sites is critical in determining whether arthroscopy can be performed. Potential anterolateral portal injury to the superficial peroneal nerve branches is an important consideration.

Imaging

Standard radiographs of the ankle are required for the initial assessment of the fracture pattern in order to assist in preoperative planning. Isolated posterior malleolar injuries or proximal fibular tenderness should prompt obtaining radiographs of the tibia-fibula to evaluate for a Maisonneuve injury. Computed tomography (CT) of the ankle is warranted if there is suspicion for intra-articular involvement. In addition, CT can also further evaluate for chondral lesions that are often missed with standard radiographs. Black et al reported that operative strategy of treating ankle fractures was changed in 24% of cases after CT review including alterations in medial malleolar or posterior malleolar fixation and fixation of an anterolateral plafond fracture.[7] Some surgeons have considered using magnetic resonance imaging (MRI) as an imaging modality to evaluate cartilage injuries, but hematoma and soft tissue edema can diminish its utility in the traumatic setting.[5]

SURGICAL PLANNING

Identifying the fracture pattern and planning which reduction instruments and hardware may be needed for reduction and fixation are crucial prior to performing the surgical procedure. Considerations should be based on surgeon's preference and fracture pattern. These fractures are fixed with a combination of plates/screws or intramedullary devices. If there is suspicion of an intra-articular fracture, osteochondral lesion, or ligament injury, obtaining the appropriate arthroscopic equipment will be necessary for evaluation and management. In addition, if there is concern for a syndesmotic injury, it is important to have appropriate stabilizing devices available (ie, suture button devices or screws).

SURGICAL TECHNIQUE AND CASE EXAMPLE

A 44-year-old male patient presented to the emergency department after sustaining a fall off of a ladder. Initial radiographic imaging demonstrated a left trimalleolar ankle fracture (Fig. 43.1A and B). Due to increased swelling and skin blistering, the patient was treated with an external fixator (Fig. 43.2A through C). A postoperative CT scan was performed for further assessment of the fracture pattern and for preoperative planning of definitive surgical fixation (Fig. 43.3A and B).

Several days later, the patient returned to the operating room for definitive fixation. He was placed in a supine position on the operating table. A nonsterile tourniquet was placed on the upper thigh and a bump placed under the ipsilateral hip to allow for appropriate internal rotation and access to the fibula. Padding was placed underneath the knee affording the ability to utilize a distraction device

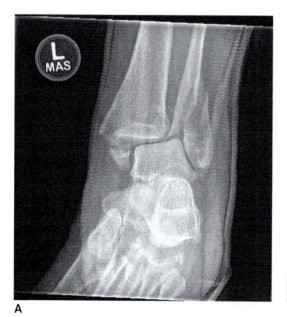
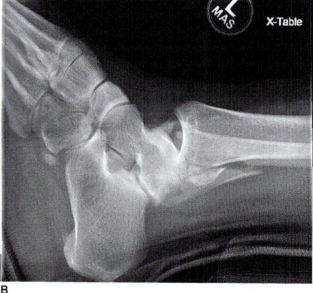

FIGURE 43.1 A, B. Case example of initial radiographic images demonstrating a left trimalleolar ankle fracture.

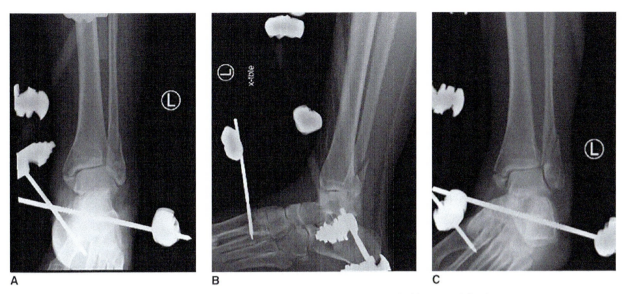

FIGURE 43.2 A-C. Radiographic images demonstrating left ankle fracture treated with external fixation.

for arthroscopy. Surgeon preference dictates whether the patient is then placed in a well-leg holder in order to allow for counter pressure when a noninvasive distractor is used for the ankle (Fig. 43.4). While it is reasonable to use an ankle distractor, the authors find that the ankle joint is readily accessible without distraction in patients with unstable ankle fractures. Regardless of whether distraction is used or not, a pad or blankets are placed under the operative leg to allow for unobstructed lateral fluoroscopic images. The leg is then sterilely prepared and draped followed by exsanguination and inflation of the tourniquet.

The arthroscopic portion of the case commences prior to fixation of the fracture. The anteromedial portal is established, just medial to the anterior tibial tendon at the level of the joint. A 2.7-mm 30° arthroscope is placed through the anteromedial portal. The anterolateral portal may then be established (Fig. 43.5). Care should be taken to avoid the superficial peroneal nerve as this portal is established in the "soft spot" lateral to the peroneus tertius. Proper placement of the portal can be confirmed with direct visualization from the anteromedial portal by first inserting a needle at the intended site. A shaver may then be inserted through the anterolateral working portal. With regard to arthroscopic fluid management, either a low flow and pressure (25 to 35 mm Hg) automated system or gravity flow may be used. This is to minimize fluid extravasation into tissues that may already be compromised.

With portals now established, the fracture hematoma that is frequently encountered may be evacuated. The ankle is then inspected, performing a standard 21-point diagnostic arthroscopy.[8] Any

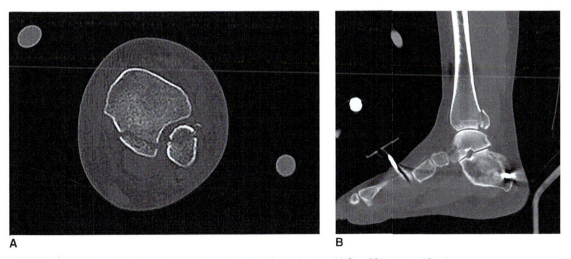

FIGURE 43.3 A, B. Postreduction computed tomography status post left ankle external fixation.

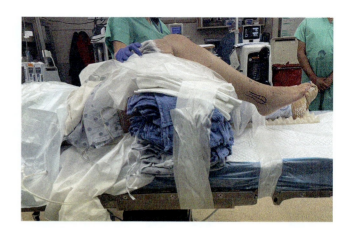

FIGURE 43.4 Patient is positioned in supine position with bump under ipsilateral hip. Towels are utilized to create a bump under the knee for optimal position of the foot and ankle during distraction for arthroscopy.

loose bodies or unstable osteochondral lesions may be addressed through removal and/or débridement (Fig. 43.6). Partial-thickness chondral lesions may be débrided to remove any unstable edges. Full-thickness cartilage lesions can undergo débridement and microfracture (Fig. 43.7). The instruments are then switched in order to evaluate and address the medial aspect of the joint. Any debris or soft tissue that may be causing a medial sided block to reduction may be débrided or excised. The arthroscopic drive-through test may then be performed. This test is considered positive if a 2.9-mm shaver can be advanced posteriorly between the medial malleolus and the talus and indicates instability of the talus.[9] This may be from an isolated syndesmotic injury, a bimalleolar equivalent lateral malleolus fracture with a deltoid injury, or a combination of the two. It has been reported that

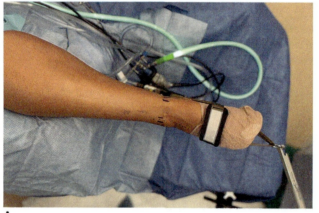

A

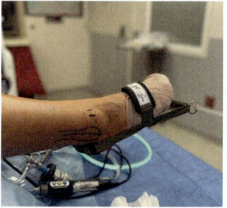

B

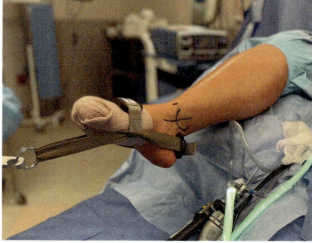

C

FIGURE 43.5 **A.** Anteromedial and anterolateral portals are marked with care to avoid the superficial peroneal nerve. **B, C.** The distal fibula and the medial malleolus are marked.

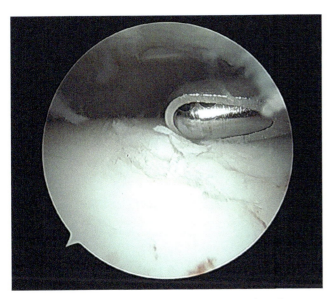

FIGURE 43.6 Arthroscopic evaluation of chondral fissuring.

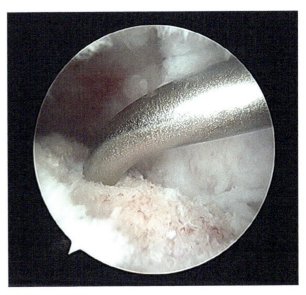

FIGURE 43.7 Microfracture during arthroscopic assisted ankle fracture fixation.

arthroscopic measurement of medial clear space may be more accurate than fluoroscopic examination.[10] The syndesmosis may then be inspected, and subluxation of the fibula relative to the tibia can be assessed (Fig. 43.8).[11,12] The articular surface can be evaluated for further assessment of fracture displacement (Fig. 43.9).

The arthroscopic instruments are then withdrawn, and exposure, reduction, and fixation of the fracture are undertaken as per surgeon preference (Figs. 43.10A through C, 43.11, and 43.12). Following fracture fixation, fluoroscopic stress views are taken to assess the stability of the syndesmosis (Fig. 43.13). This can then be correlated with repeat arthroscopic examination. If the tibiofibular clear space widens with stress testing, then further fixation of the syndesmosis is warranted. This can be performed with either tri- or quadricortical screws or with dynamic fixation using a suture-based construct. Following syndesmotic fixation, the ankle can be arthroscopically assessed to evaluate syndesmotic stability. Figure 43.14 demonstrates final radiographic imaging. Wounds are then closed as per surgeon preference, and the patient is placed in a well-padded splint.

In unique cases involving the posterior malleolus, posterior arthroscopy can be utilized. In these situations, the patient is placed in a prone position with the feet off the edge of the bed. A thigh tourniquet is utilized. The standard anatomic landmarks including the medial/lateral malleolus, Achilles tendon, and sural nerve are marked and identified. Posteromedial and posterolateral portals

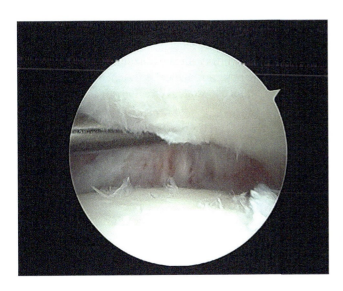

FIGURE 43.8 Evaluation of syndesmosis during arthroscopic-assisted fracture fixation.

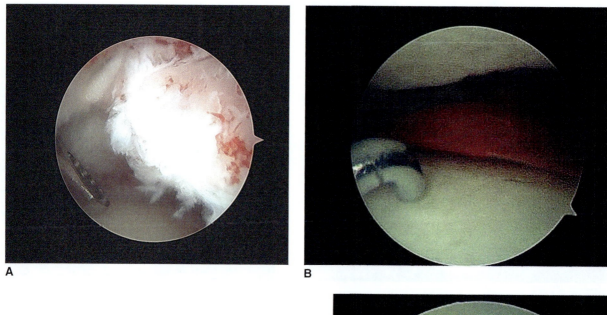

FIGURE 43.9 **A.** Evaluation of intra-articular fracture with arthroscopy during fracture fixation. **B, C.** Another case example of arthroscopic images demonstrating hematoma formation and intra-articular fragment.

are created using the tip of the lateral malleolus to gauge the location tangential to the Achilles tendon. An accessory posterolateral portal approximately 2 to 3 cm proximal to the standard posterolateral portal can also be useful in assisting with arthroscopic reduction.[13] Martin et al conducted a prospective clinical study and demonstrated good to excellent clinical outcomes following posterior arthroscopic reduction and internal fixation for the posterior malleolar fragment in trimalleolar ankle fractures.[14] Therefore, this technique may be an effective strategy in achieving anatomic intra-articular reduction.[14]

PEARLS AND PITFALLS

Tables 43.1 and 43.2 describe technical pearls and common pitfalls, respectively, during ORIF.[15]

POSTOPERATIVE MANAGEMENT

Postoperative care is similar to traditional ankle ORIF performed without utilization of arthroscopy. The postoperative protocol should be adjusted based on surgeon preference, fracture pattern, and the stability of fixation. Patients with talar or tibial cartilage injury that requires additional microfracture

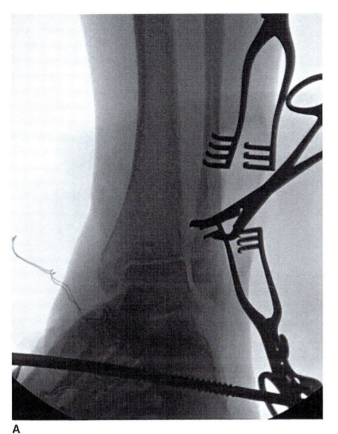
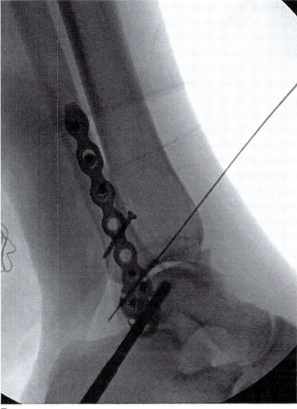
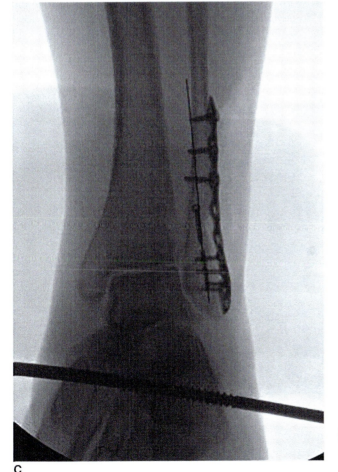

FIGURE 43.10 A-C. Intraoperative fluoroscopic images demonstrating reduction and definitive fixation of the fibula using distal fibula locking plate and interfragmentary screws.

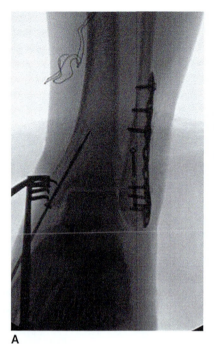 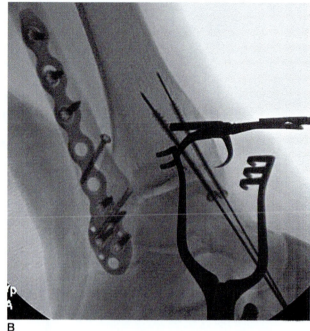

FIGURE 43.11 A, B. Intraoperative images of the reduction and definitive fixation of the medial malleolus using percutaneous cannulated partially threaded screws.

treatment typically start ROM as early as 3 weeks. Patients will be kept non–weight bearing in a well-padded splint for 2 weeks (Fig. 43.15A through C). At 2 weeks, sutures are removed and patients will transition to a fracture boot. At 6 weeks, depending on their fracture status and follow-up plain films, the patient will progress their weight-bearing status with physical therapy to maintain ROM (Fig. 43.16A and B).

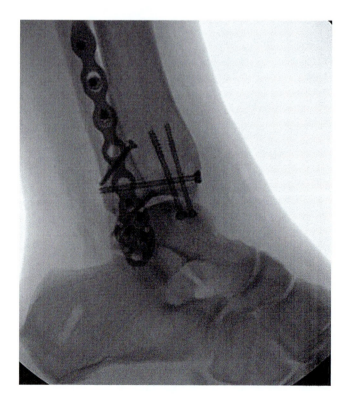

FIGURE 43.12 Intraoperative images of the reduction and definitive fixation of the posterior malleolus with percutaneous anteroposterior cannulated partially threaded screw.

43 Arthroscopic-Assisted Open Reduction and Internal Fixation Ankle

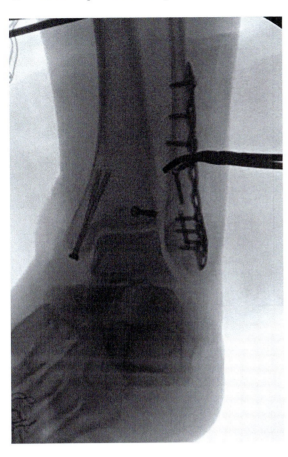

FIGURE 43.13 Intraoperative image with stress view to assess syndesmotic stability demonstrating stable syndesmosis.

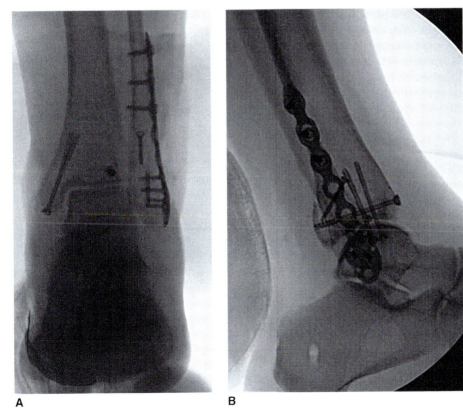

FIGURE 43.14 A, B. Final intraoperative fluoroscopic images.

TABLE 43.1 Technical Pearls

- Position the patient in the supine position. The ipsilateral hip can be elevated using a bump to provide easier access to the lateral fibula. This position will afford the ability to evaluate and manage injuries arthroscopically.
- Place a thigh tourniquet to avoid challenges of fracture reduction from the Achilles complex being contracted from a calf tourniquet. In addition, the tourniquet may allow for better visualization during arthroscopic work.
- Use a low pressure automated system (25-35 mm Hg) or gravity flow to minimize fluid extravasation into potentially compromised soft tissues.
- Arthroscopically evaluate and address cartilage injuries and loose bodies that may prevent adequate reduction.
- When addressing the syndesmosis, the surgeon should evaluate with the drive-through sign. If the shaver passes easily, the drive-through sign is positive, and further fixation of the syndesmosis is indicated. After syndesmotic fixation, perform the drive-through test again. If the drive-through sign is again positive, the test should raise suspicion that the syndesmosis or fixation is inadequate.
- Do not forget to directly visualize the deltoid ligament complex arthroscopically to rule out a deltoid injury.
- Monitor total arthroscopic time to minimize fluid extravasation in the surrounding soft tissues to prevent wound complications.

RESULTS AND COMPLICATIONS

Open reduction and internal fixation (ORIF) affords orthopedic surgeons the ability to directly visualize and treat intra-articular injury during the time of ankle fracture fixation. It allows for assessment of intra-articular reduction, and the ability to address concomitant injuries often missed on plain radiographs. Chen et al conducted a systematic review of adult patients undergoing ORIF for ankle fractures and reported that the most common concomitant injuries included chondral lesions (63.3%), deltoid ligament injuries (60.9%), and syndesmotic injuries (77.9%).[16] Hintermann et al conducted a prospective study in 288 patients and reported a 79% rate of articular injury with associated ankle fractures.[3] In addition, previous studies have also demonstrated an increase in the diagnostic effectiveness when utilizing arthroscopy in the evaluation of associated syndesmotic injuries particularly when compared with standard radiographs.[12,15] Loren and Ferkel reported a rate of 45.8% of syndesmotic disruption when evaluating ankle fractures arthroscopically.[17]

Several studies have attempted to compare traditional ORIF with ORIF. Thordarson et al conducted a prospectively randomized trial evaluating ankle fractures treated with and without arthroscopy. The authors concluded that there was no difference in SF-36 scores or lower extremity scores between the two groups and that in the short term, the addition of arthroscopy did not appear to negatively impact patient outcomes.[2] A systematic review by Gonzalez et al identified ankle arthroscopy as a tool in treating intra-articular lesions associated with ankle fractures but demonstrated that the literature has not shown that treatment of these intra-articular injuries provides any improvement in outcomes over standard ORIF.[18] In addition, there had been few prospective randomized controlled studies comparing these two operative techniques demonstrating that ORIF improves clinical outcomes over traditional ORIF, and therefore, further research is needed to determine the benefits clinically.

TABLE 43.2 Common Pitfalls

- Soft tissue swelling and fracture displacement can make identification of landmarks and arthroscopic portal location difficult.
- Be cautious of anatomy when establishing arthroscopic portals. Commonly injured structures include the following:
  - Anteromedial portal: tibialis anterior and saphenous nerve/vein
  - Anterolateral portal: intermediate dorsal cutaneous branch of the superficial peroneal nerve
- Perform the drive-through sign with minimal force to avoid cartilage injury to the medial malleolus and the medial talar dome.
- Limit débridement of anterior synovial tissue to limit bleeding that may obstruct visualization.
- If using a well-leg holder and noninvasive distraction, ensure that when the extremity is resting on the operative table, it is adequately positioned for the reduction and fixation portion of the case.

43 Arthroscopic-Assisted Open Reduction and Internal Fixation Ankle 687

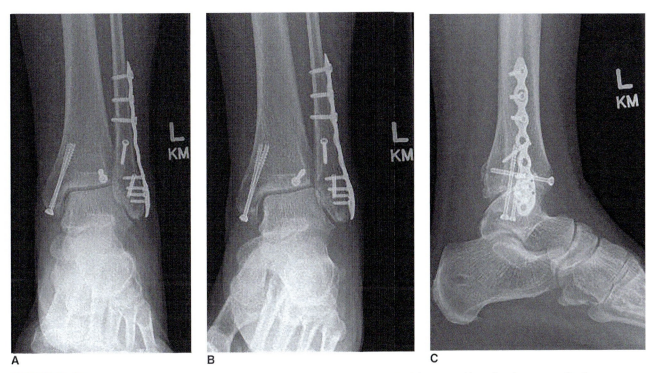

FIGURE 43.15 A-C. Postoperative radiographic imaging demonstrating well-aligned fracture with no hardware complications approximately 2 weeks postoperative from surgery. Patient was following standard postoperative protocol of 2 weeks non–weight bearing in a splint then transitioned into a fracture boot.

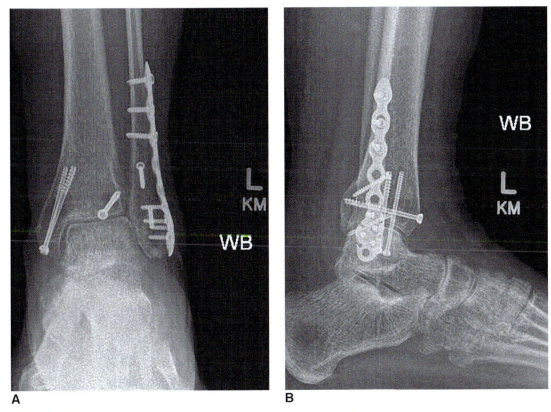

FIGURE 43.16 A, B. Radiographic imaging 3 months postoperatively following trimalleolar ankle fracture open reduction and internal fixation with well-healed fracture with hardware in place after weight bearing for 2 months.

Complications typically associated with ankle ORIF include wound dehiscence, superficial infection, deep vein thrombosis, pulmonary embolism, failed ORIF requiring reoperation, and rarely compartment syndrome.[19] A large database analysis of patients undergoing ankle fracture fixation with and without arthroscopic assistance revealed that there is no increase in complication rate or reoperation rate with the use of arthroscopy.[17] Therefore, utilizing arthroscopy during the surgical management of ankle fractures may not add any additional risk to patient outcomes.

Use of Needle Arthroscopy

Recent advances in technology of arthroscopy have afforded surgeons with the opportunity to manage patients with more minimally invasive approaches. Needle arthroscopy has gained increased attention utilizing a small 1.9-mm arthroscope that is semirigid. Previous studies have shown that there is an overall rate of articular cartilage injury of 31% when utilizing the standard arthroscope in the ankle joint; therefore, the smaller instrumentation can help reduce this risk.[19-21] In addition, there is less equipment as arthroscopic towers are not required in the operating room. Future research is warranted to better understand the benefits of using needle arthroscopy in the treatment of ankle fractures, but this new technology may offer an alternative strategy in the evaluation and management of intra-articular pathology associated with ankle fractures.

CONCLUSION

The use of arthroscopy to assist in the evaluation and management of ankle surgical fixation affords the orthopedic surgeon the ability to directly visualize and potentially address intra-articular injuries without formal arthrotomy. This chapter provided an overview for the use of ORIF in the surgical management of ankle fracture and presented surgical tips and tricks for success.

REFERENCES

1. Leontaritis N, Hinojosa L, Panchbhavi VK. Arthroscopically detected intra-articular lesions associated with acute ankle fractures. *J Bone Joint Surg Am.* 2009;91(2):333-339.
2. Thordarson DB, Bains R, Shepherd LE. The role of ankle arthroscopy on the surgical management of ankle fractures. *Foot Ankle Int.* 2001;22(2):123-125.
3. Hintermann B, Regazzoni P, Lampert C, et al. Arthroscopic findings in acute fractures of the ankle. *J Bone Joint Surg Br.* 2000;82(3):345-351.
4. Ono A, Nishikawa S, Nagao A, et al. Arthroscopically assisted treatment of ankle fractures: arthroscopic findings and surgical outcomes. *Arthroscopy.* 2004;20(6):627-631.
5. Braunstein M, Baumbach SF, Regauer M, et al. The value of arthroscopy in the treatment of complex ankle fractures—a protocol of a randomised controlled trial. *BMC Musculoskelet Disord.* 2016;17:210.
6. Kong C, Kolla L, Wing K, et al. Arthroscopy-assisted closed reduction and percutaneous nail fixation of unstable ankle fractures: description of a minimally invasive procedure. *Arthrosc Tech.* 2014;3(1):e181-e184.
7. Black EM, Antoci V, Lee JT, et al. Role of preoperative computed tomography scans in operative planning for malleolar ankle fractures. *Foot Ankle Int.* 2013;34(5):697-704.
8. Ferkel RD. *Foot and Ankle Arthroscopy.* Wolters Kluwer; 2017.
9. Schairer WW, Nwachukwu BU, Dare DM, et al. Arthroscopically assisted open reduction-internal fixation of ankle fractures: significance of the arthroscopic ankle drive-through sign. *Arthrosc Tech.* 2016;5(2):e407-e412.
10. Chiang CC, Lin CFJ, Tzeng YH, et al. Arthroscopic quantitative measurement of medial clear space for deltoid injury of the ankle: a cadaveric comparative study with stress radiography. *Am J Sports Med.* 2022;50(3):778-787.
11. Guyton GP, DeFontes K III, Barr CR, et al. Arthroscopic correlates of subtle syndesmotic injury. *Foot Ankle Int.* 2017;38(5):502-506.
12. Watson BC, Lucas DE, Simpson GA, et al. Arthroscopic evaluation of syndesmotic instability in a cadaveric model. *Foot Ankle Int.* 2015;36(11):1362-1368.
13. Martin KD, Unangst AM, Englert CR. Posterior ankle arthroscopic reduction with internal fixation. *Arthrosc Tech.* 2016;5(6):e1261-e1265.
14. Martin KD, Tripp CT, Huh J. Outcomes of posterior arthroscopic reduction and internal fixation (PARIF) for the posterior malleolar fragment in trimalleolar ankle fractures. *Foot Ankle Int.* 2021;42(2):157-165.
15. Sherman TI, Casscells N, Rabe J, et al. Ankle arthroscopy for ankle fractures. *Arthrosc Tech.* 2015;4(1):e75-e79.
16. Chen XZ, Chen Y, Liu CG, et al. Arthroscopy-assisted surgery for acute ankle fractures: a systematic review. *Arthroscopy.* 2015;31(11):2224-2231.
17. Loren GJ, Ferkel RD. Arthroscopic assessment of occult intra-articular injury in acute ankle fractures. *Arthroscopy.* 2002;18(4):412-421.
18. Gonzalez TA, Macaulay AA, Ehrlichman LK, Drummond R, Mittal V, DiGiovanni CW. Arthroscopically assisted versus standard open reduction and internal fixation techniques for the acute ankle fracture. *Foot Ankle Int.* 2016;37(5):554-562.
19. Yasui Y, Shimozono Y, Hung CW, et al. Postoperative reoperations and complications in 32,307 ankle fractures with and without concurrent ankle arthroscopic procedures in a 5-year period based on a large U.S. healthcare database. *J Foot Ankle Surg.* 2019;58(1):6-9.
20. Vega J, Golanó P, Peña F. Iatrogenic articular cartilage injuries during ankle arthroscopy. *Knee Surg Sports Traumatol Arthrosc.* 2016;24(4):1304-1310.
21. Takao M, Uchio Y, Naito K, et al. Diagnosis and treatment of combined intra-articular disorders in acute distal fibular fractures. *J Trauma.* 2004;57(6):1303-1307.

44 Minimally Invasive Open Reduction and Internal Fixation Calcaneus

Alexander B. Peterson, Max P. Michalski, and David B. Thordarson

INDICATIONS AND CONTRAINDICATIONS

Indications

The indication for minimally invasive open reduction and internal fixation (ORIF) of a calcaneus fracture is articular displacement, often defined as a step-off greater than 2 mm, as well as clinically significant displacement of the tuberosity or anterior process.

These indications are not without controversy. Much debate has been had regarding the proper management of intra-articular calcaneus fractures. Conservative management of a displaced intra-articular fracture results in malunion of the calcaneus. The classic malunion is characterized by loss of calcaneal height, varus hindfoot deformity, lateral wall displacement with gross widening of the heel, superior displacement of the tuberosity, and displaced articular fragments of the calcaneocuboid (CC) and subtalar joints.[1,2] Decreased calcaneal height leads to a loss of talar declination with associated anterior ankle impingement and decreased dorsiflexion. Additionally, the Achilles tendon is effectively shortened, resulting in diminished plantarflexion power. Varus malalignment of the tuberosity produces altered gait mechanics via secondary stiffness of the transverse tarsal joint. Lateral wall displacement can lead to peroneal tendon subluxation, irritation of the sural nerve, and painful subfibular impingement.[3] Articular incongruity potentiates development of posttraumatic arthritis, as well as impingement at the CC articulation. Furthermore, the morphologic changes can produce difficulty with shoe wear after healing.[4] It is clear why anatomic reduction of the calcaneal fracture would be beneficial.

However, during the 20th century, high complication rates and generally poor outcomes created a negative view of acute open treatment.[5] As recently as 2007, a 15-year follow-up study, using the technique of Soeur and Remy, declared that ORIF possessed no advantage over closed treatment, with regard to patient function, calcaneal height, and posttraumatic arthritis.[6] As equipment and surgical techniques improved, so did the reported outcomes of open treatment. Multiple studies since the mid-1990s have suggested that superior outcomes may be achieved with ORIF, when directly compared to nonoperative treatment. Surgical management restores Böhler angle and calcaneal height, allowing for improved ankle dorsiflexion motion and plantarflexion strength.[7-10] Furthermore, current outcomes have shown decreased heel width in operative cohorts, with fewer shoe wear issues.[8,9] Radiographic follow-up of open and closed treatment indicates lower rates of subtalar arthrosis following ORIF, requiring fewer subsequent fusions.[11] Csizy et al showed an odds ratio of 5.86 for subtalar fusion after nonoperative treatment, when compared to ORIF.[12] Most importantly, multiple studies demonstrated comparatively better function and postoperative pain scores with operative management.[7,10,13,14] Of note, certain subgroups obtain greater improvement with ORIF, including patients aged 20 to 29 years, females, young males, those with comminuted fractures, low initial Böhler angle (0° to 14°), near-anatomic postoperative reductions, Essex-Lopresti severe joint-depression fractures, Sanders type II fractures, patients with less physically demanding jobs, and those without worker's compensation claims.[7]

Subtalar arthritis and the need for late arthrodesis are frequent complications of both ORIF and closed treatment. In addition to ORIF having a lower conversion rate to arthrodesis, the long-term follow-up of patients requiring fusion for posttraumatic arthritis after ORIF shows superior functional outcomes and decreased wound complications, when compared to fusion after nonoperative management.[11,15]

The specific indication for minimally invasive incisions, over the traditional extensile lateral approach (ELA), is debated. Minimally invasive incisions encompass both percutaneous techniques as well as the limited sinus tarsi approach. For the purposes of this text, the discussion of minimally invasive incisions will primarily refer to the limited sinus tarsi approach. The primary advantage of minimally invasive surgery (MIS) for calcaneal fixation is a decreased rate of wound complications, which has been demonstrated by recent studies directly comparing MIS and ELA techniques. Kline et al compared the outcomes of 79 ELA and 33 minimally invasive cases. They reported 29% wound complication rate within the ELA cohort (9% requiring operative débridement), contrasted by 6% in the minimally invasive group (0% requiring operative débridement).[16] Kwon et al, in a retrospective review of 405 cases, similarly reported a 32.1% wound complication rate with ELA technique, and 8.3% with a minimally invasive sinus tarsi approach.[17] Weber et al, in a smaller series, showed a 7.7% wound complication rate with ELA, and zero wound complications with MIS.[18] Not only has the MIS approach demonstrated superior outcomes with regard to wound complications, but it has also produced similar outcomes as ELA with regard to patient-reported outcomes and quality of reduction.[16,18] Fortunately, follow-up outcomes of patients who experienced early soft tissue complications after ORIF with ELA did not differ from patients who avoided such complications.[19]

Contraindications

Though not absolute, one of the strongest contraindications to calcaneal ORIF is a Sanders type I, or nondisplaced, fracture. In the absence of articular incongruity, or notable malalignment of the tuber, the risk of surgical complications generally outweigh the benefits.[4,20] Additional relative contraindications are primarily related to the avoidance of devastating wound complications or the consideration of extenuating circumstances, such as severe polytrauma precluding operative intervention. Ding et al, in one of the largest reviews of its kind, provided data on relative rates of wound complications following calcaneal ORIF. Diabetes (OR = 6.23), surgical duration greater than 3 hours (OR = 6.63), tobacco use (OR = 5.79), and Sanders type IV fractures (OR = 5.6) were some of the greatest risk factors.[21] Additional frequently referenced contraindications include severe swelling, unresolved fracture blisters, grossly contaminated open injury, advanced peripheral vascular disease, delayed presentation, and drug abuse.[4,20]

PREOPERATIVE PLANNING

Initial Management

The initial evaluation of patients with calcaneal fractures, whether in the emergency department or clinic setting, should be comprehensive. Common mechanisms of calcaneal injury are motor vehicle accidents and fall from height. As such, concomitant injuries are commonly present, notably of the foot, ankle, knee, and spinal column. A high index of suspicion for visceral injury and head injury should be maintained.[22] Typically, intra-articular fractures characterized by the Essex-Lopresti classification as joint-depression injuries can be immobilized in a well-padded splint in a neutral ankle position until soft tissues allow for formal incisions. Severe tongue-type fractures, on the other hand, may put the posterior skin envelope at risk via pressure-induced necrosis. These injuries should be addressed urgently, with transient immobilization in plantarflexion in a well-padded anterior slab bulky splint, while offloading the heel. Per standard protocol, open fractures are addressed with early antibiotic prophylaxis and urgent débridement.

Imaging Review

All patients with calcaneal fractures undergo evaluation with radiographs and computed tomography (CT). Radiographs include three standard views of the foot, a Harris axial heel view, as well as routine ankle views. Given the high rate of concomitant injury, all sites demonstrating clinical

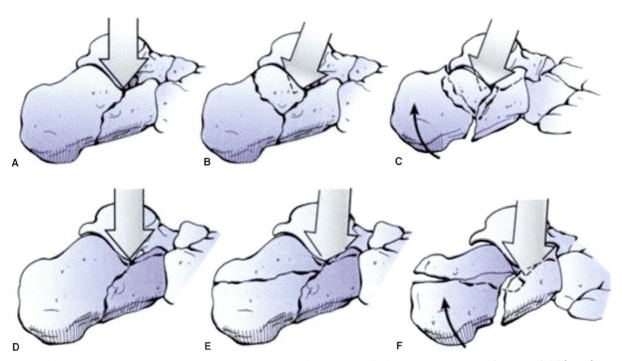

FIGURE 44.1 The Essex-Lopresti classification identifies two distinct types of intra-articular calcaneal fractures. Axial force from a downward driven talus creates a primary fracture line. The secondary fracture line of joint-depression injuries exits just posterior to the posterior facet **(A-C)**. The secondary fracture line of tongue-type injuries exits posteriorly through the tuberosity **(D-F)**.

concern, such as the knee and axial spine, should undergo imaging during the initial trauma workup. A CT scan of the ankle, with coronal cuts in the plane of the subtalar joint, is invaluable for evaluating the fracture pattern. In the absence of CT, radiographic Broden views of the subtalar joint can provide useful information about articular displacement. Thorough preoperative review of all imaging is essential to understanding the optimal route to successful operative management.

Initial review of radiographs should focus on ruling out concomitant injuries of the foot and ankle. The calcaneus fracture itself is then thoroughly analyzed. Lateral radiographs reveal the secondary fracture line, which exits posterior to the posterior facet in Essex-Lopresti joint-depression–type fractures, and through the posterior tuberosity in tongue-type fractures (Fig. 44.1). Articular depression can be assessed by measuring Böhler angle (normal is 20° to 40°) and the angle of Gissane (Fig. 44.2). The presence of a double density at the posterior facet is indicative of a sagittal split in the articular surface with depression, generally of the lateral articular fragment (Fig. 44.3).[4] Superior displacement of the tuberosity is assessed with the talo-tuber angle and distance.[2] The axial heel radiograph, or Harris projection, shows varus and shortening of the tuber and can provide

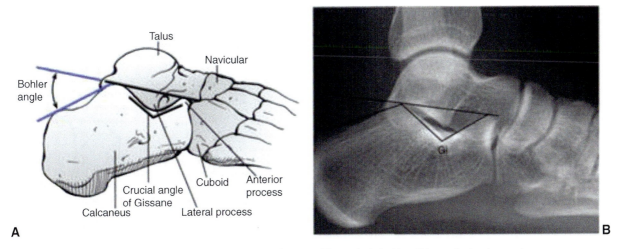

FIGURE 44.2 Böhler angle **(A)** and the critical angle of Gissane **(B)** can help in identifying articular depression.

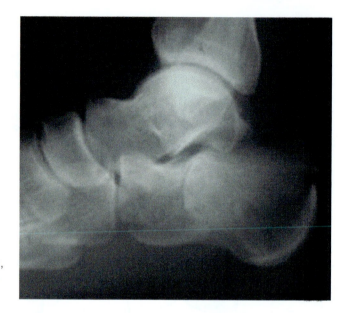

FIGURE 44.3 The double density sign, indicative of a split, partially depressed posterior facet subchondral surface.

information about the integrity of the sustentaculum tali.[23] Medial and lateral wall comminution may also be appreciated. Anteroposterior (AP) and oblique foot radiographs show displacement of the anterior process and involvement of the CC joint.

Careful evaluation of the CT images is crucial for detailed preoperative planning and provides another opportunity to rule out concomitant injury in the foot and ankle. Sagittal images are reviewed for articular fragment displacement, as well as overall shortening of the tuber. Coronal images at the posterior facet are utilized for defining the Sanders classification and understanding the needed articular reduction sequence (Fig. 44.4). Furthermore, subfibular impingement from lateral wall blowout can be defined, as can increased width of the heel. The surgeon should be cognizant of these laterally displaced fragments during application of a plate, making sure to avoid an intraosseous

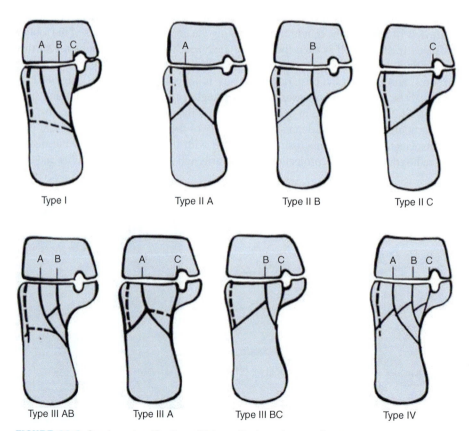

FIGURE 44.4 Sanders classification of intra-articular calcaneus fractures.

location. Sustentaculum fractures, which have been reported to be present in 44% of intra-articular calcaneal fractures, can be seen most clearly on coronal slices. In over 20% of fractures, the medial facet experiences subluxation or dislocation through displacement of the sustentaculum tali.[24] Axial images illustrate the varus deformity. They also show fracture patterns in the anterior process and involvement of the CC joint. Additionally, medial and lateral wall comminution can be visualized. Occasionally, medial fragments need to be addressed intraoperatively.[23] Peroneal dislocation is an often overlooked but relatively frequent element of calcaneal fractures. Imaging studies have reported the incidence of peroneal displacement to be approximately 30%, with intraoperative evaluation showing an incidence of 11.6%.[3,25] A fleck sign, or an avulsion fragment off the fibula, can be seen on the AP radiograph, while the frank peroneal displacement is visualized on axial CT cuts with soft tissue windows.

Timing of Surgery

The status of the soft tissues is almost always the key factor when deciding the timing of definitive fixation. Calcaneal fractures are often secondary to high-energy trauma, such as motor vehicle accidents and falls from height. These mechanisms, in conjunction with the tenuous soft tissue envelope of the hindfoot, make intra-articular calcaneal fractures prone to severe swelling and fracture blisters.[4,26,27] Swelling is traditionally assessed by the "wrinkle test." As soon as the typical skin wrinkle pattern can be visualized with dorsiflexion and eversion, and there is no pitting edema, a formal incision may be performed.[4] Operating before swelling abates is feared to result in difficult closure and subsequent wound complications. Fracture blisters develop within 24 to 48 hours and are secondary to cleavage at the dermal-epidermal junction. They can be filled with clear fluid or blood, with blood indicative of deeper injury.[26] They may be left intact or unroofed. Prior studies have described treating unroofed blisters with daily Silvadene wound care. Blister beds should be re-epithelized prior to surgery, with an average delay of 12 days. Incisions through the blister beds are associated with soft tissue complications and infection, particularly in diabetic patients.[27]

Kwon et al reported on the effect of surgical timing and wound complications with both ELA and minimally invasive sinus tarsi incisions.[17] When utilizing the ELA technique, there was a 32.1% wound complication rate, which was unaffected by the timing of surgery. The MIS technique was associated with increased wound complications when performed more than 2 weeks from injury, with a rate of 15.2%, whereas ORIF prior to 1 week resulted in a 2.1% rate of complication. Additional studies have shown similar trends.[28,29] This suggests that, when possible, minimally invasive ORIF should be performed as early as possible.

If soft tissues or severe concomitant injury will not allow for early fixation, an alternative approach involves the placement of a temporary medial external fixator. Shortly after injury, the fixator can be applied, with pins in the tuberosity, medial distal tibia, and medial midfoot. Early provision reduction of the tuberosity is obtained, with restoration of calcaneal height and length, and correction of varus. Kim et al have published good results with this technique. When compared to standard delayed fixation, they reported shorter time to definitive fixation, equivalent restoration of Böhler angle, and superior articular reduction.[30]

SURGICAL TECHNIQUE

- Regional anesthesia is performed, including single-shot popliteal and saphenous nerve blocks. MAC anesthesia is administered. General anesthesia, with or without peripheral nerve blocks, is a valid alternative and may be preferred, dependent on positioning and other patient factors.
- A standard thigh tourniquet is applied. Alternatively, a sterile calf tourniquet can be utilized. It is placed on the proximal leg, avoiding compression of the common peroneal nerve at the fibular neck. This is the routine practice of one of the authors. When peripheral nerve blocks are utilized, the leg tourniquet avoids the discomfort associated with thigh tourniquets, limiting the requirements for anesthesia. The surgeon must keep in mind that a calf tourniquet indirectly tensions the tendons crossing the ankle, which can affect forces related to fracture displacement and reduction.
- The patient is placed in the lateral decubitus position, with the help of gel rolls or bean bag positioner. An axillary roll is placed.
- Supine positioning is also acceptable when performing a limited sinus tarsi approach and may be preferred in the event of concomitant injuries, such as unstable spine fractures, pulmonary injury, or traumatic brain injury.

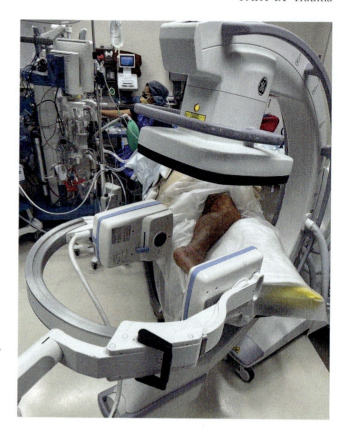

FIGURE 44.5 Dual fluoroscopy set up. The standard C-arm allows for lateral images, while the mini fluoroscopy unit provides axial heel views. Originally described by Kwon et al.

- In the event of bilateral calcaneal fractures, it is acceptable to address both sides while in the supine or prone position. Alternatively, each side may be sequentially addressed via lateral decubitus positioning.
- The mini fluoroscopy unit is routinely used, as it is the preference of the senior author who feels it is less cumbersome while allowing equal quality imaging compared to standard C-arm fluoroscopy.
- Alternatively, when in the lateral decubitus position, a dual fluoroscopic set up has been proposed for optimized workflow. Abousayed et al described the use of a large C-arm for lateral images, and a mini C-arm for axial heel images (Fig. 44.5).[31]
- Incisions are marked out. The limited sinus tarsi approach is marked from the tip of the fibula, heading toward the 4th metatarsal base. It is 3 to 4 cm in length. Fluoroscopy is helpful in the setting of moderate to severe swelling. Localize and mark the sinus tarsi as well as the CC joint (Fig. 44.6).

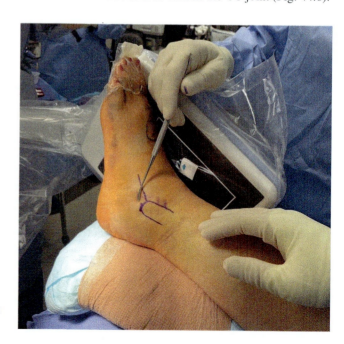

FIGURE 44.6 Fluoroscopy is helpful for accurate incision placement, as swelling and fracture displacement can distort the surface anatomy.

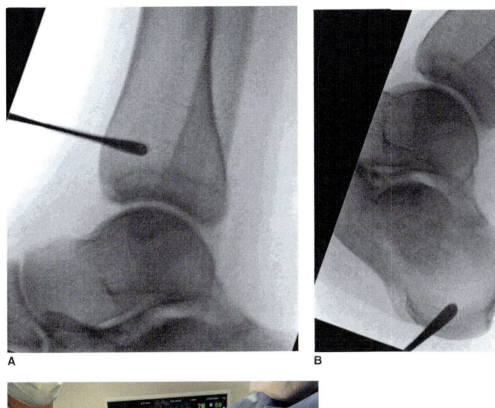

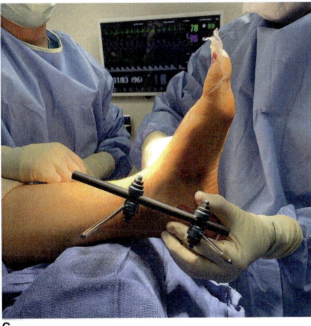

FIGURE 44.7 A and B: Fluoroscopy is used to ensure appropriate pin placement. **C:** Clinical appearance of the medial distractor with radiolucent bar in place.

- Prior to formal incision, a medially based two-pin external fixator can be placed to gain initial reduction of the tuberosity and to indirectly disimpact the posterior facet fracture. 5.0-mm self-drilling, self-tapping Schanz pins are driven into the medial aspect of distal tibia and the safe zone of the calcaneal tuberosity (Fig. 44.7).[32] Fluoroscopy is used to confirm pin placement and guide the reduction. It is necessary to check both the lateral and axial views. The calcaneal pin is firmly grasped and manipulated to effect reduction on the calcaneal tuberosity. The aim is to restore calcaneal height, length, and width and to correct the varus deformity via traction, valgus, and lateral translation forces. Pin-to-bar connecters are locked to secure the reduction (Fig. 44.8). Alternatively, a single laterally based calcaneal Schanz pin can be used to apply the reduction force, followed by temporary fixation with multiple large diameter wires, but it requires a skilled assistant for this method (Fig. 44.9).
- If the tuberosity is not adequately reducing, the aforementioned distraction technique can be performed after sufficiently mobilizing the fracture fragments through the sinus tarsi approach.

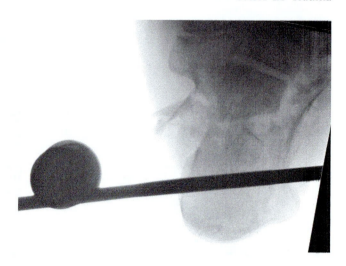

FIGURE 44.8 The medial external fixator is used to obtain and hold the reduction of the tuberosity.

- The approach is performed through the previously planned skin marks. After incising the skin, sharp versus scissor dissection is performed to lift the fat overlying the sinus tarsi and split the underlying extensor digitorum brevis muscle, taking care to protect the sural nerve as well as the peroneal tendons. Interosseous ligaments are sectioned as needed. The sinus tarsi is accessed, and the posterior facet is visualized. The calcaneofibular ligament (CFL) may be sectioned for improved access. It has been shown that disrupting the CFL without repair does not lead to late instability.[33] A rongeur can be useful to débride overlying traumatized adipose and connective tissue that may block visualization of the joint. It is often helpful to gain visualization of the anterior process and CC joint.
- The peroneal tendons are inspected for injury and dislocation. In the event of peroneal displacement, the tendons may be encountered directly under the incision (see ▶ Video 44-1). These can be addressed after ORIF.[34]
- The soft tissues are elevated from the lateral wall fragments. Properly developing this interval will help to avoid intraosseous plate placement. Perform prior to hardware placement as this can put significant stress on your reduction.
- Major fracture lines are further mobilized, as necessary. A Cobb or Freer elevator are useful tools. If necessary, this step can be performed prior to reducing the tuberosity.
- Provided the medial external fixator has sufficiently decompressed the articular surface, the posterior facet fracture is now addressed. Using the talus as a template, the articular fragments are sequentially reduced, starting with the most medial fragment. In cases of severe impaction, a lamina spreader can provide the distraction force needed to elevate the fragment up to the talar

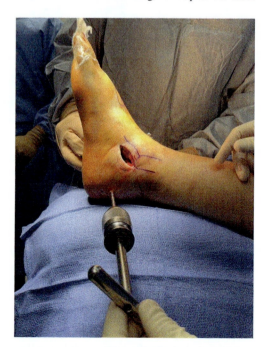

FIGURE 44.9 A single laterally based 5.0-mm Schanz pin can be used as an alternative to the medial distractor. Once reduction is obtained, 2.0-mm K-wires are used to temporarily maintain the reduction by inserting them from posterior and up the medial aspect of the calcaneus taking care not to enter the area of the depressed lateral fragment.

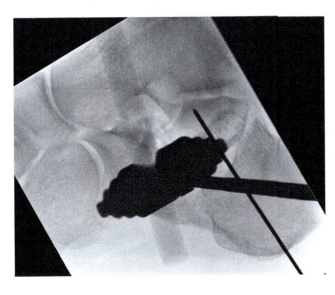

FIGURE 44.10 A retrograde K-wire is used to temporarily hold the reduction on a previously depressed lateral articular fragment from the posterior facet.

articular surface. Once reduced, fragments are temporarily pinned in position with 0.062 K-wires. Medial fragments may be pinned with oblique wires, or retrograde wires from the tuberosity up to, or through, the subtalar joint (Fig. 44.10). Once the most lateral articular fragment has been reduced, additional K-wires may be placed from lateral to medial into the sustentaculum tali.
- Bone voids that remain after elevation of the depressed fragments can be filled through impaction of finely ground cancellous bone chips.
- Major fractures of the anterior process are addressed as needed. Reduction can be held with K-wires, with fixation obtained by the anterior screws of the sinus tarsi plate, and/or independent lag and positional screws. Antegrade fully threaded screws placed from the posterior tuberosity into the anterior process can provide further rigidity.
- Once all provisional reductions have been performed, a calcaneus-specific, locking plate can be inserted into the wound along the lateral wall. Adjust its position such that at least two screws can be placed in the anterior process, the subchondral bone of the posterior facet, and the posterior tuberosity. Pin the plate in position with olive wires. Fluoroscopy is used to confirm plate placement (Fig. 44.11). Assess the axial view to ensure that the plate is superficial to the lateral cortex and not intraosseous (Fig. 44.12). Screws are then placed into the plate. Medially directed pressure is applied to the plate to assist in compressing free elements of the lateral wall and to fully seat the plate down to bone. An initial nonlocking screw can assist with drawing the plate to the lateral wall. Locking screws are placed into select holes on the plate to achieve the desired fixation. Ideally, posterior facet screws gain purchase in the sustentaculum tali medially. Fully threaded screws may be used in a lag-by-technique fashion at the posterior facet if additional compression is desired. These may be placed outside of the plate, if the fracture requires it. The screws of the posterior tuberosity generally require a separate incision. Incision placement is guided by fluoroscopy or plate-specific guides, if available. Ensure that the screws of the anterior process avoid the CC joint. Avoid long screws below the posterior facet, as these can damage medial tendons, most notably the flexor hallucis longus as it runs plantar to the sustentaculum tali.
- Lateral and axial views are intermittently assessed to confirm maintained fracture reduction, appropriate placement of the plate, and that there are no intra-articular screws. Broden views are helpful for assessing articular step-offs or intra-articular hardware.[35]
- When fixation is complete, the medial fixator is removed.
- Subtalar motion is assessed for bony blocks to motion (see ▶ Video 44-2).
- Additional soft tissue injuries are addressed, including peroneal tendon or retinacular tears.[34]
- Assess hallux motion to ensure no injury to the FHL tendon.
- Wounds are copiously irrigated and hemostasis obtained.
- Closed in layered fashion. 2-0 Monocryl or Vicryl is used to close a deep layer, including the fascia overlying the extensor digitorum brevis and fat pad. The subcutaneous layer is closed with interrupted 3-0 Vicryl or Monocryl. Skin is closed with 3-0 nylon.
- Drains are not routinely used.
- Sterile dressings are applied, followed by a well-padded short leg splint in neutral dorsiflexion.

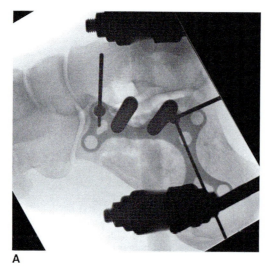
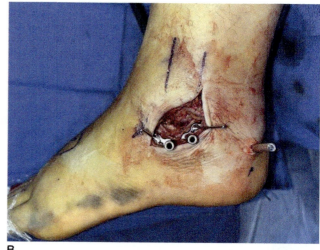
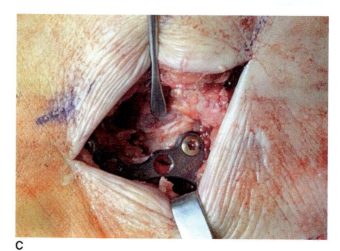

FIGURE 44.11 A, B: After reduction is obtained, the plate is applied and fluoroscopic imaging confirms an appropriate size and position. **C:** A freer elevator is pointing to the anatomically reduced posterior facet fragment.

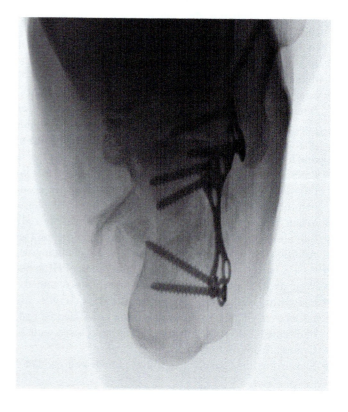

FIGURE 44.12 An axial heel view shows appropriate placement of the plate. Lateral comminution is compressed under the plate. Medial comminution was partially debulked. The remaining fragments were structurally insignificant. Note that the central two screws would have had better purchase in the sustentaculum.

PEARLS AND PITFALLS

- Be patient when it comes to compromised soft tissues. To minimize wound complications, it is best to delay surgery until the soft tissue envelope is ready for an incision. Closely evaluate swelling and blistering. Await the return of wrinkles. Decompress blisters and allow the underlying dermis to reepithelialize prior to ORIF.
- Bluntly dissecting with a Cobb elevator through the major fracture lines mobilizes difficult fragments in the setting of delayed ORIF.
- Double check lateral plate placement on the axial view to ensure it is not intraosseous. Late removal of an intraosseous plate is not a simple task.
- When possible, place screws into the sustentaculum tali (the constant fragment) for enhanced stability.
- Avoid screw overpenetration of the medial cortex to reduce the risk of tendon and neurovascular injury.
- Assess peroneal tendons for subluxation preoperative and intraoperatively. Stabilize them as necessary.
- Be cognizant of potential wound complications in the postoperative period. Infection and delayed wound healing are not rare. Maintain close follow-up for concerning wounds. Employ wound care, oral antibiotics, and surgical débridement when appropriate.

POSTOPERATIVE MANAGEMENT

- Drains are not routinely utilized.
- With effective peripheral nerve blocks, patients safely discharge home the day of surgery.
- In the early postoperative period, the patient is made non–weight bearing in a well-padded short leg splint. Elevation is encouraged.
- Two-week postoperative visit: The wound is assessed, and sutures removed if appropriate. A controlled ankle motion boot is applied, and gentle range of motion (ROM) is allowed. Non–weight bearing is continued. It is the preference of one author to use a cast to help ensure bony consolidation, soft tissue rest, and patient compliance.
- Six-week postoperative visit: Radiographs are obtained, including three standard views of the foot and an axial heel (Harris) view. ROM exercises are continued. If a cast was utilized, it is removed at the 6-week mark. Weight bearing as tolerated is initiated at 8 to 10 weeks, and the patient transitions to supportive shoes as comfort permits.
- Twelve-week postoperative visit: Repeat radiographs are obtained to assess for union before releasing remaining activity restrictions.

RESULTS AND COMPLICATIONS

A small group of studies have reported specifically on the results of the minimally invasive approach to calcaneal ORIF.[16-18,36,37] In terms of functional outcomes, American Orthopedic Foot and Ankle Society (AOFAS) hindfoot scores range from 86 to 87.2. Outcomes were rated as good or excellent in 84.2% patients, while in another study, the subjective satisfaction rate was 94%. Pain outcomes by visual analog scale rating were 0.8 to 3.5, which were lower than or equal to pain following ELA. Radiographic outcomes demonstrated a significant restoration of Böhler angle to mean values between 24° and 29°. When reported, average time to union was consistently between 12 and 13 weeks. Malunion ranged from 0% to 36%, while there were zero cases of nonunion. One study reported on the radiographic incidence of subtalar arthrosis at 1 year postoperatively, which was found to be 33%. Rates of subsequent subtalar fusion ranged from 0% to 5.2%. Wound complication rates specific to the minimally invasive sinus tarsi approach occurred at a rate of 0% to 14%. As discussed above, this is a greater rate than expected with nonoperative management but less than ELA. The rate of sural nerve injury was 0% to 3%, and in no case did it require surgical management. The current body of evidence suggests that the MIS technique can deliver equivalent patient function and fracture reduction quality when compared to ELA, while reducing the rate of surgical wound complications.

The management of calcaneus fractures has evolved tremendously over the last half century. Intra-articular injuries produce a fracture pattern that is morphologically and biomechanically disadvantageous. In an ideal scenario, anatomic restoration of the injury would be performed to avoid the negative outcomes associated with malunion. As discussed above, in select cohorts, operative management can lead to improved function, decreased pain, lower rates of arthritis, and fewer conversions to subtalar arthrodesis. Furthermore, among patients requiring subtalar arthrodesis, there are better functional scores and reduced complications after prior ORIF. Of course, surgical wound complications are an ever-present concern following ORIF of calcaneus fractures. Fortunately, MIS techniques have proven effective at reducing this negative outcome, when compared to traditional extensile approaches. Like with all complex issues, successful treatment requires a combination of appropriate patient selection, thorough preparation, well-executed technique, and diligent postoperative management.

REFERENCES

1. Banerjee R, Saltzman C, Anderson RB, Nickisch F. Management of calcaneal malunion. *J Am Acad Orthop Surg*. 2011;19(1):27-36.
2. Ghorbanhoseini M, Ghaheri A, Walley KC, Kwon JY. Superior tuber displacement in intra-articular calcaneus fractures. *Foot Ankle Int*. 2016;37(10):1076-1083.
3. Toussaint RJ, Lin D, Ehrlichman LK, Ellington JK, Strasser N, Kwon JY. Peroneal tendon displacement accompanying intra-articular calcaneal fractures. *J Bone Joint Surg Am*. 2014;96(4):310-315.
4. Sanders R. Intra-articular fractures of the calcaneus: present state of the art. *J Orthop Trauma*. 1992;6(2):252-265.
5. Lindsay W, Dewar F. Fractures of the os calcis. *Am J Surg*. 1958;95(4):555-576.
6. Ibrahim T, Rowsell M, Rennie W, Brown A, Taylor G, Gregg P. Displaced intra-articular calcaneal fractures: 15-year follow-up of a randomised controlled trial of conservative versus operative treatment. *Injury*. 2007;38(7):848-855.
7. Buckley R. Operative compared with nonoperative treatment of displaced intra-articular calcaneal fractures. *J Bone Joint Surg A*. 2002;84:1733-1744.
8. Jiang N, Lin Q-r, Diao X-c, Wu L, Yu B. Surgical versus nonsurgical treatment of displaced intra-articular calcaneal fracture: a meta-analysis of current evidence base. *Int Orthop*. 2012;36(8):1615-1622.
9. Leung K, Yuen K, Chan W. Operative treatment of displaced intra-articular fractures of the calcaneum. Medium-term results. *J Bone Joint Surg Br*. 1993;75(2):196-201.
10. Thordarson DB, Krieger LE. Operative vs. nonoperative treatment of intra-articular fractures of the calcaneus: a prospective randomized trial. *Foot Ankle Int*. 1996;17(1):2-9.
11. Howard J, Buckley R, McCormack R, et al. Complications following management of displaced intra-articular calcaneal fractures: a prospective randomized trial comparing open reduction internal fixation with nonoperative management. *J Orthop Trauma*. 2003;17(4):241-249.
12. Csizy M, Buckley R, Tough S, et al. Displaced intra-articular calcaneal fractures: variables predicting late subtalar fusion. *J Orthop Trauma*. 2003;17(2):106-112.
13. Ågren P-H, Wretenberg P, Sayed-Noor AS. Operative versus nonoperative treatment of displaced intra-articular calcaneal fractures: a prospective, randomized, controlled multicenter trial. *J Bone Joint Surg Am*. 2013;95(15):1351-1357.
14. Zhang W, Lin F, Chen E, Xue D, Pan Z. Operative versus nonoperative treatment of displaced intra-articular calcaneal fractures: a meta-analysis of randomized controlled trials. *J Orthop Trauma*. 2016;30(3):e75-e81.
15. Radnay CS, Clare MP, Sanders RW. Subtalar fusion after displaced intra-articular calcaneal fractures: does initial operative treatment matter? *J Bone Joint Surg Am*. 2009;91(3):541-546.
16. Kline AJ, Anderson RB, Davis WH, Jones CP, Cohen BE. Minimally invasive technique versus an extensile lateral approach for intra-articular calcaneal fractures. *Foot Ankle Int*. 2013;34(6):773-780.
17. Kwon JY, Guss D, Lin DE, et al. Effect of delay to definitive surgical fixation on wound complications in the treatment of closed, intra-articular calcaneus fractures. *Foot Ankle Int*. 2015;36(5):508-517.
18. Weber M, Lehmann O, Sägesser D, Krause F. Limited open reduction and internal fixation of displaced intra-articular fractures of the calcaneum. *J Bone Joint Surg Br*. 2008;90(12):1608-1616.
19. De Groot R, Frima A, Schepers T, Roerdink W. Complications following the extended lateral approach for calcaneal fractures do not influence mid-to long-term outcome. *Injury*. 2013;44(11):1596-1600.
20. Allegra PR, Rivera S, Desai SS, Aiyer A, Kaplan J, Gross CE. Intra-articular calcaneus fractures: current concepts review. *Foot Ankle Orthop*. 2020;5(3):2473011420927334.
21. Ding L, He Z, Xiao H, Chai L, Xue F. Risk factors for postoperative wound complications of calcaneal fractures following plate fixation. *Foot Ankle Int*. 2013;34(9):1238-1244.
22. Worsham JR, Elliott MR, Harris AM. Open calcaneus fractures and associated injuries. *J Foot Ankle Surg*. 2016;55(1):68-71.
23. Galluzzo M, Greco F, Pietragalla M, et al. Calcaneal fractures: radiological and CT evaluation and classification systems. *Acta Biomed*. 2018;89(Suppl 1):138.
24. Gitajn IL, Toussaint RJ, Kwon JY. Assessing accuracy of sustentaculum screw placement during calcaneal fixation. *Foot Ankle Int*. 2013;34(2):282-286.
25. Ketz JP, Maceroli M, Shields E, Sanders RW. Peroneal tendon instability in intra-articular calcaneus fractures: a retrospective comparative study and a new surgical technique. *J Orthop Trauma*. 2016;30(3):e82-e87.
26. Lim EV, Leung JPF. Complications of intraarticular calcaneal fractures. *Clin Orthop Relat Res*. 2001;391:7-16.
27. Strauss EJ, Petrucelli G, Bong M, Koval KJ, Egol KA. Blisters associated with lower-extremity fracture: results of a prospective treatment protocol. *J Orthop Trauma*. 2006;20(9):618-622.
28. Ho C-J, Huang H-T, Chen C-H, Chen J-C, Cheng Y-M, Huang P-J. Open reduction and internal fixation of acute intra-articular displaced calcaneal fractures: a retrospective analysis of surgical timing and infection rates. *Injury*. 2013;44(7):1007-1010.
29. Tennent T, Calder P, Salisbury R, Allen P, Eastwood D. The operative management of displaced intra-articular fractures of the calcaneum: a two-centre study using a defined protocol. *Injury*. 2001;32(6):491-496.

30. Kim GB, Park JJ, Park CH. Intra-articular calcaneal fracture treatment with staged medial external fixation. *Foot Ankle Int*. 2022;43(8):1084-1091.
31. Abousayed MM, Toussaint RJ, Kwon JY. The use of dual C-arms during fixation of calcaneal fractures: a technique tip. *Foot Ankle Spec*. 2014;7(3):207-209.
32. Kwon JY, Ellington JK, Marsland D, Gupta S. Calcaneal traction pin placement simplified: a cadaveric study. *Foot Ankle Int*. 2011;32(6):651-655.
33. Wang C-S, Tzeng Y-H, Lin C-C, Huang C-K, Chang M-C, Chiang C-C. Radiographic evaluation of ankle joint stability after calcaneofibular ligament elevation during open reduction and internal fixation of calcaneus fracture. *Foot Ankle Int*. 2016;37(9):944-949.
34. Ehrlichman LK, Toussaint RJ, Kwon JY. Surgical relocation of peroneal tendon dislocation with calcaneal open reduction and internal fixation: technique tip. *Foot Ankle Int*. 2014;35(9):938-942.
35. Looijen RC, Misselyn D, Backes M, Dingemans SA, Halm JA, Schepers T. Identification of postoperative step-offs and gaps with Broden's view following open reduction and internal fixation of calcaneal fractures. *Foot Ankle Int*. 2019;40(7):797-802.
36. Kikuchi C, Charlton TP, Thordarson DB. Limited sinus tarsi approach for intra-articular calcaneus fractures. *Foot Ankle Int*. 2013;34(12):1689-1694.
37. Nosewicz T, Knupp M, Barg A, et al. Mini-open sinus tarsi approach with percutaneous screw fixation of displaced calcaneal fractures: a prospective computed tomography–based study. *Foot Ankle Int*. 2012;33(11):925-933.

45 Posterior Tibial Tendon Transfer

Ajay N. Gurbani and Nelson F. SooHoo

INDICATIONS AND CONTRAINDICATIONS

Posterior tibial tendon transfer is most commonly used to address weakness of ankle dorsiflexion resulting in foot drop. Foot drop can occur secondary to a variety of pathologies, including neurologic and traumatic causes.[1] Neurogenic causes include sciatic or peroneal nerve palsy, central nervous disorders such as multiple sclerosis, and peripheral neuropathies including Charcot-Marie-Tooth disorder. Traumatic etiologies include muscle loss or secondary compartment syndromes resulting in loss of muscle function.[2-4] Foot drop can result in significant gait disturbance and disability for patients.

The initial management of foot drop includes physical therapy to focus on strengthening, heel cord stretching, and use of an ankle-foot orthosis (AFO). Particularly in the case of acute nerve injury, a period of expectant management is indicated as many patients regain some or all of their neurologic function.[5] Persistent foot drop can be managed nonoperatively, but this generally requires chronic use of an AFO for optimal function.[1,6] Traditionally, posterior tibial tendon transfer is reserved for patients who have symptoms for at least 1 year without evidence of recovery of dorsiflexion strength and dissatisfaction with bracing. Since its original description, a variety of modified techniques of posterior tibial tendon transfer have been reported in the literature, and there is no consensus regarding the superiority of one single approach.[7-10]

The indications for posterior tibial tendon transfer include patients with dorsiflexion weakness resulting in foot drop without anticipated neurologic recovery. Patients must have a functioning posterior tibial tendon muscle-tendon unit, typically with at least 4 out of 5 graded strength prior to transfer. Patients should have a supple foot and ankle, accompanied by full passive range of motion, with the exception of a degree of equinus contracture that can be addressed at the time of surgery.

Relative contraindications for this procedure include significant weakness of the posterior tibial tendon unit, as a loss of one grade of muscle strength after transfer is largely anticipated. Successful surgery will allow the patient to have functional gait without the use of an AFO, although active dorsiflexion strength postoperatively may vary.[11,12] Additionally, posterior tibial tendon transfer is contraindicated in patients who demonstrate rigid contracture or severe arthritis of the ankle, as this would preclude function of the transferred tendon. Care must also be taken to rule out an incomplete nerve injury with likelihood of improvement in dorsiflexion strength prior to proceeding with this surgery.[1,11,12]

PREOPERATIVE PLANNING

Preoperative evaluation of patients includes a thorough physical examination, assessing for deformity and neurovascular status. Standing alignment is assessed along with a thorough assessment of joint mobility to confirm suitability of a planned posterior tibial tendon transfer. Sensory evaluation is performed, with careful assessment of the potential level of any neurologic injury. Gait is also assessed, and patients may demonstrate a steppage or circumduction gait pattern.

A thorough motor examination is of key importance when considering a patient for posterior tibial tendon transfer. Lack of dorsiflexion strength should be confirmed on exam. Additionally, evaluation of the peroneal tendons and eversion strength is performed, as this may help dictate the insertion point of the transferred tendon. This evaluation also helps guide decisions regarding concomitant procedures, such as the Bridle modification, which includes transfer of the peroneus longus tendon to the anterior compartment.[9] Decreased eversion strength would favor insertion of the transfer in the lateral cuneiform as opposed to the middle cuneiform. Additionally, intact strength of the posterior tibialis as well as gastrocnemius-soleus complex must be confirmed prior to the planned surgery.

Standing radiographs of the foot and ankle are obtained to evaluate alignment and for the presence of associated deformity or arthritic changes. An electromyogram and nerve conduction study can be performed at various time points to confirm the level and degree of neurologic injury, as well as to evaluate for potential regeneration. As part of the preoperative discussion, it is important for the surgeon to clearly discuss expectations after surgery, as alterations in the patient's arc of motion with reduced plantarflexion are expected. Additionally, given that many patients will have sensory deficits in the setting of neurologic injury, it is important for the surgeon to clarify that these are not expected to improve with surgery.

SURGICAL TECHNIQUE

The authors' preferred technique is to transfer the posterior tibial tendon through the interosseous membrane to the dorsum of the foot using a modified four incision technique as first described by Hsu and Hoffer.[10] The patient is placed supine on the operating room table with a bump under the ipsilateral hip. A tourniquet is placed on the operative thigh. The operative limb is exsanguinated and the tourniquet is inflated. First, attention is paid to potential equinus contracture. If the patient does not achieve 5° to 10° of passive ankle dorsiflexion, then a percutaneous tendoachilles lengthening or gastrocnemius recession is performed.

Next, an incision is made at the insertion site of the posterior tibial tendon on the navicular. Dissection is carried out through the subcutaneous tissue and the posterior tibial tendon sheath is incised in line with the incision. The posterior tibial tendon is then released from its insertion sharply using scalpel as distal as possible. Additional length can be obtained by including the distal periosteum, which is a continuation of the posterior tibial tendon insertion, in the harvest. The tendon edge is then tagged with suture in an atraumatic fashion (Fig. 45.1).

Next, a second incision is performed overlying the distal medial leg, approximately 6 to 10 cm proximal to the tibiotalar joint (Fig. 45.2). The dissection is carried just off the medial border of the tibia, directly over the posterior tibial tendon. The flexor fascia is incised in line with the incision. The posterior tibial tendon is identified and pulled through to this incision. Often, there are adhesions that need to be released in the retromalleolar region to allow mobilization of the tendon to this incision.

A third incision is made lateral to the anterior tibial crest at the same level as the proximal medial incision. These incisions are relatively proximal at 6 to 10 cm above the joint to allow proximal release of the interosseus membrane through the lateral incision (see Fig. 45.2). This is intended to minimize binding of the transfer. Deeper dissection is carried out, and the superficial peroneal nerve and contents of the anterior compartment are retracted laterally. A right-angle clamp is utilized to create a path for the tendon from the medial incision posterior to the tibia in blunt fashion, taking care to stay just directly posterior to the tibia and deep to the neurovascular structures. The right-angle clamp is directed through the interosseous membrane to the anterolateral incision. The interosseous membrane is split longitudinally through the anterolateral incision, taking care to avoid injury to the anterior neurovascular bundle. The posterior tibial tendon is passed using tagging sutures through to the interosseus membrane using the right-angle clamp. At this stage, it should be confirmed that the tendon is able to slide freely, and enlargement of the opening within the membrane can be performed as needed to ensure there is enough excursion to reach the desired point of insertion.

Next, a fourth incision is made overlying the planned insertion point for the tendon transfer. It is the authors' preference to select this based on the patient's preoperative peroneal muscle strength. For patients with preoperative peroneal muscle weakness (rated as grade 3 or lower), a transfer is planned to the lateral cuneiform. For patients with intact peroneal muscle strength, the transfer is

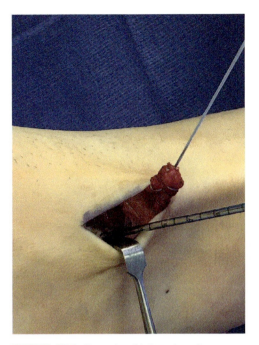

FIGURE 45.1 Posterior tibial tendon after harvest, with the end of the tendon tagged with suture to be utilized for passing.

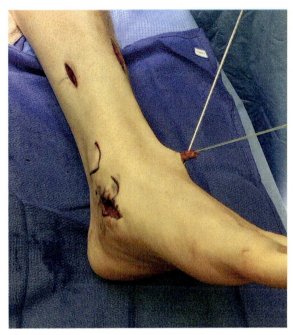

FIGURE 45.2 Location of proximal incisions are demonstrated, located approximately 6 to 10 cm proximal to the tibiotalar joint line. (Reprinted from SooHoo NF, Schon LC, Coughlin MJ. Disorders of tendons. In: Haskell A, Coughlin M, eds. *Coughlin and Mann's Surgery of the Foot and Ankle*. 10th ed. Elsevier; 2023:1220. Copyright © 2024 Elsevier. With permission.)

inserted onto the middle cuneiform. Fluoroscopy is utilized for incision planning over the selected insertion site.

A curved tendon passer is passed subcutaneously from the fourth incision and utilized to retrieve and pass the posterior tibial tendon to the desired insertion site with the tagging sutures (Fig. 45.3). The authors do not generally pass the tendon deep to the extensor retinaculum to avoid injury or binding of the other anterior tendinous and neurovascular structures. The tension is adjusted to maintain the ankle at approximately 10° of dorsiflexion.

The tendon is then secured to the insertion site in the middle or lateral cuneiform with a suture button technique. A pin is placed and localized over the appropriate cuneiform using intraoperative fluoroscopy (Figs. 45.3 and 45.4). A cannulated drill is then used to create a unicortical tunnel for the tendon insertion (Figs. 45.5 and 45.6). Next the suture button is passed through the plantar cortex and toggled 90° to allow tensioning of the transfer (Fig. 45.7). The tendon is tensioned with the foot in slight dorsiflexion and the sutures tied (Figs. 45.8 and 45.9). Intraoperative fluoroscopy is used to confirm placement of the suture button (Figs. 45.10 and 45.11). Alternatively, an interference screw may be used. Final resting tension is confirmed, as well as appropriate excursion of the tendon prior to closure of incisions.

PEARLS AND PITFALLS

- Adequate dorsiflexion is critical to the success of this procedure, and any potential equinus contracture should be addressed first.
- Careful evaluation of preoperative peroneal muscle strength can be utilized to select an appropriate insertion site for the transfer or consideration for additional procedures to address eversion weakness including the Bridle modification.
- Care should be taken to harvest the posterior tibial tendon as distal as possible to preserve potential length. This can include harvest of the distal periosteum as an extension to provide additional length for the transfer.
- The suture button technique is helpful in providing stable fixation, particularly in cases in which the distal tendon available for implantation is of marginal length or quality for tenodesis screw fixation.

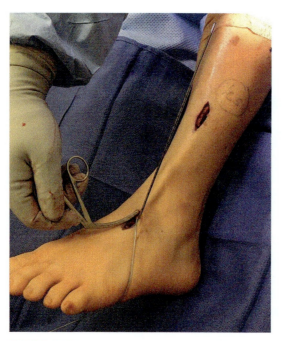

FIGURE 45.3 A curved tendon passer is utilized to pass tendon to the desired insertion site from the proximal lateral incision in a subcutaneous fashion. (Reprinted from SooHoo NF, Schon LC, Coughlin MJ. Disorders of tendons. In: Haskell A, Coughlin M, eds. *Coughlin and Mann's Surgery of the Foot and Ankle*. 10th ed. Elsevier; 2023:1220. Copyright © 2024 Elsevier. With permission.)

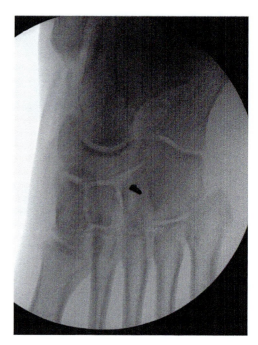

FIGURE 45.4 A pin is utilized to localize the desired insertion site fluoroscopically, which is the lateral cuneiform in this case.

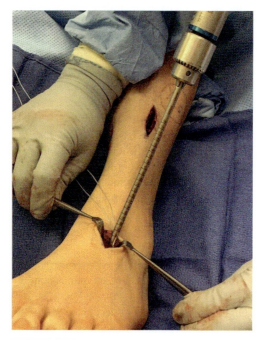

FIGURE 45.5 A cannulated drill is utilized to prepare the unicortical tunnel for insertion of the tendon transfer. (Reprinted from SooHoo NF, Schon LC, Coughlin MJ. Disorders of tendons. In: Haskell A, Coughlin M, eds. *Coughlin and Mann's Surgery of the Foot and Ankle*. 10th ed. Elsevier; 2023:1220. Copyright © 2024 Elsevier. With permission.)

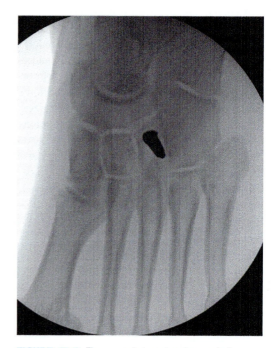

FIGURE 45.6 Fluoroscopic imaging demonstrating the pathway of the tunnel. (Reprinted from SooHoo NF, Schon LC, Coughlin MJ. Disorders of tendons. In: Haskell A, Coughlin M, eds. *Coughlin and Mann's Surgery of the Foot and Ankle*. 10th ed. Elsevier; 2023:1220. Copyright © 2024 Elsevier. With permission.)

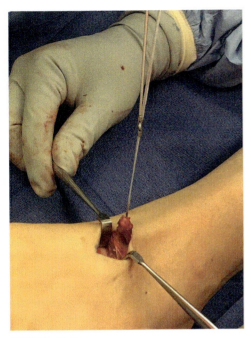

FIGURE 45.7 The suture button is demonstrated here prior to passage in the tunnel. (Reprinted from SooHoo NF, Schon LC, Coughlin MJ. Disorders of tendons. In: Haskell A, Coughlin M, eds. *Coughlin and Mann's Surgery of the Foot and Ankle*. 10th ed. Elsevier; 2023:1220. Copyright © 2024 Elsevier. With permission.)

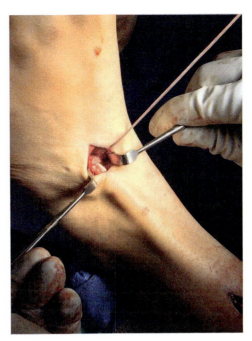

FIGURE 45.8 Once passed through the tunnel, the suture button is toggled 90° to allow for tensioning of the transfer.

POSTOPERATIVE MANAGEMENT

Initial postoperative management includes a period of non–weight bearing with immobilization in a short leg splint for 2 weeks. Patients are seen postoperatively at the 2-week mark for inspection of the surgical wounds and suture removal. At this stage, the patient is transitioned to a short leg walking cast until 4 to 6 weeks postoperatively.

At 4 to 6 weeks after surgery, patients transition to full weight bearing in an AFO and begin physical therapy. Physical therapy includes strengthening, stretching, and manual mobilization or

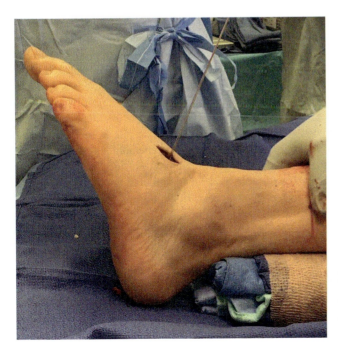

FIGURE 45.9 The sutures are demonstrated here prior to final tightening of the tendon transfer. (Reprinted from SooHoo NF, Schon LC, Coughlin MJ. Disorders of tendons. In: Haskell A, Coughlin M, eds. *Coughlin and Mann's Surgery of the Foot and Ankle*. 10th ed. Elsevier; 2023:1220. Copyright © 2024 Elsevier. With permission.)

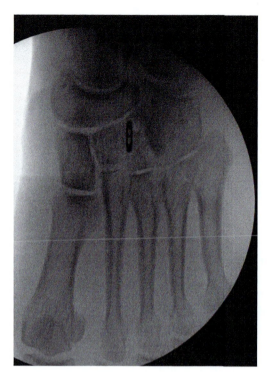

FIGURE 45.10 Oblique fluoroscopic image demonstrating position of the suture button after passage through the lateral cuneiform.

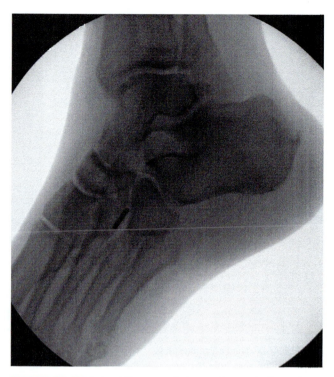

FIGURE 45.11 Lateral fluoroscopic image demonstrating suture button sitting flush against plantar cortex of the lateral cuneiform. (Reprinted from SooHoo NF, Schon LC, Coughlin MJ. Disorders of tendons. In: Haskell A, Coughlin M, eds. *Coughlin and Mann's Surgery of the Foot and Ankle*. 10th ed. Elsevier; 2023:1220. Copyright © 2024 Elsevier. With permission.)

massage as indicated. Gentle active range of motion without resistance is begun 8 to 10 weeks postoperatively. Rehabilitation also focuses on gait training and proprioceptive exercises at this stage. Formal physical therapy is carried out for a minimum of 2 months, and often longer, depending on patient progress. Patients are instructed to use an AFO for 3 months postoperatively. Impact activities including sports, running, and jumping are restricted until the 6-month mark.

RESULTS AND COMPLICATIONS

The surgical goals of posterior tibial tendon transfer include active dorsiflexion past neutral, the ability to ambulate without a brace, and return to desired activity level.[13] However, similar to the heterogeneity of techniques reported, there is a varied presentation of results of this procedure in the literature. While reported outcomes are generally favorable, there is also no consensus as to the definition of a successful outcome.[3,13]

Yeap et al presented a case series of 12 patients who underwent posterior tibial tendon transfer, with 10 patients rating their results as "good" or "excellent."[13] However, despite 11 patients obtaining a clinical motor grade of 4 or 5, dorsiflexion strength testing by dynamometer often revealed 30% torque generated as compared to the contralateral leg, comparable to results reported in other series.[6,14,15] In this series, 10 out 12 patients were able to achieve ambulation without a brace.[14] Posterior tibial tendon transfer can be used as part of correction of cavus foot deformity with procedures including calcaneal osteotomy, medial column correction, and soft tissue release. Dreher et al utilized three-dimensional gait analysis to evaluate the results of posterior tibial tendon transfer in patients undergoing correction of Charcot-Marie-Tooth foot deformity. They found correction of foot drop during gait, with improved dorsiflexion during the swing phase, but with resultant loss of active plantarflexion at push off.[16]

More recently, Cho et al found that despite similar limited restoration in dorsiflexion strength as seen in other series, there was significant improvement in functional outcomes and ability to ambulate unassisted without an orthosis at final follow-up, with only 1 out of 17 patients requiring use of a brace for occupational activity.[6] This is consistent with the results seen in other studies.[6,14,15,17]

Potential complications of posterior tibial tendon transfer include tendon scarring and adhesion to the extensor retinaculum. This risk may be reduced through the use of a subcutaneous transfer, though this is debated.[4,6] Other complications include failure of the transfer through loss of distal fixation or loosening, which has been managed with revision and shortening of the tendon in the literature with reported acceptable outcomes.[13,17] The suture button technique presented here is intended to minimize the risk of pullout as well as provide stable fixation in cases where the tendon length is marginal. Another key concern of the long-term effects of posterior tibial tendon transfer is the progressive development of arch collapse and flatfoot deformity. The magnitude of this potential risk is unclear. While there have been case reports of this complication occurring in the literature, there has been mixed results in larger case series. Some authors have presented changes in arch structure and hindfoot at final follow-up, and others have reported no such changes—the general consensus is that these changes are typically not clinically significant if they occur.[6,14-19]

In summary, posterior tibial tendon transfer can be an effective treatment option for patients with persistent foot drop that persists without evidence of recovery. Careful preoperative assessment and patient selection is critical to success of this procedure. Patients should be counseled on persistent dorsiflexion weakness; however, improvement in function and satisfactory gait without the need for bracing is expected in most patients.

REFERENCES

1. Jaivin JS, Bishop JO, Braly WG, Tullos HS. Management of acquired adult dropfoot. *Foot Ankle Int*. 1992;13(2):98-104.
2. Mont MA, Dellon AL, Chen F, Hungerford MW, Krackow KA, Hungerford DS. The operative treatment of peroneal nerve palsy. *J Bone Joint Surg Am*. 1996;78(6):863-869.
3. Schweitzer KM, Jones CP. Tendon transfers for the drop foot. *Foot Ankle Clin*. 2014;19(1):65-71.
4. Jeng C, Myerson M. The uses of tendon transfers to correct paralytic deformity of the foot and ankle. *Foot Ankle Clin*. 2004;9(2):319-337.
5. Poage C, Roth C, Scott B. Peroneal nerve palsy: evaluation and management. *J Am Acad Orthop Surg*. 2016;24(1):1-10.
6. Cho BK, Park KJ, Choi SM, Im SH, SooHoo NF. Functional outcomes following anterior transfer of the tibialis posterior tendon for foot drop secondary to peroneal nerve palsy. *Foot Ankle Int*. 2017;38(6):627-633.
7. Watkins MB, Jones JB, Ryder CT Jr, et al. Transplantation of the posterior tibial tendon. *J Bone Joint Surg*. 1954;36A:1181-1189.
8. Carayon A, Bourrel P, Bourges M, et al. Dual transfer of the posterior tibial and flexor digitorum longus tendons for drop foot: a report of 31 cases. *J Bone Joint Surg*. 1967;49A:144-148.
9. McCall RE, Frederick HA, McCluskey GM, Riordan DC. The Bridle procedure: a new treatment for equinus and equinovarus deformities in children. *J Pediatr Orthop*. 1991;11(1):83-89.
10. Hsu JD, Hoffer MM. Posterior tibial tendon transfer anteriorly through the interosseous membrane: a modification of the technique. *Clin Orthop Relat Res*. 1978;(131):202-204.
11. Pinzur MS. Principles of balancing the foot with tendon transfers. *Foot Ankle Clin*. 2011;16(3):375-384.
12. Bluman EM, Dowd T. The basics and science of tendon transfers. *Foot Ankle Clin*. 2011;16(3):385-399.
13. Yeap JS, Singh D, Birch R. A method for evaluating the results of tendon transfers for foot drop. *Clin Orthop Relat Res*. 2001;383:208-213.
14. Yeap JS, Birch R, Singh D. Long-term results of tibialis posterior tendon transfer for drop-foot. *Int Orthop*. 2001;25(2):114-118.
15. Steinau HU, Tofaute A, Huellmann K, et al. Tendon transfers for drop foot correction: long-term results including quality of life assessment, and dynamometric and pedobarographic measurements. *Arch Orthop Trauma Surg*. 2011;131: 903-910.
16. Dreher T, Wolf SI, Heitzmann D, Fremd C, Klotz MC, Wenz W. Tibialis posterior tendon transfer corrects the foot drop component of cavovarus foot deformity in Charcot-Marie-Tooth disease. *J Bone Joint Surg Am*. 2014;96(6):456-462.
17. Agarwal P, Gupta M, Kukrele R, Sharma D. Tibialis posterior (TP) tendon transfer for foot drop: a single center experience. *J Clin Orthop Trauma*. 2020;11(3):457-461.
18. Vertullo CJ, Nunley JA. Acquired flatfoot deformity following posterior tibial tendon transfer for peroneal nerve injury: a case report. *J Bone Joint Surg Am*. 2002;84(7):1214-1217.
19. Omid R, Thordarson DB, Charlton TP. Adult-acquired flatfoot deformity following posterior tibialis to dorsum transfer: a case report. *Foot Ankle Int*. 2008;29(3):351-353.

46 The Malerba Osteotomy and First Metatarsal Dorsiflexion Osteotomy

Elizabeth A. Cody

INTRODUCTION

The Malerba osteotomy and first metatarsal dorsiflexion osteotomy are two procedures commonly performed together to address cavovarus deformities. The Malerba osteotomy is a Z-type lateralizing calcaneal osteotomy useful for addressing the varus hindfoot,[1] while the first metatarsal dorsiflexion osteotomy addresses excess first ray plantarflexion. The first metatarsal dorsiflexion osteotomy may be performed alone for a relatively mild deformity with a flexible hindfoot deformity. The Malerba osteotomy is useful for more moderate or severe deformities or in the presence of a rigid hindfoot. Each may be performed individually, together, or in combination with additional procedures, with the exact procedures performed tailored to address each individual case.[2] In the setting of a subtle cavus deformity, these procedures may increase the success rate of soft tissue procedures—such as lateral ligament reconstruction or peroneal tendon repair—when performed concomitantly.

INDICATIONS AND CONTRAINDICATIONS

Because of the multiple potential etiologies of the deformity, each cavus foot must be evaluated individually. A careful understanding of the underlying disease process is critical to treatment. In forefoot cavus, plantarflexion of the first metatarsal drives the hindfoot into varus. First metatarsal plantarflexion may be innate or progressive over time, driven by muscular imbalance as in the case of Charcot-Marie-Tooth disease. Radiographically, forefoot cavus is demonstrated by an elevated talo-first metatarsal angle, with normal being 0° and anything greater than 4° being abnormal.[3] In cases where the first ray plantarflexion is not fully passively correctable, a dorsiflexion osteotomy is indicated to elevate the medial column and eliminate this underlying cause of the global deformity.

To determine if hindfoot varus is forefoot driven, the Coleman block test may be performed to evaluate the flexibility of the hindfoot. The patient stands with a wooden block of appropriate thickness placed under the lateral column of the foot. The first ray is allowed to rest on the floor. If the hindfoot remains flexible, it will correct to a neutral or valgus position.[4] In this situation with a more subtle deformity, a first metatarsal dorsiflexion osteotomy alone may be sufficient for deformity correction. A lateralizing calcaneal osteotomy is required if the hindfoot cannot correct to neutral or beyond with the Coleman block test.

Contraindications to these joint-sparing procedures include severe, rigid deformities or arthritic change, both of which are better managed with arthrodesis. Patients with a concomitant hallux valgus deformity or first tarsometatarsal (TMT) joint arthritis may be better managed with a dorsiflexion-producing first TMT joint fusion instead of an osteotomy. For patients with severe peroneal pathology and weakness, a calcaneal osteotomy is unlikely to be sufficient for correction of varus hindfoot deformity, in which case subtalar fusion is a more reliable option. The surgeon must proceed with caution if there is a suspicion of a progressive underlying neurologic lesion. The underlying disease pattern must be understood along with the associated potential for deformity recurrence. Focal neurologic lesions may be signaled by rapidly progressive deformity, marked asymmetry between sides, and long-tract signs.

PREOPERATIVE PLANNING

The location of the pain and any functional impairment should be determined, such as pain from lateral foot overload, frequent ankle sprains, and eversion weakness. Lateral foot overload may manifest as pain in the fifth metatarsal head or fifth metatarsal base, or as a history of fifth metatarsal fracture. A detailed physical examination should be performed, including evaluation of standing alignment and walking. Evaluation of standing alignment can show the "peekaboo heel" sign (Fig. 46.1).[5]

Range of motion of the hindfoot and ankle should be assessed. Joint stiffness or pain suggestive of degenerative changes should be noted. The flexibility of the hindfoot can be assessed manually be attempting to bring the hindfoot into valgus and can also be assessed with the Coleman block test as noted above. Dorsiflexion tightness with the knee flexed and extended should be documented. Manual muscle strength testing should be performed. In particular, the peroneal tendons should be carefully assessed, including individual strength assessment of both peroneus brevis (foot eversion) and peroneus longus (first ray plantarflexion). Pain or weakness during this testing is suggestive of peroneal pathology. Ankle stability should be assessed, including anterior drawer testing and varus stress testing at 90° of ankle dorsiflexion. Weight-bearing radiographs of the foot and ankle are important to assess alignment, degenerative arthritis, joint instability, bony anomalies, and stress fractures. Stress views can be useful to evaluate instability, if needed.

Thorough preoperative counseling of patients is essential. Patients need to understand what surgery can accomplish, and that their condition may change over time even after a successful operation. The first metatarsal dorsiflexion osteotomy and Malerba osteotomy are joint-sparing procedures intended to restore more normal function, but patients should be aware of the potential need for additional surgical interventions.

SURGICAL TECHNIQUE

Spinal anesthesia is generally recommended, with a popliteal nerve block for postoperative pain control. However, other anesthetic options may be preferable in some cases, depending on patient factors, patient or surgeon preferences, and the anesthesiologist's and institutional capabilities. The patient is positioned in the "sloppy lateral" position, about halfway between straight supine and lateral, using a beanbag and lateral posts (Fig. 46.2). From this position, the lateral calcaneus is easily

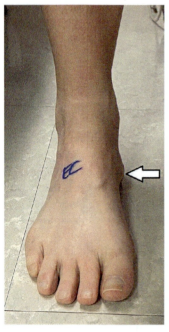

FIGURE 46.1 The "peekaboo heel" sign, in which the heel is visible medially when the patient stands facing forward, is a clinical indicator of a varus hindfoot.

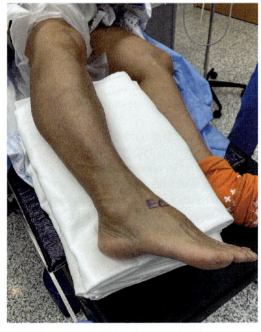

FIGURE 46.2 The patient is positioned in the "sloppy lateral" position using a beanbag. A foam pillow or stack of blankets can be used to elevate the foot.

accessed for the Malerba osteotomy. To access the dorsal first metatarsal, the table can be tilted and the leg externally rotated. Ensuring the ability to externally rotate the leg sufficiently to access to the medial side is important for any other concomitant procedures that may need to be performed, such as capsular releases or tendon lengthenings. A proximal thigh tourniquet is used.

Malerba Osteotomy

An oblique incision is made over the lateral calcaneus from the superior calcaneus overlying the retrocalcaneal bursa to the soft spot distal to the plantar fascia origin. Careful dissection is carried down to bone to avoid injury to the sural nerve, which may be gently retracted dorsally if encountered. The peroneal sheath remains anterior to the osteotomy. An elevator is used to elevate the periosteum off the lateral calcaneal wall for exposure. Small Hohmann retractors are placed at the proximal and distal edges of the calcaneus, roughly aligned with the planned proximal and distal osteotomy cuts. A self-retaining retractor may be inserted around the Hohmann retractors for additional exposure.

The Malerba osteotomy is a Z-shaped osteotomy, with the two vertical limbs oriented parallel to each other and at 90° to the horizontal limb. Two small (1.25), parallel K-wires are inserted at the two corners of the Z, spaced about 2 cm apart, to help guide the cuts (Fig. 46.3). The wires are cut short and their positioning checked on fluoroscopy to ensure appropriate positioning of the osteotomy (see Fig. 46.3). A micro sagittal saw is used to start each of the three limbs of the cut, taking care to stay parallel to the parallel wires. Once the cuts have been partially completed, the K-wires are removed.

Before completing the cuts, the lateral wedge resection should be started. This is done from the horizontal limb. These horizontal limb cuts should be performed so as to converge medially, to allow for a wedge resection. Generally, a 4- to 10-mm lateral wedge is resected, depending on the amount of deformity correction desired (Fig. 46.4). In some cases, the surgeon may choose to also perform lateral wedge resections from the vertical limbs to enable rotation of the tuberosity in a second plane for additional deformity correction. All cuts are completed carefully and the lateral wedge is removed. An osteotome may be used to help complete the osteotomy. A laminar spreader is inserted in the osteotomy site and distracted maximally to help relax the soft tissues around the osteotomy (Fig. 46.5).

The tuberosity is then rotated and shifted laterally to achieve deformity correction. A pointed reduction clamp can be used to compress the cut bone surfaces together (Fig. 46.6). Axial fluoroscopy views can be used to assess the amount of lateral translation and rotation. The position of the hindfoot is assessed visually to ensure adequate correction of deformity. Two 4.5- to 7.5-mm cannulated compression screws are inserted for fixation. Lateral and axial fluoroscopy views should be

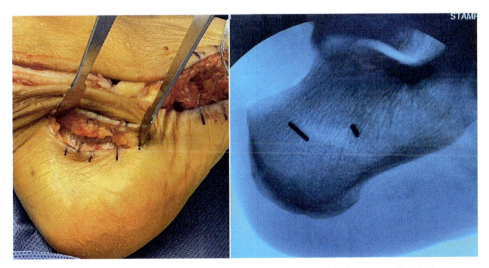

FIGURE 46.3 The Malerba osteotomy is a Z-shaped osteotomy, with the two vertical limbs oriented parallel to each other and at 90° to the horizontal limb. Two small (1.25), parallel K-wires are inserted at the two corners of the Z, spaced about 2 cm apart. The wire positioning is checked on fluoroscopy, and then the wires are used as landmarks to help guide the cuts.

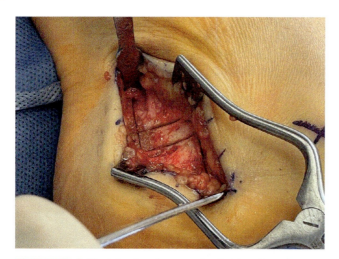

FIGURE 46.4 The lateral wedge resection is taken from the horizontal limb of the cut. The two horizontal limb cuts should be performed so as to converge medially, to allow for a wedge resection. Generally, a 4- to 10-mm lateral wedge is resected, depending on the amount of deformity correction desired.

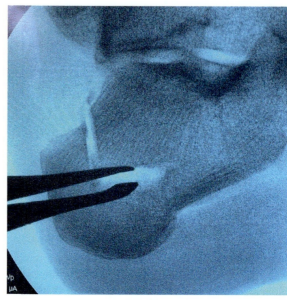

FIGURE 46.5 After completing the cuts and resecting the lateral wedge, a laminar spreader is inserted in the osteotomy site. The laminar spreader is distracted maximally to ensure completion of the cut and help relax the soft tissues around the osteotomy.

used to confirm wire positioning prior to drilling and screw insertion (Fig. 46.7). Prominent lateral bone can be shaved down using a rongeur and/or rasp if necessary. Closure is performed according to surgeon preference.

First Metatarsal Dorsiflexion Osteotomy

An approximate 4-cm dorsal incision is made over the proximal first metatarsal, extending just slightly proximal to the TMT joint. Careful dissection is carried down to the extensor hallucis longus (EHL) tendon. The dorsomedial cutaneous branch of the superficial peroneal nerve is protected

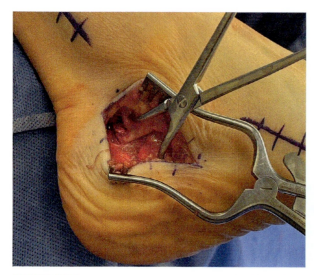

FIGURE 46.6 The tuberosity is rotated and shifted laterally to achieve deformity correction. A pointed reduction clamp can be used to compress the cut bone surfaces together.

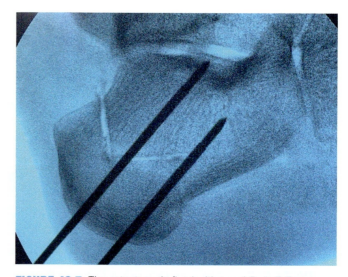

FIGURE 46.7 The osteotomy is fixed with two 4.5- to 7.5-mm cannulated compression screws. Lateral and axial fluoroscopy views should be used to confirm wire positioning prior to drilling and screw insertion.

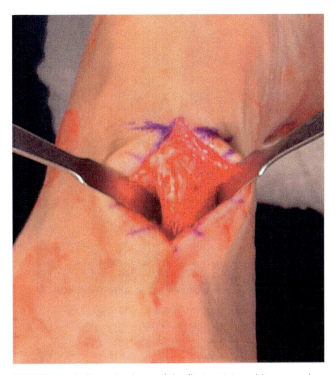

FIGURE 46.8 Once the base of the first metatarsal is exposed, small Hohmann retractors are inserted for exposure and to protect the soft tissues while making the osteotomy cuts.

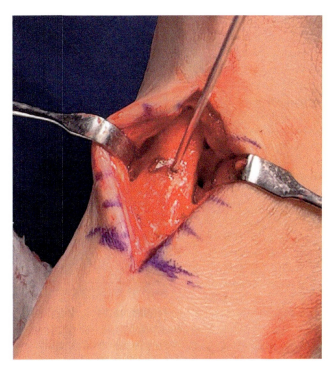

FIGURE 46.9 A K-wire is inserted in line with the planned osteotomy and its positioning checked on fluoroscopy to confirm an appropriate trajectory. The cut should be at least 1.5 cm from the first tarsometatarsal joint.

if encountered. The EHL tendon is mobilized to retract medially. Medial and lateral periosteal flaps are elevated at the base of the first metatarsal. Small Hohmann retractors are inserted for exposure and to protect the soft tissues (Fig. 46.8). A K-wire is inserted in line with the planned cut and its positioning checked on fluoroscopy (Fig. 46.9). The cut should be at least 1.5 cm from the first TMT joint.

A dorsal wedge resection is then completed using a sagittal saw (Fig. 46.10). Care is taken to leave a plantar cortical hinge intact. Given the proximal location, this is a powerful osteotomy, and often a small (2 to 3 mm) wedge resection is sufficient. With the wedge removed, the osteotomy is then closed down dorsally by applying pressure under the first metatarsal head. The plantar surface of the foot should be assessed to ensure adequate dorsiflexion of the first metatarsal. Additional bone may be resected if needed. The osteotomy may then be fixed with a single screw, small plate,

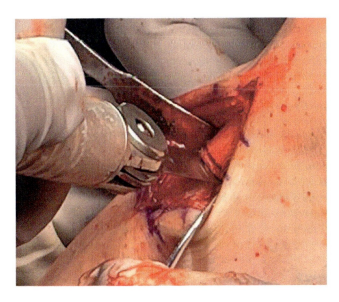

FIGURE 46.10 A dorsal wedge resection is completed using a sagittal saw. Extreme care should be taken to leave the plantar hinge intact.

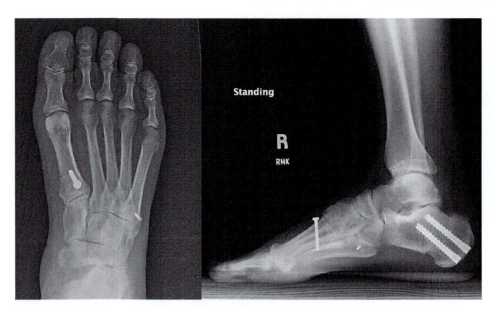

FIGURE 46.11 Anteroposterior (*left*) and lateral (*right*) views of the foot 6 weeks following Malerba osteotomy and first metatarsal dorsiflexion osteotomy. The oblique angle of the metatarsal cut can be seen on the lateral view, with one 3.5-mm cortical screw for fixation. The angled cut enables easier screw placement. The cut may also be made perpendicular to the shaft with a staple or plate used for fixation.

or staple, depending on surgeon preference (Fig. 46.11). Once the wedge has been closed down, the contour of the bone is altered such that staples will not always sit flush and plates may need to be bent to fit appropriately.

PEARLS AND PITFALLS

Malerba Osteotomy

- When lateral ankle incisions are necessary (such as for peroneal pathology), there is a potential for wound dehiscence. The two incisions should be parallel, with at least a 4-cm skin bridge. Attempts to address both procedures through one incision usually result in a very long incision that is not ideal for either procedure and requires extensive exposure and risk of injury to adjacent structures such as the sural nerve.
- To prevent loss of reduction during screw insertion, the second wire should not be overdrilled until after the first screw has been inserted.
- With a large lateral wedge resection, there will be some proximal translation of the calcaneal tuberosity, which may be helpful for deformity correction (Fig. 46.12).
- This is a very stable osteotomy that generally heals rapidly. Although other concomitant procedures often preclude early weight bearing, in the rare circumstance when the procedure is performed alone, weight bearing may be initiated as early as 4 weeks postoperatively.

First Metatarsal Dorsiflexion Osteotomy

- Leaving the plantar cortex intact increases the stability of the osteotomy and allows for easier reduction and fixation. The osteotomy heals reliably when the plantar cortex is left intact. Extreme care should be taken to ensure this is done.
- Avoid removing too much bone—start initially with a small wedge resection, and take more in small increments if needed. An excessive dorsal wedge resection increases the risk of over shortening and creating transfer metatarsalgia. If additional resection is needed, run the micro sagittal saw along the osteotomy removed an additional amount corresponding to the kerf of the blade. With the osteotomy closed down, the metatarsal heads should be palpated plantarly to ensure an appropriate amount of correction.

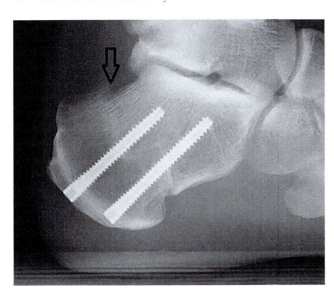

FIGURE 46.12 With a large lateral wedge resection, there will be some proximal translation of the calcaneal tuberosity, which may be helpful for deformity correction.

- If there is over shortening or an excessively long second metatarsal, performing a second metatarsal shortening osteotomy may assist forefoot balancing and prevent postoperative transfer metatarsalgia.
- If there is hypermobility of the first TMT joint, correction can be obtained through a first TMT fusion instead of the dorsiflexion osteotomy.
- If the osteotomy is unstable or the plantar cortex is inadvertently violated, additional K-wires between the first and second rays and the middle cuneiform can be used to provide supplemental fixation.

POSTOPERATIVE MANAGEMENT

The patient is placed in a non–weight-bearing well-padded short leg splint and returns to clinic at 12 to 14 days for suture removal. Non–weight bearing in a walking boot is maintained for the next 4 weeks. Active range of motion may be initiated once the splint has been removed. Casting is an alternative, although the added immobilization may prolong recovery. Radiographs should be checked at 6 weeks prior to starting weight bearing. Partial weight bearing is initiated at 6 weeks and gradually progressed over the next 2 weeks. Once fully weight bearing, the patient transitions out of the boot into regular shoes. Longer immobilization may be necessary for any concomitant procedures.

Physical therapy can generally be started at 6 weeks postoperatively. A focused home exercise program should be developed for peroneal strengthening, which is particularly important for patients who have undergone any work on their peroneal tendons.

RESULTS AND COMPLICATIONS

Outcome reports in the literature for the Malerba osteotomy and first metatarsal dorsiflexion osteotomy are rare. Most outcome reports focus on more comprehensive cavovarus foot reconstructions. Sammarco and Taylor[2] described results from 15 patients (21 feet) who underwent osteotomies of the calcaneus and one or more metatarsals for symptomatic cavovarus foot deformity. Presenting complaints were metatarsalgia, ankle instability, and ulceration beneath the second metatarsal head. Improvement in clinical scores was reported, with maintained or improved ankle, hindfoot, and midfoot motion in most patients. Complications included nonunion in 3 of 66 (5%) metatarsal osteotomies. Only one patient experienced a recurrent varus hindfoot deformity. The authors concluded that a lateral sliding elevating calcaneal osteotomy combined with dorsolateral closing wedge osteotomies of one or more metatarsal bases in the cavus foot can provide a pain-free, plantigrade foot with a lower arch and a stable ankle without sacrificing motion.

The most common potential complications related to cavus foot correction are nerve injury, nonunion or delayed union, persistent deformity, and recurrent deformity. Neurologic deficits following lateralizing calcaneal osteotomy occur in up to 34% of cases, with a majority of deficits resolving over time.[6] There is insufficient information on the incidence of sural nerve injury. Iatrogenic traction and laceration injuries can occur, or the correction can become incarcerated in scar tissue. Most symptoms resolve with conservative management. If a persistent painful neuroma occurs, proximal resection and burial is typically successful.

Tibial nerve deficits are more common following lateralizing calcaneal osteotomy. Acute tarsal tunnel syndrome is a known complication following lateralizing calcaneal osteotomy.[7,8] This is theoretically due to increased traction on the tibial nerve with lateralization of the tuberosity, together with decreased volume of the tarsal tunnel as the tuberosity is lateralized.[9,10] Some authors have suggested performing tarsal tunnel release at the time of cavovarus foot reconstruction to decrease the risk of iatrogenic tarsal tunnel syndrome,[8] although this is likely unnecessary in the case of more subtle deformities. A cadaveric study on the Malerba osteotomy has shown that major branches of the tibial nerve are in close proximity to the osteotomy site; therefore, care should be taken to limit medial penetration of the saw.[9] If a tarsal tunnel release is performed at the time of surgery, it should be performed prior to the calcaneal osteotomy, as increased rates of nerve symptoms have been reported when the release was performed after the osteotomy.[6]

Inadequate correction with the Malerba osteotomy is another potential complication and is preventable. At times, it is difficult to judge the degree of correction intraoperatively. Judicious overcorrection of hindfoot varus should be attempted. Intraoperative axial alignment radiographs can be used intraoperatively to ensure adequate correction.

Recurrence of deformity, whether related or not to neurologic disease progression, may create a progressive or recurrent cavus deformity, necessitating triple arthrodesis. All patients undergoing a joint-sparing cavus foot correction must be counseled that additional treatment such as triple arthrodesis may eventually be required.

REFERENCES

1. Malerba F, De Marchi F. Calcaneal osteotomies. *Foot Ankle Clin.* 2005;10(3):523-540, vii.
2. Sammarco GJ, Taylor R. Combined calcaneal and metatarsal osteotomies for the treatment of cavus foot. *Foot Ankle Clin.* 2001;6(3):533-543, vii.
3. Shereff MJ. Radiographic analysis of the foot and ankle. In: Jahss MH, ed. *Disorders of the Foot.* 2nd ed. WB Saunders; 1990:91-108.
4. Younger AS, Hansen ST Jr. Adult cavovarus foot. *J Am Acad Orthop Surg.* 2005;13(5):302-315.
5. Deben SE, Pomeroy GC. Subtle cavus foot: diagnosis and management. *J Am Acad Orthop Surg.* 2014;22(8):512-520.
6. VanValkenburg S, Hsu RY, Palmer DS, Blankenhorn B, Den Hartog BD, DiGiovanni CW. Neurologic deficit associated with lateralizing calcaneal osteotomy for cavovarus foot correction. *Foot Ankle Int.* 2016;37(10):1106-1112.
7. Walls RJ, Chan JY, Ellis SJ. A case of acute tarsal tunnel syndrome following lateralizing calcaneal osteotomy. *Foot Ankle Surg.* 2015;21(1):e1-e5.
8. Krause FG, Pohl MJ, Penner MJ, Younger AS. Tibial nerve palsy associated with lateralizing calcaneal osteotomy: case reviews and technical tip. *Foot Ankle Int.* 2009;30(3):258-261.
9. Cody EA, Greditzer HG IV, Macmahon A, Burket JC, Sofka CM, Ellis SJ. Effects on the tarsal tunnel following Malerba Z-type osteotomy compared to standard lateralizing calcaneal osteotomy. *Foot Ankle Int.* 2016;37(9):1017-1022.
10. Bruce BG, Bariteau JT, Evangelista PE, Arcuri D, Sandusky M, DiGiovanni CW. The effect of medial and lateral calcaneal osteotomies on the tarsal tunnel. *Foot Ankle Int.* 2014;35(4):383-388.

47 Reconstruction in Charcot-Marie-Tooth Disease

Norman Espinosa, Anish R. Kadakia, and Georg C. Klammer

INTRODUCTION

Among all hereditary neuromuscular disorders, Charcot-Marie-Tooth (CMT) is the most common with a prevalence estimated to be 4 individuals in every 10,000, which results in 200,000 cases in the European Union. In the United States, 1 in every 2,500 is affected.[1] Based on these data, almost 3 million people worldwide are affected by the disease. The disease is named after two French and one British scientist who were first to describe it.

Clinical Phenotype

Charcot-Marie-Tooth represents a genetically heterogenous disorder with a common clinical phenotype including distal predominance of limb-muscle wasting, weakness, and sensory impairment as well as a distal to proximal progression over time (Fig. 47.1).[2] This phenotype is finally the result of an axonal degenerative process that mainly involves the largest and longest fibers leading to a motor-sensory neuropathy. While CMT reveals multiple genotypes, the phenotypic expression of the disease reveals two clinical presentations: a cavovarus foot deformity and variable degree of muscle imbalance resulting in a nonplantigrade foot deformity. The nonplantigrade foot deformity itself is the result of an imbalance between agonists and antagonists and extra-recruitment of active muscle units in order to compensate.

Symptom onset typically occurs in the first or second decade of life and is continuous with a slow progressive character. The clinical presentation is variable among all patients and can often be attributed to the muscular condition. Due to this variability, every patient needs a precise preoperative assessment in order to tailor a proper treatment strategy.

Pathophysiology

One of the intriguing findings in CMT is its progressive alteration of foot geometry, which frequently starts with plantarflexion of the first metatarsal. One of the reasons for this early geometric change is secondary to weakness of the tibialis anterior (ATT) muscle unit, which is overpowered by a relatively stronger peroneus longus (PL) muscle.[3,4] As a result, the forefoot moves into pronation and forces the hindfoot to supinate or to alter into varus. This supination at the hindfoot is accelerated by the fact that the strong invertors (tibialis posterior muscle: PTT) are overpowering the evertors. Once supination or varus has taken place at the hindfoot, the triceps surae starts to act as an additional deforming force due to its medialized pulling vector (Fig. 47.1A).

During walking, the weak ATT will be compensated by the extensor hallucis longus (EHL) and extensors digitorum longus, which in turn cause clawing of the greater and lesser toes (Fig. 47.1B). This effect, in addition, promotes further plantarflexion of the first metatarsal.

While in the beginning stages of CMT, the deformity might be flexible as a whole, prolonged duration of the disease will end up in a rigid deformity (Fig. 47.1C and D). This includes an external rotation of the ankle unit (talus, tibia, fibula) and internal rotation, plantarflexion, adduction, and inversion of the remaining bones in relation to the talus.[4] Equinus can be present but is not a main characteristic in patients with CMT (Fig. 47.1A through E).

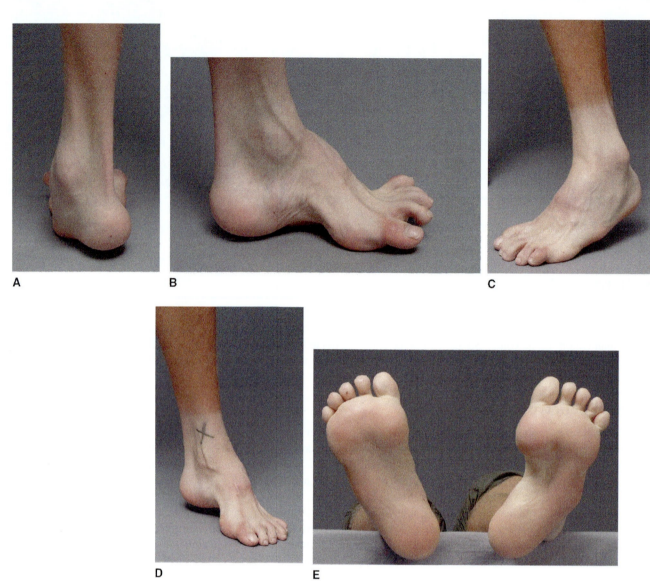

FIGURE 47.1 **A.** Depicted is the photograph of the left hindfoot in a 34-year-old male patient suffering from Charcot-Marie-Tooth disease. The hindfoot is fixed in varus. In addition, the heel is positioned in equinus, making it impossible to touch ground. Please note: the pulling vector of the Achilles tendon is medialized and acts as an additional invertor. **B.** Shown is the medial aspect of the same patient presented in **(A)**. The first ray is plantarflexed. The plantar fascia is short and contracted and the longitudinal arch elevated. Please note: the lesser toes are clawed. **C.** On the anterolateral aspect, it is visible how prominent the fibular tip has become due to the increased inversion of the hindfoot. **D.** Again, as depicted in **(B)**, the plantarflexion of the first ray becomes visible as well as the equinus position. Please note: the remarkable atrophy of the lower leg muscles. **E.** Direct view onto the plantar aspect of the left foot. The midfoot area is adducted. The contraction of the plantar fascia is verified.

Primary Goals of Treatment

The primary goals of treatment are as follows[4]:

- Restoring a stable and plantigrade foot and ankle
- Relief of pain
- Improvement of shoe wear
- Better balance control at standing and walking

INDICATIONS

The indication for any surgery in a patient with CMT disease depends on the amount of subjective disability reported by the patient.

Unfortunately, there is no information available in the literature when to embark on surgery. Most patients present with a huge delay, at a stage, when pain, functional impairment, and loss of quality of life have become predominant.

Many CMT patient may have tried braces, which could have helped them. But, when no plantigrade foot can be achieved and pain persists, surgery may be warranted.

An early intervention may prevent or halt certain progression of deformities and could reduce impairment, but in younger patients, it would be more preferable to choose an incremental strategy rather than to apply an extensile surgery.

- Failed conservative treatment
- Flexible and not arthritic deformity that would allow for a joint preserving approach
- Major impairment of daily activities
- Arthritic deformity that would allow correction through arthrodesis

CONTRAINDICATIONS

- Deformities, which are well corrected and molded in braces and/or orthotics may obviate the need for surgery
- Precarious skin conditions
- Infection
- Impaired peripheral arterial perfusion
- Diabetic syndrome

PREOPERATIVE PLANNING

History

The preoperative assessment starts with a thorough history of the patient's complaints.[5] Essential questions refer to the age of onset of deformity and disease and whether it is progressive or not. Pain can be caused by neuropathy itself or due to biomechanical alterations, which in turn results in physical overload of certain skeletal areas within the foot.

In addition, patients should be asked about a neurological assessment and, if done so, what type of CMT has been identified. In cases of uncertain diagnosis, genetic testing is of advantage to distinguish between an idiopathic cavovarus foot and CMT foot. A dynamic electromyogram can be helpful when planning muscle-tendon transfers.

Examination

Physical examination is always done with a full appreciation of the entire patient, with special focus on the lower limb region (from the pelvis to the foot). The patient is visually inspected under static (standing and sitting) as well as dynamic (walking) conditions. Observations of any atrophy of the lower limbs should be noted.

The axis of the hindfoot (intersection of the Achilles tendon with the calcaneal tuberosity) and the position of the hindfoot in relation to the mid- and forefoot are assessed. Medial rotation of the forefoot in relation to the hindfoot may indicate contracted soft tissues (Fig. 47.1A and B). Any fixed plantarflexion of the first ray should be assessed in the frontal plane (Fig. 47.1B). During walking, compensatory recruitment of the long hallux and lesser toe extensors in the presence of a weak ATT should be noted. The amount of active dorsiflexion is assessed by this method. If so, the physician should verify whether there are any lesser toe deformities present. When patients wear braces, it could be of interest to test what kind of correction is offered by those means. Thus, it is helpful to watch the patient walking with and without their orthosis to estimate the disability.

Plantar foot sensation can be tested by means of a Semmes-Weinstein monofilament, tuning fork, or pin prick.

In the presence of gait impairment, a Rhomberg test and toe proprioception may help to identify the contribution of sensory dysfunction. Additionally, the reflexes of the lower leg should be examined.[6]

Muscle strength can be assessed by means of the Medical Research Council (MRC) manual motor testing.[7] The scale starts at its lowest value of 0 (no strength) and rises up to its highest value

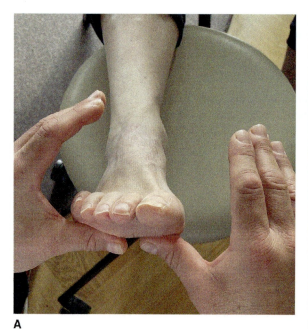 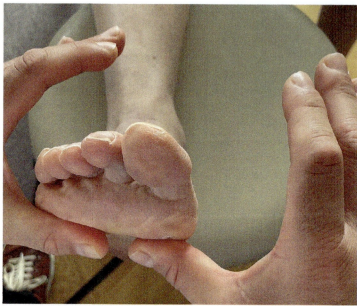

FIGURE 47.2 A. Depicted is how to clinically assess the "hyperactivity" of the first ray. The examiner starts with the right thumb under the right metatarsal head (and vice versa for the opposite foot) while supporting the second through fifth metatarsal heads with the left hand. **B.** The patient is then asked to forcefully plantarflex the foot. In patients with a hyperactivity of the peroneus longus muscle, the first ray becomes significantly plantarflexed in relation to the others and the forefoot starts to pronate.

of 5 (full strength). In order to assess any muscular imbalance, it is recommended to test every agonist and antagonist unit. However, it is important to be aware that the cavovarus deformity of the foot may impair proper evaluation of the individual muscle units.[8,9] Subtle dorsiflexion weakness is better assessed by upright heel walking than in a sitting position.

If there are deforming muscle forces present, it is important to figure out whether it would make sense to transfer them in order to improve sites where weak or paralyzed muscles exist. A muscle transfer results in loss of 1 to 2 MRC grades.[4] Therefore, a muscle, which is considered to be dynamically transferred, should not be less than MRC grade 4. When tenodesis is planned, that is, a rigid nondynamic fixation, the grade of muscle strength becomes irrelevant. Thus, in those specific cases, this rule is of no importance.

Specific Tests

- According to the Consensus Group Statement by members of the CMT Association,[6] the ATT can be tested as follows:
  - Foot hold in slight plantarflexion. Metatarsophalangeal joints locked by hands of examiner. Active dorsiflexion of the ankle.
- As described by Vienne et al,[10] the activity and force of the PL can be assessed as follows:
  - Foot hold in neutral position. The examiner places his/her thumbs underneath the first metatarsal head and second through fifth metatarsal heads. Active plantarflexion of the ankle. Pronation of the foot, that is, a remarkable plantarflexion of the first ray in relation to the other metatarsals indicates a powerful PL muscle (Fig. 47.2A and B).

When planning a correction of cavovarus in CMT patients, the corrective potential of the hindfoot varus needs to be evaluated properly. This is absolutely mandatory, because this reduction potential also dictates surgical strategy. However, this can be difficult to ascertain. Due to the altered anatomical structures of the foot and ankle in CMT, it might not be possible to correct the varus into neutral. This is specifically the case in rigid deformities.[9] In addition, any contracture of soft tissues may impair proper reduction as well.

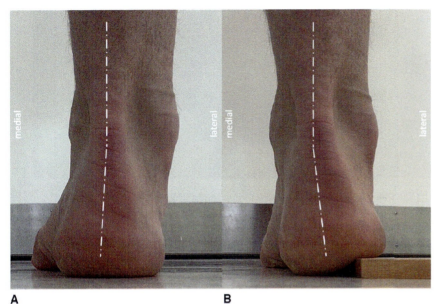

FIGURE 47.3 The image represents the technique of how to perform the Coleman block test. A hyperflexed first ray pushes the hindfoot into varus upon weight bearing (forefoot-driven hindfoot varus **(A)**). In the Coleman block test **(B)**, a wood block is placed underneath the heal and the lateral border of the foot while the medial rays (first to third) are left hanging over the medial border of the block. On full weight bearing, this allows the foot to compensate for a fixed hyperflexion of the medial rays and thus a flexible hindfoot is allowed to remain in physiological valgus.

As mentioned by many authors, the flexibility of the varus position at the hindfoot can be tested by the "Coleman" block test.[11] This test is crucial to determine whether a deformity would be forefoot driven, that is, flexible or not (Fig. 47.3). However, as reported earlier, due to various reasons the Coleman block test may not depict the true nature of the deformity. Therefore, the result of the exam could be biased and should not be used as the sole test in order to direct surgical treatment.

More recently, a consensus group proposed to test the reducibility of the hindfoot manually while the patient is seated.[6] By so doing the examiner may feel how the deforming forces could be counteracted and whether soft tissue releases will be necessary.

In addition, the integrity of the medial and lateral ligamentous apparatus should be clinically assessed.

Imaging Studies

The authors always require conventional radiographs including standing anteroposterior, lateral, and mortise views of the ankle as well as dorsoplantar, oblique, and lateral views of the foot. In addition, a hindfoot alignment view should be added to assess the amount of varus. Recent studies found a more accurate assessment of hindfoot alignment when using the long-axial view instead of the popular hindfoot alignment view (Saltzman-view).[12,13] This is due the lower susceptibility of the long-axial view to rotatory errors during performance of the radiograph.

On the lateral view of the foot, an increased lateral talo-first metatarsal (Meary) angle, decreased talar declination, increased calcaneal pitch, and decreased lateral talocalcaneal angle can be identified. The lateral view of the foot also allows identification of the break of the cavus arch, which is considered the sagittal apex of the deformity (Fig. 47.4).

Alterations of the talocalcaneal and talo-first metatarsal angles can be assessed on the dorsoplantar and oblique views. Even on those radiographs, an apex in the transversal plane can be identified, dictating the course of surgery.

In addition, a computed tomography (CT), either non–weight bearing or weight bearing, is helpful to gather a full three-dimensional image of the deformity and allows a more precise planning of the surgery.[9,14]

The weight-bearing CT depicts more accurately the deformity under loading conditions. Therefore, when planning surgery, specific alteration within the CMT foot can be better realized. This is of great help with regard to treatment.

Magnetic resonance imaging (MRI) provides an excellent tool to investigate the integrity of the soft tissues (especially the muscle units) and cartilage. When available, it should be considered.[15] The authors use MRI in order to assess the amount of fatty infiltration. The greater fatty infiltration is present, the less optimal the functional result after tendon transfers.

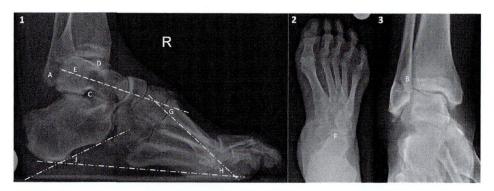

FIGURE 47.4 Typical pes cavovarus malalignment in a 53-year-old patient suffering of CMT as appreciated in standard weight-bearing radiograph series (foot dorsoplantar (1) and lateral (2) views and ankle anteroposterior (AP) (3)). Attention should be given to the following typical findings: Indicators of rotational deformity with external rotation of the tibia: posteriorly positioned fibula (A), increased overlap of distal fibula with distal tibia (B), sinus tarsi see through (or "bullet hole sinus tarsi" sign (C), and double talar dome sign (D). Horizontal orientation of the talus axis on the lateral view (E) and on the AP view reduced talocalcaneal angle less than 25° (talocalcaneal parallelism if angle less than 5°—in the selected patient example even negative angle) resulting in talocalcaneal overcoverage (F). Cavus deformity is indicated by the Meary (talus first metatarsal) angle greater than 5° (G), anterior cavus is depicted by an increase of the first metatarsal declination angle greater than 23° (H) and hindfoot-driven deformity by an increased calcaneal pitch angle greater than 30° (J).

Positioning of the Patient

The patient is placed in a supine position. The ipsilateral buttock is supported by a wedge-shaped pillow resulting in a slight internal rotation of the leg. This allows a better approach to the calcaneus. A buttress on the contralateral side, placed over the pelvis and hips, protects the patients from falling off the table.

The authors always use a thigh tourniquet and do not recommend the use of a below the knee tourniquet. The latter increases the risk of common peroneal nerve injuries and prevents free muscular mobility, which is important to have during surgery.

SURGICAL TECHNIQUE

The longer a deformity is present, the harder it will be to correct. Thus, it would be preferable to follow a joint-sparing strategy in order to prevent fusions, which in turn means that early correction of the deformity should be considered. On the other hand, surgery bears intrinsic risks and patients may be informed that it will take a long time until adequate recovery. Besides this, the progressive character of CMT blurs the future expectations. No one can predict whether the surgical result will remain stable or not.

Any surgical planning in patients suffering from CMT is nonstandardized and should, therefore, be done in an individual manner.

Surgical planning is based on the following aspects (Fig. 47.5)[4,16]:

- Apex of deformities
- Muscle imbalances
  - Mild deformities
  - Severe deformities
- Flexible versus fixed deformity
- Forefoot-driven hindfoot deformity
- Hindfoot-driven deformity
- Combination of forefoot and hindfoot-driven deformity

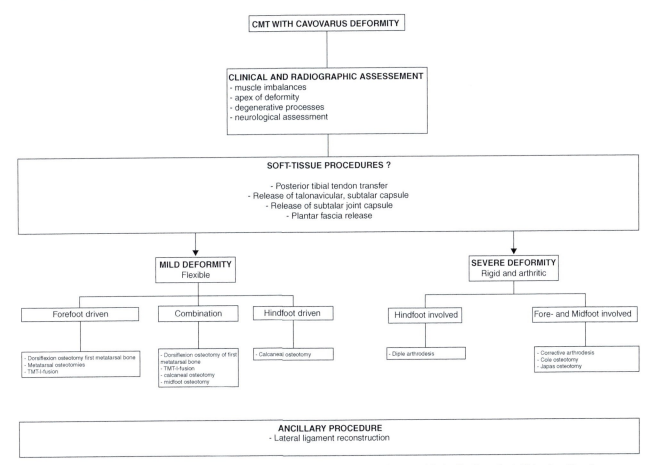

FIGURE 47.5 Depicted is the algorithm of the authors of how to approach a Charcot-Marie-Tooth patient. This algorithm has been adopted and modified according to Kaplan et al.[42] (From: Kaplan JRM, Aiyer A, Cerrato RA, et al. Operative treatment of the cavovarus foot. *Foot Ankle Int.* 2018;39(11):1370-1382. Reprinted by permission of SAGE Publications, Inc.)

Addressing the Primary Deforming Forces in CMT

The posterior tibial muscle with its tendon (PTT) is seen as a major deforming force in patients suffering from CMT. When clinical assessment confirms the PTT as a deforming force, it should be released and transferred.[4,6,17]

- *Transfer of the PTT* (Fig. 47.6)
    The first incision is made medially over the navicular tuberosity where the insertion of the PTT is found. The sheath is identified and opened until exposing the PTT (Fig. 47.6A). The PTT can then be detached from its insertion (Fig. 47.6B). With a scissor, the synovial attachments are released to allow an easy pull-through the more proximal incision.
    The second skin incision is made over the junction of the middle and distal third of the distal tibia. The course of the incision is over the medial border of the tibia. The PTT can be found located laterally to the flexor digitorum longus muscle. The PTT is then pulled through this proximal portal (Fig. 47.6C).
    The third skin incision is made 4 to 5 cm anterior and proximal to the ankle joint line. After meticulous subcutaneous dissection, the extensor retinaculum is exposed. The extensor tendons are retracted laterally. The interosseus membrane becomes visible should be carefully incised in a longitudinal fashion along the lateral border of the tibia (Fig. 47.6D).
    The PTT is now rerouted through the interosseus membrane. Take care to open the interosseus membrane liberally, because the PTT should be smoothly transferred. Transfer from posterior to anterior is achieved by means of a blunt and curved clamp. The PTT is held with the clamp and moved from superior-posterior-medial to distal-anterior-lateral. It is important to make sure that the neurovascular bundle will not be entrapped.

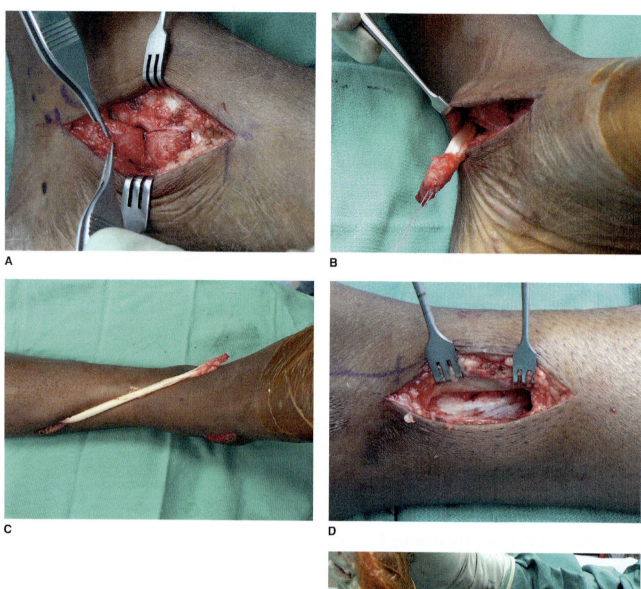

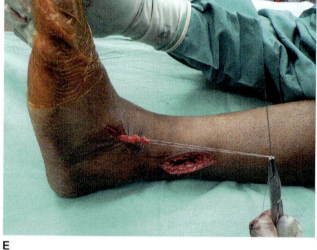

FIGURE 47.6 **A.** The posterior tibial tendon (PTT) is approached through a medial skin incision, after dissection of the tendon sheath. **B.** The PTT is detached from its insertion at the navicular bone. **C.** The second skin incision is made over the junction of the middle and distal third of the distal tibia. The course of the incision is over the medial border of the tibia. The PTT can be found located laterally to the flexor digitorum longus muscle. The PTT is then pulled through this proximal portal. **D.** Through a third incision, the interosseous membrane is prepared. The interosseus membrane becomes visible and should be carefully incised in a longitudinal fashion along the lateral border of the tibia. **E.** A fourth skin incision is made over the lateral and middle cuneiform bones. The PTT should be transferred deep to the extensor retinaculum.

A fourth skin incision is made over the lateral and middle cuneiform bones. The PTT should be transferred deep to the extensor retinaculum. A surgeon should be aware of the fact that muscle force will be lost due to this technique. Alternatively, a subcutaneous approach could be followed, which increases force of the transferred tendon. Fixation is performed by interference screws or transosseous tunnels. In order to provide appropriate tension, the ankle is hold neutrally in 5° of dorsiflexion.

If dorsiflexion is still preserved, the PTT should not be transferred but the weak lateral peroneus brevis (PB) augmented by means of a PL to PB transfer.[10,17,18]

- *Peroneus longus to brevis tendon transfer (Fig. 47.7)*
    A small or long lateral skin incision (depending on surgical need) is made over the distal third of the course of the peroneal tendons (Fig. 47.7A). This spot is found just where the PB is commencing to insert into the base of the fifth metatarsal.
    Subcutaneous dissection is performed and the PB tendon identified. The PL tendon can be reached underneath the PB (Fig. 47.7B). Its tendon sheath needs to be opened and exposes the PL tendon at the location where it enters the cuboidal canal. Two small Langenbeck hooks are used to protect the soft tissues, especially the PB tendon. With the ankle and foot held in maximal plantar flexion, a tendon retractor is inserted to engage with the PL tendon and to pull it distally. This maneuver allows tensioning of the PL tendon. The assistant assures the position of the PL tendon. At this point, the PL can be sutured side to side onto the PB tendon. The PB is connected more proximally onto the PL in order to increase the stability of the construct. The authors do not resect a segment of the PB tendon. It is the authors' preference to use a resorbable 1-0 suture. Distal to this suture, the PL is cut and the stump interwoven within the PB tendon (Pulvertaft technique) (Fig. 47.7C and D). In cases where the retinaculum needs to be detached, the latter should be repaired (Fig. 47.7E).

Addressing Contracted Medial Soft Tissues

With long-standing deformity, the probability that medial soft tissue structures become contracted and rigid increases. On the dorsoplantar view of the foot, this can be appreciated as a medial overcoverage of the talar head by the navicular. Thus, release of those structures should be considered in order to correct deformity at the junction between the hind- and midfoot.[6,17]

- *Release of the medial talonavicular joint capsule and spring ligament*
    A medial skin incision is made over the insertion of the PTT. In a case where a PTT transfer is considered, the same incision will be used to achieve this intervention.
    The talonavicular capsule and spring ligament are identified underneath the PTT and split. The authors use a scalpel to perform this. The talonavicular capsule and the spring-ligament are split in line. More proximally, the medial capsule of the subtalar joint is identified at the level of the anteromedial joint area and split. By using a blunt raspatory, the medial exit of the sinus tarsi is identified. Here, at this level, the anterior margin of the posterior talocalcaneal facet and its joint capsule can be found and split. As important landmarks for identification of the subtalar joint line serve the flexor digitorum longus tendon and posterior tibial tendon. The subtalar joint line is found dorsal to them.

Addressing the Contracted Plantar Fascia

The first metatarsal bone is frequently fixed in plantarflexion while the hindfoot progresses into varus with increased calcaneal pitch. The distance between fore- and hindfoot narrows, resulting in contracture of the plantar fascia. This process worsens when the lesser toes start to claw, increasing the windlass mechanism. Thus, a plantar fascia release often adds substantially to the correction.[19]

- *Plantar fascia release (Fig. 47.8)*
    The plantar fascia is approached through a medial skin incision. The incision itself is done at the level where the plantar skin blends into the dorsally located skin of the hindfoot (Fig. 47.8A). This is done at the level of the insertion site of the aponeurosis.
    The fatty tissue is retracted with a Langenbeck retractor until exposure of the fascia is achieved (Fig. 47.8B). Two small and long Langenbeck retractors are inserted dorsally and plantarly to the fascia. Either a Metzenbaum scissor or scalpel is used to cut the plantar fascia completely (Fig. 47.8C).

Addressing the Plantarflexed First Metatarsal

As mentioned above, the plantarflexed first metatarsal creates a force that pronates the foot and results in a counteracting supination of the hindfoot. This is also called a forefoot-driven hindfoot varus. The plantarflexion of the first metatarsal finds its origin in the overpull of the PL. Therefore, the first step in those deformities is to address both the malalignment of first metatarsal in the sagittal

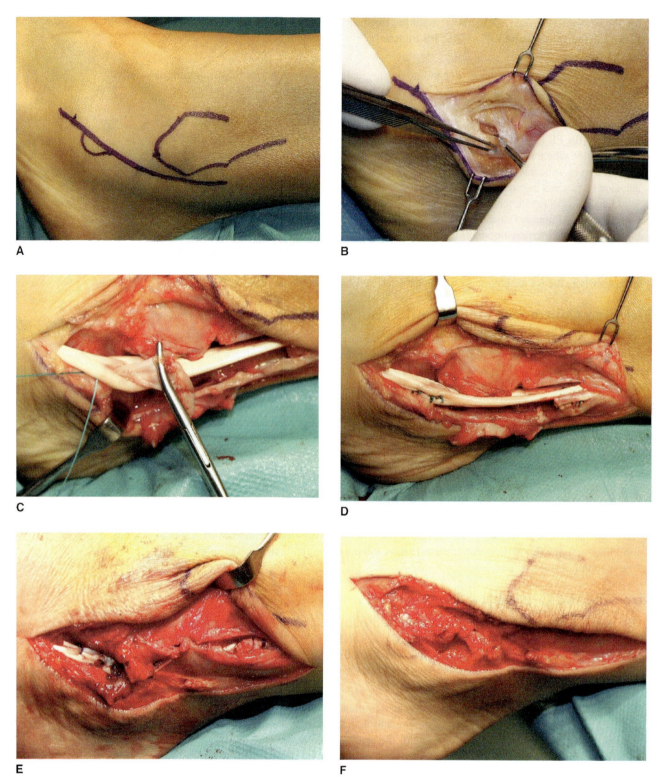

FIGURE 47.7 **A.** A lateral skin incision is made along the course of the peroneal tendon sheath. **B.** After subcutaneous preparation, the tendon sheath is exposed. At times, in order to access the tendons behind the fibula, the retinaculum needs to be detached. **C.** Depicted is the concept of Pulvertaft technique in order to fix the PL to the PB tendon. **D.** Final picture after side to side suture in combination with a Pulvertaft technique. Both tendons have been brought back to their anatomical place. **E.** The peroneal retinaculum has been repaired to ensure proper guidance of the peroneal tendons. **F.** A final clinical picture demonstrates complete closure of the remaining retinaculum more proximally along the length of the fibula.

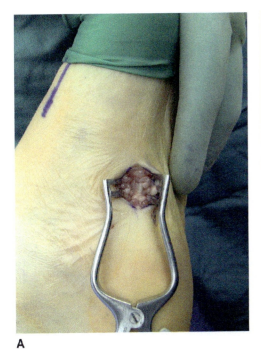
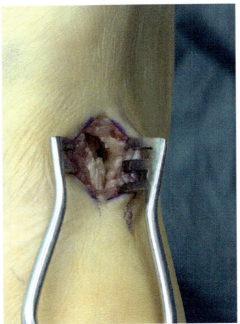
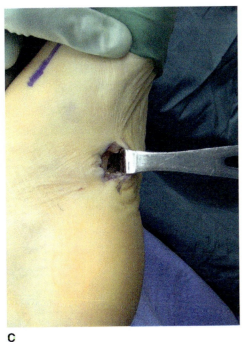

FIGURE 47.8 A. The plantar fascia is best approached through a skin incision between the plantar and dorsal skin of the foot. **B.** Depicted is the prepared plantar fascia ready to be cut. **C.** It is recommended to split the plantar fascia completely in order to provide a good correction, that is, release of deformity.

plane (dorsiflexion osteotomy at the base) and to remove the driving force by transferring the PL tendon to the PB. By so doing the lateral hindfoot will be augmented while the medial column is relieved.[4,11,20]

- *Dorsiflexion osteotomy at the base of the first metatarsal bone (Fig. 47.9)*
  - The authors prefer a medial or dorsal skin incision over the midline of the first metatarsal shaft. Take care not to injure the sensory branch of the superficial peroneal nerve.
  - The exposure is continued medially to the EHL tendon until reaching the shaft of the first metatarsal (Fig. 47.9A).
  - Two Hohmann retractors are inserted dorsal laterally and plantar medially.
  - A dorsal wedge of the proximal third of the first metatarsal bone is resected (Fig. 47.9B and C). Take care not to violate the plantar cortex of the bone. After bone-wedge removal, the distal part of the first metatarsal bone is pushed dorsally to close the osteotomy (Fig. 47.9D).

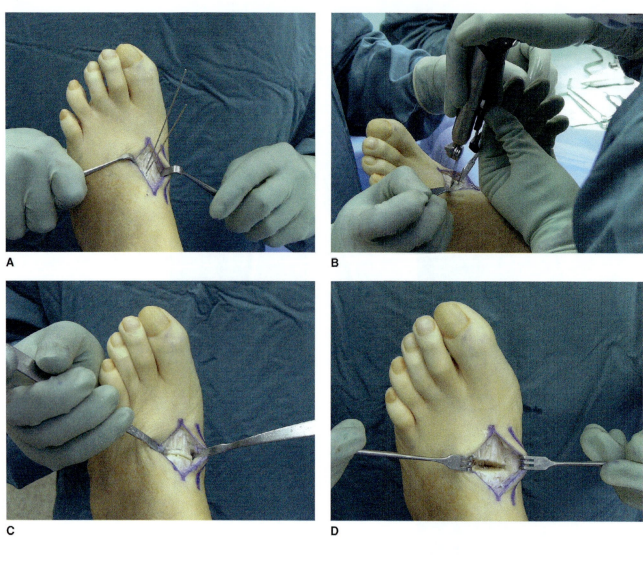
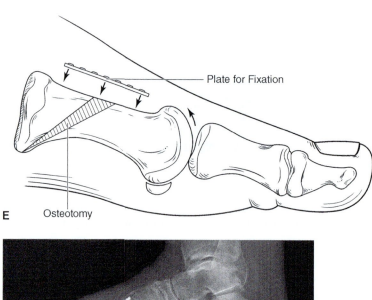
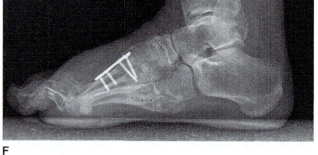

FIGURE 47.9 **A.** For an elevating osteotomy, the first metatarsal is approached from dorsal. Two Hohmann retractors or Langenbeck hooks can be used to protect the skin. The use of two K-wires can help to mark the osteotomy lines. **B.** The osteotomy is carried by means of an oscillating saw. **C.** Depicted is the dorsal wedge after osteotomy. **D.** The bony wedge has been removed. The osteotomy is now closed and fixed by means of small screw or dorsal plate. **E.** Schematic drawing of the elevating first metatarsal base osteotomy. Please note: the plantar cortex should not be penetrated or fractured. **F.** A postoperative lateral view of a right hindfoot after dorsal closing wedge and elevating first metatarsal osteotomy.

47 Reconstruction in Charcot-Marie-Tooth Disease

- Fixation can either be performed by a single 2.4-mm titanium screw or a small 2.4-mm titanium plate (Fig. 47.9E and F).
- It is important to check the correction: for this purpose, the surgeon needs to look from the front onto the first through fifth metatarsal heads. They should be in line after correction. Specific attention is put on the second and third metatarsal heads. If they are also plantarflexed, a corrective elevating osteotomy may be required.
- The combination of a dorsiflexion osteotomy of the first metatarsal bone and PL to PB transfer may correct a flexible varus deformity of the hindfoot. However, sometimes even with those surgeries a residual varus may persist, which then requires a calcaneal osteotomy.

Addressing the Calcaneal Varus Deformity

A calcaneal osteotomy is indicated when an intrinsic deformity of the calcaneus persists or if the varus hindfoot persists, even after performance of the forementioned procedures.

The primary goal is to lateralize the weight-bearing axis, to normalize ankle joint contact pressures and to improve function. By so doing the abnormal pulling vector of the Achilles tendon will be altered creating a valgus moment at the hindfoot, which acts as correcting force.

Depending on the severity of calcaneal varus, different types of osteotomies are available.[9,20-22]

- *Simple lateralizing calcaneal osteotomy (frontal plane correction; Fig. 47.10)*:
  - This osteotomy is indicated when only a frontal plane correction is needed, that is, in slight varus deformities.
  - A slightly curved incision is made over the lateral aspect of the calcaneus, starting 1 cm anterior to the Achilles tendon insertion and ending up distally over the insertion of the plantar aponeurosis (Fig. 47.10A).
  - The authors do not expose the sural nerve because any intervention close to this nerve could result in injury. Using Langenbeck hooks, the skin is protected. The dissection of soft tissues is continued until reaching the bony surface. Two Hohmann forceps are inserted dorsally and plantarly to the calcaneal tuberosity. By means of an oscillating saw, the osteotomy is performed. The saw is gently pushed and released in order to maintain control. The contralateral hand grasps the entire hindfoot. This helps to feel the penetration of the medial calcaneal cortex (Fig. 47.10B).
  - A 20-mm osteotome is inserted to open the osteotomy. Afterward, a laminar spreader is inserted and opened. This allows inspection of the medial soft tissues.
  - The posterior calcaneal tuberosity can be shifted laterally until the adequate amount of correction is reached. With dorsiflexion of the ankle, the osteotomy becomes temporarily fixed (tension band effect). The osteotomy can now be fixed by means of one 7.0-mm or two 5.5-mm screws.
- *Biplanar lateralizing calcaneal osteotomy (frontal and transversal plane correction)*:
  - This osteotomy type is needed in cases where the calcaneal bone reveals a frontal and transversal plane alteration. The approach is the same as illustrated in section A. The difference lies in the resection of a lateral bony wedge. This allows not only a shift of the tuberosity but also a rotation of it (Fig. 47.11A and B).
- *Triplanar calcaneal osteotomy (frontal, transversal, and sagittal plane correction)*:
  - This is the most powerful osteotomy of all and needs careful consideration depending on the amount of correction needed (Fig. 47.12A). As shown by Krause et al, the Z-shaped osteotomy with lateralization led to significant peak pressure reduction in a pes cavovarus model.[21]
  - A lateral skin incision is done. The authors perform a curved skin incision behind the anatomical course of the sural nerve. After subcutaneous dissection, the lateral wall of the calcaneus is exposed. A small soft tissue retractor offers help to keep the soft tissues spread apart.
  - A Z-shaped osteotomy is performed with an oscillating saw. The Z starts proximally at the level of superior-posterior calcaneal tuberosity and is driven perpendicularly approximately 10 to 15 mm in a plantar direction (Fig. 47.12B). After this step, a horizontal cut is continued from posterior to anterior (approximately 30 to 40 mm). Finally, a last cut is performed perpendicular to the horizontal cut and in a plantar direction. Whenever an additional correction in the frontal plane is needed, a wedge can be removed at the level of the intermediate horizontal osteotomy line.
  - Fixation can be achieved with two 3.5-mm or 5.5-mm screws (Fig. 47.12C).

Addressing a Severe Midfoot Arch

In very severe cases, where the midfoot is involved resulting in a very high and distorted arch, a midfoot osteotomy might be indicated. However, this is rarely necessary.

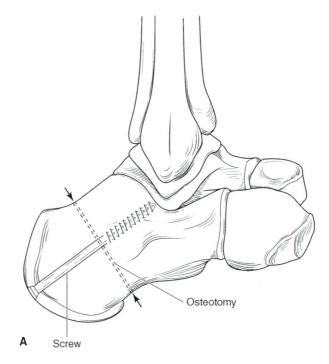
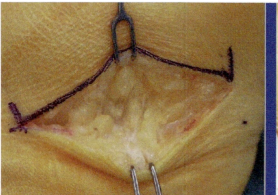
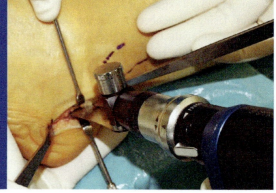
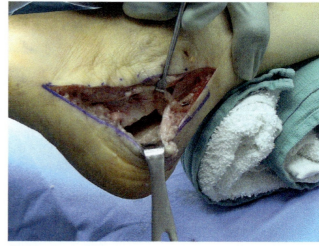

FIGURE 47.10 A. Schematic drawing of the simple lateralizing calcaneal osteotomy. One singe screw inserted plantarly is sufficient because fixation strength will be given by the tension-band mechanism exerted through the Achilles tendon pull. **B.** Intraoperative images regarding the approach as well as the technique outlined in the text. By means of an oscillating saw, the osteotomy is performed. During the osteotomy, the saw is gently pushed and released in order to maintain control. The contralateral hand grasps the entire hindfoot. This helps to feel the penetration of the medial calcaneal cortex. **C.** Depending on the amount of correction and additional surgeries, the skin incision can be enlarged in order to address not only the calcaneus but also the peroneal tendons, lateral ankle ligaments, and calcaneocuboid joint.

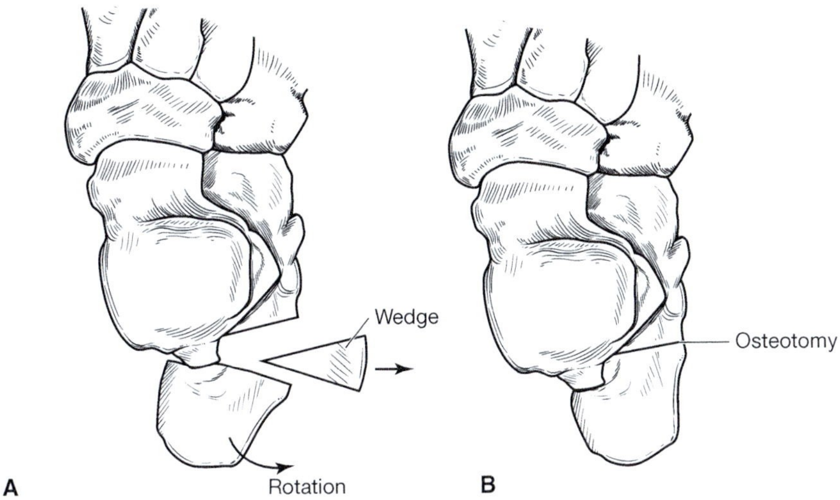

FIGURE 47.11 A, B. A lateral closing-wedge calcaneal osteotomy is shown in this line drawing. It is by its nature a biplanar correction.

The most important aspect in the preoperative planning is to identify the correct apex of deformity.

With an apex found at the level of the naviculocuneiform joints, a V-shaped osteotomy, as described by Japas, can be considered (Fig. 47.13).[23] Of note, it must include a plantar fascia release.

One of the advantages of a Japas osteotomy is the potential to correct in multiple planes. Besides this, it also preserves length of the foot. The Japas osteotomy is a V-shaped osteotomy through the midfoot without resection of a bone wedge. By so doing the forefoot can be elevated and rotated around the proximal mid- and hindfoot block.

In contrast to the Japas osteotomy, the Cole osteotomy includes removal of a dorsal wedge of bone, which runs through the midfoot.[24] As with in the Japas osteotomy, the Cole osteotomy should be done at the most prominent apex of deformity. While the Cole osteotomy is technically simple to perform, nonunion and shortening of the foot pose important risks to consider.

The Cole osteotomy becomes effective in patients who present with the apex of the sagittal foot deformity in the midfoot and should then be done through the navicular-cuneiform joints medially and cuboid laterally.

Addressing the Severe, Rigid, and Arthritic CMT Foot

Patients with CMT in whom a very rigid deformity is present, which cannot be reduced by extensile soft tissue release or osteotomies or in whom arthritic conditions have developed, may need fusions of the affected joints. Those also includes patients with severely altered foot and ankle anatomy that preclude proper reduction of the bones and joints.

Originally, triple arthrodesis has been used to address any arthritic condition at the talonavicular, subtalar, and calcaneocuboid joint.[20,25-27] One of the difficulties is that in the presence of aberrant bone anatomy, this procedure becomes difficult, requiring additional resection of bone wedges. A triple arthrodesis also stiffens the hindfoot. Therefore, the authors prefer a so-called DIPLE arthrodesis where only the talonavicular and subtalar joint will be fused.[28,29] This allows preserved motion at the calcaneocuboid joint level.

If, due to completely abnormal anatomy, an adequate reduction of the Chopart joint is not possible, the authors prefer resections at the level of the calcaneocuboid joint in order rotate the mid- and forefoot laterally. It is important to be aware of the three-dimensional correction.

However, even a fusion needs soft tissue intervention performed at the same time.

Addressing Specific Apices

In some patients, the apex of the deformity in the forefoot is not only located at the level of the first metatarsal bone but more proximally at the level of the first-tarsometatarsal joint (TMT). In those

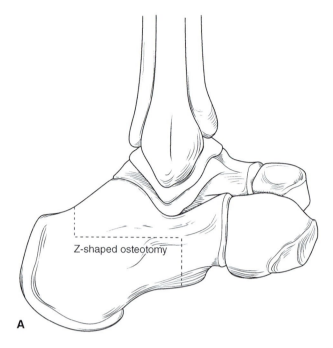
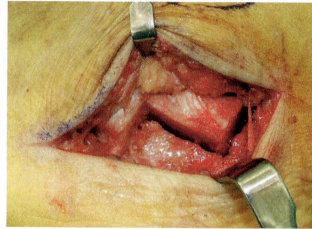

FIGURE 47.12 **A.** Depicted is a line drawing of the concept of a Z-shaped, three-dimensional osteotomy. **B.** Intraoperative photograph of a Z-shaped osteotomy. **C.** Postoperative lateral view of a calcaneus after Z-shaped osteotomy. Please note: the fixation might differ from others because none of the screws runs perpendicular to the osteotomy line.

cases, a dorsal closing-wedge osteotomy in conjunction with a first TMT fusion should be considered.[5] The osteotomy should be done through the first TMT joint.

Addressing Claw Toe Deformities

The claw toe correction is explained in detail in another section of the book. Usually, standard techniques can be used. The extensor tendons can be tenotomized or lengthened and sometimes a flexor to extensor transfer is needed. In flexible claw toes, a tendon transfer can be considered. In rigid deformities, a proximal interphalangeal fusion should be done. In case of a clawed great toe, the interphalangeal joint is fused (by a single screw) and the tendon of the EHL is transferred into the distal metatarsal through a transverse drill hole.

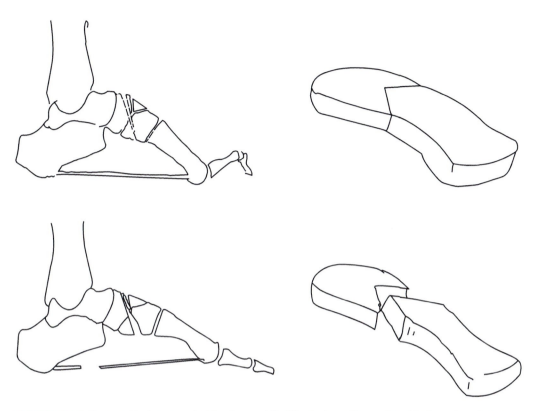

FIGURE 47.13 Illustrated is the concept of the Japas midfoot V osteotomy. As mentioned in the text, a plantar fascia release is necessary to achieve best correction.

PEARLS AND PITFALLS

General Thoughts on Reconstruction

- There is no general rule whether to start the reconstruction at the forefoot or hindfoot. The authors try to identify whether a plantarflexed first metatarsal is present. Most often this factor causes the forefoot-driven hindfoot varus. Thus, the reconstruction will start in the forefoot. Once this is achieved, any other correction at the hindfoot can be better estimated so as not to overcorrect the hindfoot, that is, having a direct implication on how much the calcaneus needs to be corrected.
- Under anesthesia, the mobility and flexibility of the foot and ankle can be tested. This has a direct impact on surgical treatment.

Tendon Transfers

- Understanding the muscle imbalance is crucial when planning any CMT reconstruction.
- Whenever a tendon transfer is needed, it is important to note that the muscle force should be at least M4. The authors even require M5 to qualify the muscle to be transferred.
- When a PTT transfer is needed, the authors very liberally create a large split of the interosseous membrane (at least the thumb of the surgeon should pass through) to allow free excursion.
- While the PTT can be pulled through the interosseus membrane from anterior, the authors use a technique that pushes the tendon from posterior to anterior through.
- In a PL to PB tendon transfer, the authors first pull the PL distally and connect it side to side to the PB tendon before cutting it at the level of the cuboidal tunnel.
- Tendon transfer cannot correct rigid deformities or contracted soft tissues. Thus, they always are executed together with osteotomies, fusions and soft tissue releases.
- Please note that any tendon transfer will need an adaptation by the patient, that is, the patient must "learn" how to use it. This capability diminishes with increasing age.

Plantar Fascia Release

- Stay close to the calcaneus in order not to injure the lateral plantar nerve. The lateral plantar nerve runs deep to the abductor.

Osteotomies

- Always identify the apex or apices of deformity.
- When performing a calcaneal osteotomy, both hands need to be used: one hand holds the entire hindfoot while the other hand operates the saw. This technique increases the surgeon's awareness when performing the calcaneal osteotomy because excessive penetration of the saw blade would also harm his or her hand. Thus, a psychological factor is added to avoid too aggressive handling of the osteotomy.
- When using an oscillating saw to perform the calcaneal osteotomy, the authors do gentle pushing actions in order to cut the bone. The oscillation of the saw and a pushing action exerted by the surgeon ensures adequate control.
- In cases in which the second metatarsal bone requires an osteotomy as well, it is preferable to perform the dorsal skin incision lateral to the midline of the first metatarsal shaft (CAVE: more proximally the dorsal pedis artery). This allows approach of the first and second metatarsal shafts through one incision.

Arthrodesis

- When performing a triple arthrodesis, the cuboid should always be pushed dorsally to avoid any plantar protrusion, which can result in pain.
- A laminar spreader helps to open up the subtalar joint.
- A Hintermann spreader is preferred to open up the talonavicular and calcaneocuboid joints.
- Whenever possible, try to preserve the calcaneocuboid joint (DIPLE arthrodesis).

POSTOPERATIVE MANAGEMENT

The postoperative management consists of non–weight-bearing cast immobilization with the foot and ankle held in a slight dorsiflexed and everted position for 2 weeks. Ambulation is facilitated by using crutches. During the hospital stay, the patient receives instructions by the physical therapist.

Suture removal takes place 2 weeks postoperatively. From the third postoperative week on, the patient is allowed to partially bear weight in the cast (25 kg) and will continue with this for an additional 4 weeks.

Six weeks postoperatively, a clinical and radiological check-up is done. Once healing of the soft tissues and bones is confirmed, a structured, physical therapy program is started. The program should include mobilization, strengthening exercises, proprioceptive training (although of course impaired), and regaining control over balance.

RESULTS AND COMPLICATIONS

Literature on the outcome of surgical reconstruction of cavovarus feet in CMT patients is limited to smaller case series, often only short- to mid-term follow-up and devoid of a control group. Evidence on the natural history or effect of conservative treatment can hardly be found.[30] Due to the continuous muscle imbalance, untreated deformities in these patients likely will progress and conservative treatment often fails.[31,32] First-line treatment nevertheless remains nonoperative including the use of an orthosis (ground-reaction ankle-foot orthosis) as long as the foot can be brought passively into a plantigrade position.[6] Deformities show a high degree of heterogeneity at the time of surgery (eg, severity, flexibility, degree of muscle weakness, phenotypic variability, or secondary changes such as instability or osteoarthritis) and correction may be attempted by variable combinations of surgical steps.[30] Therefore, the appreciation of reported outcomes between case series is flawed. Correction will never be completed to normal. Even if a correction appears complete, plantar pressure distributions has shown not to be normalized in a pedobarographic study.[33]

Charcot-Marie-Tooth patients undergoing cavovarus foot corrections often are young at time of surgery. Traditionally joint fusions, commonly triple arthrodesis, were used to achieve correction. High rates of subsequent midfoot osteoarthritis were reported after triple arthrodesis after a midterm follow-up of at mean 13 years. Facing the fact that the average age of these patients at time of follow-up was only 27 years, this is even more of a concern.[34] It, therefore, might not surprise that in a series of 30 triple arthrodesis at an average of 21 years postoperatively, 77% of CMT patients were reported to have a fair or poor outcome.[35] Similarly poor objective results were found by Wukich and Bowen; however, 86% of patients were nevertheless satisfied at 12 years follow-up.[36] Recurrence of the deformity due to continuous neuromuscular imbalance was suggested even after fusions[34]; however, other authors could not confirm progression over time.[37] Reoperation rates after triple arthrodesis have been reported to range from 36% to 50%.[38]

Consequently, the focus on cavovarus foot correction has turned to joint-sparing procedures. There is general consent that an earlier joint-sparing intervention in a flexible deformity will lead to more satisfactory results and decrease the risk of progression. However, evidence to support this is scarce.[6,39,40]

Tejero et al compared the functional results in CMT patients (52 feet) in whom joint-sparing techniques with those who underwent joint fusions. Arthrodesis was limited to rigid deformities after soft tissue release in an older patient population (on average, 15 years) with more advanced disease. Outcome at a follow-up of 1 year was assessed with the FADI functional score (Foot Ankle Disability Index) and improved in both groups. However, the increase was significantly higher in the joint-sparing group.[40] It would be of interest to see how the scores in the joint-sparing group develop by the time they reach the age of the patients that were fused. Reoperation rates were higher in the joint fusion group (3/29 versus 5/23 patients), mainly due recurrences of the deformity, nonunion, and development of osteoarthritis.

A similar joint-sparing approach with dorsiflexion osteotomy of the first metatarsal, tendon transfers for muscle rebalancing and calcaneal osteotomy in case of residual hindfoot varus was used by Leeuwesteijn et al in 33 patients.[11] After a mean follow-up time of greater than 2.5 years (range 13 to 153 months), 90% of patients were satisfied with the correction, 84% considered their foot function increased, and callosities had diminished in 81%. The FFI (foot function index) improved significantly for pain (from on average 29.3 to 14.8 points, max 100 points, $p = 0.005$) and disability (37.8 to 23.5 points, $p = .001$). In two patients, subsequent triple arthrodesis had to be undertaken due progressive deformity. Longer-time results after on average 26.1 years were published by Ward et al in a series of 41 feet in 25 patients.[38] Beside dorsiflexion osteotomy of the first metatarsal, their technique included PL to brevis transfer, plantar fascia release and EHL transfer to the neck of the first metatarsal, and in selected cases lateralization of the ATT.[38] Moderate to severe osteoarthritis was observed in 11 of the 41 feet. However, no patient had required triple arthrodesis. FFI subscores at last follow-up were 35.0 points for pain, 40.5 points for disability, and 22.1 points for activity limitations (higher scores indicate more loss of function). Twenty percent of the patients underwent subsequent surgery—almost half of those (3/7) an additional transfer of the ATT, which led the authors to adopt the transfer as part of their standard procedure. Faldini and coworkers presented their results in 2015.[41] They were able to demonstrate that plantar fasciotomy, midtarsal osteotomy, the Jones procedure, and dorsiflexion osteotomy of the first metatarsal lead to adequate correction of flexible cavus feet in 24 patients suffering from CMT disease in the absence of fixed hindfoot deformity. They were also able to show that the fact of modest outcome improvement could be attributed to the lack of motor balance.

In summary, the limited literature available does support earlier intervention in patients with cavovarus foot deformities due to CMT using joint-sparing techniques. Muscular rebalancing seems to play a major role to improve outcomes. Compared to triple arthrodesis, complication rates including adjacent joint osteoarthritis seem more favorable with a joint-sparing approach.

REFERENCES

1. Martyn CN, Hughes RA. Epidemiology of peripheral neuropathy. *J Neurol Neurosurg Psychiatry*. 1997;62(4):310-318.
2. Pareyson D, Marchesi C. Diagnosis, natural history, and management of Charcot-Marie-Tooth disease. *Lancet Neurol*. 2009;8(7):654-667.
3. Mann RA, Missirian J. Pathophysiology of Charcot-Marie-Tooth disease. *Clin Orthop Relat Res*. 1988;234:221-228.
4. Louwerens JWK. Operative treatment algorithm for foot deformities in Charcot-Marie-Tooth disease. *Oper Orthop Traumatol*. 2018;30(2):130-146.

5. Espinosa N, Klammer G. Failed cavovarus reconstruction: reconstructive possibilities and a proposed treatment algorithm. *Foot Ankle Clin*. 2022;27(2):475-490.
6. Pfeffer GB, Gonzalez T, Brodsky J, et al. A consensus statement on the surgical treatment of Charcot-Marie-Tooth disease. *Foot Ankle Int*. 2020;41(7):870-880.
7. Krause FG, Wing KJ, Younger AS. Neuromuscular issues in cavovarus foot. *Foot Ankle Clin*. 2008;13(2):243-258, vi.
8. An T, Haupt E, Michalski M, Salo J, Pfeffer G. Cavovarus with a twist: midfoot coronal and axial plane rotational deformity in Charcot-Marie-Tooth disease. *Foot Ankle Int*. 2022;43(5):676-682.
9. Michalski MP, An TW, Haupt ET, Yeshoua B, Salo J, Pfeffer G. Abnormal bone morphology in Charcot-Marie-Tooth disease. *Foot Ankle Int*. 2022;43(4):576-581.
10. Vienne P, Schöniger R, Helmy N, Espinosa N. Hindfoot instability in cavovarus deformity: static and dynamic balancing. *Foot Ankle Int*. 2007;28(1):96-102.
11. Leeuwesteijn AE, de Visser E, Louwerens JW. Flexible cavovarus feet in Charcot-Marie-Tooth disease treated with first ray proximal dorsiflexion osteotomy combined with soft tissue surgery: a short-term to mid-term outcome study. *Foot Ankle Surg*. 2010;16(3):142-147.
12. Buck FM, Hoffmann A, Mamisch-Saupe N, Espinosa N, Resnick D, Hodler J. Hindfoot alignment measurements: rotation-stability of measurement techniques on hindfoot alignment view and long axial view radiographs. *AJR Am J Roentgenol*. 2011;197(3):578-582.
13. Reilingh ML, Beimers L, Tuijthof GJM, Stufkens SAS, Maas M, van Dijk CN. Measuring hindfoot alignment radiographically: the long axial view is more reliable than the hindfoot alignment view. *Skeletal Radiol*. 2010;39(11):1103-1108.
14. Sangoi D, Ranjit S, Bernasconi A, et al. 2D manual vs 3D automated assessment of alignment in normal and Charcot-Marie-Tooth cavovarus feet using weightbearing CT. *Foot Ankle Int*. 2022;43(7):973-982.
15. Zanetti M, Saupe N, Espinosa N. Postoperative MR imaging of the foot and ankle: tendon repair, ligament repair, and Morton's neuroma resection. *Semin Musculoskelet Radiol*. 2010;14(3):357-364.
16. Socha Hernandez AV, Deeks LS, Shield AJ. Understanding medication safety and Charcot-Marie-Tooth disease: a patient perspective. *Int J Clin Pharm*. 2020;42(6):1507-1514.
17. Chen ZY, Wu Z-Y, An Y-H, Dong L-F, He J, Chen R. Soft tissue release combined with joint-sparing osteotomy for treatment of cavovarus foot deformity in older children: analysis of 21 cases. *World J Clin Cases*. 2019;7(20):3208-3216.
18. Burkhard MD, Wirth SH, Andronic O, Viehöfer AF, Imhoff FB, Fröhlich S. Clinical and functional outcomes of peroneus longus to brevis tendon transfer. *Foot Ankle Int*. 2021;42(6):699-705.
19. Kiskaddon EM, Meeks BD, Roberts JG, Laughlin RT. Plantar fascia release through a single lateral incision in the operative management of a cavovarus foot: a cadaver model analysis of the operative technique. *J Foot Ankle Surg*. 2018;57(4):681-684.
20. Dreher T, Beckmann NA, Wenz W. Surgical treatment of severe cavovarus foot deformity in Charcot-Marie-Tooth disease. *JBJS Essent Surg Tech*. 2015;5(2):e11.
21. Krause FG, Sutter D, Waehnert D, Windolf M, Schwieger K, Weber M. Ankle joint pressure changes in a pes cavovarus model after lateralizing calcaneal osteotomies. *Foot Ankle Int*. 2010;31(9):741-746.
22. An TW, Michalski M, Jansson K, Pfeffer G. Comparison of lateralizing calcaneal osteotomies for varus hindfoot correction. *Foot Ankle Int*. 2018;39(10):1229-1236.
23. Japas LM. Surgical treatment of pes cavus by tarsal V-osteotomy. Preliminary report. *J Bone Joint Surg Am*. 1968;50(5):927-944.
24. Tullis BL, Mendicino RW, Catanzariti AR, Henne TJ. The Cole midfoot osteotomy: a retrospective review of 11 procedures in 8 patients. *J Foot Ankle Surg*. 2004;43(3):160-165.
25. Barg A, Ruiz R, Hintermann B. Triple arthrodesis for correction of cavovarus deformity. *Oper Orthop Traumatol*. 2017;29(6):461-472.
26. Santavirta S, Turunen V, Ylinen P, Konttinen YT, Tallroth K. Foot and ankle fusions in Charcot-Marie-Tooth disease. *Arch Orthop Trauma Surg*. 1993;112(4):175-179.
27. Mann DC, Hsu JD. Triple arthrodesis in the treatment of fixed cavovarus deformity in adolescent patients with Charcot-Marie-Tooth disease. *Foot Ankle*. 1992;13(1):1-6.
28. Knupp M, Zwicky L, Lang TH, Röhm J, Hintermann B. Medial approach to the subtalar joint: anatomy, indications, technique tips. *Foot Ankle Clin*. 2015;20(2):311-318.
29. Knupp M, Stufkens SA, Hintermann B. Triple arthrodesis. *Foot Ankle Clin*. 2011;16(1):61-67.
30. Beals TC, Nickisch F. Charcot-Marie-Tooth disease and the cavovarus foot. *Foot Ankle Clin*. 2008;13(2):259-274, vi-vii.
31. Barton T, Winson I. Joint sparing correction of cavovarus feet in Charcot-Marie-Tooth disease: what are the limits? *Foot Ankle Clin*. 2013;18(4):673-688.
32. Sammarco VJ. Complications of lateral ankle ligament reconstruction. *Clin Orthop Relat Res*. 2001;391:123-132.
33. Chan G, Sampath J, Miller F. The role of the dynamic pedobarograph in assessing treatment of cavovarus feet in children with Charcot-Marie-Tooth disease. *J Pediatr Orthop*. 2007;27(5):510-516.
34. Angus PD, Cowell HR. Triple arthrodesis. A critical long-term review. *J Bone Joint Surg Br*. 1986;68(2):260-265.
35. Wetmore RS, Drennan JC. Long-term results of triple arthrodesis in Charcot-Marie-Tooth disease. *J Bone Joint Surg Am*. 1989;71(3):417-422.
36. Wukich DK, Bowen JR. A long-term study of triple arthrodesis for correction of pes cavovarus in Charcot-Marie-Tooth disease. *J Pediatr Orthop*. 1989;9(4):433-437.
37. Saltzman CL, Fehrle MJ, Cooper RR, Spencer EC, Ponseti IV. Triple arthrodesis: twenty-five and forty-four-year average follow-up of the same patients. *J Bone Joint Surg Am*. 1999;81(10):1391-1402.
38. Ward CM, Dolan LA, Bennett DL, Morcuende JA, Cooper RR. Long-term results of reconstruction for treatment of a flexible cavovarus foot in Charcot-Marie-Tooth disease. *J Bone Joint Surg Am*. 2008;90(12):2631-2642.
39. Boffeli TJ, Tabatt JA. Minimally invasive early operative treatment of progressive foot and ankle deformity associated with Charcot-Marie-Tooth disease. *J Foot Ankle Surg*. 2015;54(4):701-708.
40. Tejero S, Chans-Veres J, Carranza-Bencano A, et al. Functional results and quality of life after joint preserving or sacrificing surgery in Charcot-Marie-Tooth foot deformities. *Int Orthop*. 2021;45(10):2569-2578.
41. Faldini C, Traina F, Nanni M, et al. Surgical treatment of cavus foot in Charcot-Marie-tooth disease: a review of twenty-four cases: AAOS exhibit selection. *J Bone Joint Surg Am*. 2015;97(6):e30.
42. Kaplan JRM, Aiyer A, Cerrato RA, Jeng CL, Campbell JT. Operative treatment of the cavovarus foot. *Foot Ankle Int*. 2018;39(11):1370-1382.

48 Salvage of Over/Undercorrected Neuromuscular Foot

Shuyuan Li and Mark S. Myerson

INDICATIONS AND CONTRAINDICATIONS

Recurrence and under or overcorrection are the two main complications of treating neuromuscular deformities. In addition to inadequate or overaggressive prior treatment, complications could be the result of the progressive nature of some neuromuscular disorders and unbalanced growth in children causing new deformities. Using clubfoot as an example, even with prior successful treatment, it is difficult to predict long-term outcomes.[1,2] According to the literature, approximately 1 in 3 clubfoot patients suffer relapse following the Ponseti technique and standard bracing protocols. The relapses have a weak positive correlation with increasing follow-up but tend to slow down after the initial growth years.[3] Although Turco reported that only 14% of patients who underwent a posteromedial release had poor results, with overcorrection accounting for 70% of inferior outcomes, this is likely to be understated.[4,5] These deformities include equinus, cavovarus, varus/valgus ankle angulation, a valgus calcaneus, a flat-top talus, midfoot abduction or adduction, a dorsal bunion, and flexible or rigid toe deformities. Neuromuscular deformities seem to be better tolerated by patients compared to posttraumatic deformities, perhaps because patients have accepted the deformity over the long term and do not have high expectations for what should be considered a functional foot and ankle. It is common to see patients presenting for treatment in late adulthood having managed fairly well for years.[6] Moreover, even though a patient with a reasonably treated deformity can function well in daily life, in most cases, the foot will never look normal clinically nor radiographically. For example, 25 operatively treated stiff clubfeet were analyzed at a mean age of 21 years, and it was found that despite reasonable functional results at skeletal maturity, there were radiographic abnormalities in all feet with significantly decreased foot and ankle mobility.[15] There is no clear explanation for this, and it is not known if these abnormal or untreated radiographic features will progressively put the patient at risk for degenerative changes in these involved joints.[7-10]

CONCEPTS OF TREATMENT

Managing an over/undercorrected neuromuscular deformity is much more complicated than treating an original deformity, regardless of etiology. Nonoperative options such as shoe modification or bracing can be tried if the foot is flexible, but for a rigid deformity, splints and braces are not recommended since they do not have any capacity to correct the deformity and can cause skin problems. In this scenario, surgery is often needed even if the patient does ambulate, and the goal of treatment is only to make the foot shoe able (Fig. 48.1).

The goal of treatment is always to obtain a plantigrade and functional foot. However, the criteria for what constitutes a functional foot varies due to lack of motion in feet with neuromuscular deformities of long duration and unsuccessful prior treatments. In addition to malalignment, severe tendon scarring may be present. This may make it impossible to use these for transfer and tenotomy may be the only alternative. In pediatric patients, maximizing growth potential and balancing limb length should also be considered. In adults, obtaining a shoe-able plantigrade foot with reasonable function is adequate even if the foot is smaller and the leg is shorter than the contralateral side.

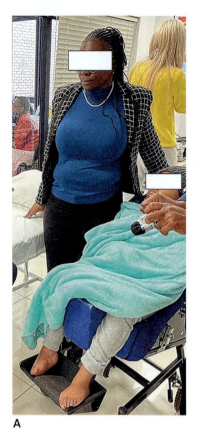
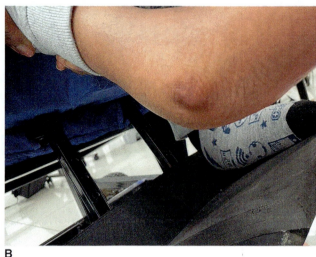

FIGURE 48.1 This is a 13-year-old child with cerebral palsy who is nonambulatory with a healed ulcer on the lateral side of the foot caused by pressure on the wheel chair **(A, B)**.

The concepts for treatment are similar to those for an untreated deformed foot, including correcting malalignment(s), balancing soft tissue tension, and muscle power. However, revision surgery must be very carefully planned with consideration for scarring, poor blood supply, poor bone quality, and limited number of tendons that can be transferred for dynamic or static purposes. Although all of our surgical procedures on global humanitarian programs have to be done acutely,[11,12] if available, consideration for gradual correction such as Ponseti casting for equinovarus or reverse Ponseti casting for calcaneovalgus deformities or external fixation can be considered.[12-16]

Most of the time, deformities are three dimensional and often associated with more than one apex requiring multiplanar correction. In general, if the deformity is not severe and there is some motion particularly of the ankle present, a combination of osteotomies, tendon transfers, and soft tissue balancing is recommended. In cases with severe multiplanar or rigid deformities, or a paralytic foot with no usable muscle power, arthrodesis in a stable plantigrade position is preferable. With the use of modern external fixation techniques, talectomy and naviculectomy are performed less frequently.[17,18] However, they are very reliable one-stage limb-saving procedures for treating severe deformities particularly in cases with no motion in either the ankle or hindfoot, and in particular in syndromic deformities when there are severe rigidity and lack of muscle function in the limb[18-21] (Fig. 48.2).

PREOPERATIVE PLANNING

Management of Equinus Deformity

Equinus can result from prior insufficient correction or caused by muscle and/or soft tissue imbalance that developed slowly during growth. It is thought that in adolescents if the ankle dorsiflexion is less than 10°, growth spurts can lead to shortening of the Achilles tendon.[15,22-24] In an equinus ankle, the capsule and tendons along the back of the ankle joint are all tight, which include the Achilles, the flexor tendons, and the peroneal tendons. When multiple prior surgeries have been performed leading to a fixed equinus associated with various combinations of adductus and varus, the contracture and scarring can be so severe that it is impossible to lengthen the Achilles and the other flexor tendons. Moreover, the quality of the Achilles can be variable, ranging from normal

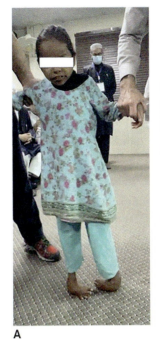
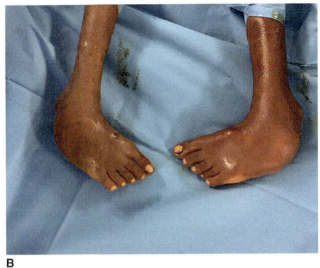
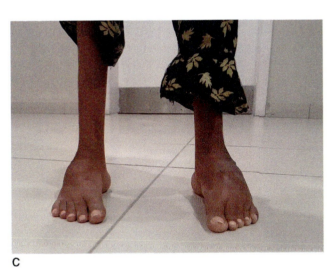
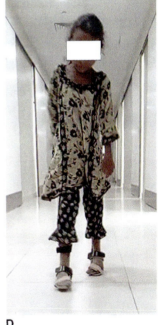

FIGURE 48.2 This is a 3-year-old child with arthrogryposis, bilateral hip dislocations, weak lower limb muscles, and rigid cavovarus feet associated with rigid ankle deformities **(A, B)**. Bilateral talectomies were performed **(C, D)**, and she was ambulatory at 2 months following surgery in a brace.

collagen fibers to ossific scar tissue. If the Achilles is soft and healthy, lengthening while preserving some of the gastrocnemius function is possible. If it is stiff and scarred, it is impossible to lengthen while expecting any meaningful function of the gastrocnemius. In this scenario, in both children and adults, a talectomy may be necessary to bypass the contracture of the Achilles. One must anticipate a significant leg length discrepancy following a unilateral talectomy that averages 2.5 cm, and approximately 3 cm if a tibiocalcaneal (TC) arthrodesis is performed. If bilateral deformities are present, this decision-making is easier since both limbs will be shorter, and leg length discrepancy will not be a concern.[25,26] Equinus deformity in the child should be approached more carefully by avoiding talectomy and/or arthrodesis wherever possible. However, bear in mind the situation of a very severe equinovarus deformity where the patient is already walking on the lateral border of the foot and fibula such that when the foot is corrected, there is actually an increase in functional limb length and the concern for shortening may not be relevant.

Transfer of the anterior or posterior tibial tendon (PTT) is indicated for either a rigid equinus or equinovarus deformity. Even if posterior tibial muscle power is not excellent, the tendon can still be transferred to remove its deforming force. If there is no functioning muscle to consider for a tendon transfer to power dorsiflexion, then a tenodesis should be considered using one of the extensor tendons. This is typically performed using the extensor digitorum longus to simply statically hold up the ankle.

In paralytic or unreducible rigid ankle equinus, an arthrodesis (ankle, tibiotalocalcaneal or talectomy with TC arthrodesis) is preferable. It is important to note that, due to the long-standing stretching and disuse of the long extensors, active dorsiflexion of the forefoot will rarely be present. Therefore, after the ankle is recovered from equinus to neutral, a static and/or dynamic equinus of the midfoot or forefoot may persist. A dynamic equinus forefoot following correction of the ankle and hindfoot can be passively pushed up into a neutral position but will often drop back down into equinus because of a lack of active function of the dorsiflexor muscles. In such cases, a tendon transfer can be used as a dynamic or static force to help correct the mid and forefoot equinus.[27] This tendon transfer can be either active (ie, a transfer) or static (ie, a tenodesis). It is difficult to know before and even during surgery whether these transferred muscles will function actively or work only as a tenodesis since it may be difficult to detect muscle function preoperatively.

Flat-Top Talus Deformity

A flat-top talus is a typical feature of a clubfoot deformity but can be seen as a result of remodeling causing equinus or equinovarus ankle and hindfoot deformities. Anterior ankle impingement is always associated with a flattop talus, and dorsiflexion of the ankle is limited due to the talus or even the navicular impinging with the anterior lip of the distal tibia (Fig. 48.3). Plantarflexion of the ankle may be present even in severe cases with altered motion since the ball and socket configuration is lost and the joint opens as a hinge. Many adults adjust to the stiffness well and do not seek treatment.

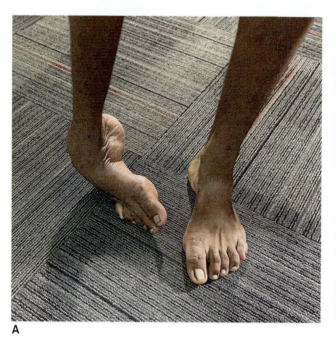
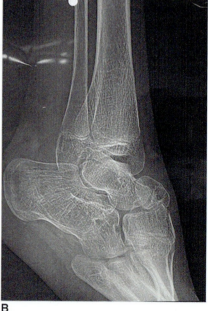

FIGURE 48.3 A 13-year-old with a severe equinovarus deformity **(A)** associated with a flat-top talus and the foot deformity noted on the lateral radiograph **(B)**. A supramalleolar osteotomy with an anterior closing wedge was performed, combined with a posterior tibial tendon transfer, a plantar fasciotomy, and hindfoot osteotomies to improve the position of the foot.

48 Salvage of Over/Undercorrected Neuromuscular Foot

If a flat-top talus is present *in a child* associated with a fixed equinus deformity and limited dorsiflexion, a good treatment is an anterior closing wedge osteotomy of the distal tibia to regain dorsiflexion.[28] This has a similar outcome as an anterior distal tibial epiphysiodesis performed in children with residual or recurrent equinus deformity but is much easier to control acutely.[29] Although a tibial osteotomy will be able to reduce impingement by providing more dorsiflexion room for the talus, one must realize that removing too much bone will not help with dorsiflexion. The goal of the procedure is not to increase range of motion but rather to place the foot in a better position. If a large wedge is removed, the plafond is severely sloped and can cause anterior subluxation of the talus. However, due to the rigidity of the ankle deformity, this subluxation does not commonly occur[4,6,28,30] (Fig. 48.4).

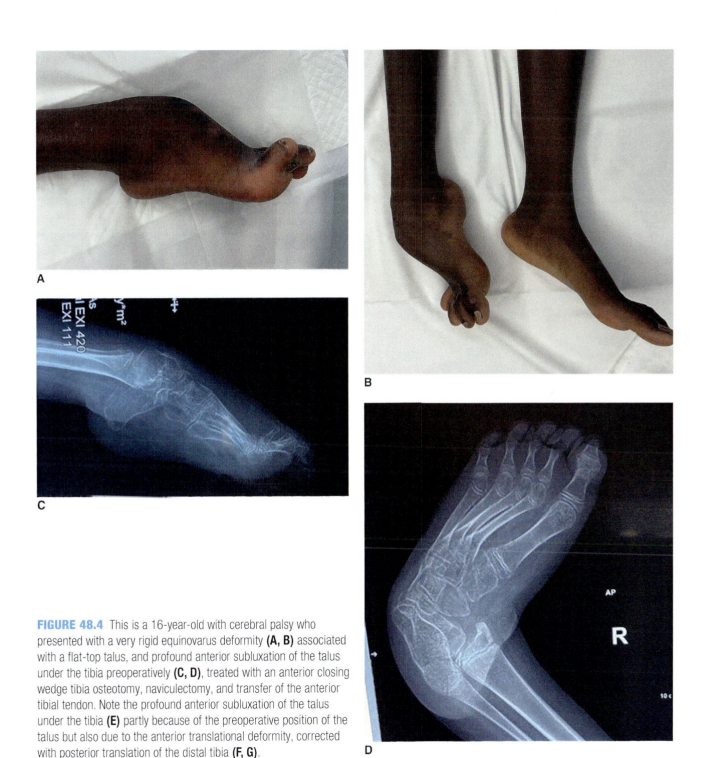

FIGURE 48.4 This is a 16-year-old with cerebral palsy who presented with a very rigid equinovarus deformity **(A, B)** associated with a flat-top talus, and profound anterior subluxation of the talus under the tibia preoperatively **(C, D)**, treated with an anterior closing wedge tibia osteotomy, naviculectomy, and transfer of the anterior tibial tendon. Note the profound anterior subluxation of the talus under the tibia **(E)** partly because of the preoperative position of the talus but also due to the anterior translational deformity, corrected with posterior translation of the distal tibia **(F, G)**.

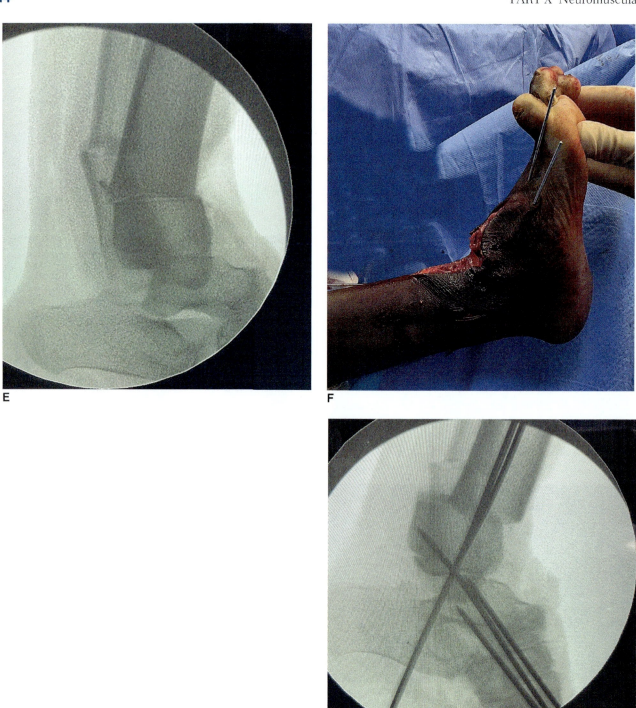

FIGURE 48.4 *(Continued)*

Hindfoot Varus

Heel varus is commonly seen in recurrent deformities caused by a relative overpull of the PTT and anterior tibial tendons (ATT), weakness of the peroneus brevis, and residual eversion rotation of the subtalar joint. Contracture of the plantar fascia and Achilles tendon will add to the development of a cavus hindfoot. With time, contracture on the medial side will worsen and the hindfoot will gradually lose its flexibility. On the lateral side, the peroneal tendons can be torn or degenerated, which will exacerbate the deformity. Treatment includes plantar fascia release, tenotomy or transfer of the PTT, and a lateralizing calcaneus osteotomy for mild deformities, combined with an osteotomy of the cuboid and arthrodesis of the naviculocuneiform joints in the presence of a cavus midfoot. For severe cases that cannot be corrected by the latter procedures or cases with both cavovarus deformity and late-stage arthritis, a subtalar joint arthrodesis with derotation or a triple arthrodesis are needed.[15,31] The decision to perform an arthrodesis may be made preoperatively but is often an intraoperative decision based on rigidity of the hindfoot following manipulation of the foot under anesthesia.

Midfoot Adduction and Abduction

Midfoot adduction is caused by relative over function of the PTT and/or ATT and weakness of the peroneus brevis. Correction of the skeletal deformity is rarely sufficient, and we believe that balancing muscle power is the foundation of treatment. A laterally based midfoot osteotomy with or without derotation may be necessary to realign the foot. The type of osteotomy will depend on the magnitude of adduction and can be done either with a closing wedge osteotomy of the cuboid or in more severe cases a closing wedge arthrodesis of the calcaneocuboid joint. In patients with years of cavoadductovarus deformity, it is common to see hypertrophy of the skin on the lateral side of the foot. After correcting the adductus, even though the foot looks aligned radiographically, the residual hypertrophied soft tissue will give a false impression that the adductus is inadequately corrected (Fig. 48.5).

Midfoot abduction is rarely seen in overcorrected clubfeet but can be caused by aggressive medial release. In children, we prefer to correct the abduction with a lengthening through the cuboid combined with a closing wedge osteotomy of the medial cuneiform although a calcaneal lengthening can be performed even for the rigid hindfoot. In adult patients, the treatment is similar to managing the rigid abduction in a flatfoot deformity. In general, a triple arthrodesis with or without calcaneal lengthening is preferable since it can address both the valgus deformity in the hindfoot and the abduction in the midfoot.

Metatarsus Elevatus

In patients with a relatively overactive ATT, first metatarsal elevation and associated limited dorsiflexion of the first metatarsophalangeal (MP) joint are often seen due to a weak peroneal longus tendon, a strong ATT, and subsequent contracture of the flexor hallux brevis (FHB) and plantar fascia. In these cases, plantarflexion of the first MP joint and the elevation of the first metatarsal head will cause a dorsal prominence of the joint and a dorsal bunion. There is limitation of dorsiflexion of the hallux MP joint similar to that associated with functional hallux rigidus. A dorsal bunion occurs in clubfoot cases when the balance between the ATT and the peroneal longus tendon is lost with weakness in the longus and relative overpowering of the medial column by the ATT.[6,32-34] The elevation of the first metatarsal increases the tightness of the plantar fascia and the FHB tendon, both of which pull the first MP joint into plantarflexion. As a result, the plantarflexed hallux turns into a deforming force, worsening the first metatarsal elevation. Soft tissues on the plantar side of the joint gradually contract and with increasingly more limited dorsiflexing function of the first MP joint. More load is then shifted to the plantar surface of the hallux IP joint during the propulsive phase of gait, ultimately leading to instability and arthritis of the IP joint. The flexor hallucis longus (FHL) does not contribute to this deformity, since it attached to the base of the distal phalanx and plantarflexes the interphalangeal joint, while in a dorsal bunion caused by an elevated first metatarsal, the interphalangeal joint is always dorsally extended to some as a result of excess loading on the hallux. In managing dorsal bunion deformities caused by an elevated first metatarsal, transferring the deforming force, that is, the ATT, is essential. The tendon is usually transferred laterally to either the middle or lateral cuneiform depending on the magnitude of the deformity (Fig. 48.6). Sometimes, the peroneus brevis is overactive and contracted in an overcorrected clubfoot deformity with prior medial sided release. In these cases, the peroneal brevis tendon can be lengthened or transferred to the peroneal longus to strengthen the plantarflexion function of the latter. The tendon transfer is ideal to slightly weaken the eversion (as there is no PTT function) but must be supplemented with either a plantarflexion osteotomy of the first metatarsal or an arthrodesis of the first TMT joint in plantarflexion. As described above, contracture of the FHB, plantar capsule, and plantar fascia all contribute to the plantarflexion of the MP joint. As always, outcomes of treating a paralytic deformity are more pre-

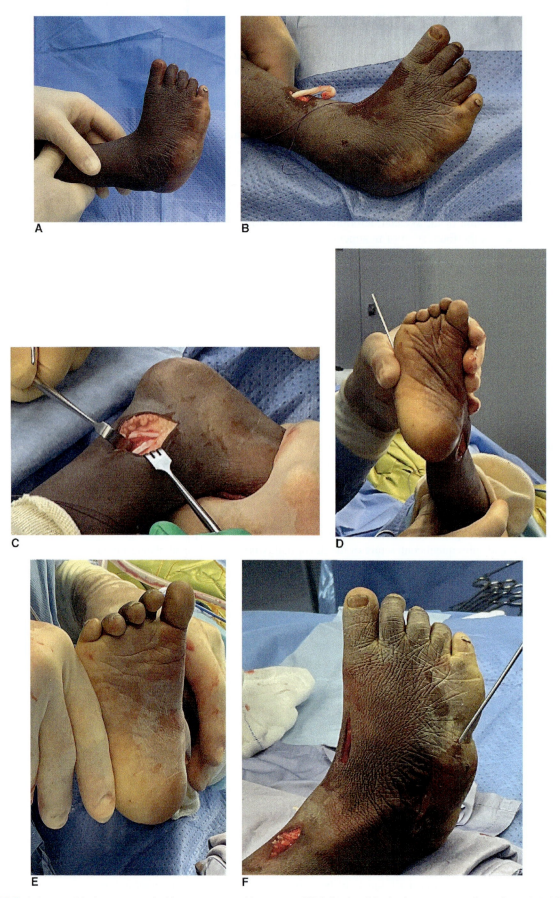

FIGURE 48.5 A 4-year-old who presented with severe cavoadductovarus **(A)** following failed prior treatments for unilateral clubfoot deformity. This was treated with a lateral transfer of the anterior tibial tendon, a lengthening of the posterior tibial tendon, and a closing wedge osteotomy of the cuboid **(B-D)**. Despite excellent alignment, the foot appears to remain slightly adducted. However, this is the result of soft tissue hypertrophy laterally and not malalignment **(E, F)**.

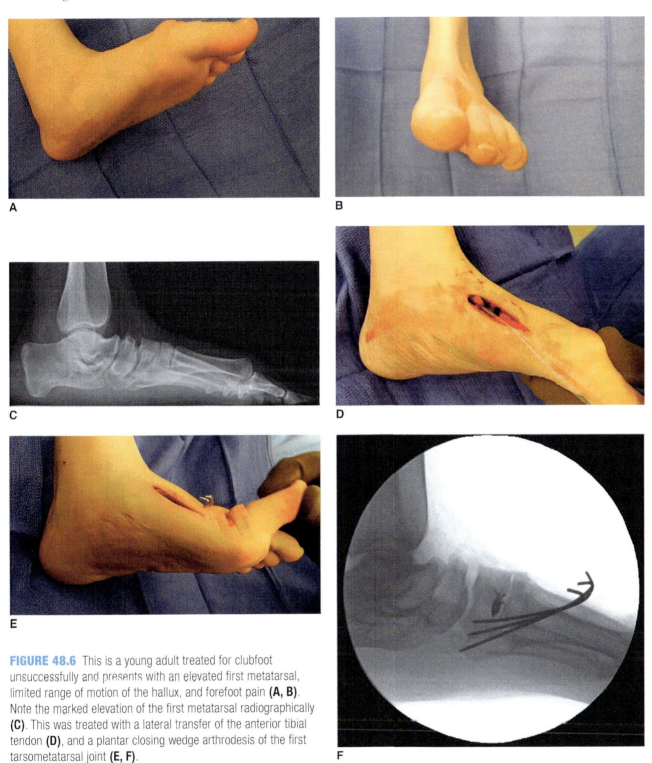

FIGURE 48.6 This is a young adult treated for clubfoot unsuccessfully and presents with an elevated first metatarsal, limited range of motion of the hallux, and forefoot pain **(A, B)**. Note the marked elevation of the first metatarsal radiographically **(C)**. This was treated with a lateral transfer of the anterior tibial tendon **(D)**, and a plantar closing wedge arthrodesis of the first tarsometatarsal joint **(E, F)**.

dictable than treating a spastic deformity. In the latter situation, one should always be careful with performing aggressive bony and soft tissue procedures to prevent overcorrection (Fig. 48.7).

Hindfoot and Ankle Valgus

Hindfoot valgus is one of the most common features of an overcorrected clubfoot.[35] Previous aggressive lengthening or tenotomy of the PTT, and release of the subtalar joint with transection of the interosseous talocalcaneal ligament,[5,36,37] can all potentially result in a hindfoot valgus deformity.

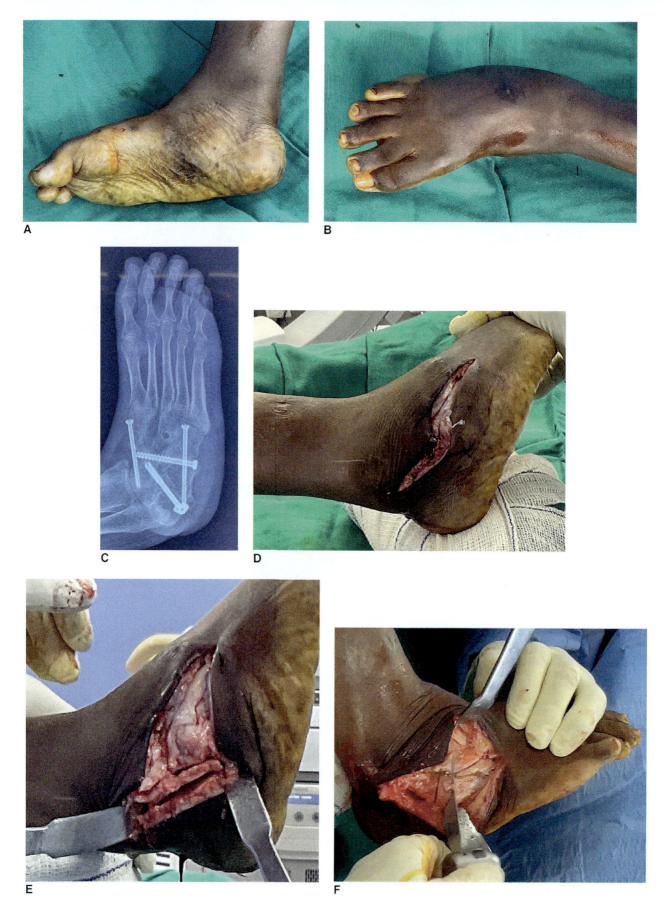

FIGURE 48.7 This is a young adult with spastic cerebral palsy who underwent a prior triple arthrodesis unsuccessfully and presented with a rigid hindfoot malunion in equinovarus **(A-C)**. Following percutaneous hardware removal, an extensile lateral incision was used to approach the hindfoot for revision arthrodesis **(D)**. There were two apices to the deformity, one in the subtalar joint, and the other in the transverse tarsal joint. The calcaneus was first approached as close to the subtalar joint as possible to perform a wedge resection to correct the heel varus **(E)**. This was then followed by a large wedge resection from the calcaneocuboid joint **(F)**, followed by temporary pin fixation **(G)**. The final intraoperative image presented **(H)**.

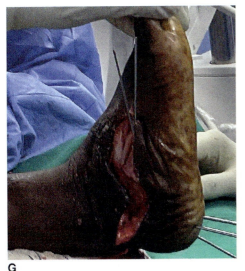
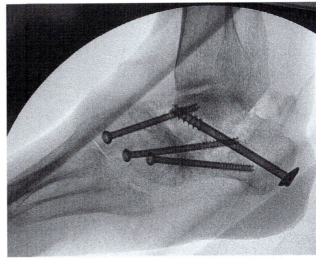

FIGURE 48.7 *(Continued)*

A valgus hindfoot will shift the insertion of the Achilles to the lateral side of the axis of the ankle and subtalar joints, converting the Achilles into a deforming force that pulls the hindfoot into more valgus. Load shear will increase in the lateral compartment of the ankle. In many cases, this leads to valgus deformity of the ankle in children due to bone remodeling of the lateral distal tibial epiphysis. In adult patients, cartilage damage on the lateral side of the distal tibial dome and/or the deltoid ligament degeneration on the medial side can occur.[4,6,28,38] While distal tibial valgus can be associated with overcorrection, we have also seen the valgus ankle as a compensation for a varus heel in the growing child.[38,39]

In cases of significant hindfoot valgus, tenderness at the tip of the fibula or over the peroneal tendons are signs of calcaneofibular impingement. The hindfoot alignment and foot posture should be evaluated for calcaneofibular impingement during stance and heel rise. With the patient in the sitting position check ankle motion, tightness of the Achilles and gastrocnemius, hindfoot flexibility, midfoot flexibility and stability, forefoot supination, and muscle power. Tenderness in the anterior aspect of the ankle joint during dorsiflexion could be a sign of anterior ankle impingement. Sometimes, the navicular is commonly dorsomedially subluxated from the talonavicular and naviculocuneiform joints and can even abut against the anterior tibia. In addition to the ankle and/or hindfoot valgus, calcaneofibular impingement, anterior tibial impingement, flat-top talus, dorsomedial subluxation of the navicular, midfoot adduction, medial column instability, first metatarsal elevation, and degenerative changes should all be evaluated radiographically both before and during surgery. Evaluation of strength of each muscle will help understand the dynamic imbalance and cause of the deformity since prior lengthening can cause reduced power, scarring, and limited tendon excursion. There is often very limited function of the PTT owing to a prior posteromedial release or tendon transfer. The authors have found that these medial scars are very difficult to explore, and it is generally fruitless to try and identify the old PTT. A hindfoot arthrodesis is generally required in the adult patient, but one should aim for realignment and not selective joint arthrodesis. In a child, however, selective osteotomies with tendon transfers are ideal to realign the foot and the ankle. The flexibility of the ankle valgus may need to be examined under fluoroscopy. Correction of the valgus ankle is always obtained with a supramalleolar osteotomy using a medial closing wedge or dome osteotomy. In pediatric patients with open epiphyses, guided medial growth control of the epiphysis is sometimes necessary to supplement the osteotomy depending on age and potential for remaining growth. We use either a 3.5-mm screw into the medial malleolus or a plate that contours specifically over the medial ankle (Fig. 48.8).

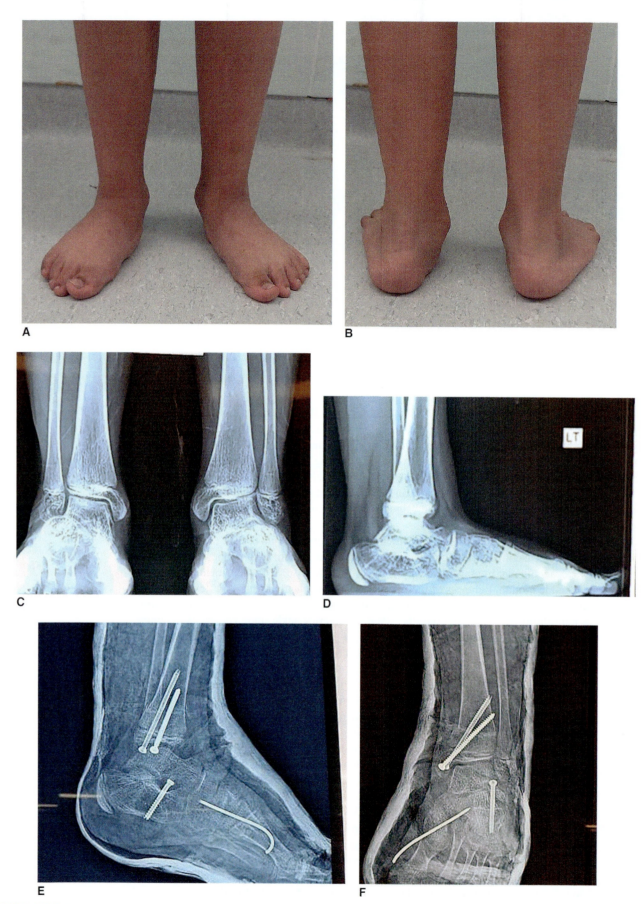

FIGURE 48.8 This is a 12-year-old with bilateral flatfeet who had underwent prior treatment with an arthroerisis which failed. He has severe flatfoot deformities **(A, B)** and on the preoperative imaging note the valgus deformity of the ankle **(C, D)**. It was felt necessary to correct the ankle deformity with a medial closing wedge supramalleolar osteotomy, but a concern remained for recurrent deformity given his age and potential for continued medial physeal growth. For this reason, a guided growth screw was added to the osteotomy **(E, F)**.

SURGICAL TECHNIQUES

Tendon Transfer

In a recurrent clubfoot or cavovarus foot with varus and adductus contracture, the ATT and PTT are deforming forces and the peroneal tendons are weak. The ATT is the antagonist of the peroneal longus and draws the foot into inversion, dorsiflexion, and adduction. Generally, only one tendon (invariably the PTT) needs to be transferred, but in severe equinoadductovarus, both tendons may require transfer. The transfer of both tendons depends on their function, for example, in severe clubfoot deformities the transfer of the PTT may not be sufficient to correct the adductus and the ATT can be transferred slightly laterally into the middle cuneiform and the PTT into the lateral cuneiform or cuboid depending on the magnitude of the deformity. For correction of an equinovarus deformity, it is always preferable not only to remove the PTT as a deforming force but also to take advantage of the transferred tendon as a potential dorsiflexor of the foot. Where to attach the transferred PTT depends on the foot deformity and function. The transferred tendon can be reattached to the middle cuneiform, lateral cuneiform, or even the cuboid in severe midfoot adductus and varus deformities. The more lateral the tendon is inserted, the more eversion and abduction and less dorsiflexion power it will have. If one is concerned about overcorrection in the child, then transfer the tendon into the middle cuneiform instead of further laterally.[40,41]

Harvesting the PTT may not be easy because of prior scarring if a posteromedial release was used. Since it is never clear what has been previously done surgically, we initiate the incision at the level of the medial malleolus and try to find the tendon in its sheath. From here, one can work distally by opening the sheath as far as possible. Because of scarring, one may not be able to harvest the entire tendon. However, it is essential to attempt to obtain as long a piece of tendon as possible for the interosseous transfer. Prior to transfer it is important to assess the function of the posterior tibial muscle by evaluating the mobility of the tendon, which normally has a soft feel with excursion of about 8 mm. Once the tendon has been dissected free and sutured, examine if there is any residual adduction contracture. If so, transferring the ATT, the releasing medial capsule of the talonavicular joint, and sometimes releasing the abductor may be necessary. Essentially, the foot must be balanced both statically and dynamically to avoid recurrence. At times, one may not be able to perform a transfer of the PTT when it is severely scarred and adherent to the surrounding soft tissues. Severe scarring precludes its use as a transfer, and a tenotomy of the PTT is often necessary. The peroneal tendons are also unlikely to be functioning in advanced cases. However, one can perform a longus to brevis transfer in an effort to aid eversion and balance of the hindfoot.

In cases with a calcaneovalgus deformity, there is generally no gastrocnemius nor posterior tibial muscle function. These are associated with overlengthening of the Achilles tendon or more commonly, myelomeningocoele. In these cases, the ATT is harvested as distally as possible and transferred posteriorly through the interosseous membrane to insert into the posterior tuberosity of the calcaneus. If too short, then the tendon can be transferred into the Achilles tendon. In addition to the transfer of the ATT, these calcaneus deformities are often associated with a valgus of the ankle and the hindfoot. As described above, an osteotomy of the tibia may be necessary as well as a transfer of both peroneal tendons into the calcaneus to assist with plantar flexion of the foot. This is illustrated in Figure 48.9 in a child with a severe calcaneovalgus deformity. To begin balancing, the foot an anterior incision is made to detach the ATT and to perform an anterior ankle capsulectomy. These ankles are often in valgus as a result of chronic compression of the epiphysis and a medial closing wedge supramalleolar osteotomy of the tibia and fibula is then performed. Depending on the magnitude of the deformity, the peroneal tendons are then detached distally and prepared for transfer into the calcaneus. The ATT is passed posteriorly through the interosseous membrane and with the peroneal tendons inserted into the calcaneus (Fig. 48.9).

Anterior Tibia Closing Wedge Osteotomy

In cases with a flat-top talus or when the Achilles tendon has lost all elasticity due to contracture and scarring, the equinus deformity cannot be corrected. In this situation, one has to be careful with repeated attempts to lengthen the Achilles tendon since it generally fails. Due to the flat-top talus, no further meaningful dorsiflexion can be obtained. A good option is to perform a closing wedge anterior distal tibial osteotomy. While the concept is to change the position of the foot relative to the distal tibia, this does not increase movement of the ankle joint.[4,6,28,30]

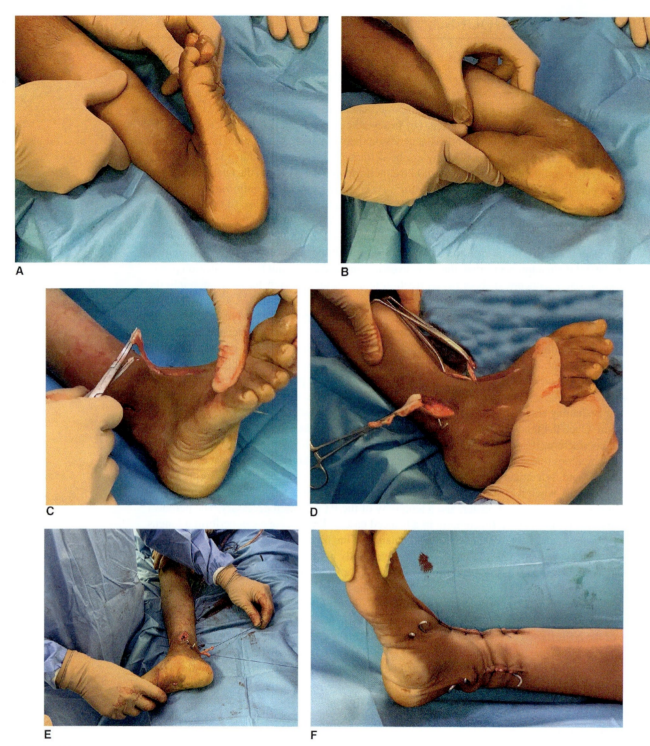

FIGURE 48.9 This is a 13-year-old with an untreated calcaneovalgus deformity resulting from myelomeningocele. Note the marked deformity in both calcaneus and valgus **(A, B)**. The procedure began with a medial closing wedge osteotomy of the tibia, followed by detaching the anterior tibial tendon as far distally as possible **(C)** for transfer through the interosseous membrane. The peroneal tendons were then released distally **(D)** and transferred into the calcaneus laterally **(E)**. The final appearance of the foot is noted **(F)**.

In the skeletally mature patient, the bone cut is made as far distally as possible in the metaphysis while leaving just enough room distally for application of a T-shaped or L-shaped plate. In a child, the osteotomy is performed about 2 to 3 cm proximal to the ankle joint and fixed with two crossed 2.5-mm smooth pins. We start the osteotomy with a smaller wedge, approximately 2 mm thick at the base, and then determine how much dorsiflexion can be obtained to ideally achieve a neutral position of the ankle (Fig. 48.10). It is important to translate the distal tibia posteriorly following the

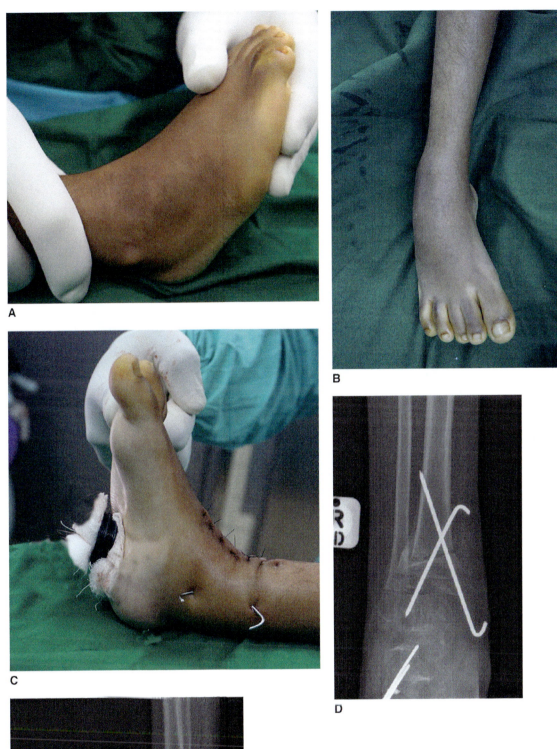
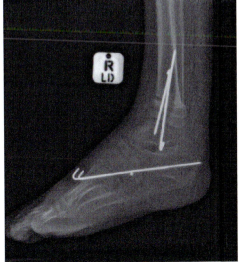

FIGURE 48.10 This child presented with severe rigid equinovarus deformity **(A, B)** following prior attempts at Ponseti correction and no motion was present in the ankle. A transfer of the posterior tibial tendon, an anterior closing wedge osteotomy of the tibia, and a closing wedge osteotomy of the cuboid were performed **(C-E)**.

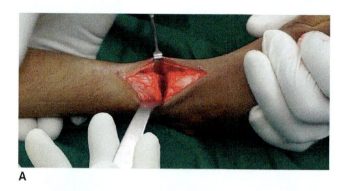
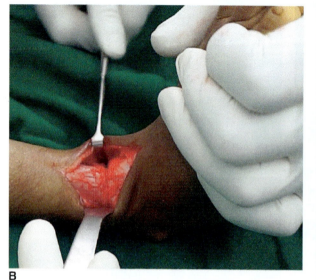
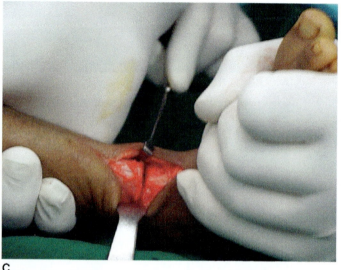

FIGURE 48.11 The technique for the anterior closing wedge osteotomy is presented with wedge resection **(A)**, closing of the wedge **(B)**, and posterior translation of the distal segment to maintain alignment **(C)**.

wedge resection in order to center the ankle and the foot under the tibia and avoid secondary translational deformities (Fig. 48.11). In all cases, an osteotomy of the fibula is also required. Usually, the authors will make a small oblique cut on the distal fibula approximately at the same level as the tibial osteotomy and let the fibular slide across the osteotomy and follow the tibia. The fibula osteotomy does not require fixation. The increase in the slope of the distal tibia (lateral distal tibial articular angle) is an obvious complication of the procedure but very rarely causes a problem with further subluxation due to the rigidity of the ankle.

Midfoot Osteotomy for the Cavus Foot

Many severe cavus deformities can be corrected without an arthrodesis of the hindfoot. The procedure begins with a plantar fasciotomy and a transfer of the PTT. An extensile lateral incision is then used to perform a triplanar (closing wedge, lateral translation, cephalad translation) of the calcaneus tuberosity. The peroneus longus is transferred to the peroneus brevis and from the lateral side a vertical osteotomy is made in the center of the cuboid. An incision is then made over the dorsocentral foot and a dorsolateral biplanar closing wedge arthrodesis is performed through the naviculocuneiform joints, which is very helpful to derotate the midfoot[42-47] (Fig. 48.12).

Triple Arthrodesis

A triple arthrodesis is an option for correcting both severe under or overcorrected hindfoot deformities but is more effective when some range of motion is present in the ankle and can be used in adolescents only when skeletal maturity is reached. In a severe cavovarus deformity, due to soft tis-

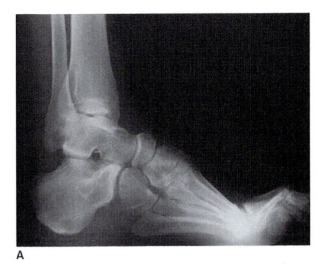 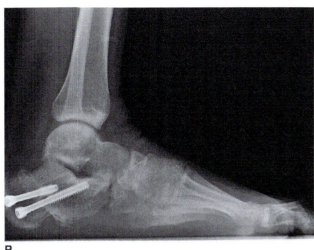

FIGURE 48.12 This is a common cavus foot associated with Charcot-Marie-Tooth disease, and despite the magnitude of the deformity **(A)**, there was sufficient flexibility in the hindfoot to perform the correction with a transfer of the posterior tibial tendon, a plantar fasciotomy, a triplanar osteotomy of the calcaneus, a transfer of the peroneus longus to brevis, an osteotomy of the cuboid, and a biplanar wedge arthrodesis of the naviculocuneiform joints **(B)**.

sue contracture, adduction of the Chopart joint and the fixed varus of the subtalar joint, much larger bone wedges will need to be removed from these joints than one may be accustomed to doing with a standard triple arthrodesis.

For correction of all types of varus deformities, we prefer to avoid a medial incision. If a tenotomy of the PTT is necessary, it can be performed percutaneously behind the medial malleolus instead of over the medial foot. The entire triple arthrodesis can be performed through an extensile lateral approach beginning at the distal fibula and ending at the base of the fourth metatarsal. Beginning with the calcaneocuboid joint, a wedge is resected, followed by débridement and wedge resection of both the subtalar and the talonavicular joints. It is often possible to extend the saw cut through the calcaneocuboid joint directly across the navicular and the head of the talus. However, this may have to be cut separately depending on the size of the wedge required for correction. Once these wedges have been removed, it is often easier to shift the foot into a neutral position. The heel should be placed in a few degrees of valgus, and there should be no residual pressure under the lateral border of the foot. A useful tip is to push up under the fifth metatarsal and cuboid during fixation in order to correct the supination deformity across the midfoot. Screw fixation is preferable, with the size, type, and number of screws being left to surgeon preference. The medial screw(s) are inserted percutaneously, depending on access to the navicular. The authors would like to emphasize that even after a triple arthrodesis is performed, if there is muscle imbalance, transferring away or at least a tenotomy of the PTT is still needed. This is due to the fact that the PTT has a broad attachment distal to the navicular and can gradually pull the foot back into adductovarus despite the arthrodesis of the transverse tarsal joints (Fig. 48.13).

Talectomy

When considering a talectomy without arthrodesis, one can consider an anterior approach to the ankle. This is more useful for deformities, which are predominantly locked in equinus without midfoot adductus and do not necessitate many additional procedures. By removing the talus from the anterior approach, both malleoli can be left intact, which may serve to provide some stability to the periarticular tissues as the calcaneus gradually scars into position. The authors have found that the anterolateral approach for performing an isolated talectomy is quite versatile, since one has the opportunity to obtain a complete lateral exposure, extending the incision distally to include the calcaneocuboid joint and the peroneal tendons as necessary. The extensile lateral approach commences behind the fibula and advancing toward the fifth metatarsal. If one is certain that a TC arthrodesis will be performed, then the distal fibula can be resected to gain access to the talectomy and for preparation of the joint surfaces. It is also easy to mold the anterior tibia and the navicular to include a tibionavicular arthrodesis and most importantly, access to the lateral foot for a wedge resection of the calcaneocuboid joint.

All ligaments and capsules connecting the talus to the adjoining bones are divided, trying to avoid injury to the articular surfaces, particularly in children. It is generally not possible to maximally invert the foot and expose the talus without cutting the calcaneofibular ligament. The main ligament that anchors the talus is the talocalcaneal interosseous ligament, which is easier to cut from the lateral approach, thereby freeing up lateral attachments and subsequently dislocating the foot to

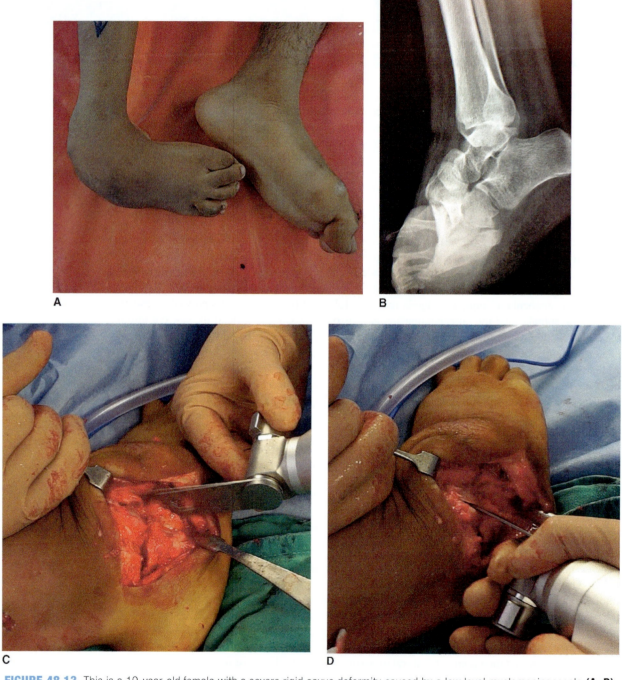

FIGURE 48.13 This is a 19-year-old female with a severe rigid cavus deformity caused by a low level myelomeningocoele **(A, B)**. An extensile lateral incision is used and a large biplanar wedge is removed from all three of the triple joints **(C, D)** and the foot derotated into a neutral position **(E)**. In addition to the triple arthrodesis, a plantar fasciectomy and a transfer of the PTT and a resection of the fifth metatarsal was performed **(F)**.

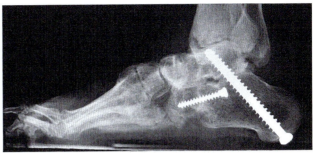
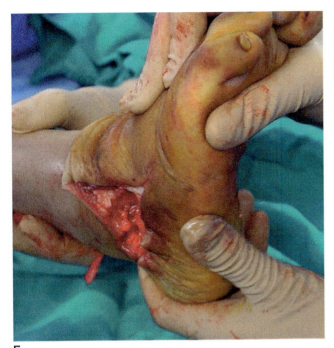

FIGURE 48.13 (Continued)

remove the talus. This is not as easy if an anterior approach is used. After freeing up the lateral ligaments, the foot can be manipulated into more equinus and varus. By holding the talus with a large towel clamp, the medial capsule of the subtalar joint and the deep portion of the deltoid ligament as well as the posterior ankle and posteromedial calcaneal capsule are cut. A posterior capsulotomy is easier to perform under direct vision noting, however, the position of the FHL and the neurovascular bundle posteromedially. It is important to remove the entire talus and not leave any small bone fragments behind, which can lead to secondary deformity.

The foot should now be quite mobile and can easily reach a neutral position without any residual equinus or adductovarus. By manipulation, the foot is positioned under the tibia ensuring that there is no residual equinus nor any tension in the posterior ankle capsule. Division of the anterior inferior tibiofibular ligament in the syndesmosis has been described to widen the ankle mortise and more easily fit the calcaneus underneath the tibia. It is essential that the foot is positioned correctly, and it should be translated slightly posteriorly under the tibia to provide a longer lever arm to give mechanical advantage to the gastrocnemius soleus.[48] Adequate posterior capsular release needs to be performed to facilitate translating the foot posteriorly. At times, this requires additional release as well as tenotomy of the Achilles tendon if contracture still exists. As the foot is moved posteriorly, the tip of the medial malleolus will be positioned immediately adjacent to the navicular and the tip of the fibula just posterior to the calcaneocuboid joint. One has to trim the anterior distal tibia or the dorsal and medial navicular if one is performing a tibionavicular arthrodesis. The latter procedure is only occasionally necessary in conjunction with a TC arthrodesis and never with an isolated talectomy.

In a TC arthrodesis, once positioned, the foot is fixed to the tibia with two 3-mm Steinman pins. The first is introduced from the posterior and inferior calcaneus through the anterior cortex of the distal tibia, and the second is inserted vertically through the calcaneus into the tibia. Any tendon transfer dorsally should be completed following the TC arthrodesis.

The authors prefer a talectomy without arthrodesis since the residual motion is generally painless and functional. Talectomy without arthrodesis creates an ankylosis between the tibia and calcaneus. It has the ability to bear full body weight and is a very reasonable procedure despite limb shortening.[17,18,25,26,49] The decision is based on stability of the hindfoot following temporary pin fixation and the age of the patient, since it is unlikely that an arthrodesis is necessary in childhood.

Removal of the talus is generally never sufficient to correct all deformity, since this will correct mostly equinus and only to a lesser extent changes in the transverse tarsal joints. Frequently, the adduction deformity of the Chopart joints is too severe to permit correction without additional correction at the calcaneocuboid joint to abduct the foot. We have found that even with talectomy and TC arthrodesis, the foot may still drop into equinus if there are no functioning dorsiflexors. Either a tenodesis or tendon transfer can be considered to correct any residual equinus (Fig. 48.14).

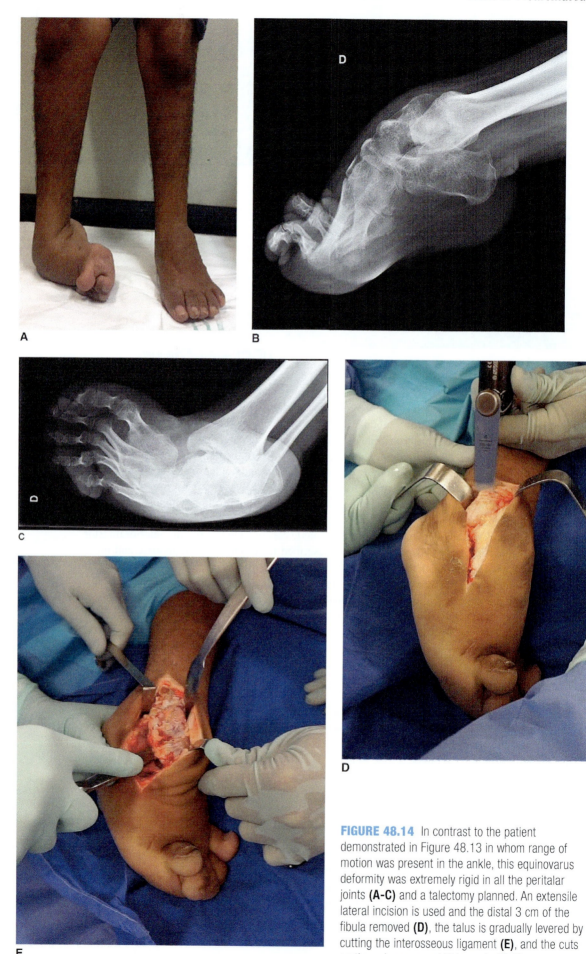

FIGURE 48.14 In contrast to the patient demonstrated in Figure 48.13 in whom range of motion was present in the ankle, this equinovarus deformity was extremely rigid in all the peritalar joints **(A-C)** and a talectomy planned. An extensile lateral incision is used and the distal 3 cm of the fibula removed **(D)**, the talus is gradually levered by cutting the interosseous ligament **(E)**, and the cuts on the calcaneus and tibia made **(F, G)**.

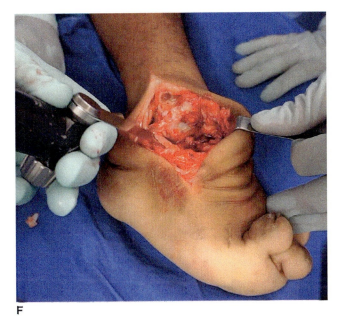

F

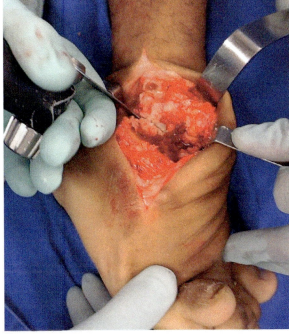

G

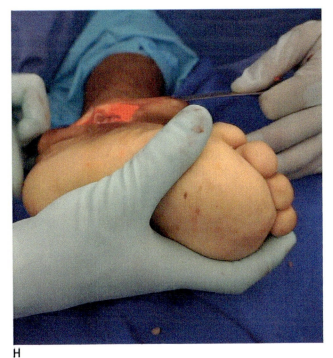

H

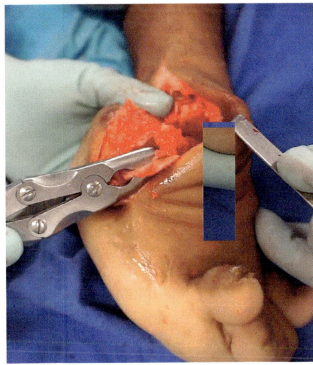

I

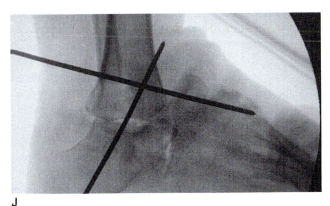

J

FIGURE 48.14 *(Continued)* The foot is then manipulated into neutral noting a persistent adductovarus deformity **(H)**, and a large wedge is removed from the calcaneocuboid joint **(I)**. Note that the foot is moved posteriorly as much as possible and in order to obtain improved correction, the anterior distal tibia and the navicular are prepared for arthrodesis in addition to the tibiocalcaneal fixation **(J)**, noted in the final clinical and radiographic appearance **(K, L)**.

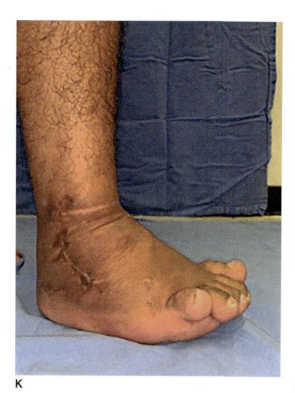
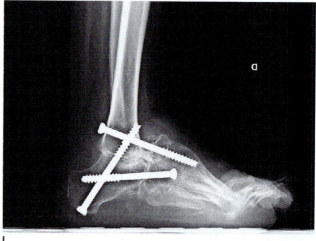

FIGURE 48.14 *(Continued)*

The Use of External Fixation

There has been a trend recently to use external fixation to correct severe primary or recurrent clubfoot deformities. This has the advantage of correcting deformities gently and gradually.[50-53] In severe deformities with significant soft tissue contracture, it can slowly bring the alignment to normal and avoid performing aggressive one stage surgery, reducing the number of combined procedures, compromising neurovascular status, or causing wound closure problems.[54] It is also an ideal treatment for patients with a history of multiple surgeries and poor skin. Although these techniques can correct the skeletal deformity, they are not able to address muscle imbalance. A study showed unexpectedly fair or poor results in 86% of feet treated with the Ilizarov method.[55] Among these, half required surgical correction for recurrent deformity. Another potential problem is the progressive development of claw toes caused by tightened FHL and FDL tendons in gradual equinocavovarus correction. In order to prevent this complication, the toes need to be fixed at the index procedure by running K-wires from the tips, crossing the MP joints into the metatarsals. At times, a tenotomy of the long flexor tendons are still required in cases with severe equinocavovarus deformities.

Additional Procedures

The above-described procedures will correct the majority of hindfoot and midfoot deformities. However, following correction, the forefoot deformities will generally worsen, since a flexion contracture of the toes or elevation (following correction of valgus) or plantarflexion of the first metatarsal (following a hindfoot varus correction) may now be present. When there is contracture of the long flexor tendons as the foot is dorsiflexed, one can choose a lengthening at the musculotendinous junction or through the tendon depending on the magnitude of contracture. If severe scarring is present posteromedially, then lengthening is not possible and tenotomies should be performed. A closing wedge osteotomy at the base of the first metatarsal or a first TMT joint arthrodesis with elevation is used to address the severe plantarflexed first metatarsal after the hindfoot varus is corrected. Vice versa, a Cotton osteotomy or first TMT joint arthrodesis with plantarflexion will help to bring a fixed forefoot supination down after a valgus hindfoot is restored to neutral.

At the completion of the above procedures, the tourniquet must be let down to ensure adequate perfusion to the foot. This is frequently compromised because of the magnitude of equinocavovarus deformity correction, the inevitable traction on the medially sided neurovascular bundle, hypoplasia of the dorsalis pedis artery, or prior scarring around the posteromedial ankle from prior surgeries. If perfusion does not return immediately, apply warm moist cloths to the foot and ankle and wait for 10 minutes. It is also useful to drop the foot down slightly off the side of the table to a dependent position. If circulation does not improve following 10 minutes, we recommend applying nitroglycerin paste. This promotes vasodilatation and may sufficiently improve venous return such that the ischemia is resolved. If not, use a Doppler ultrasound to mark out the tibial artery. If there is an appreciable change at the level of the ankle, open posteromedially and perform a complete tarsal tunnel release. When releasing the tibial nerve and artery, it is important to trace the bundle distally beyond its bifurcation to the medial and lateral branches since the flexor retinaculum may be constricting either or both vessels.

PEARLS AND PITFALLS

- There is a wide spectrum of neuromuscular disorders causing various deformities in the foot and ankle and in general they fall into either a paralytic or spastic category.
- Except for complete paralysis associated with a flail foot, muscle imbalance is always present leading not only to deformity but also followed by secondary soft tissue contracture.
- Depending on the involved muscles as well as duration and severity of disease, there are varied presentations even within the same type of neuromuscular disease and an individualized treatment plan for each patient is needed.
- General principles for deformity correction include releasing contracted soft tissues, balancing muscle power, and correcting structural alignment.
- Regardless of how well the structural malalignment has been corrected, deformities will recur in the long run with either an under or an overcorrection if muscle power is not balanced.
- Recurrence and under or overcorrection are two main types of complications in treating neuromuscular deformities. This is due to a lack of muscle balancing, the progressive nature of many neuromuscular disorders, and inadequate planning during the previous treatment/surgical attempt(s).
- The goal for managing these complications is to obtain a plantigrade foot with increased function and less pain. The principles of treatment include releasing contracted soft tissue, balancing muscle power through tendon transfer, and correcting the structural alignment through osteotomies or arthrodesis. The authors have gained considerable experience in managing these complications on our global humanitarian programs where there is very limited or no access to a full spectrum of treatment alternatives.

POSTOPERATIVE MANAGEMENT

Patients' social situation, ability, access to serial treatments, occupation, and goals for ambulation and other functions in life are other important factors to consider in planning treatment. It is essential that we maintain adequate follow-up for these patients and that there is regular communication between our team and the local host surgeons. One advantage that helps us monitor these patients is that they are able to stay in hospital in many regions of the world for a prolonged period of time until they are ambulatory with or without support. Although we would ideally want to monitor progress with follow-up radiographs, this is frequently not possible nor available. The postoperative management of these cases in underserved regions of the world is very difficult and is one of the most important criteria that we use to determine if a program is feasible. Many of these patients travel from rural regions to an accessible hospital where these humanitarian programs are held and there may be little if any specialized care available during the follow-up period. This is made more complicated by the fact that there are limited fixation options and frequently pins are used instead of plates and screws. Furthermore, we have to ensure that the pins are monitored for skin inflammation and removed at the appropriate time. There are frequently no devices available (wheelchair, ambulatory supports), and this becomes relevant when patients, especially children, are treated, and/or if bilateral surgery is performed. As noted in the introduction, we perform bilateral surgery wherever possible so as to minimize the need for the patient or family to return for additional surgery in the future. In younger children, this is a little easier since they can be carried but still remains challenging. Regardless of whether these are primary or revision surgeries and whether an equinovarus or calcaneovalgus deformity is corrected, as a broad generalization, pins are left in place for 4 weeks in children, the cast is changed, and weight bearing begins with 4 more weeks of immobilization.

Although we are accustomed to using physical therapy postoperatively in the western world following foot and ankle surgery, this is rarely available in underserved regions globally. The same applies to the use of braces such as an ankle foot orthosis. If, for example, a paralytic deformity is corrected, one needs to anticipate the potential, for example, of recurrent equinus deformity and ensure that adequate tendon transfers are performed to maintain a plantigrade foot.

RESULTS AND COMPLICATIONS

The spectrum of complications for treating clubfoot and calcaneovalgus deformities is wide. Revision surgery must be very carefully planned with consideration for scarring, poor blood supply, poor bone quality, and limited number of tendons that can be transferred for dynamic or static purposes. Overcorrected and recurrent clubfoot are two challenging circumstances with overlapping features such as valgus ankle, flap top talus, and dorsal bunion. In severe cases, it is difficult to differentiate an adaptive change from a residual, recurrent, or overcorrected deformity. Therefore, each case should be examined carefully to understand the issue in each segment of the foot and ankle and its static and dynamic causes. Only then can an individualized treatment plan following general rules for correcting deformities in foot and ankle be worked out. We have highlighted a few of the approaches that have been commonly used. There are more options that are not covered in this paper. Procedures should be combined on a case by case basis. In adult patients, some aggressive methods such as an arthrodesis or talectomy can be used for a more reliable outcome since there are no concerns for violating growth. In addition to correcting malalignment, always remember to balance the static tension of soft tissue and power of the muscles in order to achieve the goal of reconstructing a plantigrade, shoeable foot, and ankle with low risk of recurrence. Patients' social situation, ability, access to serial treatments, occupation, and goals for ambulation and other functions in life are other important factors to consider in planning treatment.

It is important to understand that what most of these patients need is to be able to wear a shoe and have a foot that is plantigrade. In the context of our expectations for outcomes of treatment in the western world, many of these results may not be acceptable but are not even considered by the patients to be a complication. Over the years, we have identified an unusual phenomenon that has been confirmed by other orthopedic specialties working in these environments, which is an extremely low rate of postoperative infection. We have tried to understand this in the context of the local environment, since the conditions in these hospitals and operating rooms frequently do not meet the standards for infection control that we are accustomed to in the western world. It may have to do with limited prior antibiotic exposure, natural resistance, or an immunity to infection, but we are not certain of the exact reason to explain this phenomenon. We frequently use percutaneous pins for stabilization and it is quite rare that these need to be removed because of superficial or deep infection. More of a potential problem is wound dehiscence as the result of correction of very severe deformities. This, however, is not as common as one might expect due to the approach to correction at the apex of the deformity so that closure is rarely performed under tension. Despite the frequent use of pins for fixation, we rarely encounter non or malunion, perhaps because many of these patients are children. However, even in adults, this is not a common problem and as a result, we have learned to do "more with less."

REFERENCES

1. Rampal V, Chamond C, Barthes X, et al. Long-term results of treatment of congenital idiopathic clubfoot in 187 feet: outcome of the functional "French" method, if necessary completed by soft-tissue release. *J Pediatr Orthop.* 2013;33(1):48-54.
2. Steinman S, Richards BS, Faulks S, et al. A comparison of two nonoperative methods of idiopathic clubfoot correction: the Ponseti method and the French functional (physiotherapy) method. Surgical technique. *J Bone Joint Surg Am.* 2009;91(Suppl 2):299-312.
3. Agarwal A, Rastogi A, Rastogi P. Relapses in clubfoot treated with Ponseti technique and standard bracing protocol—a systematic analysis. *J Clin Orthop Trauma.* 2021;18:199-204.
4. Knupp M, Barg A, Bolliger L, et al. Reconstructive surgery for overcorrected clubfoot in adults. *J Bone Joint Surg Am.* 2012;94(15):e1101-e1107.
5. Turco VJ. Resistant congenital club foot—one-stage posteromedial release with internal fixation. A follow-up report of a fifteen-year experience. *J Bone Joint Surg Am.* 1979;61(6a):805-814.
6. Zide JR, Myerson M. The overcorrected clubfoot in the adult: evaluation and management—topical review. *Foot Ankle Int.* 2013;34(9):1312-1318.

7. Church C, Coplan JA, Poljak D, et al. A comprehensive outcome comparison of surgical and Ponseti clubfoot treatments with reference to pediatric norms. *J Child Orthop*. 2012;6(1):51-59.
8. Docquier PL, Leemrijse T, Rombouts JJ. Clinical and radiographic features of operatively treated stiff clubfeet after skeletal maturity: etiology of the deformities and how to prevent them. *Foot Ankle Int*. 2006;27(1):29-37.
9. Hamel J, Hörterer H, Harrasser N. Radiological tarsal bone morphology in adolescent age of congenital clubfeet treated with the Ponseti method. *BMC Musculoskelet Disord*. 2021;22(1):332.
10. Mehrafshan M, Rampal V, Seringe R, et al. Recurrent club-foot deformity following previous soft-tissue release: midterm outcome after revision surgery. *J Bone Joint Surg Br*. 2009;91(7):949-954.
11. Eidelman M, Kotlarsky P, Herzenberg JE. Treatment of relapsed, residual and neglected clubfoot: adjunctive surgery. *J Child Orthop*. 2019;13(3):293-303.
12. Li S, Myerson MS. Managing severe foot and ankle deformities in global humanitarian programs. *Foot Ankle Clin*. 2020;25(2):183-203.
13. Dragoni M, Farsetti P, Vena G, et al. Ponseti treatment of rigid residual deformity in congenital clubfoot after walking age. *J Bone Joint Surg Am*. 2016;98(20):1706-1712.
14. Dobbs MB, Morcuende JA, Gurnett CA, et al. Treatment of idiopathic clubfoot: an historical review. *Iowa Orthop J*. 2000;20:59-64.
15. Radler C, Mindler GT. Treatment of severe recurrent clubfoot. *Foot Ankle Clin*. 2015;20(4):563-586.
16. Thomas HM, Sangiorgio SN, Ebramzadeh E, et al. Relapse rates in patients with clubfoot treated using the ponseti method increase with time: a systematic review. *JBJS Rev*. 2019;7(5):e6.
17. Holmdahl HC. Astragalectomy as a stabilising operation for foot paralysis following poliomyelitis; results of a follow-up investigation of 153 cases. *Acta Orthop Scand*. 1956;25(3):207-227.
18. Joseph TN, Myerson MS. Use of talectomy in modern foot and ankle surgery. *Foot Ankle Clin*. 2004;9(4):775-785.
19. Mirzayan R, Early SD, Matthys GA, et al. Single-stage talectomy and tibiocalcaneal arthrodesis as a salvage of severe, rigid equinovarus deformity. *Foot Ankle Int*. 2001;22(3):209-213.
20. Gursu S, Bahar H, Camurcu Y, et al. Talectomy and tibiocalcaneal arthrodesis with intramedullary nail fixation for treatment of equinus deformity in adults. *Foot Ankle Int*. 2015;36(1):46-50.
21. Yalçin S, Kocaoğlu B, Berker N, et al. Talectomy for the treatment of neglected pes equinovarus deformity in patients with neuromuscular involvement. *Acta Orthop Traumatol Turc*. 2005;39(4):316-321.
22. David BH, Olayinka OA, Oluwadare E, et al. Predictive value of Pirani scoring system for tenotomy in the management of idiopathic clubfoot. *J Orthop Surg (Hong Kong)*. 2017;25(2):2309499017713896.
23. Chandirasegaran S, Gunalan R, Aik S, et al. A comparison study on hindfoot correction, Achilles tendon length and thickness between clubfoot patients treated with percutaneous Achilles tendon tenotomy versus casting alone using Ponseti method. *J Orthop Surg (Hong Kong)*. 2019;27(2):2309499019839126.
24. Lampasi M, Abati CN, Stilli S, et al. Use of the Pirani score in monitoring progression of correction and in guiding indications for tenotomy in the Ponseti method: are we coming to the same decisions? *J Orthop Surg (Hong Kong)*. 2017;25(2):2309499017713916.
25. El-Sherbini MH, Omran AA. Midterm follow-up of talectomy for severe rigid equinovarus feet. *J Foot Ankle Surg*. 2015;54(6):1093-1098.
26. Letts M, Davidson D. The role of bilateral talectomy in the management of bilateral rigid clubfeet. *Am J Orthop (Belle Mead NJ)*. 1999;28(2):106-110.
27. Malik SS, Knight R, Ahmed U, et al. Role of a tendon transfer as a dynamic checkrein reducing recurrence of equinus following distal tibial dorsiflexion osteotomy. *J Pediatr Orthop B*. 2018;27(5):419-424.
28. Knupp M, Barg A, Bolliger L, et al. Surgical treatment of overcorrected clubfoot deformity. *JBJS Essent Surg Tech*. 2014;3(1):e4.
29. Ebert N, Ballhause TM, Babin K, et al. Correction of recurrent equinus deformity in surgically treated clubfeet by anterior distal tibial hemiepiphysiodesis. *J Pediatr Orthop*. 2020;40(9):520-525.
30. Swann M, Lloyd-Roberts GC, Catterall A. The anatomy of uncorrected club feet. A study of rotation deformity. *J Bone Joint Surg Br*. 1969;51(2):263-269.
31. Brodsky JW. The adult sequelae of treated congenital clubfoot. *Foot Ankle Clin*. 2010;15(2):287-296.
32. Yong SM, Smith PA, Kuo KN. Dorsal bunion after clubfoot surgery: outcome of reverse Jones procedure. *J Pediatr Orthop*. 2007;27(7):814-820.
33. Johnston CE II, Roach JW. Dorsal bunion following clubfoot surgery. *Orthopedics*. 1985;8(8):1036-1040.
34. McKay DW. Dorsal bunions in children. *J Bone Joint Surg Am*. 1983;65(7):975-980.
35. Burger D, Aiyer A, Myerson MS. Evaluation and surgical management of the overcorrected clubfoot deformity in the adult patient. *Foot Ankle Clin*. 2015;20(4):587-599.
36. Cohen-Sobel E, Caselli M, Giorgini R, et al. Long-term follow up of clubfoot surgery: analysis of 44 patients. *J Foot Ankle Surg*. 1993;32(4):411-423.
37. Simons GW. The complete subtalar release in clubfeet. *Orthop Clin North Am*. 1987;18(4):667-688.
38. Stevens PM, Otis S. Ankle valgus and clubfeet. *J Pediatr Orthop*. 1999;19(4):515-517.
39. Stevens PM, Kennedy JM, Hung M. Guided growth for ankle valgus. *J Pediatr Orthop*. 2011;31(8):878-883.
40. Agarwal A, Jandial G, Gupta N. Comparison of three different methods of anterior tibial tendon transfer for relapsed clubfoot: a pilot study. *J Clin Orthop Trauma*. 2020;11(2):240-244.
41. Bibbo CS, Jaglan S. Tendon transfers for equinovarus deformity in adults and children. *Foot Ankle Clin*. 2011;16(3):401-418.
42. Blakeslee TJ, DeValentine SJ. Management of the resistant idiopathic clubfoot: the Kaiser experience from 1980-1990. *J Foot Ankle Surg*. 1995;34(2):167-176.
43. Kuo KN, Jansen LD. Rotatory dorsal subluxation of the navicular: a complication of clubfoot surgery. *J Pediatr Orthop*. 1998;18(6):770-774.
44. Miller JH, Bernstein SM. The roentgenographic appearance of the "corrected clubfoot". *Foot Ankle*. 1986;6(4):177-183.
45. Swaroop VT, Wenger DR, Mubarak SJ. Talonavicular fusion for dorsal subluxation of the navicular in resistant clubfoot. *Clin Orthop Relat Res*. 2009;467(5):1314-1318.
46. Wei SY, Sullivan RJ, Davidson RS. Talo-navicular arthrodesis for residual midfoot deformities of a previously corrected clubfoot. *Foot Ankle Int*. 2000;21(6):482-485.
47. Myerson MS, Myerson CL. Managing the complex cavus foot deformity. *Foot Ankle Clin*. 2020;25(2):305-317.
48. Hsu LC, Jaffray D, Leong JC. Talectomy for club foot in arthrogryposis. *J Bone Joint Surg Br*. 1984;66(5):694-696.

49. Cooper RR, Capello W, Talectomy. A long-term follow-up evaluation. *Clin Orthop Relat Res*. 1985;201:32-35.
50. de la Huerta F. Correction of the neglected clubfoot by the Ilizarov method. *Clin Orthop Relat Res*. 1994;301:89-93.
51. Franke J, Grill F, Hein G, et al. Correction of clubfoot relapse using Ilizarov's apparatus in children 8-15 years old. *Arch Orthop Trauma Surg*. 1990;110(1):33-37.
52. Paley D. The correction of complex foot deformities using Ilizarov's distraction osteotomies. *Clin Orthop Relat Res*. 1993;293:97-111.
53. Wallander H, Hansson G, Tjernström B. Correction of persistent clubfoot deformities with the Ilizarov external fixator. Experience in 10 previously operated feet followed for 2-5 years. *Acta Orthop Scand*. 1996;67(3):283-287.
54. Ferreira RC, Costa MT, Frizzo GG, et al. Correction of severe recurrent clubfoot using a simplified setting of the Ilizarov device. *Foot Ankle Int*. 2007;28(5):557-568.
55. Freedman JA, Watts H, Otsuka NY. The Ilizarov method for the treatment of resistant clubfoot: is it an effective solution? *J Pediatr Orthop*. 2006;26(4):432-437.

Index

Page numbers followed by an "*f*" denote figures; those followed by a "*t*" denote tables.

A

AAORIF. *See* Arthroscopy-assisted ORIF (AAORIF)
Achilles lengthening, 156–157
Achilles tendinopathy, 377–378
Achilles tendon, 377, 381, 383, 386
  allograft, 485–486, 486*f*
  débridement, 377, 386
  rupture, 377, 385–386
Achilles tendon rupture repair
  minimally invasive, 403–416
    approach, 405, 406*f*
    background/etiology, 403–404
    closure, 409
    complications of, 411–413
    contraindications to, 403
    indications for, 403
    instrumentation, 405–406, 406*f*
    knotless calcaneal fixation, 408–409, 410*f*
    knotted technique/midsubstance repairs, 409
    operative technique, 405–409
    preoperative planning in, 404–405
    rehabilitation, 411
    results of, 411–413
    suture locking, 407–408
    suture passing, 406–407, 407*f*–409*f*
    traumatic laceration, 413, 414*f*
ADAPTIS porous coated technology, 227
Additive Orthopaedics, 617–619
AITFL fibers. *See* Anterior inferior tibiofibular ligament (AITFL)
Akin osteotomy, 1–18, 14*f*, 15*f*
  closure and dressing, 14, 15*f*
  complications of, 16
  concentrated bone marrow aspirate, 12
  contraindications to, 1–2
  crossing screws, 12
  indications for, 1–2
  intramedullary implants, 12
  postoperative management in, 15–16
  preoperative planning for, 2–4, 3*f*, 4*f*
  results of, 16
  surgical technique of, 4–14, 5*f*, 6*f*, 7*f*, 8*f*, 9*f*, 10*f*, 11*f*, 13*f*, 14*f*
Akin proximal phalanx medial closing wedge osteotomy, minimally invasive surgical bunionectomy, 42, 45*f*–46*f*
American Orthopaedic Foot and Ankle Society (AOFAS), 337
  hallux, 16
  scores, 217
Ankle arthrodesis (AA), 234
  approach, 529–530, 529*f*–530*f*
  arthroscopic, 567–576
  cases, 574*f*, 575*f*, 576
  closure, 533
  complications of, 575–576
  contraindications, 527, 567–569
  external fixation
    advantages, 539–540
    complications of, 558–559
    contraindications to, 539–540
    indications for, 539
    postoperative management in, 557–558
    preoperative planning in, 540
    surgical technique of, 541–548, 542*f*–543*f*
  indications, 527, 567–569
  internal fixation, 532–533, 533*f*–534*f*, 535*f*
  joint preparation, 530, 532*f*
  joint reduction, 531–532
  outcomes, 536
  patient positioning, 529
  pearls and pitfalls in, 533–534, 574–575
  postoperative management in, 535–536, 575
  preoperative planning for, 528–529, 528*f*, 571
  results of, 16, 536, 575–576
  surgical technique of, 571–574, 574*f*–575*f*
Ankle arthroscopy, ankle fracture late syndesmosis repair, 671
Ankle distraction arthroplasty (ADA)
  ankle hinged frame, 515–516, 517*f*
  application, 516–518
  circular external fixator spanning, 513
  complications, 523, 523*f*
  contraindications, 514
  indication, 514
  pearls, 522, 524*f*
  pitfalls, 522, 523*f*
  postoperative management, 523
  in posttraumatic ankle arthritis, 513–514
  preoperative planning, 514
  results, 523–525
  with routine microfracture or subchondral drilling, 514–515, 515*f*
  technical considerations, 515, 516*f*
  wire placement for hinge, 516–518, 518*f*
Ankle fracture late syndesmosis repair
  ankle arthroscopy, 671
  assessing final reduction, 671
  deltoid ligament repair, 671
  fibula fracture reduction/fibular malunion, 671
  fibular approach, 671
  indications and contraindications, 663–664
  intraoperative contralateral fluoroscopy, 670
  postoperative management, 672
  preoperative imaging, 670
  preoperative planning, 664
  results and complications, 672–673
  surgical technique
    ankle positioning, 665, 665*f*
    clamping and indirect reduction, 666–667, 667*f*
    cotton and the external rotation stress tests, 664, 665*f*
    debridement, 669–670, 670*f*
    direct open reduction, 667–668
    fluoroscopy, 668–669
    implant choice, 669
    intraoperative evaluation of reduction, 668, 668*f*
    screw trajectory, 666, 666*f*
    syndesmotic arthrodesis, 670

Ankle instability, with triple arthrodesis, 494
Ankle joint capsule, 204
Ankle stability, Malerba/first metatarsal dorsiflexion osteotomy, 712
Ankle-foot orthosis (AFO), 703
Anterior chamfer, Salto Talaris ankle replacement system, 151–153, 153f–154f
Anterior distal tibial angle (ADTA), 577
Anterior face and tip of fibula, 289–291, 290f
Anterior inferior tibiofibular ligament (AITFL), 202–204
Anterior talofibular ligaments (ATFL), 289–291, 290f, 494
Anterior tibia closing wedge osteotomy, over/undercorrected neuromuscular foot, 751–754, 753f–754f
Anterior tibial tendon (ATT), over/undercorrected neuromuscular foot, 740–742, 745, 751
Anteromedial portal, in arthroscopic ankle arthrodesis, 572
Antibiotic prophylaxis, 499
AOFAS scores, 334
APEX 3D total ankle (Paragon 28)
　age, 164
　ankle, and foot radiographs, 164
　for Arc/Chamfer, 167
　for Arc/Flat, 167
　computer tomography scans, 164
　contraindications, 163–164
　coronal plane deformity, 164
　for Flat/Chamfer, 167
　for Flat/Flat cuts (tibia/talus), 167
　indications, 163
　postoperative management, 176
　preoperative assessment, 164
　surgical technique
　　alignment guide, 165–168, 166f, 167f, 168f
　　approach, 165, 165f–166f
　　external tibial alignment guide, 165–168
　　final implant placement through closure, 172–174, 174f, 175f
　　patient-specific instrumentation, 176
　　positioning, 165
　　talar cut, preparation and sizing, chamfer, 169–172, 172f–173f
　　talar cut, preparation and sizing, flat top, 172
　　tibial cut, 168, 169f
　wound complications, 177
ARC tibia trial, 169–170, 170f
Arthritis, with triple arthrodesis, 491
Arthroscopic ankle arthrodesis, 567–576. *See also* Ankle arthrodesis, arthroscopic
Arthroscopic bone grafting, of cystic talar osteochondral lesions, intact cartilage cap, 303–306, 306f

Arthroscopic débridement and microfracture/drilling, osteochondral lesions of the talus (OLTs), 317
Arthroscopic débridement, of small talar chondral lesions, 302, 303f–304f
Arthroscopic repair, of acute talar osteochondral lesions, 302, 305f
Arthroscopic treatment, large cystic talar osteochondral lesions, 306–307, 307f
　with bone autograft, 306–307, 307f, 308f, 309f
　with bone marrow aspirate concentrate, 306–307, 307f, 308f, 309f
　extracellular matrix cartilage allograft, 306–307, 307f, 308f, 309f
　with matrix-induced autologous chondrocyte implantation, 308–309
Arthroscopy for dorsal impingement and cheilectomy, 140
Arthroscopy-assisted ORIF (AAORIF)
　anteromedial and anterolateral portals, 679, 680f
　arthroscopic assisted ankle fracture fixation, 679–681, 681f
　to assess syndesmotic stability, 681, 685f
　chondral fissuring, 679, 681f–682f
　distal fibula and the medial malleolus, 679, 680f
　due to swelling and skin blistering, 678, 679f
　foot and ankle during distraction, 678–679, 680f
　fracture displacement, 679–681, 682f
　indications and contraindications, 677
　left ankle fracture treated with external fixation, 678, 679f
　left trimalleolar ankle fracture, 678, 678f–679f
　needle arthroscopy, 688
　pearls and pitfalls, 682, 686t
　postoperative management, 682–684, 687f
　postreduction CT status post left ankle external fixation, 678, 679f
　preoperative planning
　　imaging, 678
　　soft tissue status, 677
　　surgical planning, 678
　reduction and definitive fixation of the medial malleolus, 681, 684f
　reduction and definitive fixation of the posterior malleolus, 681, 684f
　results and complications, 686–688
　syndesmosis, evaluation of, 679–681, 681f
　wound closure, 681, 685f
Articular cartilage lesions, 299
Augmentation, 382
Avascular necrosis (AVN), 179
　of the base of the phalanx and flexor hallucis longus tendon injury, 127
　talus, 615–616, 618f–619f, 626

Axiom talar implant, cobalt chromium alloy (Co-Cr-Mo), 273

B

Baumann procedure, 421f
Bilateral Thompson test, 368
Biologic augmentation, 344–345
Biplanar lateralizing calcaneal osteotomy, Charcot-Marie-Tooth, 731, 733f
Biplanar plating, hallux valgus, 77f, 97
Black metallic cutting block (Arc/Chamfer), 167, 167f
Böhler angle, in calcaneal fractures, 691–692, 691f
Bone autograft, arthroscopic treatment, large cystic talar osteochondral lesions, 306–307, 307f, 308f, 309f
Bone graft
　in ankle arthrodesis, 542
　calcaneal, 5, 6f
Bone marrow aspirate (BMA)
　harvesting, 344–345, 344f, 345f
　intramedullary screw fixation, 338–340
Bone marrow aspirate concentrate (BMAC), 306–307, 307f, 308f, 309f
　iliac crest, 354, 354f
　intramedullary screw fixation, 338–340
Bone marrow stimulation (BMS), 300–301
　complications, 314
　of small talar chondral lesions, 302, 303f–304f
Bone milling
　anatomical considerations, 209, 211f
　arc relation to implant position, 209, 210f
　and implant insertion, 209–213
　joint line tracing, 209
　rail guide placement., 212–213, 212f–213f
　router placement, 209
　Silhouette guide placement, 209, 211f
　talar resection, 209
　tibial slope, 209
　trial implant placement and stability testing, 213, 213f
　trial talus implant, 209
　Z-retractor, 211, 212f
Bone removal tools, 223
Bridle modification, posterior tibial tendon transfer, 704
Broström lateral ankle ligaments repair, 323

C

Cadaveric model, 126–127
Cadence implant, features of, 251
Cadence total ankle replacement
　anterior or posterior subluxation, 253
　bone preserving chamfer cut talus component, 253
　contraindications, 251
　flat cut talus, 253
　indications, 251
　neutral coronal and sagittal alignment, 260

Index

physical therapy, 259
postoperative management, 259
preoperative evaluation, 251–253
preoperative templating with physical or digital templates, 252–253
residual plantar flexion or dorsiflexion, 261
results and complications, 261–262
surgical technique, 253
  alignment block and cut guide, 254
  angle bisector, 256, 256f
  capsule incision, 253, 254f
  Chaput tubercle, 256
  Corner osteotome, 256, 256f
  deep dissection, 253, 253f
  distal tibia resection height, 254–255
  distal/proximal location, distal tibia cut guide, 254–255, 255f
  fine-tune alignment with sequential images, 254
  laminar spreaders, 257, 257f
  lateral fluoroscopy with trial components, 258, 258f
  lateral projection fluoroscopy, 254
  midline incision, 253
  revision or talus deformity/bone loss, 257
  rotational alignment, 256
  small *versus* large talar cut guide, 257
  superficial peroneal nerve, 253, 253f–254f
  talar sizer holder, 258
  talar trial, 258
  talus implantation, 258
  tibia resection, 256
  tibial alignment guide, 254, 254f
  tibial resection template, 254–255, 255f
surgical treatment, 251
tibial components, 253
Calcaneal fractures
  imaging of, 691–692, 691f–692f
  minimally invasive reduction and fixation of
    radiographic evaluation for, 690–692
    room setup for, 693
    Schanz pin in, 695, 696f
    surgical incisions in, 694, 694f
    tongue-type fractures in, 691–692, 691f–692f
  open reduction and internal fixation of
    advantage, 690
    angle of Gissane, 691–692, 691f
    Böhler angle, 691–692, 691f
    complications, 699–700
    contraindications, 690
    double density sign, 691–692, 692f
    Essex-Lopresti joint-depression–type fractures, 690–693, 691f–692f
    indication, 689–690
    initial management, 690
    pearls and pitfalls, 699

postoperative management, 699
results of, 699–700
Sanders classification, 692–693, 692f
surgical technique, 693–697, 695f–696f
timing of surgery, 693
Calcaneal osteotomy
  complications, 479
  lateral displacement, 471–472
  minimally invasive approaches, 472
  pearls and pitfalls, 478, 479f
  postoperative management, 478
  preoperative planning, 472–473, 472f
  results, 479
  subtalar fusion, 458, 460f, 461f
  surgical technique, 473–476, 474f–475f
Calcaneal varus deformity, Charcot-Marie-Tooth, 731, 732f, 733f, 734f
Calcaneocuboid joint, in triple arthrodesis, 501, 507, 508f
Calcaneus, 420–423
Callus formation, in Lapidus procedure, for hallux valgus, 3
Cancellous autograft, harvesting BMA and, 344–345, 344f, 345f
Capsular imbrication, 12
Cartilage regenerative techniques, 313
Center of rotation and angulation (CORA), supramalleolar osteotomy, 577
Chaput osteotomy, 323
Charcot-Marie-Tooth (CMT) disease
  clinical phenotype, 719
  contraindications, 721
  indication, 720
  Malerba/first metatarsal dorsiflexion osteotomy, 711
  pathophysiology, 719, 720f
  pearls and pitfalls
    arthrodesis, 736
    osteotomies, 736
    plantar fascia release, 736
    tendon transfers, 735
  postoperative management, 736
  preoperative planning
    history, 721
    imaging studies, 723, 724f
    physical examination, 721–723, 722f, 723f
    primary goals of treatment, 720
  results and complications, 736–737
  surgical technique
    algorithm, 724, 725f
    calcaneal varus deformity, 731, 732f, 733f, 734f
    claw toe deformities, 734
    contracted medial soft tissues, 727
    contracted plantar fascia, 727, 729f
    plantarflexed first metatarsal, 727–731, 730f
    primary deforming forces, 725–727, 726f
    severe midfoot arch, 731–733, 735f

severe, rigid, and arthritic foot, 733
specific apices, 733–734
Charcot-Marie-Tooth disorder, 703
Cheilectomy
  advantages of, 113
  complications of, 126–127
  contraindications to, 115–116
  indications for, 115–116
  postoperative management in, 126
  preoperative planning for, 116, 116f, 117f
  proximal phalanx osteotomy, 115–127, 119f–120f
  results of, 126–127
  surgical technique of, 117–125, 119f–120f
Chronic Achilles tendon ruptures, 367
  donor site morbidity, hamstring autograft harvest, 375
  FHL tendon transfer augmentation, 374, 374f
  incision locations, 370–371, 371f
  indications and contraindications, 367
  management, 367
  postoperative management, 375
  preoperative planning, 368–369
  results and complications, 375
  surgical technique, 369–370
Chronic ankle instability (CAI), varus malalignment, 285–286
Clamping and indirect reduction, ankle fracture late syndesmosis repair, 666–667, 667f
Claw toe deformities, Charcot-Marie-Tooth, 734
Closing wedge osteotomy, proximal phalangeal, 113–127
Cobey hindfoot alignment, 419
COFAS 1–3 tibiotalar arthritis, 567, 568f, 569t
Coleman block test, 711
  Malerba/first metatarsal dorsiflexion osteotomy, 712
Collateral ligament repair, crossover toe, 633–636, 635f–636f
Compression, tibiotalocalcaneal (TTC) arthrodesis, 606, 609f
Computed tomography (CT)
  of ankle arthrodesis, 540
  of calcaneal fractures, 690–693
  of tibiotalocalcaneal arthrodesis, 540
  tibiotalocalcaneal (TTC) arthrodesis, 596
Contracted medial soft tissues, Charcot-Marie-Tooth, 727
Contracted plantar fascia, Charcot-Marie-Tooth, 727, 729f
Contractures, equinus, with progressive collapsing foot deformity, 419, 427
Controlled ankle motion/movement (CAM) boot, 176, 228, 248, 346
Conventional weight-bearing radiographs and WBCT, PCFD, 432, 432f, 436, 437f

Copious irrigation, 14
Corner osteotome, Cadence total ankle replacement, 256, 256f
Coronal plane alignment, INBONE II in ankle arthroplasty, 222
Coronal plane deformity, Paragon 28 APEX 3D fixed-bearing total ankle replacement, 164
Cotton and the external rotation stress tests, ankle fracture late syndesmosis repair, 664, 665f
Cotton osteotomy, 418
　complications, 435
　contraindications, 430–431
　indications, 430, 430f, 431f
　pearls and pitfalls, 435, 435f
　postoperative management, 435
　preoperative planning, 431–432, 431f, 432f
　results, 435
　surgical technique, 432–434, 432f, 433f, 434f
Coughlin-Shurnas grading for hallux rigidus, 130, 131t
Crossover toe
　contraindications, 631, 631t
　diagnosis, 629
　indications, 631
　nonoperative treatments, 629–630, 630f
　operative treatments, 630, 631t
　pitfalls in, 643–644
　postoperative management, 641–642
　preoperative planning, 631–632, 632f
　results and complications, 642–643
　severe hallux valgus deformity and coronal plane deviation, 629, 630f
　surgery for, 3, 5
　surgical techniques, 632–641, 633f
　　correction of hammertoe deformity, 639, 640f
　　metatarsophalangeal joint soft tissue release, 633, 634f
　　percutaneous distal metatarsal osteotomy, 637–639, 637f–639f
　　plantar plate and collateral ligament repair, 633–636, 635f–636f
　　resection arthroplasty, 640
　　residual deformity, 640–641

D

Débridement, ankle fracture late syndesmosis repair, 669–670, 670f
Decision analysis model, 337–338
Deformity, with triple arthrodesis, 491, 493–494, 495f–496f
Degenerative first MTP joint arthritis, 53–54
Deltoid ligament repair, ankle fracture late syndesmosis repair, 671
Dermodesis, residual deformity, crossover toe, 641
Direct open reduction, ankle fracture late syndesmosis repair, 667–668

Distal chevron osteotomy, 37
　fluoroscopic localization, percutaneous incision site, 34–37, 35f–36f
　Sawbones model, 37, 39f
　Shannon burr, 37, 37f–38f
Distal metatarsal articular angle, method of correction of, 20–21, 20f–22f
Distal soft tissue release, hallux valgus, 93
Distal tibial cut, Salto Talaris ankle replacement system, 149–150, 149f–150f
Distal tibial osteotomy, 578
Dome osteotomy, 578
Dome osteotomy, supramalleolar osteotomy, 586, 588f, 589f
Dorsal cheilectomy, 129
Dorsal tarsometatarsal joint plating, 70–72
Dorsiflexion osteotomy, Charcot-Marie-Tooth, 727, 730f
Dorsomedial incision, first TMT joint, 7–9, 8f, 9f, 10f, 11f
Double arthrodesis, 510
Dressing sterile, in ankle arthrodesis, 552, 552f
Duble-row technique, 381
Dwyer osteotomy, 471–472

E

Endoscopic calcaneoplasty, insertional Achilles tendinopathy, 392–393, 392f, 393f
Endoscopic FHL tendon transfer, insertional Achilles tendinopathy, 396–398, 397f, 398f, 399f
Endoscopic single row achilles tendon reinforcement or augmentation, 393–395, 394f, 395f
Endoscopic single row achilles tendon reinforcement or augmentation, insertional Achilles tendinopathy, 393–395, 394f, 395f
Endoscopic suture bridge achilles tendon reinforcement or augmentation, insertional Achilles tendinopathy, 395–396, 396f
End-stage ankle arthritis (ESAA), 567, 569t
Equinus contractures with progressive collapsing foot deformity, 419, 427
Equinus deformity, management of over/undercorrected neuromuscular foot, 740–742
Evans procedure, 420
　for calcaneal osteotomy, 478
Exactech Vantage fixed-bearing total ankle replacement
　3D-printed custom cutting guides, 235
　age, 234
　ankle arthrodesis, 234
　anterolateral tibia, 248–249
　balancing procedures, ankle and foot, 235, 235t
　contraindications, 233

　coronal angulation, 235
　coronal plane deformity, 234
　deformity, 234
　design, 233, 234f
　indications, 233
　limb malalignment, 235
　low-profile design, 235
　peri-implant cysts and lucencies, 248–249
　postoperative management, 248
　preoperative planning, 235
　results and complications, 248–249
　rotational assessment, 235
　sagittal deformity, 235
　severe osteoporosis, 234
　surgical technique, 236–246
　　angel wing, 237, 238f
　　anterior approach, 236, 236f
　　anteroposterior fluoroscopy, 237, 238f
　　external alignment guide, 237, 237f, 238f
　　flat-cut talus, 240–242, 243f
　　gap check tool, 239, 240f
　　implant insertion, 244–245, 245f–246f
　　patient-specific instrumentation, 245–246
　　positioning, 236
　　preparation, 239–240, 239f–240f
　　radiographs and wound closure, 246, 247f
　　rounded talus, 239–240, 239f–240f
　　size-specific talar cutting block, 240
　　talar cut and sizing, 239–242, 239f–240f
　　tibial cut, 239
　　tibial sizing and preparation, 242, 244f, 245f
　　tibialis anterior, 236
　　varus/valgus position, 237
　　weight-bearing radiographs, 235
Extensile lateral approach (ELA), 690
Extensor digitorum brevis (EDB), 500, 501f, 509, 509f
Extensor hallucis longus (EHL)
　Kinos Axiom Total Ankle System, 265
　tendon, 7, 8f, 51, 236
Extensor hallucis longus, INFINITY total ankle arthroplasty, 180
Extensor retinaculum, 236
　INBONE II in ankle arthroplasty, 227
　Kinos Axiom Total Ankle System, 265
External alignment guide, Vantage fixed-bearing total ankle replacement, 237, 237f, 238f
External fixation
　ankle arthrodesis, 541–548, 542f–543f
　over/undercorrected neuromuscular foot, 760
　tibiotalocalcaneal arthrodesis, 553–557, 554f, 555f, 556f, 557f
　tibiotalocalcaneal (TTC) arthrodesis, 610
　traditional, for ankle arthrodesis using, 552–553, 553f

Index

External tibial alignment guide, Paragon 28 APEX 3D fixed-bearing total ankle replacement, 165–168, 166f, 167f, 168f
Extracellular matrix cartilage allograft (EMCA), 306–307, 307f, 308f, 309f
Extracorporeal shockwave therapy, 377

F

Ferkel-Sgaglione CT classification, 299, 300t, 300f
FFI (foot function index), 737
FHL tenosynovitis, 361
Fibula fracture reduction/fibular malunion, ankle fracture late syndesmosis repair, 671
Fibular approach, ankle fracture late syndesmosis repair, 671
Fibular osteotomy, 203, 204f
 SMO, 521
Fibular reduction and adjunct procedures, 214, 214f, 215f
Fibular reflection and talar sizing, 203–204, 205f
Fifth metatarsal, ORIF
 anatomic classification schemes, 337
 cancellous autograft, 346
 contraindications, 337–338
 harvesting BMA and cancellous autograft, 344–345, 344f, 345f
 indications, 337–338
 postoperative management, 346
 preoperative planning, 338, 339f
 results and complications, 347
 surgical techniques, 338–343, 342f–343f, 345–346
First metatarsal dorsiflexion osteotomy
 complications, 717–718
 contraindications, 711
 indications, 711
 pearls and pitfalls, 716–717
 postoperative management, 717
 preoperative planning, 712
 results, 717–718
 surgical technique, 714–716, 715f–716f
First ray hypermobility, cotton, medial cuneiform dorsal opening wedge osteotomy, 431
First tarsometatarsal arthrodesis
 complications, 440
 contraindications, 436
 indications, 436
 pearls and pitfalls, 440
 postoperative management, 439
 preoperative planning, 436–437, 437f
 results, 440
 surgical technique, 437–439, 438f, 439f
 using an interposition bone block
  complications, 449, 450f
  contraindications, 440
  indications, 440
  pearls and pitfalls, 448–449, 450f
  postoperative management, 448
  preoperative planning, 440–441
  results, 449, 450f
  surgical technique, 441–448, 442f, 443f, 444f, 445f, 446f, 447f, 448f
First tarsometatarsal (TMT) joint
 arthritis, 711
 ligament release, 56, 58f
 planing, 56, 58f
 surgical approach, 56, 57f–58f
Fixed-bearing Salto Talaris prosthesis, 161
Flatfoot deformity, 29
Flexor digitorum brevis release, hammertoe deformity, crossover toe, 641, 642f
Flexor digitorum longus (FDL)
 tendon, Hamstring peroneals, 275
 transfer, 420, 427
  to navicular, with PCFD, 422f
Flexor hallucis longus (FHL), 13, 211
 Hamstring peroneals, 275
 tendon, 51, 239
 tendon transfer, 367, 377
  augmentation, 374, 374f, 382, 384f, 385f
  complications, 385
  pearls and pitfalls, 385
  postoperative management, 385
  results in, 385–386
  tendon-splitting approach, 379, 381
Flexor to extensor transfer residual deformity, crossover toe, 641
Fluoroscopy, ankle fracture late syndesmosis repair, 668–669
Foot drop, 703
Foot function index (FFI), 737
Foot morphology and radiographic alignment, 338
Forefoot cavus, 711
Fracture displacement, arthroscopy-assisted ORIF, 679–681, 682f
Frame application and deformity correction lateral approach total ankle arthroplasty
 coronal assessment, 208
 frame assembly, 208, 209f
 frame positioning and talar alignment, 206–207, 207f
 intact deep deltoid ligament, 208
 laminar spreader, 207
 medial gutter débridement, 207–208
 operative extremity, 206
 sagittal deformity correction, 208, 210f
 talar alignment, 207–208
 tibial plafond, 208
 varus deformity, 208, 208f–210f
Functional instability and pain, 285

G

Gait analysis, cotton, medial cuneiform dorsal opening wedge osteotomy, 431, 431f

Gait evaluation, in triple arthrodesis, 493
Gap check tool, Vantage fixed-bearing total ankle replacement, 239, 240f
Gastrocnemius recession, 156–157, 421f, 499
 Silfverskiold test, 165
Goniometer, 116, 116f
Gould modification, lateral ankle ligament repair, 295
Gracilis hamstring tendon, peroneals, 276–277, 277f
Graft reconstruction technique, 370–374, 371f, 372f, 373f
 chronic Achilles tendon ruptures
  autograft harvesting, 369
  donor site morbidity, hamstring autograft harvest, 375
  FHL tendon transfer augmentation, 374, 374f
  gracilis and semitendinosus grafts, 370
  indications and contraindications, 367
  Langenbeck retractor, 369–370
  management, 367
  postoperative management, 375
  preoperative MRI and incision placement, 368, 368f
  preoperative planning, 368–369
  results and complications, 375
  sartorial fascia, 369–370
  surgical technique, 369–370
  incision locations, 370–371, 371f
Graft transfer, 333
Graft-augmented repair (reconstruction), 291–294
 graft choices, 291, 292f–293f

H

Haglund deformity
 causes, 377
 complications in, 385–386
 contraindications, 377–378
 indications, 377–378
 minimally invasive techniques for, 378–379
 pearls and pitfalls, 385
 postoperative management, 385
 preoperative planning, 378–379, 378f, 379f
 results in, 385–386
 tendon-splitting approach, Haglund excision, 379, 380f, 381f, 382f, 383f
Hallux rigidus, 113, 129
 cheilectomy for, 113–127
 grading systems, 114f–115f, 116
 Moberg osteotomy for, 113–127
 nonoperative treatment in, 113
 progression of, 126–127

Hallux valgus, 19
- deformity, 20–21, 20f–22f
- intrinsic and extrinsic causative factors, 19
- recurrent after scarf first metatarsal osteotomy, 29
- with and without metatarsus adductus
  - accessory articulating facet, 95–96
  - biplanar plating, 77f, 97
  - bone healing and early weight bearing, 94–95
  - complications, 98–99
  - contraindications, 53–54
  - distal soft tissue release, 93
  - dorsal plate fixation, 70–72, 74f
  - excessive compression with instruments, 96–97
  - first MTP–sesamoid arthritis, 95
  - hallux valgus correction surgery, 95
  - indications, 53
  - intercuneiform stabilization, 94
  - intraoperative fluoroscopic imaging, 95
  - medial metatarsal head resection, 97
  - medial metatarsal prominence, 66–69, 71f
  - medial plate fixation, 72, 75f
  - phalanx osteotomy, 94
  - postoperative management, 98
  - preoperative planning, 54–56
  - provisional fixation interference with screw fixation, 72, 76f
  - resection and preparation of subchondral bone, 69f, 93
  - results and complications, 98
  - surgical technique, 56–93
  - tarsometatarsal cuts, 66
  - 3 to 4 intermetatarsal base release, 94
  - 3-in-1 cut guide, 60–61, 93
  - TMT joint morphology, 95–96

Hallux varus, after scarf osteotomy, 29
Hammertoe deformity, correction of crossover toe, 639, 640f
Hamstring peroneals
- cadaveric studies, 275
- contraindications, 276
- indications, 276
- peroneal muscles, 275
- postoperative management, 281
- preoperative planning, 276
- results and complications, 281–282
- surgical technique, 276–278
  - curvilinear incision, 277–278, 277f
  - distal bone to tendon fixation of excess graft, 278, 280f
  - gracilis hamstring tendon, 276–277, 277f
  - hamstring graft, 276–277, 277f
  - peroneal retinaculum, 277–278
  - Pulvertaft maneuver, 278, 279f–281f
  - retinaculum repair over peroneal tendon, 278, 281f
  - sartorial fascia, 276–277, 277f
  - torn peroneus brevis tendon, 277–278, 278f
  - tubularization of hamstring graft, 278, 281f

Harvesting BMA and cancellous autograft, 344–345, 344f, 345f
Harvesting hamstring autograft, 369–370, 369f, 370f
Hindfoot and ankle valgus over/undercorrected neuromuscular foot, 747–749, 750f
Hindfoot and midfoot malalignment syndromes, 56
Hindfoot deformity, causes of, 491
Hindfoot valgus, 496, 498, 504
- deformities, 494, 497f
- with progressive collapsing foot deformity, 418–419
- radiographs for, 496, 497f
- subtalar joint, 504

Hindfoot varus, 496, 505f
- over/undercorrected neuromuscular foot, 744–745

Hintermann osteotomy, 424
Hip knee ankle alignment radiograph (HKA), 219–220
Hohmann retractor, 424
Hoke percutaneous tendo-Achilles lengthening, 420f–422f
Home run screw, in arthroscopic ankle arthrodesis, 573–574
Hybrid fixation, tibiotalocalcaneal arthrodesis, 595–596
Hypermobility of MTC joint, 3–4, 3f

I

Iliac crest bone marrow and bone graft harvest technique, 354, 355f–356f
INBONE II in ankle arthroplasty
- complications, 228–230
- congenital foot and ankle deformities, 231f, 232
- contraindications, 219
- deep infection, 230
- end-stage tibiotalar arthritis, 219
- impingement, 230
- INVISION total ankle revision componentry, 232
- postoperative care, 228
- posttraumatic population, 219
- preoperative deformity and origination, 220
- preoperative evaluation, 219–220
- surgical technique
  - ADAPTIS porous coated technology, 227
  - approach, 220
  - bone ingrowth versus ongrowth, 227
  - bone removal tools, 223
  - coronal plane alignment, 222
  - extensor retinaculum, 227
  - INIFINITY system, 227
  - instrumentation, 220–227
  - joint stability and hematoma control, 227
  - M4 purple ring extraction handle, 224–225, 224f–225f
  - operating room set up, 220
  - Peck drill advancement with control of INBONE PSI jig, 224–225, 225f
  - polyethylene component, 227, 228f
  - prophecy stem guide block, 224–225
  - PSI guide placement on tibia and talus, 220–222, 221f, 222f
  - Ray-tech type sponge, 220–222
  - reamer attachment, 226, 226f
  - sagittal radiographic alignment, 223
  - screw tipped joystick insertion with curette aid, 223, 224f
  - stem insertion using straight tamp, 226–227, 227f
  - subcutaneous tissue and epidermis, 227
  - tibia sizing, 226–227, 226f–227f
  - talus vascular perfusion, 232
  - trapezoidal design tapering cuts, 230

INBONE total ankle arthroplasty systems. See INFINITY total ankle arthroplasty
Incisional healing issues, 229–230
Incisional neuroma, 4
INFINITY total ankle arthroplasty
- chamfer cut, 186–187
- contraindications, 179
- indications, 179
- patient-specific cutting jigs, 179, 180f
- postoperative management, 197–198
- preoperative planning, 179–180
- results and complications, 198
- Stryker continuum, 186–187
- surgical technique, 180–195
  - AP fluoroscopic shot, 181–182
  - bicortical pins, 180–181
  - bone retrieval instrument, 185–186, 185f
  - Bovie electrocautery and curette, 186, 186f–187f
  - Corner protectors, 183–184, 184f
  - "coupling" the cuts, 185
  - extensor hallucis longus, 180
  - Kocher clamp, 184–185
  - patient positioning, 180
  - patient-specific guide system, 186, 187f
  - polyethylene with inserter, guide rods and nuts, 195, 196f
  - Talus with intact cartilage and soft tissue, 186, 186f–187f
  - 3D-printed replica, anterior tibia surface, 180, 181f, 182f
  - tibia resect-through guides, 184–185
  - tibialis anterior, 180
  - talar dome resection, 188–189, 189f
  - talus cutting jig, 188–189, 188f–189f
  - talus trial implant, 189–192
  - 3D-printed guides, 179
  - tibial impactor, 192, 193f, 194f

INIFINITY system, 227
Insertional Achilles tendinopathy

Index

arthroscopic instruments, 390–391, 391f
contraindications, 389–390
distal midline Achilles portal, 391, 392f
endoscopic calcaneoplasty, 392–393, 392f, 393f
endoscopic FHL tendon transfer, 396–398, 397f, 398f, 399f
endoscopic single row achilles tendon reinforcement or augmentation, 393–395, 394f, 395f
endoscopic suture bridge achilles tendon reinforcement or augmentation, 395–396, 396f
indications, 389–390
patient positioning, 390, 391f
pearls and pitfalls, 400
postoperative management, 398
preoperative planning, 390
results and complications, 398
wound and dressing, 398
Insertional tendinopathy, 377
Instability, with triple arthrodesis, 491
Instrumentation, minimally invasive, Achilles tendon rupture repair, 405–406, 406f
Intermetatarsal (IM) 1–2 angle
  chevron osteotomy, 20–21, 21f
  in Lapidus procedure, Akin osteotomy, 6, 6f
Intermetatarsal angle (IMA)
  lateral metatarso-sesamoid ligament release (percutaneous/open), 110
  proximal rotational metatarsal osteotomy, 101, 105f
  severe hallux valgus deformities, 31
Intermetatarsal incision, in Lapidus procedure, Akin osteotomy, 6, 6f
Internal fixation, ankle arthrodesis, 532–533, 533f–534f, 535f
Intra-articular calcaneus fractures, 689
Intramedullary nail, tibiotalocalcaneal (TTC) arthrodesis, 595, 604, 608f–609f
Intramedullary screw technique, 338–343, 342f–343f, 345
Intraoperative fluoroscopy, posterior tibial tendon transfer, 705, 708f
INVISION total ankle revision componentry, 232

J

Joint Line Reference Internal/External (I/E) Pointer, 166
Joint preparation
  ankle arthrodesis, 530, 532f, 572, 573f
  tibiotalocalcaneal arthrodesis, 600, 601f, 602f
Joint reduction, ankle arthrodesis, 531–532
Joint stability and hematoma control, INBONE II in ankle arthroplasty, 227
Joint stiffness, Malerba/first metatarsal dorsiflexion osteotomy, 712
Jones fractures, 337

K

Kinos Axiom Total Ankle System
  contraindications, 263
  indications, 263
  normal ankle joint kinematics, 263, 263f
  preoperative planning, 264, 264f
  surgical technique, 264, 264f
    alignment guide placement, 265–269, 266f
    custom implants, 267–269, 268f–269f
    design rationale and implant features, 272–273
    final implant insertion, 271, 271f, 272f
    patient-specific resection guides, 267–269, 268f–269f
    positioning and approach, 265, 265f
    postoperative protocol, 272
    preoperative standing ankle radiographs, 267, 267f
    talonavicular joint, 265
    tibial and talar cuts, 268f, 269, 269f
    tibial and talar sizing, final bony preparation, 269–271, 270f
    tibial component, titanium alloy, 273
Kirschner wire (K-wire) fixation
  in calcaneal fracture reduction and fixation, 696–697, 697f
  in hallux valgus deformity, 13
  in Moberg osteotomy, 122, 123f, 127
  in scarf osteotomy, 22
Knotless calcaneal fixation, minimally invasive, Achilles tendon rupture repair, 408–409, 410f

L

Lapicotton procedure, 481–482
Lapicotton technique of bone block fusion, 429
Lapidus
  Akin osteotomy, 1–18
    closure and dressing, 14, 15f
    complications of, 16
    concentrated bone marrow aspirate, 12
    contraindications to, 1–2
    crossing screws, 12
    indications for, 1–2
    intramedullary implants, 12
    postoperative management in, 15–16
    preoperative planning for, 2–4, 3f, 4f
    results of, 16
    surgical technique of, 4–14, 5f, 6f, 7f, 8f, 9f, 10f, 11f, 13f, 14f
  complications, 440
  contraindications, 436
  indications, 436
  osteotomy, 101
  pearls and pitfalls, 440
  postoperative management, 439
  preoperative planning, 436–437, 437f
  results, 440
  surgical technique, 437–439, 438f, 439f
Lateral ankle ligament repair
  with allograft, 291, 292f–293f
  anatomic repair and reconstruction, 296
  anterior talofibular ligament, 285, 286f
  approach, 288
  augmented with synthetic graft, 291–294, 294f
  closure, 291
  concomitant peroneal tendon injury, 295–296
  contraindications, 285
  correction of malalignment, 295
  determination of readiness for return to sport, 296, 296t
  dynamic ultrasound examination, peroneal tendons and lateral ligaments, 286
  equipment/implants and positioning, 288
  fixation, 289–291, 290f
  fluoroscopic exam, 288, 295
  focused physical examination, 285–286, 287f
  Gould modification, 295
  indications, 285
  intra-articular derangements, 296
  magnetic resonance imaging, 286
  nonanatomic reconstructions, 287–288
  palpation, 285–286
  postoperative protocols, 296, 296t
  preoperative planning, 285–286
  range of motion, subtalar joint, 285–286
  and reconstruction, 275–283
  results and complications, 296
  surgical technique, 287–294
  suture bulk, 295
  tunnel localization, 295
  weight bearing foot and ankle radiographs, 286
Lateral ankle ligament repair or reconstruction, 285
Lateral ankle sprains, 285
Lateral approach total ankle arthroplasty
  advantages, 199
  contraindications, 200
  curved tibial and talar bone resection, 199
  fibular osteotomy, 199
  global deformity on examination, 201
  indications, 200
  inherent gap balancing, 199–200
  mild to severe deformity corrections, 199–200
  multiplanar deformities, 199–200
  neurovascular examination, 201
  nonoperative treatments, 201
  peroneal artery, perforating branches, 199
  postoperative management, 216–217
  preoperative planning, 201
  recovery of motion, 217
  results and complications, 217–218
  sagittal plane conformity, conical arthroplasty surfaces, 199–200
  secondary surgery for gutter débridement, 217

Lateral approach total ankle arthroplasty (*Continued*)
  short-term and midterm follow-up, 218
  stabilizing implant rails, 199
  supplemental bony and soft tissue procedures, 199–200
  surgical technique
    anesthesia, 201–202
    closure, 214–216, 215f
    fibular reduction and adjunct procedures, 214, 214f, 215f
    frame application and deformity correction, 206–208
    lateral dissection and fibular osteotomy, 202–206, 203f
    milling and implant insertion, 209–213
    preoperative positioning and incision, 201–202, 202f
    room setup, 201–202
  symptomatic relief, 201
  Tendon deficits, 201
Lateral chamfer and plug hole, Salto Talaris ankle replacement system, 154–156, 155f–156f
Lateral closing wedge, supramalleolar osteotomy, 590, 592f
Lateral column lengthening (LCL), 481–482, 489
  for progressive collapsing foot deformity, 417–428
Lateral displacement calcaneal osteotomy (LDCO)
  contraindications, 472
  indications, 471
Lateral dissection and fibular osteotomy
  AITFL fibers, 203–204
  ankle joint capsule, 204
  fibular osteotomy, 203, 204f
  fibular reflection and talar sizing, 203–204, 205f
  lateral tibial overhang removal, 205, 205f
  longitudinal incision, 202
  medial arthrotomy and débridement, 205–206, 206f
  peroneal retinaculum, 202
  posterior inferior tibiofibular ligament fibers, 203–204
  posterior talofibular ligament off the talus, 203–204
  provisional fibular plating, 202, 204f
Lateral first MTP joint release, 59, 59f
Lateral locking plate, tibiotalocalcaneal (TTC) arthrodesis, 610
Lateral malleolar osteotomy, 324f, 333
Lateral malleolus osteotomy, 333
Lateral molecular osteotomy, 323, 324f
Lateral talus center migration (LTCM), 577
Lengthening calcaneal osteotomy (LCL), 418
  complications in, 427–428
  contraindications for, 418–419
  indications for, 418
  results in, 427–428

Lesser toes MTP plantar plate tears
  cephalic fragment and K-wire, 651, 652f
  clincal findings, 649t
  clinical and radiological results, 656, 657f–658f
  contraindications, 647–649
  indications and contraindications, 647–649, 649f–650f
  lateral and medial soft tissue reefing, 655f–656f, 656
  mattress suture and luggage tag passer, 652, 652f
  pearls and pitfalls, 659–660
  postoperative dressings, 656, 657f
  postoperative management, 659
  preoperative planning, 649–651, 650f
  results and complications, 659
  "S" shape dorsal incision, 651, 652f
  snake-headed NINJA instrument, 652–653, 653f
  straight handheld suture passer, 653, 653f
  ugly technique, 652
  Weil metatarsal osteotomy, 651, 654, 655f–656f
Longitudinal capsulotomy, lesser toes MTP plantar plate tears, 651

M

Magnetic resonance imaging (MRI)
  of Achilles tendon rupture, 405
  in ankle arthrodesis, 540
  in tibiotalocalcaneal arthrodesis, 540
Malalignment, of tibia, 577
Malerba osteotomy, 472
  complications, 717–718
  contraindications, 711
  indications, 711
  pearls and pitfalls, 716–717, 717f
  postoperative management, 717
  preoperative planning, 712
  results, 717–718
  surgical technique, 713–714, 713f, 714f
Malunion, after calcaneal fracture reduction and fixation, 699
Mann osteotomy, 101
Matrix-induced autologous chondrocyte implantation (MACI), 308–309, 311f
Mechanical instability or laxity, 285
Medial arthrotomy and débridement, 205–206, 206f
Medial capsulorrhaphy, hallux in varus and plantar flexion, 26, 27f
Medial closing wedge, supramalleolar osteotomy, 583–586, 587f
Medial cuneiform, 429
  osteotomy, 418
Medial cuneiform dorsal opening wedge osteotomy
  complications, 435
  contraindications, 430–431
  indications, 430, 430f, 431f
  pearls and pitfalls, 435, 435f
  postoperative management, 435

  preoperative planning, 431–432, 431f, 432f
  results, 435
  surgical technique, 432–434, 432f, 433f, 434f
Medial displacement calcaneal osteotomy (MDCO), 418
  complications in, 427–428
  contraindications, 418–419, 471
  dynamic component, 471
  flexor digitorum longus (FDL) tendon transfer, 471
  functions, 471
  indications, 418, 471
  results in, 427–428
  technique, 420–424, 423f
Medial distal tibial angle (MDTA), of ankle, 577
Medial eminence resection
  in Lapidus procedure, Akin osteotomy, 12, 13f
  minimally invasive surgical bunionectomy, 34–37, 35f–36f
Medial incision, in Lapidus procedure, Akin osteotomy, 6–7, 7f
Medial/lateral (M/L) alignment, 167, 167f
Medial malleolar osteotomy, 320, 321f, 322f, 333
Medial malleolar tunnel, 486
Medial malleolus, 483, 487f–488f
  osteotomy closure, 330, 332f
  stress fracture, 228
Medial opening wedge, supramalleolar osteotomy, 580, 581f, 582f, 583f
Medial talonavicular joint capsule and spring ligament, Charcot-Marie-Tooth, 727
Metatarsal and cuneiform joint surfaces, instability of, callus formation and, 3
Metatarsal shaft resection, minimally invasive surgical bunionectomy, 41, 44f
Metatarsophalangealinterphalangeal (MTP-IP) score, 16
Metatarsophalangeal joint soft tissue release, crossover toe, 633, 634f
Metatarsus adductus
  arthrodesis site preparation., 86, 88f
  combined hallux valgus and metatarsus adductus corrections, 76–79, 78f–79f
  compression wire fixation, 87–93
  correction of, 76–93, 78f–79f
  fluoroscopic assessment after definitive fixation, 87–93, 91f
  hallux valgus deformity, 1, 3–4
  metatarsus adductus correction and bone apposition, 87–93
  second and third tarsometatarsal (TMT) joint preparation, 79–82, 80f, 81f, 83f
Metatarsus elevates, over/undercorrected neuromuscular foot, 745–747, 747f–748f
Metatarsus primus varus, hallux valgus deformity, 1
Microfracture, 317–318

Index

Micronized cartilage, 306–307, 307f, 308f, 309f
Microreciprocating saw technique, calcaneal osteotomy, 479
Midfoot abduction, over/undercorrected neuromuscular foot, 745, 746f
Midfoot adduction, over/undercorrected neuromuscular foot, 745, 746f
Midfoot osteotomy for cavus foot, over/undercorrected neuromuscular foot, 754, 755f
Midline anterior ankle approach, 180
Minimally invasive chevron Akin (MICA), 31
Minimally invasive ORIF calcaneus
   advantage, 690
   contraindications, 690
   indication, 689–690
   pearls and pitfalls, 699
   postoperative management, 699
   preoperative planning
      angle of Gissane, 691–692, 691f
      Böhler angle, 691–692, 691f
      double density sign, 691–692, 692f
      Essex-Lopresti joint-depression–type fractures, 690–693, 691f–692f
      initial management, 690
      Sanders classification, 692–693, 692f
      timing of surgery, 693
   results and complications, 699–700
   surgical technique, 693–697, 695f–696f
Minimally invasive surgery (MIS) cheilectomy, 131–135, 135f–136f, 420
   biplanar fluoroscopy, 133
   blunt trocar and cannula, 134
   bunionectomy, 31–51
      closure and dressings, 42–46, 48f
      complications, 50–51
      contraindications, 31–32
      fixation using percutaneous cannulated screws, 31
      indications, 31
      outpatient procedure, 33
      popliteal nerve block for perioperative pain control, 33–34
      postoperative management, 46, 49f
      preoperative planning, 32–33
      reduction and fixation, 37–46, 40f–41f
      results, 50–51
      surgical technique, 33–46
   contraindications, 130
   extensor hallucis longus (EHL) tendon, 132
   for Haglund deformity, 378–379
   indications, 130
   instrumentation
      beaver blade, 32
      head shifting tool, 32
      irrigation, 32
      periosteal elevators, 32
      screws, 32
      Shannon burr, 33, 37f–38f
      Wedge burr, 33
   lateral osteophytes, 134
   mild to moderate hallux rigidus with dorsal osteophytes, 129
   with Moberg osteotomy, 135–137, 138f
   osteotomy, 136
   postoperative management, 139, 139f
   preoperative planning, 130, 131f
   procedure-specific tools and instruments, 129
   results and complications, 139–141
   small joint arthroscopy, 131–132
   surgical technique, 131–137, 135f–136f
Moberg osteotomy
   complications of, 126–127
   contraindications to, 115–116
   indications for, 115–116
   minimally invasive surgery (MIS) cheilectomy, 135–137, 138f
   postoperative management, 126
   preoperative planning, 116, 116f, 117f
   results of, 126–127
   surgical technique of, 117–125, 119f–120f
Mobile-bearing prosthesis, 161
Modified Broström lateral ankle ligaments repair, 323
Modified Mason Allen or Krackow 2 or 4 core strand repair, 406–407
Morton extension, 129
MOXFQ scores, 140

N

Navicular stress fractures, 349, 481–483, 484f, 485–486, 487f–488f, 488
   chronic fracture or nonunion, 354–355
   classification system, 350, 350t, 350f–351f
   contraindications, 350–351
   CT imaging, 352, 353f
   diagnosis, 351
   dorsal approach, 355
   dorsal hindfoot, ankle sprain, 352, 353f
   extrinsic factors, 349
   female sex, 349
   indications, 350–351
   intrinsic factors, 349
   MRI, 352
   nonsurgical management, 350–351, 351t
   non–weight-bearing (NWB) protocols, 350–351
   "N-spot," 351, 352f
   optimal screw position, 355
   pathogenesis, 349
   postoperative management, 357
   preoperative planning, 351–354
   regional anesthesia, 354
   results and complications, 357
   sclerotic fracture edges, 355, 355f–356f
   surgical technique, 354–357
   type II and III fractures in athletic individuals, 351
Navicular tuberosity tunnel, 486
Naviculocuneiform (NC) joint, 429
Needle arthroscopy, arthroscopy-assisted ORIF, 688
Nerve injury, after calcaneal osteotomy, 479
Neuritis, sural, Achilles tendon repair, 413
Neurogenic causes, posterior tibial tendon transfer, 703
Nonunion
   after calcaneal fracture reduction and fixation, 699
   with progressive collapsing foot deformity, 419

O

Open reduction and internal fixation (ORIF)
   5th metatarsal
      anatomic classification schemes, 337
      cancellous autograft, 346
      contraindications, 337–338
      harvesting BMA and cancellous autograft, 344–345, 344f, 345f
      indications, 337–338
      plantar plating, surgical technique, 345–346
      postoperative management, 346
      preoperative planning, 338, 339f
      results and complications, 347
      surgical techniques, 338–343, 342f–343f
   of navicular stress fractures. See Navicular stress fractures
Orthotics, foot deformity, 357
Os trigonum resection
   arthroscopic technique, 359
   contraindications, 359
   diagnosis and preoperative planning, 360–361
   indications, 359
   lateral or medial approach, 361
   mini-open technique, 361
   MRI, 360, 360f–361f
   nonoperative treatment, 359
   open medial os trigonum excisions, 365
   osseous and soft tissue structures, 359
   physical examination, 361
   postoperative management, 363–364
   radiographs, 360, 360f
   results and complications, 364–365
   sural nerve injury, 364
   surgical technique, 361–362, 361f, 362f
Osteochondral autologous transfer systems (OATS)
   contraindications, 318
   indications, 318
   plain radiographs, 318, 319f
   postoperative management, 334
   preoperative planning, 318–320
   recipient site preparation, 323, 325f, 326f
   results and complications, 334
   surgical technique, 320–333, 321f, 322f, 325f, 326f, 328f, 329f, 331f, 332f
   talar dome surface, 320
   talar osteochondral lesions, treatment, 317–335

Osteochondral graft harvesting, ipsilateral superior lateral femoral condyle, 327, 328f
Osteochondral graft transfer, 327–330, 329f, 331f
Osteochondral lesions of the talus (OLTs), 299
  Anderson MRI classification, 299, 301f
  arthroscopic débridement and microfracture/drilling, 317
  arthroscopic technique, 301–302, 311–312
  autografts, 318
  contraindications, 299
  CT classification, 299, 300t
  graft and patch hypertrophy, 314
  indications, 299
  management, 317
  MRI classification, 299, 301t
  postoperative management, 312–313
  preoperative planning, 300–301
  rehabilitation protocol, 313
  repair and regeneration, 299–315
  small joint instrumentation, 301–302
  small joint 2.7-mm 30° and 70° arthroscopes, 301–302
  soft tissue distraction, 301, 302f
  surgical technique, 301–309
  traditional open surgery, 310–311, 310f, 311f
  treatment strategies, 313
Osteophytes, 254
  in hallux rigidus, 113, 114f
Osteotomies, 418
  proximal phalangeal, 113–127
  Salto Talaris ankle replacement system, 145–148, 147f–148f
  scarf, 19–29
Osteotomy angulation, proximal rotational metatarsal osteotomy, 102t, 104
Over/undercorrected neuromuscular foot
  above-described procedures, 760
  with cerebral palsy, 739, 740f
  indications and contraindications, 739
  pearls and pitfalls, 761
  postoperative management, 761–762
  preoperative planning
    hindfoot and ankle valgus, 747–749, 750f
    hindfoot varus, 744–745
    management of equinus deformity, 740–742
    metatarsus elevatus, 745–747, 747f–748f
    midfoot adduction and abduction, 745, 746f
  results and complications, 762
  surgical techniques
    above-described procedures, 760
    anterior tibia closing wedge osteotomy, 751–754, 753f–754f
    external fixation, 760
    midfoot osteotomy for the cavus foot, 754, 755f
    talectomy, 755–757, 758f–759f
    tendon transfer, 751, 752f
    triple arthrodesis, 754–755, 756f

P

Pain
  after calcaneal fracture reduction and fixation, 699
  degenerative changes, Malerba/first metatarsal dorsiflexion osteotomy, 712
PAIS. See Posterior ankle impingement syndrome (PAIS)
Paragon 28 APEX 3D fixed-bearing total ankle replacement, 163
  age, 164
  ankle, and foot radiographs, 164
  computer tomography scans, 164
  contraindications, 163–164
  coronal plane deformity, 164
  indications, 163
  postoperative management, 176
  preoperative assessment, 164
  surgical technique
    alignment guide, 165–168, 166f, 167f, 168f
    approach, 165, 165f–166f
    external tibial alignment guide, 165–168
    patient-specific instrumentation, 176
    placement of final implant through closure, 172–174, 174f, 175f
    positioning, 165
    talar cut, preparation and sizing: chamfer, 169–172, 172f–173f
    talar cut, preparation and sizing: flat top, 172
    tibial cut, 168, 169f
  wound complications, 177
PARS jig, minimally invasive, Achilles tendon rupture repair, 405–406, 406f
Patient Reported Outcomes Measurement Information Score (PROMIS) domain, 282
  physical function, 16
PCFD. See Progressive collapsing foot deformity (PCFD)
Peck drill advancement with control of INBONE PSI jig, 224–225, 225f
Per Lauge-Hansen mechanistic theory, 663
Percutaneous chevron/Akin (PECA) vs open scarf and Akin, 50–51
Percutaneous distal metatarsal osteotomy, crossover toe, 637–639, 637f–639f
Percutaneous extracapsular chevron and Akin (PECA), 31
Peroneal retinacular procedures, 202, 288
Peroneal tendon disorders, 275
Peroneus brevis reconstruction, semitendinosus allograft, 276
Peroneus longus to brevis tendon transfer, 727, 728f
Phalanx osteotomy, 94
Pin fixation, in tibiotalocalcaneal and ankle arthrodesis, 543f
Plantar fascia release, 727, 729f
  Charcot-Marie-Tooth, 727, 729f
Plantar or plantar lateral plating, 345–346
Plantar plate, crossover toe, 633–636, 635f–636f
Plantarflexed first metatarsal, Charcot-Marie-Tooth, 727–731, 730f
Plastic resection sizing block, 168, 169f
Plate fixation, Lapidus procedure, Akin osteotomy, 9–12, 11f, 13f
Plate prominence, first TMT joint, 99
Plumb line method, 56, 56f
Poly Insertion Tool, 174, 175f
Polyethylene trial, 189–192, 191f, 194–195, 195f
Posterior ankle impingement syndrome (PAIS), 359
  arthroscopic technique, 359
  contraindications, 359
  diagnosis and preoperative planning, 360–361
  indications, 359
  MRI, 360, 360f–361f
  nonoperative treatment, 359
  open medial os trigonum excisions, 365
  osseous and soft tissue structures, 359
  physical examination, 361
  postoperative management, 363–364
  radiographs, 360, 360f
  results and complications, 364–365
  sural nerve injury, 364
  surgical technique, 361–362, 361f, 362f
Posterior chamfer, Salto Talaris ankle replacement system, 151, 152f–153f
Posterior inferior tibiofibular ligament fibers, 203–204
Posterior talofibular ligament off the talus, 203–204
Posterior tibial muscle with tendon (PTT), 725–727, 726f, 728f
  dysfunction. See Progressive collapsing foot deformity (PCFD)
  over/undercorrected neuromuscular foot, 740–742, 745, 751
Posterior tibial tendon transfer
  contraindications, 703
  indications, 703
  pearls and pitfalls, 705
  postoperative management, 707–708
  preoperative evaluation, 703–704
  results and complications, 708–709
  surgical technique, 704–705, 706f–708f
Posterolateral portal, in arthroscopic ankle arthrodesis, 572
Posteromedial (PM) osteochondral lesion of the talus, 312, 312t
Posttraumatic ankle arthritis, for ADA, 514

Index

Precontouring, first TMT joint, 99
Pre-op templating, ankle replacement surgery, 147
Primary deforming forces, Charcot-Marie-Tooth, 725–727, 726f
Progressive collapsing foot deformity (PCFD), 481–482
  clinical observation, 429, 430f
  complications in, 427–428
  contraindications to, 418–419
  cotton osteotomy
    complications, 435
    contraindications, 430–431
    indications, 430, 430f, 431f
    pearls and pitfalls, 435, 435f
    postoperative management, 435
    preoperative planning, 431–432, 431f, 432f
    results, 435
    surgical technique, 432–434, 432f, 433f, 434f
  Expert Consensus Classification System, 417
  indications for, 418–419
  lapicotton
    complications, 449, 450f
    contraindications, 440
    indications, 440
    pearls and pitfalls, 448–449, 450f
    postoperative management, 448
    preoperative planning, 440–441
    results, 449, 450f
    surgical technique, 441–448, 442f, 443f, 444f, 445f, 446f, 447f, 448f
  Lapidus
    complications, 440
    contraindications, 436
    indications, 436
    pearls and pitfalls, 440
    postoperative management, 439
    preoperative planning, 436–437, 437f
    results, 440
    surgical technique, 437–439, 438f, 439f
  lateral column lengthening for, 417–428
  medial displacement calcaneal osteotomies for, 417–428
  postoperative management in, 427
  preoperative planning for, 419
  results of, 427–428
  subtalar fusion
    active and passive range of motion testing, 454
    advanced imaging, 454–457
    calcaneal osteotomy, 458, 460f, 461f
    contraindications, 454
    incisions, 457, 457f
    indication, 453–468
    pearls and pitfalls, 466
    physical examination, 454
    postoperative management, 464

  preoperative evaluation, 454
  radiographic evaluation, 454, 455f–456f
  reduction and fixation, 459, 461f, 462f, 463f, 464f, 465f
  results and complications, 466
  subtalar joint preparation, 458, 458f, 459f
  treatment of, 417
  triple arthrodesis for, 511
PROMO (proximal rotational metatarsal osteotomy)
  complications, 111
  contraindications, 101–104
  definition, 101
  indications, 101–104
  lateral sesamoids displacement, 110
  medial ray pronation, 101
  osteotomy, 101, 102t
  postoperative management, 111
  preoperative planning, 104
  progressive pronation
    in radiographs, 101, 102f–104f
    in weight-bearing computerized tomography, 101, 102f, 103f, 104f
  progressive pronation, in radiographs and WBCT, 101, 102f–104f
  results, 111
  results and complications, 111
  surgical technique, 104–108, 109f–110f
  tarsometatarsal joint, 101–104
PROPHECY patient-specific instrumentation, INFINITY total ankle arthroplasty. See INFINITY total ankle arthroplasty
Provisional fibular plating, 202, 204f
Proximal dome osteotomy, 101
Proximal phalangeal osteotomy
  with cheilectomy
    complications of, 126–127
    contraindications to, 115–116
    indications for, 115–116
    postoperative management, 126
    preoperative planning, 116, 116f, 117f
    results of, 126–127
    surgical technique of, 117–125, 119f–120f
  residual deformity, crossover toe, 640–641
Proximal phalanx osteotomy with cheilectomy
  complications of, 126–127
  contraindications to, 115–116
  indications for, 115–116
  postoperative management, 126
  preoperative planning, 116, 116f, 117f
  results of, 126–127
  surgical technique of, 117–125, 119f–120f
Proximal rotational metatarsal osteotomy (PROMO)

  complications, 111
  contraindications, 101–104
  definition, 101
  indications, 101–104
  lateral sesamoids displacement, 110
  medial ray pronation, 101
  osteotomy, 101, 102t
  postoperative management, 111
  preoperative planning, 104
  progressive pronation
    in radiographs, 101, 102f–104f
    in weight-bearing computerized tomography, 101, 102f, 103f, 104f
  results, 111
  results and complications, 111
  surgical technique, 104–108, 109f–110f
  tarsometatarsal joint, 101–104
PSI guide placement on tibia and talus, 220–222, 221f, 222f

R

Radiographs
  in ankle arthritis, 567, 569f–570f
  crossover toe, 631–632, 632f
  Lapidus procedure, for hallux valgus deformity, 1–4
  posterior tibial tendon transfer, 704
  for triple arthrodesis, 496
Range of motion (ROM), 493
  for Moberg osteotomy, 115–116, 125f
  MTP joint, 3–4
  in TTR, 616
Ray-tech type sponge, 220–222
Reciprocating saw technique, calcaneal osteotomy, 479
Recurrent ankle sprains, 285
Rehabilitation, minimally invasive, Achilles tendon rupture repair, 411
Resection arthroplasty, crossover toe, 640
Residual bone in joint, 66, 68f
Residual deformity, crossover toe, 640–641
  dermodesis, 641
  flexor to extensor transfer, 641
  proximal phalangeal osteotomy, 640–641
  toe amputation, 641, 642f
restor3d, 617–619
Resurfacing techniques, 300–301
Retrocalcaneal bursitis, 378
Revision/talus deformity/bone loss, Cadence total ankle replacement, 257
Rotational and medial to lateral translation, Salto Talaris ankle replacement system, 148, 149f
Rounded talus, Vantage fixed-bearing total ankle replacement, 239–240, 239f–240f

S

Salto mobile-bearing design, fixed-bearing Salto Talaris prosthesis, 161

Salto Talaris ankle replacement system
  contraindications, 145
  development, 143
  extramedullary alignment guide, 147
  indications, 145
  postoperative management, 161
  preoperative planning, 145, 146f
  results and complications, 161
  surgical technique, 145–159
    Achilles lengthening, 156–157
    anterior chamfer, 151–153, 153f–154f
    approach, 145–146
    bone graft, 159, 159f
    distal tibial cut, 149–150, 149f–150f
    gastrocnemius recessions, 156–157
    lateral chamfer cut guide, 154–156, 155f–156f
    lateral ligament repairs, 156–157
    medial releases, 156–157
    positioning, 145
    posterior chamfer, 151, 152f–153f
    postoperative cast, 159, 159f
    rotational and medial to lateral translation, 148, 149f
    talar pin guide, 150–151, 151f
    talar trial components, 156–158, 157f
    tibial alignment, 147–148, 147f–148f
    tibial component, 158–159, 158f–159f
  "sweet spot" during trialing, 145
  tibial implants, 143–144, 144f
Salto Talaris prosthesis, fixed-bearing, 161
Saltzman hindfoot alignment, 419
Saxena classification, 350, 350t
Scarf first metatarsal osteotomy
  complications of, 28–29
  contraindications to, 19–20
    general anesthesia or regional anesthesia, 22
  indications for, 19–20
  modifications, 19
  nonoperative management, 19
  pitfalls in, 26–27
  postoperative management in, 28
  preoperative planning for, 20–28, 20f–22f
  results of, 28–29
  surgical technique of, 22–26, 27f–28f
Scarf osteotomy, first metatarsal. See Scarf first metatarsal osteotomy
Schantz pin, in calcaneal fracture reduction and fixation, 695, 696f
Screw fixation
  Lapidus procedure, 13
  for talonavicular (TN) arthrodesis, 508f
Screw trajectory, ankle fracture late syndesmosis repair, 666, 666f
Semmes-Weinstein monofilament, 721
Sesamoid arthritis, 95
Shannon burr, calcaneal osteotomy, 478–479, 479f
Shoes, for hallux valgus, 15–16
Silfverskiöld test, 165, 390, 494
Simple lateralizing calcaneal osteotomy, Charcot-Marie-Tooth, 731, 732f

Soft tissue dissection, 165
Soft tissue handling technique, 229–230
Soft tissue ischemia and necrosis, 229–230
Spring ligament reconstruction (SLR)
  complications in, 489
  contraindication in, 481–482
  indications in, 481–482
  pearls and pitfalls, 488
  postoperative management, 488
  preoperative planning in, 482–483
  results in, 489
  surgical technique, 483–486, 487f–488f
Stenosing tenosynovitis, 361
Step-by-step rehabilitation program, 390
Sterile dressings, in ankle arthrodesis, 552, 552f
Strayer procedure, 421f
Stress fracture of first metatarsal, 29
Stryker INBONE II total ankle arthroplasty system
  complications, 228–230
  congenital foot and ankle deformities, 231f, 232
  contraindications, 219
  deep infection, 230
  end-stage tibiotalar arthritis, 219
  impingement, 230
  INVISION total ankle revision componentry, 232
  postoperative care, 228
  posttraumatic population, 219
  preoperative deformity and origination, 220
  preoperative evaluation, 219–220
  surgical technique, 220–227
    ADAPTIS porous coated technology, 227
    approach, 220
    bone ingrowth versus ongrowth, 227
    bone removal tools, 223
    coronal plane alignment, 222
    extensor retinaculum, 227
    INIFINITY system, 227
    instrumentation, 220–227
    joint stability and hematoma control, 227
    M4 purple ring extraction handle, 224–225, 224f–225f
    operating room set up, 220
    Peck drill advancement with control of INBONE PSI jig, 224–225, 225f
    polyethylene component, 227, 228f
    prophecy stem guide block, 224–225
    PSI guide placement on tibia and talus, 220–222, 221f, 222f
    Ray-tech type sponge, 220–222
    reamer attachment, 226, 226f
    sagittal radiographic alignment, 223
    screw tipped joystick insertion with curette aid, 223, 224f
    stem insertion using straight tamp, 226–227, 227f
    subcutaneous tissue and epidermis, 227
    tibia sizing, 226–227, 226f–227f

  talus vascular perfusion, 232
  trapezoidal design tapering cuts, 230
Subchondral bone
  fenestration, fusion, 66, 69f
  resection and preparation of, hallux valgus, 69f, 93
Subchondral cysts, 513–514
Subcutaneous tissue and epidermis, INBONE II in ankle arthroplasty, 227
Subtalar arthritis, 690
Subtalar fusion
  joint preparation, 458, 458f, 459f
  progressive collapsing foot deformity
    active and passive range of motion testing, 454
    advanced imaging, 454–457
    calcaneal osteotomy, 458, 460f, 461f
    contraindications, 454
    incisions, 457, 457f
    indication, 453–468
    pearls and pitfalls, 466
    physical examination, 454
    postoperative management, 464
    preoperative evaluation, 454
    radiographic evaluation, 454, 455f–456f
    reduction and fixation, 459, 461f, 462f, 463f, 464f, 465f
    results and complications, 466
Subtalar (ST) joint distraction
  mechanism of action, 513–514
  surgical technique, 519–521, 519f, 520f
Subtalar joint, in triple arthrodesis, 500–501, 500f, 501f, 502f, 504–505, 505f, 506f
Superficial deltoid ligaments
  reconstruction, 481–482, 487f–488f
Superficial peroneal nerve (SPN), 236
  Cadence total ankle replacement, 253, 253f–254f
Supplemental fixation, tibiotalocalcaneal (TTC) arthrodesis, 609, 610f–612f
Supramalleolar osteotomy (SMO), 577–594
  with ankle distraction arthroplasty (ADA), 517f
  center of rotation of angulation (CORA), 577
  contraindications to, 577
  dome osteotomy, 586, 588f, 589f
  indications for, 577
  intraoperative complications of, 592–593
  lateral closing wedge, 590, 592f
  medial closing wedge, 583–586, 587f
  medial opening wedge, 580, 581f, 582f, 583f
  postoperative complications of, 593
  postoperative management for, 592
  preoperative planning for, 577–580, 578f, 579f
  results of, 592
  reverse dome, 590, 591f
  surgical technique, 521

Index

Sural nerve injury, calcaneal fracture reduction and fixation, 699
Sural neuritis, 296
   Achilles tendon rupture repair, 413
Surface under the cumulative ranking curve (SUCRA), 412
Suture locking, minimally invasive, Achilles tendon rupture repair, 407–408
Suture passing, minimally invasive, Achilles tendon rupture repair, 406–407, 407f–409f
Symptomatic osteochondral lesions of the talus, 317
Syndesmotic arthrodesis, ankle fracture late syndesmosis repair, 670

T

Talar alignment, Salto Talaris ankle replacement system, 150–151, 151f
Talar Chamfer Trial and Poly trial, 171, 173f
Talar tilt angle, of ankle, 577
Talar trial components, Salto Talaris ankle replacement system, 156–158, 157f
Talectomy, over/undercorrected neuromuscular foot, 755–757, 758f–759f
Talocalcaneal interosseous ligament (TCIL), 482
Talonavicular coverage angle (TNC), 482–483, 489
Talonavicular (TN) joint, 481–483, 482f, 489
   Kinos Axiom Total Ankle System, 265
   in triple arthrodesis, 502–503, 503f, 505–507, 507f, 508f
Talus
   avascular necrosis, 615–616, 618f–619f, 626
   deformity/bone loss, Cadence total ankle replacement, 257
   implantation, Cadence total ankle replacement, 258
   and polyethylene trial, 189–192, 191f, 194–195, 195f
Talus vascular perfusion, INBONE II in ankle arthroplasty, 232
Tarsometatarsal (TMT) joint arthrodesis
   bone extraction, 66, 67f
   compression, 66–69
   morphology, hallux valgus, 95–96
   unicortical biplanar plate fixation in, 94–95
Tegner scores, 334
Tendinopathy, 377
Tendinosis, 377
Tendo-Achilles lengthening (TAL), 417–418
   versus gastrocnemius recession, 616
   Silfverskiold test, 165
Tendon augmentation techniques, Achilles tendon rupture repair, 413–414

Tendon injury, 51
Tendon transfer, over/undercorrected neuromuscular foot, 751, 752f
Tendon-splitting approach, Haglund excision through, 379, 380f, 381f, 382f, 383f
Thompson test, 367, 374
3D printing services, total talus replacement, 617–619
Tibia axis to talar ratio (T-T ratio), 577
Tibial alignment guide (TAG)
   Paragon 28 APEX 3D fixed-bearing total ankle replacement, 165–168, 166f, 167f, 168f
   Salto Talaris ankle replacement system, 147–148, 147f–148f
Tibial impaction handle, and under lateral fluoroscopy, 172–174, 174f
Tibial implants, Salto Talaris ankle replacement system, 143–144, 144f
Tibial resection template, Cadence total ankle replacement, 254–255, 255f
Tibial sizing and preparation, Vantage fixed-bearing total ankle replacement, 242, 244f, 245f
Tibial trial, 189, 190f–191f
Tibialis anterior (ATT) muscle unit, 719
   Kinos Axiom Total Ankle System, 265
Tibiocalcaneal (TC) arthrodesis, over/undercorrected neuromuscular foot, 740–742
Tibiotalocalcaneal (TTC) arthrodesis
   approaches and dissection, 598, 599f, 600f, 601f
   complications, 613–614
   contraindications, 596
   external fixation
      advantages, 539–540
      complications of, 558–559
      contraindications to, 539–540
      indications for, 539
      postoperative management in, 557–558
      preoperative planning in, 540
   hindfoot intramedullary nail, 595
   hybrid fixation, 595–596
   indication, 596
   pearls and pitfalls in, 611–612
   postoperative management, 612–613, 612f–613f
   preoperative planning, 596–597, 597f
   results, 613–614
   ring external fixation, surgical technique of, 553–557, 554f, 555f, 556f, 557f
   surgical technique
      approaches and dissection, 598, 599f, 600f, 601f
      compression, 606, 609f
      external fixation, 610
      intramedullary nail steps, 604, 608f–609f
      joint preparation, 600, 601f, 602f
      lateral locking plate, 610
      positioning, 597, 597f, 598f

      reduction and alignment, 602, 604f–605f
      supplemental fixation, 609, 610f–612f
Tibiotalocalcaneal fusion. See Tibiotalocalcaneal (TTC) arthrodesis
TIDAL Technology, 273
Toe amputation, residual deformity, crossover toe, 641, 642f
Torg's classification, 338
Total ankle arthroplasty (TAA), 163
Total talus replacement (TTR)
   expected outcomes, 626
   history and physical examination, 616–619
   imaging, 617, 617f
   implants, 617–619, 618f–619f
   indications, 615–616
   postoperative care, 624f, 625–626
   surgical technique, 619–624, 620f, 621f, 622f, 623f
Traditional external fixation, for ankle arthrodesis, 552–553, 553f
Transmalleolar and transtalar drilling, 302, 304f
Transtalar drilling, of osteochondral lesion of medial dome of talus, 303–305, 306f
Trial implant placement and stability testing, 213, 213f
Triplanar calcaneal osteotomy, Charcot-Marie-Tooth, 731, 734f
Triplanar first tarsal-metatarsal corrective arthrodesis, 56–75, 57f–58f
   and metatarsus adductus correction, 54–56, 55f, 56f
Triplanar hallux valgus correction procedure, 54, 56
   and metatarsus adductus correction techniques, 54
Triple arthrodesis, 491–511
   contraindications to, 492
   cross-sectional imaging, 496–498
   indications, 491
   outcomes, 511
   over/undercorrected neuromuscular foot, 754–755, 756f
   pearls, 509–510
   pitfalls and complications, 510, 510f
   postoperative care, 510–511
   preoperative planning, 492–498
      ankle instability, 494
      deformity, 493–494, 495f–496f
      gait evaluation, 493
      patient's history, 492
      physical examination, 492–494
      range of motion (ROM), 493
      strength, 494
   radiographs for, 496, 497f
   relative contraindications, 492
   surgical preparation, 498
   surgical technique, 498–509
      calcaneocuboid joint, 501, 507, 508f
      closure, 509

Triple arthrodesis *(Continued)*
  gastrocnemius recession, 499
  general principles, 498
  reduction and fixation, 504, 504f
  setup and positioning, 498–499
  subtalar joint, 500–501, 500f, 501f, 502f, 504–505, 505f, 506f
  surface preparation, 503–504, 504f
  talonavicular joint, 502–503, 503f, 505–507, 507f, 508f
Tubularization of hamstring graft, 278, 281f
Tunnel fracture, 296

U

Ultrahigh molecular weight polyethylene (UHMWPE), 195

V

Valgus deformities, 164
Vantage fixed-bearing total ankle replacement
  age, 234
  ankle arthrodesis, 234
  anterolateral tibia, 248–249
  balancing procedures, ankle and foot, 235, 235t
  contraindications, 233
  coronal angulation, 235
  coronal plane deformity, 234
  deformity, 234
  design, 233, 234f
  indications, 233
  limb malalignment, 235
  low-profile design, 235
  peri-implant cysts and lucencies, 248–249
  postoperative management, 248
  preoperative planning, 235
  results and complications, 248–249
  rotational assessment, 235
  sagittal deformity, 235
  severe osteoporosis, 234
  surgical technique, 236–246
    angel wing, 237, 238f
    anterior approach, 236, 236f
    anteroposterior fluoroscopy, 237, 238f
    external alignment guide, 237, 237f, 238f
    flat-cut talus, 240–242, 243f
    gap check tool, 239, 240f
    implant insertion, 244–245, 245f–246f
    patient-specific instrumentation, 245–246
    positioning, 236
    radiographs and wound closure, 246, 247f
    rounded talus, 239–240, 239f–240f
    size-specific talar cutting block, 240
    talar cut and sizing, 240–242, 243f
    talar cut, preparation and sizing, 239–240, 239f–240f
    tibial cut, 239
    tibial sizing and preparation, 242, 244f, 245f
    tibialis anterior, 236
    varus/valgus position, 237
  3D-printed custom cutting guides, 235
  weight-bearing CT, 235
  weight-bearing radiographs, 235
Varus ankle arthritis, 164, 577, 578f
Varus/Valgus, 147–148, 147f–148f
Viper Tip Peg Punch Paddle, 170–171, 171f
Visual analogue scale (VAS), 140, 217, 334
Vitamin D, 419
Vulpius procedure, 421f

W

4WEB Medical, 617–619
Weight-bearing computed tomography (WBCT), 482
  in Lapidus procedure, for hallux valgus, deformity, 3–4, 4f
Weil metatarsal osteotomy, lesser toes MTP plantar plate tears, 651, 654, 655f–656f
Wire fixation, Moberg osteotomy, 122, 125, 125f
Wound closure, after Achilles tendon repair, 409

Z

Zimmer Trabecular Metal, 199
Z-shaped osteotomy, 19